The Occupational Environment — Its Evaluation, Control, and Management 3rd Edition

Edited by
Daniel H. Anna, PhD, CIH, CSP

A Publication of the American Industrial Hygiene Association®
Fairfax, VA

The information presented in this book was developed by occupational hygiene professionals with backgrounds, training, and experience in occupational and environmental health and safety, working with information and conditions existing at the time of publication. The American Industrial Hygiene Association (AIHA®), as publisher, and the authors have been diligent in ensuring that the materials and methods addressed in this book reflect prevailing occupational health and safety and industrial hygiene practices. It is possible, however, that certain procedures discussed will require modification because of changing federal, state, and local regulations, or heretofore unknown developments in research. As the body of knowledge is expanded, improved solutions to workplace hazards will become available. Readers should consult a broad range of sources of information before developing workplace health and safety programs.

AIHA® and the authors disclaim any liability, loss, or risk resulting directly or indirectly from the use of the practices and/or theories discussed in this book. Moreover, it is the reader's responsibility to stay informed of the policies adopted specifically in the reader's workplace and any changing federal, state, or local regulations that might affect the material contained herein.

Specific mention of manufacturers and products in this book does not represent an endorsement by AIHA®.

ISBN: 978-1-935082-15-6

AIHA®

2700 Prosperity Avenue, Suite 250
Fairfax, Virginia 22031

Tel: (703) 849-8888
Fax: (703) 207-3561
E-mail: Infonet@aiha.org
http://www.aiha.org

AIHA® Stock Number: BIHT10-566

Foreword

By John Howard, MD

I am pleased that the American Industrial Hygiene Association (AIHA®) has published the Third Edition of *The Occupational Environment—Its Evaluation, Control, and Management*, first published by the National Institute for Occupational Safety and Health (NIOSH) in 1973. Once again, *The Occupational Environment* will serve as a primary and comprehensive reference for occupational and environmental health practitioners and students throughout the world.

Today, we in the occupational safety and health community are challenged by having to know about, and respond to, hazards and risks that were largely unanticipated 40 years ago when the Occupational Safety and Health Act was enacted into law. Indeed, 40 years ago, an industrial hygiene practitioner might have had command of the entire body of knowledge in occupational hygiene without reliance on reference texts. Now, that achievement is only for the very few. The scope of risks in the occupational environment has multiplied and even the historical ones have become more complex to control. Now, most of us need to rely on a comprehensive resource like *The Occupational Environment*.

The Third Edition of *The Occupational Environment: Its Evaluation, Control, and Management* will assist professionals to address today's critical issues by including updated and new chapters on air contaminants, risk assessment, sampling, occupational exposure limits, biological monitoring, engineered nanoparticles, prevention through design, internationalization of hazard communication, and many other topics of interest. The ultimate achievement of The Occupational Environment will be in making the occupational environment as safe and healthful as it can be for the protection of workers.

I would especially like to acknowledge the contributions of the many expert chapter contributors, the editor, and the work of the AIHA, in developing the Third Edition. All of your efforts will help to ensure that the occupational and environmental health practitioners of now and of the future will be able to achieve the highest level of skill to address old and new problems in the occupational environment.

John Howard, MD
Director, National Institute for Occupational Safety and Health
U.S. Department of Health and Human Services
September 2011

Preface

By Daniel H. Anna, PhD, CIH, CSP

Since the publication of the Second Edition of *The Occupational Environment: Its Evaluation, Control, and Management* in 2003, the role of the industrial hygienist has continued to evolve and expand. The scope of responsibilities for most industrial hygienists now includes at least some aspects of safety, environmental, sustainability, quality, security, emergency response, or part of another ancillary discipline. But, even with all of these changes, one thing has remained constant — the need for qualified, trained professionals who can anticipate, recognize, evaluate, and control potential health hazards that arise in and from the workplace. The increasing reliance on technology, the expanding world of nanotechnology, the continuing globalization of business and industry, and the changing definition of "workplace" all contribute to the complexities of potential exposures and the challenges of assessing risk of exposure. Terms like exposure risk assessment and management have become part of the language used to describe traditional industrial hygiene responsibilities to a broader international audience.

The evolution of the profession played a role in the development of this edition, and, in turn, hopefully the revised content will play a significant role in preparing IHs for success in the continually evolving work environment. It was essential to incorporate changes because this book serves as a primary textbook for courses that help to prepare future IH, EHS and other related professionals. Beyond the classroom, this book has traditionally served as a fundamental reference for a broad range of topics within the scope of IH related competencies. But with the increasing complexities of the profession and the increasing scope of competencies required to protect worker health, this book can only serve as the starting point for many of the topics presented. In many chapters, the authors have added recommended resources to consult for additional information.

Nearly 120 authors contributed to this edition. New chapters were added to address nanotechnology, professional ethics, IH issues in construction, and the AIHA® Value Strategy. Almost half of the chapters were written or revised by new authors. Most of the other chapters had significant changes and updates to the content.

The most obvious physical difference in this edition is the split into two volumes. Many users of the previous edition commented on the book being "entirely too big" to transport. The decision to divide the book into two parts resulted from the user feedback and the fact that this edition has too many pages to reliably bind into a single volume. Separating the content was a tremendous challenge; countless iterations were considered. In the end the chapters were grouped loosely around chemical hazards, physical hazards and management/program aspects. Many of the relationships between chapter content and chapter location have been maintained from the previous editions. Although this edition is provided in two volumes, it should be considered a single book.

It is an honor to be associated with this edition, to be the first person to read all of the chapters, and to know how many people will benefit from the wealth of information contained in *The Occupational Environment — Its Evaluation, Control and Management.*

Acknowledgments

The most significant contributions to this book came from nearly 120 authors that voluntarily contributed chapters to this edition. Since the first edition of the AIHA Press version of "The Occupational Environment" was published in 1997, this book has become a primary reference for industrial hygienists and an essential textbook used in industrial hygiene and other EHS academic programs. Without their willingness to share their expertise and time to write and revise the technical chapters for this book, development of this outstanding resource for IH and other EHS professionals would not have been possible. A sincere thank you is also extended to the AIHA® Volunteer Groups, and countless AIHA® members and other affiliated professionals who provided thorough technical reviews of the chapters. The peer review process is an essential part of validating the technical content and, by default, the knowledge base for the profession. A special thank you also goes out to the authors and editor of the previous editions; they developed the framework for this and all future editions.

A few individuals from the AIHA® staff deserve individual recognition. Words cannot describe the significant contributions Katie Robert made to this project, including, among her other responsibilities, editing, formatting and preparing content for publication. Katie was an outstanding colleague and friend throughout this project. She kept the project progressing by using her amazing ability to balance "nagging" with an understanding about how my day job sometimes interfered with progress. Jim Myers worked long hours on the layout of the chapters and the design and overall appearance of the book. His work was especially appreciated during the last few months prior to publication as the number of submitted chapters increased and the deadlines shortened. Finally, thanks to Sheila Brown for assisting with the editing of some chapters when the backlog in the queue started to build.

Most of the work on this edition occurred while I was a faculty member at Millersville University. Thank you to the Faulty Grants Committee and the administration at Millersville University for recognizing the significance of this publication and providing some release time from my course load that allowed me to focus on this project. I also want to thank the many students who provided input about the book from their perspective; their comments helped shape many of the changes seen in this edition.

On a personal level, no one was more understanding about my time commitment to this project than my wife Laura. She provided encouragement from the beginning and continued support throughout the project, in spite of having to endure far too many stories, complaints, and frustrated moments. And, my son Nik, whose entire life has occurred during this project, has already said that he will be happy when there is nothing to review "before we go play."

About the Editor

Daniel H. Anna, PhD, CIH, CSP

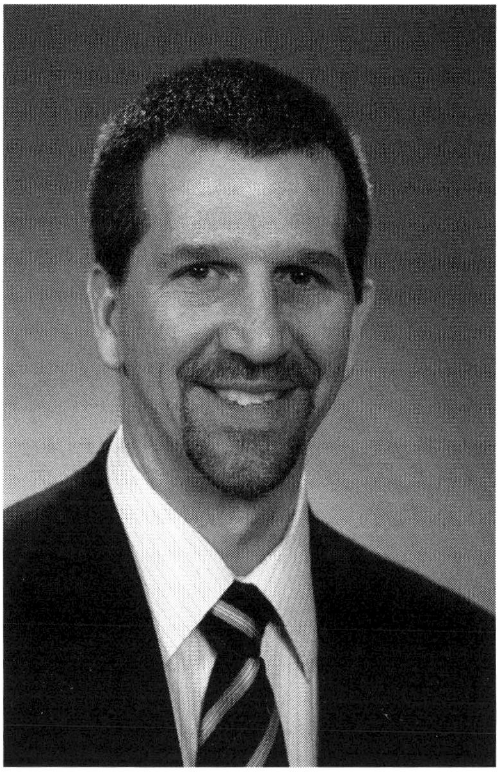

Dr. Anna is currently a Senior Industrial Hygienist and Assistant Group Supervisor at the Johns Hopkins University Applied Physics Laboratory (APL) in Laurel, MD. Prior to joining APL, he spent nearly 15 years at Millersville University (Millersville, PA), where he was a Professor and Program Coordinator in the Occupational Safety & Environmental Health program. In addition, he has worked an industrial hygienist in the petrochemical industry and as an independent consultant. Dr. Anna received a Bachelor of Science in Safety Science from Indiana University of Pennsylvania, a Master of Science in Industrial Hygiene from Texas A&M University, and a PhD in Industrial Health from the University of Michigan. Dr. Anna is a Certified Industrial Hygienist and a Certified Safety Professional. He has been an active member of AIHA® since 1991. He is a graduate of the inaugural Future Leaders Institute in 2005, and has served in leadership roles in the Central Pennsylvania Local Section, on several AIHA® technical committees, and as a Director and the Secretary on the AIHA® Board of Directors.

Contents

Section 5: The Human Environment

Section 6: Methods of Controlling the Work Environment

Section 7: Program Management

The Occupational Environment — Its Evaluation, Control, and Management 3rd Edition

Volume 2

AIHA
Protecting Worker Health

Outcome Competencies

After completing this chapter, the reader should be able to:

1. Define underlined terms used in this chapter.
2. Recall the physics of sound.
3. Discuss the physiology of hearing.
4. Explain acceptability criteria.
5. Apply noise measurement techniques.
6. Employ noise abatement technology.
7. Implement a hearing conservation program.
8. Discuss vibration effects, measurement, and control.
9. Discuss ultrasound effects, measurement, and control.

Key Terms

A-weighted response • acceleration • accelerometer • acoustic trauma • acoustical absorption • air conduction • amplitude • annoyance • antivibration • audiogram • audiometer • audiometric testing • bandwidths • bone conduction • C-weighted response • conductive hearing loss • constrained-layer damping • criteria for Fatigue Decreased Proficiency (FDP) • decibels • directivity • displacement • dissipative mufflers • dosimeter • earmuffs • FFT (fast Fourier transform) spectrum analyzer • flat response • formable earplugs • free-layer damping • frequency • Hand-Arm Vibration Syndrome (HAVS) • hearing protective device (HPD) • lagging • mass loading • noise enclosures • noise-induced hearing loss • noise-induced permanent threshold shift (NIPTS) • noise-induced temporary threshold shift (NITTS) • Noise Reduction Rating (NRR) • occupational vibration • octave bands • periodic vibration • personnel enclosure • premolded earplugs • random vibrations • Raynaud's Phenomenon of Occupational Origin • reduced comfort • resonance • reverberant field • root-mean-square (rms) • semi-inserts • sensorineural hearing loss • sound absorption coefficient • sound intensity analyzers • sound intensity level • sound level meter (SLM) • sound power level • sound pressure level • sound propagation • sound shadow • standing waves • subharmonics • tinnitus • total absorption • transmission loss (TL) • ultrasound • velocity • vibration-induced damage • vibration-induced white finger (VWF) • vibration isolators • vibration transmissibility ratio • wavelength • whole-body vibration

Prerequisite Knowledge

College level algebra, college level physics, introduction to calculus.

Key Topics

- I. Physics of Sound
  - A. Sound Pressure Level
  - B. Sound Intensity Level
  - C. Sound Power Level
  - D. Combining and Averaging Sound Levels
  - E. Frequency
  - F. A-, C-, and Z-Weighting
  - G. Sound Propagation
- II. Physiology of Hearing
  - A. Anatomy
  - B. Auditory Sensitivity
  - C. Audiometry
  - D. Classification of Hearing Loss
  - E. Effects of Excessive Noise Exposure on the Ear
- III. Acceptability Criteria
  - A. Hearing Loss Criteria
  - B. Other Considerations
- IV. Noise Measurements
  - A. Sound Measuring Devices
  - B. Sound Measurement Techniques
- V. Control of Noise Exposure
  - A. Justification for Performing Noise Control
  - B. Administrative Controls
  - C. Engineering Controls
- VI. Hearing Conservation Programs
  - A. Sound Survey
  - B. Engineering and Administrative Controls
  - C. Hearing Protection Devices
  - D. Audiometric Testing
  - E. Employee Training and Education
  - F. Record Keeping
  - G. Program Evaluation
- VII. Vibration in the Workplace — Measurements and Control
  - A. Effects of Vibration
  - B. Terminology
  - C. Criteria
  - D. Measurement of Vibration
  - E. Conducting the Workplace Measurement Study
  - F. Control of Occupational Vibration
- VIII. Ultrasound
  - A. Uses of Ultrasound
  - B. Ultrasound Paths
  - C. Effects of Ultrasound
  - D. Exposure Criteria
  - E. Measurement
  - F. Exposure Controls

Noise, Vibration, and Ultrasound

24

By Robert D. Bruce, PE, INCE.Bd.Cert; Arno S. Bommer, INCE.Bd.Cert; Charles T. Moritz, INCE.Bd.Cert; Kimberly A. Lefkowitz, INCE and Noel W. Hart, INCE

Overview

Excessive exposure to noise, vibration, and ultrasound can be harmful to humans. For at least 100 years, it has been known that excessive exposure to noise can result in permanent hearing loss. Also, since about 1918 it has been clear that excessive exposure to vibration might cause permanent damage to workers' hands and fingers and, recently, it was concluded that exposure to ultrasound should be limited. In each case, techniques to reduce these exposures have quickly followed recognition of the problem. Still, even though knowledge of and solutions to these problems have been available for some time, workers continue to incur noise-induced hearing loss and vibration-induced damage.

The design profession and the manufacturers and packagers of equipment are entrusted with the responsibility of designing machines, processes, and systems that do not adversely impact the health and safety of the working public. If they are unable to design safe machines, processes, and systems, it is their responsibility to notify the user of the potential danger and to provide information about how the user can be protected. It is, in turn, the occupational hygienist's responsibility to ensure that the sound, vibration, and ultrasound created by machines, processes, and systems comply with health and safety standards. In some companies, occupational hygienists are also responsible for ensuring that new equipment meets the noise limits in the purchase order. As will be discussed later in this chapter, the hygienist's first task often is to quantify the exposure (both magnitude and duration) of the worker to the physical agent. When the exposures exceed the values allowable under applicable standards or regulations, the hygienist is often called on to select and provide the appropriate controls (i.e., administrative controls, engineering controls, or personal protective equipment).

In this chapter, two physical agents are discussed: sound (noise and ultrasound) and vibration. Since noise is the most prevalent complaint of workers in society today, much of this chapter will focus on noise. First, there is a brief discussion of the physics of sound and the physiology of hearing. Next, noise criteria, noise measurements, control of noise, and hearing conservation programs are examined. The chapter closes with a discussion of vibration and ultrasound.

Physics of Sound

Introduction

Sound is a disturbance that propagates as a wave of compressions and rarefactions through an elastic medium. The speed at which the sound propagates (c) is a function of the medium's elasticity and density and can be calculated from the following equation:

$$c = \sqrt{\frac{\text{elasticity}}{\text{density}}} \qquad (24\text{-}1)$$

For a solid, the elasticity of a material is represented by Young's Modulus. For a gas, the elasticity is the product of the pressure and the ratio of the specific heat at constant pressure to the specific heat at constant volume. For air at sea level, the equation for the speed of sound reduces to:

$$c = 20.05\sqrt{T} \qquad (24\text{-}2)$$

Where:

T = absolute temperature in Kelvin (°C+273.2)

At 21°C, the speed of sound in air is 344 m/sec. In solids and liquids, where the ratio of elasticity to density is higher than in air, sound travels much faster. For example, the speed of sound in water is about 1,500 m/sec and in steel it is about 5,000 m/sec.

The frequency (f), amplitude, and wavelength (λ) of a sound wave are shown in Figure 24.1. The frequency (measured in hertz or cycles per second and abbreviated Hz), wavelength (in e.g., meters), and speed of sound (c, in e.g., m/sec) are related in the following equation:

$$\lambda = \frac{c}{f} \qquad (24\text{-}3)$$

The wavelength of sound is important, for example, in designing noise control treatments because sound-absorptive treatments should be at least 1/4 wavelength thick for optimum absorption (though thinner treatments may also be effective depending on the specific material properties). In 21°C weather at sea level, sound at 125 Hz has a wavelength of about 2.75 m while sound at 2,000 Hz has a wavelength of only 0.17 m. For high-temperature air such as in gas turbine exhausts, the speed of sound increases and thus the wavelength of sound is longer. To be effective at high temperatures, sound absorptive treatments need to be very thick (8" to 16"), especially for low frequencies.

Sound Pressure Level

The dynamic range of human hearing sensitivity is large: humans can detect changes in atmospheric pressure (sound waves) less than 20 μPa (1 Pa = 1 N/m^2) in magnitude while still being able to withstand pressure changes greater than 20 Pa in magnitude. As a result of this very large dynamic range, sound is often described in terms of a logarithmic quantity, the sound pressure level. Sound is carried by the instantaneous pressure fluctuations (above and below

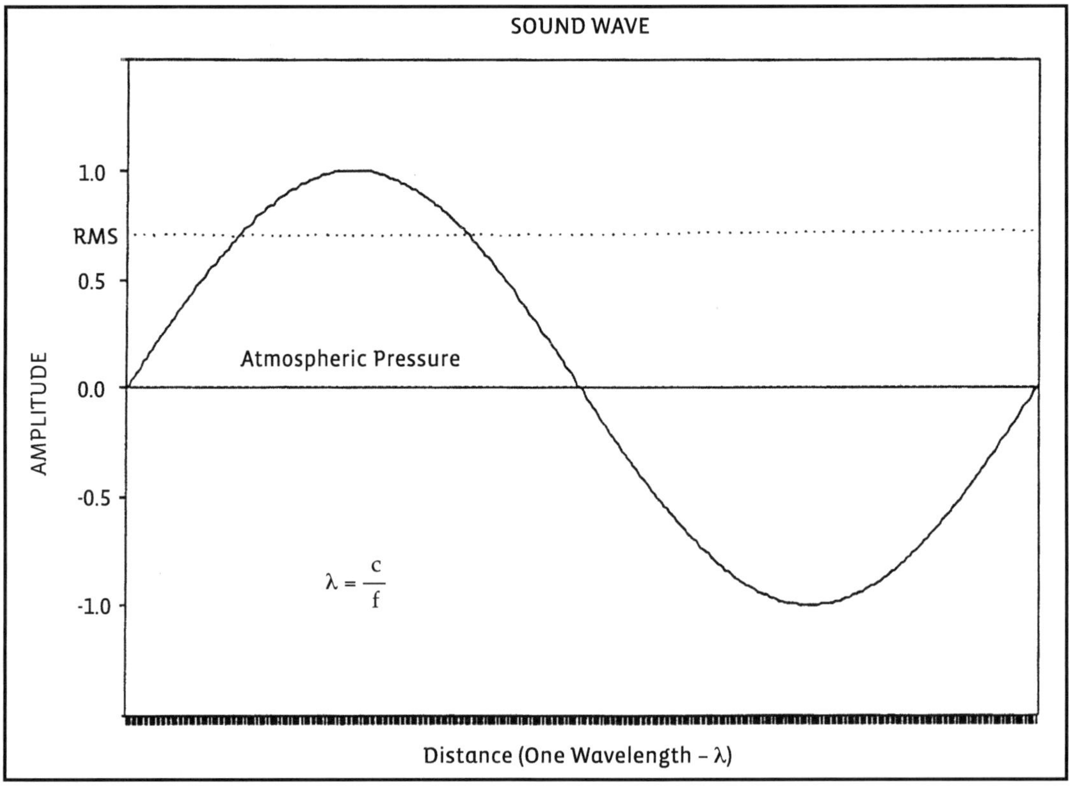

Figure 24.1 —Frequency, amplitude and wavelength of a sound wave.

atmospheric pressure.) The sound pressure level equation is given below, where P is the instantaneous sound pressure in Pa and P_{ref} is the reference pressure defined as 20 μPa.

$$L_P = 10 \log_{10} \left[\frac{P}{P_{ref}} \right]^2 \qquad (24\text{-}4)$$

The units of sound pressure level are decibels, abbreviated dB.

In calculating acoustical levels, logarithms are always base 10. The normal dynamic range of human hearing is from about 20 μPa to greater than 20 Pa; the equivalent range in decibels is from 0 dB (the approximate threshold of hearing) to greater than 120 dB (near the threshold of pain).

Since most sounds are made of waves with the peaks above atmospheric pressure roughly equal in number but opposite in amplitude to the troughs below atmospheric pressure, the average pressure is atmospheric pressure and the average fluctuation is 0. To calculate a more meaningful average, the sound-pressure disturbances (positive or negative) are squared (resulting in a positive number), and then the square root is taken of the average of these squared pressure changes. The result is the root-mean-square (rms) sound pressure. Alternatively, to determine the level of the individual sound impulses, the peak sound pressure above atmospheric pressure can be measured instead of the rms average value.

Sound Intensity Level

The sound intensity level (L_i) is similar to the sound pressure level (L_p) except that L_i is a vector quantity, having both amplitude and direction. For example, a sound wave producing an L_p of 90 dB can have a L_i ranging from +90 dB to -90 dB depending on the direction of the sound wave propagation relative to the direction that the sound measurement probe is pointing. In an ideal diffuse, reverberant field with sound waves traveling equally in all directions, the sound intensity will be 0.

Although the L_i does not correspond to the loudness of a sound (the L_p is more comparable to loudness), it is useful as an analytical measurement and is necessary to accurately determine the sound power level as described in the following section.

Sound Power Level

Sound pressure level or sound intensity level data can be used to calculate the sound power level of an acoustic source. Sound power is analogous to the electrical power rating of a light bulb and is also measured in watts. Whereas the sound pressure, like the amount of illumination provided by a light bulb, varies as a function of distance and room conditions, the sound power, like the power rating of a light bulb, is independent of distance and of any room conditions. The sound power level is defined as:

$$L_W = 10 \log_{10} \left[\frac{W}{W_{ref}} \right] \qquad (24\text{-}5)$$

Where:

W = acoustic power in watts; and
W_{ref} = reference acoustic power, 10^{-12} watts. Prior to about 1960 in the United States, a W_{ref} of 10^{-13} watts was used in some publications.

Since sound power is equal to the intensity times the area over which the intensity is measured, the L_w of a sound source is calculated by adding the average L_i, measured over an imaginary surface enveloping the source, to 10 times the logarithm of the area (in square meters) of the measurement surface. The imaginary measurement surface must completely surround the sound source and have no sound-absorptive materials within its boundaries. These surfaces are often shaped hemispherical or conformal (every point on the imaginary measurement surface equal distance from the equipment). The formula is:

$$L_W = L_i + 10 \log_{10}(A) \qquad (24\text{-}6)$$

Where:

A = measurement surface area in m^2

For spherical area:

$$A = 4\pi r^2 \qquad (24\text{-}7)$$

For hemispherical area:

$$A = 2\pi r^2 \qquad (24\text{-}7b)$$

Where:

r = radius of sphere or hemisphere

When only L_p data are available, they are either presumed to be equal to the L_i or a correction factor is estimated. L_p will be much higher than L_i if the sound measurements are made at a reverberant location.

Combining and Averaging Sound Levels

The decibel scale is logarithmic, which means that the combined sound level of 10 items each producing 70 dB at 10 m will be 80 dB, not 700 dB. Be sure to add the sound pressures represented in decibels, not the decibels themselves. To add sound pressure levels together, sound intensity levels together, or sound power levels together, the following equation should be used:

$$L_{total} = 10 \log_{10} \left[\sum_{1}^{n} 10^{(L_n/10)} \right] \qquad (24\text{-}8)$$

Although the equation above works well for spreadsheet and other computer applications, it is difficult to use when summing levels quickly without a computer or calculator. A shortcut, shown in Table 24.1, can be used to estimate the sum of different sound levels.

For example, if three noise sources each have a sound power level of 100 dB, their total sound power level using the short-cut method is 100 $+_{log}$ 100 = 103; 103 $+_{log}$ 100 = 105 dB. (The notation "$+_{log}$" indicates the shortcut method of logarithmic addition using the information in Table 24.1.) Using Equation 24-8, the total sound power level of the three sources would be 104.8 dB.

Table 24.1 — Short Cut Decibel Addition

Difference Between Two Levels to be Added	*Amount to Add to Higher Level to Determine Sum*
0–1 dB	3 dB
2–4 dB	2 dB
5–9 dB	1 dB
10 dB	0 dB

Sound pressure levels at different positions around most equipment are likely to vary by at least 3 dB. To calculate the average sound pressure level (in dB), it is necessary first to average the sound pressures (in Pa) and then to determine the sound pressure level of the average sound pressure.

Mathematically, the formula is:

$$L_{P(AVG)} = 10 \log_{10} \left[\frac{1}{n} \sum_{1}^{n} 10^{(LP_n/10)} \right] \qquad (24\text{-}9)$$

For example, the average of the following eight sound pressure levels (80, 80, 80, 81, 81, 81, 82, and 88 dB) is 83 dB.

Frequency

Most people can hear sounds ranging from very low frequencies below 30 Hz (the rumble of the largest organ pipes) to very high frequencies near 15,000 Hz (e.g., the "mosquito" ringtone for cell phones). Most sounds have components at many different frequencies. For measurement purposes, this broad range of frequencies is normally divided into nine octave bands. An octave is defined as a range of frequencies extending from one frequency to exactly double that frequency. Each octave band is named for the center frequency (geometric mean) of the band. The center, lower, and upper frequencies for the commonly used octave bands are listed in Table 24.2.

For more detailed acoustical analysis, the octaves can be divided into one-third octave bands. For even more detail, narrow-band analyzers can measure the levels in bandwidths of less than 1 Hz. Narrow-band analysis is especially useful in tracking different tones (relatively high levels at a single frequency) produced by different equipment items.

A-, C-, and Z-Weighting

Although octave-band sound level data are necessary for designing noise control treatments, a single-number description of the sound is often convenient. Most sound level meters provide the option of quantifying the combined sound at all frequencies with several different "weighting" filters: the "A-weighted" response, the "C-weighted" response, and the "flat" response, which is now termed the "Z-weighted" response.

Table 24.2 — Commonly Used Octave Bands

Name of Octave Band (Center Frequencies (Hz)	*Defining Frequency (Hz)*		*A-Weighting of Octave Band (dB)*	*C-Weighting of Octave Band (dB)*
	Lower	*Upper*		
31.5	22.4	45	-39.4	-3.0
63	45	90	-26.2	-0.8
125	90	180	-16.1	-0.2
250	180	355	-8.6	0.0
500	355	710	-3.2	0.0
1000	710	1400	0.0	0.0
2000	1400	2800	+1.2	-0.2
4000	2800	5600	+1.0	-0.8
8000	5600	11,200	-1.1	-3.0

The most common single-number measure is the A-weighted sound level, often denoted dBA. The A-weighted response simulates the sensitivity of the human ear at moderate sound levels. Low-frequency sounds are significantly reduced in level (-26.2 dB at 63 Hz), and high-frequency sounds are slightly increased (+1.2 dB at 2,000 Hz). The A-weighting and C-weighting values at the standard octave bands are shown in Table 24.2.

After this weighting, the levels at all frequencies are summed logarithmically to determine the A-weighted sound level. In addition to being a good estimate of the perceived loudness at moderate levels, there is also a good correlation between the A-weighted sound level and the potential loss of hearing from prolonged noise exposure. Because of this, the A-weighted sound level is used for many applications from community noise ordinances to occupational noise exposure regulations. Table 24.3 presents typical A-weighted sound levels for different sounds.

The C-weighted response simulates the sensitivity of the human ear at high sound levels. It has less weighting applied than the A-weighting filter (for example, only -1 dB at 63 Hz). The Z-weighted response includes the entire audible frequency spectrum without any weighting.

Sound Propagation

An ideal point source, in the absence of sound reflections or absorption, will produce sound pressure levels at a distance "r" (in meters) according to the following equation:

$$L_P = L_W + 10 \log_{10}\left[\frac{Q}{4\pi r^2}\right] \qquad (24\text{-}10)$$

The term r is the distance from the center of the acoustical source, which can be estimated by assuming it is at the center of the machine — but not the edges of the machine. The term $1/4\pi r^2$ is the reciprocal of the spherical area through which sound is radiated. The factor Q can be considered a directivity factor. Q = 1 where there are no reflecting surfaces nearby and sound radiates spherically. Q = 2 where the sound source is near the floor with the sound radiating hemispherically, producing twice the sound energy (+3 dB) at the same distance compared with spherical radiation. If the source is near the intersection of the floor and a wall, the sound radiates in a one-quarter-spherical pattern and Q = 4. If the source is located directly in the corner of a room, it will radiate sound in a one-eighth-spherical

Table 24.3 — Typical A-Weighted Sound Levels

Sound Source and Measurement Location	*A-Weighted Sound Pressure Level*
Pneumatic chipper at operator's ear	120 dBA
Accelerating motorcycle at 1 m	110 dBA
Shouting at 1.5 m	100 dBA
Loud lawnmower at operator's ear	90 dBA
School children in noisy cafeteria	80 dBA
Freeway traffic at 50 m	70 dBA
Normal male voice at 1 m	60 dBA
Copying machine at 2 m	50 dBA
Suburban area at night	40 dBA
Air conditioning in auditorium	30 dBA
Quiet natural area with no wind	20 dBA
Anechoic sound testing chamber	10 dBA

pattern and Q = 8. These Q values represent a simplified presentation of directivity, and sound sources may have directional sound radiation patterns of their own without considering reflections. Alternatively for a measurement surface with a shape that is not a section of a sphere, the reciprocal of the enveloping measurement surface area (1/A) can be substituted for $Q/4\pi r^2$.

In most indoor spaces, sound levels near a sound source will decrease with distance from the center of the source as defined in the preceding formula. At moderate distances from the source, multiple sound reflections from room surfaces will increase the sound level above what would be calculated using the formula. At greater distances, sound levels will remain constant regardless of additional distance from the source; this area is defined as the reverberant field. The sound level in the reverberant field depends on the sound power level of the sound source and the amount of sound absorption in the room. The formula for the sound level inside a building is:

$$L_P = L_W + 10 \log_{10} \left[\frac{Q}{4\pi r^2} + \frac{4}{TA} \right] \qquad (24\text{-}11)$$

Where:

TA = total absorption in the room in m^2, calculated by summing the products of each surface's area with its sound absorption coefficient.

Readers who are familiar with acoustics will notice that Equation 24-11 is written using only the total sound absorption rather than the room constant which is the total sound absorption divided by the quantity: "1-the average statistical absorption coefficient." This approximation has been developed due to the differences between the Sabine sound absorption coefficient, which is reported by manufacturers of acoustical products, and the statistical absorption coefficient, which is used in the theoretical development of Equation 24-11. Those differences are such that R is approximately TA when the available sound absorption coefficients are used to calculate TA.[1]

Since the sound absorption values of surfaces in rooms vary significantly at different frequencies, reverberation calculations should be made in octave bands, not using the A-weighted sound level. For sound propagation inside rooms with large volumes or over long distances outdoors, there is significant sound reduction in the 4,000 and 8,000 Hz octave bands due to atmospheric sound absorption. Additional details on the effects of sound absorption are presented in the section of this chapter on the control of noise exposure.

Physiology of Hearing

Introduction

The function of the hearing mechanism is to gather (outer ear), transmit (middle ear), and perceive (inner ear and brain) sounds from the environment. The frequency range of the young human ear typically extends from 20 Hz to 20,000 Hz. Hearing sensitivity is greatest during childhood. As people get older, their ability to hear high frequency sound decreases due to aging, noise exposure, and drugs. From a practical standpoint, many adults have difficulty perceiving sounds above 14,000 Hz.

The translation of acoustical energy into perceptions involves the conversion of sound pressure waves first into mechanical vibrations and then into electrochemical activity in the inner ear. This activity is transmitted by the auditory nerve to the brain for interpretation.

Anatomy

Sound can be perceived through air-conducted or bone-conducted pathways. With air conduction, sound waves pass into the external ear and cause movement of the tympanic membrane (ear drum). The tympanic membrane excites the bones of the middle ear, which produce signals that are processed in the inner ear. With bone conduction, vibrations travel through the skull to the inner ear or are re-radiated as sound in the external or middle ear. Bone conduction occurs, for example, when one taps your jaw. The sound one perceives is not coming through the ears but through the skull. Under ordinary conditions, bone conduction is much less significant than air conduction in the hearing process. Sound perception via air conduction is the most efficient and common route and is discussed in more detail.

External Ear

A cross section of the ear is shown in Figure 24.2. The ear can be divided into three sections: an external portion (outer ear), an air-filled middle ear, and a fluid-filled inner ear. The external ear consists of the pinna, the external auditory meatus (earcanal), and the tympanic membrane (eardrum). The pinna aids in the localization of sound and increases the sound level at the tympanic membrane at some frequencies.

The external auditory canal extends from near the center of the pinna to the tympanic membrane. The canal is about 26 mm in length and about 7 mm in diameter. The ear canal protects the tympanic membrane and acts as a resonator, providing about 10 dB of gain to the tympanic membrane at around 3,300 Hz.

The tympanic membrane separates the external ear from the middle ear. This almost cone-shaped, pearl-gray membrane is about 10 mm in diameter. The distance the membrane moves in response to the sound pressure waves is incredibly small, as little as one billionth of a centimeter.[2]

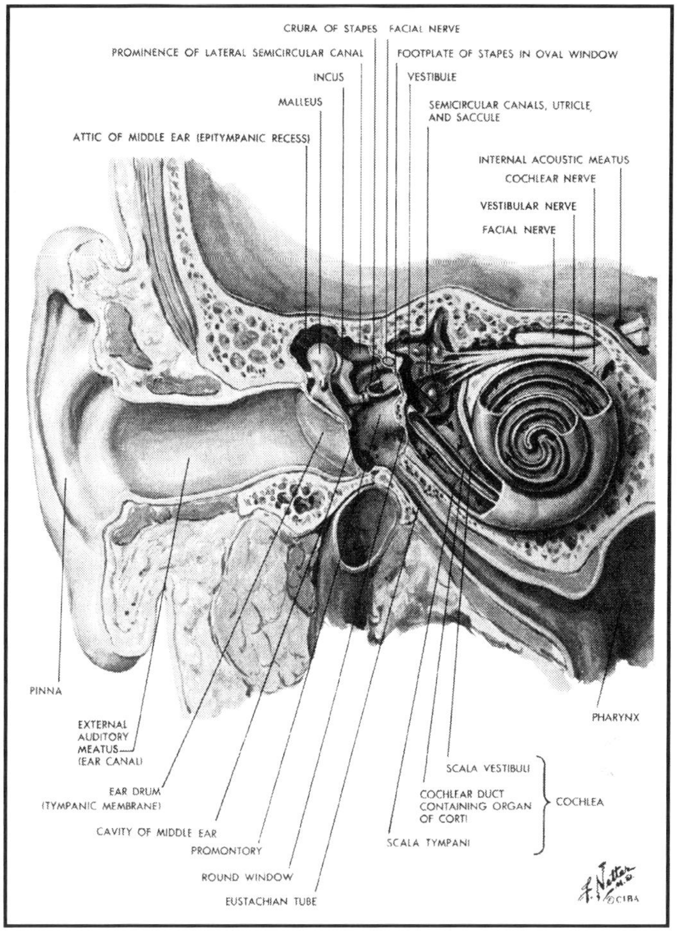

Figure 24.2 — Pathway of sound conduction showing anatomic relationships. (© 1990 by Novartis Medical Education, Summit, NJ). Reproduced with permission from *Atlas of Human Anatomy* by F.H. Netter, MD. All rights reserved.)

Middle Ear

The middle ear, located between the tympanic membrane and the inner ear, is an air-filled space containing the ossicles, which transfer vibration from the outer ear to the inner ear. The middle ear is an impedance matching system, effectively converting sound in the air to motion in the fluid in the inner ear. The ossicles are the three smallest bones in the human body: the malleus (hammer), the incus (anvil), and the stapes (stirrup). The handle of the malleus attaches to the eardrum and articulates with the incus, which is connected to the stapes. The malleus and the incus vibrate as a unit, transmitting the energy from the tympanic membrane to the footplate of the stapes, which pushes the oval window in and out. Due to the lever action of these bones, the displacement is decreased, but the force from the sound wave is increased by a factor of approximately three.

Not shown in Figure 24.2 are two intratympanic muscles, the tensor tympani and the stapedius. These two muscles help maintain the ossicles in their proper position and help to protect the internal ear from excessive sound levels. When the ear is exposed to sound levels above 80 dB,[3] the tensor tympani and stapedius muscles contract, decreasing the energy transferred to the oval window. This protective reflex, identified as the "aural reflex," does not react fast enough to provide protection against impulsive sounds, nor do the muscles stay contracted long enough to provide protection from long-term steady-sound exposures.

The Eustachian tube connects the anterior wall of the middle ear with the nasopharynx. It is about 38 mm in length and consists of an outer osseous (bony) portion (one-third of the tube which opens into the middle ear) and an inner cartilaginous part (two-thirds of the tube which opens into the throat). The lumen of the osseous portion is permanently opened while that of the cartilaginous portion is closed except

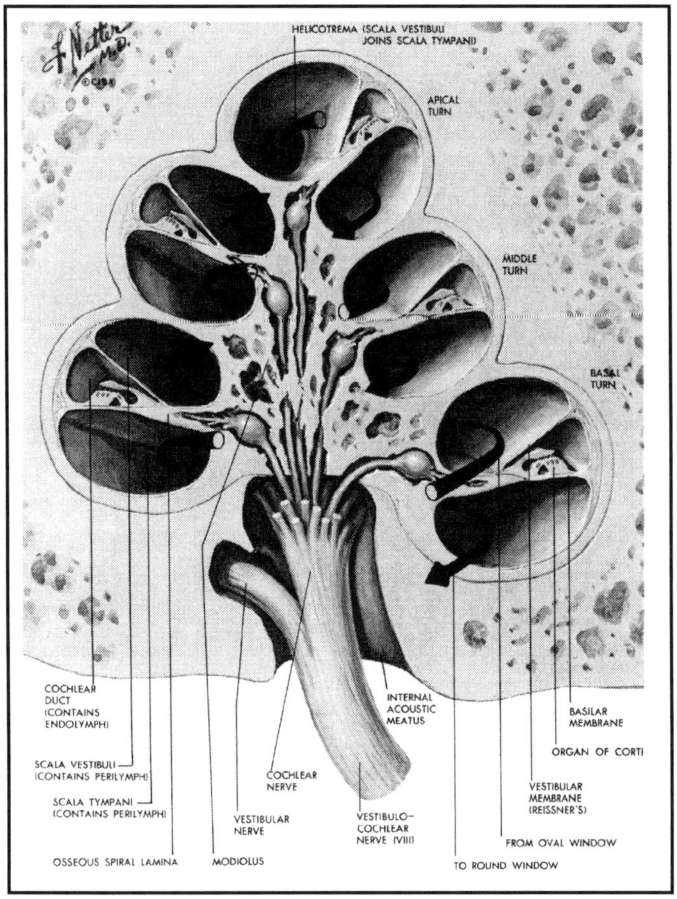

Figure 24.3 — Cross section of the cochlea. (© 1992 by Novartis Medical Education, Summit, NJ). Reproduced with permission from *Clinical Symposia*, Vol. 44, No. 3; illustrated by F.H. Netter, MD. All rights reserved.)

during certain periods. The act of swallowing, for example, opens the cartilaginous portion of the Eustachian tube up to the middle ear and equalizes the atmospheric pressure on either side of the tympanic membrane. This equalization of pressure is necessary for optimal hearing.

Inner Ear

The inner ear is a complex system of ducts and sacs that house the three semicircular canals (used for balance) and the cochlea. The cochlea, shown in Figure 24.3, resembles a snail shell which spirals for about two-and-three-quarter turns around a bony column called the modiolus. Within the cochlea are three canals: the scala vestibuli, the scala tympani, and the scala media or cochlea duct. A bony shelf, the spiral lamina, together with the basilar membrane and the spiral ligament, separate the upper scala vestibuli from the lower scala tympani. The cochlear duct is cut off from the scala vestibuli by Reissner's vestibular membrane.

The scala media is a triangular-shaped duct that contains the organ of hearing, the organ of Corti. The basilar membrane, narrowest and stiffest near the oval window, widest at the apex of the cochlea, helps form the floor of the cochlear duct. On the surface of the basilar membrane are found phalangeal cells that support the critical "hair cells" of the organ of Corti. The hair cells are arranged in a definite pattern with an inner row of about 3,500 hair cells and three to five rows of outer hair cells numbering about 12,000. The cilia of the hair cells extend along the entire length of the cochlear duct and are imbedded in the undersurface of the gelatinous overhanging tectorial membrane (see Figure 24.4). In general, the hair cells at the base of the cochlea respond to high-frequency sounds while those at the apex respond to low-frequency sounds.

The movement of the stapedial footplate in and out of the oval window moves the fluid in the scala vestibuli (see Figure 24.5). This fluid pulse travels up the scala vestibuli but causes a downward shift of the cochlear duct with distortion of Reissner's membrane and a displacement of the organ of Corti. The activity is then transmitted through the basilar membrane to the scala tympani. At the end of the cochlea, the round window acts as a pressure relief point and bulges outward when the oval window is pushed inward.

The vibration of the basilar membrane causes a pull, or shearing force, of the hair cells against the tectorial membrane. This "to and fro" bending of the hair cells activates the neural endings so that sound is transformed into an electrochemical response. This response travels through the vestibulocochlear nerve and the brain interprets the signal as sound.

Auditory Sensitivity

To convert acoustical energy in air to a fluid-borne signal, the ear must resolve the impedance matching problem that exists. Without such a solution, only about 0.1% of the airborne sound would enter the liquid medium of the inner ear, whereas the other 99.9% would be reflected away from its

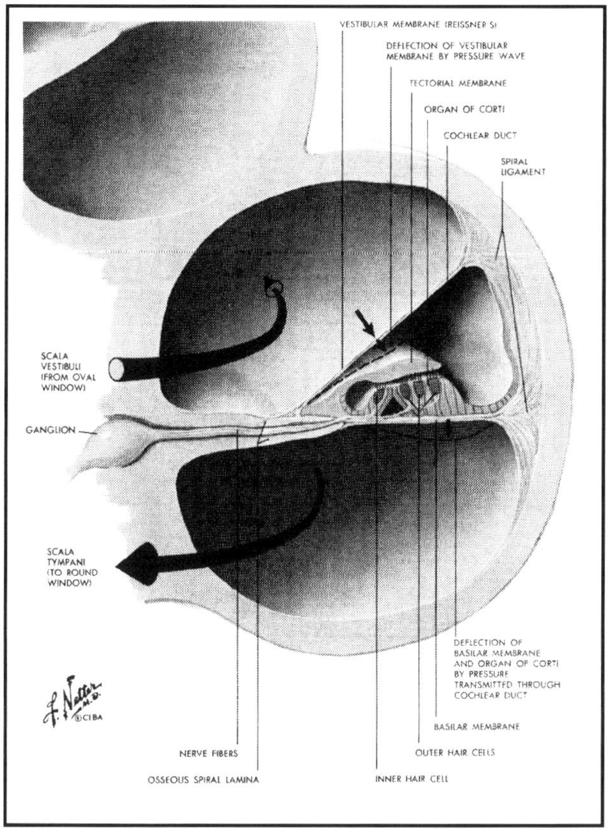

Figure 24.4 — Transmission of sound across the cochlear duct stimuilating the hair cells. . (© 1992 by Novartis Medical Education, Summit, NJ). Reproduced with permission from *Clinical Symposia*, Vol. 44, No. 3; illustrated by F.H. Netter, MD. All rights reserved.)

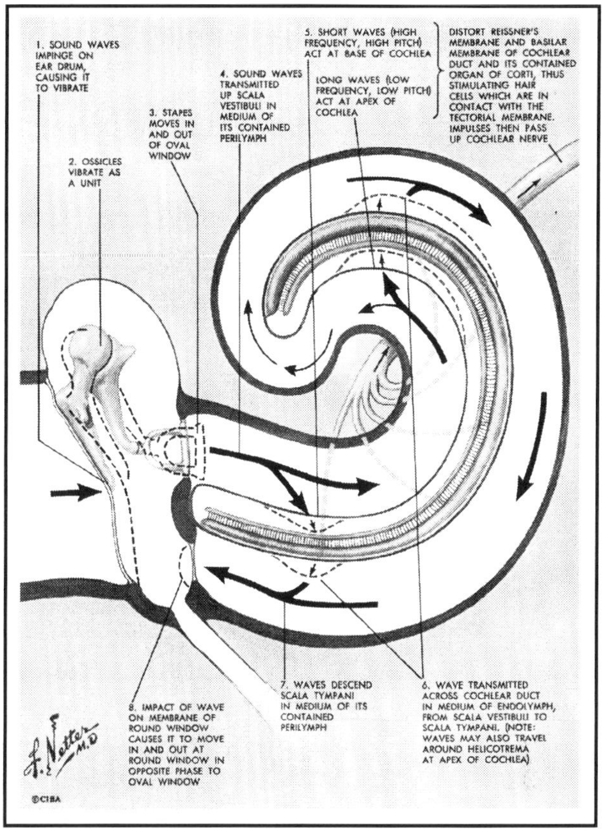

Figure 24.5 — Transmission of vibrations from the eardrum through the cochlea. (© 1970 by Novartis Medical Education, Summit, NJ). Reproduced with permission from *Clinical Symposia*, Vol. 22, No. 4; illustrated by F.H. Netter, MD. All rights reserved.)

surface. This represents a 30 dB decrease in the liquid level vs. the airborne level. In other words, the intensity of vibration in the fluid of the inner ear would be 30 decibels less than the intensity present at the external ear.

The middle ear has two arrangements to narrow this potential energy loss. First is the size differential between the comparatively large eardrum and the relatively small footplate of the stapes. The eardrum has an effective area that is 14 times greater than that of the stapedial footplate. This effect increases the force of pressure from the eardrum onto the footplate of the stapes so that there is approximately a 23 dB increase of sound intensity of the fluid of the inner ear. Also, the lever action of the ossicles increases the force by about 2.5 dB. Thus, the impedance matching mechanism of the middle ear accounts for a 25.5 dB increase in the intensity of sound pressure at the air-liquid interface.

Audiometry

The pure tone audiometer is the fundamental tool used in industry to evaluate a person's hearing sensitivity. It produces tones at 500, 1,000, 2,000, 3,000, 4,000, and 6,000 Hz. Many audiometers include a tone at 8,000 Hz and some also include tones at 125 Hz and 250 Hz. The intensity output from the audiometer can vary from 0 dB to about 110 dB and is often marked "hearing loss" or "hearing level" on the audiometer.

The zero reference on the audiometer ("0 dB hearing level") is the average level for normal hearing for different pure tones and varies according to the "standard" to which the audiometer is calibrated. Reference levels have been obtained by testing the hearing sensitivity of young healthy adults and averaging the sound level at specific frequencies at which the tones were barely perceptible. If a person has a 40 dB hearing loss at 4,000 Hz, it means that the intensity of a tone at 4,000 Hz must be raised 40 dB above

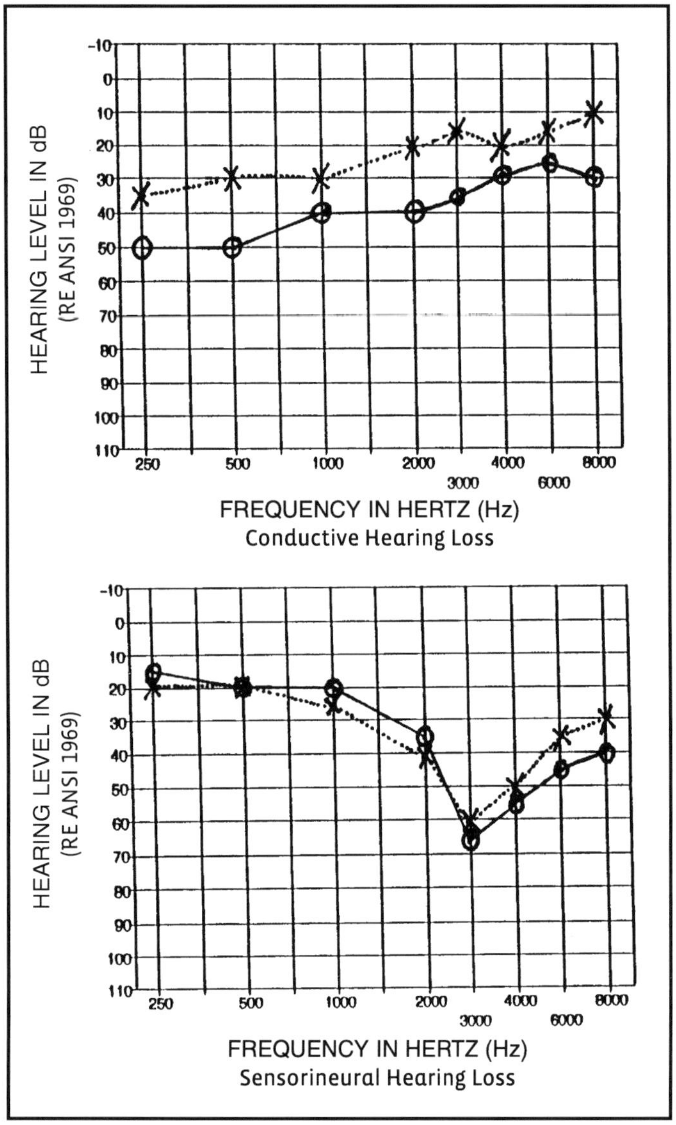

Figure 24.6 — Audiograms showing conductive and sensorineural hearing loss.

the "standard" to be perceived by that person. Since the threshold of hearing is different for different frequencies, the sound pressure level required to produce 0 dB hearing level will also be different for different frequencies.

The audiogram serves to record the results of the hearing tests. The level of the faintest sound audible is plotted for each test frequency. In conductive hearing losses, the low frequencies show most of the threshold elevation, whereas the high frequencies are most often affected by sensorineural losses. A "dip" in the range of 3,000 to 6,000 Hz is often an indication of noise-induced hearing loss. However, older individuals might have noise-induced hearing loss, but this dip might not show due to presbycusis effects at higher frequencies. Examples of audiograms that indicate conductive and sensorineural losses are shown in Figure 24.6.

The recording of an audiogram is deceptively simple, yet for valid test results one must have a properly calibrated audiometer, a proper test environment, and an Occupational Hearing Conservationist certified by the CAOHC.[4] When a marked hearing loss is encountered, more sophisticated tests by an audiologist or physician are required to diagnose the site and cause of the hearing loss.

Classification of Hearing Loss

The three main types of hearing loss are conductive hearing loss, sensorineural hearing loss, and a combination thereof.

Conductive Hearing Loss

Any condition that interferes with the transmission of sound to the cochlea is classified as a conductive hearing loss. Pure conductive losses do not damage the organ of Corti or the neural pathways.

A conductive loss can be due to wax (cerumen) in the external auditory canal, a large perforation in the eardrum, blockage of the eustachian tube, interruption of the ossicular chain due to trauma or disease, fluid in the middle ear secondary due to infection, or otosclerosis (i.e., fixation of the stapedial footplate). A significant number of conductive hearing losses are amenable to medical or surgical treatment.

Sensorineural Hearing Loss

A sensorineural hearing loss is almost always irreversible. The sensory component of the loss involves the organ of Corti, and the neural component implies degeneration of the neural elements of the auditory nerve.

Exposure to excessive noise causes irreversible sensorineural hearing loss. Damage to the hair cells is of critical importance in the pathophysiology of noise-induced hearing loss. Invariably, degeneration of the nerve fibers accompany severe injury to the hair cells. Sensorineural hearing loss can also be attributed to various causes, including presbycusis, viruses (e.g., mumps), some congenital defects, and drug toxicity (e.g., aminoglycosides).

Effects of Excessive Noise Exposure on the Ear

Excessive noise exposure to the ear can cause a noise-induced temporary threshold shift (NITTS), a noise-induced permanent threshold shift (NIPTS), tinnitus, and/or acoustic trauma.

Noise-Induced Temporary Threshold Shift (NITTS)

NITTS refers to a temporary loss in hearing sensitivity. This loss can be a result of the short-term exposure to noise or simply neural fatigue in the inner ear. With NITTS, hearing sensitivity will return to the pre-exposed level in a matter of hours or days (without continued excessive exposure).

Noise-Induced Permanent Threshold Shift (NIPTS)

NIPTS refers to a permanent loss in hearing sensitivity due to the destruction of sensory cells in the inner ear. This damage can be caused by long-term exposure to noise or by acoustic trauma.

Tinnitus

The term "tinnitus" is used to describe the condition in which people complain of a sound in the ear(s) in the absence of actual sounds around them. The sound is often described as a hum, buzz, roar, ring, or whistle. This sound is produced by the inner ear or neural system. Tinnitus can be caused by non-acoustic events such as a blow to the head or prolonged use of aspirin. However, the predominant cause is long-term exposure to high sound levels, though it can be caused by short-term exposure to very high sound levels such as firecrackers or gunshots. If tinnitus occurs immediately following a noise exposure, it means that the exposure was potentially damaging to hearing and if it is experienced repeatedly, it will likely result in permanent hearing loss. Many people experience tinnitus during their lives. Often the sensation is only temporary, though it can be permanent and debilitating. Diagnosis and treatment of tinnitus can be difficult because tinnitus is subjective and cannot be measured independent of the subject. Tinnitus can be quantified in patients by having them match the tone of their tinnitus with another adjustable tone presented to them.

Acoustic Trauma

Acoustic trauma refers to temporary or permanent hearing loss due to a sudden intense acoustic event such as an explosion. The results of acoustic trauma can be a conductive or sensorineural hearing loss. An example of a conductive loss is when the event causes a perforated eardrum or destruction of the middle ear ossicles. An example of a sensorineural loss due to acoustic trauma is when the event causes temporary or permanent damage to the hair cells of the cochlea.

Acceptability Criteria

Introduction

The acceptability of noise can be judged by whether the level of the noise and exposure to the noise can cause hearing loss, annoy people, or interfere with speech communication, hearing or emergency warning signals.

Hearing Loss Criteria

Noise-induced permanent threshold shift affects 10–20 million workers in this country alone.[5,6] If employees are exposed to high noise levels each workday for a working lifetime without adequate hearing protection, they can develop a permanent, irreversible hearing loss.

Figure 24.7 illustrates the impact of noise exposure on hearing. The figure presents the hearing level distribution for four sets of workers.[7] One set is a non-noise-exposed group. The median hearing level as a function of frequency of this non-noise-exposed group is shown in each of the three graphs as the dashed line near the top of each graph. The other three sets of workers (one set for each of the three graphs) were exposed to average daily noise levels of 85 dBA, 90 dBA, and 95 dBA, respectively. The mean age and mean exposure time for these workers are also shown. In addition to the median levels for the noise-exposed workers, the cumulative distribution of the data is also shown. For example, at 4,000 Hz, exposure to a noise level of 90 dBA resulted in a median hearing level of about 40 dB, whereas exposure to a noise level of 85 dBA resulted in a median hearing level of only about 30 dB.

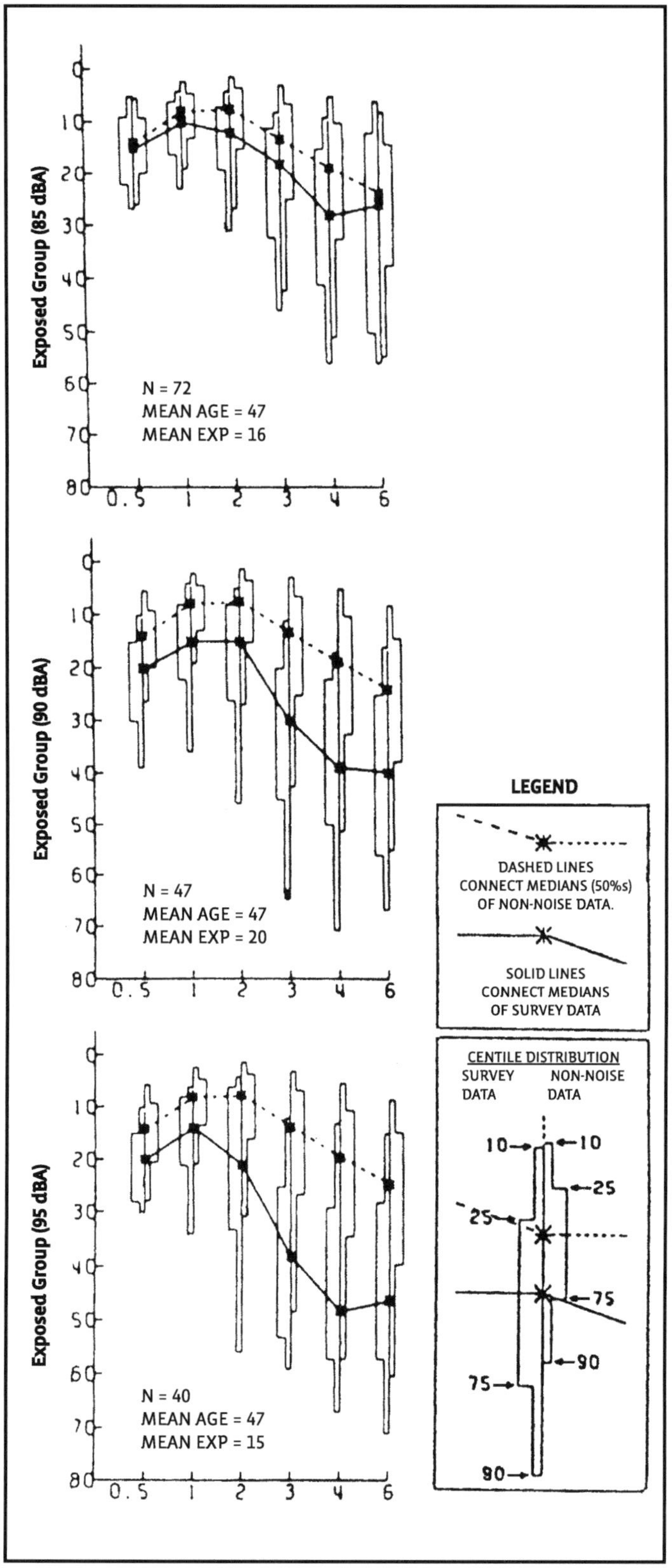

Figure 24.7 — Hearing level distribution for workers aged 43 to 51 exposed to daily average noise levels of 85, 90, and 95 dBA and for workers not exposed. (Adapted from Reference 7).

Federal Regulations

The noise exposure of employees in most occupations and industries is regulated by at least one federal agency. In the following paragraphs, the regulations of the following agencies are summarized:

- Occupational Safety and Health Administration (OSHA)
- Mine Safety and Health Administration (MSHA)
- Federal Railroad Administration (FRA)
- U.S. Coast Guard (USCG)
- Federal Highway Administration (FHWA)
- U.S. Department of Defense (DOD).

Occupational Safety and Health Administration. The U.S. Department of Labor enacted the first specific regulation in the United States for protecting the hearing of civilian employees by amending the Walsh-Healey Act to incorporate a limitation on the noise exposure of workers covered by that act. OSHA was created by Congress in

Table 24.4 — OSHA's Noise Exposure Limits[8]

OSHA's Table G-16. Permissible Noise Exposures for Determining the Need for Engineering or Administrative Controls

Duration (hr/day)	*Sound Level (dBA)*
8	90
6	92
4	95
3	97
2	100
11/2	102
1	105
1/2	110
1/4	115

OSHA's Table G-16a. Permissible Noise Exposure for Determining the Need for Hearing Conservation Program

A-weighted Sound Level	*Duration Reference Hours*
80	32
85	16
90	8
95	4
100	2
105	1
110	0.50
115	0.250
120	0.125
125	0.063
130	0.031

the Occupational Safety and Health (OSH) Act of 1970 and authorized to protect workers against material harm. The current OSHA noise exposure regulation, 29 CFR 1910.95, limits the noise exposure of most civilian employees working in the manufacturing, utilities, and service industries to the values given in Table 24.4.[8] It should be noted that the current OSHA regulation is basically the same as the original regulation but with a thorough definition of what OSHA means by a "continuing, effective hearing conservation program." This regulation has an exchange rate or doubling rate of 5 dB. In other words, as the sound level is increased by 5 dB, the permissible duration time is decreased by 50%.

Exposure to continuous steady-state noise is limited to a maximum of 115 dBA, while exposure to impulse or impact noise is limited to 140 dB peak unweighted sound pressure level.

If workers are exposed to different A-weighted sound levels during the day, the total noise dose (D) is computed with the formula:

$$D = \frac{C_1}{T_1} + \frac{C_2}{T_2} \ldots + \frac{C_n}{T_n} \qquad (24\text{-}12)$$

Where:

C_n = employee's exposure time at a particular noise level; and
T_n = total time allowed at that noise level.

A dose of 1.0 (100%) is equivalent to a time-weighted average (TWA) of 90 dBA. The equation for TWA is:

$$TWA = 16.61 * \log_{10}(D) + 90\text{dBA} \qquad (24\text{-}13)$$

Where:

D = total noise dose.

For determining the need for engineering or administrative procedures, only the exposures to sound levels ≥90 dBA are used in the calculation, as noted in Table 24.4. If the dose is greater than 1.0 (100%) (TWA >90 dBA), feasible administrative or engineering controls must be initiated to reduce the TWA to not greater than 90. For determining the need for hearing conservation programs, all sounds at or above 80 dBA are used in the calculation. If the calculated dose exceeds 0.5 (TWA >85 dBA), employees must be included in a comprehensive hearing conservation program that includes sound monitoring, feasible administrative or engineering controls, audiometric testing, hearing protection, employee training and education, and record keeping. The details of this program are delineated in the current OSHA noise regulation.[8]

Some workers are not covered by the provisions of 29 CFR 1910.95. OSHA provides for the protection of construction workers through 20 CFR 1926.52.[9] The major difference between 1910.95 and 1926.52 is that in the construction industry no protection is required for TWAs between 85 dBA and 90 dBA, and the specific provisions of the hearing conservation program are not listed in detail. As a result, construction workers are more likely to be exposed to noisy operations without proper hearing protection.

Another example of workers not covered by all of the detailed requirements of the hearing conservation portion of CFR 1910.95 are the employees of oil and gas well drilling and servicing operations.[10] Also, civilian employees of other federal agencies are not covered by the OSHA regulations. In accordance with Executive Order 12196, however, they are supposed to be covered by regulations issued by their respective agencies.[11] These regulations were to be as protective as the OSHA regulation. It is unclear which agencies, if any, issued such regulations.

In addition to construction workers, oil and gas well drilling and servicing operations, most civilian federal employees, and a number of other workers are not covered by the OSHA regulation. These include farm workers who are employed by farms with fewer than 10 workers, crew members on all commercial vessels, trainmen, mine workers, and civilian and military employees of the U.S. Department of Defense. Table 24.5 provides a list of the worker types, the federal agencies responsible for the administration of their noise limits, the acoustical aspects of their regulations, and a reference for the information. The following considerations are considered:

- Exchange rate, either 3 dB (equal energy) or 5 dB (OSHA),

- Action level above which a hearing conservation program is required,
- Permissible exposure level and the reference time period,
- Threshold (the lowest level included in the noise dose calculation),
- Maximum continuous sound, often 115 dBA,
- Maximum impulse noise, often 140 dB, and
- Mandatory hearing protection program, either yes or no.

These regulations are discussed in the following sections.

Mine Safety and Health Administration. There are two categories in the mining industry: coal mining and metal and nonmetal mining—both of these industries are divided into surface mining and underground mining. The mining regulation requires hearing conservation programs including audiometric testing for miners with TWAs greater than 85 dBA.[12] The program emphasizes using engineering controls and requires provision of double hearing protection (earplugs plus earmuffs) when the TWA is greater than 105 dBA.

Federal Railroad Administration. The FRA regulation limits noise exposures to 90 dBA for 8 hrs using the 5 dB-exchange rate. Since trainmen often work 12-hour shifts and since this is the maximum allowable work load, the practical limit is 87 dBA for a 12-hour exposure. Hearing protection is mandatory above 90 dBA and has to be offered to employees with exposures greater than 85 dBA. In addition, noise levels inside the cab of locomotives built after October 29, 2007 must not exceed 85dBA.[13,14]

U.S. Coast Guard. Since crew members on commercial vessels are exposed to sound levels continuously for a 24-hour period, the

Table 24.5 — Summary of Occupational Noise Regulations in the U.S.

	Acoustical Requirements								
Agency and Worker Types	*Exchange Rate*	*Action Level (dBA)*	*Permissible Exposure Level (dBA)*	*Hours Allowed at Sound Level in B and C*	*Threshold in dBA*	*Maximum Continuous Sound (dBA)*	*Maximum Impulse Noise (dBA)*	*Mandatory Hearing Conservation Program*	*References*
OSHA									
Manufacturing, Utilities, and Service Sectors	5	85	90	8	80*	115	140	Yes	8
Construction Workers	5	90	90	8	90	115	140	Yes**	9
Other Agencies' Civilian Employees	5		90	8	80	115	140	No	11
MSHA									
Mining Metal, Nonmetal, and Coal; Underground and Surface	5	85	90	8	90	115	140	Yes#	12
FRA									
Trainmen	5	85	90	8##	80	115	140	Yes	13,14
DOT									
Crew Members on all Commercial Vessels	5		82	24	80	115	140	No	15
Motor Vehicles	–		90	–	–	–	–	No	16
DOD	3	85	85	8	80	130	140	Yes	17

* 80 dBA for hearing conservation; 90 dBA for engineering and administrative controls.
**This regulation does not provide any details for a hearing conservation program.
At 105 TWA, both ear plugs and muffs are required.
For 12 hr shifts, 87 dBA.

Coast Guard has developed a criteria of L_{eff}[24] of 82 dBA.[15] This is equivalent to an exposure of 90 dBA for 8 hours and to less than 80 dBA for the remaining 16 hours (since the time at noise levels less than 80 dBA is not counted in the calculation). Although hearing protection is strongly encouraged, a mandatory hearing protection program with all of the provisions of the OSHA regulation is currently not required.

Federal Highway Administration. The FHWA limits all vehicle interior noise levels to 90 dBA.[16] In effect, this places a limit on the noise exposure of truck drivers, bus drivers, and other drivers.

U.S. Department of Defense. The different branches of the DOD (principally the Army, Air Force, and Navy) have from time to time used different action levels and different exchange rates (3, 4, and 5 dB) for evaluating noise exposure. Currently, the Army, Air Force, and Navy use a 3 dB exchange rate with an 8-hour TWA of 85 dBA as the action level at which civilians and military personnel are included in an audiometry program.[17]

Hearing Damage Risk Recommendations. Other organizations have developed recommendations for limiting noise exposure in order to prevent hearing loss.

U.S. Environmental Protection Agency (EPA). Among other responsibilities, the EPA is charged with protecting the public with an adequate margin of safety under its enabling legislation. The EPA recommended an L_{eq}(8 hours) of 85 dBA and a future regulation of 80 dBA.[18] Inherent in the use of an L_{eq} measure of the noise level is the use of a 3 dB exchange rate.

National Institute for Occupational Safety and Health (NIOSH). In 1972, NIOSH recommended an 85 dBA TWA standard with a 5 dB exchange rate for occupational noise exposures.[19] In 1998, NIOSH released a criteria document[20] in which it recommends:

- Limiting noise exposure to 85 dBA TWA for 8 hours
- Using a 3 dBA exchange rate
- Reducing the expected performance (NRR) of hearing protectors
  - 25% for muffs,
  - 50% for formable (presumably including foam) plugs, and
  - 70% for all other plugs
- Starting hearing conservation program at an 8-hour TWA of 82 dBA
- Using hearing protection for any noise exposure over 85 dBA.

International Institute of Noise Control Engineering (I-INCE). The I-INCE has issued a report discussing noise in the workplace. It recommends a TWA of 85 dBA and a 3 dB exchange rate.[21]

American Conference of Governmental Industrial Hygienists (ACGIH®). ACGIH gives threshold limit values (TLVs®) for noise.[22] No exposure to continuous, intermittent, or impact noise in excess of a peak C-weighted sound level of 140 dB is allowed. Exposures are based on a 3 dB exchange rate. The recommended TLVs® range from 80 dBA for a 24-hour period to 139 dBA for 0.11 seconds. Exposures in excess of these values require personnel to be included in a hearing conservation program.

Most nations use 85 dBA as the permissible exposure limit. Many use 90 dBA for compliance with requirements for engineering controls. With the exception of the civilian United States regulations and Chile, Brazil, and Israel, other nations use a 3 dB exchange rate rather than the 5 dB rate.[23]

These recommendations by EPA, NIOSH, I-INCE, and ACGIH®—along with the practice of many countries—are likely to influence future corporate policies and government regulations in the United States. Although researchers continue to discuss the merits of these different noise criteria, this is certain: each individual accumulates hearing loss at his or her own rate, and the higher the noise level and longer the exposure time, the greater the probability of permanent hearing loss.

Sound Exposure

Recently, it has been proposed that occupational noise exposures be considered in terms of sound exposure which has the units of Pascals squared seconds and has been abbreviated as PASQUES.[24] Rather than express a worker's noise exposure by saying he was exposed to 80 dBA for 8 hrs per day for 2,000 hours per year for 40 years, one would say that his sound exposure was 11.5 million PASQUES. This quantity is arithmetic instead of logarithmic. If he were exposed to 90 dBA instead of 80 dBA, his exposure would be 115 million PASQUES. Alternatively, if he were exposed to 4 million PASQUES in 20 years and then to 3 million PASQUES in the remaining 20 years, then his 40-year exposure would be 7 million PASQUES.

Other Considerations

Besides hearing loss, there are other concerns about noise such as speech interference and annoyance.

Speech Interference

Face-to-face voice communication and telephone usage are affected by noise levels. For situations in which speech communication is important (e.g., control rooms) the background sound level should be limited to 55 dBA.[25] Although it is possible to communicate at higher background sound levels for short periods, it is very difficult to maintain a high vocal output throughout a work shift.

When exposed to sound levels above about 45–50 dBA, a talker will raise his or her voice by 3–6 dB for each 10 dB increase of noise. In Table 24.6, the column labeled "shouting" represents the maximum normal output from a talker. This communication is just-reliable, which means trained listeners would score 70% on a word list composed of phonetically balanced monosyllabic words.[26] Parenthetically, if you have to shout to be understood at a distance of 1 m, the sound level is high enough to warrant the use of hearing protection.

High noise levels can also interfere with the audibility and clarity of emergency warning devices.

Annoyance

Annoyance is usually associated with community noise concerns; however, employees in occupational environments can also be annoyed by sounds. Methods are available for estimating community responses to sounds,[27] but there are no methods for estimating individual responses. Noises with tonal sounds, aperiodic sounds, screeches, rumbles, and whines can interfere with the performance of tasks requiring concentration; these sounds can also be annoying. In general, when the sound level of an intermittent broad-band noise is about 10 dBA above the background sound levels, it is likely to annoy listeners. Tonal sounds and other "attention-getting" sounds might cause annoyance at lower levels.

Noise can interfere with a person's ability to perform tasks. Conflicting data suggests that noise can disrupt or enhance performance. Obviously, task interference from noise is a multifaceted issue, and the effects of other variables influence the studies.[28]

Table 24.6 — Speech Communication in Noisy Environments

Distance between Listener and Talker		*Maximum Background Sound Level in dBA for Just-Reliable Communion when "Shouting"*
feet	*meters*	
1	0.3	98
1.6	0.5	93
3.3	1	84
6.6	2	78
13.2	4	71
26.4	8	66

Noise Measurements

Introduction

The measurement of sound and vibration has been greatly facilitated by advances in the electronics and computer industries. Today, the occupational hygienist can carry instruments for measuring the noise dose, the octave band sound pressure level, the vibration of a surface, and the sound intensity of a source along with a portable computer in a briefcase. The ease of making measurements has resulted in an increase in the number of possible measurements. Whenever sound or vibration is measured, it is imperative to remember the question: Why are these measurements being made? Distractions are numerous and one must not forget this question while making measurements. This section will focus on measurement systems, noise measurements for OSHA compliance, and noise and vibration measurements for evaluating sound sources.

Sound Measuring Devices

For the purpose of evaluating personnel noise exposures, the A-weighted sound level is needed at the ear of the person being monitored. For determining the source of a noise (e.g., part of a machine or system), it may be necessary to measure the sound pressure, sound intensity, and/or the vibration of the equipment at different frequencies. This section will discuss the instrumentation that hygienists can use to measure noise and vibration.

Sound Level Meters

The basic instrument for the occupational hygienist or engineer investigating noise levels is the sound level meter (SLM). The SLM consists of a microphone, preamplifier, amplifier with calibrated gain, frequency weighting filters, meter response circuits, and an analog meter or digital readout all conveniently packaged together in one unit. Most meters will have an output jack where the signal can be connected to a computer for logging or data export. There are three levels of precision available, classified by the American National Standards Institute (ANSI) as Types 0, 1, and 2.[29] Type 0 is a laboratory standard; Type 1 is for precision measurements in the field; and Type 2 is for general purpose measurements. Type 1 instruments have an accuracy of ±1 dB and Type 2 instruments have an accuracy of ±2 dB. A Type 2 meter is the minimum requirement by OSHA for sound measurement equipment and is usually sufficient for surveys by hygienists, but when designing cost-effective noise control treatments, a Type 1 meter is usually preferred.

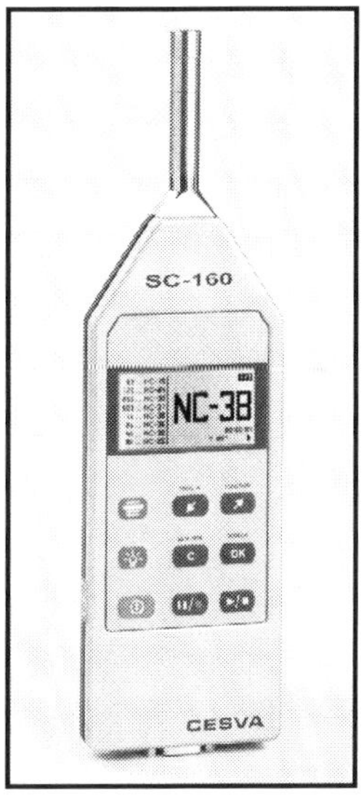

Figure 24.8 — An integrating and logging Type 2 sound level meter capable of octave band measurements. (Courtesy CESVA).

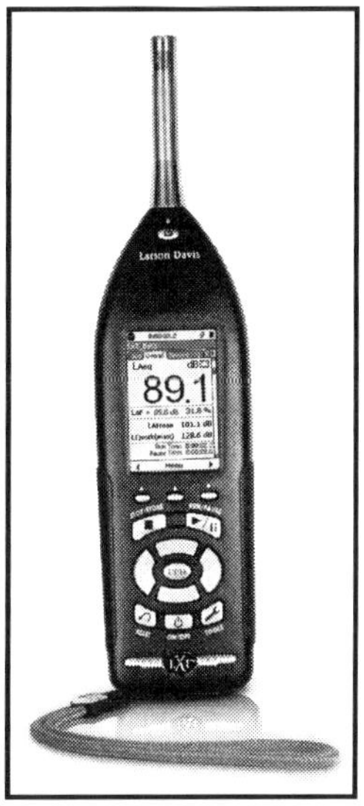

Figure 24.9 — An easy to use integrating and logging Type 2 sound level meter capable of one-third octave and octave band measurements designed with the IH in mind. (Courtesy Larson-Davis).

Most SLMs provide at least two options for frequency weighting: A and C. Some also provide a flat response. The term Z weighting has been applied to the flat response on newer units because it specifies a frequency range along with allowed deviations. Most SLMs have two response characteristics: slow and fast. With the fast response, the meter very closely follows the sound level as it changes. Slow response tends to be more sluggish and gives an "average" of the changing sound level. The OSHA regulation requires measurements to be made with the slow meter response.

Some meters have an "impulse" response or a "peak" response for transient or impulsive sounds. The peak value can also refer to the maximum value of the SLOW or FAST weighted waveform depending on the meter.[30] The impulse response is an integrated measurement and should not be used when measuring peak levels for OSHA compliance. With the impulse response, the meter initially responds very quickly to sounds of short durations, but it decays slowly in order to facilitate reading the value. On some meters with a digital display, the indicated impulse level can remain at the value until the user resets the meter. The peak value can also be displayed until the meter is reset.

In many situations the noise level varies with time such that reading a single number from a meter is difficult. An integrating SLM measures the sound level over a period and calculates the integrated sound level (e.g., L_{eq} [3 dB exchange rate] or L_{osha} [5 dB exchange rate]). Examples of integrating SLMs with an A-scale reading and the ability to measure peak values are shown in Figures 24.8 and 24.9.

Dosimeters

Noise dosimeters are a special type of sound level meter that measures the noise dose. Noise dose is given as a percentage of an allowable maximum dose of 100% which would be 90 dBA for 8 hours. OSHA specifies a total daily allowable time weighted average level (L_{TWA}) that is calculated from the noise dose, D, in the following equation for a 5 dB exchange rate:

$$L_{TWA} = L_{PEL} + (16.61)\log(D/100) \qquad (24\text{-}14)$$

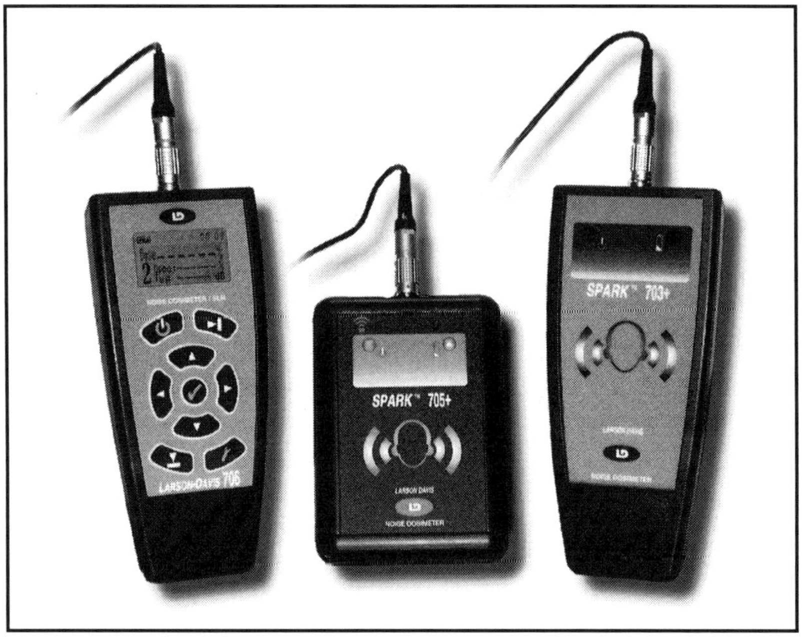

Figure 24.10 — Wearable, logging noise dosimeters. (Courtesy Larson-Davis).

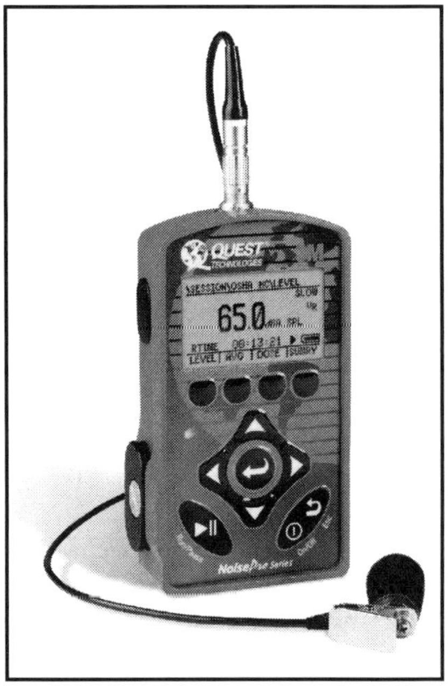

Figure 24.11 — Another wearable, logging dosimeter. (Courtesy Quest).

L_{PEL} is the level in dB. Many instruments can be used as a sound level meter to measure the sound level in an area, or as a dosimeter to calculate the daily noise dose based on a full work shift of measurements. Most dosimeters can also calculate a projected dose based on a shorter, exemplary sample. Different noise dose criteria, exchange rates, and thresholds can be selected, such as an 85 dBA criterion, 5 dB exchange rate and an 80 dBA threshold. The dosimeter can be programmed to sample from, say, 8 a.m. to noon, then 1 p.m. to 5 p.m., and can be locked to protect the data from potential tampering by unauthorized personnel. The dosimeter can be interfaced with a computer for data retrieval or it can be connected directly to a printer to print detailed reports of sound level fluctuations over time. Figures 24.10 and 24.11 are examples of dosimeters.

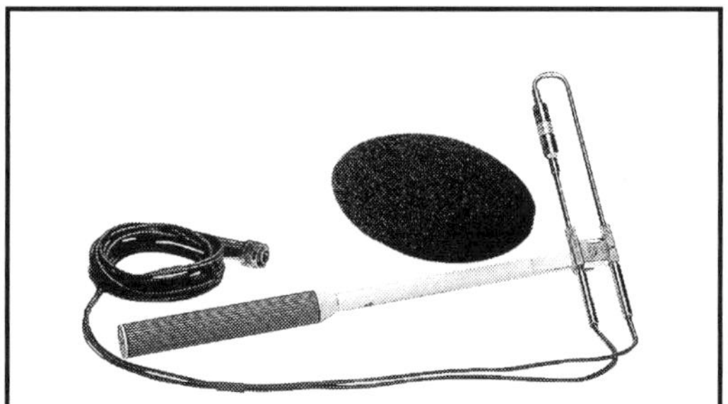

Figure 24.12 — Intensity probe for measuring sound intensity. (Courtesy Rion).

Sound Intensity Meters

Sound intensity analyzers can be used to identify specific noise sources and to determine compliance with purchase specifications limiting the sound power level. While the sound pressure level indicates the level of the sound (but not the direction from which the sound is coming), sound intensity is a measure of both the magnitude and direction of the sound energy. Noise sources can be pinpointed and their sound powers can be rank-ordered using sound intensity, even in occupational environments that are often reverberant. Figure 24.12 shows a sound-intensity probe.

Narrow-Band Analyzers

Measuring the A-weighted sound level is usually sufficient for determining employee noise exposures and determining compliance or violation with some community noise ordinances. However, to analyze sound sources and develop noise control treatments, the frequency content of the sound must be determined. For example, a noise control treatment will have different effects in controlling a low-frequency hum, a mid-frequency whine, or a high-frequency squeal. Usually, the audible frequency spectrum is divided into nine octave bands of frequency ranging from 31.5 Hz to 8,000 Hz. For a more detailed analysis, the spectrum is

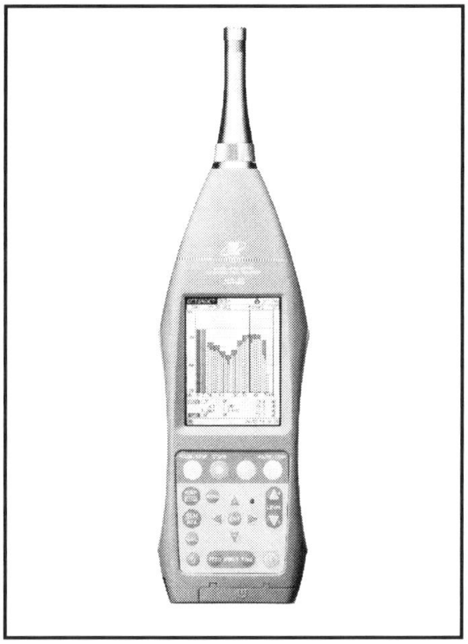

Figure 24.13 — An integrating and logging Type 1 sound level meter capable of one-third octave and octave band measurements. (Courtesy Rion).

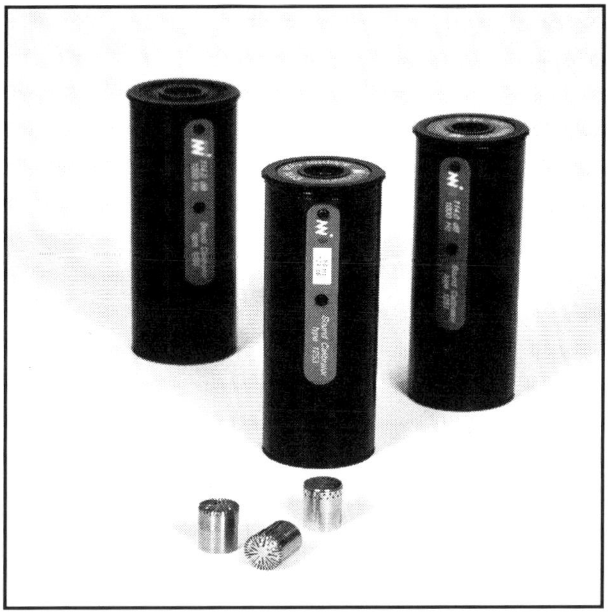

Figure 24.14 — Acoustic calibrators. (Courtesy MMF).

measured in one-third octave bands. Usually a Type 1 (precision) SLM is used for octave and one-third octave band analysis. Figure 24.13 shows a Type 1-integrating SLM that can measure levels in octave or one-third octave bands.

Another approach is to use a FFT (fast Fourier transform) spectrum analyzer to divide the spectrum into even smaller bands. This type of analysis can be used to identify tones that can be traced to specific pieces of equipment. For example, if a tone appears at 29.2 Hz (1750 rpm), the noise source is probably related to a rotating equipment item such as an electric motor, many of which operate at 1750 rpm. A dual-channel analyzer is part of a sound intensity instrumentation system.

Audio Recorders

Although it is good practice to perform both measurements and analysis in the field, sometimes it is either inconvenient to move the analysis instrumentation to the site or there is too much data to analyze in "real time." For these situations, an instrumentation recorder can be quite helpful. Sound and vibration data can be recorded in the field and played back in the laboratory for analysis. Since the frequency response and dynamic range of the device can influence the recording, these parameters should be considered. Various types of recorders are available that can record from one to many channels of data. Many devices allow you to specify sampling rate, which is directly related to the dynamic range of the recording, the higher the sampling rate, the greater the dynamic range and frequency response for the same length of time. In addition to external recording options, many SLMs include their own recording option, either onto a connected computer or a memory card inserted into the meter itself.

Calibrators

For accurate measurements, it is necessary to calibrate the SLM before each set of measurements and then check the calibration during the day (approximately every 4 hours) and after the measurements are complete. For dosimeter measurements, calibration before and after a shift is normally sufficient. Figure 24.14 illustrates one type of acoustic calibrator. The calibrator applies a known sound pressure level to the microphone, and the SLM is adjusted to read the proper level. With many calibrators, a correction must be made for the altitude above sea level because this affects the barometric pressure. In general, the correction is needed only at higher altitudes (lower barometric pressures) such as 1,500 m. This correction can be determined from the instruction

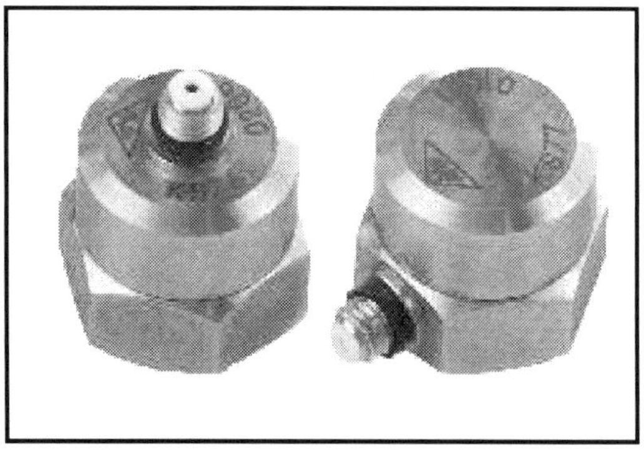

Figure 24.15 — Single axis accelerometer (Courtesy Norsonic).

manual or from a barometer included with the calibrator. Only the calibrator designed to calibrate a particular type and size of microphone should be used. In addition to this regular calibration check, sound meters and calibrators should be inspected, calibrated, and certified annually by qualified companies.

Vibration Instruments

Since noise is radiated from vibrating surfaces of machinery, it may be of interest to measure the vibration of the surface. Accelerometers are the most common transducer used for vibration measurements.

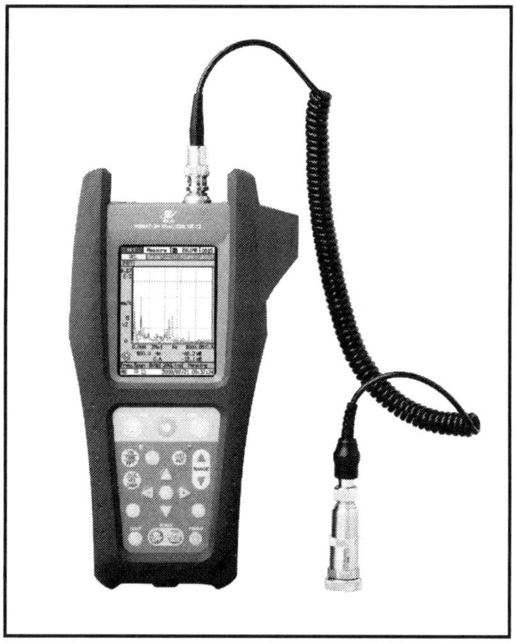

Figure 24.16 — A single box solution vibration meter capable of FFT analysis and data logging over several common frequency ranges (Courtesy Rion).

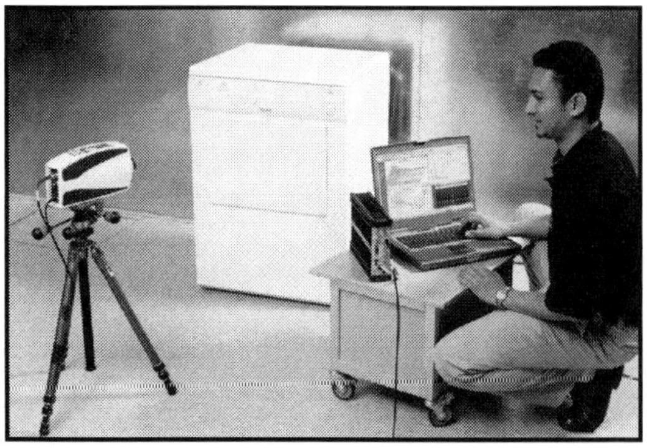

Figure 24.17 — Laser Doppler vibrometer measuring vibration levels on a laundry machine (Courtesy Bruel & Kjaer).

Figure 24.15 shows two accelerometers. They have an electrical output that varies according to the acceleration of the surface on which the accelerometer is mounted. The output is normally proportional to charge, being a piezoelectric element, but many accelerometers have built-in charge-to-voltage convertors, making it proportional to voltage. It is essential to match the type of preamplifier to the output of the accelerometer, either voltage or charge. The accelerometer can be temporarily attached to the surface by using a thin layer of non-drying, air-conditioning-duct-sealing compound (putty), beeswax, superglue, or a magnetic mount. Care should be taken not to make measurements at the resonance frequency of the accelerometer or the mounting. For accuracy at high frequencies or for permanent mounting, a threaded steel stud and a thin film of petroleum jelly should be used. A vibration meter is the simplest setup, usually having the preamplifier built into the device. The vibration meter shown in Figure 24.16 allows for measurement of acceleration, velocity, or displacement. By examining the spectrum of the vibration signal, one can determine which surfaces are radiating particular sounds. A newer and arguably more accurate method of vibration measurement is the laser Doppler vibrometer (LDV) shown in Figure 24.17. An LDV works by utilizing a laser to measure the Doppler shift of a vibrating surface. From the shift, the LDV derives the velocity, acceleration, or displacement. Because the device makes no physical contact with the measurement surface no extraneous damping from the measurement device occurs. Additional information about vibration measurements will be presented later in this chapter in the section on vibration.

Sound Measurement Techniques

Sound measurements for the purpose of occupational hearing conservation are focused on determining the duration of employee exposure to various sound levels. Sometimes, occupational hygienists are also called on to investigate and solve community noise problems. Although the criteria will be different, the principles of noise measurements are the same.

OSHA Compliance Survey

An OSHA compliance survey is performed in an industrial facility to identify areas with hazardous levels of noise and to determine the employees who should be included in a hearing conservation program. For example, in the United States, employees covered by 29 CFR 1910.95 with TWAs greater than 85 dBA should be included in a hearing conservation program. Since most measuring dosimeters are Type 2 and accurate to ±2 dB, a conservative approach is to include those persons within 2 dB of the action level.

The sound level meter is the primary instrument used in task-based monitoring and provides backup information to verify the noise dose calculated by the dosimeter. It is used to identify areas where sound levels exceed the action level and to identify equipment items or areas that control an employee's noise dose.

Sufficient details on the equipment operating conditions and worker locations must be documented to explain any changes in sound levels or noise doses when the survey is repeated.

The basic plan for determining compliance is:

- Tour the facility and develop a detailed understanding of the operation of the facility and its noise sources. Take this tour with someone who is familiar with the plant and its operations. During this tour, speak with knowledgeable personnel about operations and maintenance requirements. Make notes on a floor plan of the area if possible.
- Identify workers and their locations and estimate the length of time they spend in different areas or how long they use particular tools, etc.
- Perform an A-weighted sound level survey of the facility, marking the A-weighted sound levels on the floor plan and noting which equipment is on or off.
- Compare the sound levels in the facility with the locations of personnel, as reported to you and as observed by you.
- Identify employee groups based on their exposure to noise in common areas. Use dosimeters to measure the noise exposures of individuals within these different groups.
- Compare the noise doses as determined by the dosimeter with doses calculated using the measured noise levels and the estimated exposure times.
- Evaluate any discrepancies and re-measure as necessary.
- Include individuals with TWAs greater than 80 dBA in a hearing conservation program. (OSHA requires placing those exposed to 85 dBA or greater in a hearing conservation program, but 80 dBA is considered a better practice.)
- Develop noise control treatments where feasible for equipment that causes employees to have a TWA greater than 85 dBA. (OSHA requires this procedure for TWAs greater than 90 dBA.)

This generalized approach can be used to quantify the noise exposures of workers in most industrial facilities.

Before making measurements, the SLM must be calibrated properly. The time, date, location, and other pertinent information should be recorded on a data sheet; Figure 24.18 is an example of a useful data sheet for recording octave band measurements. For OSHA-related measurements, the instrument should be set to measure the A-weighted level with slow meter response. The meter should be held with the microphone at ear height (approximately 1.5 m). The average meter reading should be recorded at each position. If there is significant fluctuation (more than ±3 dB) the minimum and maximum readings, and the central tendency, should be recorded. Care should be taken to ensure that the relevant noise source is operating normally and that other sources that normally do not operate are switched off.

Noise exposure calculations based on area levels and time estimates are susceptible to many potential inaccuracies, especially if there is high worker mobility, the sound level fluctuates, or there is significant impulsive sound. Workers can carry noise dosimeters during their normal work shift to document their noise exposure. For OSHA-related measurements, the dosimeter should be calibrated and the proper settings should be entered for the weighting (A), meter response (slow), threshold (80 dBA), exchange rate (5 dBA), and criterion (90 dBA). The instrument can be worn in a pocket or attached to the user's belt, and the microphone should be attached to the shoulder, pointing upward, approximately 0.15 m (6 in) from the ear. OSHA stipulates the microphone must be located within a 30 cm (1 ft) radius of the center of the head.[30] The

CORPORATION NAME
ADDRESS

Sheet ____ of ____

Project Description:

Sketch of Site (with distances to noise sources):

Job Number: *Initials:*

Location:

Date:

Quantity measured:
SPL ACC VEL DISP dB re: ______

Time	Cal, dB	Temp	%RH	Wind Sp	Dir

CONDITIONS:	Time	Pos.	Octave Band Center Frequency, Hz									A-wt
			31.5	63	125	250	500	1000	2000	4000	8000	

NOTES:

Figure 24.18 — Sample data sheet.

dosimeter manufacturer will often provide detailed operating instructions.

It is best to conduct individual monitoring on each employee with any noise exposure higher than 85 dBA. If an employee's work schedule varies significantly from day to day, dosimetry should be conducted for several days. If many workers perform essentially the same tasks, it may be possible to obtain a representative sample without measuring everyone.[31] Care must be taken in selecting the sample size to ensure that there is high confidence the highest exposures are documented. If there is any doubt on how representative any noise exposure data is, it is best to err on the side of making additional measurements.

Identifying and Locating Noise Sources

In identifying offending noise sources, the hygienist should first use his or her ears. Since all conventional hearing protection devices are most effective at high frequencies, care must be taken not to ignore these less audible sounds when wearing hearing protection.

Ideally, when investigating noise sources (not noise exposures), all pieces of equipment should be turned off except the equipment under investigation, though in occupational situations this often is impossible to do. If there are several sound sources in a reverberant space, the offending source might be difficult to isolate. In this case, a 1/1- or 1/3-octave band filter set will help to locate the source, since there usually will be excessive sound in a particular band. In some cases, a narrow-band analyzer will be necessary to identify tones that are characteristic of the particular piece of equipment. As noted earlier, another method for analyzing sound sources is to measure sound intensity. Although the equipment is sophisticated and expensive, an intensity analyzer can be used to isolate a source in a reverberant space better than a sound level meter.

Compliance of Equipment with Purchase Noise Specification

Purchase specifications limiting the noise emissions of new or reconditioned equipment can reduce noise exposure in occupational environments. Usually the specification requires that the equipment meet a certain maximum sound level at a distance of 1 m away or at a particular operator position under specified operating conditions. The criterion may be A-weighted sound levels, octave-band sound pressure levels, or sound power levels.

Many national and international standards can be referenced in a purchase specification; however, some of these standards do not provide the hygienist with the information needed to determine the noise exposure. The purchase specification must tie the sound level requirements to a specific location, preferably the operator position, and to the normally loaded operating conditions for the equipment.

Control of Noise Exposure

Introduction

Noise exposures must be controlled whenever they exceed government or company noise requirements. Usually the best first step to reduce noise is to develop a written noise control plan. The plan can include the following items:

- Determine current noise exposures of employees.
- Implement a hearing conservation program with audiometric testing and available hearing protection for all employees with time-weighted average noise exposures greater than 85 dBA.
- Reduce noise exposures for employees with TWAs of 90 dBA or above, when feasible, with engineering or administrative controls.
- Determine the cost-effectiveness of different noise control options for reducing noise exposures. Details on noise control treatments are discussed in this section.
- Develop guidelines for the purchase of new and replacement equipment, for the modification of existing facilities, and for the design of new facilities. These guidelines should include the purchase of quiet equipment and the design of building surfaces to absorb sound and to prevent excessive sound transmission. Often, it is much less expensive to prevent the noise problems from the start than to reduce excessive noise in completed facilities.

Justification for Performing Noise Control

The primary reasons for reducing noise levels in an occupational environment are hearing protection, legal liabilities, speech communication, safety, productivity, and annoyance.

Hearing Protection

For more than 100 years, the business community has had access to the knowledge that excessive exposure to high noise levels can cause permanent hearing loss. Frequently this knowledge is not distributed throughout a company and, as a result, noise control is given a low priority. The individuals charged with completing construction projects on time and within budget often do not know efficient ways to reduce noise. Many times their solution is to put some money aside for future measurements and ill-defined retrofit solutions. This is an inefficient way to perform noise control.

High sound levels produce greater risk of dangerous noise exposures than lower noise levels. For example, no significant hearing loss would be expected for most workers who spend a working lifetime at sound levels less than the equivalent of 80 dBA for an 8-hour day. On the other hand, if the workers were to spend this time at 95 dBA, typical high-frequency hearing losses of greater than 30 dB could occur.

Hearing protective devices provide only 9 to 15 dBA of reliable protection for most workers. Workers exposed to TWAs above 100 dBA while wearing hearing protection can still incur substantial hearing loss over a lifetime since the protected ears would still be exposed to TWAs higher than 85 dBA.

Legal Liabilities

In most industrialized countries, hearing conservation is required by regulatory statute. For example, under 29 CFR 1910.95, OSHA requires that all employee exposures to noise be controlled to a TWA of 90 dBA or less. Although the 1983 Hearing Conservation Amendment spells out the detailed requirements of an acceptable hearing conservation program for exposures greater than the equivalent of 85 dBA, it does not indicate that hearing protection is an acceptable form of noise control when the TWA is greater than 90 dBA. Engineering controls (reducing noise levels around people) and administrative controls (removing people from noisy areas and buying quiet equipment) are the only acceptable permanent solutions under this regulation. Although hearing conservation programs can be very effective in reducing the risk of hearing impairment of workers, the only completely effective method is to reduce the noise of all sound sources to acceptable levels. Obviously, this will require a concerted effort on the part of owners and vendors.

If a company fails to protect a worker's hearing, then the company may face fines and lawsuits over the work conditions and future hearing loss of workers.

Speech Communication

Speech communication can be improved dramatically by reducing sound levels. Although it generally is not appreciated, most maintenance personnel and operators depend on speech communication for receiving much of their instructions and information and for working safely and efficiently. If two people were attempting to communicate in an 84 dBA environment, they could speak in a normal voice only if they were 1 m (3 ft) or less apart.

In a situation in which communication is crucial (e.g., during an emergency situation or in a control room) the ambient sound level will need to be much lower to achieve acceptable speech communication throughout an area or room. To compound issues, communication in a moderately noisy environment is more difficult for workers who have incurred some hearing loss.

Safety

Reduced noise levels increase safety by aiding communication and by making it easier to hear alarms or other audible signs of danger. Emergency warning systems must be designed to produce sound levels 10–15 dB above the background sound level. With very high sound levels, high-powered, closely spaced emergency warning speakers must be used.

Annoyance and Productivity

Lower noise levels mean lower annoyance, and in many cases this means better productivity and a safer workplace.

Annoyance can also result from wearing hearing protection for extended periods of time. Earmuffs can be very uncomfortable due to the perspiration that develops under the muffs in warm climates or in enclosures or buildings. Lower noise levels can also improve employee concentration.

When residences are located near industrial facilities, the residents may find occupational noise annoying.

Administrative Controls

Administrative noise control measures consist of either relocating people away from noisy areas or redistributing noise exposures such that many employees are given acceptably low exposures instead of a few employees having excessive exposures. These types of controls are conceptually simple but are often difficult to implement and document; thus, they are seldom used.

Clearly, the best administrative program is to eliminate the source of the noise by purchasing quieter equipment and processes. This can also be considered an engineering control as discussed in the following section.

Engineering Controls

When administrative controls cannot be used to reduce noise exposures, engineering noise controls can be used. The simplest (though not necessarily cheapest) option is to replace noisy operations with quieter equipment, quieter processes, or quieter materials. Equipment can also be relocated. Some equipment manufacturers have options for quieter models. Intrinsically quieter equipment is often more efficient, easier to maintain, and less costly than equipment retrofitted with treatments. When purchasing quieter equipment, precise noise specifications should be used to ensure that the guaranteed sound levels are for the equipment operating under normal loads and conditions.

When quieter equipment cannot be purchased, noise control treatments can be applied to the equipment. The rest of this section addresses different types of noise control treatments. Before determining which treatment is most appropriate for a particular situation, the source of the noise problem should be analyzed to determine the mechanisms of sound generation and propagation and the proximity of employees. If there are multiple sound sources, they should be rank-ordered according to their A-weighted sound levels, ease of solving the problem, number of employees impacted, or some composite rating such as the Noise Control Priority Factor(32) or the Priority Number.(33) A range of possible treatments can then be considered. Often, operational and maintenance concerns will eliminate some options. The remaining options can then be evaluated in detail for cost-effectiveness. It is often most effective to install simple treatments for the loudest sound sources first. It should then be easier to analyze noise from other sound sources and to develop appropriate additional noise control treatments. Although a hygienist can accomplish much with a simple A-weighted sound level meter and a basic understanding of noise control concepts, acoustical consultants are often necessary when complicated measurements or treatment designs are required.

Most occupational noise sources can be separated into two general mechanisms by which the sound waves are generated: surface motion of a vibrating solid, and turbulence in a fluid (including air). Some noise sources include combinations of these two mechanisms. Noise control for sources with a vibrating surface include reducing: 1) the driving force, 2) the response of the surface to the driving forces, and 3) the radiation efficiency of the vibrating surfaces.

Noise control for fluid turbulence generally involves reducing turbulence by reducing pressure drops, reducing velocities, and smoothing flow.

Once sound is transmitted to the air, it can be reduced by treating the sound path using the following types of treatments: 1) sound absorption, 2) equipment enclosures, 3) personnel enclosures, 4) shields or barriers, 5) lagging, and 6) mufflers.

Each of these different types of noise control treatments is discussed in detail in the following sections.

Reduce Driving Force

Driving forces in mechanical equipment may be repetitive or nonrepetitive. These forces can be reduced by decreasing the speed, maintaining the dynamic balance, providing vibration isolation, and, in the case of impact operations, increasing the duration of the impact while reducing the force.

The repetitive forces on a machine are often caused by imbalance or eccentricity in a rotating member. These forces strengthen with an increase in rotational speed, and this usually results in higher noise levels from the machine. As a result, machines should be selected to operate at slower speeds when this requirement does not conflict with other operational needs.

All rotating mechanical equipment should be in proper dynamic balance to minimize the level of repetitive forces. Proper preventive maintenance of bearings and proper lubrication and alignment of equipment are vital. When machines are balanced improperly or when bearings are worn, it is possible for the noise levels to increase as much as 10 dBA above the sound levels of normal operation.

Resilient materials such as rubber, neoprene, and springs can reduce noise by reducing vibration propagation to structures; the design of vibration isolation treatments are discussed in the vibration section of this chapter. Resilient materials installed at impact sites can be used to reduce impact forces. For example, a neoprene-lined bin can be used instead of a bare metal bin to catch small metal parts. This treatment has worked on stock guides, chutes, tumbling barrels, and hoppers and works particularly well when the falling parts do not have sharp edges. The noise levels can be reduced by 10–20 dBA by these treatments.

Many metal fabricating operations (e.g., forging, riveting, shearing, and punching) use impacts to process material. Due to the short duration of the impact, large forces are required. The noise level is a function of the maximum amplitude of the force that is applied; consequently, a lesser force applied over a longer period will produce less noise.

Reduce Response of Vibrating Surface

Often, the easiest method to reduce the response of a vibrating surface is to increase its damping. A vibrating surface, such as a panel, converts some energy of motion into heat energy as it flexes. The rapidity with which the vibration energy is dissipated is directly related to the damping. A structure with little damping, such as a bell, will continue to vibrate for a long time after it is excited. A highly damped structure will not ring if struck, but will quickly convert the energy to heat. For a given driving force, a highly damped surface will vibrate much less than a lightly damped surface similar in mass and stiffness. Consequently, a highly damped surface will radiate less sound than a surface with low damping.

Before treating a vibrating surface to reduce the noise, the designer needs to determine which surfaces are radiating high levels of noise. This issue is sometimes obvious. Large, flat, unsupported surfaces are likely to be more important radiators of noise than small or stiff surfaces. If a machine is small, it may be expedient to treat all vibrating surfaces. If the machine is large or if the treatment is complicated, this might not be cost-effective, and it may be important to first determine which surfaces make the greatest contributions to the area noise levels.

Increasing the damping of a surface is most effective when the surface is vibrating at or near a resonance frequency. Damping material should be added where the panel has the greatest amplitudes of vibration; damping applied in the center of a vibrating panel with fixed edges is much more effective than damping applied near the edges. Significant noise attenuation can be achieved by treating as little as 50% of the surface area; however, without detailed knowledge of the panel vibration, 80–100% coverage is recommended.

The two types of commonly applied damping treatments are free-layer damping (also called extensional damping) and constrained-layer damping. In free-layer damping, a layer of nonhardening viscoelastic material, usually in the form of tapes, sheets, tiles, mastics, or sprays, is adhered to the surface. Constrained-layer damping involves the use of a laminated construction consisting of two or more sheet metal layers, each separated by and adhesively bonded or mechanically attached to a viscoelastic layer. If the metal layers in a constrained layer damping treatment are bolted together, the bolts must be appropriately isolated from the metal panels using neoprene grommets. Because of possible damage to exposed damping surfaces in many occupational environments, the metal exterior surface of constrained-layer damping may be preferable to the less durable exterior surface of free-layer damping. Note that the effectiveness of the damping treatment will be independent of the side of the panel that is treated, so damping can be placed away from harmful exposures or hidden for aesthetics.

In addition to reducing the vibration of a surface at resonance frequencies, damping treatments also reduce the transmission of high-frequency sound through the panel, but only if the entire panel has been treated.

The temperature of the surface on which the damping material is to be applied must be known since the properties of damping materials are highly dependent on temperature. Resistance to chemicals, oil, and other environmental considerations may also be important in the selection of a damping material. Detailed information on damping materials is available from the individual manufacturers. Liquid mastics and elastomeric damping sheets are the most common damping materials. High-temperature damping materials (up to 320°C [600°F]) are also available for applications such as steel muffler shells, high-speed blower housings, steel piping systems, gearboxes, fan housings, and turbine exhausts.

As a basic guideline, free-layer damping treatments should be at least as thick as the surface to which they are applied and are usually not greater than twice the thickness. The greater the ratio of the damping thickness to the panel thickness, the greater will be the noise attenuation. However, once the damping material thickness becomes more than twice the panel thickness, the increases in performance with additional thickness are significantly reduced.

For free-layer damping, viscoelastic materials are usually preferred since the performance of a treatment can be estimated using the manufacturer's product literature. Although the noise attenuation provided by a damping treatment is very difficult to predict accurately, the attenuation may be estimated from:

$$\text{Noise Attenuation} = B \log_{10}\left(1 + \frac{\eta_c}{\eta_i}\right) \qquad (24\text{-}15)$$

Where:

- B = 20 for structures vibrating at resonance;
- B = 10 for structures with broad-band excitation;
- η_c = composite damping loss factor; and
- η_i = damping loss factor present initially in the structure.

As shown, the composite damping (η_c) must be considerably greater than the initial damping (η_i) to achieve significant reduction. The composite damping loss factor (η_c) from bonding a viscoelastic layer to a structural plate may be estimated from:

$$\eta_c = \frac{\eta_d}{1 + \dfrac{E * H / (e * h)}{3 + 6h / H + 4(h / H)^2}} \qquad (24\text{-}16)$$

Where:

- E = modulus of elasticity of the plate (N/m^2);
- e = modulus of elasticity of the damping material;
- H = thickness of the plate (m);
- h = thickness of the damping treatment (m); and
- η_d = loss factor of the damping material.

The ratio of the moduli of elasticity (e/E) is presumed to be much less than 1 in the derivation of this equation. Representative values of E and η_d are presented in Table 24.7.[34] Since the properties of damping materials vary significantly as a function of frequency and temperature, the values given in this table are presented as general ranges only. The manufacturer's data for specific materials and applications should be obtained before performing final calculations.

The loss factor of a panel before treatment (η_i) is sensitive to construction techniques and edge conditions. It can be measured by striking the panel and measuring the resonant response as a function of frequency. Using a narrow band analyzer, the frequency of each peak and the frequency of each point 3 dB down at each side of the peak is determined. The initial loss factor can be calculated by dividing the difference

Table 24.7 — Representative Values of Sound Speed, Density, Modulus of Elasticity, and Loss Factor for Common Building and Damping Materials[34]

Materials	*Speed (m/sec)*	*Density r (kg/m³)*	*Modulus of Elasticity E (N/m²)*	*Lost Factor (dimensionless)*
Aluminum	5150	2700	7.2×10^{10}	0.0001–0.01
Lead	1200	11,000	1.6×10^{10}	0.002–0.015
Steel	5050	7700	20×10^{10}	0.0001–0.01
Plexiglas	1800	1150	$.37 \times 10^{10}$	.0002
Plywood	—	600	$.37 \times 10^{10}$	0.01–0.04
Damping Materials	—	—	$7 \times 10^5 - 7 \times 10^8$	0.1–1.0

in frequency of the 3-dB-down points by the peak frequency. If the loss factor of the panel is low (e.g., <0.01) before treatment, noise attenuations on the order of 10–30 dB can be achieved.

In one application, the lower section of a rubber compounding mill was encased in a metal shell. Functioning as a sounding board, the metal shell radiated the vibration from the motor, gear, and roll of the mill. The vibration was damped by an application of free-layer damping material to the inner surface of the metal shell. The octave band noise attenuation achieved was:

Octave-Band Center Frequencies (Hz)							
63	125	250	500	1000	2000	4000	8000
11 dB	8 dB	14 dB	10 dB	6 dB	7 dB	9 dB	11 dB

Design equations for constrained-layer treatments have been derived,[34] but they involve complex frequency and wavelength dependencies and, due to space limitations, are not presented here. Because of the complexities involved, design of constrained-layer treatments often require the assistance of an experienced professional.

One successful case history involved noise that was produced by almost continuous impacts between stock material and the tubes that fed the stock to screw machines. A viscoelastic damping material was sandwiched between inner and outer tubes. At 4000 rpm with 13 mm (1/2 in.) stock, the noise measured 0.3 m (1 ft) from the middle of the stock tube was reduced as follows:

Octave-Band Center Frequencies (Hz)							
63	125	250	500	1000	2000	4000	8000
12 dB	15 dB	15 dB	14 dB	20 dB	29 dB	34 dB	30 dB

Reduce Radiation Efficiency by Reducing Area of Vibrating Surface

Sound can be radiated from a surface when at least one dimension of the surface is longer than one-fourth of the wavelength of the sound. Thus, low-frequency sound requires larger surfaces for radiation than high-frequency sound.

It sometimes is possible to reduce the sound radiated from a surface by reducing the total area or by dividing a large surface into a number of smaller sections. When possible, perforated or expanded metal can be used in place of solid panels (presuming that the panel itself is not part of an acoustic enclosure).

Use Directivity of Source

Many occupational sources radiate more sound in one direction than in another. This behavior is called the sound directivity. Directive sources include stacks, intake, and exhaust openings on fans and blowers, enclosure openings, and large vibrating metal panels. Occasionally it is possible to orient a source such that a particular location receives less sound than other locations around the source. For stacks, the directivity effects at different angles compared with a source that radiates spherically (equally in all directions) are presented in Table 24.8.[35]

The values in this table can be added to the L_p determined by Equation (24.10) in which Q=1 for an elevated stack to determine the L_p at different angles to the stack.

In the reverberant sound field inside a building, the directivity of the source cannot normally be used to reduce the sound. The only exception is if the source can be oriented such that the sound radiates directly toward a sound-absorptive material.

Reduce Velocity of Fluid Flow

High-velocity fluid flow can generate noise problems in air-ejection systems, vents, valves, and piping. The noise is generally caused by turbulence in the fluid flow. Although reducing velocities will reduce turbulence and noise, this is often not a practical option.

Consideration should be given to using mechanical part ejectors in place of the air-ejection systems. Quiet nozzles sometimes can be used for air-ejection systems. It also is possible to reduce air velocities in conjunction with more accurate aiming of the nozzles. For exhaust vents on air-operated equipment, small silencers can be installed to reduce the noise.

If the ratio of the absolute pressures upstream and downstream of a valve is 1.9 or greater, the flow through the valve will be choked (sonic). Large pressure drops across valves can be avoided by using diffusers to reduce the pressure upstream of the valve. Valve manufacturers can generally provide sound level data for their valves based on the operating conditions, and some manufacturers have options for quieter valves. Due to their small size and heavy construction, little noise is radiated from the valve bodies themselves; most of the noise is radiated from the piping or vents downstream of the valves. Mufflers can sometimes be installed downstream of valves, or the piping can be lagged as described later in this section.

Increase Sound Absorption

Most rooms are neither perfectly reflective nor perfectly absorptive. Sound levels decrease at a rate of 6 dB per doubling of distance (from the center of the source) at locations close to small sound sources in most rooms (as they do outdoors or in an anechoic chamber). They then approach a constant level at greater distances from sound sources (as they do in reverberation chambers).

To predict the attenuation of sound in a room, it is first necessary to determine the total amount of sound absorption in the room (TA). This is determined by multiplying the surface area of each interior surface material by the material's coefficient of absorption. The coefficient of absorption is the ratio of the sound energy absorbed by a material to the sound energy incident upon the material. An extremely absorptive material such as thick glass fiber will have an absorption coefficient (α) of close to 1.0 (all of the sound is absorbed). An extremely sound reflective surface such as sealed concrete will have a sound-absorption coefficient of close to 0.0 (all of the sound is reflected). Sometimes, manufacturers of sound-absorptive materials will quote values greater than 1.0; this is a result of the absorption test conditions, and a maximum value of 1.0 should be used in equations.

Table 24.8 — Directivity of a Stack (in dB) by Angle Compared with Spherical Radiation[35]

	Octave Band Center Frequencies (Hz)							
Angle	*63*	*125*	*250*	*500*	*1000*	*2000*	*4000*	*8000*
45°	+5	+5	+6	+6	+6	+7	+7	+7
60°	+2	+2	+2	+2	+1	0	-1	-2
90°	-3	-4	-6	-8	-10	-12	-14	-16
135°	-4	-6	-8	-10	-13	-16	-18	-20

Materials have different absorption coefficients at different frequencies. Absorption coefficients also vary with material thicknesses. Table 24.9 presents octave-band sound-absorption coefficients for various materials.[35–40]

The formula for calculating the total absorption of a room is:

$$TA = S_1\alpha_1 + S_2\alpha_2 \ldots + S_n\alpha_n \qquad (24\text{-}17)$$

Where:

TA = total absorption in metric Sabins (1 metric Sabin equals the sound absorption of 1 m^2 of perfectly absorptive material, α=1.0)

S_1, S_2, S_n = areas in m^2 of each interior surface

α_1, α_2, α_n = corresponding coefficients of absorption for these surfaces

The sound absorption of openings in a room must also be considered when calculating the total absorption. The absorption coefficient of an opening such as an open door or window is 1.0. A 2 m^2 open window will therefore add 2 metric Sabins to the total absorption. Also, the air volume can contribute to the sound absorption. This generally has to be taken into account only

Table 24.9 — Sound-Absorption Data for Common Building Materials(35–40)

Material	Sound-Absorption Coefficient 125 Hz	250 Hz	500 Hz	1000 Hz	2000 Hz	4000 Hz
Walls						
Sound-reflecting:						
Brick, unglazed, unpainted	0.03	0.03	0.03	0.04	0.05	0.07
Brick, glazed or painted	0.01	0.01	0.01	0.02	0.02	0.03
Concrete block, painted	0.10	0.05	0.06	0.07	0.09	0.08
Cork on brick or concrete	0.02	0.03	0.03	0.03	0.03	0.02
Glass, typical window	0.35	0.25	0.18	0.12	0.07	0.04
Gypsum board, ½-in. paneling	0.29	0.10	0.05	0.04	0.07	0.09
Metal*	0.05	0.02	0.01	0.02	0.02	0.02
Plaster, gypsum or lime, on brick or tile	0.01	0.02	0.02	0.03	0.04	0.05
Plaster, gypsum or lime, on lath	0.14	0.10	0.06	0.05	0.04	0.03
Plywood, 3/8-in. paneling	0.28	0.22	0.17	0.09	0.10	0.11
Wood, ¼-in. paneling, with air space behind	0.42	0.21	0.10	0.08	0.06	0.06
Sound-absorbing:						
Concrete block, coarse, unpainted	0.36	0.44	0.31	0.29	0.39	0.25
Medium weight drapery, 14 oz/sq. yd., draped to half area	0.07	0.31	0.49	0.75	0.70	0.60
Fiberglass fabric curtain, 8½ oz/sq. yd., draped to half area	0.09	0.32	0.68	0.83	0.39	0.76
Shredded wood fiberboard, 2-in. thick on concrete	0.32	0.37	0.77	0.99	0.79	0.88
Foams: (Acoustical open cell)						
1-in., 2 lb/cu. ft. polyester	.16	.25	.45	.84	.97	.87
2-in., 2 lb/cu. ft. polyester	.24	.49	.81	.91	.98	.97
Glass fiber:						
1-in., 3 lb/cu. ft.	.23	.50	.73	.88	.91	.97
1-in., 6 lb/cu. ft.	.26	.49	.63	.95	.87	.82
Floors						
Sound-reflecting:						
Concrete, terrazzo, marble or glazed tile	0.01	0.01	0.01	0.02	0.02	0.02
Cork, rubber, linoleum, or asphalt tile on concrete	0.02	0.03	0.03	0.03	0.03	0.02
Wood	0.15	0.11	0.10	0.07	0.06	0.07
Wood parquet on concrete	0.04	0.04	0.07	0.06	0.06	0.07
Sound-absorbing:						
Carpet, heavy, on concrete	0.02	0.06	0.14	0.37	0.60	0.65
Carpet, heavy, on foam rubber	0.08	0.24	0.57	0.69	0.71	0.73
Indoor-outdoor carpet	0.01	0.05	0.10	0.20	0.45	0.65
Ceilings						
Sound-reflecting:						
Concrete	0.01	0.01	0.02	0.02	0.02	0.02
Gypsum board, ½-in. thick	0.29	0.10	0.05	0.04	0.07	0.09
Plaster, gypsum or lime, on lath	0.14	0.10	0.06	0.05	0.04	0.03
Plywood, 3/8-in. thick	0.28	0.22	0.17	0.09	0.10	0.11
Sound-absorbing:						
Suspended acoustical tile, ¾-in. thick, 16-in. air space above	0.76	0.93	0.83	0.99	0.99	0.94
Thin, porous sound-absorbing material, ¾-in. thick (mounted to structure)	0.10	0.60	0.80	0.82	0.78	0.60
Thick, porous sound-absorbing material, 2-in. thick (mounted to structure) or thin material with 1-in. air space behind	0.38	0.60	0.78	0.80	0.78	0.70
Sprayed cellulose fibers, 1-in. thick on concrete	0.08	0.29	0.75	0.98	0.93	0.76
Air Absorption						
Air, per 1000 m^3-@ 50% RH	0	0	0	3.0	7.5	23.6

* Absorption coefficients for metal were estimated by the authors of this chapter. Low-frequency absorption coefficients will depend on the metal thickness.

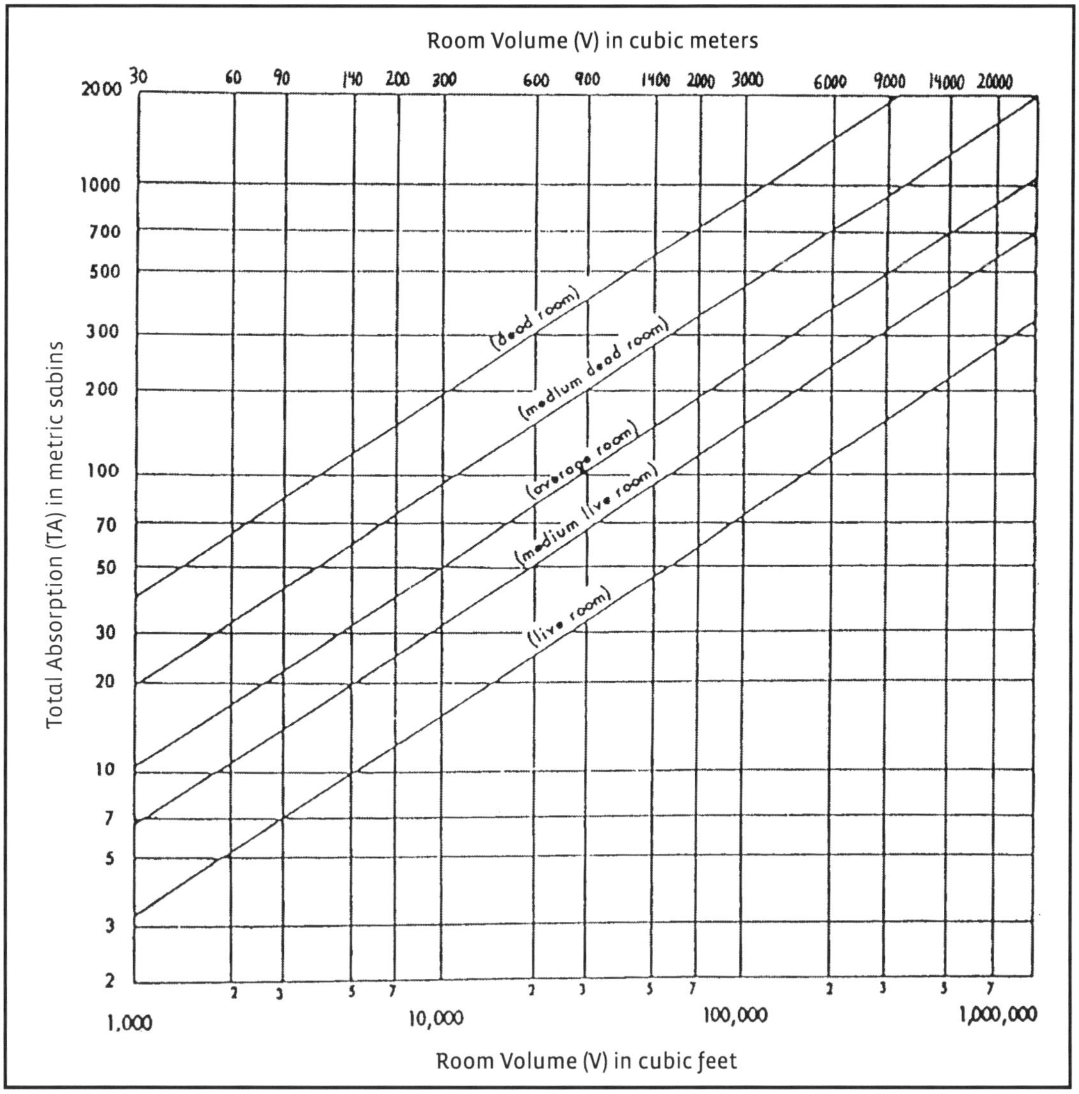

Figure 24.19 — Total room absorption for typical rooms. (Adapted from Reference #34).

with the higher octave band frequencies (2,000, 4,000, and 8,000 Hz) in large rooms.

Example: Calculating Total Absorption at 1,000 Hz

The 1,000 Hz total absorption for a room with 80 m^2 of concrete (α = 0.02), 210 m^2 of sheet metal (α = 0.02), 60 m^2 of windows (α = 0.12), 40 m^2 of open windows (α = 1.0), and 150 m^2 of 25 mm thick acoustical foam (α = 0.98) is: (80 * 0.02) + (210 * 0.02) + (60 * 0.12) + (40 * 1.0) + (150 * 0.98) = 200 metric Sabins.

As an alternative to the equation, TA can be approximated by using Figure 21.19 and estimating the relative reverberation of a room.

Example: Calculating Sound Levels in a Reverberant Space

As discussed previously in this chapter, the relationship between the sound pressure level (L_p) and the sound power level (L_w) is given in Equation 24-18 as:

$$L_w = L_{pa} + 10 \log_{10} (A) \qquad (24\text{-}18)$$

Where:

L_w = sound power level;
L_{pa} = average sound pressure level; and
A = surface area in square meters of the imaginary shell around the equipment where the L_p measurements were made.

This formula is accurate in non-reverberant sound fields such as those found outdoors or in close proximity to the equipment. Inside a reverberant room, sound propagates in accordance with the following formula:

$$L_p = L_w + 10 \log_{10} \left[\frac{Q}{4\pi r^2} + \frac{4}{TA} \right] \quad (24\text{-}19)$$

Where:

- Q = directivity factor (use 2 for a source near a surface such as the floor);
- r = distance from the acoustic center of the source (in meters);
- TA = total absorption in room (in metric Sabins); and
- L_w = sound power level.

This equation is presented graphically in Figure 24.20. Note that if the total absorption is very high, as in an anechoic chamber (where 4/TA becomes very small), this equation approaches the earlier simplified equation for outdoor sound radiation: sound levels decrease at a rate of 6 dB per doubling of the distance from the source. Also note that absorption (TA) has little effect on the sound pressure level at distances close to the sound source. This area is called the acoustic near-field. At greater distances from the source in a reverberant room, the sound level approaches a constant level. This area, called the reverberant field, is the area where sound levels are controlled by the amount of absorption in the room, not the distance from the sound source.

For a location in the reverberant field of a sound source, sound reduction can be achieved by increasing the amount of sound absorption in the room. The purpose of this method of noise control is to reduce the reverberant buildup of sound in a room, and ideally, to achieve the same attenuation of sound over distance that is achieved outdoors (6 dB per doubling of distance). In most cases, the maximum reduction that can be achieved by adding absorption to a room is 3–8 dBA. Employees may appreciate this improvement more than an equal decibel improvement of source noise control since a less reverberant space is usually a more pleasant work environment. This noise control technique is only practical when the room is originally reverberant and the sound receiver is located a sufficient distance from the sound source (in the reverberant field).

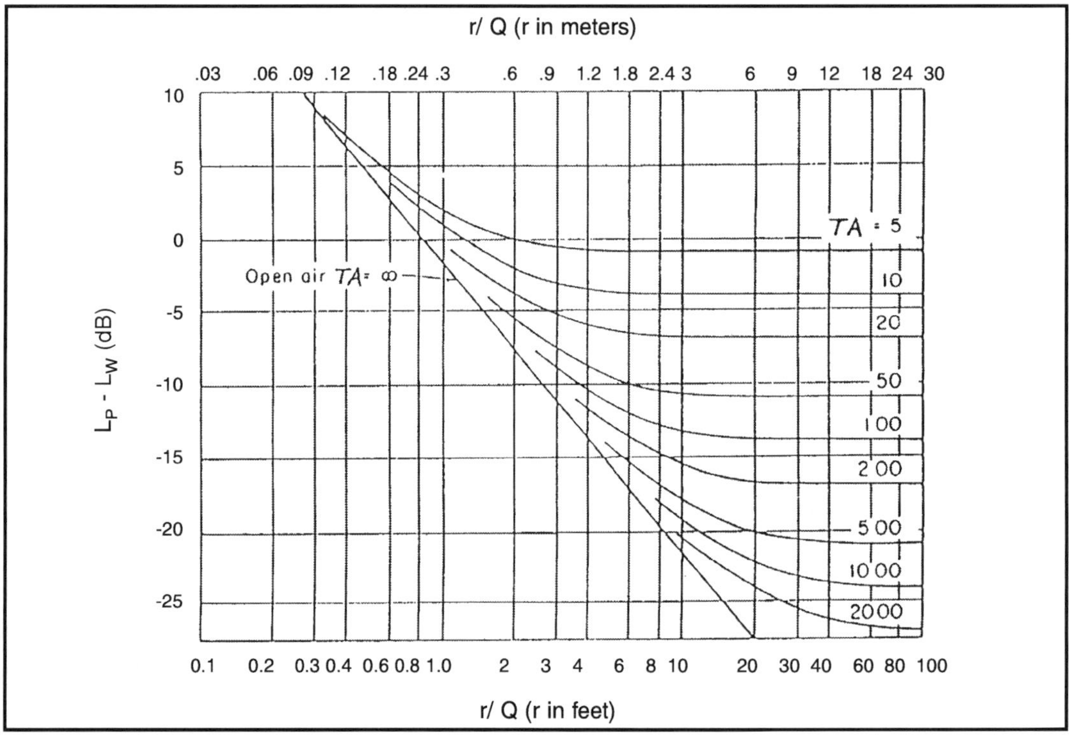

Figure 24.20 — Curves for determining the LP relative to LW in a room with total absorption (TA) at a distance (R) from a source of directivity (Q). (Adapted from Reference #34).

The amount of noise attenuation (NA) at a position in the reverberant field that can be achieved by adding sound absorption to a room is determined by using the following formula for each relevant octave band:

$$NA = 10 \log_{10} \left[\frac{TA_2}{TA_1} \right] \quad (24\text{-}20)$$

Where:

NA = noise attenuation in dB;
TA_1 = TA before treatment; and
TA_2 = TA after treatment.

When increasing room absorption to reduce sound levels, it is important to determine which octave band frequencies need reduction and to choose absorptive materials that are highly absorptive in those frequencies. For example, thicker sound absorptive treatments are necessary for reducing low-frequency sound levels.

Example: Room Treatment by Increasing Sound Absorption

Room:	13 m × 14 m × 4 m
Volume:	728 m^3
Ceiling:	Plaster - 182 m^2
Floor:	Concrete - 142 m^2
Floor:	Carpet - 40 m^2
Walls:	Painted Brick - 216 m^2
Frequency of interest:	1,000 Hz

The total absorption (TA_1) at 1,000 Hz before treatment is equal to:

Ceiling - Plaster	182 × 0.05 =	9.1
Floor - Concrete	142 × 0.02 =	2.8
Floor - Carpet	40 × 0.37 =	14.8
Walls - Brick	216 × 0.02 =	4.3
Air Absorption	.73 × 3.0 =	2.2
Total	**33.2 metric Sabins**	

The ceiling is to be covered with acoustical tile having an absorption coefficient of 0.80 at 1,000 Hz. The total absorption (TA_2) after treatment is equal to:

Ceiling - Tile	182 × 0.80 =	45.6
Floor - Concrete	142 × 0.02 =	2.8
Floor - Carpet	40 × 0.37 =	14.8
Walls - Brick	216 × 0.02 =	4.3
Air Absorption	.73 × 3.0 =	2.2
Total	**169.7**	

The noise attenuation at a location far from a sound source (in the reverberant field) is calculated as follows:

NA =

$$10 \log_{10} \frac{TA_2}{TA_1} = 10 \log_{10} \frac{169.7}{33.2} = 7.1 \text{ dB} \quad (24\text{-}21)$$

The results can be quite different for other frequencies; therefore, similar calculations must be repeated for all octave band frequencies of interest. In one case history, 10 automatic wire-cutting machines at a facility were located in an alcove measuring 6 m × 18 m. The operator did not have to tend the machines constantly. The ceiling was wood, the floor was concrete, three walls were brick, and one side was open to a large storage area. The addition of acoustical absorption to this area was recommended because there were multiple noise sources and very little absorption initially, and because the operator was far from the noise sources. Acoustical absorption was applied to the ceiling and to one wall. An area of 128 m^2 was covered. After the area was treated, the employees commented that the working conditions had improved considerably. There was no noise attenuation in the frequencies below 300 Hz. In the upper octave bands, the L_p was reduced from 4 dB to 12 dB (depending on frequency) near the machines. At 6 m from the center of the machines, (the operator location in the reverberant field), the attenuation was between 15 dB and 20 dB in the upper octave bands.

Equipment Noise Enclosures

Noise enclosures reduce the noise of a sound source by completely surrounding the source with a barrier material. The sound energy must then propagate through the wall of the enclosure before reaching the area outside. The three primary design concerns for enclosures are: use of a good barrier material for the enclosure, application of sound absorption to the interior of the enclosure, and avoidance of enclosure leaks. The ability of the barrier to prevent transmission of sound is quantified as its transmission loss (TL). The amount of sound absorption in an enclosure is quantified as its total absorption, as defined in the previous section. The purpose of the absorption is to prevent the sound level inside the enclosure from building up due to reverberation. The estimated noise attenuation at a location outside the enclosure that is achieved by enclosing a noise source is calculated by using the following formula:

$$NA = TL - 10 \log_{10} \left[\frac{S}{TA} \right] \qquad (24\text{-}22)$$

Where:

The floor was concrete
NA = noise attenuation in dB;
TL = transmission loss of enclosure material;
S = exterior surface area of the enclosure in m^2; and
TA = total absorption inside the enclosure in metric Sabins.
(S/TA can be considered an absorption correction.)

Sound absorption coefficients are given in Table 24.9, and Table 24.10 lists the measured TL of common building materials.[36,37,40] As shown in Equation 24-22, the noise attenuation of an enclosure depends largely on the TL of the barrier material. This material must normally be constructed of material weighing at least 5 kg/ m^2 (1 lb/ft^2) and must be durable enough to withstand any expected abuse. If the interior is completely lined with a perfectly absorptive material, such that the total absorption (TA) equals the exterior surface area (S), then NA = TL. If TA is only half of S (because only half the interior is treated or because the entire interior is treated with a material with an absorption coefficient of 0.5), then NA = TL – 3. If the interior of the enclosure has no sound absorptive treatment, then the enclosure might achieve very little noise attenuation. Also, the problems caused by any small leaks in the enclosure will be exacerbated by the increased reverberant sound levels in an untreated enclosure. In many cases, 25–50 mm (1–2 in.) thick glass fiber or acoustical foam is used as the absorptive material. Whenever the enclosed equipment leaks oil, water, or chemicals, it is important to protect the sound absorptive material with thin films (1 mil or 25 µm) of materials such as Mylar® or Tedlar®. In addition to the enclosure barrier TL and the sound absorption inside the enclosure, several other design elements need to be considered:

- No significant leaks can be allowed in the surface of the enclosure in order to achieve a noise attenuation ≥10 dB. All joints or cracks must be completely sealed. Access and maintenance panels must close and seal tightly.
- The enclosure must be completely vibration-isolated from the enclosed equipment. Any direct structural connection will transmit vibration to the enclosure, which will then radiate sound in the enclosure to the outside room. If a connection is necessary, it must be vibration-isolated (e.g., by using a flexible connection).
- Auxiliary cooling may be required to prevent enclosed equipment from overheating. Any ventilation ducts, with or without fans, must be treated with sound-absorptive materials and must be oriented to prevent a direct line of sight from worker positions into the enclosed equipment. (See the subsequent section on partial enclosures.)

Example: Design of Full Enclosure

Since transmission loss data and sound absorption coefficient data are often only given for the 125–4,000 Hz octave bands, this example only considers those octave bands. Most acoustical problems are in this frequency region, but if a problem arises in the 31.5, 63, or 8,000 Hz octave bands, the same formulas apply and TL and sound absorption data can be estimated.

The first step in designing an enclosure is to determine the acoustical requirements. This can be done by subtracting the octave band noise criterion from the measured octave band sound levels at a position of concern. The differences are the required noise attenuation of the enclosure in each of the octave bands. If the criterion is only for an A-weighted sound level, it will first be necessary to create an octave band spectrum goal equal to the A-weighted criterion. The following table shows calculations of the required NA.

Table 24.10 — Transmission loss data for common building constructions(36,37,40)

Building Construction	*125 Hz*	*250 Hz*	*500 Hz*	*1000 Hz*	*2000 Hz*	*4000 Hz*
			Transmission Loss (dB)			
Walls						
Interior:						
2-in. solid plaster on metal lath (18 psf)	20	22	22	27	36	42
2 × 4 wood studs 16-in. o.c. with ½-in.gypsum board both sides (6 psf)	10	28	33	42	47	41
2 × 4 wood studs 16-in. o.c. with ⅝-in. gypsum board both sides - one side screwed to resilient channels. 3-in. glass-fiber batt insulation in cavity (6.5 psf)	32	42	52	58	53	54
6-in. concrete block wall, painted (34 psf)	37	36	42	49	55	58
8-in. concrete block wall with ¾-in. wood furring, gypsum lath and plaster both sides (67 psf)	43	47	47	55	58	60
2½-in. steel channel studs with ⅝-in. gypsum board both sides (11 psf)	15	24	38	48	40	42
Construction above with glass-fiber insulation in cavity	23	35	44	53	45	43
2⅝-in. steel channel studs with 2 layers ⅝-in. gypsum board one side, 1 layer other side (8 psf)	22	26	40	51	44	47
Construction above with glass-fiber insulation in cavity	28	38	50	57	50	50
2⅝-in. steel channel studs with 2 layers ⅝-in. gypsum board both sides (10 psf)	27	34	48	55	50	57
Construction above with glass-fiber insulation in cavity	33	44	55	60	55	60
Exterior:						
4½-in. brick with ½-in. plaster each side (55 psf)	34	34	41	50	56	58
9-in. brick with ½-in. plaster each side (100 psf)	41	43	49	55	57	60
Two wythes of plastered 4½-in. brick, 2-in. air space with glass-fiber in cavity (90 psf)	43	50	52	61	73	78
2 × 4 wood studs 16-in. o.c. with 1-in. stucco on metal lath on outside and ½-in. gypsum board on inside (8 psf)	21	33	41	46	47	51
6-in. concrete with ½-in. plaster both sides (80 psf)	39	42	50	58	64	67
Floor-Ceilings						
2 × 10 wood joists 16-in. o.c. with ½-in. plywood subfloor, $^{25}/_{32}$ in. oak on floor side, and ⅝-in. gypsum board on ceiling side (10 psf)	23	32	36	45	49	56
Construction above with 3-in. glass-fiber batt insulation in cavity	25	36	38	46	51	57
4-in. thick reinforced concrete slab (53 psf)	48	42	45	56	58	66
14-in. precast concrete tees with 2-in. slab, and 2-in. concrete topping (75 psf)	40	45	49	52	60	68
6-in. thick reinforced concrete slab with ¾-in. T & G wood flooring on 1½-in × 2-in. wooden battens on 1-in. thick glass-wool quilt (83 psf)	38	44	52	55	60	65
18-in. steel joists 16-in. o.c. with 1⅝-in. concrete on ⅝-in. plywood nailed to joists and heavy carpet on underlay. On ceiling side, ⅝-in. gypsum board nailed to joists (20 psf)	27	37	45	54	60	65
Roofs						
Corrugated steel, 24-gauge with 1⅜-in. sprayed cellulose insulation on ceiling side (1.8 psf)	17	22	26	30	35	41
2½-in. sand gravel concrete (148 pcf) on 28-gauge corrugated steel supported by 14-in. steel bar joists, with ½-in. gypsum plaster on metal lath and ¾-in. metal furring channels 13½-in. o.c. on ceiling side (41 psf)	32	46	45	50	57	61

Table 24.10 — Transmission loss data for common building constructions (continued)[36,37,40]

	Transmission Loss (dB)					
Building Construction	*125 Hz*	*250 Hz*	*500 Hz*	*1000 Hz*	*2000 Hz*	*4000 Hz*
Doors						
2½-in. acoustical door with 12-gauge steel facing	43	49	48	55	57	44
1¾-in. hollow wood core door, no gaskets or closure, ¼-in. air gap at sill	14	19	23	18	17	21
Construction above with gaskets and drop seal	19	22	25	19	20	29
1¾-in. solid wood core door with gaskets and drop seal (4.3 psf)	29	31	31	31	39	43
1¾-in. hollow 16-gauge steel door, glass-fiber filled core with gaskets and drop seal (6.8 psf)	23	28	36	41	39	44
Glass						
⅛-in. single plate-glass pane	18	21	26	31	33	22
¼-in. single plate-glass pane with rubber gasket	25	28	30	34	24	35
$>^9/_{32}$ in. laminated glass pane (i.e., viscoelastic layer sandwiched between glass layers)	26	29	33	36	35	39
¼- + ⅛-in. double plate-glass window with 2-in. air space	18	31	35	42	44	44
Construction No. 38 with 4-in. air space	21	32	42	48	48	44
Panels						
lead sheet - Z|zn in.	28	32	33	32	32	33
lead sheet - Z|, in.	30	31	27	38	44	33
20 g aluminum sheet, stiffened	11	10	10	18	23	25
22 g galvanized sheet steel	8	14	20	23	26	27
20 g galvanized sheet steel	8	14	20	26	32	38
18 g galvanized sheet steel	13	20	24	29	33	39
16 g galvanized sheet steel	14	21	27	32	37	43
18 g fluted steel panels stiffened at edges	30	20	22	30	28	31
¼-in. plywood	17	15	20	24	28	27
¾-in. plywood	24	22	27	28	25	27
⅛-in. lead vinyl curtains	22	23	25	31	35	42

Octave Band Sound Pressure Level

	125	250	500	1000	2000	4000	dBA
Sound Level	96	91	93	87	86	81	94
Criterion Required	92	86	81	77	74	72	85
NA	4	5	12	10	12	9	-

Next, it is important to determine the size of the enclosure and the amount of absorption that can be applied to the interior of the enclosure. In each octave band, the total absorption (TA) and the absorption correction (10 log(S/TA)), must be calculated. This absorption correction and a safety factor of 3–5 dB should then be added to the required NA to get the required TL. The safety factor allows for differences between the performance achieved in a laboratory and those typically achieved in the field. In this example, the exterior surface area of the enclosure is 5 m² and the interior is completely treated with a material with the sound absorption coefficients listed in the following calculation table:

Octave Band Center Frequencies

	Surface Area (m²)	125	250	500	1000	2000	4000
Absorption Coefficient	5	0.23	0.45	0.68	0.96	1.00	0.98
Total Area and Absorption	5	1.15	2.25	3.4	4.8	5.0	4.9
10 log (S/TA)		6	3	2	0	0	0
Required NA		4	5	12	10	12	9
Safety Factor		5	5	5	5	5	5
Required TL		15	13	19	15	17	14

After the required TL has been determined, a barrier material and thickness meeting all of the octave band TL requirements can be chosen from Table 24.10. If the criterion is for an A-weighted sound level and not for octave band levels, then an acceptable material will not have to meet every octave band TL requirement as long as the resulting treated octave band sound levels add up to an A-weighted spectrum that meets the criterion.

In one case study at an industrial facility, noise from a steam turbine that was used to drive a boiler feed pump significantly exceeded the exposure criterion and was especially annoying due to its tonal nature. To lower the noise, the turbine was enclosed in 1.6 mm thick (16 gauge) steel, lined with 25 mm (1 in.) thick glass fiber with a density of 48 kg/m³ (3 lb/ft³). The noise attenuation was 14 dB in the 4,000 Hz octave band in which the loudest tones occurred, thus solving the noise problem.

Partial Enclosures

Sometimes a complete enclosure around a noise source is not possible. For example, openings in an enclosure are often required for maintenance, controls, drive shafts, ventilation, or process flow. In these cases, a partial enclosure can be built to achieve some noise control. Partial enclosures are constructed similarly to complete enclosures; they have good barrier materials on the outside and sound absorption on the inside, but because of their openings they normally provide less than 10 dBA of noise attenuation.

Since sound will not be significantly attenuated by propagating through direct openings to the outside, paths to the outside should be convoluted and treated with sound-absorptive surfaces when possible. If sound is forced to reflect off sound-absorptive walls before reaching the outside, the sound level can be reduced significantly. Convoluted paths are normally only possible with ventilation openings, but even a straight opening into a partial enclosure (such as an opening around a conveyor belt) can be treated to reduce sound levels by making a long, narrow tubular duct with sound-absorptive walls. The following items should be considered in the design of a partial enclosure:

- Any openings in an enclosure should be directed away from personnel locations; otherwise, there will be little or no sound reduction at the operator positions.
- The number and area of openings in an enclosure should be minimized.
- The interior of the enclosure should be treated with as much sound-absorptive material as possible.
- Partial enclosures work best at reducing high-frequency sounds where the dimensions of the enclosure surfaces are at least several times longer than the wavelength of the sound waves.

The noise attenuation provided by a partial enclosure can be estimated by using the following equation:

$$NA = 10 \log_{10} \frac{TA}{OS} \quad (24.23)$$

Where:

NA = noise attenuation in dB;
OS = area of the openings in square meters; and
TA = total absorption inside the enclosure (including the openings) in metric Sabins.

The NA will be limited to no more than the TL of the barrier material. To achieve the noise attenuation calculated in the formula above, the barrier material of the partial enclosure must have a transmission loss (TL) value at least 10 dB greater than the noise attenuation calculated for the partial enclosure. If the opening in the enclosure is pointing toward the employee, the noise attenuation at his or her location will probably be at least 3 dB less than that calculated above, depending on the directivity of the noise source.

Personnel Enclosures

When there are multiple noisy sound sources in a room and a low number of operators, it is sometimes useful to enclose the employees instead of the equipment. The equipment room will still be loud, but the operators will be in a relatively quiet enclosure. This personnel enclosure can include equipment controls and windows for observing operations of the equipment. The noise reduction from the outside of the enclosure to the inside can be calculated with the following equation:

$$NR = TL_C - 10 \log_{10} \left[\frac{1}{4} + \frac{S_t}{TA} \right] \quad (24\text{-}24)$$

Where:

NR = noise reduction in dB
TL_C = composite transmission loss of the enclosure walls, roof, etc.
S_t = area of enclosure surfaces between noisy and quiet sides (in m²)
TA = total absorption inside the interior of enclosure in metric Sabins

This equation can also be used to determine the NR of a wall separating a noisy room from a relatively quiet room. Like equipment enclosures, personnel enclosures are limited by the TL of the walls and roof and the sound absorption inside the enclosure. The TL of a personnel enclosure is normally more difficult to calculate than the TL of a machine enclosure since it often includes windows, doors, ventilation, and different roof and wall structures. The composite TL of an enclosure consisting of several materials is determined by the following equation:

$$TL_C = 10\log_{10}\left[\frac{S_t}{S_1*10^{(-TL_1/10)} + S_2*10^{(-TL_2/10)} \ldots + S_n*10^{(-TL_n/10)}}\right] \quad (24.25)$$

Since small openings and building elements with low TL values significantly reduce the effectiveness of the entire enclosure, it is important to pay close attention to all components when designing an enclosure. The number and sizes of windows should be minimized, and if possible, laminated or double-layered glass (with as deep an air gap as possible) should be used. Doors should be equipped with seals around all four edges. The walls and roof should also be carefully sealed. Any ventilation ductwork running from the inside of the enclosure to the outside should have an interior lining of sound-absorptive material and should include 90° bends to reduce sound transmission. The interior should be treated with an abundance of sound-absorptive materials. Although carpet is sometimes used on the floor, it is usually effective at absorbing only high-frequency noise (above 2,000 Hz). Therefore, the walls and ceiling should be treated with good high- and low-frequency sound-absorptive materials.

Example: Design of a Personnel Enclosure

A personnel enclosure is proposed for a large manufacturing area. The existing sound levels in the area where the enclosure will be located and the desired goal for the interior of the enclosure are listed below:

Octave-Band Center Frequencies

	125	250	500	1000	2000	4000	dBA
Existing Sound Level	85	89	87	84	78	71	89
Enclosure Design Goal	72	66	61	57	54	52	65
Required	NR	13	23	26	27	24	19

The enclosure will be 2 m wide × 4 m long × 2 m high. The floor will be carpeted, the ceiling will have acoustical tile, and the walls will have some sound-absorptive panels as well as a door and windows. The total absorption (using the absorption coefficients from Table 24.9) and required TL are calculated below:

Octave-Band Center Frequencies

	Surface Area (m²)	125	250	500	1000	2000	4000
Carpet Abs. Coefficient	8	0.02	0.06	0.14	0.37	0.60	0.65
Carpet Absorption		0.2	0.5	1.1	3.0	4.8	5.2
Ceiling Abs. Coefficient	8	0.76	0.93	0.83	0.99	0.99	0.94
Ceiling Absorption		6.1	7.4	6.6	7.9	7.9	7.5
Plywood Wall Abs. Coefficient	12	0.28	0.22	0.17	0.09	0.10	0.11
Plywood Wall Absorption		3.4	2.6	2.0	1.1	1.2	1.3
Treated Wall Abs. Coefficient	8	0.23	0.54	0.60	0.98	0.93	0.99
Treated Wall Absorption		1.8	4.3	4.8	7.8	7.4	7.9
Window/Door Abs. Coefficient	4	0.35	0.25	0.18	0.12	0.07	0.04
Window and Door Absorption		1.4	1.0	0.7	0.5	0.3	0.2
Total Area (S_t) and Abs. (TA)	32	12.9	15.8	15.2	20.3	21.6	22.1
$10\log(1/4+S_t/TA)$		4	4	4	3	2	2
Required NR		13	23	26	27	24	19
Safety Factor		5	5	5	5	5	5
Required Composite TL		22	32	35	35	31	26

Note that S_t is the total surface of the walls and roof and does not include the floor, which is not exposed to exterior noise.

S_t would be further reduced if a wall or the roof of the enclosure was not exposed to noise, for example if the enclosure was placed against a wall.

In the following table, the composite TL is calculated for the enclosure using TL values from Table 24.10. As shown, this can be fairly complicated to do by hand. One way of reducing the work is to put the calculations in a spreadsheet computer program. The easiest (though least precise) method is to choose roof and wall materials with TL values greater than the required amount for the composite TL and then to try to get windows and doors that do not reduce the composite TL significantly.

In the above example, the proposed wall is made of 64 mm (2½ in.) steel channel studs with 16 mm (5/8 in.) gypsum board on both sides and glass fiber insulation in the cavity. The roof is constructed similarly except with wooden studs and a resilient channel. The door is a glass-fiber filled 1.6 mm thick (16 gauge) steel door equipped with gaskets and a drop seal. The window is 6 mm (1/4 in.) single plate glass. Note that the weak composite TL in the 2000 Hz octave band is caused by the low TL for the window at that frequency. This shows that a significant weakness in any building element, even if it is not large in area, can reduce the composite TL of the entire enclosure.

	Octave-Band Center Frequencies						
	Surface Area (m^2)	125	250	500	1000	2000	4000
TL of Wall	20	23	35	44	53	45	43
$S \times 10^{(-TL/10)}$		0.100	0.0063	0.0008	0.00010	0.0006	0.001
TL of Roof	8	32	42	52	58	53	54
$S \times 10^{(-TL/10)}$		0.005	0.0005	0.00005	0.00001	0.00004	0.00003
TL of Window	2	25	28	30	34	24	35
$S \times 10^{(-TL/10)}$		0.063	0.0032	0.0020	0.00080	0.008	0.0006
TL of Door	2	23	28	36	41	39	44
$S \times 10^{(-TL/10)}$		0.010	0.0032	0.0005	0.00016	0.00025	0.00008
Total $S \times 10^{(-TL/10)}$		0.178	0.0132	0.0033	0.00107	0.00889	0.00171
Composite TL	32	23	34	40	45	36	43
Required TL		22	32	35	35	31	26

Shields or Barriers

Barriers placed between an employee and noisy equipment can be an effective means of lowering noise exposure. A barrier causes a "sound shadow" at the receiver with a consequent attenuation of Lp. Since sound diffracts more than light around an edge, the shadow zone is only partially shielded from the noise. Mid- and high-frequency sound is diffracted less than low-frequency sound; therefore, barriers are more effective for shielding from mid- and high-frequency sound sources. The attenuation of a barrier can be calculated as a function of the difference in the length of the sound path imposed by the barrier. The sound path difference is given by:

$$d = \sqrt{S^2+h_s^2} + \sqrt{R^2+h_t^2} - \sqrt{(S+R)^2+(h_t-h_s)^2} \qquad (24.26)$$

Where:

d = difference between the path length from the source to the receiver over a barrier and the straight line-of-sight path between the source and receiver without the barrier;

S = distance to the barrier from the source (m);

R = distance to the barrier from the receiver (m);

h_s = height of the barrier above the source (m); and

h_r = height of the barrier above the receiver (m).

These variables are illustrated in Figure 24.21. In Table 24.11, an estimate of the attenuation or insertion loss of a barrier is given as a function of the path difference (d) and the frequency. These values are for an ideal barrier with no reflecting surfaces nearby. It can be seen in the table that the insertion loss due to a barrier ranges from 5–24 dB. For the greatest insertion loss, the path difference should be maximized; thus, the barrier should be as tall as possible and placed as near the source or receiver as possible (not halfway between).

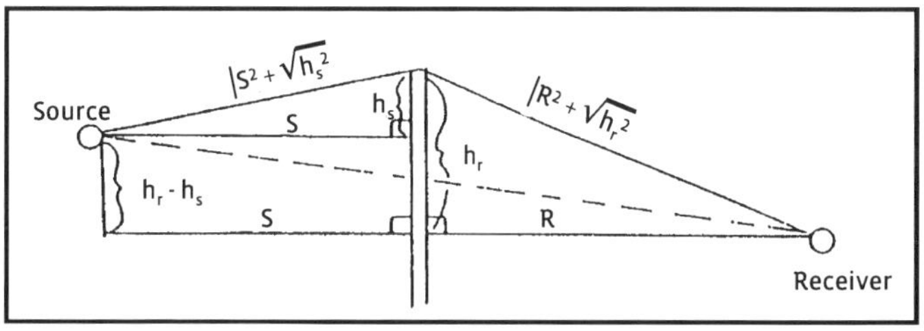

Figure 24.21 — Variables used for calculation of barrier insertion loss.

Table 24.11 — Insertion loss (in dB) of an ideal barrier based on the path difference

Path Difference	Octave Band Center Frequency (Hz) 31.5	63	125	250	500	1000	2000	4000	8000
3 mm	5	5	5	5	5	5	6	6	7
6 mm	5	5	5	5	5	6	6	7	9
10 mm	5	5	5	5	5	6	7	8	10
15 mm	5	5	5	5	6	6	8	9	12
20 mm	5	5	5	5	6	7	8	10	13
30 mm	5	5	6	6	6	8	9	12	15
60 mm	5	5	6	6	8	9	12	15	18
0.1 m	5	6	6	7	9	11	14	16	19
0.15 m	5	6	7	8	10	13	16	18	21
0.2 m	6	6	8	9	11	14	17	20	23
0.3 m	6	7	9	10	13	16	18	21	24
0.6 m	7	8	11	13	16	18	21	24	24
1 m	8	9	12	14	17	20	23	24	24
1.5 m	9	11	14	16	19	22	24	24	24
2 m	10	13	15	18	21	24	24	24	24
3 m	1	14	16	19	22	24	24	24	24
6 m	14	16	19	22	24	24	24	24	24
9 m	15	18	21	24	24	24	24	24	24

If a barrier is used indoors, reflections off ceilings and walls will probably reduce its performance. Generally, indoor barriers are most effective when the exposed individual is in the direct field of the noise source. A rough estimate of the insertion loss of a barrier with a ceiling above the barrier can be derived by considering only the sound path that is reflected off the ceiling to the receiver in the barrier shadow zone. The insertion loss is calculated as:

$$IL = 10 \log_{10}\left[\left(\frac{dc}{dl}\right)^2 * \frac{1}{(1-\alpha)}\right] \qquad (24\text{-}27)$$

Where:

IL = difference between the level of the direct sound path without a barrier and that of the sound path reflected off the ceiling;

dc = path length in meters that the sound travels to the ceiling and down to the receiver position behind the barrier;

dl = line-of-sight distance in meters from the source to the receiver without a barrier; and

α = absorption coefficient of the ceiling (if this is 1.0, there will be no sound reflection and no need for this calculation).

This equation should be used to calculate the sound level of reflected sound paths off any walls, ceilings, or other surfaces that directly reflect sound from a source to a receiver around a barrier. There may be several such paths. The total expected sound level at the receiver position should be calculated by using Table 24.11 to calculate the sound level at the receiver position from the diffracted sound path over the barrier and Equation 24-27 to calculate the sound level at the receiver position from each reflected sound path. The resulting diffracted and reflected sound levels should then be added logarithmically (Equation 24-27) to get the total L_p.

A few other factors should be considered during the design of barriers to be installed in occupational environments:

- The transmission loss of the barrier itself should be at least 10 dB greater than the expected insertion loss of the barrier. This prevents noise transmitted through the barrier from having an appreciable contribution at the receiver position.

- For outdoor barriers, care must be taken to consider reflections off nearby buildings or large equipment. As for the case of indoor barriers, reflected noise will lower the barrier performance to less than that estimated in Table 24.11.
- All significant diffracted paths should be considered. For example, the sound levels calculated for diffracted paths around the sides of a free-standing barrier should be added to the sound level from the refracted path over the barrier and the reflected paths.
- Table 24.11 is derived with the noise source considered as a point source. For many large sources, such as cooling towers, the position of an appropriate source radiation point is not obvious. One approach is to divide the surface of the large source into many point sources, make separate calculations for each point, and then add the results together. A conservative and less time-consuming approach is to place the source point at the top of the equipment.
- If two barriers or a barrier and a wall are situated in parallel with the sound source between them, noise reflected back and forth between the two surfaces can "walk up" the barrier and lower the insertion loss. This potential can be minimized by choosing a barrier that is acoustically absorptive on the side facing the sound source.

Example: Calculation of Barrier Insertion Loss

A sound source inside a building produces a level of 98 dB in the 1,000 Hz octave band at an operator position 9 m (30 ft) distant (horizontally). The sound is radiated from an inlet duct, the top of which is positioned 3.4 m (11 ft) above the floor. The operator is usually standing, and his or her ear height is taken as 1.5 m (5 ft). A barrier is to be erected between the noise source and the operator. Because of access requirements, the barrier will be placed 1.8 m (6 ft) from the source. The barrier height is 3.7 m (12 ft). The ceiling height is 6 m (20 ft) and covered with thermal insulation that has an absorption coefficient of 0.5 at 1,000 Hz. Assume that there are no reflected or diffracted sound paths around the side edges of the barrier. Calculate the insertion loss of the diffracted path over the barrier and the loss of the reflected path off the ceiling.

The path difference over the barrier is calculated to be d = 0.15 m (0.5 ft). The insertion loss of the barrier therefore is about 13 dB at 1,000 Hz as read from Table 24.11; thus, the L_p would be reduced to 98 – 13 = 85 dB by the barrier, assuming there are no other sound pathways or significant sound sources in the near vicinity. To calculate the ceiling path length, it helps to draw a scale sketch of the source, barrier, receiver, and ceiling in elevation. Choose a ceiling reflection point such that the angle between the ceiling and the sound path from the source is the same as the angle between the ceiling and the sound path to the receiver (a mirror-like reflection) as shown in Figure 24.22. For this example, the total reflected ceiling path length is 11.5 m (37.6 ft). The line-of-sight distance is about 9.3 m (30.6 ft). The reduction along the ceiling pathway from Equation 24-27 is 5 dB. The contribution from the ceiling path, therefore, is 98 – 5 = 93 dB. The L_p at the receiver is the result of the combination of the barrier and ceiling contributions of 85 +log 93 = 94 dB, a reduction of only 4 dB. The barrier reduction of 13 dB is overshadowed by sound reflected off the ceiling.

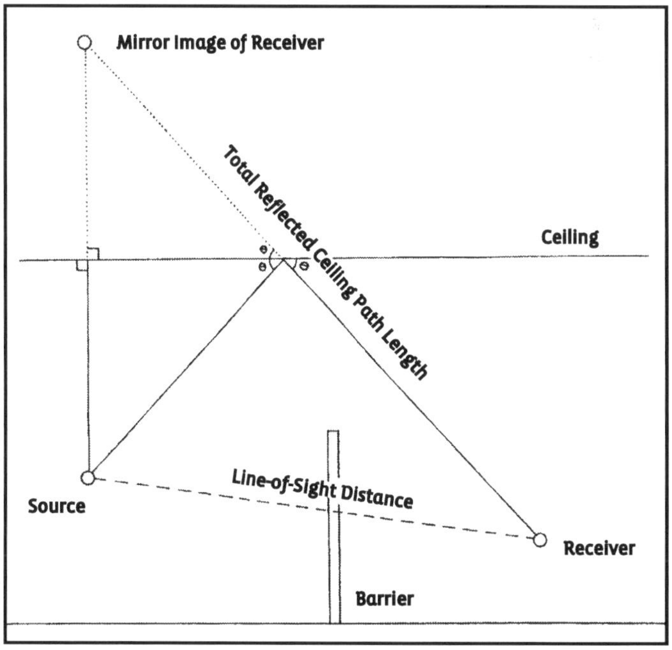

Figure 24.22 — Calculation of sound reflection over a barrier.

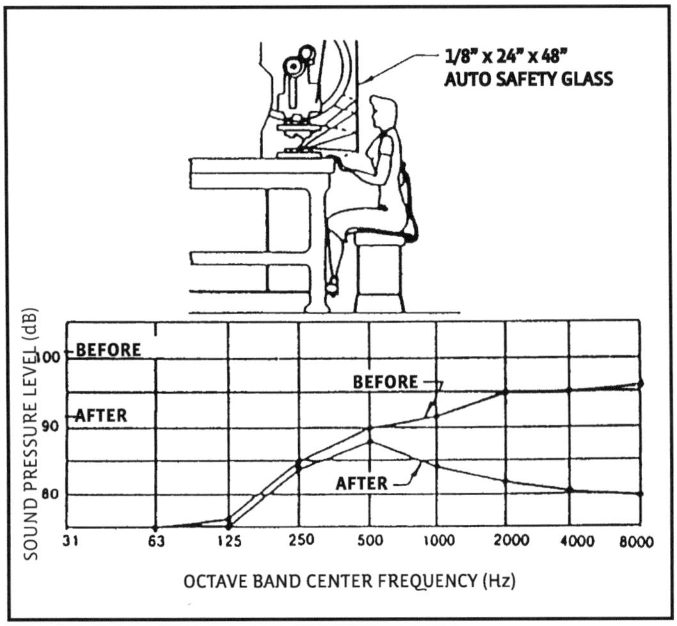

Figure 24.23 — Noise levels before and after installation of a glass shield. (Adapted from Reference #37).

If the absorption coefficient were increased to 0.98 at 1,000 Hz, the reduction reflecting off the ceiling path would be 19 dB for an Lp of 79 dB. The summed level would be 79 +log 85 = 86 dB. For this latter case, the barrier performance would not be appreciably compromised by the ceiling reflection.

The placement of shields between an employee and a noise source can be an effective treatment, especially if the noise is high frequency and the employee and noise source are close to the shield. A shield used on a punch press is illustrated in Figure 24.23. Safety glass (6 mm [1/4 in.] thick) was installed between the operator and the press. Lps before and after treatment are presented in the figure. The designer should be aware that in situations in which multiple units are in close proximity, noise from nearby units might make this type of treatment ineffective.

Lagging

It is sometimes impractical to enclose a noise source because of its shape, operations access requirements, or insufficient space. Damping may not be practical if the excitation frequency is different than the panel resonances or if the panel is thick (recall that damping treatments should generally be as thick as the panel to which they are attached). In these situations an enclosure-like treatment attached directly to the vibrating surface can be effective. This treatment is commonly referred to as "lagging." It is a common treatment for piping.

High-frequency sound radiation can be reduced by wrapping a surface with a sound-absorptive material such as glass fiber or acoustical foam. Sound below about 1,000 Hz will be little affected, however. A significant improvement can be attained by covering the absorptive wrapping with an air-tight limp barrier material. This barrier can be asphalt paper, neoprene sheeting, lead, loaded vinyl, etc.—the heavier and more limp, the better. Increasing the thickness of the sound-absorptive layer generally also improves the noise attenuation; especially at frequencies below 1,000 Hz. Manufacturers offer lagging materials in the form of foam/vinyl composites as well as other material combinations.

With lagging, the outer layer acts like the walls of an enclosure, and the sound-absorptive layer provides both vibration isolation for the outer layer and also sound absorption for the space between the outer layer and the sound-radiating surface. Lagging treatments will generally be effective above the frequency given by the following equation:[34]

$$f = \frac{63}{\sqrt{wd}} \qquad (24\text{-}28)$$

Where:

f = limiting frequency in Hz;
w = limp barrier surface weight in kg/m^2; and
d = thickness of the absorptive layer in meters.

Below the frequency given by this equation, the insertion loss will be essentially zero. In fact, when this treatment is applied to a small pipe, the sound levels in this low-frequency region may increase a few dB over the untreated condition due to the increase in the size of the sound-radiating surface. The insertion loss of a lagging treatment increases above the frequency defined by Equation 24-28 and may attain 30–45 dB in the highest frequencies, though 15–20 dB is more common.

Lined Ducts and Mufflers

In some situations the noise of HVAC systems becomes an important contribution to the employee noise environment. Ventilation ducts can also be significant noise transmission pathways between noisy and quiet areas. Ducts may also be used as intakes to and discharges from noisy equipment. Noise traveling through ducts can be attenuated by the application of various sound-absorptive duct linings. A simple formula to estimate the attenuation of sound through straight ducts of a regular cross section lined with absorption is:

$$NA = 1.05\alpha^{1.4} \frac{P}{S} \qquad (24\text{-}29)$$

Where:

- NA = noise attenuation in dB/m of duct length;
- α = absorption coefficient for the lining material;
- P = lined perimeter of the duct in meters; and
- S = cross-sectional area in m^2.

This formula is most accurate for low frequencies and/or narrow ducts such that $f < 34/w$[34] where "w" is the duct width in meters. At higher frequencies, the attenuation will be less than calculated due to the "beaming" of sound straight down the duct without reflecting off the side walls. This formula can also be applied to parallel baffle sound absorbers with accuracy sufficient for many occupational noise problems. Noise attenuation of the parallel baffles generally increases as the distance between the baffles decreases. Of course, muffler performance data from the manufacturer is always preferable.

Blocking the line-of-sight between the source and receiver is an effective element of noise attenuation. Bends or staggered absorbers at 90° along a duct will greatly increase the noise attenuation, particularly at high frequencies. It might be necessary in these cases to evaluate the resulting increase in back pressure. Figure 24.24 presents sketches and trends in the noise attenuation of various arrangements of lined ducts.

Dissipative and reactive mufflers can be used to control noise from exhausts or

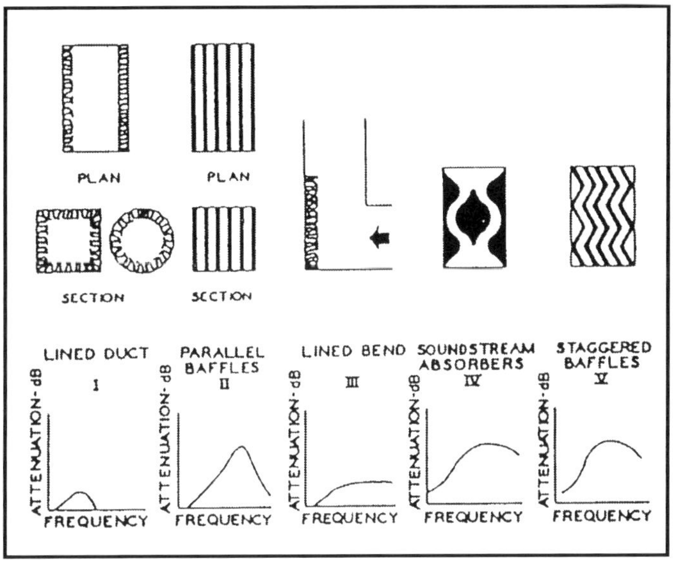

Figure 24.24 — Examples and general acoustic performance of lined ducts and mufflers. (Adapted from Reference #37.)

intakes. Dissipative mufflers have an absorptive lining inside the muffler. In general, these mufflers provide broad-band noise attenuation (attenuation across a wide band of frequencies) with the maximum attenuation being a function of the thickness of the lining as well as its acoustical properties. Dissipative mufflers are generally used to reduce the noise from fans, blowers, and product entrances and exits from enclosures. A reactive muffler provides attenuation by a series of cavities and side branches with abrupt cross-sectional area changes. The resulting impedance changes reflect the sound back toward the source. These mufflers are likely to have superior performance over a narrow band of frequencies. They are often used with internal combustion engines and fluidborne noise sources.

The design of reactive mufflers is beyond the scope of this chapter. They are usually effective only over a narrow range of frequencies. It might be safer to design an absorptive muffler with a broader frequency response, if possible. However, if the noise is produced in a narrow frequency range and is unlikely to change based on different operations, a reactive muffler may be specified. Since reactive mufflers are complicated to design, they should be purchased with a performance guarantee.

In Figure 24.25, there is a sketch of a combination parallel-baffle dissipative

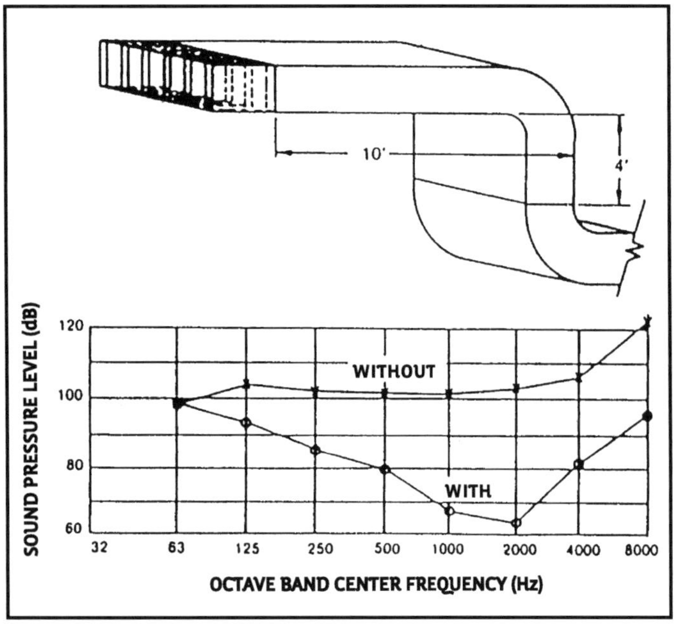

Figure 24.25 — Noise levels with and without muffler, (Adapted from Reference #37).

muffler and elbow. This arrangement was attached to the compressor intake of a 5 MW (7000 hp) gas turbine. Six parallel baffles were constructed of 1.2 mm (18 gauge) perforated steel, each 89 mm (3.5 in.) wide and filled with glass fiber. The duct was 2.1 m × 2.4 m (7 ft. × 8 ft.), and the elbow was constructed of 6 mm (1/4 in.) unlined plate. L_ps measured with and without the muffler installed are presented in the figure.

As an example, the discharge of a filter-bag separator of a pneumatic conveying system handling synthetic fiber fluff produced objectionable noise in the filter area. An absorptive muffler was not desired because of the potential for becoming clogged with fibers from the exhaust stream. A reactive muffler was installed and provided the following values of noise attenuation:

Octave-Band Center Frequencies (Hz)				
63	125	250	500	1000
12 dB	23 dB	13 dB	11 dB	10 dB

In this section, a wide variety of noise control treatments were presented with the intent that occupational hygienists will become familiar with ways to reduce employee noise exposure.

Hearing Conservation Programs

Introduction

The OSHA hearing conservation amendment provides a good outline of the minimum requirements for an effective hearing conservation program.[41] This includes sound monitoring, feasible administrative or engineering controls, audiometric testing, hearing protection, employee training and education, and record keeping. The true test of an effective program, however, is in the results of the employees' hearing tests.

This section briefly discusses the main requirements for an effective hearing conservation program. Although developing a program might seem straightforward, maintaining an effective program is quite challenging. Many texts have been written to provide assistance.[42–45]

Sound Survey

As noted earlier under the noise measurements section, a sound survey is performed to identify areas with hazardous levels of noise and to determine who should be included in a hearing conservation program. ANSI has requirements for Type I or Type II sound measurement equipment[46–48] and ANSI S12.19-1996 provides specific guidelines for performing noise measurements to determine occupational noise exposure.[49] These measurement procedures were discussed in the measurement section earlier in this chapter.

Engineering and Administrative Controls

Reducing the noise level to below the action level or limiting workers' exposure by reducing their time in noisy areas should be the primary methods of protecting workers' hearing.[50,51] Engineering and administrative controls combined with hearing protection may be the only way to prevent hearing loss. Also, though a decrease in the sound level of 3–5 dBA might not sound significant, this decrease can double the allowable noise exposure time. Ideally, hearing protection should be considered an interim solution while striving toward long-range goals such as purchasing quieter equipment and using cost-effective noise control solutions.

Unfortunately, there are many work locations where feasible solutions have not been available to reduce noise levels. Consequently, hearing protection remains an important means of conserving employee hearing.

Hearing Protection Devices

A good hearing protective device (HPD) is an effective means to reduce the sound exposure of persons either before engineering or administrative noise controls can be administered or when these controls are not yet feasible. The best HPD for a given situation is the one that is consistently and properly worn by the employee. Selection of an appropriate HPD depends on necessary attenuation; audibility of speech and warning signals; compatibility with other safety equipment; care and cleaning requirements; comfort; cost; ease of use; personal preference; temperature and humidity; and visibility (i.e, the HPD is visible so it is easy to monitor compliance with HCP policy).

All of these factors should be evaluated thoroughly before choosing the types of HPDs that will be made available. Workers should be given several choices of appropriate HPDs. Purchasing agents should also be informed of the reasoning behind the selection of the HPDs so they do not inadvertently purchase a lower-cost product they believe is equivalent. The main types of hearing protectors are illustrated in Figure 24.26.[52] "Roll-down" foam earplugs, premolded earplugs, formable earplugs, earmuffs, and semi-insert hearing protectors are discussed in the following sections.

"Roll-Down" Foam Earplugs

"Roll-down" foam earplugs can be made from polyvinyl chloride (PVC) or polyurethane (PU). These earplugs are among the most comfortable and protective hearing protective devices available, and because of this, they are the most widely used earplug. Once thought of as disposable, they have been used for extensive periods of time (a week or more) without any problems.

One disadvantage is that the "roll-down" requires employees to have clean hands, and thus in some environments, they may not be appropriate. These plugs are now available in multiple sizes, so care must be taken by the employer not to provide only the smallest size; smaller plugs in regular-sized ears are more comfortable, but provide less noise reduction.

Premolded Earplugs

Premolded earplugs, such as the V-51R, E•A•R Express™ Pod Plug, Howard Leight Quiet® plug, or multiflanged plugs are preformed and are simply inserted in the ear. They are generally made from soft rubber-like materials. Their main advantages are that they can be inserted and removed easily without touching the portion of the plug that is inserted in the ear canal, and they can be worn easily with other safety equipment such as hard hats and safety glasses. Although laboratory attenuation data can be excellent, good field attenuation can be challenging due to their sensitivity to individual fit. To provide adequate attenuation, they need to seal well and be sized to ensure a proper fit.

Formable Earplugs

Formable earplugs (e.g., fiberglass down, silicone putty, and cotton wax) are formed by the user prior to inserting them into the ear canals. They are less sensitive to individual fit since they can expand or conform to match an individual's anatomy. To provide adequate attenuation, formable earplugs need to seal well and should be sized to ensure a proper fit.

Earmuffs

Although the first earmuffs available did not provide as much attenuation as earplugs, muffs now provide as much attenuation as the best earplugs when worn properly. Proper fitting is still important with earmuffs but is not quite as individualistic as with plugs. Consequently, muffs offer more consistent protection, although performance can decrease when the user wears glasses. Although muffs usually last much longer, they generally are more expensive than plugs, and in hot, humid environments they can be uncomfortable to wear for long periods due to sweat accumulation under the muffs. One notable advantage with muffs is that it is easy to check for employee compliance.

Active noise reduction earmuffs work on the principle of creating a sound wave equal in magnitude but opposite in phase to the

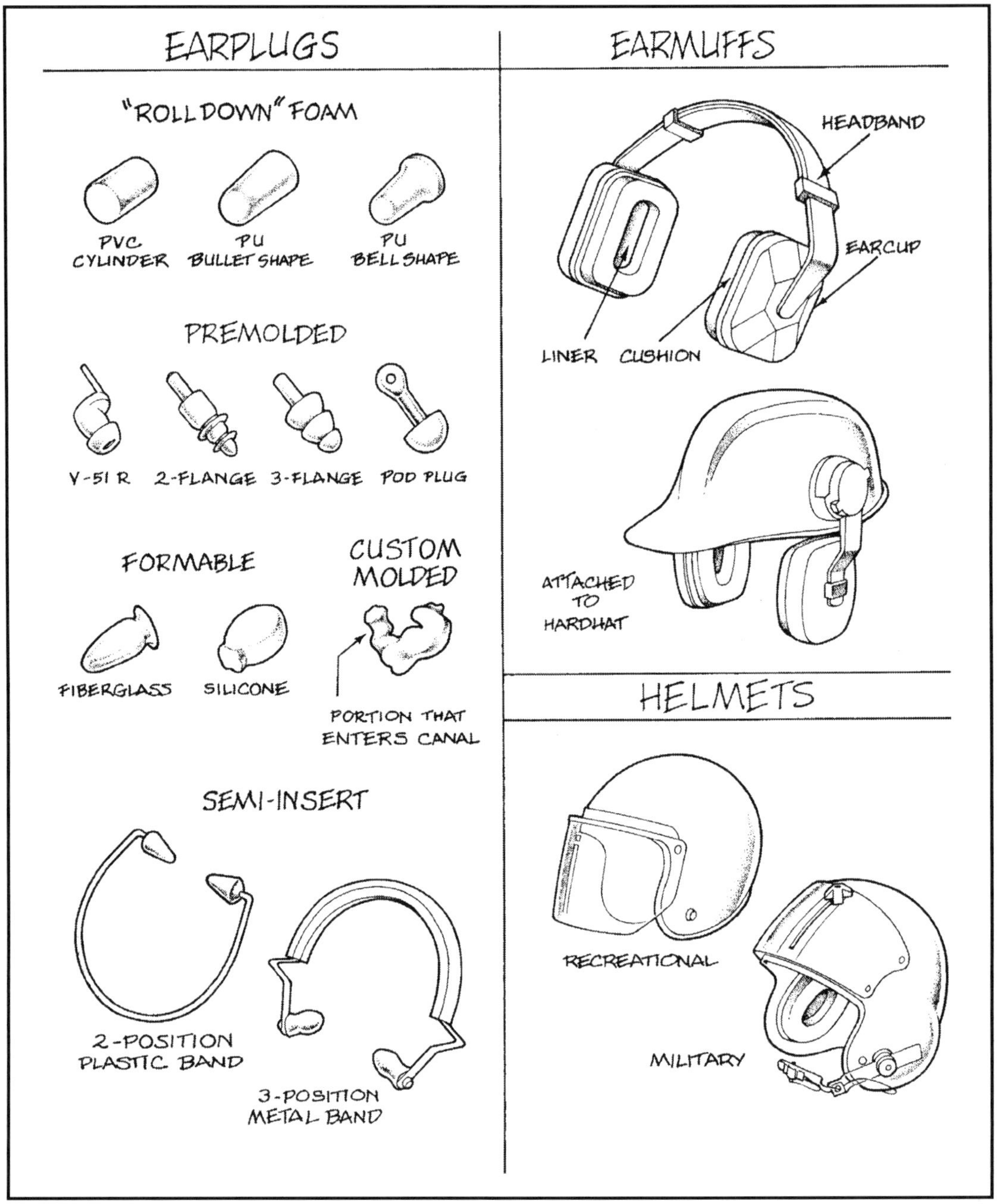

Figure 24.26 — Types of hearing protection. (Adapted from Reference #52).

noise. When the two sound waves combine, the sound is significantly reduced. Active noise reduction muffs work best for lower-frequency sounds (e.g.<250 Hz). These systems can be expensive. In environments with extremely high low-frequency sound levels (e.g., in military aircraft) the active noise reduction muff can be used effectively to provide speech communication using the intercom system.

Semi-Inserts

Semi-inserts are a cross between earplugs and earmuffs. They use earplug-like devices attached to the ends of a headband that are pressed into the ear canal. They are moderately comfortable but do not provide as much attenuation as most muffs or plugs. These devices are primarily intended for intermittent use in moderately noisy environments.

HPD Attenuation Ratings

The EPA requires that hearing protectors be labeled with their Noise Reduction Rating (NRR).[53] The NRR is a single-number rating of the hearing protection. The higher the NRR, the higher is the attenuation for a specific ideal situation (laboratory-fit of HPD). Unfortunately, the data do not provide reliable estimates of the attenuation provided to employees, so consequently, adjustments must be made.

To determine the protected A-weighted sound level at a worker's ear, the effective NRR is subtracted from the C-weighted sound level or the effective NRR is subtracted from the A-weighted sound level plus 7 dB. According to OSHA, the effective NRR is equal to one-half the laboratory NRR.[54] NIOSH recently recommended that instead of reducing the estimated attenuation of all types of hearing protectors by one-half, muffs should be reduced by 25%, formable earplugs by 50%, and premolded earplugs by 70%.[20,55]

Instead of using the NRR, the manufacturers' octave-band attenuation values from the NIOSH compendium of hearing protection devices can be used.[55] The octave-band attenuation values are then subtracted from the measured octave-band sound pressure levels at the worker's ear to determine the expected octave-band sound level (and the A-weighted sound level) in the ear.

Since all of these procedures are based on the NRR, it should be recognized that the expected sound levels are, at best, good estimates.

Audiometric Testing

An audiometric testing program is an integral part of the hearing conservation program. The audiometric test records provide the only data that can be used to determine whether the program is preventing noise-induced permanent threshold shifts (NIPTS). Audiometric tests should be performed by a licensed or certified audiologist, an otolaryngologist or other physician, or a technician certified by the Council for Accreditation of Occupational Hearing Conservationists (CAOHC). A technician who performs audiometric tests must be responsible to an audiologist, otolaryngologist, or physician. Audiograms should be obtained annually. All employees whose noise exposure exceeds the action level (a TWA of 85 dBA for OSHA compliance), should be included in an audiometric testing program. In some cases it might make sense to include all plant personnel in an audiometric testing program to detect and prevent all causes of hearing loss, not only hearing loss from occupational noise.[45]

Performing audiometric testing after a period of quiet provides an accurate representation of any NIPTS incurred. However, audiometric testing can also be used to measure NITTS as a means of education before any NIPTS is incurred. By testing workers during the work shift or at the end of a work shift and noting any threshold shift, workers who are not wearing their HPDs properly can be identified.[56] Of course, these workers will need to be retested after a period of quiet to ensure that the threshold shift is only temporary.

Employee Training and Education

All persons involved in the hearing conservation program must be educated annually on the effects of noise on hearing, proper use of hearing protection, advantages and disadvantages of different types of hearing protection, purpose of audiometric testing, and their individual audiometric results. This training should include not only the noise-exposed workers but management, supervisors, audiometric technicians, issuers of HPDs, and anyone else involved in the hearing conservation program. Although each group will need a slightly different training focus (management will need to understand any legal responsibilities and supervisors will need to understand how to enforce HPD use), everyone involved needs to understand the risks of noise-induced hearing loss and their particular roles in maintaining an effective program.[57]

Numerous resources are available for use in training programs[57–61]; training, however, does not have to take the form of videotapes or lectures to be effective. Audiometric testing of workers at the beginning and end of one workday while educating the workers about TTS and its consequences has proved to be very effective. In one case, worker use of hearing protectors increased from 35% to 80% after an education program and the posting of pre-shift and post-shift audiograms.[62]

Record Keeping

Detailed records must be kept of employee's audiometric test records as well as plant noise exposure, types of hearing protection worn by the employee, documentation of employee training, documentation of technician training and certification, audiometer calibration data, and any other medical or audiological test results or examinations. Also, a record of the employee's recreational noise exposure may be useful. Plant sound survey data and engineering or administrative noise control records likewise need to be maintained. This is not only for review by audiologists and physicians, but also for protection against worker's compensation claims or other legal action. Audiometric records for each worker should be maintained during the worker's employment, but it is recommended that records be kept for the worker's lifetime to protect against possible future legal action.

Program Evaluation

It is important to evaluate the effectiveness of a hearing conservation program. Checklists such as those recommended by NIOSH[63] used in conjunction with audiometric database analysis can ensure that all aspects of a program are monitored. NIOSH recommends that an effective program have a significant threshold shift incidence rate of 5% or less.[19] A significant threshold shift in this case is defined as an increase of 15 dB in hearing threshold, not corrected for age, at any of the audiometric test frequencies (500, 1,000, 2,000, 3,000, 4,000, or 6,000 Hz) that is repeated for the same ear and frequency in back-to-back tests.

OSHA defines a significant threshold shift as a shift of 10 dB or greater, corrected for age, between the most recent audiometric test and the baseline in the average hearing threshold levels at 2,000, 3,000, and 4,000 Hz for either ear. If the average hearing threshold shift exceeds 25 dB, the hearing loss becomes recordable as a work-related injury or illness. The forms for record keeping (OSHA Form 300, 301, and 300A) were updated. In 2003, employers were required to record cases of occupational hearing loss as an "injury" (single event acoustic trauma) or "other illness" (long term noise exposure), as appropriate. After 2004, employers will need to record hearing loss cases in a separate column.[64–66]

Another method of evaluation is through database analysis.[67] By analyzing a database of workers' audiometric test records, hearing trends for different groups can be examined, or individuals can be compared with the reference group. If, for example, workers in a particularly noisy area of a plant show increased hearing loss, this might be an indication that a different hearing protector or engineering noise controls are needed. If one worker shows a significant threshold shift and there are no shifts for all other workers in his or her area, it might be an indication that he or she is using the HPD incorrectly or is receiving excess noise off the job. The ANSI Technical Report for evaluating the effectiveness of hearing conservation programs recommends use of audiometric data base analysis for programs having more than 30 participants and provides recommended criteria for various statistical parameters.[68]

Vibration in the Workplace—Measurements and Control

Introduction

Human exposure to vibration is normally divided into whole-body vibration and hand-arm vibration. Although these two different types of vibration exposure usually result in different effects and responses, workers can be exposed to both types simultaneously.[69] For example, when a jack-hammer operator holds the tool away from his body, supporting and guiding it only by his limbs, he is exposed to hand-arm vibration; however, if he leans against the jack hammer with his abdomen, he is exposed to whole-body vibration as well.

In 1974, NIOSH estimated that 8 million workers were exposed to occupational vibration in U.S. industries.[70] Of these, about 6.8 million were exposed to whole-body vibration and 1.2 million to hand-arm vibration. The majority of those exposed to whole-body vibration were truck and bus drivers, heavy equipment operators, and aircraft pilots. Those exposed to hand-arm vibration include operators of gasoline-powered chain saws, string trimmers, and pneumatic tools. Table 24.12 provides a detailed listing of the various occupations and types of vibration exposures.[71,72]

Table 24.12 — Vibration exposure in U.S. industries[71,72]

Industry	*Type of Vibration*	*Common Vibration Sources*
Agriculture	Whole Body	Tractor operation
Automotive Assembly	Hand-Arm	Pneumatic tools
Boiler Making	Hand-Arm	Pneumatic tools
Construction	Whole Body and Hand-Arm	Vehicles, pneumatic tools
Diamond cutting	Hand-Arm	Vibrating hand tools
Forestry	Whole Body and Hand-Arm	Tractors, chainsaws
Foundries	Hand-Arm	Vibrating cleavers, pneumatic tools
Furniture Manufacturing	Hand-Arm	Pneumatic chisels
Grounds Maintenance	Hand-Arm	String trimmers, chainsaws
Iron and Steel	Hand-Arm	Vibrating hand tools
Lumber	Hand-Arm	Chainsaws
Metal Working	Whole Body and Hand-Arm	Drills, sanders, grinders, stand grinding
Mining	Whole Body and Hand-Arm	Vehicles and rock drills
Shipyards	Hand-Arm	Pneumatic hand tools
Stone dressing	Hand-Arm	Pneumatic hand tools
Textile	Hand-Arm	Sewing machines, looms
Transportation	Whole Body	Vehicle operation

Effects of Vibration

Hand-Arm

Prolonged exposure to hand-arm vibration can lead to a condition known as Raynaud's Phenomenon of Occupational Origin, vibration-induced white finger (VWF), or hand-arm vibration syndrome (HAVS).[73–75] The first symptoms are intermittent tingling and/or numbness of the fingers which does not interfere with work or other activities.[75] The worker may later experience attacks of finger blanching (turning white) usually confined at first to a single fingertip. With added vibration exposure, attacks may extend to the base of the finger. Cold often triggers these attacks, but other factors are involved, such as body temperature, metabolic rate, vascular tone, and emotional state. Attacks usually last 15–60 minutes, but in advanced stages they may last as long as two hours. Recovery from attacks can also be painful. With additional vibration exposure, the symptoms of HAVS become more severe and include increasing stiffness of the finger joints, loss of manipulative skills, and loss of blood circulation, which can lead to gangrene and tissue necrosis. At this point, there are no long-term medical treatments for HAVS.[76]

Whole-Body

Whole-body vibration can cause both physiological and psychological effects ranging from fatigue and irritation to motion sickness (kinetosis) and to tissue damage. Much of whole-body vibration research is rooted in military settings (e.g., pilots, ship motion studies, tank ride studies). Some work has taken place in the occupational setting, principally in transportation and with on- and off-road vehicles. Since it is potentially dangerous to expose human subjects to high acceleration levels in the laboratory, researchers have simulated high-level exposures using animals and then extrapolated to potential biological effects on humans. Because of the difficulty of obtaining hard epidemiology and medical data, human performance studies have been concerned primarily with performance decrements or comfort reduction at low vibration levels.

The most frequently reported adverse effects of whole-body vibration are lower-back pain, early degeneration of the lumbar spinal system, and herniated lumbar discs.[77]

Terminology

Periodic Vibration

Vibration is considered periodic if the motion of a particle repeats itself considerably over time. The simplest form of periodic vibration is called simple harmonic motion, which can be represented by a sinusoidal curve similar to the sound wave shown in Figure 24.1 earlier in this chapter. The motion of any vibrating particle can be characterized at any time by its:

- Displacement from the equilibrium position;
- Velocity, or rate of change of displacement; or
- Acceleration, or rate of change of velocity.

For simple harmonic motion, these three characteristics of motion are related mathematically. Any characteristic may be converted into another using either integration or derivation.

Displacement

The displacement (X) of a particle from its reference position under influence of harmonic motion can be described mathematically as:

$$X = X_{peak} \sin(2\pi f t) = X_{peak} \sin(\omega t) \qquad (24\text{-}30)$$

Where:

X_{peak} = maximum displacement;
f = frequency in Hz;
t = time in seconds; and
ω = angular frequency (equal to $2\pi f$).

Displacement is most significant in the study of the deformation and bending of structures.

Velocity

As a particle displaces up and down, it moves with a characteristic velocity (V). The velocity is the time rate of change of displacement and can be determined mathematically for simple harmonic motion by taking the derivative of Equation 24-30.

$$V = \omega X_{peak} \cos(\omega t) = V_{peak} \cos(\omega t) \qquad (24\text{-}31)$$

Velocity is often measured in preventative maintenance programs for rotating machinery.

Acceleration

The acceleration of a particle (A) is the time rate of change of the velocity. The acceleration is determined mathematically for simple harmonic motion by taking the derivative of Equation 24-31.

$$A = -\omega^2 X_{peak} \sin(\omega t) = A_{peak} \sin(\omega t) \qquad (24\text{-}32)$$

The minus sign indicates that the acceleration is a one-half cycle (180°) out of phase with reference to the displacement. For occupational vibration, the acceleration is the most important quantity since it is proportional to the forces applied to the hand, arm, or whole body, and it is believed that the forces are the source of damage.

RMS

Peak values are useful for pure sinusoidal vibration; however, because workplace vibration is complex and contains many vibration frequencies, the root-mean-square value is used. The RMS average is given by Equation 24-33 and is calculated by summing the squares of the acceleration values measured over time, dividing by the measuring time, and then taking the square root of the resulting value.

$$A_{RMS} = \sqrt{\frac{1}{T}\int_0^T A^2(t)dt} \qquad (24\text{-}33)$$

The RMS value of the acceleration is directly related to the energy content of the vibration being measured.

Resonance

Resonance is a condition in which the movement of the human body (or any other mechanical system) acts in concert with an externally generated vibration force, resulting in an amplification of the resulting vibration movement. In other words, parts of the human body like to vibrate more at certain frequencies than at other frequencies. At these resonant frequencies the body amplifies the vibration and exacerbates the occupational vibration problem. Resonance frequencies for the whole-body occur in the 4–5 Hz range.[78] Resonance frequencies for the hand-arm system tend to be higher in frequency, in the 150–300 Hz frequency range. In structures, resonant vibration can cause large displacements that can cause severe damage, such as the Tacoma Narrows Bridge collapse in 1940.

Random Vibration

Random vibrations occur quite frequently in nature and may be defined as motion in which the vibrating particles undergo irregular motion cycles that never exactly repeat themselves. Because of their aperiodicity, random vibrations result in energy over a broad-frequency spectrum. A mechanical shock pulse is an example of random vibration. Note that for a pulse or a random signal the measured acceleration signal cannot be integrated to obtain the velocity or displacement as with a periodic signal.

Vibration Transmissibility Ratio

In many cases, it is desirable to know how much vibration is transmitted through structures (e.g., vehicle seats or gloves). In other words, how well does the driver's seat remove, transmit, or amplify the vibration coming up from the floor of the vehicle to the driver's buttocks? The vibration transmissibility ratio is the ratio of the vibration output (vibration at the seat) to the vibration input (vibration at the floor of the vehicle). A transmissibility ratio of 1 means there is no change in the level of vibration between the input and output; a ratio >1 indicates an amplification of the original vibration; a ratio <1 indicates a reduction or attenuation of the original vibration.

Criteria

The acceptability of hand-arm or whole-body vibration is judged on whether the level of vibration exposure can potentially cause damage to the body or decrease performance. Until recently guidelines for hand-arm vibration were generally concerned with potential damage to the body, and guidelines for whole-body vibration were more concerned with performance degradation. Most new standards include potential damage limits or suggestions for both types of vibration. European Directive 2002/44/EC lists both exposure limits and action levels for each type of vibration.(79) Because the effects of vibration depend on a number of factors in addition to the magnitude, and because of the tentative nature of the current guidelines, the user must thoroughly understand the standard or guide before comparing criteria with measured data. Failure to do so might result in inaccurate interpretation and results.

Hand-Arm

The etiology of hand-arm vibration disorders is not well understood. The frequency spectrum, amplitude, and exposure duration are important in evaluating hand-arm vibration, but so are worker posture, particular part of the hand exposed, the temperature, the noise level, and any other conditions that could affect the worker's circulatory system (e.g., disease, smoking, chemical exposure).

Three hand-arm vibration consensus standards or guides are currently in use in the United States:

- ISO 5349-1–2001: Guidelines for the measurement and assessment of human exposure to hand-transmitted vibration —
  - Part 1: General requirements(80)
  - Part 2: Practical guidance for measurement at the workplace(81)
- ANSI S2.70–2006 Guide for the Measurement and Evaluation of Human Expoure to Vibration Transmitted to the Hand
- ACGIH's® "Hand-Arm (Segmental) Vibration Syndrome (HAVS)" section in its TLVs® Handbook.(82)

Also, the NIOSH hand-arm criteria document(83) provides a work practices and medical monitoring approach without including a numerical exposure recommendation. OSHA has not adopted any of these standards.

When analyzing sound for hearing conservation, the concern generally is with the sound level in decibels at frequencies between 20 Hz and 10,000 Hz. In hand-arm vibration, the concern is mostly with the RMS acceleration in meters per second squared at frequencies between 5 Hz and 1,500 Hz.

The three hand-arm vibration standards are discussed in the following sections.

ISO 5349-1-2001. Because the etiology of hand-arm vibration disorders is not well-understood, in part because of a limited amount of data, this standard by the International Organization for Standardization (ISO) presents recommended methods for measuring, analyzing, and reporting hard-arm vibration data. It does not, however, include an exposure criterion as part of the standard. Guidance for acceptable hand-arm vibration exposure and various health effects of vibration exposure are provided in

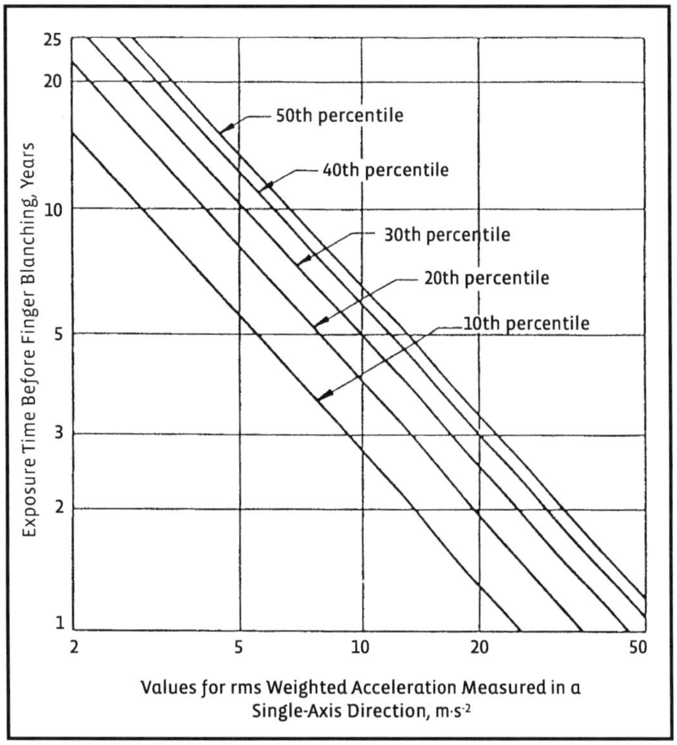

Figure 24.27 — Exposure time for different percentiles of population group exposed to vibrations in three coordinate axes. (Adapted from Reference #84).

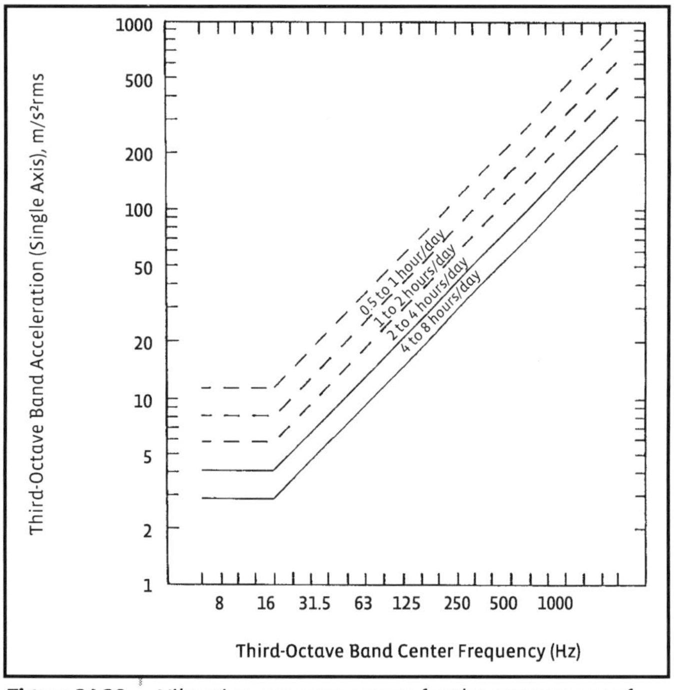

Figure 24.28 — Vibration exposure zones for the assessment of hand-transmitted vibration. (The zones of daily exposure time are for RMS accelerations of discrete frequency vibration and for narrow-band or broad-band vibration analyzed as third-octave band RMS acceleration. The values are for the dominant single-axis vibration generating compression of the flesh of the hand. The values are for regular daily exposure and for good coupling of the hand to the vibration source.) (Adapted from Reference #85.)

the Annexes. Hand-arm vibration exposure is provided in Annex A, where the time before the onset of finger blanching can be compared with the weighted vibration level for different percentiles of a population (as shown here in Figure 24.27).[84] Guidelines for procedures to prevent HAVS are presented in Annex E of the ISO standard. These preventative measures include physical examinations, use of low-vibration tools, careful maintenance, worker training and education, use of gloves, and having the worker grip the tool with the least amount of force necessary.

ISO 5349-2-2001. Part 2 of ISO 5349 builds upon part 1 by detailing specified measurement locations and procedures in the workplace. The annexes contain specific examples of accelerometer mounting methods and locations for many different types of tools ranging from pneumatic hammers to lawn trimmers.

ANSI S.270-2006. The ANSI standard is similar to the ISO standard in that it presents recommended methods for measuring, analyzing, and reporting hand-arm vibration data, but it does not include an exposure criterion as part of the standard. Guidance for acceptable hand-arm vibration exposure is provided "for information only" in the standard's appendices. In addition to analyzing the weighted vibration level, exposure curves are provided for one-third octave band levels (as shown here in Figure 24.28). If the actual acceleration levels and exposures exceed the allowable exposure time and if there is good coupling between the worker's hands and the vibration source, the worker might be at risk for developing HAVS.

Hand-Arm (Segmental) Vibration Syndrome. The ACGIH® document specifies that measurements shall be made according to the procedures ASNI S2.70-2006 or ISO 5349. Unlike the other two standards, ACGIH® provides threshold limit values for hand-arm vibration. The TLVs® for vibration in the Xh, Yh, or Zh axis (the subscript h signifies hand-arm vibration) are shown here in Table 24.13.

ACGIH® also recommends use of antivibration (AV) tools and gloves, proper work practices (such as keeping the worker's hands warm), and a medical surveillance program.

The European Union has set the hand-arm standardized 8-hour exposure as defined in ISO 2631-1–1997 to an action level of 2.5 m/s^2 and a maximum exposure limit of 5 m/s^2.

Whole-Body

The main criteria document for whole-body vibration is ISO 2631-1–2001.[86] The American National Standards Institute issued the ISO 2631 standard as ANSI S3.18–2002[87] and the ACGIH® TLVs® for whole-body vibration[88] are also drawn from this document. With whole-body vibration, measurements are made in the back-to-chest (ax) side-to-side (ay) and foot-to-head (az) directions. Criteria for Fatigue Decreased Proficiency (FDP), reduced comfort (RC), and exposure limits (EL) are provided in Figure 24.29 (az axis) and Figure 24.30 (ax and ay axis).

The FDP boundaries represent the ability of a person to work at task(s) under vibration exposure without the vibration interfering with the worker's ability to perform. The RC boundaries are concerned with preservation of comfort during vibration exposure. The EL attempts to preserve health and safety of workers during vibration exposure.

Table 24.13 — ACGIH® Threshold Limit Values (TLVs®) for exposure of the hand to vibration in the Xh, Yh, or Zh axis[22]

Total Daily Exposure Duration	*Maximum Frequency-Weighted, RMS, Component Acceleration (which shall not be exceeded in any axis)*
4 hr–<8 hr	4 m/sec^2
2 hr–<4 hr	6 m/sec^2
1 hr–<2 hr	8 m/sec^2
<1 hr	12 m/sec^2

The European Union has set the whole body standardized 8-hour exposure as defined in ISO 5349-1-2001 to an action level of 0.5 m/s^2 and a maximum exposure limit of 1.15 m/s^2. The vibration dose can also be used. If this is the case the action level is 9.1 m/s$^{1.75}$ and the exposure limit is 21 m/s$^{1.75}$.[79]

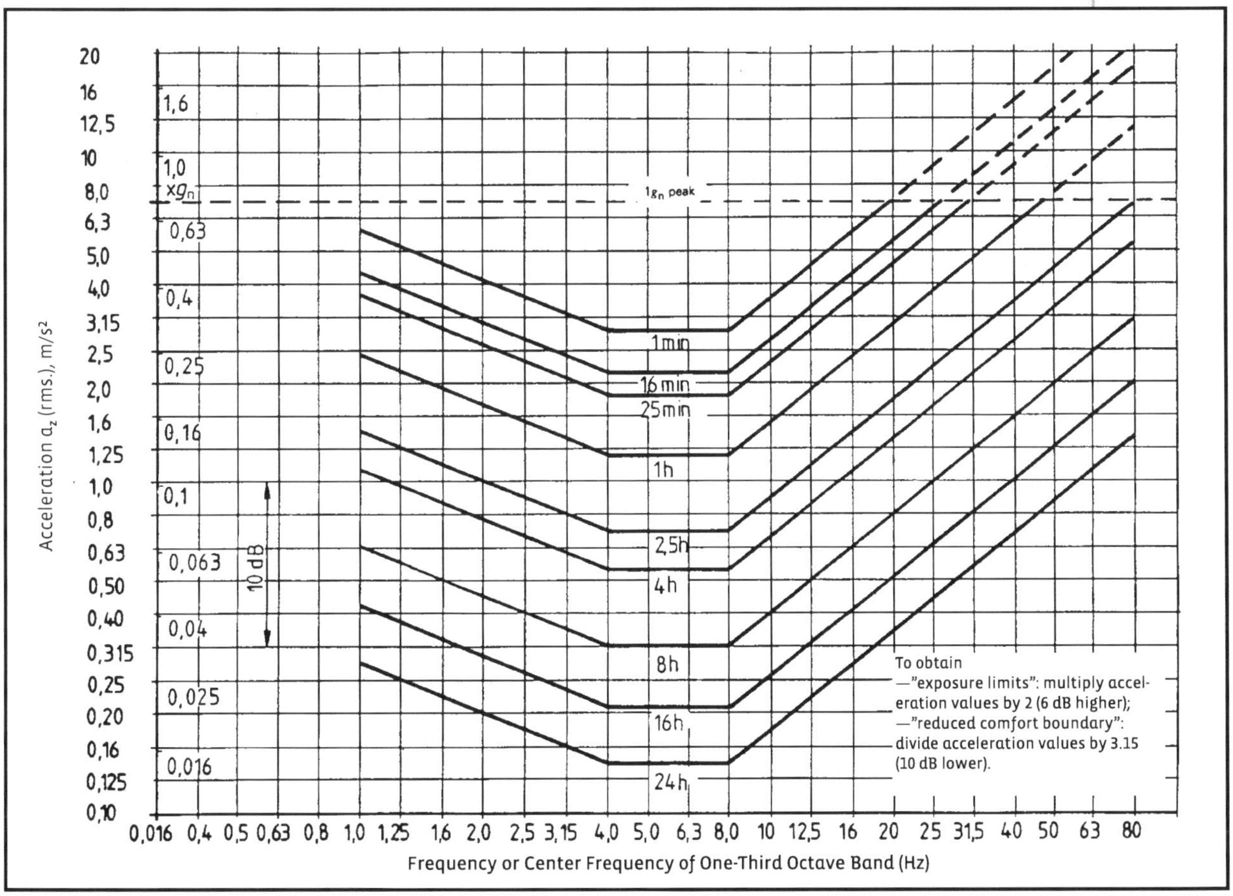

Figure 24.29 — Longitudinal (az) acceleration limits as a function of frequency and exposure time: "Fatigue-decreased proficiency boundary." (Adapted from Reference #86.)

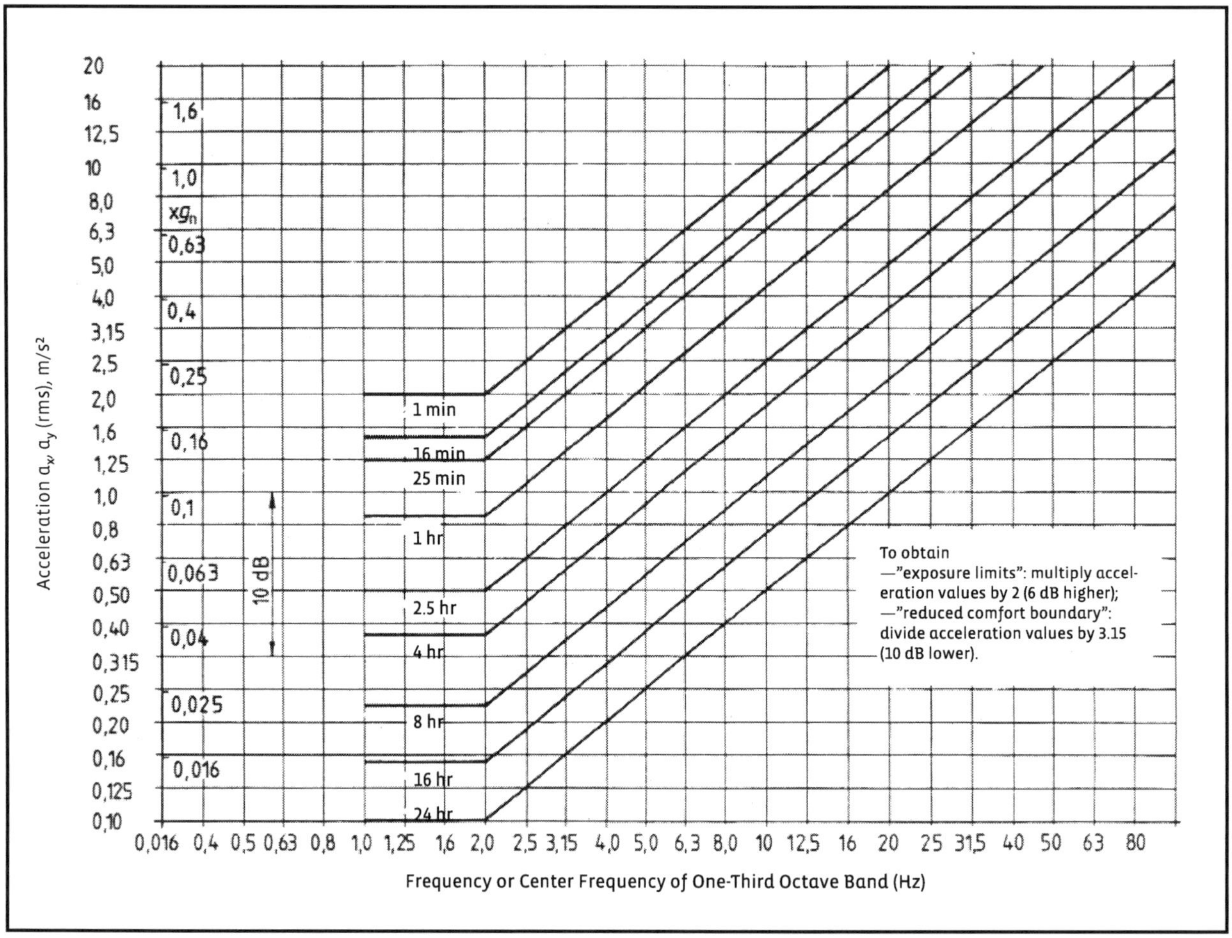

Figure 24.30 — Transverse (ax, ay) acceleration limits as a function of frequency and exposure time: "fatigue-decreased proficiency boundary." (Adapted from Reference #86).

Measurement of Vibration

A variety of component systems consisting of mechanical, electrical, and optical elements are available to measure vibration. The most common system uses a vibration transducer to transform the mechanical motion into an electrical signal, an amplifier to enlarge the signal, an analyzer to measure the vibration in specific frequency ranges, and a calibrated metering.

Vibration Transducers

Accelerometers are the most common type of vibration transducer, and they produce an output signal proportional to the acceleration. The output signal is either charge or voltage sensitive depending on the accelerometer and any internal electronics. Two piezoelectric discs produce a charge on their surfaces due to the mechanical strain on the asymmetric crystals composing the discs. The strain is in the form of vibration inertia from a moving mass atop the discs. The upper limit of the accelerometer's useful frequency range is determined by the resonant frequency of the mass and the stiffness of the whole accelerometer system. The lower limit of the frequency range varies with total capacitance of the system determined by the cable length and the properties of the connected amplifiers. The accelerometer's sensitivity and the magnitude of the charge developed across the output terminals depends on the properties of the materials used in the piezoelectric discs and the weight of the mass. The mechanical size of the accelerometer, therefore, determines the sensitivity of the system; the smaller the accelerometer, the lower the sensitivity. In contrast, a decrease in size results in an increase in frequency of the accelerometer's resonance and thus a wider useful range. Other factors to consider in the selection of a suitable accelerometer include the transverse sensitivity (which is the sensitivity to accelerations in a plane perpendicular to the plane of the discs) and the environmental conditions during the accelerometer's operation (primarily temperature, humidity, and varying ambient pressure). Charge based units are generally more robust due to their simplicity, but require more complicated and expensive preamplifiers.

Since the acceleration, velocity, and displacement for nonrandom vibration are all interrelated by differential operations, all of the variables can be measured with an accelerometer.

The laser Doppler vibrometer (LDV) represents a newer method of measuring vibration free of the mounting, heat and mass loading problems inherent with accelerometers. It uses a laser beam to measure the velocity of the targeted surface. While the LDV can be the most expensive type of vibration measurement system, they can acquire data very quickly and can be used to measure the vibration on surfaces where conventional accelerometers cannot.

Preamplifier

The preamplifier is introduced in the measurement circuit for two reasons: 1) to amplify the weak output signal from the accelerometer, and 2) to transform the high output impedance of the accelerometer to a lower, acceptable value. It is possible to design the preamplifier in either of two ways: one in which the preamplifier output voltage is directly related to the input voltage (a voltage amplifier) or one in which the output voltage is proportional to the input charge (a charge amplifier).

The major difference between the two types of amplifiers is in their performance characteristics. When a voltage amplifier is used, the overall system is very sensitive to changes in the cable length between the accelerometer and the preamplifier, whereas changes in cable length produce negligible effects on a charge.[89] The input resistance of a voltage amplifier will also affect the low-frequency response of a system.

Measurement

Since vibration is a vector quantity and therefore has magnitude and direction, it is mandatory when specifying or taking vibration measurements, comparing data, etc., to define both of these quantities. Vibration can appear in six directions at any one given measurement point: three linear perpendicular vector components (x, y, and z) and three rotational components (pitch, yaw, and roll). For human vibration work, only the linear motion components are measured.

Measurement coordinate systems are defined and standardized for both hand-arm and whole-body vibration. The coordinate systems are shown in Figures 24.31 and 24.32. To avoid confusion, whole-body measurement components are denoted as ax, ay, and az, whereas hand-arm measurement components are denoted as Xh, Yh, and Zh. Hand-arm vibration measurements can be

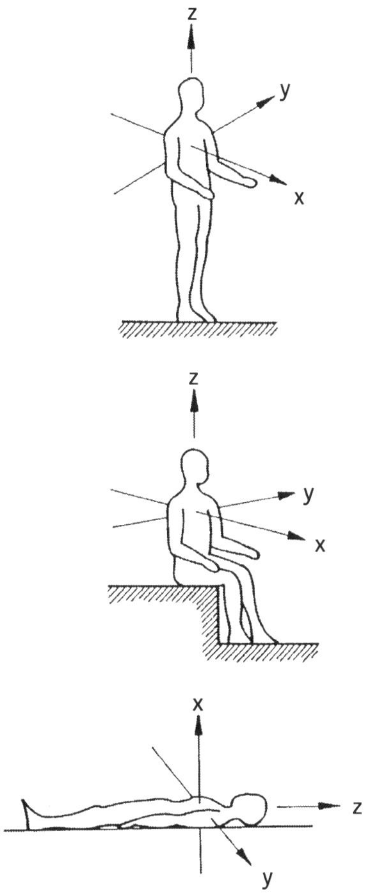

a_x, a_y, a_z = acceleration in the directions of the x-, y- and z-axes
x-axis = back-to-chest
y-axis = right side to left side
z-axis = foot- (or buttocks) to-head

Figure 24.31 — Basicentric coordinate system for whole-body vibration. (Adapted from Reference #86).

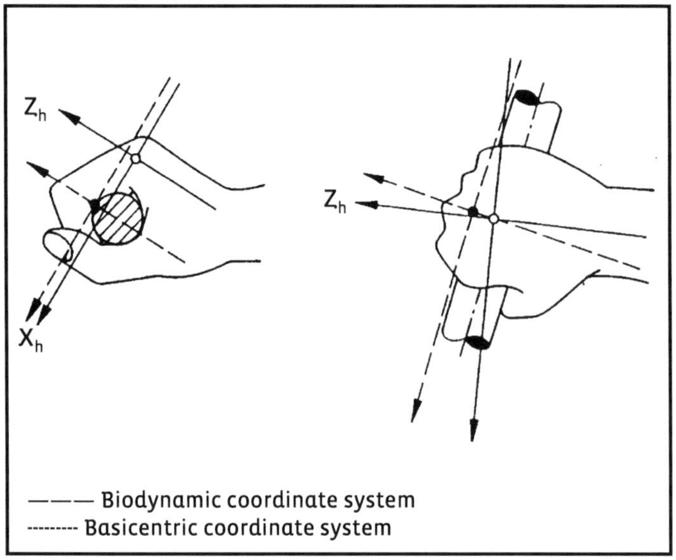

Figure 24.32 — Biodynamic and basicentric coordinate systems for hand-arm vibration. (Adapted from References #84 and #85).

made using one of two coordinate systems depending on the accelerometer mounting: a basicentric system if measurements are made on the handle of the tool nearest the position where the worker grips the tool, or a biodynamic system if the measurements are made on the third metacarpal.

The particular work situation and measurement requirements determine which type of accelerometer to use. The weight or mass of the accelerometer must be as small as possible in relation to the structure to be measured. An accelerometer that is too heavy will weigh down the surface and give inaccurate results, which is called mass loading. To avoid mass loading, the general rule is that the accelerometer's mass should be no more than one-tenth of the effective mass of the surface to which it is mounted.

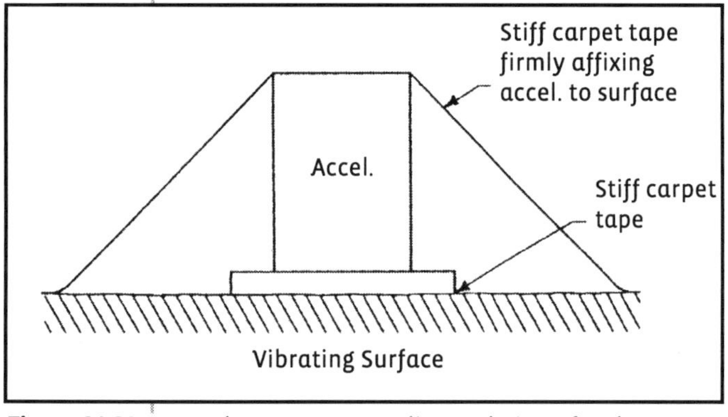

Figure 24.33 — Accelerometer mounding technique for the measurement of vibration impinging on the surface of the human body. (Adapted from Reference #69).

The dynamic amplitude range of the device must accommodate the maximum acceleration level anticipated. For example, a 10 g (98 m/sec^2) accelerometer should not be used to measure a 100 g (980 m/sec^2) acceleration source, since the accelerometer would be destroyed very quickly. Similarly, a 100 g accelerometer is not used to measure a 1 g signal because the accelerometer would be insensitive to small signals and, thus, small changes would not be detected. Also, the frequency response of the accelerometer must match the range of the frequency spectrum that is measured.

Accelerometer Mounting

Proper mounting of an accelerometer to a structure means the device is rigidly affixed to the vibrating source in line with the direction of vibration. If the accelerometer is not rigidly affixed, it will produce a false output signal. With poor mounting, the tendency is to lower the natural frequency of the system, thereby reducing the effective bandwidth (window) of the accelerometer. If the device is not in line with the vibration, a component of the vibration will not be measured due to misalignment.

Many accelerometers come with threaded studs that can be screwed directly into the structure. Another mounting method is to use a thin layer of beeswax between the accelerometer and the test structure. Epoxy or cyanoacrylate cement can also be used; however, soft glue should not be used because the soft material acts as a mechanical low-pass filter.

In some instances, the accelerometer can be mounted using a strong permanent magnet that is affixed to a metal test structure. A probe-type fixture, where the accelerometer is simply held against the surface, is not recommended for human vibration analysis.

To mount an accelerometer to the hand, the skin surface must be thoroughly cleaned. The accelerometer is then taped to the hand using stiff carpet tape as shown in Figure 24.33.[69]

When measuring vibrating pneumatic hand-tools, or whenever the acceleration level is expected to be high, other mounting techniques need to be used. Figure 24.34 shows three mounting techniques for measuring the vibration on the handle of a pneumatic grinder.[89] The accelerometer is mounted to an automotive hose clamp or removable bracket that is firmly attached to the tool handle where the worker grasps the tool. Alternatively, a section of the handle can be milled flat, a mounting screw tapped, and the accelerometer screwed into the handle. Also available are special adapters that are placed between a worker's hand (Figure 24.35) and the tool or between a worker's buttocks and his seat (Figure 24.36).

Conducting the Workplace Measurement Study

Before performing any vibration measurements, it is important to understand the role vibration plays in the work process. It is important to walk through the entire process and spend time observing how workers work, especially with a vibrating process. It is also important to meet with the appropriate participants (workers, management, labor, occupational hygienists) and describe what will be done, how it will be done, and how much disruption will be caused by the measurements.

If possible, a video camera should be used to record each step of the overall work process and particularly the actual work process involving vibration. In vibration processes, there is usually a repetition in work cycles that can be broken down into many steps. Depending on the variability of the levels, average readings might be required. It is recommended that observations be made of experienced workers rather than inexperienced workers. New workers on the job may have had little training and may not have developed good work habits.

Control of Occupational Vibration

Occupational vibration can be controlled by modifying work practices, such as limiting exposure time, gripping a tool with less force, purchasing low-vibration equipment, wearing AV gloves, and by using engineering controls such as damping or isolation. It is often necessary to use several techniques to minimize the effects of harmful vibration.

Modifying Work Practices

Because the effects of vibration depend on factors such as worker posture, ambient temperature, and exposure level and time,

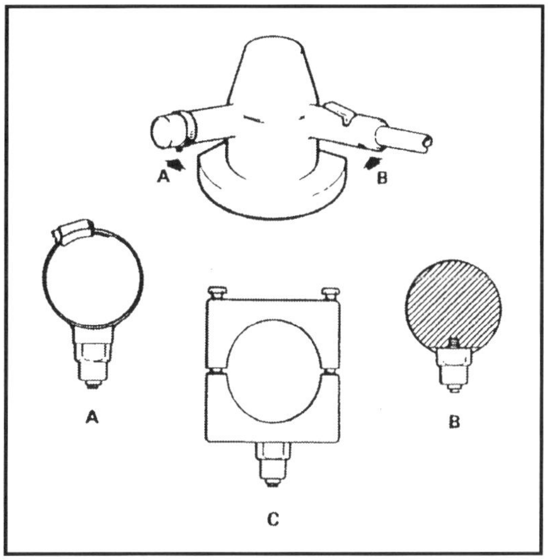

Figure 24.34 — Mounting techniques for measuring the vibration on the handle of a pneumatic grinder. (Adapted from Reference #90).

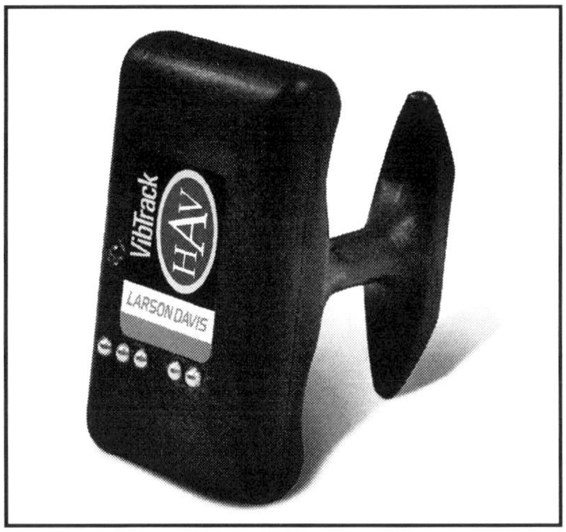

Figure 24.35 — Integrated measurement and data logging system for hand-arm vibration conforming to ISO 5349. (Courtesy Larson-Davis).

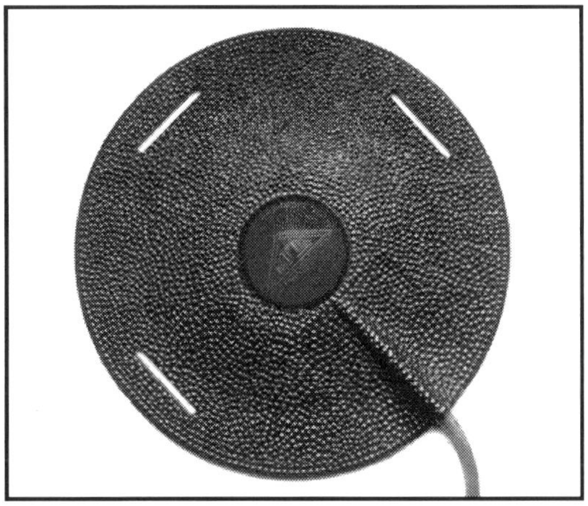

Figure 24.36 — Specialized tri-axial accelerometer for measuring human vibration on seating surfaces. (Courtesy MMF).

the effects of hand-arm or whole-body vibration can be reduced significantly by modifying work practices. The following AV work practices for hand-arm vibration can be used[91,92]:

- Use both AV tools and AV gloves.
- Use work breaks (e.g., 10 minutes per continuous exposure hour) to avoid constant vibration exposure.
- Measure and monitor the vibration of tools so that tools with increased acceleration levels due to age and wear can be replaced or repaired.
- Screen all workers regularly for HAVS through a specialized medical exam.
- Advise workers to have several pairs of warm AV gloves available and require that the gloves and warm clothing be worn.
- Advise workers to reduce smoking while using vibrating hand tools to avoid the vasoconstrictive effects of nicotine.
- Advise workers to grasp the tool as lightly as possible to reduce mechanical coupling to the hands.
- Have a physician examine workers if symptoms of tingling, numbness, or signs of white or blue fingers appear.

The following work practices should help minimize the effects of whole-body vibration[93]:

- Limit the time spent by workers on a vibrating surface to no more than is absolutely necessary to perform the job safely.
- Maintain smooth access roads for workers operating off-highway equipment
- Have machine controls moved off vibrating surfaces (whenever possible).
- Isolate vibrating equipment from surfaces where workers are stationed.
- Have work breaks to avoid constant vibration exposure (e.g., 10 min/hr).
- Maintain vibrating machinery to prevent development of excessive vibration.
- Have a physician consult with workers who have a history of, or who are currently suffering from, musculoskeletal problems (especially the lower spine) before they are exposed to whole-body vibration.

Training courses on the effects of occupational vibration and on proper use and maintenance of equipment are important in heightening the awareness of the problem by workers, management, labor, occupational hygienists, and medical personnel.

Low-Vibration Tools

As in noise control, the most effective place to control vibration exposure is at the source. For hand-arm vibration, AV tools can be purchased. Since the early 1970s, for example, gasoline-powered chain saw manufacturers have been aware of HAVS and have designed a series of AV chain saws. Where AV saws were used extensively, there was a lower prevalence of HAVS. Today, nearly all gas-powered chain saw manufacturers have at least one AV saw in their product line. In some cases, acceleration levels have fallen from the 20–30 g range to less than 1 g.

These saws must be maintained and their vibration isolators replaced periodically to keep the vibration levels low. This same expertise was applied by many manufacturers to other professional tools such as gas-powered string trimmers, edgers, and other tools used in gardening and grounds keeping. In the pneumatic tool industry, many manufacturers now offer AV tools or tools with AV grips.

Keep in mind that because most pneumatic AV designs are new, their long-term effectiveness in reducing HAVS are not yet known.

AV Gloves

AV gloves use special vibration isolation materials such as Sorbothane® brand elastomer or Viscolas® brand elastomer. The amount of protection afforded by AV gloves varies as a function of frequency and gripping force. Although workers should be encouraged to wear AV gloves and to keep their hands warm and dry, the amount of protection gloves provide is difficult to predict. In one study using chipping hammers, researchers measured a 41%–67% decrease in acceleration levels at the workers' hands.[94] In another study, increased vibration levels were measured in some frequencies.[95] ISO's 10819–1996 standard now provides guidelines with which gloves marketed in Europe must comply to be considered "anti-vibration" gloves.[96]

Vehicle Seats

For whole-body vibration, special seats can help isolate the worker from the vibration of the vehicle. For many years, manufacturers of heavy equipment, farm vehicles, and over-the-road trucks and buses offered and installed reduced-vibration or suspended seats for operators; in some cases, these suspended seat designs are offered as options in lieu of a cheaper, more rigid seat. As a rule, these special seats do help in removing undesirable vibration from the operator's lower trunk and they should be used when available. There are three difficulties with these seats, however: 1) the operator must adjust the seat to his or her body weight, and many workers do not understand the need to do so; 2) these seats must be serviced and maintained according to the manufacturer's specifications; and 3) these seats have limited isolation and damping at low frequencies.

Engineering Control of Occupational Vibration

From an engineering standpoint, vibration can be diminished by reducing the driving force, reducing the response of the vibrating surface, isolating the vibrating source, or utilizing active control methods. Each of these techniques and their limitations are discussed in the following sections.

Reduce Driving Force

As with sound, vibration can be reduced by decreasing the driving force. These forces can be reduced by decreasing the speed, maintaining the dynamic balance, or in the case of impact operations, increasing the duration of the impact while reducing the forces. Sometimes these options are only practical in designing new equipment; however, mechanical vibration can often be reduced by proper balancing of rotating machinery and proper maintenance of machinery. For pneumatic hand tools, the driving force can be reduced by using the smallest tool possible for the job.

Reduce the Response of the Vibrating Surface

The most common method to reduce the response of a vibrating surface is to increase its damping. Damping reduces the response to resonant vibrations in the structure but does not reduce the response to a driven force such as a hammer blow. The amount of vibration reduction from damping depends on the thickness of the damping material, the method in which the damping material is applied, and the surface temperature. Since the driving forces are most often the concern in occupational vibration problems, damping alone is rarely a solution.

Vibration Isolation

Vibration isolators decouple structures, such as the human hand from a pneumatic tool or a driver from a vehicle, by using "soft" connections. Vibration energy is absorbed by the isolator instead of being transmitted to the user. The transmissibility ratio (the ratio of the vibration output to the vibration input) varies depending on the resonant frequency of the isolator and the frequencies being isolated. Figure 24.37 shows the transmissibility vs. frequency ratio (driving frequency divided by natural frequency) for different amounts of damping in a system. To be effective, the resonant frequency of the vibration isolators must be less than one-half the lowest frequency to be isolated. Forces at driving frequencies near the isolator resonance are amplified by an amount dependent on the damping.

The resonant frequency of the isolator (fn) can be calculated using Equation 24-34.

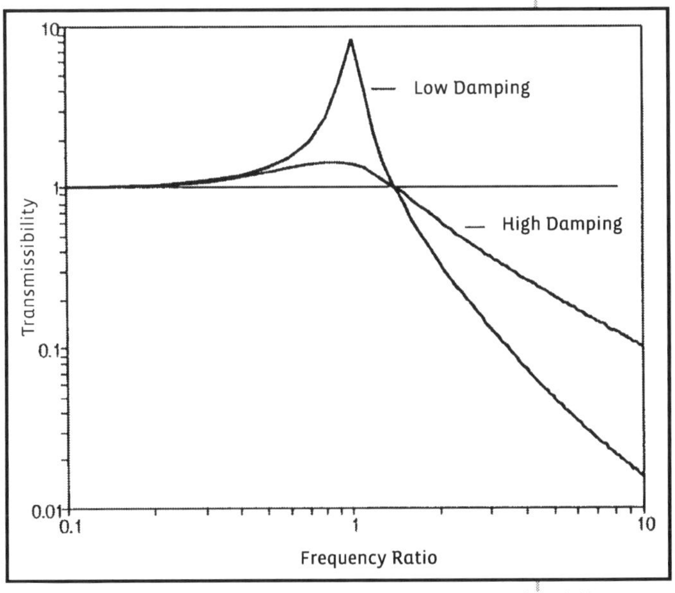

Figure 24.37 — Transmissibility vs. frequency ratio for different amounts of damping.

$$f_n = 0.5\sqrt{\frac{1}{\delta_{st}}} \quad (24\text{-}34)$$

Where:

δ_{st} = static deflection in meters under load, such as the weight of a driver sitting on a seat. A reduction in transmissibility can take place only by allowing the isolator to deflect by motion. Thus, certain space clearances must be provided for the isolated equipment.

Active Controls

Recent developments in real time signal processing technology and piezoelectrics has led to the development of the first generation of active vibration control methods. These controls attempt to effectively cancel out vibrations by using an excitation source to create an identical vibration with the opposite phase.

Ultrasound

Ultrasound is commonly defined as sound with frequencies above the range audible to the human ear. Although the audible range varies from person to person, the division between audible sound and ultrasound is often placed at 20 kHz. Ultrasound can be broken into three main categories:

- "Low-frequency Ultrasound" — ranging from 16 kHz to 100 kHz
- "Mid-frequency Ultrasound" — ranging from 100 kHz to 1 Mhz
- "High-frequency Ultrasound" — ranging from 1 Mhz to 10 Mhz

Most of the effects on hearing are present in the low-frequency ultrasound range. In addition to ultrasonic waves in the air, ultrasonic energy in liquids (liquidborne ultrasound) can also be a hazard.[97]

Uses of Ultrasound

In the past several decades, uses of ultrasound have increased rapidly in industry, hospitals, the military, and the home. These uses may produce harmful levels of ultrasound. The most common exposures to ultrasound are through the air and through liquids. Often, liquid-borne ultrasound is the most hazardous when direct contact is involved.

Low-frequency ultrasound in air is used for cleaning, welding, emulsifying, alarms, and pest control. Low-frequency ultrasound is also used in liquids for cleaning (e. g. jewelry and metal) and for air treatment (e.g. humidifiers and cleaners). High-frequency ultrasound is commonly found in medical settings. Mid-frequency ultrasound is often used for therapeutic techniques such as induced hyperthermia. Table 24.14 is a listing of established and promising ultrasound applications in industry.

Ultrasound Paths

Airborne Ultrasound

Like sound at audible frequencies, the velocity of ultrasound in air is about 344 m/sec. Unlike low-frequency (below 500 Hz) sound that can curve around corners with very little loss in amplitude, high-frequency (above 2 kHz) sound propagates in a very directional manner. Indeed, the higher the frequency the more directional the sound propagation. Because of this, barriers effectively block high-frequency sounds resulting in shadow zones, areas where the sound source cannot be detected. In the ultrasound range, a barrier as thin as a piece of paper can create shadow zones. For this reason, only a small portion of high-frequency sound will enter the ear canal unless the sound is transmitted directly toward its entrance. Standing waves (areas of closely spaced high and low levels near a sound reflective surface) are also common for high-frequency sounds. Some adverse effects have been seen from exposure to airborne ultrasound, including headache, sore throat, and dizziness. These effects are often considered psychological and can vary between individuals.

Liquidborne Ultrasound

The velocity of sound in water is approximately 1,500 m/sec. Ultrasound within liquids is generally diffuse and uniform in level when the liquid is contained within sound reflective walls. Because the human body is made of mostly water, when any part of the human body is in direct contact with liquid in which ultrasound is present, it easily travels into the body and experiences very little attenuation. This can be dangerous because

Table 24.14 — Ultrasonics in Industry — Established uses, promising applications, and recent developments[105,117]

Application/Frequencies	*Description of Process*	*Intensity Range*
Cleaning and degreasing/ 20-50 kHz	Cavitated cleaning solution scrubs parts immersed in solution	<1–6 W/cm^2
Soldering and braising	Displacement of oxide film for bonding without flux	1–50 W/cm^2
Plastic welding/about 20 kHz	Welding soft and rigid plastic	About 100 W/cm^2
Metal welding/10–60 kHz	Welding similar and dissimilar metals	About 2000 W/cm^2
Machining/about 20 kHz	Drilling; rotary machining; impact grinding using slurry	
Extraction/about 20 kHz	Extracting juices and chemicals from flowers, fruits, and plants	About 500 W/cm^2
Atomization/20–300 kHz	Fuel atomization to improve combustion efficiency	
Emulsification and dispersion	Mixing and homogenizing liquids, slurries, and cream	
Defoaming and degassing	Separation of foam and gas from liquid	
Foaming of beverages	Displacing air by foam in containers prior to capping	
Electroplating	Increasing plating rates and producing more uniform deposits	
Erosion	Cavitation erosion tests, deburring, and stripping	
Drying	Drying powders, foodstuff, pharmaceuticals, paper, and plastic	
Control and measurements	Interruption or deflection of beam; Doppler effect	
Drilling and braiding	Slurry used between sonically vibrated tool and workpiece	
Nondestructive testing	Pulse-echo exploration for flaws and gauging thickness	
Agglomeration and precipitation	Separating solids from gases producing larger particles	
Impregnation of porous materials	Increased density, absence of gas inclusions	
Degassing of melts (metal glass)	Improvement of material density; refinement of grain structure	
Mixing of slurry (pulp)	Improvement of consistency	
Agitation of chemicals	Maintaining uniform solutions and concentration	
Accelerating chemical reactions	Aging of liquors; tanning of hides; extractions	
Food treatment	Destroying molds and bacteria; tenderizing, removing starch	
Metal insertion into solid plastic	Vibrating metal softens plastic as it is inserted	
Measuring fluid flow particle size	Noncontacting measuring method	

the levels at which liquidborne ultrasound is present can be very high, resulting in burning at the contact site, damage to the nervous system, or cellular damage to the ear and eyes.[98]

Effects of Ultrasound

Physiological effects of Airborne Exposure

Wide ranges of effects have been reported for ultrasound exposure, including annoyance, feelings of discomfort and fullness in the ears, malaise, fatigue, nausea, vestibular dysfunction, tinnitus, and headache.[99] Most exposures to ultrasound in the workplace are the result of ultrasound processes being performed by the worker in the same room. Table 24.15 lists examples of physiological effects of ultrasound exposure.

Von Gierke[100] found that subharmonics of incident sounds between 3.5 Hz and 23 kHz formed from ultrasonic frequencies on the eardrums of animals. If this phenomenon also occurs in human ears, hearing damage from ultrasound exposures could occur as a result of audible subharmonics (integer

Table 24.15 — Physiological effects of ultrasound (as noted)

HUMAN		*SMALL ANIMALS*
Death (calculated)[101]	--- 180 dB ---	
	--- 170 dB ---	
Loss of equilibrium[113]		
		Death (rabbits)[113]
Dizziness[113]		
	--- 160 dB ---	
Mild warming (body surface)[105]		
		Body temperature rise (hairless mice)[114]
	--- 150 dB ---	
Mild heating (skin clefts)[105]		Death (mice, rats, guinea pigs)[105]
	--- 140 dB ---	Body temperature rise (haired mice)[114]
	--- 130 dB ---	
	--- 120 dB ---	Mild biological changes (rats, rabbits)[111]
No physiological changes[115]		
	--- 110 dB ---	
No hearing loss occupational exposure[112]	--- 100 dB ---	

fractions [e.g., ½] of the ultrasonic frequency) without these subharmonics existing (and being measurable) in the work area. Parrack supported this theory by reporting temporary threshold shifts for humans as a result of ½-order subharmonics generated within the ear for a wide range of frequencies.[101] Airborne ultrasound exposure can also affect parts of the body other than the ear, through localized heating of tissue. Fortunately, the acoustic impedance of air is significantly different from that of the body, resulting in only a small fraction of the incident airborne ultrasound being absorbed by the body; the rest is reflected. Because of this impedance mismatch, airborne levels must be extremely high to cause damage to inner body parts.

In summary, the potential of permanent hearing impairment from exposure to ultrasound is not known definitely. Noise-induced hearing impairment is much less likely to result from ultrasound than from audible sound exposures. Subharmonics of ultrasound are most likely to cause noise-induced hearing impairment or other problems, but these subharmonic levels may not be detectable in normal noise measurements.

Annoyance of Airborne Exposure

The adverse effects of airborne ultrasound include, but are not limited to, headache, sore throat, dizziness, and nausea. These responses, sometimes collectively called ultrasonic sickness, are highly variable among individuals. Exposed individuals may experience these symptoms while the sound levels are low or inaudible. High-level ultrasound can cause changes in vestibular function, which may explain dizziness as a symptom. These reactions are considered temporary and are often considered psychological; however, they should be taken seriously and exposure levels should be reduced.

Direct Contact with Liquidborne Ultrasound

Because acoustic impedances are better matched between liquids and the body than between air and the body, the human body can absorb a much higher percentage of incident ultrasound when in direct contact with a transducer or a liquid medium. Such exposure results in localized tissue heating and other damage. Therefore, workers must be prohibited from touching transducers or immersing any part of their body in a liquid while an immersed transducer is operating.

Ultrasound can decrease the surface tension of solvents, which results in higher concentrations of vapor. The air around these operations must be monitored regularly until it is determined that the exposure to the solvent vapor is safe.

Exposure Criteria

It is very difficult to develop a meaningful hearing conservation guideline for ultrasound exposures for three reasons: First, the sensitivity of the ear significantly varies over the wide range of ultrasound frequencies. Second, the measurement of exposure and the assessment of the effects of airborne ultrasound are difficult. Finally, ultrasound is used in liquid as well as air media so there is potential danger from contact with either the source (a transducer) or liquid medium.

Table 24.16 shows ultrasound exposure limits proposed in the United States and other countries. The objectives of the different limits vary. Some recommendations intend to prevent objective physiological effects (primarily hearing impairment) while others intend to limit subjective effects. With the exception of the U.S. Air Force's 85 dB limit across all frequency bands, most of the exposure limits allow higher levels at higher frequencies (≥20 kHz).

The first known document to set high-frequency exposure limits above 10 kHz in the United States was Air Force Regulation 161- 35 (1973).[(102)] This document, "Hazardous Noise Exposure," deals with whole-body effects. Hearing protection is required when the sound level in any one-third octave band above 10 kHz exceeds 85 dB. A limit of 30 minutes each working day is set for levels at or above 150 dB in the same bands. Although this regulation is still in effect, the required use of hearing protection for exposures above 85 dB is very conservative; therefore, the USAF may adopt the levels proposed first by Parrack[(101)] and later by ACGIH®.[(103)]

ACGIH® first published its recommended TLVs® for ultrasound in 1988.[(103)] ACGIH® published higher ceiling values in 1998 that are significantly different than most other standards and are not presented in this chapter.[(104)] Another valuable guideline is the Canadian Safety Code-24, *Guidelines for the safe Use of Ultrasound, Part II — Industrial and Commercial Applications*.[(105)]

There are several reasons why ultrasound exposures were not included in many of the existing health and safety regulations:

- Most of the current rules, regulations, and guidelines on noise were in the

Table 24.16 — Various occupational exposure limits (in dB)

	Sound Pressure Levels in One-Third Octave Bands Proposed By (*)							
Frequency in kHz	*1*	*2*	*3*	*4*	*5*	*6*	*7*	*8*
8	90	75	--	--	--	--	--	--
10	90	75	--	--	--	80	--	--
12.5	90	75	75	85	--	80	--	--
16	90	75	85	85	--	80	--	75
20	110	75	110	85	105	105	75	75
25	110	110	110	85	110	110	110	110
31.5	110	110	110	85	115	115	110	110
40	110	110	110	85	115	115	110	110
50	110	--	110	--	115	115	110	110

* Legend:
1-Japan (1971)
2-Acton (1975)
3-USSR (1975)
4-USAF (1976)
5-Sweden (1971)
6-USA ACGIH (1988)
7-INTL IRPA (1984)
8-Canada (1989)

frequency range from 125 Hz to 8 kHz. Many authorities still agree with this opinion.
- Adding the ultrasound frequency range to regulations would delay achieving consensus and publishing these documents.
- Relatively few persons were exposed to high-level ultrasound when the first noise regulations were written.
- The effects of ultrasound were not well understood and susceptibility to ultrasound was generally considered to be highly variable.
- The measurement techniques to measure ultrasound are not as well developed as those to measure audible sound and it is therefore very difficult to regulate.
- Hearing threshold levels are not normally measured above 8 kHz.

As the number of ultrasound sources continues to increase, further knowledge should be gained on the effects of exposure. ACGIH's® TLVs® presented in Table 24.17 should be used as a guideline until a regulation is adopted. Although some organizations propose a 3-dB-per-doubling, equal-energy dose response, it may be appropriate to use the daily exposure limits regardless of exposure time due to a lack of supporting data for the dose-response relationship due to adverse ultrasound effects unrelated to hearing loss.[99]

Table 24.17 — Maximum permissible exposure limits to ultrasound[17]

1/3 Octave Band (kHz)	*SPL (dB re 20μPa)*
10	80
12.5	80
16	80
20	105
25	110
31.5	115
40	115
50	115

Measurement

When measuring ultrasound, the objective of the measurements must be carefully considered (even more than with audible sound) before performing the measurements. Measurement at ultrasonic frequencies presents several problems that require special equipment and procedures differing from standard noise measurements. Many instruments are not intended for use above 10 kHz, and only a few sound level meters and analyzers can measure sound above 20 kHz. Measurements taken in liquid media involve further complications and much care must be taken to obtain accurate data.

Since ultrasound exposure limits are often given in one-third octave bands, appropriate instrumentation should be used. Objects the size of a human head can shield a microphone from ultrasound; therefore, measurements should be made either at the location of the worker's ears without the worker present or on both sides of the worker's head. Due to the extreme directionality of ultrasound, measurements should be taken at the same location with the microphone positioned at several different angles.

Higher frequency one-third octave bands include more frequency data. For a sound with a perfectly flat spectrum (equal energy per frequency), the one-third octave band levels will increase with frequency. This is not necessarily reflected in the exposure criteria.

Instrumentation

One of the most vital and yet restrictive components of any sound measurement system is the microphone. Although many rules-of-thumb were developed for microphone selection, nothing replaces the manufacturer's instruction books and the advice of those who use the instruments.

Microphones and hydrophones must be selected from the specified frequency ranges, and several different transducers may be required to cover the full spectrum. In general, a 6 mm (¼ in.) or smaller diameter microphone must be used in order to obtain a relatively flat frequency response at ultrasonic frequencies. These microphones have lower sensitivity and poorer signal-to-noise ratios at lower frequencies than larger diameter microphones. Some microphones are specifically designed for the ultrasonic ranges extending to higher frequencies with higher sensitivities. Besides frequency, the following considerations may be important in choosing ultrasound microphones and hydrophones:

- Level of sensitivity to obtain an acceptable signal-to-noise ratio

- Directional characteristics (free-field, pressure-type, random-response, etc.)
- Rugged construction to cope with environmental factors (heat, rough handling, electromagnetic fields, corrosive vapors, liquids, etc.)
- Adequate dynamic range

Since instrumentation for ultrasound measurements is generally more sophisticated, more expensive, and less familiar than comparable instrumentation for audible sound, more time should be allowed for the selection of ultrasound equipment. Sound level meters that meet OSHA's Type II minimum specifications should not be used for ultrasound measurements because there are no tolerance limits defined above 10 kHz.

The field of bioacoustics has been detecting airborne ultrasound for much longer than most areas, and they have developed some commercially available ultrasound recorders. They use a special ultrasound microphone and can record up to several hundred kHz in air. They do not perform real time frequency analysis and post-processing on the recorded signal is required to obtain one-third octave bands. An example of this setup is shown in Figure 24.38. There are also commercial frequency analyzers that can measure up to about 80 kHz. These can be used with a variety of measurement devices so it is important that the selected microphone fulfills the frequency requirements. An example of a frequency analyzer is shown in Figure 24.39.

The detection of liquidborne ultrasound is more highly developed because the Navy has been doing research on the subject for much longer than airborne ultrasound has been a concern. However, the equipment is still much more sophisticated than the traditional sound level meter and needs to be chosen with care.

Techniques

Because ultrasound is much more directional than audible sounds, measurement samples should be made with microphones oriented in different directions to account for these directional characteristics. Generally, the required number of samples increases with frequency. For each orientation, many samples might be required to account for the standing waves common in some spaces with high-frequency noise.

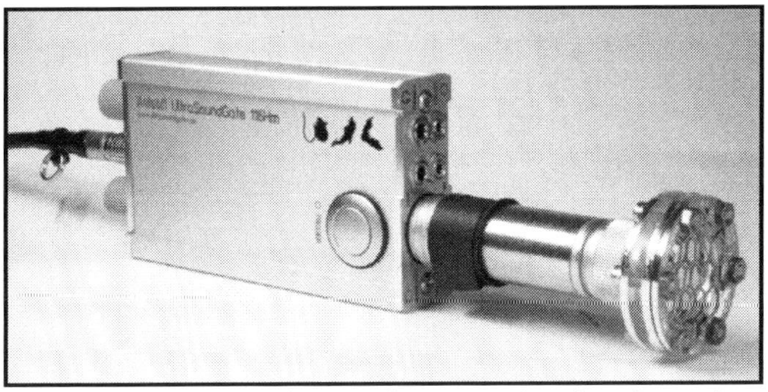

Figure 24.38 — A microphone and computer interface for use in measuring ultrasound. (Courtesy Avisoft).

More samples might also be required to account for localized areas in "ultrasound shadow zones." To determine the exposure dose, samples can be averaged over a period of time. In general, samples should be repeated at different orientations and locations until the data trends toward a stable average value.

A good rule-of-thumb is that the microphones will register the loudest levels when pointed directly at the loudest source. This will allow identification of the sources, so further measurements can be made.

Some ultrasound sources such as sewing or welding with ultrasound can be difficult to measure because they use pulsing operations with different peak levels, pulse lengths, and pulse repetition rates. Since the available damage-risk criteria does not include these parameters, the value of this exposure information is difficult to quantify. Different body locations such as the crevices between

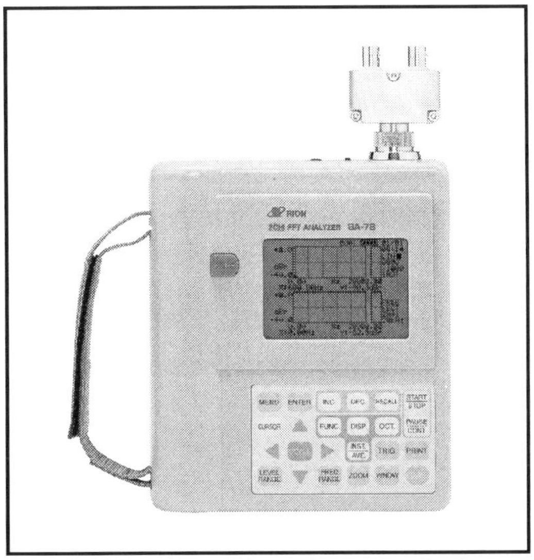

Figure 24.39 — FFT analyzer. (Courtesy Rion).

fingers are more susceptible to heating from ultrasound[105–109] and should be considered when trying to measure exposure.

In summary, ultrasound measurements may require special frequency bandwidths, numbers of samples, microphones, and microphone orientations. Considerable care must be taken in placing and orienting the microphones. Locations of reflecting surfaces and barriers must be considered and recorded as part of the measurement data. Many samples must be taken in most cases to determine a representative value because of the extreme changes in ultrasound levels that might be caused by acoustic shadows and standing waves.

High-Frequency Hearing Measurement

ANSI has no standard test procedures for measuring hearing levels at frequencies between 8 kHz and 20 kHz, and OSHA has no requirements for such tests. Although it is more difficult to conduct tests at these frequencies than at the normal audible frequencies, it is possible with specialized commercially available audiometers.

Exposure Controls

Administrative Controls

It is sometimes possible to reduce employee exposure to ultrasound by relocating work areas or ultrasound to another room. Because of the high directivity and absorption by air of ultrasound, it is possible to reduce exposure significantly by changing locations even within a room.

Engineering Controls

Engineering controls for ultrasound are often effective because of its high directivity and the high transmission loss characteristics of most materials at ultrasound frequencies. High-frequency sounds are blocked more effectively by barriers than lower frequencies, thereby creating sound shadows. Barriers can be used to isolate either the noise source or the worker. When simple barriers are insufficient due to the direction of the ultrasound or the positions of workers, complete enclosures can be built around the ultrasound source or the worker.

If the dimensions of a barrier are larger compared with the wavelength of a sound, the barrier will generally be effective in blocking the sound. Since ultrasound wavelengths are very small, any solid object with dimensions greater than 0.3 m (1 ft) will be an effective noise barrier.

Most acoustical data for noise control treatments extends to a maximum of 8 kHz. In general, transmission loss (TL) at ultrasound frequencies can be presumed to be at least as high as the TL for the highest given frequencies. Similar presumptions cannot be made for sound absorption data or silencer insertion loss data; however, un-faced porous materials such as glass fiber and acoustical foam, generally provide good absorption at ultrasonic frequencies.

Standing waves are often found around high-frequency noise sources. Standing waves can be reduced or eliminated by applying sound-absorptive treatments to the surfaces reflecting the ultrasound. Sound-absorptive values at ultrasonic frequencies vary significantly depending on the frequency and the physical properties of the materials. Even a very thin film (1/1000 in. or 25 μm) covering of sound-absorptive material will significantly reduce sound absorption at high frequencies by reflecting the ultrasound. Other treatments discussed in this chapter, such as damping and lagging, may also be appropriate for ultrasound.

Personal Protection

Little information is available on the protection levels offered by personal hearing protectors for ultrasound exposure. Methods for the measurement of hearing protector attenuation characteristics generally cover only the frequency range from 125 Hz to 8 kHz. For frequencies between 8–32 kHz, the attenuation values for 8 kHz can be used.[110] With ultrasound, extra care should be taken in inserting earplugs or putting on earmuffs to avoid any gaps or leaks through which ultrasound can pass.

Summary and Acknowledgments

The problems of overexposure to two physical agents—sound (noise and ultrasound) and vibration—have been discussed in this chapter. For each of these agents, criteria have been reviewed either in the form of governmental regulations, international standards, or recommendations from distinguished professional organizations concerned with worker health and safety. Recommendations have been presented for quantifying worker exposure to these physical agents by noise dosimetry, sound pressure level measurements, sound intensity measurements, vibration measurements, and ultrasound measurements. Also, different methods of reducing worker exposure to various physical agents have been presented in the form of engineering controls, administrative controls, and personal protective equipment and programs.

The authors are indebted to numerous individuals who contributed to the investigation of noise, vibration, and ultrasound in the occupational environment over the past 60+ years. In addition, the authors wish to recognize Jessica Arellano without whose careful attention to detail over the past year, this chapter would not have been completed.

References

1. **Embleton, T.F.W.:** Sound in Large Rooms. In *Noise and Vibration Control.* Beranek, L.L. (ed.). New York: McGraw-Hill, 1971. pp. 219–244.
2. **von Bekesy, G.:** The Ear. *Sci. Am. 197*:66 (1957).
3. **Gulik, W.L., G.A. Gescheider, and R.D. Frisina:** *Hearing: Physiological Acoustics, Neural Coding, and Psychoacoustics.* New York: Oxford University Press, 1989. p. 83.
4. **Suter, A.H.:** *Hearing Conservation Manual,* Fourth edition. Milwaukee, WI: Council for Accreditation in Occupational Hearing Conservation, 2002.
5. **Simpson, M.A., and R.D. Bruce:** *Noise in America: The Extent of the Noise Problem* (EPA Report No. 550/9-81-101). Washington, D.C.: U.S. Environmental Protection Agency/Office of Noise Abatement and Control, 1981.
6. **Suter, A.H.:** The Development of Federal Noise Standards and Damage Risk Criteria. In *Hearing Conservation in Industry, Schools, and the Military.* Lipscomb, D.M. (ed.). Boston, MA: College Hill Press, 1988.
7. **National Institute for Occupational Safety and Health (NIOSH):** Occupational Noise and Hearing: 1968–1972 (NIOSH Pub. No. 74-116). Cincinnati, OH: NIOSH, 1974.
8. "Occupational Noise Exposure," Code of Federal Regulations Title 29, Part 1910.95. 1971. [39 FR 23502, June 27, 1974, as amended at 46 FR 4161, Jan. 16, 1981; 46 FR 62845, Dec. 29, 1981; 48 FR 9776, Mar. 8, 1983; 48 FR 29687, June 28, 1983; 54 FR 24333, June 7, 1989.]
9. "Occupational Noise Exposure," Code of Federal Regulations Title 20, Part 1926.52.
10. "Occupational Noise Exposure," Code of Federal Regulations Title 29, Part 1910.95-subparagraph (o). 1971.
11. "Occupational Safety and Health Programs for Federal Employees" (Executive Order 12196; as amended by Executive Order 12223). Feb. 26, 1980.
12. "Occupational Noise Exposure," Mine Safety and Health Administration, Code of Federal Regulations, Title 30, Part 62, 1999.
13. "Occupational Noise Exposure for Railroad Operating Employees." Title 49, Part 227, Subpart B. (2007).
14. "Requirements of the Hours Service Act: Statement of Agency Policy and Interpretation," Code of Federal Regulations Title 49, Chapter II, Part 228, Appendix A. 1977. [42 FR 27596, May 31, 1977, as amended at 43 FR 30804, July 18, 1978; 53 FR 28601, July 28, 1988.]
15. **U.S. Coast Guard:** "Navigation and Vessel Inspection Circular No. 12-82: Recommendations on Control of Recessive Noise." Washington, D.C.: U.S. Department of Transportation/U.S. Coast Guard, June 1982.
16. "Vehicle Interior Noise Levels," Code of Federal Regulations Title 49, Chapter III, Part 393.94. 1973. [38 FR 30881, Nov. 8, 1973, as amended at 40 FR 32336, Aug. 1, 1975; 41 FR 28268, July 9, 1976.]
17. **U.S. Department of Defense:** "DOD Hearing Conservation Program" (DOD Instruction 6055.12). Washington, D.C.: U.S. Department of Defense, April 22, 1996.
18. **U.S. Environmental Protection Agency (EPA):** "Occupational Noise Exposure Regulation; Request for Review and Report." Washington, D.C.: U.S. Environmental Protection Agency, 1974. [39 FR 43802-43809.]
19. **National Institute for Occupational Safety and Health (NIOSH):** Criteria for a Recommended Standard ... Occupational Exposure to Noise (NIOSH Pub. No. HSM 73-11001). Cincinnati, OH: NIOSH, 1972.
20. **National Institute for Occupational Safety and Health (NIOSH):** Occupational Noise Exposure, Revised Criteria 1998, U.S. Dept. HHS (NIOSH) Pub. No. 98-126, Cincinnati, OH: 1998.
21. **Embleton, T.F.W.:** "Technical Assessment of Upper Limits on Noise in the Workplace: Final Report" Noise News International 4, 203-216, 1997.
22. **American Conference of Governmental Industrial Hygienists (ACGIH®):** Noise. In 1995–1996 Threshold Limit Values (TLVs®) for Chemical Substances and Physical Agents and Biological Exposure Indices (BEIs®). Cincinnati, OH: ACGIH®, 1995. pp. 108–110.

23. **Suter, A.H.:** Standards and Regulations, Chapter 16 in *The Noise Manual*, 5th edition, edited by E. H. Berger, L. H. Royster, J. D. Royster, D. P. Dricoll, and M. Layne, AIHA Press, Fairfax, 2000. p. 660.
24. **Bruce, R.D., A. Bommer, N. Hart, and K. Lefkowitz:** "Safe Lifetime Occupational Noise Exposure—1 Lone." Proceedings for Inter-noise 2010. April 19–21, 2010.
25. **Bruce, R.D., and E. McKinney:** "Noise Criteria for Ships and Offshore Platforms." Proceedings of Noise-Con 94, Progress in Noise Control for Industry, Fort Lauderdale, Fla., 1994. pp. 995–1000.
26. **Levitt, H., and J.C. Webster:** Effects of Noise and Reverberation on Speech. In Handbook of Acoustical Measurements and Noise Control. Harris, C.M. (ed.). New York: McGraw-Hill Inc., 1991. p. 16.10.
27. **Hoover, R.M., and R.D. Bruce:** Powerplant Noise and Its Control. In *Standard Handbook of Powerplant Engineering*. Elliott, T.C. (ed.). New York: McGraw-Hill Inc., 1989.
28. **Suter, A.H.:** Communication and Job Performance. In *Noise: A Review* (ASHA Monographs No. 28). Rockville, MD: American Speech-Language-Hearing Association, November 1992.
29. **American National Standards Institute (ANSI):** American National Standard Specification for Sound Level Meters. New York: ANSI S1.4-1983 (R2001).
30. **Earshen, J.J.:** Sound Measurement: Instrumentation and Noise Descriptors (Chapter 3). In *The Noise Manual*, 5th edition. Berger, E.H., L. H. Royster, J. D. Royster, D. P. Dricoll, and M. Layne (eds). Fairfax, VA: AIHA, 2000.
31. **Royster, L. H. et al.:** Noise Surveys and Data Analysis (Chapter 7). In *The Noise Manual*, Fifth Edition. Berger, E.H., L.H. Royster, J.D. Royster, D.P. Dricoll, and M. Layne. Fairfax, VA: AIHA, 2003.
32. **Driscoll, D.P. and L.H. Royster:** Noise Control Engineering (Chapter 9). In *The Noise Manual*, 5th edition. Berger, E.H., L. H. Royster, J. D. Royster, D. P. Dricoll, and M. Layne (eds.). Fairfax, VA: AIHA Press, 2003.
33. **Dear, T. A.:** Controlling Noise at Its Source Can Help Protect Workers' Hearing. *Occupational Health and Safety*, 1987, pp 60–64. (Discussed in Pelton, H.K., Noise Control Management. New York: Van Nostrand Reinhold, 1992.
34. **Beranek, L.L. (ed.):** *Noise & Vibration Control*. New York: McGraw-Hill Inc., 1971.
35. **Miller, L.N.:** *Noise Control for Buildings and Manufacturing Plants*. Cambridge, MA: Bolt Beranek and Newman Inc., 1981.
36. **Egan, M.D.:** *Concepts in Architectural Acoustics*. New York: McGraw-Hill Inc., 1972.
37. **Bruce, R.D., and E.H. Toothman:** Engineering Controls. In *Noise and Hearing Conservation Manual*, 4th edition. Berger, E.H., W.D. Ward, J.C. Morrill, and L.H. Royster (eds.). Akron, OH: AIHA®, 1986. pp. 417–521.
38. **National Institute for Occupational Safety and Health (NIOSH):** *Compendium of Materials for Noise Control* (DHEW Pub. No. 75-165) Cincinnati, OH: NIOSH, 1975.
39. **Acoustical and Insulatory Materials Association:** Bulletin of the Acoustical and Insulatory Materials Association. Park Ridge, IL: AIMA, 1974.
40. **Bies, D.A., and C.H. Hansen:** *Engineering Noise Control, Theory and Practice*. London, England: Unwin Hyman, 1988.
41. "Hearing Conservation Program," Code of Federal Regulations Title 29, Section 1910.95, Part C. 1971.
42. **Berger, E.H., L.H. Royster, J.D. Royster, D.P. Driscoll and M. Layne (eds.):** *The Noise Manual*, 5th edition. Fairfax, VA: AIHA Press, 2003.
43. **Lipscomb, D.M. (ed.):** *Hearing Conservation in Industry, Schools, and the Military*. Boston, MA: College Hill Press, 1988.
44. **Gasaway, D.C. (ed.):** *Hearing Conservation: A Practical Manual and Guide*. Englewood, NJ: Prentice-Hall, Inc., 1985.
45. **Sataloff, R.T., and J. Sataloff:** *Occupational Hearing Loss*, 2nd edition. New York: Marcel Dekker Inc., 1993.
46. **American National Standards Institute (ANSI):** *Specifications for Sound Level Meters* (ANSI S1.4–1983 [R1994]). New York: ANSI, 1995.
47. **American National Standards Institute (ANSI):** *Specifications for Sound Level Meters* (Supplement to ANSI S1.4–1983) (S1.4a-1985). New York: ANSI, 1985.
48. **American National Standards Institute (ANSI):** *Specification for Personal Noise Dosimeters* (ANSI S1.25–1991). New York: ANSI, 1991.
49. **American National Standards Institute (ANSI):** *Measurement of Occupational Noise Exposure* (ANSI S12.19–1996). New York: ANSI, 1996.
50. **Erdreich, J.:** Alternatives for Hearing Loss Risk Assessment. *Sound and Vib. 19(5)*:22–23 (1985).
51. **Suter, A.H.:** Noise Control: Why Bother? *Sound and Vib. 18(10)*:5 (1984).
52. **Berger, E.H.:** Hearing Protective Devices (Chapter 10). In *The Noise Manual*, Fifth edition. Fairfax, VA: AIHA Press, 2000. p. 385.
53. "Product Noise Labeling," Code of Federal Regulations Title 40, Part 211, Subpart B - Hearing Protective Devices. 1979.
54. "Guidelines for Noise Enforcement," Code of Federal Regulations Title 29, Part 1910.95(b)(1)-Instruction CPL 2-2.35. 1983.

55. **Franks, J.R., C.L. Themann, and C. Sherris:** The NIOSH Compendium of Hearing Protection Devices (NIOSH Pub. No. 94-130) Cincinnati, OH: NIOSH, 1994.
56. **Berger, E.H.:** Noise Control and Hearing Conservation: Why Do It? (Chapter 1). In *The Noise Manual*, Fifth edition. Fairfax, VA: 2000.
57. **Royster, L.H., and J.D. Royster:** Education and Motivation (Chapter 8). In *The Noise Manual*, Fifth edition. Fairfax, VA: 2000.
58. **Feldman, A.S. and C.T. Grimes:** Employee Training Programs in Occupational Hearing Conservation. In *Hearing Conservation in Industry*. Baltimore, MD: Williams & Wilkins, 1985. pp. 156–163.
59. **Berger, E.H., et al.:** "An Earful of Sound Advice about Hearing Protection." Indianapolis, IN: E•A•R Division of Cabot Corporation, 1988.
60. **Day, N.R.:** *Hearing Conservation: A Guide to Preventing Hearing Loss.* Daly City, CA: Krames Communications, 1983.
61. **Berger, E.H.:** "The Ardent Hearing Conservationist" presented at the 26th Annual Conference of the National Hearing Conservation Association, February 22–24, 2001. Raleigh, NC.
62. **Zohar, D., A. Cohen, and N. Azar:** Promoting Increased Use of Ear Protectors in Noise Through Information Feedback. *Human Factors 22*:69–79 (1980).
63. **National Institute for Occupational Safety and Health (NIOSH):** *Preventing Occupational Hearing Loss: A Practical Guide* (NIOSH Pub. No. 96-110). Cincinnati, OH: NIOSH, 1996.
64. **Megerson, S.C.:** OSHA's Final Rule for Recording Occupational Hearing Loss. *CAOHC Update, 14(3)*:1,3,10 (2002).
65. **Megerson, S.C.:** Amendments to OSHA's Final Rule for Recording Occupational Hearing Loss. *CAOHC Update 15(1)*:3 (2003).
66. Occupational Injury and Illness Recordkeeping and Reporting Requirements; Final Rule, Occupational Safety and Health Administration, Federal Register, Vol. 67, 44037-44048, July 1, 2002.
67. **Royster, J.D., and L.H. Royster:** Evaluating Hearing Conservation Program Effectiveness Audiometric Data Base Analysis (Chapter 12). In *The Noise Manual*, Fifth Edition. Fairfax, VA: AIHA®, 2000.
68. **American National Standards Institute (ANSI):** *Evaluating the Effectiveness of Hearing Conservation Programs*, ANSI Technical Report S12.13 TR-2002. New York: ANSI, 2002.
69. **Wasserman, D.E.:** *Human Aspects of Occupational Vibration.* Amsterdam, The Netherlands: Elsevier, 1987.
70. **Wasserman, D.E., D.W. Badger, T. Doyle, and L. Margolies:** Industrial Vibration — An Overview. *J. Am. Soc. Safety Eng. 19(6)*:38–43 (1974).
71. **Wasserman, D.E.:** *Occupational Diseases: A Guide to Their Recognition* (NIOSH Pub. No. 77-181). Cincinnati, OH: NIOSH, 1977.
72. **Radwin, R.G., T.J. Armstrong, and E. Vanbergeijk:** Vibration Exposure for Selected Power Hand Tools Used in Automobile Assembly. *Am. Ind. Hyg. Assoc. J. 51(9)*:510–518 (1990).
73. **Taylor, W.:** *The Vibration Syndrome.* London: Academic Press, 1974.
74. **Pelmear, P.L., W. Taylor, and D.E. Wasserman:** *Hand-Arm Vibration — A Comprehensive Guide for Occupational Health Professionals.* New York: Van Nostrand Reinhold, 1992.
75. **Taylor, W., and P. Pelmear (eds.):** *Vibration White Finger in Industry.* London, England: Academic Press, 1975.
76. **Taylor, W., and D. Wasserman:** Occupational Vibration. In *Occupational Medicine.* Zens, C. (ed.). Chicago, IL: Yearbook Medical Publishers, 1988.
77. **Hulshof, C., and B.V. Van Zanten:** Whole Body Vibration and Low-Back Pain — A Review of Epidemiological Studies. *Intl. Arch. Occup. Env. Health 59* (1987).
78. **Griffin, M.J.:** Handbook of Human Vibration. London, England: Academic Press, 1990.
79. "On the minimum health and safety requirements regarding the exposure of workers to the risks arising from physical agents (vibration)." Directive 2002/44/EC of the European Parliament. (2002).
80. **International Organization for Standardization (ISO):** *Guidelines for the Measurement and Assessment of Human Exposure to Hand-Transmitted Vibration — Part 1: General Requirements* (ISO 5349-1-2001). Geneva, Switzerland: ISO, 2001.
81. **International Organization for Standardization (ISO):** *Guidelines for the Measurement and Assessment of Human Exposure to Hand-Transmitted Vibration — Part 2: Practical Guidance for Measurement at the Workplace* (ISO 5349-2-2001). Geneva, Switzerland: ISO, 2001.
82. **American Conference of Governmental Industrial Hygienists (ACGIH®):** Hand-Arm (Segmental) Vibration Syndrome (HAVS). In *1995–1996 Threshold Limit Values® (TLVs®) for Chemical Substances and Physical Agents and Biological Exposure Indices (BEIs®).* Cincinnati, OH: ACGIH®, 1995. pp. 84–87.
83. **Henschel, A., and V. Behrens:** *Criteria for a Recommended Standard — Occupational Exposure to Hand-Arm Vibration* (NIOSH Pub. No. 89-106). Cincinnati, OH: NIOSH, 1989.

84. **International Organization for Standardization (ISO):** *Guidelines for the Measurement and Assessment of Human Exposure to Hand-Transmitted Vibration* (ISO 5349-1986). Geneva, Switzerland: ISO, 1986.
85. **American National Standards Institute (ANSI):** *Guide for the Measurement and Evaluation of Human Exposure to Vibration Transmitted to the Hand* (ANSI S3.34-1986). New York: American National Standards Institute, 1986.
86. **International Organization for Standardization (ISO):** *Evaluation of Human Exposure to Whole-Body Vibration — Part 1: General Requirements* (ISO 2631-1–2001). Geneva, Switzerland: ISO, 1985.
87. **American National Standards Institute (ANSI):** *Guide for the Evaluation of Human Exposure to Whole-Body Vibration* (ANSI S3.18-2002). New York: ANSI, 2002.
88. **American Conference of Governmental Industrial Hygienists (ACGIH®):** Whole-Body Vibration. In *1995–1996 Threshold Limit Values (TLVs®) for Chemical Substances and Physical Agents and Biological Exposure Indices (BEIs®).* Cincinnati, OH: ACGIH®, 1995. pp. 124–131.
89. **Broch, J.T.:** *Mechanical Vibration and Shock Measurements.* Glostrup, Denmark: Bruel & Kajaer, 1984.
90. Test Procedure for the Measurement of Vibration from Hand Held (Portable) Power Driven Ginding Machines (PNEUROP 6610/1983). London, England.
91. **National Institute for Occupational Safety and Health (NIOSH):** *Current Intelligence Bulletin #38: Vibration Syndrome* (NIOSH Pub. No. 83-110). Cincinnati, OH: NIOSH, 1983.
92. **Radwin, R.G.:** "Neuromuscular Effects of Vibrating Hand Tools on Grip Extensions, Tactility, Discomfort, and Fatigue." 1986. [University of Michigan, Industrial and Operations Engineering Dept./DHHS (NIOSH) Grant Reports 5-RO3-OH01852-02 and 1-T15-OH07207-01.]
93. **Wasserman, D.:** *Occupational Vibration in the Foundry* (NIOSH Pub. No. 81-114). Proceedings of the Symposium on Occupational Health Hazard Control Technology in the Foundry and Secondary Non-Ferrous Smelting Industries. Cincinnati, OH: NIOSH, 1981.
94. **Goel, V.K., and K. Rim:** Role of Gloves in Reducing Vibration: An Analysis for Pneumatic Chipping Hammer. *Am. Ind. Hyg. Assoc. J. 48(1)*:9–14 (1987).
95. **Gurram, R., S. Rakheja, and G.J. Gouw:** Vibration Transmission Characteristics of the Human Hand-Arm and Gloves. *Intl. J. Ind. Ergon. 13*:217–234 (1994).
96. **International Organization for Standardization (ISO):** *Method for the Measurement and Evaluation of the Vibration Transmissibility of Gloves at the Palm of the Hand* (ISO 10819-1996). Geneva, Switzerland: ISO, 1996.
97. **Lefkowitz, K., R. Bruce, and A. Bommer:** "Ultrasound in the Home and Workplace," Proceedings for Inter-noise 2009. August 23–26, 2009.
98. **Wiernicki, C. and W.J. Karoly:** Ultrasound: Biological Effects and Industrial Hygiene Concerns. *Am. Ind. Hyg. Assoc. J. 46*:488–96 (1985).
99. **Lawton, B.W.:** Damage to human hearing by airborne sound of very high frequency or ultrasound frequency, Institute of Sound and Vibration Research, Contract Research Report 343/2001 Southampton, 2001.
100. **von Gierke, H.E.:** Subharmonics Generated in Human and Animal Ears by Intense Sound. *J. Acoust. Soc. Am. 22*:475 (1950).
101. **Parrack, H.O.:** Effects of Air-borne Ultrasound on Humans. *Intl. Audio. 5*:294–308 (1966).
102. **U.S. Air Force:** "Hazardous Noise Exposure" (USAF Regulation 161-35). 1973.
103. **American Conference of Govern-mental Industrial Hygienists (ACGIH®):** Threshold Limit Values® and Biological Exposure Indices® for 1988–1989. Cincinnati, OH: ACGIH®, 1988. p. 107.
104. **American Conference of Govern-mental Industrial Hygienists (ACGIH®):** 1998 TLVs® and BEIs® Threshold Limit Values for Chemical Substances and Physical Agents, Biological Exposure Indices. Cincinnati, OH: ACGIH®, 1998.
105. **Bly, S.H.P., and D. Morison:** *Guidelines for the Safe Use of Ultrasound: Part II — Industrial and Commercial Applications.* Ottawa, Canada: Safety Code 24. Environmental Health Directorate, Health Protection Branch, 1991.
106. **Kelly, E. (ed.):** Ultrasonic Energy. In *Biological Investigations and Medical Applications.* Urbana, Ill.: University of Illinois Press, 1965.
107. **Kelly, E. (ed.):** *Ultrasound in Biology and Medicine* (Pub. No. 3). Washington, D.C.: American Institute of Biological Sciences, 1957.
108. **Knight, J.J.:** Effects of Airborne Ultrasound on Man. *Ultrasonics 6*:39–42 (1968).
109. **Reid, J.M., and M.R. Sikov (eds.):** *Interaction of Ultrasound and Biological Tissues. Proceedings of a Workshop at Battelle Seattle Research Center,* Nov. 8–11, 1971. (DHEW (FDA) Pub. No. 73-8008 (BRH/DBE 73-1). 1972.)

110. **Berger, E. H.:** "Attenuation of Hearing Protectors at the Frequency Extremes." Proceedings of the Eleventh International Congress on Acoustics, Paris, France, 1983. pp. 289–292.
111. **Acton, W.I.:** The Effects of Industrial Airborne Ultrasound on Humans. *Ultrasonics:* 124–268 (1974).
112. **Acton, W.I., and M.B. Carson:** Auditory and Subjective Effects of Airborne Noise from Industrial Ultrasonic Sources. *Br. J. Ind. Med. 24*:297–304 (1967).
113. **Allen, C.H., H. Frings, and I. Rudnick:** Some Biological Effects of Intense High Frequency Airborne Sound. *J. Acoust. Soc. Am. 20*:62–65 (1948).
114. **Danner, P.A., E. Ackerman, and H.W. Frings:** Heating in Haired and Hairless Mice in High-Intensity Sound Fields from 6-22,000 hertz. *J. Acoust. Soc. Am. 26*:731 (1954).
115. **Grigor'eva, V.M.:** Effect of Ultrasonic Vibrations on Personnel Working with Ultrasonic Equipment. *Soviet Phys.-Acoust. 11*:426–427 (1966).
116. **Ravizza, R., H. Heffner, and B. Masterton:** Hearing in Primitive Mammals. I: Opossum (Didelphis virginianus). *J. Audio. Res. 9*:1–7 (1969).
117. **Steinberg, E.B.:** Ultrasonics in Industry. *Proceed. IEEE 53(10)*:1292–1304 (1965).

Outcome Competencies

After completing this chapter, the reader should be able to:

1. Define underlined terms in this chapter.
2. Describe nonionizing electromagnetic radiation.
3. Review biological/health effects for ultraviolet, laser, radio-frequency radiation, and extremely low frequency fields.
4. Calculate hazard distances for laser radiation and some sources of radio-frequency radiation.
5. Review measurement fundamentals for nonionizing radiation.
6. Describe elementary control measures.

Key Terms

absolute gain • aphakes • aversion response • broad-band • cancellation • Class 1 • Class 2 • Class 2a • Class 3a • Class 3b • Class 4 • contact currents • continuous wave • current density • cutaneous malignant melanoma (CMM) • diffuse reflection • divergence • duty cycle • effective irradiance • electric fields • electric-field strength • electromagnetic spectrum • electromagnetic radiation • extremely low frequency (ELF) • far field • flash blindness • frequency • geometrical resonance • hazard distance • illuminance • induced currents • infrared (IR) • intrabeam viewing • irradiance • Lambertian surface • laser radiation • Laser Safety Officer (LSO) • luminance • magnetic fields • magnetic flux density • magnetic-field strength • microwave radiation • minimum erythemal dose (MED) • near field • nominal hazard zone (NHZ) • nonbeam hazards • nonionizing radiation • nonmelanoma skin cancer (NMSC) • optical density (OD) • optical radiation • permeability • permittivity • perturbation • phosphenes • photoconjunctivitis • photokeratitis • photometer • photon energy • photosensitivity • plane waves • power density • precautionary principle • prudent avoidance • radiance • radiant exposure • radio-frequency (RF) • radiometer • radiowaves • retinal hazard • region • reversible behavior disruption • specific absorption (SA) • specific absorption rate (SAR) • shielding effectiveness (SE) • spatial averaging • specular reflection • visible wavelength • ultraviolet (UV) • UV-A • UV-B • UV-C

Prerequisite Knowledge

Introductory college physics.

Key Topics

I. Introduction
   A. Electromagnetic Radiation
   B. Electromagnetic Spectrum
   C. Nonionizing Radiation

II. Optical Radiation and Illumination
   A. Anticipation
   B. Recognition
   C. Evaluation
   D. Control Measures

III. Laser Radiation
   A. Anticipation
   B. Laser Characteristics
   C. Types of Lasers
   D. Harmful Effects of Laser Exposure
   E. Other Safety Concerns
   F. Evaluation
   G. Laser Characteristics and Capabilities to Injure Personnel
   H. Laser Classification

IV. Radio-Frequency and Microwave Radiation
   A. Anticipation
   B. Recognition
   C. Evaluation
   D. Control Measures

V. Extremely Low Frequency Fields
   A. Anticipation
   B. Recognition
   C. Evaluation
   D. Control Measures

VI. Static Magnetic Fields

VII. Nonionizing Radiation Control Program
   A. Responsibility
   B. Medical Monitoring
   C. Information and Training
   D. Hazard Communication
   E. Self-Checks and Audits

Nonionizing Radiation

25

By Thomas P. Fuller, ScD, CIH, MSPH, MBA

Introduction

Electromagnetic Radiation

Radiation can be simply described as energy emitted from a central source traveling through space. Sometimes this energy is in the form of energetic particles, known as particulate radiation, a type of ionizing radiation. Another type of radiation has no mass, but can travel as individual packets or bundles of energy called photons. Photons propagate through space in the form of electric and magnetic fields that are coupled in a manner where they oscillate perpendicularly to one another, with the same frequencies and wavelengths. These type of radiations are known as electromagnetic radiation. A diagram demonstrating the propagation of an electromagnetic radiation is shown in Figure 25.1.

Electromagnetic radiation is the propagation, or transfer, of energy through space and matter by time-varying electric and magnetic fields. In the case of electromagnetic energy, the fields are composed of vector quantities. A vector field is any physical quantity that takes on different values of magnitude and direction at different points in space.

As depicted in Figure 25.1, the electric and magnetic fields are in time phase and space quadrature. Space quadrature means the electric and magnetic vector fields are mutually orthogonal (lie on perpendicular planes). Time phase means that the electric and magnetic field oscillations reach their peaks at the same time.

Electric fields are produced by electric charges, while magnetic fields are produced by moving charges, or a current. Electric and magnetic fields in turn will exert a force on electric charges, and this is the basis for interactions with matter. Electric fields will act on a charge regardless of its motion, while the charge must be in motion relative to the magnetic field, or vice versa, before an interaction occurs between the magnetic field and the charge.

Electromagnetic Spectrum

The electromagnetic spectrum is subdivided into named regions (see Figure 25.2). Any location on the spectrum may be characterized by wavelength, frequency, and photon energy.

Wavelength, designated lambda (λ) is the distance between the ends of one complete cycle of a wave. Frequency, designated by the letter "f" or the Greek letter nu (ν) is the number of complete wave cycles that pass a point in space in 1 second. Frequency and wavelength are related by the speed of light, c, where $f = c\lambda$.

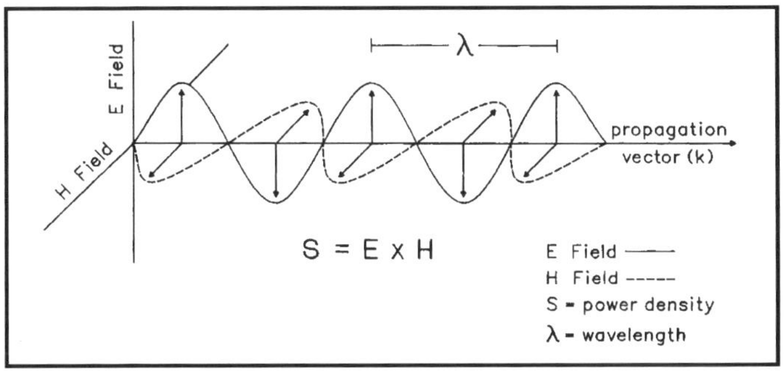

Figure 25.1 — Representation of an Electromagnetic Wave — The waves representthe electric and magnetic fields in the same phase, with the same wavelengths, but traveling perpendicularly to one another.

Photon energy describes the energy possessed by electromagnetic energy when characterized as discrete bundles or "quanta", as described by quantum theory. The unit of photon energy is the joule (J) or the electron volt (eV).

Nonionizing Radiation

Ionizing radiation refers to any particulate or electromagnetic radiation that has sufficient engergy to knock an electron out of the orbital shell of an atom. For most atoms, the ionization potential for the outer orbiting electrons is around 12.4 electron volts (eV). Thus, photons with energies less than 12.4 eV, that are not capable of ionizing and atom, are termed nonionizing radiation. Portions of the electromagnetic spectrum that are nonionizing in nature are indicated on Figure 25.2. The nonionizing spectral region includes the ultraviolet (UV), visible, infrared (IR), radio-frequency (RF), and extremely low frequency (ELF) radiation.

Quantities and units often used in the practice of nonionizing radiation safety are compiled in Table 25.1. Characteristics of the nonionizing radiation spectral region are shown in Table 25.2, and discussed elsewhere.[4–7]

As indicated in Table 25.3, wavelength is the descriptor used for UV, visible, and IR radiation and frequency is used for RF and ELF. Because these spectral regions have differences in absorption, biological effects, exposure guidelines, measurement instrumentation, and control measures; each is discussed separately in the following text.

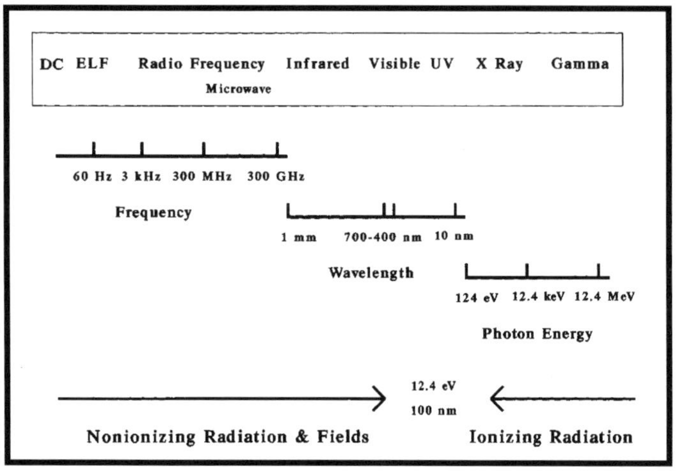

Figure 25.2 — The electromagnetic spectrum is a continuum that spans high-energy gamma radiation to non-time-varying fields (static fields). The spectrum often is divided into two regions: ionizing and nonionizing radiation. The boundary between these regions is a photon energy of 12.4 eV.

Table 25.2 — Composite Characteristics of NIR

Wavelength:	100 nm to 300,000 km
Frequency:	3.0 PHz to 1 Hz
Photon energy:	1.987 × 10-18 J to 6.6 × 10-34 J

Table 25.3 — Fundamental Characteristics

Region	*Wavelength*	*Frequency*
Ultraviolet	100-400 nm	——
Visible	400-770 nm	——
Infrared	770 nm-1 mm	——
Radio frequency	——	300 GHz-3 kHz
Extremely low frequency	——	3 kHz-3 Hz

Table 25.4 — Spectral Bands for Optical Radiation

Region	*Band*	*Wavelength*
Ultraviolet	UV-C	100-280 nm
	UV-B	280-315 nm
	UV-A	315-400 nm
Visible		400-770 nm
Infrared	IR-A	770-1400 nm
	IR-B	1.4-3.0 mm
	IR-C	3.0 mm-1 mm

Optical Radiation

Anticipation

UV, visible, and Infrared (IR)radiation are called optical radiation because they behave according to the laws and principles of geometric optics. The optical wavelengths can be divided into spectral bands, as shown in Table 25.4. The boundaries between the bands have no basis in fundamental physics and serve only as a framework for addressing biological effects.

The UV divisions are named regions. UV-A is the blacklight region, UV-B the erythema region, and the UV-C the germicidal region. The 100–180 nm region is known as the vacuum UV region, because these wavelengths are readily absorbed in air and may lead to the production of gases such as ozone. UV-B and UV-C regions are often called actinic UV, because they are capable of causing chemical reactions.

Quantities and Units

Two systems of quantities and units, radiometric and photometric, are used for optical radiation. Radiometric quantities constitute a physical system that can be used to describe the emission from, or exposure to, any optical radiation. The photometric system is a subset of the radiometric system but is based on the response of the human eye to optical radiation and is used only for visible radiation. The radiometric system is used mainly for assessing optical radiation hazards, whereas the photometric system is used for specifying exposure limits for visible radiation and lighting requirements.[5]

Table 25.1 — Important Quantities and Units

Quantity	*Symbol*	*Unit Name*	*Unit Abbreviation*
Beam size at lens	b_o	length	cm
Conductivity		siemen/meter	S/m
Contact current	I_c	milliampere	mA
Current density	J	ampere/square meter	A/m^2, mA/cm^2
Divergence	ϕ	radian[A]	rad, mrad
Duration of single pulse; allowable exposure duration	t	time	s, sec
E-field strength	E	volt/meter	V/m, V^2/m^2, kV/m
Energy	Q	joule	J
Exit beam diameter	a	length	cm, mm
Focal length	f_o	length	cm
Frequency	υ,f	hertz	Hz (GHz, MHz, kHz)
H-field strength	H	ampere/meter	A/m, A^2/m^2
Illuminance	E_e	lumen/square meter	lm/m^2 = 1 lux
		lumen/square foot	lm/ft^2 =1ft-candle
Induced currents	I_i	milliamperes	mA
Integrated radiance	L_p	joule/square centimeter × steradian	J/cm^2-sr
Irradiance	E	watt/square meter	W/m^2, mW/cm^2
Luminance	L_v	candela/square meter	cd/m^2
Luminous intensity	I_e	lumens/sr	lm/sr,
Magnetic flux density	B	tesla	T (mT, μT)
Maximum viewing angle	α_{max}	radian	rad, mrad
Minimum viewing angle	α_{min}	radian	rad, mrad
Mode field diameter	ω_o	length	μm
Numerical aperture	NA	dimensionless	--
Optical density	OD,D_λ	dimensionless	--
Permeability	μ	henry/meter	H/m
Permittivity	ε	farad/meter	F/m
Photon energy	Q_p	joule, electron volt	J, eV
Power	Φ, F	watt	W
Power density	W,S	watt/square meter	W/m^2, mW/cm^2
Pulse repetition frequency	F,PRF	hertz	Hz
Radiance	L	watt/square centimeter-steradian	W/cm^2-sr
Radiant exposure	H	joule/square meter	J/m^2, mJ/cm^2
Reflectivity	ρ	dimensionless	--
Solid angle	Ω	steradian[A]	sr
Specific absorption rate	SAR	watts/kilogram	W/kg
Specific absorption	SA	joules/kilogram	J/kg
Spectral irradiance	E_λ	watt/square centimeter-nanometer	W/cm^2-nm
Total exposure duration	T	time	s, sec
Viewing angle	α,θ	radian[A]	rad, mrad
Wave impedance	Z	ohm	Ω
Wavelength	λ	meter	m (nm, μm, mm)

[A]These quantities are mathematically dimensionless, but the units are assigned for practical purposes.

Radiometric and photometric quantities and units are shown in Table 25.1. Similar quantities from both systems include irradiance-illuminance, radiance-luminance, radiant intensity-luminous intensity, and radiant exposure-light exposure. For example, radiance is radiometric brightness (all optical wavelengths), while luminance is brightness as perceived by the eye (just visible wavelengths). Conversions between the two systems are possible but require spectral data and the use of wavelength-dependent conversion factors (called luminous efficacy), since the eye does not respond equally to all wavelengths. Spectral data are usually provided by the quantity spectral irradiance ($E\lambda$), which has units of $W/m^2/nm$ or W/m^3. Spectral irradiance is the irradiance within a narrow spectral band.

Radiance is the radiometric brightness of an extended source. It is the radiant power per solid angle per unit area, where the solid angle is usually defined as a cone (area projected from the surface of a source perpendicular to the direction of the flux).[6–8] Irradiance is the dose rate in photobiology. It describes the radiant flux that crosses a given surface (receiver), divided by the area of that surface. Radiant exposure is the photobiological dose of radiant energy. Hence, the dose in optical radiation is in joules/centimeter squared (J/cm^2), while the dose rate is in watts/ centimeter squared (W/cm^2). (Remember: $1 W = 1 J/s$ or $P = Q/t$).

Key concepts associated with illumination are luminance, luminance contrast, and illuminance. Luminance describes the brightness of an object, or the luminous intensity per unit area of surface and is expressed in units of candela per square meter (cd/m^2), where $1 cd/m^2 = 10^{-4} cd/cm^2 = 0.2919$ footlamberts (ftL). Luminance contrast (LC) refers to the percentage difference in luminance of the features of the object being viewed and is expressed by

$$LC = (B_1 - B_2)/ B_2 \times 100 \qquad (25\text{-}1)$$

where B_1 and B_2 are the brighter and darker areas, respectively. Illuminance is the luminous flux crossing a surface of a given area and is expressed in units of lumens per square meter (lm/m^2) where $1 lm/m^2 = 1 lx = 0.0929$ foot-candles (fc).

Health Effects

The target organs for UV radiation are the skin, eyes, and immune system. Skin effects that may be of importance from occupational exposures include erythema, photosensitivity, aging, and cancer. Ocular effects are photokeratoconjunctivitis, cataracts, and retinal effects.

Skin. The most common adverse response of the skin to UV is erythema or sunburn. The International Commission on Illumination (CIE) erythema reference action spectrum indicates that the skin is most sensitive (lowest effective doses) from 250 nm to about 300 nm.[9,10] The erythemal response (skin reddening) is a vascular reaction involving vasodilation and increased blood volume, and ranges from a slight reddening to severe blistering. The changes observed depend on the dose and spectral content of the incident radiation, the pigmentation and exposure history of the exposed skin, and the thickness of the stratum corneum. The erythemal response begins at 2 to 4 hr postexposure, peaks at 14 to 20 hr, and lasts for up to 48 hr. Parrish et al. determined that the minimum erythemal dose (MED) from 250 to 304 nm ranged from 14 to 47 mJ/cm^2 and increased dramatically above 313 nm.[11] Radiant exposure between 15–50 mJ/cm^2 is also referred to as the threshold dose for erythema and applies to lightly pigmented skin not recently exposed to UV radiation (not conditioned). The defense measures taken by the skin on exposure, melanogenesis and skin thickening subsequent to hyperplasia, will increase the threshold required to produce the same degree of reddening.[12]

Certain chemicals found in medications, plants, or industrial operations are photosensitizing agents. Photosensitivity includes two types of reactions: phototoxicity and photoallergy. Phototoxicity is more common and affects all individuals if the UV dose or the dose of the photosensitizer is high enough. Photoallergy is an acquired altered reactivity in the exposed skin resulting from an immunologic response.

Various lists of photosensitizing agents are available.[13,14] Agents include many medications (e.g., some acne treatments, antibiotics, oral contraceptives), some artificial sweeteners, deodorants, perfumed soaps, sunscreen agents, plants (e.g., figs, parsley, limes, parsnips, and pinkrot celery), and industrial photosensitizers including coal tar, pitch, anthracene, naphthalene, phenanthrene, thiophene, and many phenolic agents.

Skin aging (also called dermal elastosis) is associated with chronic UV exposure. It is characterized by damage to dermal connective tissues with a loss in elasticity with laxity of tissues, furrowing of skin, and irregular pigmentation.[15,16]

The carcinogenic effects of UV radiation have been studied extensively, and literature reviews are available.[17–19] Evaluating the carcinogenicity of solar and UV radiation, an International Agency for Research on Cancer (IARC) working group found that solar radiation is carcinogenic to humans and all UV regions are probably carcinogenic to humans.[17] The National Toxicology Program has listed solar radiation and exposure to sunlamps or sunbeds as a known human carcinogen.[20]

Three types of skin cancers are of concern: squamous cell carcinomas (SCC) and basal cell carcinomas (BCC) [referred to jointly as nonmelanoma skin cancer (NMSC)] and cutaneous malignant melanoma (CMM). The American Cancer Society estimates that about 1.35 million new cases of skin cancer are diagnosed annually.[21]

BCC are slow growing, superficial tumors that rarely metastasize. Risk factors for BCC include fair complexion, inability to tan, red or blonde hair, blue or green eyes, freckling, increasing age, sunburn in childhood, and outdoor occupation.[22–24] SCC are superficial tumors that can metastasize, although not common. Risk factors for SCC include sunlight exposure, average daily hours of exposure, number of blistering sunburns, sun exposure during childhood and adolescence, fair complexion. degree of freckling, hazel or blue eyes, and red or blonde hair.[25–27]

A study that examined non-solar sources of UV found no increased risk of BCC and SCC associated with sources including welding, mercury vapor lamps, and black lights.[28] The carcinogenic action spectrum for humans is known to include the UV-B region but may extend throughout the UV-A region.

The incidence of cutaneous malignant melanoma has increased rapidly in the United States and worldwide in the past 30 to 40 years with about 40,000 new cases of CMM each year in the United States. Mortality rates have increased by 191% and 84% for white males and females, respectively, from 1950–1954 through 1990–1994.[29] Although several factors, such as the presence of moles and genetic predisposition, have been associated with this disease, increased solar exposure has been implicated as a contributing factor.[30] An action spectrum for CMM in a hybrid fish suggests the involvement of not only UV-B, but also UV-A and blue light.[31,32]

UVR exposure also depresses both the systemic and local immunologic response.[33] Effects that have been observed include altered function of epidermal Langerhans cells, reduced T cells (possibly a transient effect), inhibition of natural killer cell activity, and changes in cytokine regulation.[34]

UV exposure does produce some beneficial or therapeutic effects[35], including vitamin D3 synthesis and therapy for skin conditions including vitiligo, psoriasis, mycosis fungoides, acne, eczema, and pityriasis rosea. In some treatments, photosensitizing agents are used to enhance the effect of UV radiation.[36]

Eye. UV-B and -C are primarily absorbed in the tissue of the cornea and conjunctiva. Corneal transmission ranges from 60 to 83% in the UV-A band, with much of the energy absorbed by the lens. Photokeratitis and photoconjunctivitis result from acute, high-intensity exposure to UV-B and UV-C. Commonly referred to as "arc eye" or "welder's flash" by workers, this injury results from exposure of the unprotected eye to a welding arc or other artificial sources rich in UV-B and UV-C. Sunlight exposure produces these sequelae only in environments where highly reflective materials are present such as snow ("snow blindness") or sand.

Symptoms include lacrimation, blepharospasm (twitching or spasm of certain ocular muscles), and photophobia accompanied by a sensation of sand in the eye and severe pain. These symptoms become apparent at 2–12 hr postexposure, and persist for up to 48 hr, usually without residual damage. Photochemical denaturation and coagulation of protein structures are the basic mechanisms of cell damage.[37] No increasing tolerance to subsequent irradiation develops.[12]

Threshold doses for humans range from 4 to 14 mJ/cm^2 between 220 and 310 nm.[37,38] An action spectrum has been established, and the wavelength of minimum threshold occurs at 270 nm. Reciprocity holds for exposure durations up to several hours; thus, the tissue damage depends on the total dose, and not the dose rate.

The only lenticular effect linked with UVR exposure, primarily solar radiation, is the cataract. In the United States, estimates of the number of cataract operations range up to 1 million annually and cataracts are the third leading cause of blindness.(39) Predisposing factors include age, gender, family history, nutritional status, and certain medical conditions and medications.

An action spectrum has been established for lenticular opacities in rabbits. For exposures of less than one day, threshold radiant exposures from 290 to 320 nm ranged from 0.15 to 12.60 J/cm² for transient opacities, and 0.5 to 15.5 J/cm² for permanent opacities. In both cases, the minimum threshold was 300 nm. From 325 to 395 nm cataracts could not be produced even at very high exposures. Primates were exposed only at 300 nm; the threshold radiant exposure was 0.12 J/cm².(37)

Epidemiological studies of human populations in six countries on four continents have attempted to discern if an association exists between sunlight exposure and the occurrence of cataracts, specifically senile cataracts. Although individual solar or UV radiation exposures were not measured, diverse surrogates such as UV-B counts, hours of sunlight exposure, and geographic location were used to characterize average daily exposures. Where associations were positive, relative risk or odds ratios ranged from 1.10 to 5.8, demonstrating a consistent association between UV exposure and cataracts.(40–43) In reviewing the literature, Waxler concluded that the threshold for cataracts is 2500 MEDs yearly, corresponding to daily exposures of 7 to 90 mJ/cm² for UV-B and 0.4 to 98 J/cm² for UV-A.(44) Also, there is some evidence that systemic photosensitizers, primarily drugs, may play a role in cataractogenesis.(45,46)

Exposure to UV-A and UV-B, primarily from solar radiation, has been implicated as an etiologic agent in solar retinitis, cystoid macular edema (CME), and senile macular degeneration (SMD).(47) In adults, transmission of these wavelengths through the ocular media is minimal except in an aphake (absence of the lens condition). Although originally thought to be a thermal injury, solar retinitis (also known as eclipse blindness) is a photochemical lesion resulting from absorption of UV-A and blue wavelengths. Experimental studies have determined that retinal damage occurs at lower exposures at 325 nm than at 441 nm (5.0 vs. 30 J/cm² respectively). The threshold for broad-band UV-A exposure is 0.09 J/cm².(44)

Visible Radiation

The photon energy range of visible radiation is approximately 3.1 to 1.8 eV. While this energy level is small it can be absorbed by body tissues and is sufficient to cause changes in the vibrational/rotational energies of the tissue molecules thereby producing either direct or indirect effects. A direct effect is one that results from chemical changes within a tissue due to absorption of visible photons. Light is a known direct hazard to two organs, eye and skin. An indirect effect results from chemical signals released by cells in response to exposure to visible photons. Examples are effects on biological rhythms and inhibition of melatonin synthesis by the pineal gland.

The process of vision is associated with visible radiation. Nothing is visible to humans when visible radiation is absent. Hence, the proper quality and quantity of visible radiation (illumination) is necessary in order to safely and effectively work. In fact, it is clearly understood that poor lighting of the work area will compromise safety.

Skin. Exposure to high-intensity visible wavelengths can lead to thermocoagulation of skin similar to that produced by electrical or thermal burns. Several variables influence the threshold for and the amount of damage: the incident intensity, absorption and scattering by the skin, exposure duration, area of skin exposed, and degree of vascularization of the irradiated tissue.(48) Individuals with certain diseases or genetic deficiencies are sensitive to light, but the mechanisms and action spectra are not well documented.(49) Some photosensitizing agents may have action spectra that reach into the visible region.

Eye. The human eye is highly transparent to light which is transmitted through the ocular media to the retina, with minimal absorption. These photons initiate a photochemical chain reaction in light-sensitive absorbers in the retina resulting in the sensation of vision.[12] The light intensity at the retina is a factor of 104 to 106 greater than that incident on the pupil, which is called optical gain.

Retinal effects occur through four interaction mechanisms: (1) thermal; (2) photochemical; (3) elastic or thermoacoustic transient pressure waves; and (4) nonlinear phenomena. The latter two mechanisms are seen primarily with lasers. The absorption of light by tissue produces heat. At sufficient intensities, the resulting rapid rise in temperature can denature proteins and inactivate enzymes. The thermal mechanism is the primary damage mechanism for 1 ms to 10 sec exposure durations.[6] Long-term (>10 to 100 sec) exposure to light levels above normal environmental levels may produce photochemical damage in the retina. The action spectrum mimics the spectral absorption of melanin through the lower end of the visible (500 to 400 nm) region down into the UV-A region. Photochemical damage can be enhanced by the thermal mechanism that predominates in the 500 to 1400 nm range, although there is no sharp cutoff point between the two.[50]

Exposure to intense light from sources such as the sun, carbon arc, or welder's arc without proper protection may produce temporary or permanent retinal scotomas (blind spots). Reports of injuries from observing solar eclipses date back as far as Hippocrates (460 to 370 B.C.), and sporadic references to this have been made throughout the centuries.[51] Factors affecting the degree of retinal hazard include the size, type, and spectral intensity of the source, the pupil size, retinal image quality, and the spectral transmittance of the ocular media, the spectral absorption of the retina and choroid, and the exposure duration. Thresholds for retinal damage have been determined for both incoherent and coherent optical radiation sources under a wide variety of exposure conditions. The threshold radiant exposure for retinal damage is 30 J/cm^2 for a 1000 sec exposure at 441 nm for retinal photochemical damage, corresponding to a retinal irradiance of 30 mW/cm^2. The damage may be cumulative over 2 or more days. At 633 nm, the threshold increases to 950 mW/cm^2, for the same exposure duration. Threshold retinal irradiances for broad-band sources as low as 0.93 $\mu W/cm^2$ have been reported for all-day exposures. Because of the lack of information on the human eye, exposure limits are based on data obtained primarily on rabbits and monkeys, which are extrapolated to the human eye.

Exposure to short-wavelength light, between 400 and 500 nm, can produce so-called blue effects to the retina. These effects are thermal in nature with brief exposure to intense levels of short-wavelength light. Relatively long-term exposure to lower levels of blue light can produce photochemical damage to the retina. Reviews of ocular effects of blue-light available.[52,53] As mentioned earlier, the action spectrum of malignant melanoma in hybrid fish extended through the UV spectral region and included some blue-light wavelengths.[31,32]

One of the controversial issues associated with visible radiation is the effect of illumination on job performance. The concept exists that the levels of illumination and source luminance routinely encountered in interior working environments may constitute some type of an ocular health hazard. Studies on humans and animals exposed to common interior lighting intensities have produced evidence to indicate the possibility of hazards, however such studies have not been considered conclusive. The four major findings developed at a NIOSH symposium on illumination were high levels of lighting may cause damage to the eye; poor lighting conditions can cause aesthenopia (eye strain); diseases such as glaucoma, cataracts, and retinal degeneration do not result from exposure to low levels of illumination; and if there is sufficient illumination to perform a task reasonably well, then there is sufficient light to meet safety criteria. While the cause of eye strain is not definitely known, it appears that repeated occurrences of eye strain probably do not lead to any permanent eye damage. Workers over 40 years of age will probably encounter more symptoms of eye strain, such as headaches, tired eyes, irritation, since they require more light to perform a similar job than younger workers.

There are several reasons why visual performance in workers over 40 years of age tends to become worse with time. There is a loss of accommodation around 40–45 years of age, making it harder to focus at short working distances. This phenomena is known as presbyopia. The pupils becomes smaller with age, known as senile myosis.

The amount of light reaching the retina is reduced due to absorption of shorter wavelengths in the lens and increased scatter of the light entering the eye. The optical density of the lens increases due mainly to effects of UV radiation on the lens. Finally the lens starts to fluoresce due to aging factors. The net result is reduced visual acuity, contrast sensitivity, color discrimination, and increased sensitivity to glare requiring longer period of time to recover from exposure to high luminance fields.

Symptoms of visual discomfort are red, sore, watery eyes, headaches, tiredness, poor posture, squinting, irritability, stress, decrease in work efficiency, or reading difficulties. Lighting conditions related to visual discomfort are shadow formation, flickering or pulsing sources, reduction in luminance contrast, and glare.

Glare may produce visual discomfort, often due to squinting in an effort to screen light. If glare is substantial or frequently induced, it may result in tiredness, irritability, possibly headache, and a decrease in work efficiency.[51]

Glare can be differentiated into veiling glare, discomfort glare, or blinding glare (flash blindness). Although all three are present in the case of high-intensity light, the effects of the first two are primarily evident only when the source is present. Blinding glare is especially significant where it produces afterimages that persist long after the light itself has vanished. Regardless of whether the glare source is specularly or diffusely reflected, it can cause discomfort or affect visual performance, or both. The visual discomfort or annoyance from glare is well understood and has been confirmed by many experiments. Certain experimental studies have found that people sometimes become more physically tense and restless under glare conditions. Although the cause is physical, the discomfort brought about by glare is often subjective. The evaluation of discomfort, then, must make use of subjective responses as criteria. Involved in such procedures is the concept of the borderline between comfort and discomfort.[54]

Flash blindness, a relatively new problem occurring only since the development of intense light sources brighter than the sun, is a temporary effect in which visual sensitivity and function is decreased severely in a very short time period. This normal visual response, whose complex mechanism is not well understood, is related to the eye's adaptive state and the size, spectral distribution, and luminance of the light source.[6]

Infrared Radiation

Skin. The damage to skin from IR exposure results from a temperature increase in the absorbing tissue. The increase depends on the wavelength, the parameters involved in heat conduction and dissipation, the intensity of the exposure, and the exposure duration. The most prominent effects of near-IR include acute skin burn, increased vasodilation of the capillary beds, and an increased pigmentation that can persist for long periods of time. With continuous exposure to high-intensity IR, the erythematous appearance due to vasodilation may become permanent.[55] Many factors mediate the ability to produce a skin burn. It is evident that the rate at which the temperature of the skin is permitted to increase is of prime importance. High levels of far-IR, often referred to as radiant heat, are encountered in glassblowing, foundries, and furnaces. This IR exposure can be a significant contributor to thermal stress.

Eye. IR produces thermal effects to the eye. The cornea is highly transparent to IR-A, has water absorption bands at 1.43 and 1.96 µm, and becomes opaque to IR above 2.5 µm.[56] Chronic corneal exposure to subthreshold doses may lead to "dry eye," characterized by conjunctivitis and decreased lacrimation.[56]

Moderate IR doses can result in constriction of the pupil (miosis), hyperemia, and the formation of aqueous flares. More severe exposures may lead to muscle paralysis, congestion with hemorrhage, thrombosis and stromal inflammation. Within a few days, necrosis of the iris may cause bleached atrophic areas to form. Pigmentation loss at the border of the iris follows in 2 to 4 days.[57]

Damage to the lens of the eye from IR has been investigated for many years. The term "glassworker's cataract" has become generic for lenticular opacities found in workers exposed to processes hot enough to be luminous.[12] The occupational groups at risk include glassblowers, foundry and forge workers, cooks, and laundry workers, as well as those who worked in sunlight.[56] Robinson reported that lens opacities on the posterior surface found in glassworkers were different in appearance from senile cataracts.[58] Dunn found no evidence of any ocular disturbance among glassworkers[57], and Keating et al. found no posterior cortical changes in iron rolling mill workers.[56] The incidence of posterior capsular opacities was higher, however, this differs from what is classified as a cataract.[59]

The mechanism for IR cataractogenesis has long been debated. Some results appear to support the hypothesis that the iris must be involved in IR- or heat-induced cataractogenesis, at least with regard to acute exposure conditions.

The retina is susceptible to near-IR since the ocular media are relatively transparent to these wavelengths. For extended exposures, the corneal irradiance required to produce a minimal retinal lesion at 1064 nm is almost three orders of magnitude greater than that at 442 nm.[56] Absorption of IR by the retinal pigment epithelium produces heat. If the heat is not dissipated rapidly and the temperature of the tissue rises about 20°C, irreversible thermal damage will result from the denaturation of protein and other macromolecules.[50] The size or area of the image on the retinal choroid apparatus and the absorbed retinal irradiance (dose rate) are two of the most critical factors in the production of thermal injury.

Recognition

Generation and Sources

Optical radiation sources generally fall into the following categories (1) sunlight; (2) arc or discharge lamps; (3) incandescent (warm-body) sources; (4) welding arcs; (5) lasers; and (6) light-emitting diodes (LEDs). Lasers are discussed later in this chapter. Some sources of optical radiation are compiled in Table 25.5.

The sun provides a large component of worker exposure to optical radiation since as much as one-third of the work force is exposed occupationally to sunlight. The exposure varies greatly with climate, geography, altitude, and work activities. The solar irradiance outside the atmosphere is about 135 mW/cm^2 while at sea level, the maximum is about 100 mW/cm^2.[7] The solar spectrum peaks at about 450 nm and drops off rapidly in the UV and more gradually in the IR region.

Table 25.5 — Common Exposures to Optical Radiation Sources

Sources	*Spectral Regions of Concern*	*Potential Exposures*
Sunlight	UV, visible, near-IR	farming, construction, landscaping, life guards, other outdoor workers
Arc lamps	UV, visible, near-IR	photoreproduction, optical laboratories, entertainment
Germicidal lamps	actinic UV	hospitals, laboratories, medical clinics, maintenance
Hg-HID lamps	UV-A, blue light	maintenance, industry, warehouses, gymnasiums
(Broken envelope)	actinic UV	
Carbon arcs	UV, blue light light activities	laboratories, search
Industrial IR sources	IR	steel mills, foundries, glass-making, drying equipment
Metal halide UV-A lamps	near-UV, visible	printing plants, maintenance, integrated circuit, manufacturing
Sunlamps	UV, blue light	tanning parlors, beauty salons, fitness parlors
Welding arcs	UV, blue light	construction, repair and maintenance, bypassers

Note: Table adapted from Reference 9.

UV and visible radiation are generated by electronic transitions in excited atomic systems. IR radiation is produced by changes in the vibrational, rotational, or translational energy states in molecules.

UV Radiation. Uses of UV radiation include curing materials, suntanning, photoluminescence, chemical manufacturing, treating skin disorders, germicidal applications, UV spectroscopy, and photomicrolithography. UV is an unwanted byproduct in processes such as welding, metal cutting, and glass manufacturing. A listing of selected occupations and associated UV exposure levels is available.[14]

The main UV source is the sun. Global UV radiation has two components: the sun's beam and sky radiation. Sky radiation is diffuse and caused by scattering in the atmosphere. Global UV-A is a stable component of global radiation.[60,61] Solar UV-B wavelengths less than about 295 nm are attenuated by stratospheric ozone, although wavelengths as low as 286 nm have been detected at the earth's surface.[62]

UV-B is sensitive to the angle of the sun, being greatest when the sun is overhead, from about 10 a.m. to 2 p.m., solar time[63], and the time of year.[64] Dosimetric studies with mannequins have shown that the greatest sunlight exposures are received by horizontal surfaces such as the tops of the feet, shoulders and ears, back of the neck, and the area around the nose, cheekbones, and lower lip.[65–67] Although the environmental UV irradiance is often sufficient to produce skin and eye effects for relatively brief exposure times, ocular effects generally do not develop because of shielding of the eye by the orbit, eyebrows, and eyelashes, and squinting.[68,69]

A number of outdoor occupations and activities have been evaluated for UV exposure. These include fishermen[70], construction workers[70], farmers and gardeners[71–73], landscape workers[70], physical education teachers[71], outdoor sports athletes[74,75], lifeguards[71], and airline pilots.[76]

Of the man-made sources, welding and various lamps are the major sources of occupational exposure. Some of the more hazardous welding processes include argon-shielded gas-metal arc welding (GMAW) with aluminum or ferrous alloys and helium-shielded gas tungsten arc welding (GTAW) with ferrous alloys.[6] Parameters important in determining the UV irradiance include the arc current, shielding gas, electrode wire material, base metal, and joint geometry. Weld geometry and the degree to which the arc is buried in the weld also influence UV levels.[14] Laser welding and some surface applications with carbon dioxide lasers may generate potentially hazardous actinic UV levels because of the interaction of the energetic far-infrared laser beam with metallic materials.

Lamps that may emit relatively high levels of UV include metal halide, high-pressure xenon, mercury vapor, and other high-intensity discharge lamps.[6,77–79] The spectral output of mercury vapor lamps varies with the gas pressure. Low pressure lamps emit line spectra characteristic of mercury (mostly 253.7 nm) and are used primarily for germicidal applications. Overexposure[80] and potential overexposures to users have been reported.[81,82] Medium to high-pressure lamps are used for curing and area lighting, such as in gymnasiums and parking lots. These lamps produce a bluish light and may be hazardous if viewed at close distances. Mercury lamps used for area lighting have two envelopes. The inner envelope is quartz (transparent to UV), while the outer envelope is made of materials that are largely opaque to UV. The output may produce hazardous exposures some distance from the lamp if the outer envelope is broken and the lamp continues to operate, which can occur in lamps that are not self-extinguishing. UV curing processes irradiate UV-curable materials and monomeric photosensitizers with 300 to 400 nm (predominantly 365 nm) UV to produce a hard, durable film.

UV-A, -B, and -C have been found from fluorescent lamps used in open fixtures, but UV-B and UV-C were not found when an acrylic diffuser was used with the fixture. The highest UV-B and UV-C irradiances were associated with high-output (HO) and super high-output (SHO) lamps.[83]

Medical uses include phototherapy, photochemotherapy, and disinfection and sterilization. The spectral output from some lamps used in photomedicine has been reported[84,85], and some exposures may be in excess of exposure limits.[86] Phototherapy workers have a greater risk of dying from skin cancer than medical workers who do not work with UV, but their risk is much less than medical workers who use ionizing radiation.[87]

Dentists may use UV and blue-light-curable materials. Generally, handheld applicators that are properly designed, maintained, and used will minimize exposure to the dentist. However, improper use or excessive leaks[88] may result in mouth burns to the patient.

Visible Radiation. The sun is the major source, along with various lamps, projection systems, welding arcs, and lasers (see Table 25.5). The luminance of the noonday sun is 1.6×10^5 cd/cm^2[6], while the time necessary for blue-light injury is about 90 seconds.[72] Solar blue-light exposures on the flight deck of a commercial aircraft were higher than those experienced by the general population, but within exposure guidelines.[89]

Luminance from welding arcs can be hundreds to ten thousands of candelas per centimeter square. Blue light from various types of welding ranges from 0.16 to 135 W/cm^2-sr.[6]

Xenon short-arc lamps emit relatively high levels of blue light, while low-pressure fluorescent lamps emit relatively low levels. Luminance levels for xenon short-arc lamps were around 10^4 to 10^5 cd/cm^2.[6] Evaluation of a headband-mounted xenon arc lamp used during surgery found a broadband spectrum between 400 and 680 nm. An adjustable lens system allows for variable collimation. At highest collimation, the spectral irradiance exceeded the exposure limit for retinal hazard at a distance of more than 2 m. At minimum collimation, the exposure limit was exceeded out to 0.5 m.[90]

For potential blue-light exposures to photoflood lamps used in TV studios and theaters, acceptable exposure duration varied from 1 min to 3 hr at distances between 2.25 and 10 m. Calculated values of luminance were between 30 and 1900 cd/cm^2.[91] Quartz linear lamps used for space heating are reported to emit negligible levels below 600 nm, when fitted with a ruby sleeve.[92]

Workers from NIOSH evaluated luminance levels from thermal arc spraying[93], laboratory furnaces[94] aluminum reduction potrooms[95], and glass furnaces[96] finding maximum levels of 16.7, 1.9, 0.3, and 0.93 cd/cm^2, respectively.

Light-emitting diodes (LEDs) are solid-state sources that emit noncoherent light. Exposure to LEDs, which are increasingly being used for illumination, photocuring, and other applications, has not been extensively evaluated. Effective blue-light radiances of 0.367 W/cm^2-sr for a blue LED and 0.0208 W/cm^2-sr for a green LED has been reported.[97]

Illumination. In the work environment lighting is necessary to provide for visibility of work tasks and objects and to insure safe working conditions. Illumination is the amount or quantity of light falling on a surface. The three general categories of lighting uses are ambient, task, and accent. The first two uses are of prime importance in the work environment. Finally, the use of appropriate illumination principles and designs, as well as maintenance of that equipment, affects our health, morale, comfort, and productivity.

Some key characteristics of light sources are efficiency, color rendering index and color temperature. Efficiency refers to the ability of converting energy into visible light. Color rendering index is a relative scale that rates how perceived colors of objects illuminated by a given source matches the color produced by the same object when illuminated by a reference standard light source. Finally, color temperature refers to the color of a blackbody radiator at a given temperature.

The four major types of lighting sources currently used in the workplace are incandescent, fluorescent, high-intensity discharge (HID), and low-pressure sodium. In the future, illumination sources such as photoluminescent markings, light emitting diodes, and light emitting polymers may be used in certain applications.

Incandescent light is produced by passing a current through a thin filament causing it to become hot and glow. There are three major categories of incandescent lamps: standard, reflector, and tungsten-halogen. Standard and reflector lamps are inexpensive, energy inefficient, and exhibit relatively short working lifetimes. Tungsten-halogen lamps contain gas in the glass envelope which extends the life of the filament, making the lamp last longer.

Fluorescent lamps are the most commonly used source because they operate longer, are efficient, and produce diffuse light. These operate by passing a discharge current through mercury vapor. The mercury atoms emit UVR which is absorbed by a phosphor coating on the interior of the glass envelope. The phosphor molecules are stimulated to emit light. They are available as tubes or compact modes and require ballasts for starting and circuit protection.

Disposal of ballasts/tubes must be conducted in accordance with applicable state/federal regulations since ballasts may contain polychlorinated biphenyls (PCBs) and tubes may contain small amounts of mercury.

HID lamps also produce an arc between two electrodes but the arc is shorter generating more light, heat, and pressure. The HID lamps have long life, high luminous flux per watt, and are small devices. Two limitations are warm-up time and the "restrike" period after the lamp is switched off. The different types of HID sources in order of increasing efficiency are mercury vapor, metal halide, and high pressure sodium.

High-pressure mercury vapor lamps are discharge lamps that may be used for illumination of large spaces such as gymnasiums and warehouses. Low pressure sodium lamps are the most efficacious light sources, but produce poor light quality. One disadvantage is that these lamps can explode if the sodium comes in contact with water.

The amount of illumination required for a task varies according to difficulty of the visual task and is a function of object size, contrast, luminance, and the viewing time. Small, low contrast objects that are viewed with low luminance levels in a short time are harder to see than large, high contrast objects viewed at high luminance for longer time periods. In the industrial environment size, viewing time, and contrast level, may not be easy to change-whereas the luminance can be easier to change. Unfortunately issues such as glare, veiling reflections, shadows, and color have an impact on vision requirements.

The perception of color may be difficult when nonwhite lighting is used. For example, white and yellow objects may appear the same color when illuminated by red or yellow light, while blue surfaces may appear to be black. Masking of colors can be a safety issue that requires the use of warning signs/labels that have alternate colors.

Poorly designed luminaries or poorly utilized illumination can result in difficulty in task viewing, wasted energy and light pollution (upward and outward distribution of light).

In recent years office illumination has been modified to accommodate the influence of video display terminals and the need to reduce glare from computer screens. One approach used to minimize screen glare is to locate overhead light sources on either side and slightly behind the computer. This approach can be difficult to accomplish because of room layout and number of employees working with computers in a given room. Reducing source luminance is another technique but often the ambient light levels become greatly reduced potentially creating other concerns. Other suggestions are to enhance task light by using different light sources close to the work area, controlling light levels by use of dimmers, and to purchase screens having anti-reflection coatings.

Infrared Radiation. Most of the sources discussed under visible radiation also emit IR radiation. Also, a number of IR lasers and optical wireless communications systems use IR light-emitting diodes (LEDs).[98,99]

In the NIOSH studies cited earlier, sources of IR radiation were thermal arc spraying (170 mW/cm^2)[93], laboratory furnaces (130 mW/cm^2)[94], aluminum reduction potrooms (190 mW/cm^2)[95], and glass furnaces (173 mW/cm^2).[96] Evaluation of potential exposures to glass factor ovens operating between 1130 and 1370 °C exceeded the exposure limits.[100] Peak IR-A irradiance values in the Swedish iron and steel industry were 140 mW/cm^2 while hotrolling ingots and 130 mW/cm^2 in an electrosteel plant.[101]

Quartz linear lamps with ruby sleeves were reported to pose no hazard for normal use, but the evaluators recommended that they should be switched off for maintenance tasks at distances closer than 1 m.[92] An evaluation of IR illuminators used with closed-circuit television (CCTV) surveillance systems found a value of irradiance of 10 mW/cm^2 at 5 m, with increasing levels as one approached the device. Hence, there is a potential hazard for individuals involved with installing and maintaining these systems.[102] Spot welding produced IR (800 to 1800 nm) levels between 3 and 2500 mW/cm^2.[103]

Evaluation

Exposure Guidelines

Both exposure and emission standards are employed to protect people from hazardous optical radiation. Exposure standards are used to limit the amount of optical radiation to which a worker or the general public can be exposed, regardless of the source. Emission standards apply only to specific optical radiation sources, such as high-intensity mercury vapor lamps or the laser. Such standards and guidelines are available from a number of sources, and examples of each are highlighted here. This overview is not a compendium of available standards; the reader is encouraged to seek out further sources of such information.

Ultraviolet Radiation. The American Conference of Governmental Industrial Hygienists (ACGIH®)[104], the National Institute for Occupational Safety and Health (NIOSH)[105], and the International Commission on Nonionizing Radiation Protection (ICNIRP)[106] recommend occupational exposure limits for UV radiation.

These are wavelength-dependent values of radiant exposure where the limiting value (3 mJ/cm^2) is reached at 270 nm, the most biologically-effective wavelength for corneal effects.[68] The TLVs® apply to UVR in the spectral band from 180 to 400 nm and to exposure of eye and skin to solar radiation and all artificial UVR sources except lasers. These TLVs® should not be used for photosensitive individuals or to persons concomitantly exposed to systemic or topical photosensitizing agents, or ocular exposure of aphakes. They are applicable for exposure durations from 0.1 sec to the whole working day.

These exposure guidelines are based primarily on studies of acute exposures in humans and animals including keratoconjunctivitis, erythema, and cataracts. However, the guidelines may have some limited applicability with regards to certain chronic effects.[107]

Light and Near-Infrared Radiation. ACGIH® has recommended criteria for source luminance (1 cd/cm^2), retinal thermal injury from visible light, retinal photochemical injury from blue light, retinal thermal injury from IR-A, and corneal and lenticular injury from IR-A and -B radiation.[69,104]

The TLV® for retinal injury from light depends upon the measured value of spectral radiance, the viewing duration, the angular subtense, and a weighting factor called the retinal thermal hazard function [R(λ)]. The angular subtense, α, is the mean of longest dimension (l) and shortest dimension (w) of the source (e.g., a lamp) divided by the distance to the source (r) or $\alpha = (l+w)/2r$, for small viewing angles. The spectral region for R(λ)is 380 to 1400 nm.

The blue light TLV® depends upon source (image) size and exposure (viewing) duration. For extended objects (relatively large images), the TLV® is in terms of integrated radiance for exposure durations of ten thousand seconds or less, and radiance for longer exposures. For sources where the viewing angle is small, the TLVs® are in terms of radiant exposure for exposures less than 100 seconds and irradiance for longer exposures. The blue-light hazard function [B(λ)] applies to the band between 305 and 700 nm, but the most biologically effective region is centered around 435–440 nm.

The TLV® for the IR-A and -B regions (770 to 3000 nm) protects against thermal injury to the cornea and lens (cataracts) by limiting exposure to 10 mW/cm^2 for durations of 1000 sec or more. For shorter exposure durations, the TLV® is time dependent. To protect the retina, IR sources such as heat lamps or those lacking a strong visual stimulus (defined as luminance < 0.01 cd/cm^2) require a more rigorous analysis to ensure that IR-A radiance does not exceed $0.6/\alpha$. The TLV® for the near-IR retinal thermal hazard, in terms of radiance, is dependent upon the angular subtense. This TLV® is relaxed by a factor of $t^{-0.25}$ for exposure times (t) shorter than 810 seconds.

Workers who have had their lens(es) removed (aphakes) in cataract surgery have an increased risk of retinal photochemical injury. Wavelengths in the 300 to 400 nm range can be transmitted to the retina if these workers do not have a UV-absorbing intraocular lens implant(s). The blue-light TLV® is modified in the 305 to 440 nm region using an appropriate aphakic hazard function.

Illumination. Current information about appropriate light levels are available from the Illuminating Engineering Society of North America (IESNA). The IESNA has established a generalized procedure to aid in selecting the necessary illuminance based on knowledge of space, task, and occupant characteristics. In the IESNA Handbook[108] there are seven illuminance selection criteria which are divided into three visual task groups called orientation and simple, common, and special. The illuminance for each group range from 30 to 100, 300 to 1000, and 3000 to 10,000 lux, respectively. In addition, IESNA recommends that 16 design issues be taken into consideration to achieve a high quality visual environment.

There is also some guidance about workplace lighting levels found in various sections of the OSHA regulations. Many of these state that lighting shall be adequate and provided, but do not define what is the appropriate level. However, in regulations dealing with hazardous waste site operations, labor camps [29 CFR 1910.142(g)], man lifts, and construction illumination levels are given that range from 50 to 350 lux.

Emission (Product) Standards

The U.S. Food and Drug Administration (FDA) has product standards for sources of optical radiation including high-intensity mercury vapor discharge lamps, sunlamps, and lasers. (See the section on laser safety for a discussion of the standard on products containing lasers.)

The standard on high intensity mercury vapor discharge lamps (21 CFR Part 1040.30) applies to mercury vapor and metal halide lamps. It requires lamp manufacturers to provide a label to inform the user if the lamp will self-extinguish when the outer glass envelope is broken. The sunlamp standard (21 CFR Part 1040.20) requires manufacturers to affix a warning (danger) label on each product, provide the consumer with instructions for using the sunlamp, incorporate a timer and a manual control to terminate the exposure, and include protective eyewear with each sunlamp.

Instruments

These include broadband radiometers and spectroradiometers. Broadband radiometers integrate spectral irradiance over a wide range of wavelengths (see Figure 25.3). Spectroradiometers determine spectral irradiance in successive narrow wavelength bands, and these may be weighted by a hazard action spectrum.

In general, radiometers (see Figure 25.3) are used to measure radiant power and have calibrated output in irradiance. Typically, these instruments also have an integration function that allows radiant exposure to be measured over time. The output of some radiometers used to measure actinic UV is in effective irradiance (E_{eff}) in W/cm^2, which is the irradiance of a broadband source weighted against the peak of the spectral effectiveness curve, 270 nm.

The optical sampling system may include input optics, band filters or monochromators, detectors, and the electronics package. Useful UV detectors for continuous-wave (CW) sources include photoelectric detectors (photodiodes and photomultiplier tubes) and thermal detectors (thermopiles and pyroelectric detectors). Ideally, detectors for broadband instruments should display a wavelength-independent (flat) response within the spectral region of interest with a rapid decrease outside of this

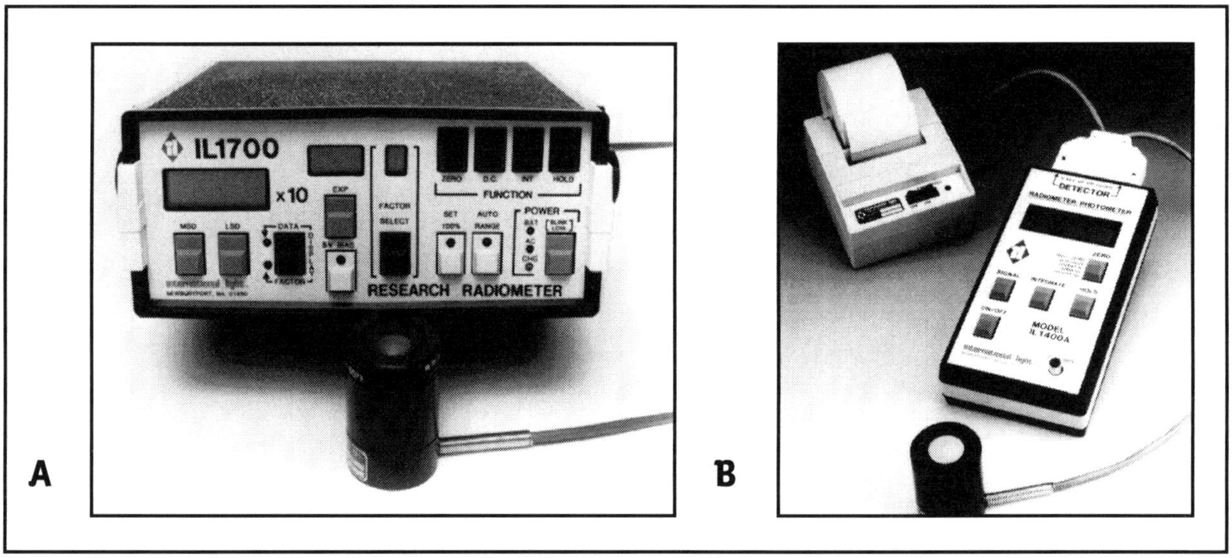

Figure 25.3 — Broadband radiometers. (a) A portable research radiometer with an optical sampling system; typically, the sampling probe incorporates three elements: diffuser, filter, and detector. (b) A handheld radiometer and optical sampling probe is shown with a small printer. (Courtesy of International Light, Inc.).

band. Some detectors have been noted to deviate from linearity at high UV levels.[109]

Filters[110,111] include bandpass, cutoff, and special filters, and attenuation filters such as neutral density. A special (weighting) filter used with portable radiometers provides spectral weighting so that transmission closely matches the exposure criteria. Some detectors may respond to visible or IR radiation, or both, and require a filter to absorb these wavelengths.

Input optics include diffusers and integrating spheres. Diffusers provide uniform illumination of the detector, make the detector-source alignment less critical, and provide a cosine response at the detector. Integrating spheres, which have been used for solar measurements, involve a hollow cavity to collect optical radiation for detection.

Monochromators are components of spectroradiometers used to measure a narrow spectral region without the use of filters. The monochromator includes an inlet slit, diffraction grating/prism, alignment linkage, internal mirrors, and an exit slit is connected to the detection system. The bandwidth or bandpass of a monochromator is the width of the transmitted spectral distribution. Bandwidth depends on the slit width and grating. Generally, smaller slit openings produce smaller bandwidth, up to the limiting bandwidth or instrument resolution.

Lighting surveys utilize meters that measure illuminance and/or luminance (see Figure 25.4). A radiometer that has been properly filtered to match the spectral sensitivity function of the fovea (denoted the CIE photopic standard observer) is called a photometer. The meter can be designed to read out in units of lux or foot-candles. Detectors used with the photometer must be cosine and color corrected, respond to the CIE photopic standard observer, and be calibrated.

There are a number of sources of error in radiometry,[114–117] the most common being susceptibility to stray source and ambient light. Ambient lighting and broad-band source emissions may exceed the spectral irradiance one is attempting to measure. Unless the instrument can reject this light, considerable error may be associated with the measurement data.[14]

A number of different UV dosimeters have been developed, with polysulphone being most common. Other types include plastics, phosphors, glasses, ceramics, films and electronic.[14,116–118]

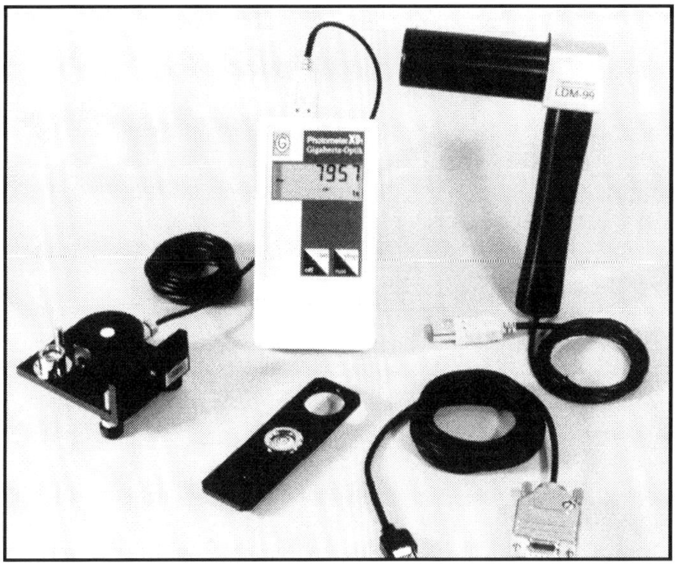

Figure 25.4 — An illuminance/luminance meter with detector used for lighting surveys. (Courtesy Gigahertz-Optik, Inc.)

Exposure Assessment

Optical Radiation. Prior to measurement, the evaluator should determine source characteristics (e.g., spectral distribution of a lamp or current of a welding arc), operator-source interaction, and the location of the source relative to reflective objects such as aluminum surfaces. Make sure that the instrument is calibrated and the spectral distribution of the source is within the calibrated response spectrum of the instrument. Allow the instrument to warm up, if required, zero the output indication, then check for zero-point drift. Broadband optical radiation exists in the work environment and may interfere with measurement. This must be taken into consideration by zeroing or filtering incident optical radiation. The evaluator should pay attention to personal safety and take any personal protective equipment that may be necessary.

When measuring, the effective irradiance, radiant exposure, radiance, or integrated radiance is read directly as the output or is calculated from the output data (see Figure 25.5). For example, the potential exposure to IR has been estimated by combining limited measurement data with calculations using the characteristics of the black body spectrum.[100]

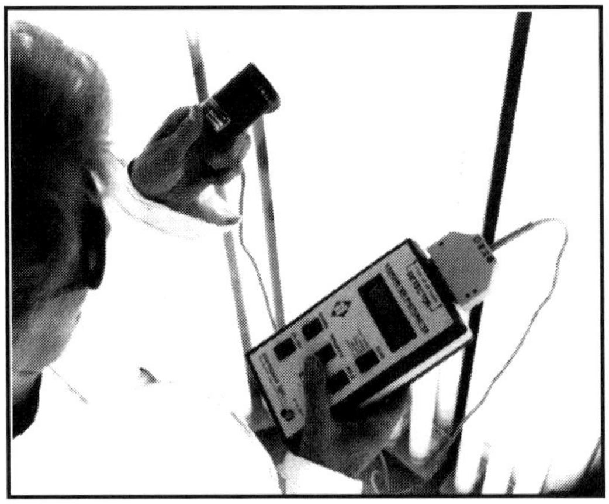

Figure 25.5 — Use of a handheld radiometer. The optical sampling probe is directed toward the source, and the irradiance (or radian exposure) is read from the display. (Courtesy International Light, Inc.).

Another example is the determination of the effective UV irradiance must be calculated for instruments that have their output in spectral irradiance (E_λ), which is a wavelength-dependent quantity, as:

$$E_{eff} = \Sigma\, E_\lambda S_\lambda D_\lambda \qquad (25\text{-}2)$$

Here, E_λ is the measured spectral irradiance in a narrow bandwidth, S_λ is the relative spectral effectiveness at a given wavelength within that band, and D_λ is the actual bandwidth in nanometers. S_λ is read from a tabular compilation of the latest booklet of TLVs® for UV radiation, and the bandwidth is a function of the instrument. This process is similar for other weighted quantities such as those using blue-light hazard or retinal burn hazard functions.

For welding arcs, the effective UV irradiance at a given distance can be estimated prior to measurement if the arc current is known. It has been found that values of measured effective irradiance do not exceed:

$$E_{eff} = ((4 \times 10^{-4}\ \text{watts/ampere}^2) \times I^2)/r^2 \qquad (25\text{-}3)$$

where I is the arc current in amperes and r is distance from the source in centimeters. This equation may be used to estimate the upper limit of the effective irradiance for arc currents from 10–20 A to greater than 700 A.[6]

For broad-band measurement data in the UV-B and UV-C, the allowable exposure duration (t) may be calculated as the quotient of the radiant exposure at 270 nm (30 J/m^2 = 3 mJ/cm^2 = 0.003 J/cm^2) and the measured value of effective irradiance, as:

$$t(s) = \frac{30\ \text{J/m}^2}{E_{eff}\ (\text{W/m}^2)} \qquad (25\text{-}4)$$

If the effective irradiance (E_{eff}) at a specific wavelength or bandwidth is known, the allowable exposure duration may be determined by using the wavelength-specific values of radiant exposure (e.g., H = 6 mJ/cm^2 at 254 nm) and irradiance, where t = H/E. (Equation 25-4 should be applied with caution if the measured quantity is not relatively constant.)

At times, collecting data at a large number of locations or distances from the source may not be practical. Here, the inverse square law may be used to estimate the radial increase or decrease of intensity of optical radiation that is an uncollimated, extended sources as:

$$E_1 = E_2 r_2^2 / r_1^2 \qquad (25\text{-}5)$$

Use of the inverse square law may provide a conservative estimate for levels of actinic UV that are readily absorbed by certain molecular species including atmospheric molecules and water vapor.[113] However, the absorption by air molecules at wavelengths greater than 200 nm is insignificant for distances of up to several hundred yards.[113] Conversely, an underestimation of the irradiance may occur if the source geometry produces a high gain, that is, if the optical power is contained in a smaller cross-sectional area or the radiation is collimated.[119]

Lighting Surveys. Lighting surveys should be performed with the workers at their work stations. All lighting sources and conditions should be those normally used and encountered, and lamps must be allowed to warm up properly. First, perform a visual inspection, noting the qualitative characteristics of the lighting environment.

The detector should be positioned at a uniform, level position as measured from the floor. Measurements may be made using a standardized grid with grid separation distances of approximately 0.5 to 1 meter. In making measurements care must be taken to eliminate any reflected light or shadows from the detector's field of view. It will be necessary to make more measurements in a space where the illumination is highly nonuniform than in a uniformly illuminated space. There are a number of lighting software programs to aid in evaluating results obtained from surveys.

Control Measures

Control measures for optical radiation must address both skin and eye. Successful engineering controls include isolation or enclosure of the process and safety subsystems such as interlocks, shutters, and alarms. Personal protection includes clothing, sunscreens and sun blocks, and the use of protective eyewear.

Engineering Controls

Barriers or enclosures may be made from a variety of efficient attenuating materials including metals, plastics, and glasses. Transmission curves of various filter materials and UV inhibitors are available.(110) Some useful UV filter materials are polyester films, cellulose acetate, and acrylics such as methyl methacrylate based polymers.(39,110,120)

Most common materials transmit little UV, although this is a function of wavelength, material thickness, and angle of incidence. Window glass (2.4 mm thick) transmits almost no UV below 300 nm; around 330 nm the transmission increases to about 50%. Data indicate that little radiation at 308 nm is reflected from the surface of glass at angles of incidence less than 60. For angles greater than this, the degree of reflection increases exponentially.(121)

Commercially available welding curtains may be made of materials that are either opaque or transparent to visible wavelengths. Opaque materials include canvas duck, asbestos substitutes, and polymer laminates. Transparent welding curtains may allow visual contact with welders, reduce arc glare, and increase general illumination levels.(122) Generally, curtains should attenuate UV and blue light to minimize potential hazards while transmitting near the peak of visual sensitivity, around 550 nm. In testing 25 transparent, colored welding curtains, NIOSH found that wavelengths less than 340 nm were highly attenuated.(122)

Many plastics, glasses, and some dyes may degrade with long-term exposure to UV radiation. Solarization, resulting from photochemical reactions, is a decrease in UV transmissivity in quartz and glass and may lead to a perceptible color change in the glass.

Doors or access panels to barriers or enclosures that contain UV radiation in excess of the applicable exposure limit should be interlocked. Interlocks can be connected to power supplies or shutter mechanisms and, in some cases, may also be connected to the exhaust ventilation systems for welding effluent or ozone.

Some lamp enclosures may be interlocked, such as self-extinguishing mercury vapor lamps. These lamps stop operating within 15 min of breakage of the outer of the two envelopes. The FDA requires that self-extinguishing mercury vapor lamps be marked with the letter "T." If the lamp is not self-extinguishing, the FDA requires that such lamps be marked with the letter "R."

Visual or audible alarms, or both, should be used where workers may access a noninterlocked enclosure that contains hazardous levels of UV. This is especially important if the source does not emit visible radiation that may indicate potential exposure.

With regards to illumination, it is important to understand that where the light goes or is directed is more important than the object that produces the light. Fixtures can distribute light upward, downward, or in many directions, with either diffuse or concentrated distribution. Downward lighting tends to emphasize floors and/or surfaces/objects whereas upward lighting emphasizes the ceiling and upper walls. Upward lighting can be used to produce diffuse components by the use of ceiling reflectors and can be a solution for minimizing computer screen glare. Fixtures which produce multidirectional distribution of light is considered to produce uniform illumination.

When considering lighting controls, it is important to appreciate the surfaces and objects that are to be illuminated. In principle lighting comes down to a simple concept of having sufficient brightness to comfortably visualize the object in the field of view without causing glare problems. However, there are situations where illumination levels need to be altered.

Skin Protection

Sun Blocks and Sunscreens. In the past decade, the availability of, and emphasis on the need for, sunblocks and sunscreens that are applied to the skin to reduce cutaneous UV exposure from solar radiation have increased considerably. A sunblock reduces exposure by reflecting and scattering the incident radiation. Zinc oxide and titanium dioxide are very effective sunblocks, reflecting up to 99% of the radiation both in the UV and visible regions, possibly into the IR region also. Although very effective, the sunblocks are messy and some people think they present an unacceptable appearance.

Sunscreens, on the other hand, absorb UV usually over a limited wavelength range in the UV-B and UV-A regions, and are considered to be drugs by the FDA.(123) The agents include para- aminobenzoic acid (PABA) and its esters, benzophenones, salicylates, cinnamates, and anthranilates. Usually in a gel or cream, the preparations have good substantivity, allowing them to bind with the stratum corneum and resist removal by perspiration during heavy activity or by water when swimming. All provide protection in the UV-B range; only the benzophenones and anthranilates provide limited protection in the UV-A region. PABA preparations can discolor clothing and can cause contact-type, eczematous dermatitis. The body's natural photoprotector, melanin, absorbs strongly in the UV-A.(124)

Sunscreens are designed to protect against UV-induced erythema and sunburn, although their efficacy in reducing the risk of cancer(125,126) and immunologic effects(127) has been questioned. The sun protection factor is the measure of effectiveness of these agents; SPF equals the ratio of the UV-B dose required to produce erythema with protection to that required without protection. Although many commercial products claim very high SPFs, protection above an SPF of 15 has not been documented.(128) To achieve a product's SPF rating, it is important to apply the proper amount of sunscreen to the skin, a fact often overlooked in use. It has also been reported that sunscreens provide less protection in the outdoor environment than suggested by label values. This was attributed to the changing ratio of UV-B to UV-A with changes in the angle of the sun throughout the day.(129)

Quick-tanning preparations containing b-carotene or carthoxanthine produce a "tan" by coloring the skin but offer no protection against UV.(49) Hawk et al. tested 55 commercial products available in the United Kingdom in 300 human volunteers.(130) Sunscreens provided good protection against UV-B but only a few products were effective in the UV-A region, mostly at the short wavelengths. Sunblocks reflected the radiation throughout the UV region far into the visible range (up to 650 nm).

Since their effectiveness in preventing melanoma has not been established, other protective measures such as hats and protective clothing, and avoidance of exposure during peak hours (10 a.m.–2 p.m. sun time) should be used.(131)

Clothing. Factors affecting UV protection of fabrics include weave, color, stretch, weight, quality, and water content.(132,133) Evaluation of transmission in one study showed that UV leaks through openings in the mesh structure of woven fabrics. Fabrics made of continuous films exhibited good attenuation. Transmission of materials ranged from 1% for a FR-8 treated breezetone to 0.0003% for a number of fabrics shown in Table 25.6.

Table 25.6 — Selected Fabrics with 0.003% Transmission of Actinic UV

Welder's leather
FR-7A® treated sateen
FR-8® treated twill
FR-8® treated denim
1006 aluminized rayon
1019 aluminized rayon
Kevlar® blend - 22 oz
11501-1 unaluminized Perox®
1000-1 aluminized Perox®
Cotton interlock knit coated with nitrile rubber latex
Leather-stained sheepskin, lightweight
Leather-chrome tanned side-split cowhide

Note: Adapted from Reference 135.

Generally, laundering of fabrics increased the attenuation(132) while wetting clothing decreased attenuation. The best protection is afforded by tightly woven, dark, unstretched, dry clothing.(14)

Australian researchers have tested the UV transmission between 280 and 400 nm of more than 2000 samples of fabrics and materials. From this research, they derived UV protection factors (see Table 25.7).(132) The UV protection factor (UPF) is defined as the ratio of the effective UV dose for unprotected skin to the effective dose for protected skin. The range of UPF values for cotton and polyester-cotton fabrics was broad, while all samples of Lycra™ exceed a UPF value of 40.[132] Analogous to the UPF, clothing protection factor (CPF) is used in the United Kingdom.

In general, thicker stockings provide greater protection than thinner stockings[134], and stretching reduces protection.[135] Most polymer gloves used for chemical protection will provide some UV protection. The degree of UV reduction can be ascertained by field measurement of the incident and transmitted UV.

Eye Protection

Hats. Hats with wide brims (> 7.5 cm) that encircle the head afford protection to the face, ears and neck. Baseball-type hats protect the forehead, nose and eyes.[136]

Optical Density. Optical density (OD or D_1) is the quantity used to specify the ability of protective eyewear to attenuate optical radiation, where:

$$D_1 = \log_{10} (ML/EL) \tag{25-6}$$

Here, D_1 is the level of attenuation necessary to reduce the measured (or calculated) level (ML) to the exposure limit (EL). For optical radiation, ML and EL will usually be in terms of irradiance or radiant exposure, but both numerator and denominator must be in the same terms. OD values are shown in Table 25.8.

Field tests of eyewear can be made to determine D_λ. This requires measuring the level at the position of the worker's eye, with and without the eyewear covering the detector. If the measured quantity were irradiance at the eye, D_λ would be determined from

$$D_\lambda = \log_{10} (E_o/E) \tag{25-7}$$

Here, E_o is the measured effective irradiance without eyewear, and E is the measured irradiance with the eyewear in place.

Recommended levels of attenuation can be found in the technical literature. For example, Parrish et al.[137] state that UV-A-opaque eyewear for environmental use (solar UV) should transmit no more than 0.1% (D_λ = 3) to the central part of the pupil.

Table 25.7 — UV Protection Factors (UPF) for Clothing

UPF	*Absorption (%)*
10	90
20	95
30	96.7
40	97.5
50	98
100	99
200	99.5

Source: Adapted from Reference 134.

The quantity used to specify the optical transmission characteristics of protective eyewear for welders is the shade number. Shade number (S#) is related to optical density by:

$$S\# = (7/3)D_\lambda + 1 \tag{25-8}$$

where a shade number of 10 equates to an D_λ of 3.857. It should be noted that D_λ in Equation 25-8 reflects broadband attenuation of optical radiation, and is not specific to a particular spectral region. Welding filters may have a single shade number with constant attenuation or be auto-darkening, where the filter rapidly switches from a low (light) shade number to a high (dark) shade number when an arc is struck. Generally, the UV attenuation of commercially available filter shades is effective[6,138], although UV entering from the rear of welding helmets may produce unacceptable exposures.[139,140]

Commercially available sunglasses are worn by outdoor workers for glare control, comfort, and fashion. Sunglasses can very in the amount of UV protection they provide. In general, sunglasses with polycarbonate lenses will attenuate UV-B well and UV-A well up to wavelengths around 360 to 380 nm, with increasing transmission beyond. Sunglasses

Table 25.8 — Optical Density (OD)

OD Value	*Attenuation*
1	10
2	100
3	1000
4	10,000
5	100,000
6	1,000,000
7	10,000,000
8	100,000,000

utilize absorptive coatings to attenuate these long UV wavelengths. Typically, tinted UV protective eyewear, not cosmetic sunglasses, are recommended for workers with outdoor jobs.

Absorbing Material. Materials commonly used in the construction of protective eyewear are glass, polycarbonate, and CR-39 plastic. Glass and polycarbonate absorb actinic UV well, while glass, polycarbonate and CR-39 may not provide sufficient attenuation in the near UV at wavelengths above about 350 nm. Hence, always ensure that the spectral transmission of the protective eyewear is compatible with the spectral distribution and intensity of the source. This information should be available from equipment and eyewear manufacturers, and some information is published in periodicals.[141,142]

Some sources of optical radiation may produce broadband emissions requiring filtration in more than one spectral region. Under these conditions, protective eyewear must be capable of attenuating all potentially hazardous wavelengths to acceptable levels. This usually requires the use of a suitable base material plus coatings or lens additives. For example, some arc lamps may be rich in actinic UV and blue light. Polycarbonate could be used to absorb the actinic UV, while amber or yellow pigments could be added to absorb the blue light. The use of pigments may reduce the luminous transmittance of the eyewear, however, which is troublesome in some environments. Didymium or cobalt blue lenses and gold or copper coated faceshields are used in the glassblowing industry to absorb UV and IR radiation.[143]

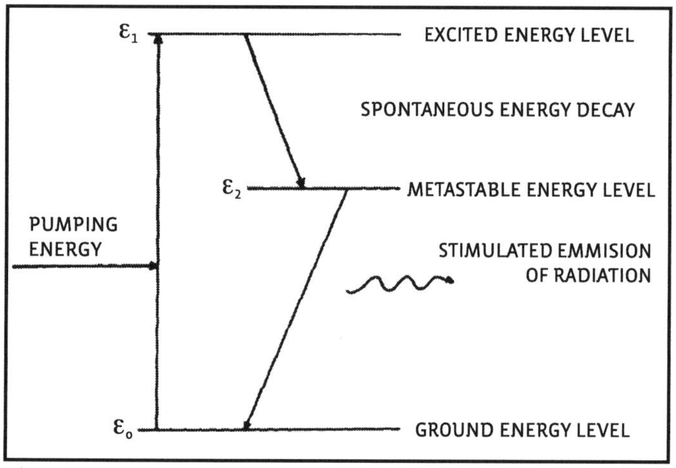

Figure 25.6 — Schematic of Laser Operations.

Other Factors. In addition to transmission data, the comfort, frame design, and fit are important factors. Leakage around frames may pose functional and measurement problems, because UV leakage as high as 25% has been found for poorly fitting eyewear.[137]

Laser Radiation

Anticipation

The term LASER is an acronym for Light Amplification by Stimulated Emission of Radiation. This is a process whereby some type of active medium results in emission of coherent, monochroatic light. Active laser mediums may be in the form of gasses, solid state materials such as glass, dydes dissolved in a solvent And semiconductor materials. When some form of excitation mechanism or energy source is applied, such as radiofrequency radiation, light, electric current, or chemical reaction, some of the orbital electrons of the active medium inside the vessel become excited and move to a higher energy state. At some point the lasing medium absorbs so much energy and so many electrons are in the excited state that a population inversion occurs. This means that some of the high energy electrons decay back down to the lower energy state through a stimulated emission of a visible or invisible photon. The wavelength, frequency, and energy of this photon will depend upon the types of gases used in the active medium, the power level and the pulse duration. A diagram representing the processes of stimulated emission or radiation is shown on Figure 25.6.

This three level energy diagram represents one of the many possible sets of energy level transitions that can result in laser action. An absorbed photon (pumping energy) results first in an electron in an excited state at e_1. However, the emitted laser photon energy corresponds to e_2 -e_0 since e_2 is the longer-lived (metastable) level.

Once the population inversion is achieved, the spontaneous decay of a few electrons from the energy level to a lower energy level starts a chain reaction via a feedback mechanism. The photons emitted spontaneously hit other atoms without being absorbed and stimulate their electrons to make the transition from the metastable energy level to the lower energy levels, emitting photons with precisely the same wavelength, phase and direction.

When this reaction is produced in an optical cavity with high reflectance mirrors on each end, the chain reaction continues and the number of photons emitted tends to continue to increase. When one of the mirrors is only partially reflective then a laser beam will be emitted. This beam then passes through an output coupler which focuses and aligns the beam as it emerges from the laser. A basic diagram of a laser optical cavity is shown on Figure 25.7.

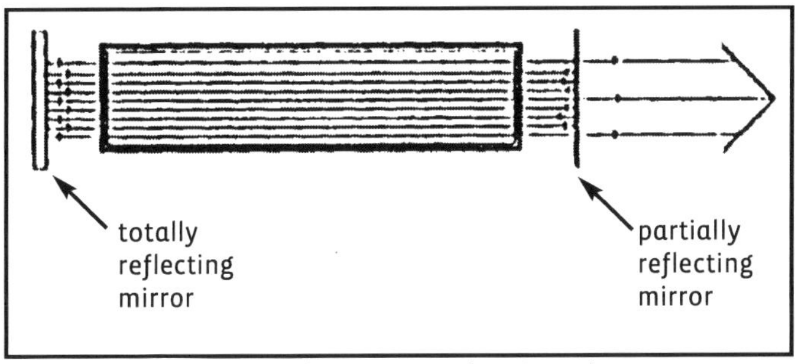

Figure 25.7 — Diagram of Laser Optical Cavity.

Laser Characteristics

The emerging laser beam takes on some special properties because of the way it is produced. Besides being very powerful, the beam is also monochromatic, directional, and coherent. By monochromatic we mean that the light emitted tends to be one color. In actuality it is one wavelength specific to the active medium and the stimulated emission photon, so it may actually be invisible, and not really a visible color. This phenomenon is special in that the light is not white, or polychromatic as would be emitted from an incandescent bulb or other broadband conventional light sources.

It is common for laser radiation to be generated and used at a fundamental frequency (wavelength). However, harmonics of the fundamental frequency may be generated by various methods, for example by the use of crystalline materials such as potassium titanyl phosphate (KTP) or lithium triborate (LBO). Harmonic generation may allow a laser with an Near-IR beam to produce a visible beam (second harmonic) or an UV-A beam (third harmonic). The conversion efficiency to the harmonic must be determined, since it may be necessary to provide safety controls for both the fundamental and harmonic frequencies, in some applications.

A useful feature of some lasers is tunability, where the wavelength can be adjusted within a given spectral region. The first type of tunable laser was the dye laser. The lasing medium is a powder dissolved in an organic solvent, which is then pumped into the optical cavity. Other methods for creating variable wavelenghts is through the uses of nonlinear optical components such as an optical parameter oscilator (OPO).

Another special characteristic of the laser beam is that it is highly directional. As the beam is emitted from the output coupler it is moving in one direction and it tends to stay in this mode as it moves through most mediums with very little divergence, or spread, of the emitted beam.

The last attribute of the laser is that the beam is coherent. This means that the photon waves tend to be in phase in space and time. This is one reason that so much energy and power can be condensed into one powerful beam.

As can be seen by the electromagnetic spectrum shown in Figure 25.8, the visible range of possible laser emissions is somewhat narrow when compared with other possibilities in the infrared and ultraviolet ranges of laser emission wavelengths. It should be noted that the visible spectrum for lasers, as defined by the ANSI standard, differs slightly from the visible spectrum under the optical radiation portion of this chapter. Laser emissions can be extremely hazardous even if they cannot be seen. Lasers that are not visible to the naked eye can be even more dangerous than those in the visible ranges.

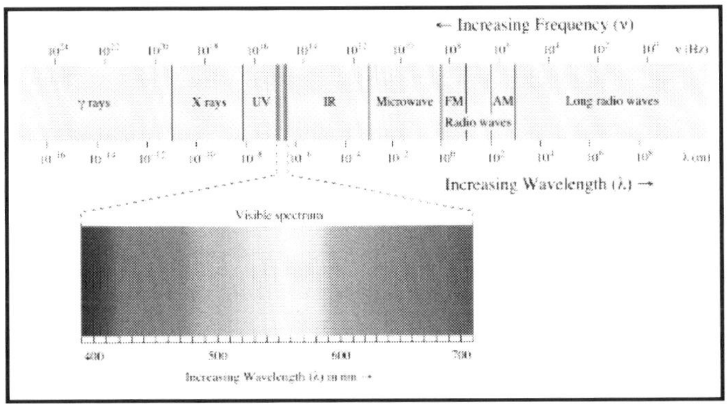

Figure 25.8 — The Electromagnetic Spectrum.

Types of Lasers

Temporal Characteristics

There are two general types of lasers. One is the type of laser that generates a continuous wave of light which is emitted as a steady beam. This type of laser has a peak power equal to the average power output and the beam irradiance is constant with time. CW lasers emit a "temporally constant power of laser light." The second type of laser is the pulsed laser. The pulsed laser has a mode of operation which consists of the emission of either a single pulse or a series of laser pulses with pulse periods ranging from a few picoseconds to seconds. Pulsed lasers may be normal pulse, Q-switched, or mode-locked.

For a frame of reference, consider that the innate human aversion response time to bright light, including visible laser light, is approximately 0.25 sec. Note that the aversion response does not occur with exposure to invisible radiation such as UV and IR. With this in mind, if a laser emits radiation for a time greater than or equal to 0.25 sec, it is defined as a CW laser. It follows that pulses are noncontinuous emissions in which the duration of each pulse is shorter than 0.25 sec.

Pulse widths, however, may be much shorter than the aversion response time. These are realized with Q-switched or mode-locked pulses. Q-switching produces pulses on the order of a few nanosecond to microseconds, while mode-locked pulses are even shorter, in the picosecond domain. Special pulsing techniques, such as cavity dumping, can produce pulses on the order of femtoseconds.

In some applications, such as information management with bar-code scanners, the laser beam may be scanned. In scanning, the output is spatially distributed (often in some form of a linear pattern) in a manner that makes it physically impossible for the entire output to enter the eye. This reduces the retinal irradiance compared to a raw (unscanned) beam.

For each type of laser the hazards are different depending upon the exposure duration, the wavelength, the output power, and the pulse duration and frequency. The wavelength is an important consideration because this is the property affecting the lasers ability to penetrate materials and it determines which part of the eye it is most likely to be affected. The wavelength will also determine if the beam is visible or invisible to the naked human eye. Protective eyewear or barriers need to specifically address the wavelength or wavelengths of interest. For example, a protective goggle that provides adequate protection for a helium neon (HeNe) laser with a wavelength of 632 nm may not (and most likely would not) be effective for a Nd:YAG laser with a wavelength of 1,064 nm.

For continuous lasers the average power and exposure duration are the primary factors in determining the laser hazard level. To effectively evaluate pulsed laser safety the following items must also be considered; Total Energy per Pulse, Peak Power, Pulse Duration, Pulse Repetition Frequency, and Radiant Exposure.

Direct Beam vs. Reflection

Ocular hazards can be the result of three different types of exposures, these are direct, diffuse, and specular as shown on Figure 25.9. Direct exposures are those in which the beam hits the eye directly. Most intrabeam exposures will be to a small beam or point source of light, called small source viewing. Most laser beams fall into this category. The direct beam may also be an extended source-one that can be resolved into a geometrical image by the eye.[8] Exposure to laser array can be even more complex with indivual emitters being a point source but the entire array being an extended source.

Reflections of laser light may also be hazardous. Reflections may be specular or diffuse, or a combination of the two. Specular reflection, which may be regarded as a type of direct viewing, occurs when the beam is incident on a mirror-like surface. Specular reflection is a wavelength-dependent phenomenon as it occurs when the size of the surface irregularities of the reflecting surface are smaller than the incident wavelength.

In practice, most slightly rough, non-glossy surfaces act as diffusing surfaces to incident laser beams. A diffusing surface acts as a plane of very small scattering sites that reflect the beam in a radially symmetric manner. The roughness of the surface is such that the surface irregularities are larger than the laser wavelength, which randomly scatters the incident beam. The reflected radiant intensity (I) depends on the incident intensity (I_0) and the cosine of the viewing angle (q) where:

$$I(r,\theta) = I_0 \cos \theta c \qquad (25\text{-}9)$$

This relationship is known as Lambert's Cosine Law and a surface behaving in this manner is referred to as a Lambertian surface. This relationship defines an ideal plane diffuse reflector.

It should be stressed that "rough" surfaces do not always act as diffuse reflectors at all wavelengths. For example, brushed aluminum, which is partially diffuse for visible wavelengths, is a good specular reflector for far infrared wavelengths, such as those emitted by a CO_2 laser.

Also, beam reflections from so-called semi-specular reflectors may include both a specular and a diffuse component. In this case, the reflection has features of a diffuse reflection, but in a preferred direction. Examples of semi-specular surfaces include epoxy paint over plywood, aluminum painted plywood, and ice.[144]

Diffuse exposures are the result of the initial beam being reflected by some surface that is rough and tends to scatter the incident beam in several directions resulting in a general reduction in the power intensity of the beam in any one direction. Diffuse reflections may also include the reflection of a laser beam as it traverses through an area of smoke or steam.

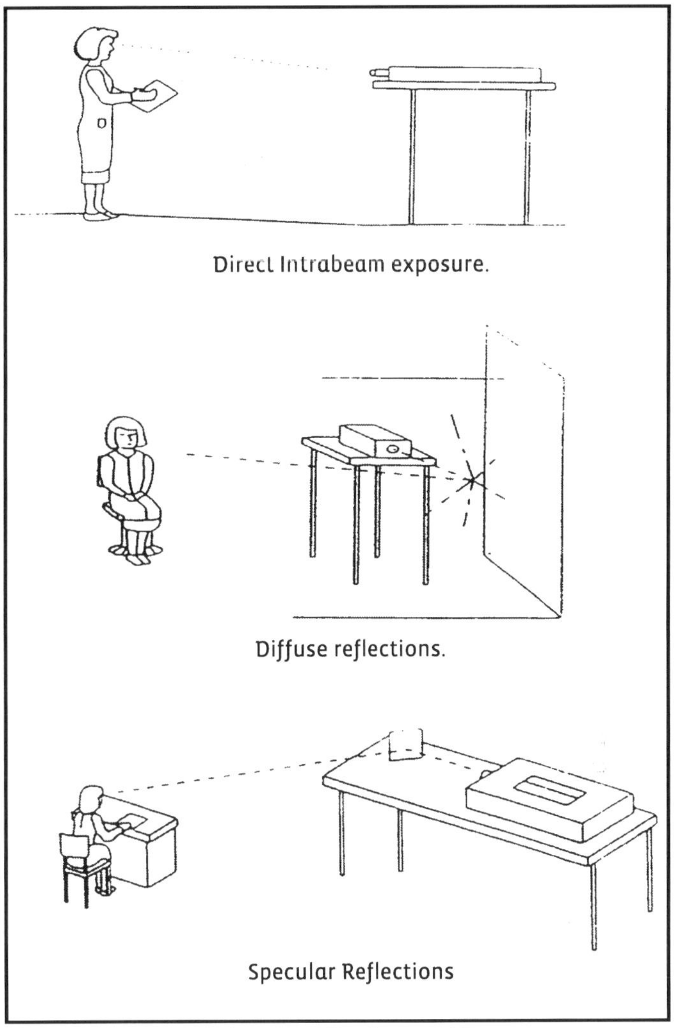

Figure 25.9 — Types of Laser Reflections and Exposures.

Quantities and Units

Laser radiation is described by irradiance and radiant exposure. The unit of irradiance usually applied to exposure considerations is the watt per centimeter square (W/cm^2); the joule per centimeter square (J/cm^2) is used for radiant exposure. By convention, irradiance is usually applied to exposures to CW lasers, and radiant exposure is used for exposure to pulsed laser beams.

The spectral character of laser radiation is described by the wavelength whose unit is the micrometer (μm).

Biological and Health Effects

The target organs for laser radiation are the skin and eyes. Generally, due to the larger surface area of the skin, it may be at greater risk of exposure than the eye. However, the eye is more vulnerable to laser radiation.

Scientific understanding of the hazards of laser radiation to these target organs is derived primarily from studies of laboratory animals. These studies, and studies of broadband optical radiation, have shown that exposure to laser radiation or radiation at laser wavelengths produces threshold effects, with the exception of some stochastic effects associated with UV radiation.

Laser-induced biological effects depend primarily on wavelength, irradiance, and exposure duration. The penetration depth into the skin and eyes is wavelength dependent. In general, actinic UV wavelengths, mid-IR and far-IR are absorbed topically, primarily by the epidermis or cornea, whereas visible and near-IR wavelengths are transmitted through the ocular media to the retina. Near-IR wavelengths also penetrate relatively deeply into the skin.

Interactions with Matter and Damage Mechanisms. Damage mechanisms may be photomechanical, thermal, or photochemical. Photomechanical effects, sometimes called photoacoustic effects, occur when brief pulses are incident on tissues. Such pulses may be generated by Q-switched or mode-locked lasers. Since P = Q/t, where t is pulse duration, which is generally less than 100 ns for Q-switched lasers, exposure produces very high peak irradiance for even modest values of pulse energy. Such exposure has been shown to produce a plasma at the site of absorption within the eye. The plasma expands rapidly, often in the form of shock waves or sonic transients, disrupting tissues as it propagates. After a short distance, the pressure waves may terminate in cavitation, as the vapor bubble collapses.[145] Photomechanical effects (also called photoacoustic effects) can destroy tissues directly and may cause hemorrhaging, with blood collecting in the vitreous. A number of accidents involving photomechanical effects to the eye have occurred, and a relatively large number of these involve neodymium:YAG (Nd:YAG) lasers.

Thermal effects affect the eye or skin, and occur in exposure times from microseconds to seconds, although microsecond pulses may produce both photomechanical and thermal effects. Thermal effects involve absorption of radiant energy by a chromophore (absorbing structure) such as melanin or hemoglobin. Absorption increases the random molecular motion and, hence, the total energy of the tissues. This is manifest in the tissues as heat, which produces damage by denaturing protein and inactivating enzymes. For threshold retinal thermal lesions, the damage is greatest at the center of the lesion, and diminishes toward the border of the lesion. All types of laser radiation can produce thermal effects, although it may not be the predominate mechanism for tissue effects for lasers emitting UV radiation.

Photochemical effects to the eye and skin primarily involve UV radiation, while retinal effects also involve visible light up to 550 nm (blue and green laser light). Photochemical damage is attributed to the photoproducts of light-induced chemical reactions or changes. An example is the UV-activated dimerization of adjacent pyrimidine molecules in a deoxyribonucleic acid (DNA) molecule, which may interfere with DNA synthesis and replication. Cellular studies with a type of UV laser, the excimer laser, determined that a wavelength of 248 nm (KrF laser) was most effective in damaging DNA, producing mutagenic and cytotoxic effects. The relative effectiveness of DNA damage decreased at 308 nm (XeCl laser), and again at 193 nm (ArF laser).[146]

Studies with test animals have established that photochemical effects occur from relatively lengthy (>10s of seconds) exposure of the eye (retina) to blue and green laser radiation.[147–149] Photochemical threshold lesions of the retina exhibit relatively uniform damage across the lesion, in contrast to thermal lesions, as discussed earlier. Photochemical effects to the skin from exposure to blue and green laser radiation have not been reported.

Eye. The major ocular structures at risk are the cornea, iris, lens, retina, and optic nerve (see Figure 25.10). The target tissue is determined by not only the exposure location but the penetration depth, which is wavelength dependent. For example, overexposure to UV laser radiation can cause photokeratitis of corneal tissues and cataracts, while exposure to visible wavelengths and near-infrared wavelengths can result in retinal lesions. Laser affects on tissue are dependent on the power density of the incident beam, the tissues ability to absorb the laser wavelength, the amount of time the beam is incident on any one spot, and the effects of circulation and conduction.

Harmful Effects of Laser Exposure

The laser radiation wavelength determines where the beam will interact with the eye anatomy. The anatomy of the eye affected by laser light incident on the eye depends upon the wavelength. For example, Far Ultraviolet and Mid and Far Infrared wavelengths each tend to be absorbed by the initial layers of the eye, either in the cornea or aqueous. Visible light and near ultraviolet and near infrared wavelengths, on the other hand, pass through the cornea and lens to directly impact with the retina.

Another phenomena associated with laser light is that the eye tends to condense the already intense light as it focuses it onto the retina. Incandescent light from an extended light source tends to be somewhat more diffuse as it hits the back of the eye and the retina.

Eye damage occurs where the incident light is absorbed (see Figure 25.11). For ultraviolet light in the wavelength ranges from 315 to 400 nm the prevalent effects are cataracts and presbyopia (farsightedness). The cataracts are a photochmical injury and do not rely on any thermal effect. For accidental exposure to UV light in the range from 100 to 315 nm the significant effects are keratoconjunctivitis and milky cornea. The cornea is also the primary inury sight for mid and far-IR wavelengths. The IR injuries are thermal in nature and their severity depends upon the depth to which the cornea is burned. Burns to the epithileal layer of the cornea may be repaired by the body but deeper burns may be permanent.

In the retinal hazard zone from 400 to 1,400 nm eye injury can be in the form of retinal damage with the negative impact on vision or on the fovea with an impact on acuity. Some of the visible affects of damaging laser light on the retina are seen by broken blood vessels in the retina and blood floating in the aqueous. For CW lasers and pulses of longer pulsewidths the effects tends to be thermal in nature. For short pulse widths, such as from Q-switched and mode locked lasers, the results is a photoacoustic injury where the high peak power causes the retina to explode and separate from the back of the eye. Retinal lesions typically result in a scatoma, or blind spot, within the field of vision. The prominance of the scatoma is related to its size and location. Lesions in the peripheral vision typically result in a less severe effect and in fact may not even be noticable. Lesions located within the central vision area, such as the macula or fovea, can result in significant loss of vision. Lesions which effect the optic disc can result in the loss of large areas of vision relative to the physical size of the lesion.

Wavelengths in the 400 to 550 nm (blue/green) region are also capable of causing photochemical injury in the form of photoretinitis. These injuries occur from longer duration exposures and have a delayed appearance similart to sunburn.

Skin exposures to laser light may lead to either acute or chronic skin injury. Acute injury is probably the easiest type to understand. The effects are either thermal, leading to localized burns or photochemical contributing to erythema which is localized skin reddening, much the same as sunburn. Both of these types of over exposures can be extremely painful and hazardous. Chronic skin injuries can result from prolonged skin exposure over long periods of time at exposure levels that are too low to induce an acute response. Chronic exposures can lead to increased incidence of photochemical responses that lead to early aging, or in the case of ultraviolet light exposures, can cause skin cancer. When working with UV

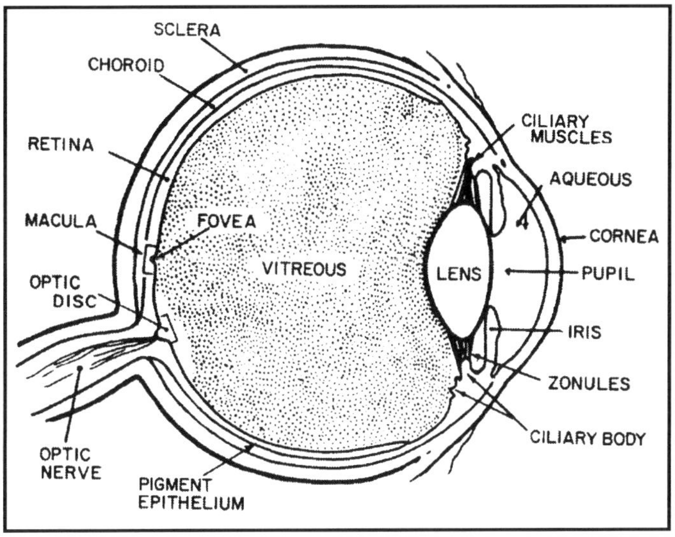

Figure 25.10 — The general structure of the eye showing the principal structures.

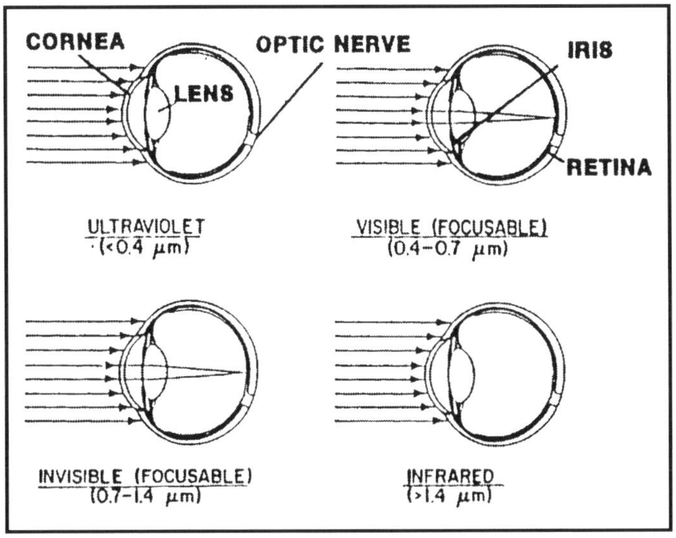

Figure 25.11 — Absorption and Transmission of Laser Light by Components of the Ocular System.

lasers it is important to review the diffuse light hazard to the skin and consider the cumulative effects of exposure over repetetive exposure periods.

Other Safety Concerns

Other safety considerations that may go into the assessment and evaluation of laser hazards include the following items; electrical hazards, skin exposure hazards, chemical, associated gas hazards and laser generated airborne contaminants. Some other special considerations include whether the laser is enclosed in an engineered system of protection, if the beam is invisible, if maintenance repair and modifications will be necessary on a routine basis, and whether there is a potential for explosion, fire, or hazardous fumes.[150]

Ancillary, or non-beam hazards assiciated with lasers include electrical hazards, shock and electrocution, are primary hazards of laser systems. Of all the ancillary hazards mentioned here, the electrical are the most significant with most deaths attributed to laser systems being electrical fatalities. General guidelines to prevent electrical shock include; not wearing metal jewelry when working with lasers, using only one hand to work on circuits, assuming that all floors are conductive when working with high voltage, checking that capacitors are discharged, shorted and grounded before allowing access to the capacitor area, periodically checking containers for deformities and leaks, using rubber gloves and insulating floor mats when available, not working alone, and having easy access to main power shutoff. As most optical workbenches are metal it is important to have appropriate grounding and bonding in place. It is also good practice to have at least a few personnel in the work area trained and certified in cardiopulmonary resuscitation (CPR), in the event that this form of first aid is needed.

Gas lasers may pose hazards from both toxic and pressure hazards. For instance, excimer lasers utilize halogen gases such as krypton chloride or hyrdogen fluoride. Additionally, a cylinder of compressed gas may become an unguided missile by rapid decompression if mishandled.

Dye lasers utilize organic dyes dissolved in a solvent. The dyes themselves tend to have hazardous properties, such as being carcinogens and/or mutagens. All of the dyes are powerful coloring agents so contact with even the innocuous dyes should be avoided.

Solvents used in dye lasers are extremely flammable. Ignition may occur via high voltage pulses or flash lamps. Direct beams and unforeseen specular reflections of high-powered lasers are capable of igniting flammable materials. Other fire hazards are associated with electrical components and beam enclosures.

Other hazards which may be associated with the operation of high power laser systems include cryogenic coolant hazards or excessive noise from high powered systems.

Airborne contaminants[151] may be generated when a powerful laser beam interacts with matter. Studies have examined this issue for metals[152–154], concrete[152], plastics[155–159], composites[160,161], glasses[162,163], wood[164], and tissues.[165–172] Airborne contaminants may also occur from the normal operation of gas lasers[173–175], whereas the skin, respiratory system, and other organs or systems may be targeted during preparation or use of dye lasers that involve handling of organic dyes and solvents.[176–178]

Plasma radiation occurs at the site of interaction of an energetic laser beam with a metal. A few studies of plasma radiation have demonstrated that the interaction of a focused beam from a CO_2 laser with various metals produces potentially hazardous levels of actinic UV and blue light near the site of interaction.[179,180] X-rays may be generated when high-energy, rapidly pulsed laser beams interact with plasmas in laboratory experiments using lasers.[181–183] X-rays may also be generated from high voltage power supplies and transformers associated with laser systems. Collateral radiation may also include radio-frequency radiation[184], and power-frequency fields.[185]

Accidents. Relative to the tremendous growth in laser applications and uses, relatively few accidents have occurred, even considering that accidents are probably highly underreported.[186,187] Lasers cited in specific accident reports include ruby[188–192], Nd:YAG[188,193–200], doubled-YAG[192], CO_2[201], argon[188,193–196,202], krypton[193], dye lasers[188,193,194,203], HeCd[188], and HeNe.[204] Relatively few eye injuries have been reported from diode lasers in laser pointers, and these occurred when individuals overcame the aversion response and stared into the beam for many seconds at close range.[205,206]

Accidents have included exposure to the direct beam, reflected beam,and a number of nonbeam accidents/incidents including fires, and electrocution and shock. Accident and incident reports may be grouped into research and development, education, medical, industrial, military, and entertainment.

Reviewing the records of reported laser incidents reveals the following: (1) Q-switched Nd:YAG lasers have been involved in a large number of the reported ocular accidents; (2) most skin injuries and fires are associated with CO_2 lasers; (3) the only deaths attributed to laser systems were from electrocution and embolism (following medical procedures); (4) performing beam alignment is a relatively high-risk task; and (5) a relatively high number of ocular accidents have occurred when eyewear was available but not worn.

Evaluation

The output power is directly related to the hazard classification of the laser in that it provides an indication of the radiant energy and radiant power that may be transferred from the laser to the eye. To a lesser extent the Irradiance (radiant energy incident on the point element of a surface), and Radiant Exposure (time integral of the irradiance) are also useful in determining laser hazards.

Depending on the combination of the factors mentioned here, a Laser is classified according to its potential hazard. Hazard classifications have undergone some changes in the past few years. The current classifications now include Class I, Class 1M, Class 2, Class 2M, Class 3R, Class 3B, and Class 4. or IIIb, and Class IV.

Laser Characteristics and Capabilities to Injure Personnel

The assigned laser classification is the primary means of determining its capability of causing personnel injury. Manufacturers are required to provide a laser classification for commercial lasers and laser systems manufactured after August, 1976. In addition to the laser classification, engineering, administrative, and personnel protective devices to minimize hazards should be evaluated and identified by the LSO. Hazard evaluations require availability of all pertinent data from the manufacture to include a minimum of the following information:

1. Power or energy output,
2. Beam diameter,
3. Beam divergence,
4. Pulse duration,
5. Pulse frequency- repetition rate,
6. Wavelength,
7. Beam profile, and
8. Maximum anticipated exposure duration.

Laser Classification

In accordance with the IEC 60825-1 Second Edition, laser hazard classifications have been developed in order to standardize evaluations and associated safety controls. Table 25.9 summarizes the hazard capabilities and the laser class.

Table 25.9 — Laser Classifications

Class	Hazard Capabilities
Class 1	Laser products that are safe during use, including long-term direct intrabeam viewing,even when exposure occurs while using optical viewing instruments (eye loupes or binoculars). Class 1 also includes high powered lasers that are fully enclosed so that no potentially hazardous radiation is accessible during use.
Class 1M	Laser products that are safe for long-term direct intrabeam viewing for the naked eye (unaided). Eye injury may occur for these products if optical viewing instruments are used within 100 mm for diverging beams and certain collimated beams.
Class 2	Laser products that emit visible radiation in the wavelength range from 400 nm to 700 nm that are safe for momentary exposures but can be hazardous for deliberate staring into the beam.
Class 2M	Laser products that emit visible laser beams and are safe for short time exposure only for the

naked (unaided eye). Eye injury may occur following exposure with optical viewing instruments for diverging beams within 100 mm from the source, or for certain collimated beams.

Class 3R — Laser products that emit radiation that can exceed maximum permissible exposures under direct intrabeam viewing, but the risk is low because of the required exposure durations.

Class 3B — Laser products that are normally hazardous when intrabeam ocular exposure occurs within the Nominal Ocular Hazard Distance (NOHD) including accidental short duration exposures. Specular reflections of Class 3B laser beams may be hazardous, although diffuse reflections are normally considered safe. Class 3B lasers may produce minor skin injuries or even pose a risk of igniting flammable materials.

Class 4 — Laser products for which intrabeam viewing and skin exposure is hazardous and for which the viewing of diffuse reflections may be hazardous. These lasers also often represent a fire hazard.

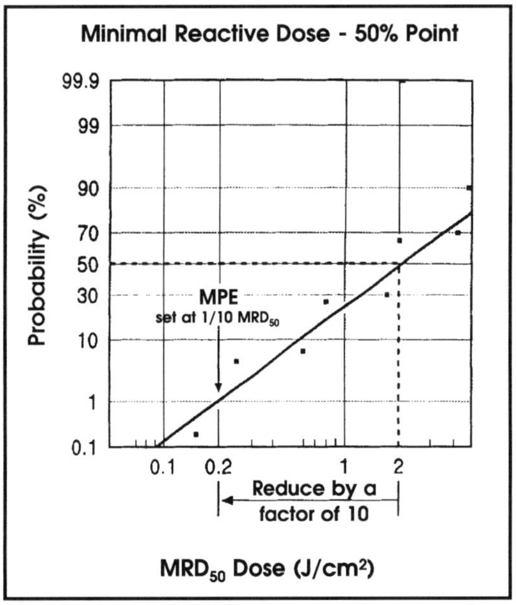

Figure 25.12 — Typical regression plot converting MRD_{50} data into MPE data. Note that the MPE is set a factor of 10 below the 50% probability point for ocular damage.

Certified laser manufacturers are required to label their products as to the Class type as of September 19, 1985 (10 CFR Part 1040).

Exposure Guidelines. Guidelines used in the United States have been published by ANSI(207), ACGIH®(104), ICNIRP(208,209), and IEC.(210) In addition to these general guidelines, there are also guidelines for specific environments including health care(211,212), optical fiber communications(213,214), education(215), and outdoor use.(216)

The guidelines include exposure limits for the eye and the skin. In general, the limits for the eye are more conservative. The limits are wavelength dependent over a range between 180 nm and 1 mm.

The exposure limit in ANSI Z136.1 is called the maximum permissible exposure (MPE). It should be emphasized that viewing a beam at MPE levels would be annoying and/or uncomfortable. It would not be hazardous, however, because MPEs are below known hazard levels. For the most part, MPEs were established in studies using animals, although there are limited data from exposure of human volunteers. In the assessment, the animal data were often displayed using a regression line on a probability graph, as shown in Figure 25.12. The data as collected are expressed in terms of probability. MPEs are based on the MRD_{50}, or laser dose level at which effects are seen in one-half of the exposures, with a tenfold safety factor.

The determination of the MPE for a specific laser should be performed using the methods outlined in ANSI Z136.1.

In addition to the Federal Laser Product Performance Standard, the Federal Aviation Administration (FAA) has published procedures for using laser in outdoor environmets (FAA Advisory Circular AC-70-1 *Outdoor Laser Operations*). In federal workplace safety standards, the Occupational Safety and Health Administration (OSHA) has addressed the use of lasers in the construction industry standard. This includes the general use of lasers (29 CFR 1926.54) and eye and face protection (29 CFR 1926.102). The relevant section of the general industry standard for personal protective equipment would also apply (29 CFR 1910) for protective eyewear. Other applicable OSHA standards have been reviewed.(217) Also, OSHA has made a number of written interpretations concerning lasers and the construction industry standard available from OSHA's homepage (http://www.osha.gov).

Some states have requirements for lasers and some states and municipalities have requirements for laser pointers.[218] In general, comprehensive regulations require that lasers must be registered with the state agency, so they should be inventoried and tracked to ensure compliance. State agencies may also request information concerning the Laser Safety Officer (LSO), and require a minimum level of competence for them. The ANSI standard provides guidance on training of LSOs.[207]

Exposure Assessment

In contrast to the classical occupational hygiene approach where the agent under investigation is measured, field measurement of laser radiation is usually not recommended because of the complexity of making meaningful measurements. For example, measurement requires alignment between the laser beam and a small aperture that covers the detector (e.g., a 7-mm aperture is used when measuring laser radiation within the retinal hazard region). As mentioned earlier, alignment is a process that involves an increased risk of accidental contact with the beam.

Instead of measurement, hazard evaluation uses numerical methods to analyze potential laser hazards. ANSI Z136.1 provides guidance on hazard evaluation, including a number of solved problems in Appendix B of the standard.[194] Also, a number of useful reviews of laser hazard analytical techniques are available.[219–230]

As a first step in this process, the evaluator should perform a survey so the numerical analysis can be meaningfully related to the workplace. This should include an assessment of possible nonbeam hazards, as well as an appraisal of beam hazards. At this time, some of the operational parameters required for the numerical analysis (see Table 25.10) may be obtained or reviewed. Sources of this information include labels on the laser product, specifications in operations and service manuals, and the manufacturer.

The next step in the hazard evaluation is determining the exposure limit (MPE), which depends on wavelength and exposure duration. There may be some cases where exposure to the beam below the exposure limit may also cause a significant hazard due to visual interference for instance if a laser beam is propogated through navigable airspace. The exposure limit is then used to determine the nominal hazard zone (NHZ), the fundamental tool of laser hazard evaluation where there is access to an open beam. Conceptually, the NHZ is the zone around the laser where the beam intensity exceeds the exposure limit, as demonstrated in Figure 25.13. As a laser beam propagates in space, it spreads out due to divergence, and it may undergo atmospheric attenuation if used outdoors. As the beam diverges, the irradiance decreases until, ultimately, it is reduced to a value equal to the exposure limit. Since this occurs at the boundary of the NHZ, persons outside the NHZ boundary are exposed below the exposure limit and considered to be in a "safe" location.

Table 25.10 — Important Laser Operational Parameters

- Wavelength
- Exposure duration
- Optical power
- Beam divergence
- Exit beam diameter
- Pulsed laser
  - Energy per pulse
  - Pulse repetition frequency
  - Pulse width
  - Average power
- Laser with lens
  - Focal length
  - Size of beam incident on lens
- Fiber optic output
  - Mode of fiber
  - Numerical aperture of fiber (multimode fiber)
  - Mode field diameter (single mode fiber)

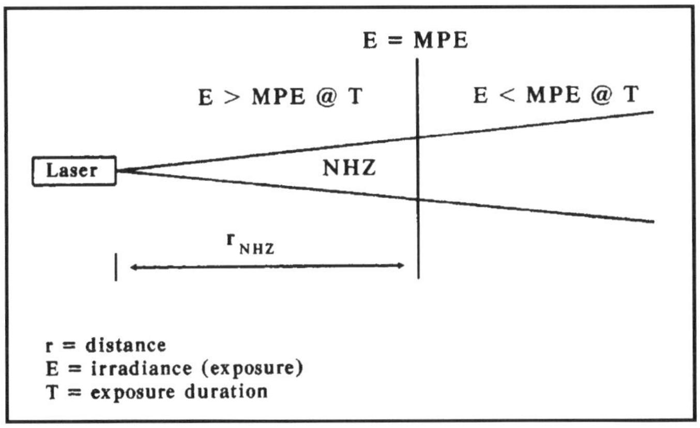

Figure 25.13 — The NHZ indicates the area or volume in space where there is the potential for overexposure.

Table 25.11 — NHZ Equations

$r = \frac{1}{\phi}\left[\left(\frac{4\Phi}{\pi\,MPE} - a^2\right)\right]^{1/2}$	Viewing the direct beam (intrabeam)
$r = \left(\frac{f_o}{b_o}\right)\left(\frac{4\Phi}{\pi\,MPE}\right)^{1/2}$	Lens on laser
$r = \left(\frac{1.7}{NA}\right)\left(\frac{F}{\pi\,MPE}\right)^{1/2}$	Multimode optical fiber
$r = \left(\frac{\omega_o}{\lambda}\right)\left(\frac{\Phi\pi}{2MPE}\right)^{1/2}$	Single mode optical fiber
$r = \left(\frac{\rho\Phi\cos\theta}{\pi\,MPE}\right)^{1/2}$	Diffuse reflection

Notes: The ANSI Z136.1 exposure limit is the maximum permissible exposure (MPE). NHZs may be determined for the eyes or skin, because exposure limits exist for both target tissues. The NHZ for the eyes is called the nominal ocular hazard distance.

Nominal Hazard Zones. The purpose of an NHZ evaluation is to define that region where control measures are required.[231] Also, knowledge of the NHZ is useful in pre-installation planning meetings and laser safety training sessions. ANSI Z136.1 requires that the LSO determine the NHZ for Class 3b and 4 lasers with limited open-beam paths and open-beam paths.[207]

Table 25.12 — NHZs for Select Lasers

		NHZ (m)		
Laser Type	*Exposure Duration*	*Direct Beam*	*Lens-on-Laser*	*Diffuse Reflection*
Argon[A]	0.25 sec	1000	—	0.5
	8 hr	2100	—	1.0
Nd:YAG[B]	10 sec	2680	134	1.3
	8 hr	7280	364	3.6
CO_2[C]	10 sec & 8 hr	564	5.6	0.6

[A]λ = 488 nm, CW, Φ = 20 W, a = 1 mm, ϕ = 1 mrad, θ = 0°, ρ = 100%, MPE (0.25 sec) = 0.0025 W/cm², MPE (8 hr) = 5.8 × 10-4 W/cm²

[B]λ = 1064 nm, pulsed, Φ = 5 W, Q = 50 mJ, a = 1 mm, ϕ = 1 mrad, θ = 0°, ρ = 100%, F = 100 Hz, t = 30 nsec (Q-switched), b_o = 5 mm, f_o = 25 cm, MPE (10 sec) = 8.89 × 10^{-5} W/cm², MPE (8 hr) = 1.2 × 10^{-5} W/cm²

[C]λ = 10.6 µm, CW, Φ = 1 kW, a = 20 mm, ϕ = 2 mrad, b_o = 2.54 cm, f_o = 12.7 cm, θ = 0°, ρ = 100%, MPE (10 sec & 8 hr) = 0.1 W/cm²

Four NHZ models have been suggested in ANSI Z136.1: intrabeam, lens-on-laser, fiber optics, and diffuse reflection.[207] These are compiled in Table 25.11. When these equations are used, it is important that the units are consistent, since this is a common source of error. In this regard, note that beam divergence is usually given in terms of milliradians, but all calculations must be performed in radians.

For a laser with constant output characteristics, the largest (worst-case) NHZ will occur for intrabeam (small-source) viewing (see Figure 25.14). In this case, the irradiance is limited only by beam divergence, unless used outdoors at distances greater than 300 m[6], where atmospheric absorption may become significant. In general, the intrabeam NHZ may extend to relatively large distances.

Most occupational uses of lasers incorporate a lens as the final component in the beam path. Typically, a converging lens focuses the beam with the effect of increasing the irradiance, which reaches a maximum in the focal plane of the lens. However, this also causes the beam to spread with an angle usually many times larger than the inherent laser beam divergence in the space beyond the focal plane. Subsequently, the irradiance decreases at relatively short distances from the focal plane, which reduces the extent of the NHZ in comparison to the intrabeam NHZ.

Generally, laser radiation spreads out rapidly when emitted from the end of an optical fiber, although beam-like qualities have been reported from fractured fibers used in the operating room.[232] Hence, the optical fiber is a beam-expanding element that is optically equivalent to a short-focus lens placed in the beam path. The effect of the optical fiber is that it shrinks the range of the NHZ, again, compared to the intrabeam NHZ.

The fourth model is for diffuse reflection of the beam. The reflected irradiance or radiant exposure from a Lambertian surface at some distant point is inversely related to the square of the distance (r) from the surface. This describes diffuse reflections from a point source. For a CW laser, this is:

$$E = \frac{\rho\phi\cos\theta}{\Pi r^2} \qquad (25\text{-}13)$$

When Equation 25-13 is rearranged to solve for distance and the exposure limit is substituted for irradiance (or radiant exposure), the equation for diffuse reflection in Table 25.11 results. In general, worst-case conditions are often used where the viewing angle is 0° (where cos θ = 1) and the reflectivity ρ is 100%. As might be expected, diffuse reflection reduces the NHZ to relatively short distances because the beam is randomly scattered.

It is important to remember that since MPEs are time dependent, it is possible to calculate more than one hazard zone (distance) for a given laser. Table 25.12 includes estimates of the NHZ for some typical laser conditions.

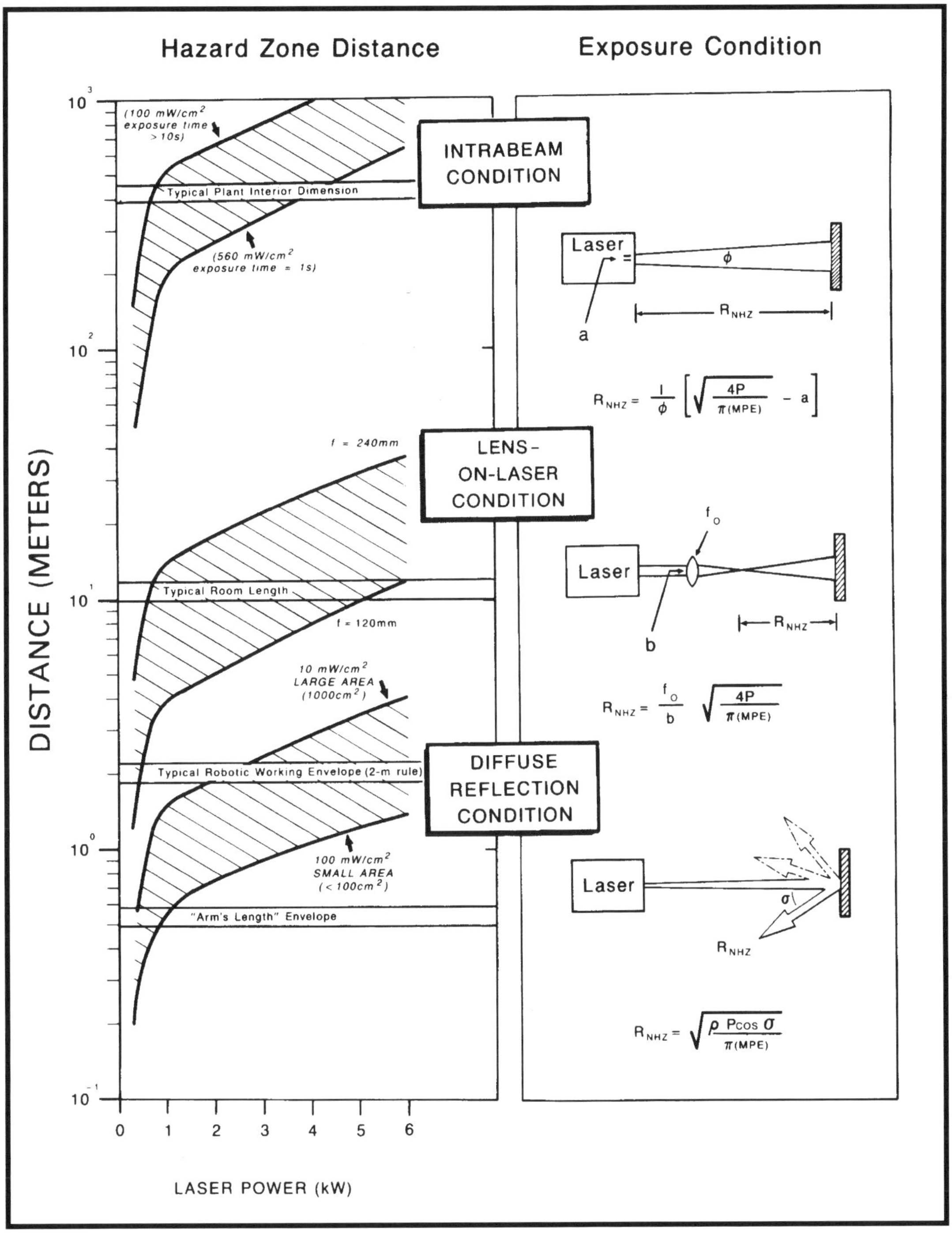

Figure 25.14 — Comparison of the extent of three NHZ models (intrabeam, lens-on-laser, and difuse reflection) for a high-power carbon dioxide laser in an industrial setting. (Note tha the equation for the intrabeam NHZ has been reformulated in the most recent versions of ANSI Z136.1.)

Control Measures

Control Measures are required if there is potential for exposure at levels above the exposure limits. In general, control measures are necessary for normal operation and maintenance of Class 3B and 4 lasers that have limited open-beam paths and open-beam paths. Accordingly, it is a good practice to use engineering controls, such as beam enclosures, whenever possible, to minimize the need for administrative and procedural control measures. Obviously, if the beam path is totally enclosed, then the potential for hazardous exposure may exist only during service, if there is an embedded Class 3B or 4 laser. If open-beam systems are necessary, the ANSI Z136.1 standard is a useful reference since it lists control measures as a function of the laser class.[207]

General

Laser control measures include the following items and activities; Engineering Controls, Administrative and Procedural Controls, Personnel Protective Equipment, Warning Signs and Labels, and special considerations. Engineering controls are the most important because they remain constant or fixed in place and ideally cannot be bypassed. Laser operations should always be enclosed to the greatest extent possible. Access ways or enclosures should be interlocked whenever practical so that the emission will be shut down whenever the access is opened. Other laser engineering controls include beam enclosures, panic buttons, key switches, and beam stops.

Administrative and procedural controls are the next most important safety controls. Administrative controls include the development of policy and procedures to ensure that entry to laser work areas is controlled, safe practices and protocols are developed and implemented, personnel are trained in general laser safety and receive hands-on training from project supervisors, and that all laser regulations and standards are being met in the laser safety program.

Given the laser classifications, there are specific laser hazard controls for each of the categories according to their hazard significance. Class 1 lasers require no controls and no user safety rules are necessary. Class 2 laser safety controls require that a person never stare into the laser beam. Only prolonged exposure to the beam presents a potential for damage. Class 3R lasers require basic engineering controls to enclose as much of the beam as possible and prevent any inadvertent exposure to the beam by unauthorized users. Additional controls for Class 3R lasers may include caution labels and warning signs for laser work areas. Class 3R lasers may also require the development of administrative procedures regarding the safe operation of the system. Class 3B lasers require danger warning labels and more stringent engineering controls such as safety system interlocks to prevent operation of the laser in the event that engineering enclosures are breached. Additionally, Class 3B lasers require the consideration and use of personnel safety devices such as laser protective eyewear or protective clothing. Any direct exposure to the Class 3B laser beam is to be avoided. Class 4 lasers present the most serious safety hazards and the engineering controls should ensure that they are only operated within a localized enclosure or in a controlled workplace. Eye and skin protection should be provided to all personnel working in the laser area. Remote firing and viewing techniques should be utilized whenever possible.

Laser hazard control measures can be designed and incorporated to address the most significant hazards. Control measures are designed to reduce the possibility of exposure to the eye and skin to hazardous levels of radiant laser energy and to the other hazards associated with the operation of the laser devices. One of the most important aspects of laser safety and control is to limit the laser power to the minimum level necessary to perform the intended task. ANSI standard Z136.1-2007, Table 10, "Control Measures for the Seven Laser Classes," should be used as a guideline in the development of safety controls.

Engineering Controls

Engineering controls are the priority means of minimizing the possibility of accidental exposures to laser hazards. If engineering controls are impractical or inadequate, then safety should be supported through the use of administrative procedures and personnel protective equipment. Engineering controls that may prove useful and effective in improving the safety of a laser or laser system are provided in the following list:

1. Protective housings with interlocks and labels,
2. Barriers, shrouds, and absorbent beam stops,
3. Fail-safe interlock systems,
4. System control master switches,
5. Permanently attached beam stops and attenuators,
6. Laser system status indicators and warning lights,
7. Laser control area warning lights,
8. Equipment labels and area warning signs and lights,
9. Equipment grounding methods,
10. Viewing portals, collecting optics, and display screens,
11. Enclosed beam paths, and
12. Emission delays.

Sample Laser Safety Warning Signs are provided in Figure 25.15.

Administrative and Procedural Controls

Administrative and procedural controls are methods and instructions which specify safety rules or work practices and which implement or supplement engineering controls and which may specify the use of personnel protective equipment. Administrative controls may include but are not limited to the following items:

1. Laser safe operating procedures,
2. Maintenance and safety inspection programs,
3. Laser registration and hazard evaluation.

The operating conditions and alignment procedures must be clearly identified and described in procedures. These procedures must include safety controls and precautions to address this laser safety program. Safety controls must address the most significant hazards even if those conditions are only evident for a fraction of operating time. The safety controls should consider, at a minimum, the following items:

1. Methods to limit access,
2. The number of lasers and laser systems in one general work area,
3. The degree of system isolation,
4. The availability of engineered controls to restrict untrained personnel,
5. Variations in beam paths and power levels,
6. The proximity of specularly reflective objects, The use of optics and lenses which could easily alter beam paths, wavelengths or beam diameter, and
8. Specific requirements for visitors.

Personnel Protective Equipment

All personnel who work in areas where there is a possibility of being exposed to hazardous level of laser radiation should be required to wear approved laser eyewear. Exceptions may be made in special cases if

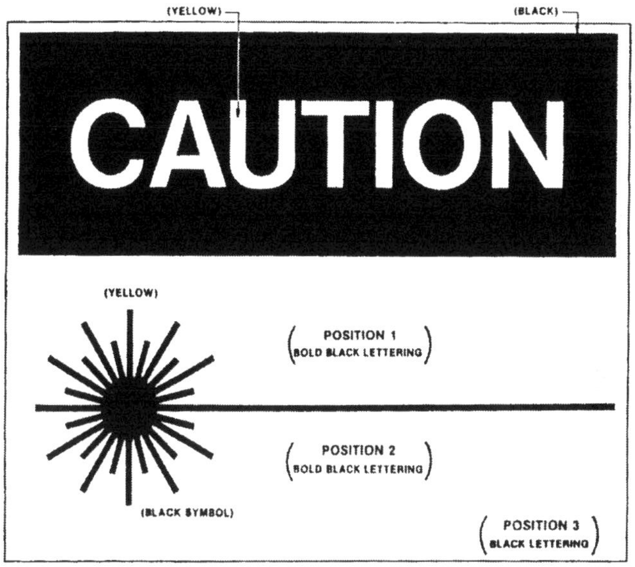

Sample Warning Sign for Class 2 and Certain Class 2M Lasers

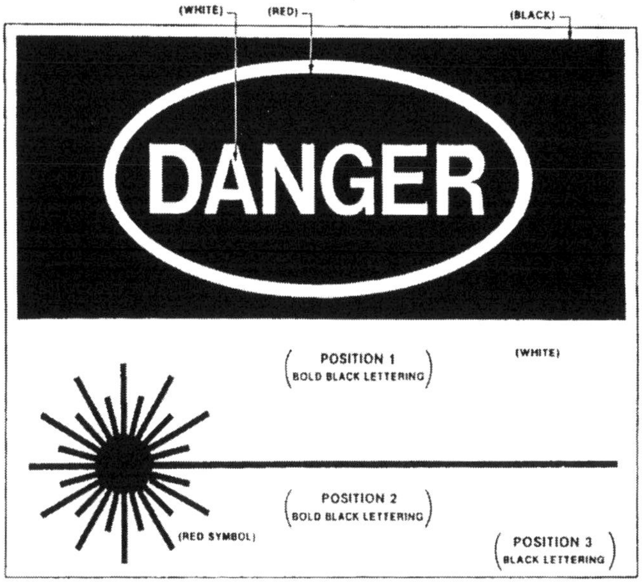

Sample Warning Sign for Class 3R, Class 3B, and Class 4 Lasers

Figure 25.15 — Laser Safety Warning Signs.

wearing protective eyewear produces a greater safety hazard than when it is not worn.

Flame resistant clothing may be appropriate for some laser installations where there is a possibility of either chronic or acute skin exposure. Loose-fitting clothing and long, loose hair could also be a hazard in a laser laboratory. Jewelry, including watches, should never be worn when working with lasers to minimize both the possibility of beam reflections and electrocution.

Personnel protective equipment includes eyewear, clothing, and gloves. The eye may be protected against harmful laser radiation by the use of protective eyewear that attenuates the intensity of laser light while transmitting enough ambient light for safe visibility (luminous transmission). The ideal eyewear provides maximum attenuation of the laser radiation while transmitting the maximum amount of ambient light. No single lens material is useful for all wavelengths or for all radiation exposures.

In choosing protective eyewear, careful consideration must be given to the operating parameters, Maximum Permissible Exposure, and wavelength. ANSI Z136.1 requires that protective eyewear be available and worn whenever hazardous conditions may result from laser radiation or laser related operations.

Laser-protective eyewear is characterized by optical density (OD or D_l; see Equations 25-5 and 25-6) and wavelength.[233,234] For example, a D_1 of 6 represents a reduction of the incident radiation by a factor of 1 million. Usually, D_1 is determined for the anticipated worst-case exposure, where there is exposure to the direct beam. The incident intensity value is calculated using the area of the limiting aperture[207], because MPEs are determined using the same values of limiting aperture.

It is possible for the eyewear to be damaged or fail (crack, melt, etc.) when exposed to high-intensity laser beams.[235–237] Hence, eyewear is used only when other control measures are inadequate. Although it does not necessarily physically damage the eyewear, a potentially hazardous phenomenon called "nonlinear optical transmittance" (dynamic bleaching) has also been observed in a small number of filter types. This occurs when the laser radiation saturates an absorber with a resulting increase in the amount of laser radiation transmitted.[238,239] Also, other researchers observed that some filter materials exhibited a spike in the initial values of power transmittance, which rapidly decayed to a steady-state value.[240]

In the U.S., the ANSI standard requires that eyewear must be marked with D_1 and wavelength so users can select the proper eyewear.[207] This becomes an important issue when more than one type of eyewear is used in an area with more than one type of laser. Eyewear should be used as directed, and stored properly. It should be inspected routinely to determine if there is pitting, crazing (fine cracks), or solarization of the lenses (degradation over time which appears as change in color or density) and if goggle straps or spectacle sideshields are in good condition.

The following example illustrates how to determine the necessary D_λ for an alignment using a 5-W argon laser, where a diffusing surface with a reflectivity of 80% is viewed at an angle of 0° for 600 sec at arm's length (assume r = 0.5 m). From Equation 25-13, the irradiance at 0.5 m is calculated to be 0.5 mW/cm^2. The MPE for 600 sec in the visible spectrum is 16.7 μW/cm^2, so the necessary optical density is 1.5, which is an attenuation of about 30 times

Protective clothing can be used to reduce the level of chronic exposure to the skin from ongoing laser operations. More importantly, protective clothing and gloves that are flame resistant can be used to prevent an acute exposure to the skin and subsequent burns. Laser burns to the skin are similar to thermal or radiant (sun) burns. Jewelry should never be worn when working with lasers, both because it presents a reflective hazard, and an electrical conductive hazard.

Laser Safety Training

Laser safety training should be required for all personnel who use Class 3B and 4 lasers. The training should be commensurate with the hazard of the laser in use and should cover topics such as:

1. Fundamentals of laser operation (physical principles, construction, etc.),
2. Bioeffects of laser radiation on the eye and skin,
3. Relations of specular and diffuse reflections,

4. Nonradiation hazards of lasers (electrical, chemical, etc.),
5. Laser and laser system classifications,
6. Control measures,
7. Overall management and employee responsibilities, and
8. Medical surveillance practices.

Laser Safety Officer (LSO)

The LSO, as described in the ANSI standard, is one who administers the overall laser safety program. Importantly, this standard defines the LSO as one with "the authority and responsibility to monitor and enforce the control of laser hazards and effect the knowledgeable evaluation and control of laser hazards."[194] Also, the LSO should receive training commensurate with the level of hazard posed by the lasers in use.

Alignment Practices. An area of particular concern in laser safety is beam alignment. In general, this should be done with the beam power as low as practical, or with an alignment laser, which is usually a low-power laser with a visible beam that is coaxial with the beam to be aligned.

Only diffuse reflections of visible beams should be viewed. Consider that the inverse square relationship with distance is valid as long as the distance is much greater than the laser spot diameter. Consequently, a diffuse surface acts as a distance-dependent attenuator that permits indirect viewing of low-powered laser beams when the reflecting spot is small. An example of this might be a point source-diffuse reflection of a relatively low-powered beam from a non-glossy business card held at arm's length. It should be stressed that diffuse viewing should be performed only when wearing the appropriate type of laser protective eyewear. So-called alignment eyewear has a relatively low value of D_1 because it is for safe viewing of a diffuse reflection. Some eyewear manufacturers label such eyewear "DVO," which stands for diffuse viewing only.

Invisible beams can be viewed using various phosphor image converter materials. These are often in the form of a "viewing card." The cards absorb the invisible optical radiation, then emit at wavelengths that are visible through protective eyewear. Since there may be significant reflections from viewing cards that are laminated with high-gloss plastics, it is best to purchase viewing cards with diffusing finishes, or to place matte-finish tape over the laminate.[241] IR beams can be observed with infrared viewers that produce a visible spot that can be seen through IR-protective eyewear.

Radio-Frequency and Microwave Radiation*

**This section written by R. Timothy Hitchcock*

Anticipation

The RF spectral region is 300 GHz to 3 kHz. Usually, microwave radiation is considered a subset of RF radiation, although an alternative convention treats radiowaves and microwaves as two spectral regions. In the latter context, microwaves occupy the spectral region between 300 GHz and 300 MHz, while radiowaves include 300 MHz to 3 kHz.

Various order-of-magnitude band designations (see Table 25.13) have been assigned to the RF and sub-RF portion of the spectrum. Frequencies in the various bands are allocated for uses including navigation, aeronautical radio, broadcasting, and citizens' radio. In addition to band designations, specific frequencies are designated for industrial, scientific, and medical (ISM) uses. ISM frequencies are 13.56, 27.12, 40.68, 915, 2450, 5800, and 24,125 MHz. Designations for frequency bands used with radar are shown in Table 25.14.

Table 25.13 — Nomenclature of Band Designations

Frequency Range	*Designation*	*Abbreviation*
<30 Hz[A]	subextremely low frequency	sub-ELF
30-300 Hz[A]	extremely low frequency	ELF
300-3000 Hz[A]	voice frequency	VF
3-30 kHz	very low frequency	VLF
30-300 kHz	low frequency	LF
300-3000 kHz	medium frequency	MF
3-30 MHz	high frequency	HF
30-300 MHz	very high frequency	VHF
300-3000 MHz	ultra high frequency	UHF
3-30 GHz	super high frequency	SHF
30-300 GHz	extremely high frequency	EHF

[A]The IEEE definition of band designations does not include VF, and defines ELF as 3-3000 Hz and <3 Hz as ultralow frequency (ULF).

Table 25.14 — Radar Letter-Band Designations

Letter Designation	*Nominal Frequency Range (GHz)*	*Specific Radar Bands (GHz)*
HF	0.003–0.03	
VHF	0.03–0.3	0.138–0.144
		0.216–0.225
UHF	0.3–1.0	0.420–0.450
		0.890–0.940
L	1–2	1.215–1.400
S	2–4	2.300–2.500
		2.700–3.700
C	4–8	5.250–5.925
X	8–12	8.500–10.680
Ku	12–18	13.4–14.0
		15.7–17.7
K	18–27	24.05–24.25
Ka	27–40	33.4–36.0
V	40–75	59–64
W	75–110	76–81
		92–100
mm	110–300	126–142
		144–149
		231–235
		238–248

Quantities and Units

Seven quantities may be used to characterize exposure to RF fields: the specific absorption rate (SAR), specific absorption (SA), electric-field strength (E), magnetic-field strength (H), power density (W or S), induced currents (I_i), and contact currents (I_c). The SAR and SA are quantities that represent exposure within tissues. E, H, and W are measures of the intensity of the fields in space, while I_i and I_c are measures of RF-induced electric currents. Additionally, the exposure limits are frequency dependent, so frequency is an important factor.

The SAR is the rate at which energy is absorbed per unit mass, or dose rate. It is the fundamental quantity of the exposure criteria, and the dosimetric quantity of choice in studies of biological effects. It is generally expressed in units of watts per kilogram (W/kg), representing the power deposited in a unit mass. This is also used for metabolic rate and, for comparison, the resting metabolic rate of an adult human being is about 1 W/kg. The SAR depends on the electric-field strength in tissues (E_i), the electrical conductivity (σ) of tissues, and the density of tissues (ρ) as in:

$$SAR = \sigma E_i^2/\rho \qquad (25\text{-}14)$$

The SA is the time integral of the SAR and, as such, is the RF dose. It is the energy absorbed per unit mass of tissue, with units of joules per kilogram (J/kg).

In general, the determination of SAR and SA does not lend itself to field evaluations of exposure but is limited to carefully controlled studies in the laboratory or numerical models. Because of this, exposure guidelines are written in terms of related quantities, called derived limits, that are more easily evaluated when determining exposure. These include E, H, and W for electromagnetic fields, which may be viewed as surrogate measures for the SAR. Hence, the exposure guidelines are in terms of frequency-dependent derived limits that will maintain the SAR at an acceptable level.

Electric-field strength and magnetic-field strength are vector quantities, but only the magnitude is reported in safety evaluations. E fields are generated by electric charges and are measured in terms of the electric potential (V) over some distance. The unit is the volt per meter (V/m). Since power is related to the square of the voltage, E^2 (V^2/m^2) is often used in exposure guidelines or in describing the output of measurement instruments.

H fields are generated by moving electric charges, such as a current (I) moving through a long, thin wire. The flux density (B) of the magnetic field at some distance (r) from the wire is

$$B = I/2\pi r. \qquad (25\text{-}15)$$

H is used for RF magnetic fields and has units of amperes per meter (A/m). Since power deposition in tissues is related to I^2, H^2 (A^2/m^2) may also be used. (To convert between B and H, use $\mu = B/H$, where μ is the magnetic permeability. For fields in air, μ is the value of the magnetic permeability of free space, μ_o, 1.257×10^{-6} henry/meter.)

Power density (W) represents the time-averaged energy flow across a surface, and typically is used when measuring microwave radiation. The unit of power density is watts per meter squared (W/m^2), although the use of milliwatts per centimeter squared (mW/cm^2) in hazard evaluation is common. (Conversion: 1 W/m^2 = 0.1 mW/cm^2.) W is related to E and H by:

$$W\ (W/m^2) = E^2/120\pi = 120\pi H^2. \qquad (25\text{-}16)$$

RF fields can induce currents within exposed tissues. These induced currents (I_i) flow through the body to ground, with a common path through the foot, which is called the "short-circuit" or foot current. The unit of electric current is the ampere (A), although the milliampere (mA) is the magnitude usually addressed in safety evaluations.

In an environment where there are RF fields, it is possible for contact with conductive objects to result in currents that flow into the body at the point of contact, which is usually the hand. If this occurs, exposure guidelines may require evaluation of contact currents (I_c) in mA.

Physical Characteristics

Understanding certain properties of an RF field is necessary to perform a hazard evaluation. These properties include near and far fields, plane waves, impedance, polarization, modulation, gain, and duty cycle.

Near and Far Fields. The antenna is the circuit element that causes the RF energy to be radiated. The transition of RF energy from the conduction state on the surface of an antenna to the radiation state in free space is not immediate but passes through the near field then into the far field (see Figure 25.16).

The reactive near field exists in the space immediately surrounding the antenna. Here, the E- and H-field components exist in a complex temporal and spatial pattern, and the energy is non-propagating or "stored." A short distance from the antenna is the radiating near field, characterized by both energy storage and propagation (radiation). Here, the spatial pattern of the beam intensities is complex and may increase or decrease with distance or may remain unchanged. Beyond the near field is a transition zone, then the far field. In the far field, there is propagation, and the power density follows the $1/r^2$ law for distance.[242,243]

Plane Waves. To understand plane waves, consider an ideal point-source antenna which emits radiation in an isotropic pattern. The radiation pattern would be spherical (uniform in all directions), so near this antenna a receiver detects curvature in the approaching field. However, if removed sufficiently far from the source, some distance into the far field, a receiver would sample only a very small area of an immense curved wavefront. In the local region of space occupied by the receiver, it would detect a flat, or planar front; hence, the name, plane waves.

Two important characteristics of plane waves are space quadrature and time phase (see Figure 25.1). Space quadrature exists when the E- and H-field vectors are at right angles to one another and to the direction of propagation. The time phase of the fields is such that the E and H vectors reach their maximum and minimum values simultaneously.

Free-Space Impedance. The impedance, Z, of free space is the quotient of E/H. In the near-field impedance must be determined. However, when plane-wave conditions exist, the free-space wave impedance is a constant value, 377 (120π) ohms (Ω), at a given point in space.

Combining the expressions for power density and impedance for a plane wave yields:

$$W\ (mW/cm^2) = E^2/3770 \qquad (25\text{-}17)$$

and

$$W\ (mW/cm^2) = 37.7H^2 \qquad (25\text{-}18)$$

which are useful formulas for conversions involving field strength and power density.

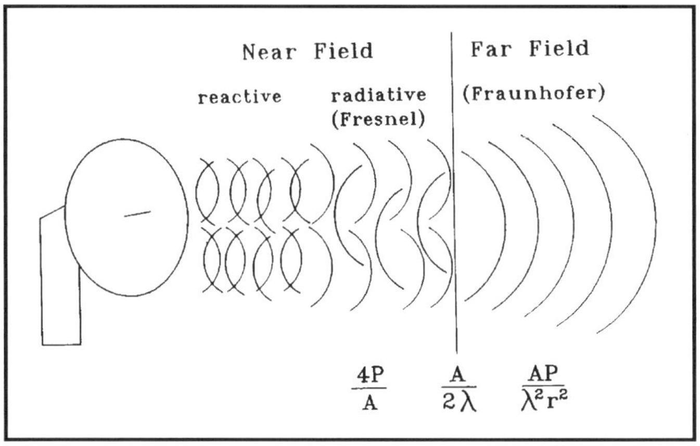

Figure 25.16 — RF emissions (shown as curved surfaces) in the regions around an aperture antenna. Near the antenna is the near field then a transition region leading into the far field. The power density in the near field and far field, and the distance to the boundary between the two zones, may be estimated from the equations. Note that radiation exists in the far field where the power density is dependent on distance, whereas the power density in the near field is not.

Polarization. Polarization is that property of an electromagnetic field describing the time-varying direction and amplitude of the electric-field vector. A field may be polarized linearly, circularly, or elliptically, or it may be unpolarized. Specifically, the type of polarization is described as the figure traced as a function of time by the amplitude of the E-field vector at a fixed location in space. An observer would view this trace along the direction of propagation.

Modulation. Modulation is the process by which some characteristic of an unmodulated carrier wave (a carrier of information) is varied by a modulating wave (called a signal). The modulating signal, which is lower in frequency than the carrier, is used to superimpose information on the carrier wave. If the amplitude of the carrier is varied, the wave is amplitude modulated (AM). If the frequency or phase of the carrier is varied, then the wave is frequency modulated (FM) or phase modulated (PM), respectively. AM and FM are used in broadcasting, while FM and PM are used in communications. Digital modulations such as time-division multiple-access (TDMA), and code-division multiple-access (CDMA) are also used in communications.

Some industrial and medical RF sources may be opportunistically amplitude modulated, with the modulating signal in the ELF spectral region. This occurs because the electric circuitry allows the imposition of the fundamental or a higher harmonic of the power frequency (50 or 60 Hz) on the RF carrier.[244,245]

Gain. Gain is a measure of the directional properties of an antenna, representing an increase in power output of the system in relation to an ideal isotropic emitter. For a point-source antenna, gain equals 1. If a reflector is placed near this antenna, it changes the radiation pattern due to collimation or focusing, and the gain is greater than 1.

Absolute gain (G) is a ratio of the actual transmitted power density in the main beam to the power density transmitted from an isotropic radiator. If the absolute gain of an antenna with area (A) operating at a given wavelength is unknown, a conservative estimate of absolute gain can be calculated from:

$$G = 4\pi A/\lambda^2 \qquad (25\text{-}19)$$

When gain is used in calculations, values of absolute gain must be used:

$$G = 10^{(g/10)} = \text{antilog}\,(g/10) \qquad (25\text{-}20)$$

where

g = gain in decibels.

Duty Cycle. Some sources may exhibit a cyclic or intermittent operation, where RF is emitted for only a fraction of the total time of operation, the "on-time," in an operational cycle. The ratio of on-time to the total time of operation (on-time plus off-time) is called the duty factor or duty cycle (DC). DC is also the product of the pulse repetition frequency (PRF) in pulses per second (Hz) and the pulse width or duration (PW) in seconds (PRF × PW).

Duty cycle is important, because it allows the determination of average power (where average power = peak power × DC), and most exposure guidelines are in terms of average power. Sources that typically have a duty cycle less than 1 include radar, dielectric sealers, induction heaters, RF welding units, some communication devices, and medical diathermy units.

Interactions with Matter

Radiofrequency radiation and microwaves are energetic photons that can travel easily long distances through space and matter. As incident photons impact with matter a variety of interactions may occur including transmission, absorption, reflection, or scatter.

In transmission the incident photon passes directly through the materials without imparting any energy or changing directions. In another case, the beam may be completely absorbed by the medium. The energy of the beam is imparted to the medium in the form of heat, vibration, or induced electric current. Absorption of an RF or microwave beam is affected by a variety of specific factors including the wavelength, the frequency, the wave polarization relative to the dimensions of the body, the dielectric properties of the absorbing material, and the physical and conductive characteristics of the environment surrounding the material.

Absorbing matter can be categorized into three basic groups depending on their electrical properties. Conductors are materials with high electrical conductivities and are highly reflective of electromagnetic radiation. Dielectric materials are electrical insulators that may both reflect and transmit RF energy. These materials may also absorb small amounts of energy. Lossy dielectrics are imperfect insulators that absorb and attenuate electromagnetic fields. Biological tissue tends to be a lossy dielectric material that becomes increasingly conductive at low frequencies.

Depending on the RF or microwave frequencies and the dielectric properties of the exposed medium the imparting photons may be scattered by reflection, diffracted, or all or a portion of the beam may be absorbed. A portion of the beam may also pass directly through the body without interacting. The actual interactions that are experienced by any given body is extremely difficult to determine due to the variations in body and anatomical geometry, the variations in tissue makeup and density, and the composition of layers of different tissues as the beam passes through the body. The differences create a multitude of interfacial reflections and deflections with the possibility of standing-wave formations between the various tissues and the air-tissue interfaces.

Microwave frequencies tend to be absorbed within the topical layers of the body or skin. As frequency decreases penetration deepens and interactions tend to occur more often in the deeper tissues.

The size and shape of the medium, or body, can have a substantial affect on the absorption of energy through a resonance phenomenon.

Biological Interactions

Radiofrequency radiation can interact with biological tissue through a variety of mechanisms. The interactions can involve both magnetic and electric fields. Interactions take place through either thermal or nonthermal means.

The biological effects of exposure to RF radiation have been studied for a variety of frequencies, power levels, and experimental models. Studies have previously focused on parameters associated with scientific, industrial, medical and communications purposes. In the past few years, with the exponential growth in the use of personal mobile communications systems, research has been expanded on the types of sources and exposures associated with these technologies.

In general, heating of the whole body or localized regions have been the focus of detrimental health effects studies. Thus, body and tissue heating has been the basis of most consensus exposure guidance. With the advance of more sophisticated laboratory techniques however, and the expanding growth of the sources, more research is focusing on possible nonthermal detrimental biological effects, including the risk of cancer.

In thermal response mechanisms the electric field creates an oscillating current within the biological tissue. This rapid transfer of energy creates molecular motion and generates localized heating of the tissues. Additional heat is created when water molecules, with large randomly oriented permanent dipole moments, are forced to orient with the field direction. The work required to rotate the viscous water dipoles results in significant energy transfer. Of course, these thermal interactions are greatly dependent on the RF frequencies, power levels, and the anatomic structure and molecular make up of the particular tissue being exposed and a great amount of additional research is still need to completely understand all thermal interactions in all body parts.

Whole body heating can occur with RF exposure and is absorbed by the body with a resultant increase in molecular rotational and translational kinetic energy. The absorbed heat is distributed throughout the body by the blood circulation and is eventually lost to the external environment. This whole body heating can raise the core body temperature to the level where it can interfere with cardiovascular and thermoregulatory functions. Body heating may also impact cognitive functions when the physiological limits of tolerance are achieved. Whole body heating has also been shown to have effects on temperature regulation in pregnant women, neonates, and in children.[246] A variety of detrimental and teratogenic effects have been demonstrated on animals an d humans in utero including reduced fetal growth and developmental defects.[247]

Nonthermal Effects

A broad range of nonthermal RF interactions have been investigated and reported but are much less understood than thermal affects on tissues. Typical radiations of a single RF photon that are less than 1 GHz do not generate enough energy to ionize a molecule (1 eV). Nor is it likely that a significantly large number of photons would hit a molecule at the same time imparting enough energy at one point to create an ionization. Therefore, the mechanisms that would be needed to cause damage in tissue would need to arise from some other mechanisms.

Excitation by molecular vibration is one interaction mechanism that has been described.[248] In complex biological complexes, such as DNA, it could be possible for RF fields to excite individual atoms to the extent that structures, or activities, could be disrupted.

RF electric fields may be able to affect a voltage drop across cell membranes due to their high electrical resistance, compared with other tissues.[249] At low frequencies it could be possible that the changes in molecular resistance could induce or inhibit normal membrane activities and responses, thus interfering with normal cellular function.

One aspect of molecular activity that must be considered in evaluating the affects of RF radiation on tissues is the normal random fluctuating electric and magnetic fields, or Brownian Motion, associated with the random motion of charged cells. These random fields that already exist within cells in tissue pose a limit on the sensitivity of the system to respond to applied RF fields. If the RF field is below a certain threshold for a given type of biological tissue, and below the given "thermal noise" that normally exists in the tissue, then it could be assumed that RF exposure levels below the thermal noise would not induce biological changes in the cells.

Effects from Electric Fields

The significance of electric field perturbations on biologic material may be most noted on the potential effects on DNA. DNA is primarily proteins that are chains of amino acids connected by peptide bonds. These protein chains in DNA and other biologic materials are often formed in loops or helices, and folded over onto themselves. The arrangement of the chain in space is named a conformation. The side chains of the amino acids are often polar. These side chains either attract or repel one another and to some extent determine the conformation and create differential potential energies and dipole moments within the tissues. Experiments have been conducted that indicate that RF exposure can induce conformational changes within the protein chains.[250,251] Based upon the results of current experiments it is not possible to determine the true significance of the changes or whether the results would be consistent for a range of exposure or RF dose rates.

Changes in binding ligands like Ca^{2+} to cell receptor proteins have been shown to result from RF exposure of cell receptors. Chiabrera found that significant changes in ligand binding could be produced by exposure to RF fields.[252] It is not exactly clear what strengths of RF fields are necessary to produce significant effect of the ligands to affect protein conformations, but evidence shows that it is likely to be below current guideline levels. It is also not clear whether the changes in binding ligands are biologically significant, per se.

RF exposure to tissues has been shown to enhance the interaction between cells. Cells are normally attracted to one another by dispersive forces. When exposed to RF fields oscillating dipole moments are produced within cells that enhance the attraction. The aggregation of the dielectric particles in a fluid that result from these increased attractions is called the Pearl-Chain Effect.[253,254] The biological significance of the pearl-chain effect is yet to be determined or demonstrated.

Studies conducted by Woodward[255] indicated that at frequencies of less than 80 MHz, the concentration of free radicals could be increased by low intensity RF fields. It is not believed that RF radiation at frequencies of 1 GHz or higher would be likely to induce elevated levels of free radicals, but due to the well established relationship between free radicals and disease, particularly cancer, this continues to be an important area for research.[256]

Health Effects

A broad range of health effects have been postulated to be associated with exposure to RF and microwave fields. Affects have been studied on animals through laboratory investigations. These types of studies allow for some level of control over exposure conditions, dose measurements, and the parameters of the electromagnetic field such as frequency, power levels, and dose durations. Limitations in these types of studies include differences in biological systems between animals and humans, differences in anatomical configurations and the wave associated dose distributions and absorption considerations due to geometric differences between animals and humans. Due to the expansive possible variations in exposure scenarios such as different frequencies, doses, and durations, many studies have used different study parameters, making it difficult to make comparisons or "fill in the holes" between one study and another.

Epidemiologic studies have been undertaken at an increasing rate in the past few years due to the public concern and apprehension with the exponentially expanding use of RF and microwave radiations for communications and other purposes. With public awareness comes concern, warranted or unwarranted, and calls for more research, and sometimes more control and precautionary approaches in the absence of data.

Neurobehavioral Effects

Some of the earliest studies of the health effects of exposure to Radiofrequency radiation involved the ability of RF exposures to induce behavioral changes in animals. Over the years other health effects associations with behavioral and neuorobiological functions have been made with RF exposure including poor concentration, sleep disruption, lack of memory, loss of sexual libido, and loss of appetite.(246)

Recent studies of impacts on cognitive performance have demonstrated conflicting results.(257,258)

Subjective symptoms of RF and microwave exposure have been noted in a variety of reports. Subjective complaints of headaches, migraines, fatigue, skin irritation and warmth have been reported.(259,260) Other reported affects include dizziness, blurred vision, malaise, confusion, and memory loss.(261) Subsequent single and double blind studies performed on different groups of so called "sensitive" individuals with true and sham exposures indicated no significant difference in groups to actually identify exposures, or feel the stated effects in relation to the exposures.(262–264)

Reproductive and Developmental Effects

Ocular Effects

In a comprehensive review of Ocular Effects of RF Energy by Elder it was determined that clinically significant ocular effects, including cataracts, have not been demonstrated in human populations exposed for long durations to low level radiofrequency fields.(265) Although some studies have shown ocular effects in rabbits and monkeys, the intensity of the doses of RF radiation (near lethal levels), use of localized near field exposures, and differences in geometrical configuration of the anatomies, it is not reasonable to assume similar effects in humans at exposure levels within existing exposure guidelines. After review of available human studies on RF and ocular cancer Elder also concluded that there is no clear association.

Cancer

A number of epidemiological studies and reviews have been published within the last few years on the relationships between cancer and RF or microwave field exposure. To date, the overall balance of evidence is not strong enough to link these radiations to the increase incidence or risk of cancer in humans.(266–269) Study problems included inconsistencey in design of the studies, lack of detail and accuracy in exposure estimates, an inabilities in study designs to deal with other confounders and relevant factors. Due to the methodological defects and other limitations of these studies there is also not enough information to soundly conclude that there are no risks or hazards associated with RF exposure, therefore studies continue. In a recent comprehensive review of studies on RF occupational, residential, and cell phone exposures to RF, the Advisory Group on Nonionizing Radiation of the British National Radiation Protection Board concluded that no relations to cancer have been shown consistently.(270)

Human data are limited and present no clear trends, so scientists have relied on animal models to establish biological effects. These effects have been extrapolated to humans and used in setting exposure limits. Animal studies have found effects in most major systems including nervous, neuroendocrine, reproductive, immune, and sensory.[5,243,271–276] The following review addresses effects on behavior, reproduction and development, and the eyes and cancer.

Interaction with Tissues. Tissues are classified as a lossy dielectric material, that is, a material that interacts with the field and absorbs considerable RF energy. RF energies are more highly absorbed in tissues of high water content (e.g., muscle) than in tissues with low water content (e.g., fat). RF interaction with tissues may be complex, with standing waves formed at the interface of tissues with different dielectric properties, such as skin-fat or fat-muscle.

In general, short-wavelength RF has a relatively shallow penetration depth into tissues such that, at frequencies of more than a few gigahertz, absorption is in the skin. Longer wavelengths may penetrate more deeply, and the body is relatively transparent to long-wavelength magnetic fields. Obviously, penetration depth may affect what organs or systems are at risk.

Numerous studies have clearly shown that absorption of RF energies produces thermal effects, although some athermal and nonthermal effects have been reported.[277–280]

RF exhibits three modes of tissue interaction at the molecular level: polar molecule alignment, molecular rotation and vibration, and the transfer of kinetic energy to free electrons and ions.[281] Alignment of polar molecules with the field is an ubiquitous mechanism that results in frictional heating.

Behavior and Nervous System Effects. Exposure guidelines are based on a few well-established effects observed in test animals. One of these is reversible behavior disruption in short-term studies, a sensitive measure of RF exposure.[282–286] In general, behavioral changes are thermal effects attributed to significant increases in body temperature due to absorbed RF energy.[285,286] Also, a few studies have evaluated the effects of RF on cognition, as reviewed by D'Andrea.[287]

There are East European and Russian reports of RF workers with certain nonspecific symptoms (also found in workers not exposed to RF and members of the public) associated with the nervous system. These effects may have clinical signs extending to the cardiovascular system, called "radiowave illness" or "microwave sickness."[288–291] Some similar symptoms have been reported in the United States medical literature in two cases of apparently acute overexposure to high-power microwaves.[292,293]

In addition to behavioral effects, combined interactions of RF fields with neuroactive drugs and chemicals have been reported in test animals.[294,295]

Reproduction and Development. Teratogenic effects have been reproducibly demonstrated at 27.12 MHz with rats, when the whole-body average (WBA) SAR was relatively high, around 10 to 11 W/kg.[296–298] These appear to be thermal effects, as a dose-response effect was seen with high rectal temperatures.[298] Developmental abnormalities were observed in rodents at 2450 MHz, with high values of WBA SAR.[299,300]

Epidemiological studies of reproductive endpoints have demonstrated no trends.[301–309] Two studies reported effects on semen quality[310,311], but a follow-up study of one report[311] found no effects on semen quality.[312] Also, a study of dielectric heater operators found no difference in semen characteristics and hormones in comparison to controls, except for follicle stimulating hormone which was significantly higher in the exposed group.[313] Other studies have evaluated exposure to female physiotherapists finding a lower than expected sex ratio of offspring[308], low birth weight[314], and no effects.[315,316] Taskinen and colleagues observed an increase in spontaneous abortion for exposure to shortwave, but multivariate analysis attributed this to confounding variables.[304]

Ocular Effects. Effects have been reported to the cornea, iris vasculature, lens, and retina. Effects to the corneal endothelium of monkeys were reported at 2450 MHz by one research group[317,318], but not by another.[319]

Historically, cataracts have been of concern because the avascular nature of the lens increases its susceptibility to heat-induced change. The most effective frequencies in test animals are 1 to 10 GHz. Acute thresholds have been determined for restrained rabbits receiving ocular exposure in the near field of a 2.45-GHz applicator.[320,321] No cataracts were observed with far-field exposure of unrestrained animals[322], even if exposures were almost lethal.[323] Studies of cataracts in people with purported RF exposure do not support a causal link[324–330] although one study suggested an aging effect on the lens.[327] A few studies have reported effects to retinal tissues[331,332], but effects have not been observed consistently.[333]

Cancer. Limited data suggest that RF may be a possible tumor promotor in animals[334,335], while other studies demonstrate no significant differences in RF-exposed groups and controls.[336–338] One study found significant differences in primary malignancies in RF-exposed rats when the tumor data for all tissue types were combined. However, no other health effects were observed in the more than 100 other endpoints evaluated.[339,340] In summary, the animal data on cancer are inconclusive.

Epidemiological studies have provided some suggestive evidence that RF energies are carcinogenic to human beings.[243,341] No differences were observed in cancer mortality in two studies of military personnel categorized as RF exposed[342,343] but a third study found a link between exposure of Polish military personnel to pulsed RF and an increased incidence of cancers of the alimentary canal, brain, and hematopoietic and lymphatic systems.[344] Another study categorized possible RF exposure of Air Force personnel on the basis of job title, finding a modest increase (39%) in brain cancer.[345]

No differences were observed between the staff at the Radiation Laboratory at the Massachusetts Institute of Technology (radar development during World War II) and the general population. A significant difference in cancer of the gall bladder and bile ducts was reported when MIT personnel were compared with a cohort of physician specialists.[346]

No link between use of handheld cellular telephones and brain cancer has been reported[268,347–349], although there are questions about latency period because cell phones have been in use for a relatively brief time which translates to short duration of exposure with regard to chronic disease. In a study of police officers, findings were statistically significant for melanoma for officers in the 10-to-60 years from hire group, but were not significant for testicular cancer in the same group.[350]

A study in Great Britain reported statistically significant results for adult leukemia, skin cancer, and bladder cancer for people living within 10 km of 1 FM radio and TV antenna.[351] However, this result was not replicated in a study of all high-power transmitters in Great Britain, although some evidence was found of a decrease in leukemia with increasing distance from the antennas.[352] Australian researchers determined a statistically significant increase in the incidence of and mortality from childhood leukemia.[353] This hypothesis-generating study needs further evaluation with a more rigorous study design.

The human studies to date have a number of limitations. One major limitation is the absence of information on doses, dose-response, or duration of exposure. Others include the classification of possible exposures on the basis of job title, a small number of cases or small sample size, little control for confounding factors, and no consistency in findings in studies reporting statistically significant associations.

Accidents, Incidents, and Other Concerns. A number of accidents and incidents have been reported. They may be categorized as ocular[354–358], nervous system[292,293,359–364], reproductive[356,365,366], skin[356,358–361,364,367–373], and cancer.[374–377] In general, it appears that exposure to high levels of RF may result in nerve damage and skin damage. Reviews of accidents are available.[243,276,378,379]

Other concerns with exposure to radiofrequency fields include possible perturbation of the field by metallic implants (e.g., metal staples, cochlear implants)[380–383] or metallic objects that are worn (e.g., jewelry, watches, metal-framed spectacles).[384] RF fields may also interfere with electronic devices such as sampling devices[385,386], medical electronics (e.g. cardiac pacemakers)[387–389], and electroexplosive devices. In some chemical sample preparation methods that utilize RF, microwaves have been reported to superheat solutions, which may lead to melting of reaction vessels or explosions.[390]

Recognition

Generation

RF energy is generated by the acceleration of charge in oscillatory circuits. Generators include RF vacuum tubes (triode, tetrode, and pentodes), microwave vacuum tubes (klystrons, magnetrons, and traveling-wave tubes), and solid-state devices (semiconductor diodes and triodes).[243]

Sources

Sources are natural (sun, galaxies, lighting, human body) and man made.[243,391–394] Man-made sources are radiators, leakage sources, or a combination. Radiators (e.g., antennas) intentionally emit RF energy into the environment. Leakage may be the consequence of poor design, lack of maintenance, or improper maintenance. Information on selected sources is contained in Table 25.15 and discussed in the following text. To allow for a meaningful evaluation, the operational frequency or frequencies of the source must be determined.

Because the operational frequencies are less than 100 MHz, evaluations of dielectric heaters must include measurement of E and H fields, Ii, and possibly Ic. These units operate in a cyclic manner requiring determination of and correction for the duty cycle. Evaluations have shown that work with unshielded or improperly shielded heaters may result in overexposure. In general, overexposures are to free fields (primarily electric)[396–398] and induced currents.[399,400]

Induction heaters are also low-frequency sources. Typically, measurements of induction heaters require duty-cycle correction.

Table 25.15 — Information on Some Important RF Sources

Source	*Frequencies (MHz)*	*Uses*	*System Components*
Dielectric heater	10-70; many at 27.12	heat, seal, weld, emboss, mold, or cure dielectric	power supply, RF generator, tuning circuitry, press, electrodes (die) materials
Induction heater	0.250-0.488	heat conductive materials via electromagnetic induction	power supply, RF generator, transmission line, induction coil
Plasma processors	0.1-27; many at 13.56	chemical milling; nitriding of steel; synthesis of polymers; modifying polymeric surfaces; deposition (sputtering) and hardening of coatings and films; and etching, cleaning, or stripping photoresist	RF generator, transmission line, reactor vessel, RF tuning and control module, vacuum pump, gas storage, and gas delivery system
Radar	EHF, SHF, UHF	detection, tracking, ranging	transmitter, waveguide, antenna, receiver, display
Broad-casting	see Table 22.19	radio, TV	transmitter transmission lines, tower, antennas
Com-munications	HF, VHF, UHF	fixed position and mobile systems used for voice/data transmission	transmitter, receiver, transmission lines, antennas
Video display terminals	VLF, LF	visual imaging component of information processing systems	Cathode-ray-tubeVDTs have been the focus of most evaluations.
Diathermy	microwave (915 or 2450) or shortwave (13.56 or 27.12)	heat therapy	generator, control console, transmission line, applicators
Electro-surgical units	0.5-100	cauterizing or coagulating tissues	generator, transmission line, surgical probe, current return cable

H-field values in excess of exposure guidelines have been reported near these devices.[401]

Measurement of E, H, Ii, and possibly Ic is required for plasma processing units, too. Generally, leakage is low, but unshielded viewing ports are a potential leakage source. Also, units configured with twin reactor vessels may leak from an open vessel while the second vessel is in use[402], and equipment attached to plasma units can act as antennas and emit RF energy.[403]

The beam emitted from radar antennas is highly directional and, in some cases, very narrow. Some antennas move horizontally (scan) or vertically (elevation), and most units are pulsed at relatively high peak powers. The combination of scanning, elevation, and pulsing (duty cycle <1) usually results in brief exposures for individuals irradiated by the beam.

Evaluations of commercial radar (airport surveillance and approach traffic control)[404], aircraft[405,406], marine[407–409], and police traffic-control radars[410–413] have not demonstrated over exposures during normal operation. However, exposure to airport radar[404] and aircraft units[405,406] may be of concern during maintenance activities. Reports have characterized overexposure from a portable military unit[292] and a military aircraft unit.[293] Evaluation of other military radars has demonstrated high RF levels when a rotating beam was stopped, which required an interlock to be disconnected.[414]

Broadcasting types and frequencies are in Table 25.16. Broadcast towers may support a single antenna or multiple, stacked antennas (FM and TV), or be the antenna (AM radio). For stacked antennas, it is possible that significant exposure may occur to maintenance personnel from antennas that are not being serviced but are still energized.[415] The hands and feet of climbing personnel may also receive high exposures, especially if the transmission line is located near the ladder. When maintenance work is performed on energized AM towers, it is possible body current may exceed the exposure limits.[416] Workers may experience spark discharge and sustained contact currents as they climb onto the tower.

Evaluations of fixed communications systems have not demonstrated overexposures of operational personnel.[392,417,418] It is possible that relatively high levels of RF may be encountered by maintenance personnel who work on satellite communications (SATCOM) systems or near energized cell-site antennas.[419] Mobile[420–422] and portable communication systems may produce relatively high RF levels very near the antennas. Hence, when the antenna is located very near the head, exposure may result in relatively high local values of SAR.[423,424] RF currents on metallic parts of the radio case may also produce relatively high levels of exposure to the face.[425,426] Reports on cellular telecommunications by expert panels are available.[427,428]

Table 25.16 — Broadcast Frequency Allocation

Type	*Carrier Frequency (MHz)*
AM radio	0.535–1.605
FM radio	88–108
Low-band VHF-TV	54–72, 76–88
High-band VHF-TV	174–216
UHF-TV	470–806

Numerous evaluations of low-frequency E and H fields from cathode-ray-tube type video display terminals (VDTs)[429,431] and televisions[271,432] have not demonstrated the potential for overexposure. RF fields may be emitted from any surface of these devices, but the magnitude decreases rapidly with distance. In general, most of the RF energy emitted by cathode-ray-tube-type VDTs/TVS resides in the VLF and/or LF band designations.

Diathermy units may operate continuously or be pulsed, and some may be amplitude modulated or have a ripple at ELF frequencies.[244,245] The leakage field of the applicator depends on the type of applicator. Relatively high levels may be found in the vicinity of the cables.[433,434] Adjustment of the equipment during operation may result in exposure to the hands.[435]

Evaluations of solid-state and spark-gap electrosurgical units (ESUs) demonstrated that field strengths increased with increasing output power and levels were higher for solid-state units.[436] Levels near the probe and unshielded leads may exceed exposure criteria.[435–437]

Evaluation

Exposure Guidelines

RF guidelines for occupational exposure are recommended by groups including the

Institute of Electrical and Electronics Engineers (IEEE)[438], the ACGIH®[104], the ICNIRP[439], the National Council on Radiation Protection and Measurements (NCRP)[440], and the Federal Communications Commission (FCC).[441] Discussions of other occupational guidelines are available.[243,442]

The NCRP, ICNIRP, and FCC have limits for members of the general public, while the IEEE recommends limits for controlled and uncontrolled environments. A major difference between these two environments is that individuals in the controlled environment (CE) are aware of the potential for exposure, whereas individuals in the uncontrolled environment (UE) have no knowledge or control over their exposure.[438] Prior to an evaluation, it must be determined which environment members of the exposed group are in, whether general public or workers, so the proper exposure limits are used.

The exposure limits are derived from a fundamental quantity of exposure called the basic limit. Current density is the basic limit at the lowest frequencies, less than 100 kHz, where electrostimulation of tissue is significant. SAR is the basic limit throughout much of the remainder of the RF region, from 100 kHz to 6 GHz.[438] SARs have been recommended for whole-body average exposure, spatial-peak exposure, and exposure to the extremities, as shown in Table 25.17. From 6 to 300 GHz, power density is used.

The exposure (derived) limits form an envelope around the human whole-body absorption spectra, as shown in Figure 25.17. The relationship between frequency and body height in this figure demonstrates that maximum absorption occurs at a given frequency for a given body height, and this concept is called geometrical resonance. For any individual, resonance (maximum absorption rate) is established when body height is about 40% of the incident wavelength, and the E-field vector is parallel with the long axis of the body.[443] The guidelines address resonance for grounded or ungrounded (free space condition) bodies. These conditions have been integrated to produce the resonance range that typically spans 30–300 MHz, the region where the exposure limits are lowest.

Because the body absorbs RF more poorly at frequencies outside the resonance region, the exposure limits increase via sloped transition regions to low- and high-frequency plateau regions. In the low-frequency region (less than about 3 MHz), the exposure limits are the highest because the body is highly sub-resonant and RF energy is poorly absorbed. In the high-frequency region (greater than a few gigahertz), RF energy absorption and hence, the limits, are at levels between the other regions. This is called the quasi-optical region because wavelength is decreasing and interaction begins to approximate that of optical wavelengths.

Note that the SAR does not vary with frequency as do the derived limits. This is because a single threshold dose rate for unfavorable biological effects (4 W/kg for reversible behavior disruption in test animals) was determined from a review of the biological database. As shown in Figure 25.18, a tenfold safety factor was applied to

Table 25.17 — Specific Absorption Rates (W/kg)

	Whole-Body Average (W/kg)	*Spatial Peak (W/kg/g)*	*Extremities (W/kg/10 g)*[A]
Controlled environment[B]	0.4	8	20
Uncontrolled environment[B]	0.08	1.6	4
Occupational	0.4[C] 0.4[D]	8[C] 10[D]	20[C] 20[D]
General population[D]	0.08	2	4

[A]Local SAR based on absorption in 10 g of tissue.
[B]From Reference 511.
[C]From Reference 106.
[D]From Reference 513.

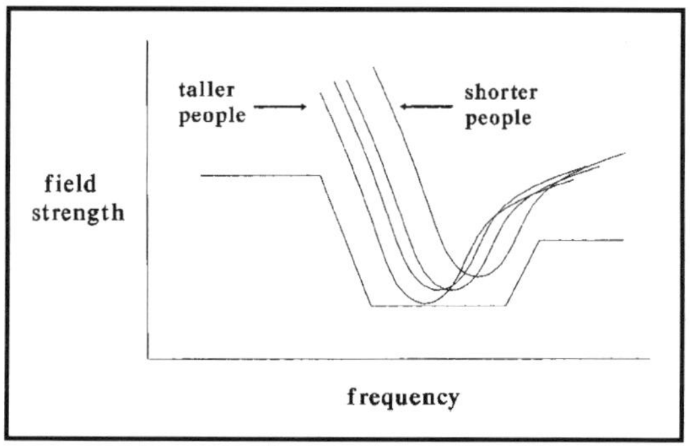

Figure 25.17 — The derived limits form an envelope around the family of RF absorption spectra for individuals of different heights. The envelope is formed by three regions where the limits plateau, and two transition (sloping) regions where the limits must be calculated.

this to produce a whole-body average SAR of 0.4 W/kg for occupational exposures and the controlled environment. The WBA-SAR for the UE or the general population (0.08 W/kg) includes an additional fivefold safety factor. Hence, this lower SAR is not based on a lower threshold dose rate for potentially hazardous effects.

In general, the averaging time for occupational and general population limits for free fields is 6 and 30 minutes, respectively. Six minutes applies to the CE except at frequencies between 15 and 300 GHz where it decreases to 10 seconds at 300 GHz, and must be calculated.[438] In general, 30 minutes is used for the extended resonance range, where limits for the UE are less than limits for the CE.

Additional criteria for induced and contact currents exist for exposure at low frequencies, typically less than 100 MHz. At these low frequencies, the body is highly conductive and RF E-fields in space induce currents within the body. It has been demonstrated that these currents may produce locally high values of SAR, so guidelines have been developed to control this type of exposure. RF energies may also couple to conductive objects, such as a vehicle body, metal fence, or metal roof, and be conducted into the body when contact is made. Since this may result in RF shock or burns there are exposure guidelines for contact currents written in terms of grasping contact with the hand.[104,438]

The magnitude of the limits for induced and contact currents is frequency dependent between 3 and 100 kHz, and the averaging time is 1 sec. Between 100 kHz to 100 MHz, the exposure limit (average value) is 100 mA in the CE with a 500 mA ceiling value and an averaging time of 6 min. The limits in the UE are 45 mA and a ceiling value of 220 mA.[438]

Although not an exposure guideline, the FDA has a performance standard for microwave ovens in 21 CFR Part 1030.[444] This includes requirements for manufacturers of these ovens, and allowable microwave leakage at the time of manufacture and throughout the service life of the oven.

Instruments

Instruments are available to measure RF fields, body currents, and contact currents. In general, these instruments are broad-band,

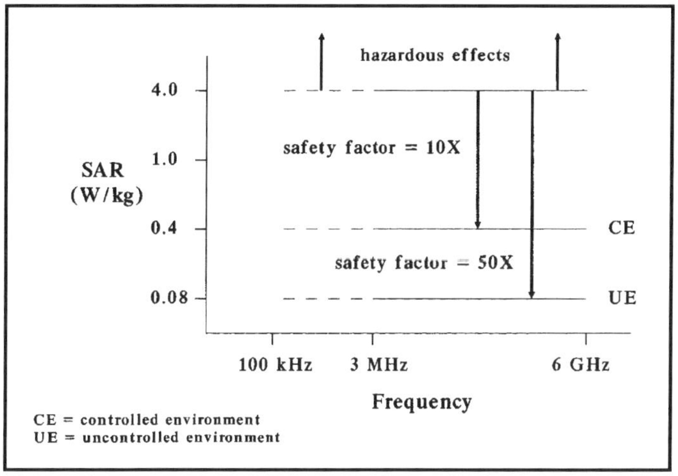

Figure 25.18 — The whole-body average SAR was determined from studies with test animals. Potentially hazardous effects occur at whole-body SARs in excess of 4 W/kg. As discussed in the text, the SARs for the controlled and uncontrolled environments were derived by the application of 10-fold safety factors, respectively. As displayed, the SAR is most meaningful between 3 MHz and 6 MHzm although in the standards it applies between 100 kHz and 6GHz.

meaning they have a wide calibrated frequency range and a frequency-independent response within this range. Some instruments, typically used for microwave oven measurements, have been designed and calibrated for 915 or 2450 MHZ, and are not broad-band instruments. All instruments should be calibrated at least annually and, if broad-band, at a number of frequencies across the frequency range.

Densitometry. The measurement of RF field strength and power density is called densitometry.[273] Densitometric measurements of fields in space are made with analog or digital survey instruments that have three components: probe, connective cable or optical fiber, and metering instrumentation, as shown in Figures 25.19 and 25.20. The probe includes antennas to couple the field into detectors. The output from the detectors is directed to the metering instrumentation where it is processed and displayed and/or logged. Output units may include V/m, A/m, V^2/m^2, A^2/m^2, $|FSU|^2$ (field-strength units squared = V^2/m^2 or A^2/m^2), W/m^2, mW/cm^2, pJ/m^3, or percentage of standard.

For the most part, linear antennas (monopoles or dipoles) are used for E-fields[444–446], and loop or coil antennas are used for H fields.[447,448] Commonly, detectors

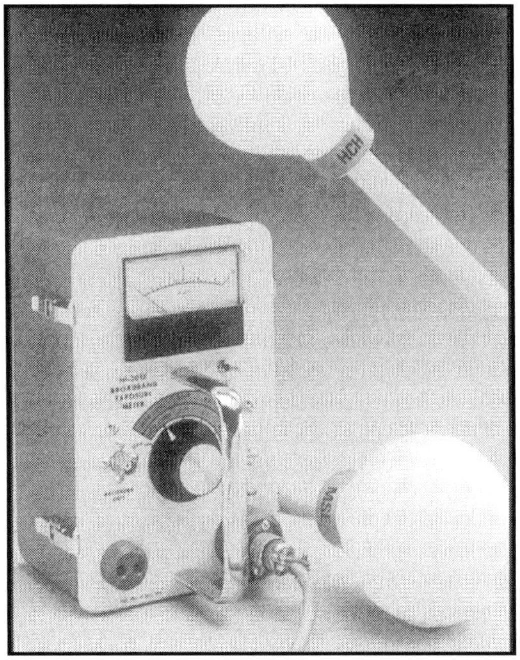

Figure 25.19 — A broadband survey meter with E- and H-field probes. The antennas and detectors (diodes) are enclosed in the polystyrene insulator. The tape at the base of the insulator is labeled for the type of probe (E field=MSE; H field=HCH) and color-coded to match one of the two scales located above the indicator knob on the meterin instrumentation. (Courtesy of Holaday Industries, Inc.)

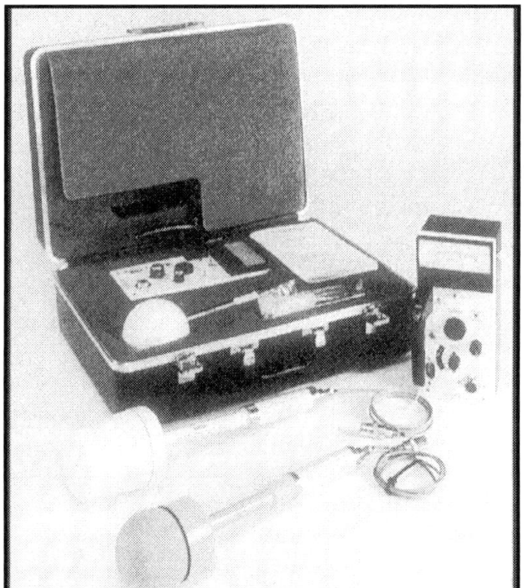

Figure 25.20 — A broadband survey meter with probes, carrying case, and operations manual. The antennas and detectors (thermocouples) are located within the RF-transparent plastic or polystyrene. Calibration factors are included under the clear plastic that covers the handle of the probe. (Courtesy of Narda Microwave)

are thermocouples or diodes(446,449), and are encased in an RF-transparent material (polystyrene, plastic) along with the antennas. Most instruments have interchangeable broad-band probes, which are color-coded or labeled to differentiate between E- and H-field response and to link the probe with a color-coordinated scale, at least on instruments with analog meters. Some newer instruments "handshake" with the probe and automatically select the proper output parameters.

Displacement current sensors have been developed for use in monitoring low-frequency E fields, such as those associated with video display terminals (see Figure 25.21). This instrument is a type of parallel-plate capacitor with two small, conductive plates electrically connected by a wire. Immersed in an RF field, a current flows between the plates and is measured by an operational amplifier.(450,451) Also, this instrument has a loop antenna for magnetic fields, located around the perimeter of the conductive plates.

Current Monitors. Two types of induced current monitors are available: stand-on and clamp-on devices (see Figure 25.22). Stand-on meters use a parallel-plate capacitor design to measure foot currents flowing to ground.(452,453) The bottom plate must

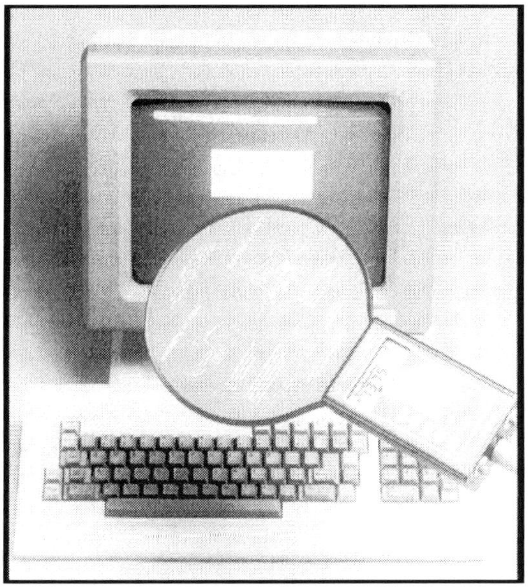

Figure 25.21 — A displacement current sensor that may be used for monitoring low-frequency E and H fields such as those emitted by video display terminals. (Courtesy of Holaday Industries, Inc.)

make contact with ground, which may be difficult in some environments, especially outdoors. Both analog and digital devices are available. A human body model antenna that may be coupled to a stand-on meter is also available. A review of the performance of two manufacturers' makes of stand-on meters is available.[454]

The clamp-on device (see Figure 25.22b) is a current transformer that determines the current flowing through an appendage such as the ankle or wrist.[416,455,456] In this configuration, the body part is the primary circuit and the measurement device includes the secondary circuit and a detector. The readout module may be on the transformer or may be remote. In the latter case, an optical fiber connects to the readout, a logging device, or both. Output is in mA or percent of standard.

A contact current monitors currents flowing through a handheld probe, which is connected to a ground plate with a connective cable (see Figure 25.23). The instrument has the impedance equivalent of the human body when making grasping contact with the hand, and output is in mA. The performance of this instrument has also been reviewed.[454]

Personal Monitors. At present, RF dosimeters are not in general use, because of difficulties in making meaningful measurements. This is partly due to RF shadowing, an effect that shields a measurement device worn near the body. The shadow develops on the side of the body facing away from the source[457,458], which introduces bias into the measurement data. Although not dosimeters, personal monitors with audible alarms that are activated when the intensity reaches some threshold value are available. In some units, the alarm threshold is preset, but in others it may be selected.

Frequency Counters. These are portable, handheld instruments that allow the user to determine or confirm the most intense single frequency associated with a source. These instruments offer broad-band operation, and high sensitivity, and they are relatively inexpensive. Care must be taken not to overload the instrument by using it too near powerful RF sources.

Exposure Assessment

This may involve measurement, numerical modeling, or both. Prior to collecting measurement data or making calculations,

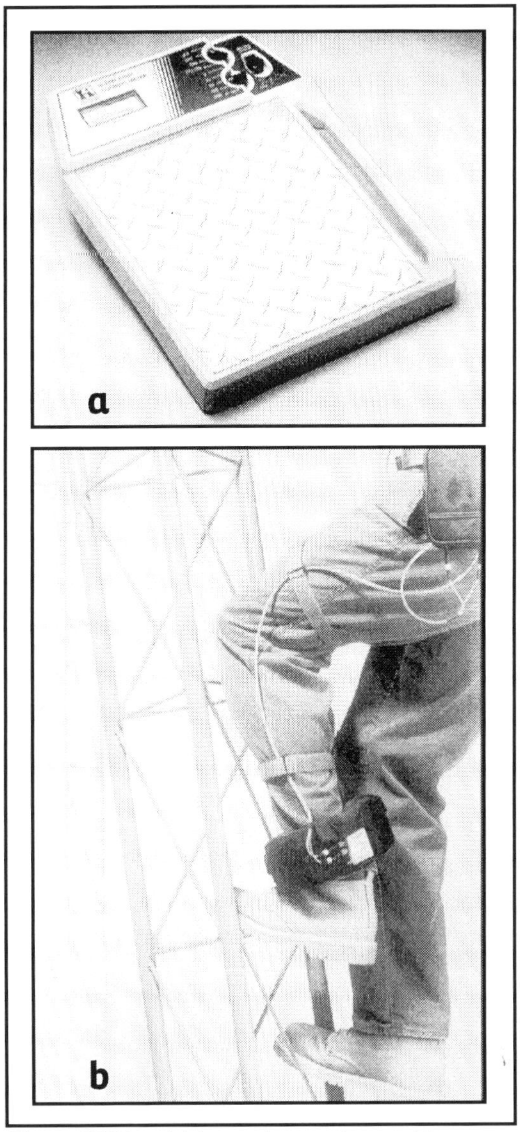

Figure 25.22 — (a) A stand-on meter used to measure the short-circuit current flowing out of the foot; (b) a clamp-on current transformer measuring currents flowing in the ankle. The unit is connected via optical fiber to a system readout device that is located on the user's waist. (Courtesy of Holaday Industries, Inc.)

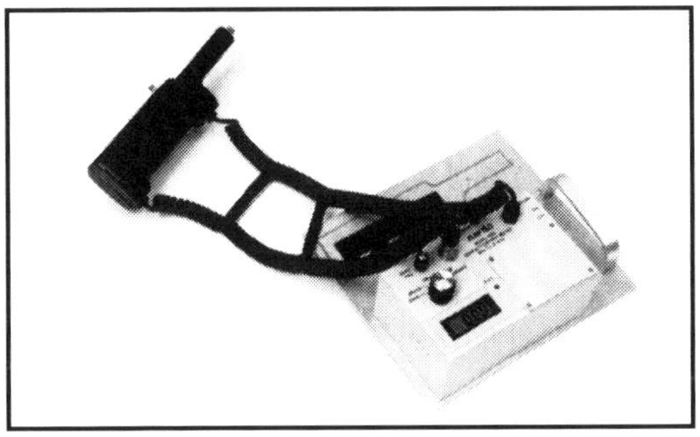

Figure 25.23 — A contact current meter showing the sampling probe, connective cable, meter, and base plate. (Courtesy of Marda Microwave)

the evaluator should be familiar with the source and tasks related to RF exposure, preferably by observation. In general, the evaluation is done under worst-case conditions, since all other conditions of exposure for a given task will be acceptable if the worst-case does not result in overexposure.

When preparing to evaluate exposure by measurement, one should be aware of potential sources of error (see Table 25.18), should determine source characteristics (see Table 25.19), and know what measurements are required (see Table 25.20). A useful guide to help prepare for an evaluation is available from the NCRP.[395]

Because all RF instruments respond properly to a finite frequency range, the operational frequency of the source must be within the calibrated frequency range of the instrument. If it is not, use an instrument that has the proper frequency range, or contact the instrument manufacturer about extending the calibrated frequency range.

Field Survey Procedures. Before making measurements, allow the instrument to equilibrate with the temperature in the survey area, then check the instrument zero in a RF-free zone. First, evaluate source emissions (look for "hot spots" and areas of worst-case leakage), then assess exposure.

To evaluate emissions, extend the probe in the direction of the source, then proceed toward the source, slowly immersing the probe in the field, so that it "sees" the field first. Move the probe in the horizontal direction and then the vertical direction across a relatively small area, probing for hot spots. A thorough evaluation will probably involve placing the probe at locations not normally occupied, and may result in determining relatively intense fields. Remember that, although source characterization may produce useful data on emissions, it should not be used to assess potential overexposure, which is the next step in the evaluation. However, if emissions are low (e.g., <1/5 the occupational limits) or not detectable (limits of detection should be <1/5 the occupational limits), it is reasonable to document the results and not perform further evaluation.[243]

Now, from the evaluation of emissions and the observations of the job, determine the possible worst-case exposure condition(s). Exposure should be evaluated without the operator being present, the operator-absent condition, since the presence of the operator's body may perturb (influence) the RF fields and their measurement. One way of doing this is spatial averaging.[438,449] This is a method of estimating average

Table 25.18 — Sources of Measurement Error

- No knowledge of operational and/or calibrated frequencies.
- Instrument responses to amplitude modulated fields or pulsed emissions.
- Perturbation of the fields to be measured by evaluator and/or instrument.
- Standing wave formation and multipath effects.
- Probe interaction with the source and reflections.
- Interaction of the leads and metering instrumentation with the field.
- Zero drift and field zeroing problems.
- Probe burnout in intense fields.

Table 25.19 — Source Characteristics

- Frequency (fundamental and harmonic content)
- Modulation (FM, AM, other)
- Polarization
- Continuous wave (CW) or pulsed
- Characteristics of pulsed sources
  - Pulse repetition frequency (PRF)
  - Pulse width or duration
  - Duty cycle (factor)
- Antenna characteristics
  - Power (effective radiated power [ERP], output)
  - Effective area
  - Diameter of aperture antenna
  - Gain
  - Beam width
  - Scan rate (angle)

Table 25.20 — Types of RF Measurements Required by C95.1-1999

Frequency	*Measurement*
300 GHz-300 MHz	E or H or W: spatial average
300 MHz-100 MHz	E & H: spatial average
100 MHz-3 kHz	E & H: spatial average[A] induced currents[B] contact currents[B,C]

[A]Consideration should be given to remote monitoring of low-frequency E fields, because the evaluator's body may significantly perturb these fields.
[B]Required by C95.1 if the measured E-field value exceeds a frequency-dependent percentage of the E-field MPE.
[C]Required only if there are conductive objects that may contain/store RF energy as an electrical current.

exposure of the whole body by collecting densitometric data across the vertical dimension of a simple linear model of the body. A typical model is a 200-cm tall dielectric "stickman," made from materials of low relative permittivity such as PVC or CPVC pipe, which is placed at the operator position.(243) If the instrument does not have a spatial-average function, a minimum of 10 equally spaced (e.g., 20-cm spacing) measurements must be made between 0 and 200 cm, then arithmetically averaged, as in Equation 25-21.

$$\text{spatial average} = \left(\frac{\sum_{i=1}^{n} X_i^2}{n} \right)^{1/2} \qquad (25\text{-}21)$$

Here, n is the number of measurements and x is either the electric or magnetic field strength. Note, when averaging field-strength units be sure to use the square of the quantity, since the SAR is power dependent. For power density, squaring the measured values is not necessary since it is already in terms of power; just sum them and divide by the number of measurements ($\Sigma W/n$).

Measurements should also be performed at the locations of the eyes and testes. The C95.1 standard allows frequency-dependent excursions (called relaxations) from the MPEs at all anatomical locations except for the eyes and testes, so the exposure limits can not be exceeded at those locations.

When collecting data, be aware of the requirements for the measurement distance, since this varies with different standards. For example, C95.1 specifies 5 cm from the generating device or 20 cm from reradiating objects(438), while the ACGIH® recommends 5 cm.(104) Because of spatial variability of the field and the rapid change of field strength with distance, large differences may occur in measurement data collected at different measurement distances.

The exposure guidelines specify that exposure data must be time-averaged. This is done manually, or with a data logger, or time-averaging module. A 6-min averaging time usually applies to occupational exposures at frequencies less than 15 GHz. Between 15 and 300 GHz, averaging time is inversely related to frequency, and must be calculated.(104,438)

If exposure is relatively uniform and continuous for the averaging time, it is not necessary to sample for the entire period. However, if the intensity of exposure varies, as might occur if the worker moves in and out of the field (e.g., when supplying parts or removing product from a manufacturing process), it will be necessary to determine a time-weighted average (TWA), where:

$$TWA = \frac{(ML_1 \times t_1) + (ML_2 \times t_2) + \ldots + (ML_n \times t_n)}{t} \qquad (25\text{-}22)$$

Here, ML is the measured level (spatial average) for a given exposure duration, t.

Hazard Calculations for Intentional Radiators. These provide an estimate of either the power density at a given distance from an antenna or the hazard distance.(242,243,392,441) Hazard distance (range) is the linear distance from the antenna at which the field intensity is reduced to the exposure limit.

To calculate the maximum power density on the beam axis (W) in the near field of an aperture antenna, use:

$$W = 16P\eta/\pi D^2 = 4P\eta/A \qquad (25\text{-}23)$$

Here, P is the antenna power (watts), η is the antenna efficiency (values ≤ 1), D is the diameter of the antenna, and A is the cross-sectional area of the antenna.

Since the near-field equations are independent of distance, it is presumed that the calculated power density exists between the source and the boundary of the near field, R_{nf}, which is estimated by:

$$R_{nf} = \frac{D^2}{4\lambda} \qquad (25\text{-}24)$$

Now, to calculate the power density in the far field, use:

$$W = GP/4\pi r^2 \qquad (25\text{-}25)$$

or $W = GP/\pi r^2$, which assumes 100% ground reflection and produces a slightly higher estimate of power density.

To estimate the hazard distance in the far field of aperture antennas, substitute the appropriate exposure limit (EL) for W, in Equation 25-25, then rearrange to solve for distance.

$$r = (GP/4\pi EL)^{1/2} \quad (25\text{-}26)$$

Again, when 100% ground reflection is assumed, the hazard distance equation becomes $r = (GP/EL)^{1/2}$. Gain, G, may be calculated as shown in Equation 25-19.

For FM and TV antennas, hazard distance formulas without and with ground reflections are, respectively:

$$r = (30\ ERP)^{1/2} / EL \quad (25\text{-}27)$$

$$r = (48\ ERP)^{1/2} / EL \quad (25\text{-}28)$$

ERP is the effective radiated power, in watts, which is the product of gain and transmitter power. Although Equations 25-27 and 25-28 can be derived in terms of power density, they are normally expressed in terms of electric-field strength for broadcast sources. So, EL is in V/m and r is in meters.

Measurement of Induced and Contact Currents. It may be necessary to measure induced and contact current at frequencies between 3 kHz and 100 MHz. Note, this does not include FM broadcast frequencies between 100 and 108 MHz (see Table 25.20). The C95.1 standard does not require measurement of currents if the measured E-field strength is below a certain percentage of the E-field MPE.[438]

To measure induced currents, stand-on instruments should be located at the position where the operator normally stands or sits. Connect the remote readout device, if one is used. Have the operator stand on the instrument and perform his or her normal function while you monitor the output. If the source is pulsed, be sure to monitor a sufficient number of work cycles to determine operator exposure. For current transformers, clamp the device around the appendage (usually the ankle, as shown in Figure 25.22b). Locate the data logger on the belt and secure the optical fiber so that it is out of the way. Switch the units on, and determine exposure. (Note that the measured value of the induced current will vary, even if the source has a relatively constant RF field, if the operator moves around, momentarily contacts conductive objects, or is joined by another individual at the work location.) Be sure to time average the data for either 1 sec (3–100 kHz) or 6 min (100 kHz to 100 MHz).

Exposure guidelines require that contact currents be measured if there are conductive surfaces or objects that can store RF electric energy, and release this on contact. To make this determination, one must be familiar with objects in the workplace and how these objects are grounded, or their lack of grounding. (Note: electrical grounding does not ensure that the machine is properly grounded for RF currents.) Conductive objects to consider include ladders, metal tables, metal handles or pulls, vehicles, fences, reinforcing bar, chains, guy wires, frames, metal roofs, and shipboard components.

Currently, only one contact current instrument is commercially available. To use this instrument, connect the sampling probe to the instrument. Select the highest range if the magnitude of the current is unknown, and locate the meter at ground potential, usually on the floor. The path of the current is through the handheld sample probe and to the meter via the connective cable. Touch the sample probe to the surface and depress the probe switch to determine the current. Remember that these numbers represent human impedance where the worker is barefoot and grasping the object with his hand.

Control Measures

Engineering Controls

Engineering controls include interlocking, shielding, bonding, grounding, filtering, and waveguides below cutoff. Good design practices include fail-safe positive-mode interlocks, built-in leakage detectors, visual "power-on" indicators, and visual and audible alarms. Interlocks are used at system access points, such as transmitter access panels. Because of the potential for faulty relays and switches, it may be prudent to use redundant relays in circuits for alarms and power-off conditions.[459] A maintenance program should be established to evaluate safety system performance periodically, including interlock checks. Lock-out/tag-out procedures for working with sources of hazardous energies must be implemented and followed. If flammable materials are used, fire/smoke detectors, alarms, and extinguishers should also be included in system specifications.[460]

Shielding and Enclosures. Incident RF fields induce currents in the surface of conductive materials such as those typically used for shielding. Shields use reflection, absorption, and internal reflection[461,462] to manage these currents and reduce the incident fields that penetrate the conductive material.

Shielding effectiveness (SE) is used to describe the capability of a material as a shield (see Table 25.21). SE is a function of losses resulting from absorption, reflection, and internal reflection. SE, in decibels (dB), is calculated by:

$$SE = 10 \log_{10} (W_i/W_t) \text{ dB} \qquad (25\text{-}29)$$

where W_i and W_t are, respectively, the incident and transmitted power density.

Shields are constructed from a single layer of a suitable material or layers of materials. Shielding materials exhibit a frequency-dependent nature in SE. Plane waves are effectively attenuated by materials that have high conductivity, low permeability, and low characteristic impedance. Generally, materials suitable for E fields produce high reflective losses. Metals that are most effective for E fields and plane waves include silver, copper, gold, aluminum, brass, bronze, tin, lead, chromium, and zinc.[463] Polymers and polymer blends containing conductive materials are also used.[464,465]

H-field shielding materials include iron, some stainless steels (SS430), steel (SAE 1045), grain-oriented silicon-iron, nickel-iron alloys such as Mu-Metal, and cobalt-iron alloys such as Vaccoflux.[463,466] Composites, made of multiple layers of materials such as copper-stainless steel-copper, copper-alloy-copper[467], and copper-plywood[468] may also be used.

RF-shielded enclosures use shielding materials to reduce leakage and penetration of RF fields. In designing an enclosure, attention is given to the selection of the base shielding material and to seams, panels, flanges, cover plates, doors, ventilation openings, cable penetrations, and grounding. Seams should be overlapped[469] and welded.[470] Panels and cover plates should be attached with conductive gaskets such as those made of Monel, neoprene, silicone, and tin-plated beryllium-copper.[471,472] Gasket materials may be fabricated into various forms including metal meshes, metal meshes on elastomer cores, knitted wire mesh, spring-finger stock, foam-backed metal composites, hollow tube (conductive neoprene), and various specialty shapes.[472,473] Periodic maintenance of gaskets will be necessary, and the frequency of maintenance depends on the environment and the type of gasket used.

Table 25.21 — Interpretation of Field Reduction Values

Attenuation (dB)	*Qualitative Description*
0–10	negligible shielding
10–30	minimum significant shielding
30–60	average shielding
60–90	above-average shielding
90–120	excellent shielding
>120	superior shielding

Waveguide Below Cutoff. A waveguide is often a hollow metal tube (circular, rectangular, or square) used to confine and guide electromagnetic waves with minimum transmission loss. Conversely, the purpose of a waveguide below cutoff is to attenuate electromagnetic waves. If there are openings in shielded enclosures for ventilation or conveyor openings in RF process equipment, RF leakage through these openings will decrease the SE of the enclosure. The use of waveguide below cutoff sleeves in the openings will help maintain the SE of the enclosure. An example is a honeycomb filter that is used to allow air movement but attenuates electromagnetic waves.[474,475] Waveguides below cutoff have also been used successfully to control leakage around conveyors in industrial microwave dryers and RF sealers.[476]

Resonant Frequency Shift. If the source operates near the whole-body, grounded-resonance frequencies, around 10 to 40 MHz, the WBA-SAR may be reduced by separating the body from ground by a small distance. The SAR reduction is achieved by effectively shifting the body into the free-space resonance absorption condition, while exposure continues to occur at grounded-resonance absorption frequencies. Shifting the body to the free-space resonance condition where resonance is around 70 MHz reduces the body's ability to absorb the lower frequency RF energy. This has been demonstrated by simulating an air gap between human subjects and ground with expanded polystyrene and hydrocarbon resin foam, both of which are electrically insulating materials.[477] Other insulating materials may also prove successful in reducing the SAR, as long as they are relatively transparent to RF E fields, as indicated by low values of relative permittivity (measure of the effect of a material on the E field relative to free space), and the separation distance is sufficiently large.[399,478,479]

Location of Equipment and Personnel. Studies have indicated that placement of a lossy dielectric, such as a person, near a flat, RF-reflective surface, can enhance the SAR. This effect was further enhanced if the person was located in a reflective corner.[443,479,480] The materials of building construction and the placement of RF devices within the building are therefore important considerations in minimizing exposures.

Administrative and Procedural Controls

Administrative controls include footwear, protective clothing and gloves, prepurchase review of sources, controlling the duration of exposure, increasing the distance between the source and workers (although this may be achieved by engineering modifications), restricting access, and placing warning signs.[243]

Footwear, Protective Clothing and Gloves. Footwear may modify absorption by volunteers exposed on a ground plane at frequencies between 0.63 and 50 MHz.[399,452,456,477,481] This is accomplished by reducing the grounding effect and shifting the body toward the free-space resonance condition, as discussed earlier. The level of reduction depends on the type of shoes and socks worn and the RF frequency. For example, the use of nylon or wool socks reduced absorption to the same extent as an air gap of comparable thickness[477], and rubber-soled shoes[399] and clogs with thick wooden soles[456] had a similar effect.

RF-protective suits are made of a base material (e.g., wool, polyester, or nylon) that is impregnated with a highly conductive metal, such as silver, or is woven with metallic stainless-steel thread.[482–486] If the metallic fibers are oriented in one direction, they may demonstrate polarization sensitivity. A mesh design, where the fibers occupy vertical and horizontal positions, is not sensitive to field polarization.[487]

Openings in RF-protective suits for the hands or feet, zippers, or facepiece may introduce the potential for RF leakage into the suit. In addition to RF penetration, other concerns include suit ignition, arcing, and standing-wave formation. If RF-protective clothing is used, it is important to ensure that adequate test data indicate the necessary attenuation will be achieved at the specified frequency or frequencies, the suit is not flammable, and no electrical safety hazard exists. Users should be trained on the proper use of the suit and to understand and recognize use limitations in their workplace.

Protective gloves may provide protection from RF-induced contact currents and spark discharge. Rubber insulated gloves can be effective in reducing low-frequency contact currents. OSHA inspectors have documented two cases in which gloves were effective in controlling spark discharge to the hands of longshoremen. In one report, workers wore fleece-lined rubber gloves where the open-circuit voltage was 100 to 330 V and the short-circuit current was 180 to 1900 mA.[488] In the second case, workers wore two pairs of gloves. The outer pair was leather, while the inner pair was rubber. The open-circuit voltage and the short-circuit current were 300 V and 300–1000 mA, respectively.[489]

Tell reported current reduction factors for gloved hands vs. bare hands at AM radio frequencies of 4 to 31 times. The magnitude of the reduction depended on the RF frequency, glove type, and hand pressure. Reduction factors varied inversely with frequency, and heavy duty leather work gloves had the greatest reduction factors, while a rubber glove had the lowest.[490]

Distance. Increasing the distance between the person and the source is probably the most frequently used control measure, but it is also the control measure that can be circumvented most easily. Workers should be informed of the extent of the zone of exclusion and the supportive rationale. Zone limits are often delineated by clearly visible methods, such as tapes, paints, or signs, or by physical delimiters such as rope, fencing, or traffic cones. Both horizontal and/or vertical distance from a source may be limited. Controlling vertical distance may be necessary to minimize exposure of maintenance personnel on radio and MW towers.

Duration of Exposure. Many exposure guidelines allow an RF energy dose (SA) of 144 J/kg for the applicable averaging time, where SAR × t_a = 144 J/kg (e.g., 0.4 W/kg × 360 sec = 0.08 W/kg × 1800 sec = 144 J/kg). Reciprocity allows the SAR to be higher if the total exposure duration (T) is less than t_a, as long as the product of the two (SAR × T) does not exceed 144 J/kg. Since the exposure limits are derived from the SAR, it follows that if the product of exposure duration and exposure intensity (e.g., measured level, ML) does not exceed some constant value (e.g., T × ML ≤ EL × t_a), the exposure is within acceptable limits. For a given exposure (ML), the allowable exposure duration (t) can be calculated from:

$$t = (EL \times t_a)/ ML \qquad (25\text{-}30)$$

where EL is the exposure limit and ML is the measured (or calculated) level. Remember, this control measure should be used only when ML exceeds EL and the exposure duration is less than t_a.

Warning Signs. The IEEE C95.2 standard recommends the design and color scheme of warning symbols for RF radiation, RF electric currents, and for touching hazards between 3 kHz and 300 GHz. Recommendations for including this symbol in a sign are made by IEEE.[491]

Work Practices. Good work practices include reducing the source operating power during "hot" maintenance and service to levels that do not result in potential overexposure. Following maintenance activities, it is important to ensure that all fasteners have been replaced and that all areas of potential leakage, such as waveguide flanges and access panels, are secure. It is important to verify that the area is clear of personnel before switching on sources that generate RF beams. Maps of areas of potential over exposures may be generated and used with area demarcation.

Extremely Low Frequency (ELF) Fields*

Anticipation

**This section was written by Robert M. Patterson and R. Timothy Hitchcock*

The ELF spectral region includes the spectral region between 3000 and 3 Hz. In this part of the spectrum the fields are slowly time-varying and the wavelengths are quite lengthy.

When the source-receptor distance for electromagnetic radiation is large compared with the wavelength, the electric and magnetic fields are linked and must be considered together (although measurement of either will suffice). This is referred to as the "far" or "radiation" zone, where there is an electromagnetic field. (See the discussion of near and far fields in the section on radiofrequency radiation.)

When the source-receptor distance is small with respect to the wavelength, the electric and magnetic fields are not linked. This is the "near" or "static" zone, where the fields are independent and can be considered as separate entities. ELF fields have wavelengths on the order of 1000 km, so one is always in the near or static zone. ELF fields are considered as separate, independent, non-radiating electric and magnetic fields at any conceivable observation point. This is referred to as the "quasi-static approximation."

Quantities and Units

Electric fields are created by electric charges. The electric field, E, is defined by the magnitude and direction of the force it exerts on a static unit charge

$$F = qE \qquad (25\text{-}31)$$

where F is force (newton), q is electric charge (coulomb), and E is electric field (V/m).

The magnitude or intensity of E describes the voltage gradient, or the difference in voltage between two points in the field. Electric field intensities near alternating current (ac) high-voltage transmission lines are in the range of kilovolts per meter (kV/m).

The magnetic flux density, B, characterizes the magnetic field strength, H, as E characterizes the electric field and is linearly related to the magnetic field through:

$$B = \mu H \qquad (25\text{-}32)$$

Here, B = magnetic flux density (tesla [T]), μ = magnetic permeability, and H = magnetic field strength (A/m).

The magnetic permeability depends on the medium; the magnetic permeability of a vacuum is designated μ_0. Air and biological matter have permeabilities essentially equal to μ_0. This means that the magnetic flux density is unchanged by these materials.

Basic Physics

Magnetic fields are created by moving charges, or currents. This applies to all fields, whether they are from magnets, power lines, or the earth. Just as the electric field is defined by the force on a unit charge, the magnetic field is defined by the magnitude and direction of the force exerted on a moving charge or current

$$F = q(v \times B) \quad (25\text{-}33)$$

where

v = velocity (m/sec).

The magnetic flux density, which may be represented by lines of induction per unit area, has units of tesla, T. One tesla is 10,000 gauss (G), a frequently used engineering unit. The microtesla (μT) is most appropriately scaled and hence, more convenient, for environmental levels. Convenient conversions are 1 μT equals 10 mG, and 1 mT equals 10 G. The static magnetic flux density of the earth is about 50 μT.

The CGS system of units, which preceded the present SI system, used units of centimeters, grams, and seconds. In the CGS system, the permeability, μ_0, is dimensionless and equal to 1. As a result, B numerically approximates H in the CGS system, and the two came to be used interchangeably. The value of μ0 in the SI system is 4×10^{-7} H/m. This factor can be used to convert true magnetic field strength (A/m) to magnetic flux density (T) in air by the expression $B = \mu_0 H$.

Interaction with Matter/People. Electric fields interact with humans through the outer surface of the body, inducing fields and currents within the body. Hair vibration or other sensory stimuli may occur in fields greater than 10 kV/m. A safety issue arises from currents induced in metal structures, which may produce shocks when humans contact the structure and provide a path to ground.

An electric field causes currents to flow in the body, as expressed by Ohm's law:

$$J = \sigma E \quad (25\text{-}34)$$

where J = induced current density (A/m²), and σ = tissue conductivity in siemens per meter (S/m).

A grounded person in an electric field experiences a short-circuit current (in this case, current flowing out of the foot to earth) of approximately[492]:

$$I_{sc} = 1.5 \times 10^{-7} f W^{2/3} E_o \quad (25\text{-}35)$$

where

I_{sc} = short-circuit current (μA);
f = frequency (Hz);
W = weight (g); and
E_o = external electric field strength (V/m).

Thus, a person weighing 70 kg would have a total short-circuit current of about 153 μA in a 10 kV/m field at 60 Hz. Deno[493], and Kaune and Phillips[494], investigated current flow in models of humans and laboratory animals exposed to 60-Hz electric fields. Their data indicate that current densities induced in a grounded, erect person exposed to a 10 kV/m vertical electric field are 0.55 μA/cm² through the neck and 2 μA/cm² through the ankles.

Time-varying magnetic fields induce electric fields, which in turn induce currents, in tissue in direct proportion to the magnetic flux density, the frequency of oscillation, and the radius of the current loop. The electric field and current flow are perpendicular to the flux density. A vertically directed flux density causes current to flow in standing humans in loops whose plane is perpendicular to the vertical axis. For a sinusoidally varying flux density and a circular current flow, the current density can be expressed as:

$$J = \sigma \pi f r B \quad (25\text{-}36)$$

where f = frequency (Hz), and r = loop radius in meters (around 0.15–0.2 m).

With average tissue conductivity equal to 0.2 S/m, the current density at the perimeter of the torso of an adult can be approximated as:

$$J = 0.1 f B \quad (25\text{-}37)$$

The maximum current density induced in the normal residential environment is of the order of μA/m². For electric arc welders it may be of the order of mA/m² or greater.

With photon energy directly proportional to frequency, it is readily apparent that ELF fields will cause neither ionization nor heating. Because the body is a relatively good conductor, the highest internal field that can be induced by an E-field strength in air is about 1 V/m, which leads to a mass-normalized rate of energy transfer of 10^{-4} W/kg, 4 orders of magnitude less than the resting metabolic rate (1 W/kg).[(495)] Pulsed magnetic fields can produce higher internal electric fields, but they are still too small to produce measurable tissue heating. Any interactions of ELF fields in air with humans are thus non-thermal.

Biological and Health Effects

The search for biological and health effects of EMF exposure has been going on at an accelerating pace for more than three decades. Results have been mixed, and their interpretation has been controversial, with little consensus on biological effects and virtually none on health effects that might arise from fields at the levels found in occupational or general community environments.

This section will focus on the synopsis and presentation of the most recent findings and determinations on various health effects made in topical review papers. This approach is being taken due to the vast number of independent studies completed in recent years in this ever expanding area os scientific research. And it is a way to highlight the key assessments and provide an indication of where health effects analyses and potential regulatory outcomes might be headed. The section closes with an overview of the epidemiological studies into possible health effects of EMF.

The previous section described how the effect of fields exerts force on charged entities, creating currents, and how the relations between fields and induced currents are quantified through the conductivity of the medium, for example, tissue. Organizations have recommended exposure limits for ELF-EMF based on the following correspondence between current density and biological effects[(496)]:

- 1–10 mA/m²; minor biological effects have been reported;
- 10–100 mA/m²; well established effects occur, including effects on the visual and nervous systems;
- 100–1000 mA/m²; stimulation of excitable tissue occurs, causing possible health hazards;
- 1000 mA/m² and above; extrasystoles and ventricular fibrillation can occur.

Recalling the approximation, J » 6 B (at 60 Hz), magnetic fields of the order of 1 mT would lead to current densities in the range of 6 mA/m².

Phosphenes. This is the sensation of flickering light within the eye. It appears to be produced by stimulation of retinal tissue and by any number of agents (e.g., pressure, mechanical shock, chemical substances, and sudden fright). If the agent inducing phosphenes is ELF fields, then it is termed electrophosphenes and magnetophosphenes, depending on the field that causes them. Phosphenes occur when the induced current density is of the order of 10 mA/m² or more. Studies have demonstrated that the sensitivity to phosphenes is greatest around 20 Hz. In general, B-field intensities must be on the order of 10 mT for the production of magnetophosphenes.

Calcium Efflux. *In vitro* experiments have examined effects on doubly-ionized, radioactive calcium. occurring in windows of field frequency and power. A chemical exposure analogy would be as if a little benzene were harmful but a greater amount were not, and a still greater amount were again harmful.

In the first of these studies[(497)], a modest increase in the exchange of calcium-45 with a physiologic bath was observed for sectioned chick brain exposed to a 147-MHz carrier wave amplitude modulated at 16 Hz. Other modulation frequencies did not produce as large an effect, and exposure to just a 16-Hz E field had the opposite effect, decreasing efflux. Later work suggested that the effect depended on the relative orientation and strength of the earth's magnetic field, and that it occurred in "windows" of field frequency and intensity and even temperature of the experimental preparation.[(498–501)]

Genetic Effects. Genetic toxicology studies have found no reliable effects, but there are scattered positive findings.[(502–504)]

Reproduction and Development. Studies with test animals have examined a variety of species with exposure to E or B fields.

There have been scattered positive findings for exposure to test animals, but no consistent, reproducible observations.[505] For example, in a multigenerational study, female miniature swine were exposed to 60-Hz E fields of 35 kV/m for 20 hr/day. When these and an unexposed control group were bred with unexposed males, the control group had a greater rate of fetal malformations than the exposed group. This result reversed in a second breeding. Breeding of the offspring produced similarly conflicting results.[506] Because of the ambiguities in the swine study, a study using a similar protocol was performed with rats (E field = 0, 10, 65, and 130 kV/m).[507] There were no significant increases in litters with malformations among the exposed group of animals.

Six laboratories in North America and Europe examined the effect of B-fields (1 μT and pulsed at 100 Hz) on chicken embryos.[508] Data from two laboratories and pooled data from all laboratories found a significant increase in abnormal embryos in the exposed groups. However, the interaction between the incidence of abnormalities and the laboratory doing the experiment was also significant, that is, the effect of exposure differed significantly among laboratories.

Flux densities of 1 or 0.61 mT at 60 Hz were used in two studies of reproductive and developmental toxicology in rats. There was a significant difference in the number of fetuses per litter in the 1-mT group in the first experiment, but this was not observed in the replicate study. There were no significant differences in fetal body weight or the incidence of malformations among the exposure groups.[509] Other researchers exposed pregnant rats (0.002, 0.2, and 1 mT at 60 Hz) and found no significant differences in developmental abnormalities.[510]

In a recent review by Juutilainen, he looked at numerous experimental studies on the effets of ELF on animal development. Overall, it was conculded that ELF electric fields up to 150 kV/m rather consistently do not suggest developmental effects. Although some studies have shown possible skeletal alterations in mammals, taken as a whole, experimental studies of adverse developmental effects of ELF have not been established.[511]

Reviews of human studies are available.[505,512] Evaluations examined residential exposure (appliances esp. electric blankets), occupational exposure other than VDT use (e.g., substations), and VDT use. End points evaluated include spontaneous abortion, congenital malformations, preterm delivery, low birth weight, and intrauterine growth retardation. A few scattered positive findings have been reported, but no trends established. However, there have been relatively few studies of exposures to sources other than to VDT operation. There are a number of methodological limitations which are addressed in the review articles cited above.

Effect on Melatonin. The possible effects of ELF fields on levels of the pineal hormone melatonin have been investigated. Animal studies have demonstrated effects on melatonin from E fields[513,514], B fields[515], and no effects.[516–519] Other effects include E-field exposure decreased serum melatonin but not pineal melatonin levels[520]; pulsed static B fields affected melatonin if exposure was during the mid- or late-dark phase, but not when exposure was during the day time or early dark phase[521]; short-term B-field exposure affected pineal and nocturnal serum melatonin, while long-term exposure affected just nocturnal serum melatonin[522]; serum melatonin was not affected by daytime E- and B-field exposure with a slow onset[523], but it was reduced by variable exposure with a rapid onset/offset.[524] The National Institute of Environmental Health Sciences (NIEHS) Working Group concluded that there is weak evidence that exposure to E and B fields alters melatonin in rodents but not in sheep or baboons.[525] In a study by Noonan, an assessment of occupational exposure to magnetic fields in case-referent studies of neurogenerative diseases indicated some support for an association between occupational magnetic field exposure and Parkinson's disease.[526]

The outcome of twelve studies on possible ELF-induced effects on melatonin in humans has been reviewed by the NIEHS. Five laboratory studies were negative, but one laboratory and six observational studies demonstrated some effects on melatonin or its urinary metabolite, 6-hydroxymelatonin sulfate (6-OHMS).[525] In later studies, no statistically significant effects were reported in female garment factory workers[527], men exposed to an electric sheet[528], and women[529] and men exposed to intense B fields at night.[530]

A decrease in nocturnal melatonin was observed in women in another study[531], while others have suggested a reduction in 6-OHMS associated with work in an electrical substation or with 3-phase fields.[532]

Cancer Studies[1]. A number of cancer types have been evaluated but the types studied most often in relation to ELF exposure are leukemia, brain cancer, and breast cancer. Experiments with test animals have examined initiation, promotion and co-promotion in models of mammary cancer, skin cancer, brain cancer, leukemia, and lymphoma. The findings are complex to interpret and do not demonstrate any clear trends. McCann and colleagues reviewed the published literature and concluded that "a weak promoting effect of Mfs [magnetic fields] under certain exposure conditions cannot be ruled out categorically based on available data."[533] Boorman et al. examined the literature on mammary cancer finding that "The totality of rodent data does not support the hypothesis that 50 or 60 Hz magnetic-field exposure enhances mammary cancer in rodents, nor does it provide experimental support for possible epidemiological associations between magnetic-field exposure and increased breast cancer risk."[534]

For human studies, evaluations have included both residential and occupational settings and children and adults. A number of useful review articles and meta-analyses are available including general[525,535–538] and topical reviews of leukemia[539–545], brain cancer[540,546,547], and breast cancer.[548–550]

In a review study of Childhood Leukemia Electric and Magnetic Fields Temporal Trends conducted by Kheifets in 2006, they looked at numerous studies with various methodologies to assess any patterns of exposure and possible relationships. They identified a relationship between the incidence in childhood cancer, including leukemia, and the average exposures to EMF. But because of so many approvimations an dassumptions in calculations the ecologic evidence could not meaningfully support a causal link.[551] In another review study in 2006, also by Kheifets, it was concluded that the fraction of childhood leukemia cases possibly attributable to worldwide ELF exposure is small.[552]

Early occupational studies, here defined as prior to 1993, often utilized job titles and information from death certificates. In general, many of these studies found no-to-modest increases in risk of leukemia and brain cancer and no dose-response effect.[540]

Early studies of childhood cancer utilized wire coding to classify residences with regards to potential magnetic field intensity, and spot measurements. Generally, these studies demonstrated a weak association with leukemia.[540]

More recent studies have utilized spot and personal measurement strategies and detailed numerical models to estimate exposure. Three studies examined the risk of power company workers in the U.S., Canada, and France (see Table 25.22). Of these, one reported no increase in risk of leukemia and brain cancer[553], while the others found an increase in risk of leukemia[554] and brain cancer.[553] A combined analysis of the data from the three studies found that the relative risk (RR) per 10 μT-yrs was 1.09 (95% confidence interval, CI = 0.98 to 1.21) for leukemia and 1.12 (95% CI = 0.98 to 1.28) for brain cancer.[541]

A meta-analysis of 38 studies of occupational B-field exposure and leukemia reported a pooled RR = 1.18 (CI = 1.12 to 1.124). The highest pooled RR (1.55, CI = 1.10 to 2.19) was for the chronic lymphocytic leukemia subtype (12 studies).[542] The NIEHS Working Group found limited evidence of an increased risk of chronic lymphocytic leukemia in workers and exposure to ELF magnetic fields.[525] The Advisory Group on

Table 25.22 — Summary of Three Power Industry Studies

Study	*Sahl et al. (1993)*[621]	*Theriault et al. (1994)*[622]	*Savitz et al. (1995)*[623]
Exposure measure	above mean (25 μT-years)	above 90th percentile (15.7 μT-years)	above 90th percentile 4.3 μT-work years or 18.8 μT-years
Brain cancer RR (95% CI)	0.81 (0.48–1.36)	1.95 (0.76–5.00)	2.29 (1.15–4.56)
Leukemia RR (95% CI)	1.07 (0.80–1.45)	1.75 (0.77–3.96)	1.11 (0.57–2.14)
AML RR (95% CI)	——	2.68 (0.50–14.50)	1.62 (0.51–5.12)

[1]Note: Because of the large number and complex nature of published studies, this section will draw largely upon findings from critical reviews published in either the peer-reviewed literature or by expert panels.

Non-ionising Radiation (AGNIR) of the United Kingdom's National Radiological Protection Board (NRPB), concluded that a review of occupational cohort studies on leukemia and ELF exposure are equivocal, at best.(537)

A pooled analysis of childhood leukemia found no increase in risk for B-fields < 0.4μT, while the RR = 2.00 (95% CI = 1.27 to 3.13) for children with residential exposure m 0.4 μT.(614) Wartenberg performed a meta-analysis for childhood leukemia finding the following RR values: 1.1 (0.9–1.3) for spot measurements, 1.2 (0.9–1.5) for calculated fields, 2.7 (0.8–8.7) for wire codes by spot measurements, and 1.6 (0.5–4.6) for wire codes by 24-hour measurements. He estimates 175 cases of leukemia by wire code data and 240 cases by spot measurements with the following assumptions: exposure causes leukemia; the studies are accurate and representative; and that exposure follows a log-linear relationship.(545) In a review of the literature, both the NIEHS Working Group and the International Agency for Research on Cancer (IARC) found limited evidence for an increased risk of childhood leukemia and residential exposure.(538)

Kheifets and colleagues have reviewed the literature on brain cancer. In meta-analyses she reported a pooled RR = 1.21 (CI = 1.11–1.33) in 1995(546) and a pooled OR = 1.16 (95% CI = 1.08–1.24) in 2001. In the latter review, Kheifets states that there is "little support for an association between residential EMF exposure and childhood or adult brain cancer."(547) In a review of three major studies of utility workers, the estimated combined RR/10 μT-yrs was 1.12 (95% CI = 0.98–1.28), as noted above.(541) Members of the NIEHS Working Group(525) and IARC(538) concluded that there was inadequate evidence of brain cancer in adults and children, while AGNIR concluded evidence from cohort studies was equivocal.(537)

The risk of breast cancer and ELF exposure has been evaluated in men and pre-, peri-, and postmenopausal women. Erren reviewed 48 published studies and included studies with estimates of RR (24 for women and 15 for men) in a meta-analysis. The average RR = 1.12 (95% CI = 1.09–1.15) for women and 1.37 (95% CI = 1.11–1.71) for men demonstrates a small increase in risk of breast cancer.(548) After reviewing the literature, other researchers have suggested that this is an area requiring further research.(549,550)

Over the years, a number of expert panels have addressed the question of ELF exposure and cancer. Three of these mentioned earlier are the NIEHS Working Group, IARC, and AGNIR. All three groups examined an extensive volume of scientific literature in their assessments. Based upon their evaluations, the NIEHS Working Group classified ELF magnetic fields as a Group 2B (possibly) carcinogen for childhood leukemia and chronic lymphocytic leukemia in workers. IARC found limited evidence for an excess cancer risk on the basis of childhood leukemia from exposure to high residential magnetic fields, and also placed ELF magnetic fields in Group 2B. IARC found inadequate evidence for all other cancer types in children and adults from exposure to ELF electric and magnetic fields.(538) AGNIR, led by Sir Richard Doll, found "some epidemiological evidence that prolonged exposure to higher magnetic fields is associated with a small risk of leukaemia in children."(537) Both IARC and AGNIR cite a value of m0.4 μT when referring to high levels of residential exposure.

In a 2001 report by the International Commission for Non-Ionizing Radiation Protection they reviewed hundereds of recent studies and analyzed the results. Overall the group found numerous methodologic problems with the study of extremely low level electromagnetic fields that make it difficult to acertain true associations between exposue and health outcomes. The study determined that there etiologic relationship between any chronic diseases and exposure to EMF. The study did find however, an association between postnatal exposures to levels above 0.4 μT and childhood leukemia.(556)

Recognition

Generation

Electric fields are generated by electric charge, while magnetic fields are produced by the motion of electric charge. In the workplace, these fields are produced by the generation, transmission, and use of electricity, and anything in this path is a potential exposure source, from the generator, to the power lines, to an electric drill or clock.

Sources

Useful reviews of sources of and exposure to ELF magnetic fields are available.(557–563) Others have examined exposure from specific sources or environments including residential[(564–568)], appliances[(569–572)], schools[(573)], office[(574–578)], medical[(579–582)], transportation[(583–587)], farming[(589)], communications and broadcasting[(589,590)], industry[(591–599)], and utilities.[(600–605)]

The strongest electric fields generally occur in power plants, where maximum levels of 15–29 kV/m have been recorded, or near transmission lines and are typically about 10 kV/m directly under the wires and 1 or 2 kV/m at the edge of the right-of-way.[(557)] Fields from building wiring, power tools, and other electrical appliances typically range only up to 100 V/m.[(604)]

Occupational sources and source characteristics are as varied as the occupational environments in which they are found. However, two basic facts may be noted: sources of strong electric fields are associated with high electrical charge, such as around high-voltage equipment, and sources of high magnetic fields are generally characterized by high currents, such as around high-amperage equipment or locations of high current flow. These sources need not be associated with heavy industry; electrical transformers and wiring located in office building vaults are non-industrial sources of high fields.

Stuchly and Lecuyer measured fields at the worker's position for 22 electric arc welding machines, which use high amounts of current. Electric fields were generally low, about 1 V/m (maximum = 300 V/m; mean = 47 V/m). Magnetic flux densities ranged from about 1 μT to a few hundred μT, and averaged 136 μT. The highest measurement was 1 mT at a worker's hand. The frequency of highest flux density was usually 60 Hz, although for some sources it was 120 or 180 Hz.[(594)]

Rosenthal and Abdollahzadeh measured flux densities in microelectronics fabrication rooms. In the aisles of the rooms, values ranged from 0.01 to 0.7 μT and averaged 0.07 μT. Higher levels were found near specific pieces of equipment. The authors estimated an 8-hr time-weighted-average exposure for a worker using the furnace to be 1.8 μT, and 0.6 μT for one using the sputterer.[(596)]

Very high flux densities were measured at the worker's position at welding machines and steel furnaces. Seventy mT was measured at an induction heater, and 10 mT was found near a spot welder.[(597)]

Bowman et al. sampled 114 work sites. "Electrical worker" environments had geometric mean electric fields of 4.6 V/m and flux densities of 0.5 μT. Secretaries had values of 2–5 V/m, 0.31 μT if they used a VDT, and 0.11 μT if they did not. For power line workers, the overhead line environment yielded geometric means of 160 V/m and 4.2 μT. A value of 5.7 μT was determined for underground lines. Other findings included 298 V/m and 3.9 μT at a transmission substation, and 72 V/m and 2.9 μT at a distribution substation. Radio and television repair shops yielded 45 V/m, while ac welding produced 4.1 μT.[(185)]

Personal exposure data have been collected for work, non-work, and sleep periods in a study of 36 Canadians – 20 utility workers and 16 office workers. The time-weighted average of 1-week's data yielded a geometric mean electric field of 10 V/m. The utility workers' geometric mean magnetic field exposure was 0.31 μT. It was 0.19 μT for the office workers. Both groups had a level of 0.15 μT while sleeping. At work, the utility workers' exposures averaged 48.3 V/m and 1.66 μT. Office workers were exposed to a geometric mean level of 4.9 V/m and 0.16 μT.[(606)]

Environmental measures of ELF-magnetic flux densities have been reported. In a study by Straume, the environmental levels of ELF were measured with a hand-held magnetic flux density meter and compared with International Commission on Nonionizing Radiation Protection basic restrictions. Average levels indicated between 0.13 μT to 0.9 μT with a peak recorded value of 37 μT.[(607)]

Other personal exposure data include: geometric mean exposure between 0.66 and 1.27 μT for captains and first officers of commercial airliners[(608)]; 8-hr geometric mean exposure of 0.53 μT for low-voltage electrical distribution workers versus 0.46 μT for high-voltage workers in a petroleum refinery[(598)]; full-shift TWA exposures of 0.498 and 0.654 μT for pharmacy workers[(582)]; levels between 0.03 and 1.3 μT for trolley transport workers[(587)]; TWA exposures between 0.02 and 8.26 μT for workers at a uranium enrichment plant; and full-shift personal exposures of 21.2 μT for manual metal arc welding and 2.3 μT for active gas welding.[(595)]

Evaluation of exposure to workers grouped into 28 occupational categories at 5 United States power companies found the highest time-averaged B-field personal exposures in electricians, linemen, and cable splicers. Also, power-plant operators, instrumentation and control technicians, and machinists may also receive relatively high B-field exposures.[605]

Evaluation

Exposure Guidelines

Limits on exposure to extremely low electric fields, magnetic fields, and contact currents have been primarily designated as voluntary guidelines or standards. These have been developed by a variety of worldwide organizations including the International Commission on Non-Ionizing Radiation Protection, the Institute of Electrical and Electronic Engineers, and the Amercian Conference of Governmental Industrial Hygienists. The limits are primarily selected to minimize the possibility of neural stimulation. They result in limitations on electric fields and current density levels that may result in tissue from exposure sources. This may also include the avoidance of annoying or startleing interactions that are experienced when exposed to certain levels of spark discharge or contact current. For the most part, limits are related to the amount of exposure induced stimulation that results in the induction of visual phosphenes that result when electric currents or magnetic fields are applied to the head. The recommended limits are als related to excitation of central and peripheral neural tissue and cardiac muscle.[439,609,610]

Ideally, exposure guidelines and standards are established on the basis of an accepted mechanism of interaction, dose-response studies in animals, and epidemiological evidence of similar effects in humans. None of this has occurred for ELF fields. No accepted, biologically plausible mechanism has been advanced to explain how fields interact with biological systems to yield observed in vitro responses, much less disease in an organism. In fact, the field parameter or parameters to be measured, because of their possible biological significance, are unknown. The traditional approaches that "more is worse" and that time-weighted-average or even peak exposures are the quantities of interest have been called into question by studies suggesting that effects occur in windows of frequency and power. The choice of exposure metric is thus made difficult by the lack of knowledge about interaction mechanisms and the lack of a clearly defined, exposure-associated health effect.

The current biological basis for the exposure guidelines includes acute effects to central nervous system tissues. Effects that are often cited include phosphenes and alterations of visual evoked potentials (VEP). These effects occur at relatively high levels of exposure. Phosphenes is a biological effect while alterations of the VEP "are not necessarily harmful."[611]

Exposure guidance, based on the current understanding of ELF-induced biological effects, has been developed by a number of countries and organizations.[611,612] This chapter will focus on guidelines published by the ACGIH®[99] and the ICNIRP.[2][439,613]

The rationale for these exposure limits is based on induced body currents. For occupational exposures, both the ACGIH® and ICNIRP recommend limiting induced current densities in the body to those levels that occur normally, that is, up to about 10 mA/m^2 (higher current densities can also occur naturally in the heart). They acknowledged that biological effects have been demonstrated in laboratory studies at field strengths below those permitted by the exposure guidelines, but both concluded that there was no convincing evidence that occupational exposure to these field levels leads to adverse health effects.

The ACGIH® guideline extends into part of the RF spectral region, which that organization calls subradiofrequency.[104] The ACGIH® TLV® for occupational exposure to ELF electric fields states that exposure should not exceed 25 kV/m for frequencies from 0 (DC) to 100 Hz. For frequencies in the range of 100 Hz to 4 kHz, the TLV® is given by

$$E_{TLV} = 2.5 \times 106 / f \text{ (V/m)} \qquad (25\text{-}38)$$

where:

E has units of V/m (rms value); and

[2]At this writing, Standards Coordinating Committee 28 of the IEEE has prepared a draft standard for human exposure to electromagnetic fields between 0 and 3 kHz. This standard will not be addressed above due to its draft status.

f = frequency in Hz.

A proviso is added for workers with cardiac pacemakers, limiting power-frequency exposures to 1 kV/m. Electromagnetic interference with pacemaker function may occur in some models at power-frequency electric fields as low as 2 kV/m.

The TLV® for magnetic fields from 1 to 300 Hz limits routine occupational (rms) exposure to ceiling values determined by

$$B_{TLV} = 60 / f \text{ (mT)} \qquad (25\text{-}39)$$

where f is the frequency in Hz. At frequencies below 1 Hz, the TLV is 60 mT. From 300 Hz to 30 kHz the ceiling value is a limit of 0.2 mT. For workers with cardiac pacemakers, the limit is 0.1 mT at power frequencies.

Because of ambiguities in the scientific understanding of the mechanism of biological interaction, the sub-RF TLVs are ceiling limits, that is, they are values not to be exceeded.[104]

ICNIRP makes recommendations for exposure limits of both workers and members of the general public to electric and magnetic fields.[439] The fundamental quantity, the current density, is called the basic restriction and the measured field quantity is the reference level. As mentioned above, the basic restriction for the occupational standard is a current density of 10 mA/m^2, while the basic restriction for the general public is 2 mA/m^2 for frequencies between 4 Hz and 1 kHz. At frequencies between 1 and 4 Hz, the current density is frequency dependent. ICNIRP does not recommend an averaging time for the ELF spectral region "because the known effects of induced and contact currents at those frequencies are acute phenomena involving a rapid response of the nervous system."[613]

Frequency-dependent reference levels are recommended both E and B. The allowable E-field strength reaches a maximum in the band between 1 and 25 Hz at values of 20 and 10 kV/m for occupational and general public exposure, respectively. Field strength then decreases with frequency before reaching another plateau. Exposure limits at 60 Hz are 8333 V/m for workers and 4167 V/m for members of the general public.

For B fields, the maximum flux density occurs at less than 1 Hz, then decreases in a frequency-dependent manner up to around 800 Hz. Exposure limits at 60 Hz are 417 and 83 μT for workers and the general public, respectively.

Instruments

Discussions of ELF EMF measurement instrumentation are available.[574,614–618] Instrument types include survey instruments and personal exposure monitors, as well as waveform capture instruments that provide spectral data. In general, instruments are broad-band and dedicated to either E-field or B-field measurement, although some instruments measure E and B fields. Antennas are a single-axis or tri-axis design. Instruments incorporating single-axis antennas are sensitive to the orientation of the antenna relative to the incident field; the tri-axis designs are isotropic.

Electric Fields. E fields are usually measured with a device shown schematically in Figure 25.24a. Called a free-body dipole probe, it measures the induced current between two halves of an isolated conducting body. In an electric field that is parallel to the axis of the box, the current flowing between the two halves is proportional to the field strength and frequency: $I = KfE$, where I is the current (A), f is the frequency (e.g., 60 Hz), E is the electric field strength (V/m), and K is a proportionality factor. Electric fields are modified or "perturbed" by conducting objects, such as persons making measurements. For this reason the device is often extended at the end of a non-conducting pole or connected to the read-out unit by a fiber optics cable.

Magnetic Fields. Instruments commonly used to measure power-frequency magnetic fields (or flux densities) are based on Faraday's law of voltage induction in a conducting coil (see Figure 25.24b). A conducting loop in a time-varying magnetic field will have a voltage (that is, an electromotive force, or emf) induced in it that is proportional to the time rate of change of the field and the area of the loop. In a sinusoidally varying field, the induced emf equals $2fnAB$, where f is the frequency, n is the number of turns in the loop, A is the area of the loop, and B is the magnetic flux density (tesla) perpendicular to the plane of the loop. The device can be made more sensitive by increasing the area or the number of loops, or both. A standard measurement procedure

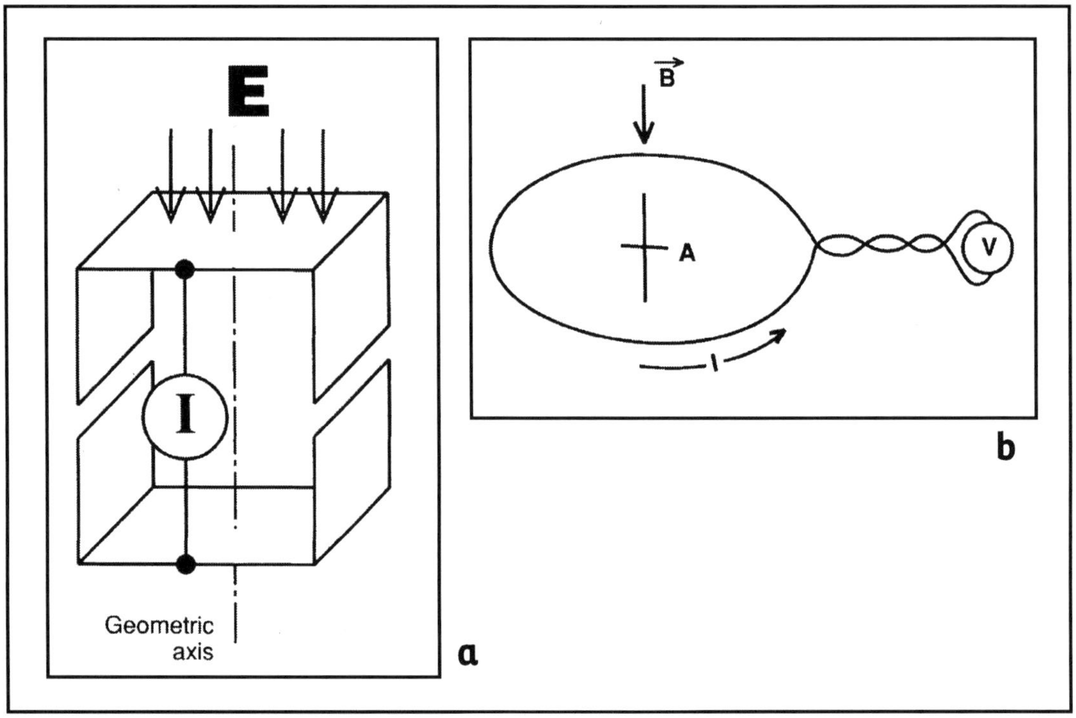

Figure 25.24 — (a) Schematic showing the principle of operation of a free-body electric-field meter. A current flows between the two halves in proportion to the electric-field strength. (b) Schematic of the principle of operation of a magnetic-field coil. The voltage induced in the coil is proportional to the magentic-flux density, its frequencym the area of the coil, and the number of loops.

is to orient the coil within the field to obtain a maximum reading.

Alternatively, the magnitude of the resultant flux density can be calculated from three measurements taken at right angles to each other:

$$B = (B_x^2 + B_y^2 + B_z^2)^{1/2} \qquad (25\text{-}40)$$

However, it is difficult for the surveyor to rotate the probe precisely around the center of the coil, leading to measurement error. More sophisticated instruments incorporate three orthogonal coils and electronic circuitry to find the resultant (i.e., they do not require special orientation). Such an instrument is shown in Figure 25.25.

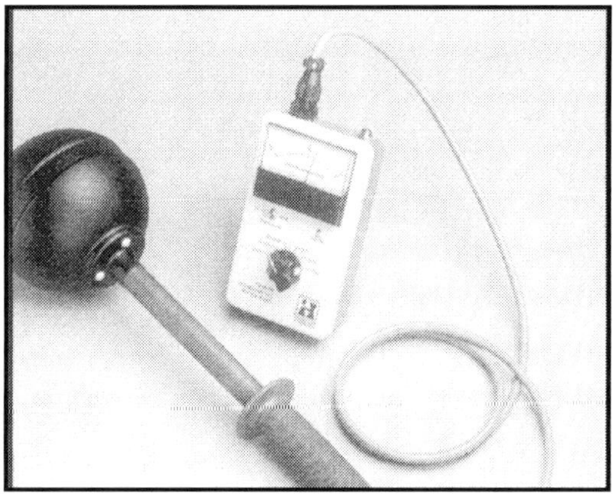

Figure 25.25 — A broadband ELF magnetic-field instrument that includes a tri-axis antenna array contained within the black plastic sphere. (Courtesy of Holaday Industries, Inc.)

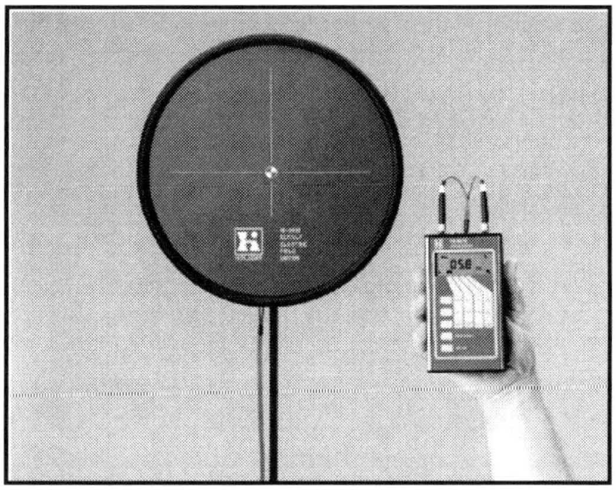

Figure 25.26 — A broadband E-field antenna connected to a datalogger with a fiber optic connection. (Courtesy of Holaday Industries, Inc.)

Many companies manufacture monitors that use the principles described here. Their products differ in how they record measurements. Some, useful mainly for surveys, indicate only the instantaneous field intensity. When connected to a device such as a chart recorder or data logger (see Figure 25.26), these instruments can collect data over time or space for later analysis.

Personal Exposure Monitors. A number of personal exposure monitors that are worn on the body have been introduced. These are most useful for magnetic fields since the human body does not perturb low-frequency magnetic fields (i.e., the body appears to be largely transparent to these fields), as it does electric fields. In general, these instruments include on-board microprocessors to control data recording and recovery. Comparisons and specifications of some personal monitors have been reviewed in the literature.[619–626]

Exposure Assessment

Field surveys include source identification and characterization, observation of the interaction of the workers with the source, followed by collection of measurement data. Various organizations and workers have suggested measurement strategies and exposure assessment. NIOSH has published a manual of measurement and computational methods.[627] Other published methods include those for the workplace[557,628–632], schools[573], office environment[577,578], utilities[601,605,633,634], transportation[629], and residence.[563,634–637]

Control Measures

Engineering Control

Methods of reducing field levels and exposure levels are receiving increasing attention. This area of inquiry and its application are generally referred to as field management. Three broadly described methods are available for reducing field levels: shielding, separation, and cancellation.

Shielding is probably the simplest way to reduce electric fields.[638] For 60-Hz fields, air has a conductivity of about 10^{-9} S/m, while the conductivity of metals is above 10^{+7} S/m. The factor of 10^{+16} greater conductivity of metals causes charge to be conducted to a grounded metal surface, terminating the field.[639] Shielding of magnetic fields can be accomplished near isolated equipment, such as transformers, but not easily. Special, conductive, high-permeability materials and designs are required. Shielding may be either passive or active. Passive shielding utilizes currents induced by ambient magnetic fields, while active shielding utilizes the purposeful generation of currents in shielding materials that where the "magnitude, direction, and phase angle create fields in opposition to the ambient fields."[640]

Separation is effective and can be useful when adequate distances can be maintained between the source of the field and the person exposed. The strength of a magnetic field from an electric current is expressed by the Law of Biot and Savart:

$$dB = K\, I\, dl \times r / r^3 \qquad (25\text{-}41)$$

where:

K = a constant;
I = current in a conductor of length dl; and
r = distance from the conductor.

Applying the Biot-Savart Law with I in amperes and r in feet, the magnetic field due to current in an effectively infinitely long wire is given by $B = 6.56\, I/r$, and for two closely spaced, parallel wires, the field is $B = 6.56\, Id/r^2$, with d being the spacing of the wires. Finally, if the current flows in a loop, the field is $B = 10.31\, Ia^2/r^3$, where a is the area of the loop.[639] Thus, magnetic field intensities decline with distance for a single wire, with the square of the distance from parallel wires such as power lines or house wiring, and with the cube of the distance from wire loops such as those in motors or on electric stoves.

Cancellation can be applied on scales from power lines to electric blanket wiring. The general principle involves having wires in proximity carry current, and produce fields, that are opposite in phase. The field from one wire then effectively cancels the field from the other at locations removed from the two.

Administrative and Procedural Control

Administrative control measures may be limited because the exposure guidelines (e.g., TLV®) are expressed as a ceiling value, and not as a time-weighted average. Thus, time limitation of exposures may not be effective.

An alternative is the administrative approach of prudent avoidance (also referred to as the precautionary principle) to limit exposures.[557] Prudent avoidance is an approach in which one chooses a low-cost, easily accomplished method to reduce exposure but makes no concerted effort in this regard. An example is the choice between walking in the vicinity of a high-strength field source or taking an equally effective, alternative route farther away from the source.

Static Magnetic Fields

Due to the recent rapid expansion in the development and use of technologies and industries using strong static magnetic fields a brief discussion will be presented here. In 2006 the World Health Organization published a health criteria document on static magnetic fields as part of the Environmental Health Criteria Program.[641] The document provided a review of current health effects and biological responses from static magnetic fields that became the basis for recommended exposure guidelines in the document.

Sources of Exposure

The earth's static magnetic field averages approzimately 50 μT, and varies between 30 to 70 μT. The magnetic flux densities under direct current transmission lines can reach 20 μT. Other sources in common residential and industrial uses may result in localizaed magnetic fields up to 0.5 mT.[642]

Other sources of high static magnetic fields include magnetic resonance (MR) medical imaging systems. MR systems generate typcial flux densities from 0.15 to 3.0 T for limited durations (typcially less than one hour).[643] Some of these types of systems may now however, achieve flux densities up to 10 T.

A wide variety of new emerging technologies also may generate strong static magnetic fields. Fields inside magnetically levitated trains may have typcial flux densities of 100 μT with certain peak values of up to several mT. Other industries with strong static magnetic fields include thermonuclear reactors, superconducting generators, and particle accelerators.

Biological and Health Effects

A timely and detailed review of scientific evidence has been completed and reported by ICNIRP.[642] Various plausible interaction mechanisms were discussed in detail including magnetic indusction,magneto-mechanico effects, and electron spin interactions. This report also provided descriptions of a variety of in vivo and in vitro studies on related health effects. The review includes results of laboratory studies with in vitro systems, lab animals, and humans. Epidemiological studies are also reported and reviewed in the ICNIRP article.

Recommended Exposure Limits

The ICNIRP recommended limits that resulted from the analysis of the latest health effects research assessment indicated that occupational exposue to the head and trunk should not exceed a spation peak magnetic flux density of 2 mT in most situations. When flux densities are restricted to the limbs, the levels can be permitted up to 8 mT.[642]

Limits of flux density exposure to the general public should not exceed 400 mT. In addition, care should be taken not to inadvertently expose members of the general public to levels over 0.5 mT when controls cannot be implemented to ensure these people do not have implanted electronic medical devices or implants with ferromagnetic materials. So as a practical note, unless the environment is controlled to exclude people with medical devices and implants, the area flux densities should be maintained below 0.5 mT.

Nonionizing Radiation Control Program

The goal of the radiation control program is to ensure that sources of nonionizing radiation minimize the risk of adverse health effects to the users. An operational nonionizing radiation control program, which will help meet this goal, should incorporate the elements compiled in Table 25.23. A few of the key features included in this table are discussed next.

Responsibility

Management must recognize the necessity of having a nonionizing radiation protection program and take ownership. The authority and responsibility to implement the program should reside with a knowledgeable (competent) person, such as the Nonionizing Radiation Safety Coordinator (NRSC).[644] It is possible that the individual responsible for the ionizing radiation program or the laser safety program (the RPO or LSO, respectively) may be assigned the responsibility for the complete nonionizing radiation safety program. The competent person should have or receive technical training commensurate with the degree of hazard presented by the workplace sources.[243]

In organizations with a variety of NIR sources, it may be prudent to establish a Nonionizing Radiation Safety (NRS) committee.[644] The responsibilities of the committee include, but are not limited to, recommending policies and procedures, providing technical advice, and reviewing qualifications of users, equipment requests, and exposure reports. In practice, there are few NRS committees, but a number of facilities do have laser safety committees, as recommended in ANSI Z136.1.[207]

Medical Monitoring

In the U.S., there are few consensus recommendations for medical monitoring for nonionizing radiation workers. ANSI Z136.1 recommends medical surveillance prior to work with Class 3b and Class 4 lasers and following accidental exposure. Workers are classified as either incidental or laser personnel. Incidental personnel should be evaluated for visual acuity, while laser personnel should receive a more comprehensive ocular examination. Skin examinations are suggested if individuals have a history of photosensitivity and work with UV lasers.[207]

NIOSH made recommendations for workers who are exposed to UV radiation. These include a review of the medical history with respect to sunlight-related conditions, and a suggestion to provide information to workers to raise their level of awareness of possible UV-related conditions.[105]

OSHA and NIOSH have supported medical monitoring for individuals who work with RF sealers and heaters.[645] The World Health Organization (WHO) recommends medical surveillance if RF exposure "would significantly exceed the [IRPA] general population limits."[276] Some organizations, primarily military and defense contractors, perform ocular surveillance exams of RF workers. These may include preplacement, termination, and accident exams.[278,646,647]

Regarding medical examinations for ELF-exposed individuals, according to WHO, "In view of the fact that there is no health effect that could be attributed specifically to ELF exposure, it is not practicable to recommend any specific medical examinations, apart from those that may be appropriate for electrical fitters and linemen in general."[4]

Table 25.23 — Elements of a Nonionizing Radiation Protection Program

- Program responsibility
- Inventory of sources
- Prepurchase approval of sources
- Hazard assessment
- Accident/incident investigation
- Control measures
- Information and training
- Hazard communication
- Medical surveillance
- Instrument calibration
- Self-checks and audits
- Documentation
- Record keeping

Information and Training

Employees should be provided with information concerning NIR sources in their workplaces, potential exposures, and operating procedures. Some organizations recommend that individuals who have a high likelihood of being exposed at or above the applicable exposure limits should receive education and training commensurate with the level of risk. For example, U.S. Department of Defense Instruction 6055.11 requires RF safety training for "personnel who routinely work directly with equipment that emits RF levels in excess" of the exposure limits.[647] Also, ANSI Z136.1 requires laser safety training of users who are at greatest risk of overexposure (i.e., users of Class 3b and Class 4 lasers). It may be prudent, however, to provide brief information sessions to individuals who have low-level exposures or where there is a low risk of exposure.

Informational and training requirements are often reviewed during the prepurchase review meeting. DOE recommends that workers be trained "prior to assignment to a job involving potential exposure to NIR and at least annually thereafter."[648]

NIR safety training should provide the exposed individuals with an understanding of the sources and exposure levels in their workplaces. This information will help place the potential exposures in perspective. Other information that might be in the training program includes company information (policy, operating procedures, medical monitoring/surveillance, intracompany contacts, etc.) and information on instrumentation, as appropriate.

Hazard Communication

Although OSHA did not extend the hazard communication law to physical agents, the concept of effective risk communication is also integral to programs dealing with physical agents. As a minimum, the nonionizing radiation safety program should familiarize exposed workers with the potential hazards of nonionizing radiation. To maximize effectiveness, the program will also proactively share information about exposure levels and the resulting risks with the workers. Such an approach helps simplify and explain otherwise complex and often confusing issues dealing with real and purported biologic effects of nonionizing radiation. Documentation of the results of any hazard evaluations should be shared with employees who use the source, and their supervisors.

The conclusions of accident investigations should be made available to employees, including the outcome of field evaluations and clinical examinations.

Self-Checks and Audits

Periodic self-checks are often performed by individuals responsible for significant sources of nonionizing radiation. These include checks of hardware and administrative controls. Periodic audits may be used by the competent person to evaluate the effectiveness of the self-check program.

Summary

Nonionizing radiation includes UV, visible, IR, RF, and ELF spectral regions and laser radiation. Sources of NIR are both naturally occurring and man-made. Because the number of man-made sources of NIR is increasing, and a larger number of these may generate more than one type of NIR, the potential for exposure to NIR is increasing.

Overexposure to NIR electromagnetic radiation and fields may cause a variety of biological and health effects. These span the spectrum from benign effects, such as constriction of the pupillary opening on exposure to light, to serious diseases, such as UV-induced skin cancer. In general, most effects are non-stochastic, with the intensity of the response varying with the magnitude of the dose or dose rate. Some stochastic effects (e.g., skin cancer) arise from UV exposure, and effects windows have been reported in *in-vitro* studies of ELF fields.

Exposure guidelines have been recommended from 180 nm in the UV-C spectral region through the ELF and sub-ELF region to fields generated by direct current (non-time-varying electric and magnetic fields). The guidelines for each spectral region are discrete, whereas the limits for laser radiation cover all optical radiation (UV, visible, and IR). Graphically depicted, the UV and RF limits are examples of envelope curve guidelines drawn around a body of effects that form the biological basis of each guideline. The RF and ELF guidelines (including sub-RF) are derived from the basic limits, SAR and current density, respectively. The guidelines are dynamic, and are revised when there is consensus concerning the available scientific evidence.

Broad-band field survey instruments are available for most NIR regions, except for some infrared and microwave wavelengths. Dosimeters or personal exposure monitors are available in the UV and ELF spectral regions, although NIR dosimetry is still a developing area at this time. Numerical modeling to predict potential exposure is useful for some sources, especially when the radiation is in the shape of a beam, as it is in lasers and some collimated microwaves.

Engineering and administrative/procedural control measures apply throughout the NIR spectrum. Shielding is an effective engineering control throughout, but is more complicated for low-frequency magnetic fields. Distance is also useful throughout, since the intensity of NIR decreases with radial distance from the source. Personal protective equipment is most useful for optical radiation.

A nonionizing radiation protection program needs management support, the involvement of a competent technical staff, and workers who are aware of the potential hazards of NIR sources with which they work. Successful implementation of such a program will minimize the risk of NIR-related health effects, meet regulatory requirements, help control insurance costs, and reduce the impact of possible negative publicity.

References

1. **International Radiation Protection Association:** Review of concepts, quantities, units and terminology for non-ionizing radiation protection. *Health Phys. 49*:1329–1362 (1985).
2. **Sutter, E.:** Quantities and units of optical radiation and their measurement. In *Dosimetry of Laser Radiation in Medicine and Biology* (SPIE Vol. IS 5), pp. 38–79. Bellingham, Wash.: SPIE Optical Engineering Press, 1989.
3. **National Council on Radiation Protection and Measurements (NCRP):** *Radiofrequency Electromagnetic Fields—Properties, Quantities and Units, Biophysical Interaction, and Measurements.* Washington, D.C.: NCRP, 1981.
4. **World Health Organization (WHO):** *Extremely Low Frequency (ELF) Fields* (Environmental Health Criteria 35). Geneva: WHO, 1984.
5. **Murray, W.E., R.T. Hitchcock, R.M. Patterson, and S.M. Michaelson:** Nonionizing electromagnetic energies. In *Patty's Industrial Hygiene & Toxicology*, vol. 3, Part B, 3rd. ed., pp. 623–727. New York: John Wiley & Sons, 1995.
6. **Sliney, D., and M. Wolbarsht:** *Safety with Lasers and Other Optical Sources.* New York: Plenum Press, 1980.
7. **World Health Organization (WHO):** *Lasers and Optical Radiation* (Environmental Health Criteria 23). Geneva: WHO, 1982.
8. **Sutter, E.:** Extended sources—concepts and potential hazards. *Optics Laser Technol. 27*:5–13 (1995).
9. **McKinlay, A.F., and B.L. Diffey:** A reference action spectrum for ultraviolet induced erythema in human skin. *CIE J. 66*:17–22 (1987).
10. **Diffey, B.L.:** Observed and predicted minimal erythema doses: A comparative study. *Photochem. Photobiol. 60*:380–382 (1994).
11. **Parrish, J.A., K.F. Jaenicke, and R.R. Anderson:** Erythema and melanogenesis of normal human skin. *Photochem. Photobiol. 36*:187–191 (1982).
12. **Matelsky, I.:** Non-ionizing radiations. In *Industrial Hygiene Highlights*, vol I. Pittsburgh: Industrial Hygiene Foundation of America, Inc., 1968.
13. **U.S. Food and Drug Administration:** *Medications that Increase Sensitivity to Light: A 1990 Listing*, by J.I. Levine (Publication no. DHHS [FDA] 91-8280). Rockville, Md.: U.S. Department of Health and Human Services, 1990.
14. **Hitchcock, R.T.:** *Ultraviolet Radiation* (Nonionizing Radiation Guide Series), 2nd ed. Fairfax, Va.: American Industrial Hygiene Association, 2001.
15. **Taylor, C.R., and A.J. Sober:** Sun exposure and skin disease. *Ann. Rev. Med. 47*:181–191 (1996).
16. **Yaar, M., and B.A. Gilchrest:** Studies of photoaging. In C.L. Galli, C.N. Hensby, and M. Marinovich, editors, *Skin Pharmacology and Toxicology*, pp. 205–209. New York: Plenum Press, 1990.
17. **International Agency for Research on Cancer (IARC):** Solar and Ultraviolet Radiation (IARC Monographs on the Evaluation of Carcinogenic Risks to Humans, vol. 55). Lyon, France: IARC, 1992.
18. **Lefell, D.J., and D.E. Brash:** Sunlight and cancer. *Sci. Am. 275*:52–59 (1996).
19. **de Gruijl, F.R.:** Skin cancer and solar UV radiation. *Eur. J. Cancer 35*:2003–2009 (1999).
20. **National Toxicology Program:** *Ninth Report on Carcinogens.* Research Triangle Park, N.C.: National Institute of Environmental Sciences, 2000.
21. **American Cancer Society:** *Skin Cancer Information.* [Online] Available at www2.cancer.org/skinGuide/index_info.html
22. **Lear, J.T., and A.G. Smith:** Basal cell carcinoma. *Postgrad. Med. J. 73*:538–542 (1997).
23. **Lear, J.T., B.B. Tan, A.G. Smith, et al.:** Risk factors for basal cell carcinoma in the UK: case-control study in 806 patients. *J. Royal Soc. Med. 90*:371–374 (1997).
24. **Lock-Andersen, J., K.T. Drzewiecki, and H.C. Wulf:** Eye and hair colour, skin type, and constitutive skin pigmentation as risk factors for basal cell carcinoma and cutaneous malignant melanoma. *Acta Derm. Venerol. 79*:74–80 (1999).
25. **English, D.R., B.K. Armstrong, A. Kricker, M.G. Winter, P.J. Heenan, and P.L. Randall:** Case-control study of sun exposure and squamous cell carcinoma of the skin. *Int. J. Cancer 77*:347–353 (1998).
26. **English, D.R., B.K. Armstrong, A. Kricker, M.G. Winter, P.J. Heenan, and P.L. Randall:** Demographic characteristics, pigmentary and cutaneous risk factors for squamous cell carcinoma of the skin: A case-control study. *Int. J. Cancer 76*:628–634 (1998).

27. **Lear, J.T., B.B. Tan, A.G. Smith, et al.:** A comparison of risk factors for malignant melanoma, squamous cell carcinoma, and basal cell carcinoma in the UK. *Int. J. Clin. Prac. 52*:145–149 (1998).
28. **Bajdik, C.D., R.P. Gallagher, G. Astrakianaskis, G.B. Hill, S. Fincham, and D.I. McLean:** Non-solar ultraviolet radiation and the risk of basal and squamous cell skin cancer. *Br. J. Cancer 73*:1612–1614 (1996).
29. **Jemal, A., S.S. Devesa, T.R. Fears, and P. Hartge:** Cancer surveillance series: Changing patterns of cutaneous malignant melanoma mortality rates among Whites in the United States. *J. Natl. Cancer Inst. 92*:8111–818 (2000).
30. **Centers for Disease Control and Prevention (CDC):** Death rates of malignant melanoma among White men—United States, 1973-1988. *Morb. Mort. Wkly Rep. 41*:20–21, 27 (1992).
31. **Setlow, R.B., E. Girst, K. Thompson, and A.D. Woodhead:** Wavelengths effective in induction of malignant melanoma. *Proc. Natl. Acad. Sci. 90*:6666–6670 (1993).
32. **Setlow, R.B.:** Relevance of in vivo models in melanoma skin cancer. *Photochem. Photobiol. 63*:410–412 (1996).
33. **National Radiological Protection Board (NRPB):** *Cellular and Molecular Effects of UVA and UVB*, by N.A. Cridland and R.D. Saunders (NRPB-R269). Chilcon, Didcot, Oxon, U.K.: NRPB, 1994.
34. **Duthie, M.S., I. Kimber, and M. Norval:** The effects of ultraviolet radiation on the human immune system. *Br. J. Dermatol. 140*:995–1009 (1999).
35. **Green, C., B.L. Diffey, and J.L.M. Hawk:** Ultraviolet radiation in the treatment of skin disease. *Phys. Med. Biol. 37*:1–20 (1992).
36. **Epstein, J.H.:** Phototherapy and photochemotherapy. *N. Engl. J. Med. 322*:1149–1151 (1990).
37. **National Institute for Occupational Safety and Health:** *Ocular Ultraviolet Effects from 295 nm to 400 nm in the Rabbit Eye*, by D.G. Pitts, A.P. Cullen, P.D. Hacker, and W.H. Parr (Publication no. HEW [NIOSH] 77-175). Cincinnati, Ohio: U.S. Department of Health, Education and Welfare, 1977.
38. **Pitts, D.G., and T.J. Tredici:** The effects of ultraviolet radiation on the eye. *Am. Ind. Hyg. Assoc. J. 32*:235–246 (1971).
39. **Taylor, H.R., S.K. West, F.S. Rosenthal, B. Munoz, H.S. Newland, H. Abbey, and E.A. Emmett:** Effect of ultraviolet radiation on cataract formation. *N. Engl. J. Med. 319*:1429–1433 (1988).
40. **Pitts, D.G., L.L. Cameron, J.G. Jule, and S. Lerman:** Optical radiation and cataracts. In *Optical Radiation and Visual Health*, pp. 5–41. Boca Raton, Fla.: CRC Press, Inc., 1986.
41. **Zigman, S.:** Recent research on near-UV radiation and the eye. In *The Biological Effects of UVA Radiation*, pp. 252–262. New York: Praeger Publishers, 1986.
42. **Dolin, P.J.:** Assessment of the epidemiological evidence that exposure to solar ultraviolet radiation causes cataract. *Doc. Ophthalmol. 88*:327–337 (1994).
43. **Delcourt, C, I. Carriere, A. Ponton-Sanchez, A. Lacroux, M.-J. Covacho, and L. Papoz:** Light exposure and the risk of cortical, nuclear, and posterior subcapsular cataracts. *Arch. Ophthalmol. 118*:385–392 (2000).
44. **Waxler, M.:** Long-term visual health problems: Optical radiation risks. In *Optical Radiation and Visual Health*, pp. 183–204. Boca Raton, Fla.: CRC Press, 1986.
45. **Dayhaw-Barker, P., D. Forbes, D. Fox, and S. Lerman:** Drug phototoxicity and visual health. In *Optical Radiation and Visual Health*, pp. 147–175. Boca Raton, Fla.: CRC Press, 1986.
46. **Lerman, S.:** Effect of UVA radiation on tissues of the eye. In *The Biological Effects of UVA Radiation*, pp. 231–251. New York: Praeger Publishers, 1986.
47. **Marshall, J.:** Ultraviolet radiation and the eye. In *Human Exposure to Ultraviolet Radiation: Risks and Regulations*, pp. 125–42. Amsterdam: Elsevier Science Publishers B.V. (Biomedical Division), 1987.
48. **Goldman, L., S.M. Michaelson, R.J. Rockwell, D.H. Sliney, B.M. Tengroth, and M.L. Wolbarsht:** Optical radiation, with particular reference to lasers. In Nonionizing Radiation Protection, 2nd ed., pp. 49–83. Copenhagen: World Health Organization, 1989.
49. **Epstein, J.H.:** Photomedicine. In *The Science of Photobiology*, 2nd ed., pp. 155–192. New York: Plenum Press, 1989.
50. **Ham, W.T., Jr., R.G. Allen, L. Feeney-Burns, and M.F. Marmor:** The involvement of the retinal pigment epithelium (RPE). In *Optical Radiation and Visual Health*, pp. 43–67. Boca Raton, Fla.:CRC Press, 1986.
51. **Geeraets, W.J.:** Radiation effects on the eye. *Ind. Med. 39*:441–450 (1970).
52. **Bullough, J.D:** The blue-light hazard: A review. *J. Illum. Eng. Soc. 29*:6–14 (2000).
53. **Kitchel, E.:** The effects of blue light on ocular health. *J. Vis. Impairment Blindness 94*:399–403 (2000).
54. **Luckiesh, M., and S.K. Guth:** Brightness in visual field at borderline between comfort and discomfort. *Illum. Eng. 44*:650–670 (1949).
55. **Moss, C.E., R.J. Ellis, W.E. Murray, and W.H. Parr:** Infrared radiation. In *Nonionizing Radiation Protection*, 2nd ed., pp. 85–115. Copenhagen: World Health Organization, 1989.

56. **National Institute for Occupational Health and Safety:** *Biological Effects of Infrared Radiation*, by C.E. Moss, R.J. Ellis, W.H. Parr, and W.E. Murray (Publication no. DHHS [NIOSH] 82-109). Cincinnati, Ohio: U.S. Department of Health and Human Services, 1982.
57. **Dunn, K.L.:** Cataract from infrared rays; "glass workers' cataract": A preliminary study. *Arch. Ind. Hyg. Occup. Med. 1*:166–180 (1950).
58. **Robinson, W.:** On bottle-maker's cataract. *Br. Med. J. 2*:381–384 (1907).
59. **Keating, G.F., J. Pearson, J.P. Simons, and E.E. White:** Radiation cataract in industry. *Arch. Ind. Health 11*:305– 315 (1955).
60. **Thorington, L.:** Spectral, irradiance and temporal aspects of natural and artificial light. *Ann. N.Y. Acad. Sci. 453*:28–54 (1985).
61. **Frederick, J.E., and A.D. Alberts:** The natural UV-A radiation environment. *Biological Responses to Ultraviolet A Radiation*, pp. 7–18. Overland Park, Kan.: Valdenmar Publishing, 1992.
62 **Garrison, L.M., L.E. Murray, and A.E.S. Green:** Ultraviolet limit of solar radiation at the earth's surface with a photon counting monochromator. *Appl. Opt. 17*:683–684 (1978).
63. **Scotto, J., T.R. Fears, and G.B. Gori:** Ultraviolet exposure patterns. *Environ. Res. 12*:228–237 (1976).
64. **Driscoll, C.M.H.:** Solar UVR measurements. *Radiat. Prot. Dosim. 64*:179–188 (1996).
65. **Diffey, B.L., M. Kerwin, and A. Davis:** The anatomical distribution of sunlight. *Br. J. Dermatol. 97*:407–410 (1977).
66. **Urbach, F.:** Geographic pathology of skin cancer. In *The Biological Effects of Ultraviolet Radiation*, pp. 635–650. New York, Pergamon Press, 1969.
67. **Diffey, B.L., T.J. Tate, and A. Davis:** Solar dosimetry of the face: The relationship of natural ultraviolet radiation exposure to basal cell carcinoma localisation. *Phys. Med. Biol. 24*:931–939 (1979).
68. **Sliney, D.H.:** The merits of an envelope action spectrum for ultraviolet radiation exposure criteria. *Am. Ind. Hyg. Assoc. J. 33*:644–653 (1972).
69. **Sliney, D.H.:** Eye protective techniques for bright light. *Ophthalmology 90*:937–944 (1983).
70. **Rosenthal, F.S., C. Phoon, A.E. Bakalian, and H.R. Taylor:** The ocular dose of ultraviolet radiation to outdoor workers. *Investig. Ophthalmol. Vis. Sci. 29*:649–656 (1988).
71. **Gies, H.P., C.R. Roy, S. Toomey, R. MacLennan, and M. Watson:** Solar UVR exposures of three groups of outdoor workers on the Sunshine Coast, Queensland. *Photochem. Photobiol. 62*:1015–1021 (1995).
72. **Larko, O., and B.L. Diffey:** Natural UV-B radiation received by people with outdoor, indoor, and mixed occupations and UV-B treatment of psoriasis. *Clin. Exp. Dermatol. 8*:279–285 (1983).
73. **Challoner, A.V.J., D. Corless, A. Davis, et al.:** Personnel monitoring of exposure to ultraviolet radiation. *Clin. Exp. Dermatol. 1*:175–179 (1976).
74. **Igawa, S., H. Kibamoto, H. Takahaski, and S. Arai:** A study on exposure to ultraviolet rays during outdoor sports activity. *J. Therm. Biol. 18*:583–586 (1993).
75. **Diffey, B.L., O. Larko, and G. Swanbeck:** UV-B doses received during different outdoor activities and UV-B treatment of psoriasis. *Br. J. Dermatol. 106*:33–41 (1982).
76. **Diffey, B.L., and A.H. Roscoe:** Exposure to solar ultraviolet radiation in flight. *Aviat. Space Environ. Med. 61*:1032–1035 (1990).
77. **McKinlay, A.F.:** Artificial sources of UVA radiation: Uses and emission characteristics. In *Biological Responses to Ultraviolet A Radiation*, pp. 19–38. Overland Park, Kan.: Valdenmar Publishing, 1992.
78. **Bergman, R.S., T.G. Parham, and T.K. McGowan:** UV emission from general lighting lamps. *J. Illum. Eng. Soc. 24*:13–24 (1995).
79. **Moseley, H.:** Ultraviolet and laser radiation safety. *Phys. Med. Biol. 39*:1765–1799 (1994).
80. **Gulvady, N.U.:** UV keratoconjunctivitis vs. established dose effect relationships. *J. Occup. Med. 18*:573 (1976).
81. **Murray, W.E.:** Ultraviolet radiation exposures in a mycobacteriology laboratory. *Health Phys. 58*:507–510 (1990).
82. **Boettrich, E.P.:** "Hazards Associated with Ultraviolet Radiation in Academic and Clinical Laboratories." Masters thesis, Department of Radiation Biology and Biophysics, University of Rochester, Rochester, N.Y., 1985.
83. **Cole, C., P.D. Forbes, R.E. Davies, and F. Urbach:** Effect of indoor lighting on normal skin. *Ann. N.Y. Acad. Sci. 453*:305–316 (1985).
84. **Diffey, B.L., and A.F. McKinlay:** The UVB content of "UVA fluorescent lamps" and its erythemal effectiveness in human skin. *Phys. Med. Biol. 28*:351–358 (1983).
85. **Fischer, T., J. Alsins, and B. Berne:** Ultraviolet-action spectrum and evaluation of ultraviolet lamps for psoriasis healing. *Int. J. Dermatol. 23*:633–637 (1984).
86. **Larko, O., and B.L. Diffey:** Occupational exposure to ultraviolet radiation in dermatology departments. *Br. J. Dermatol. 114*:479–484 (1986).
87. **Diffey, B.L.:** The risk of skin cancer from occupational exposure to ultraviolet radiation in hospitals. *Phys. Med. Biol. 33*:1187–1193 (1988).
88. **Lerman, S.:** Human ultraviolet radiation cataracts. *Ophthal. Res. 12*:303–314 (1980).

89. **Roscoe, A.H., and B.L. Diffey:** A preliminary study of blue light on an aircraft flight deck. *Health Phys. 66*:565–567 (1994).
90. **Fox, R.A., and P.W. Henson:** Potential ocular hazard from a surgical light source. *Australasian Phys. Eng. 19*:12–16 (1996).
91. **Hietanen, M.T.K., and M.J. Hoikkala:** Ultraviolet radiation and blue light from photofloods in television studios and theaters. *Health Phys. 59*:193–198 (1990).
92. **McIntyre, D.A., W.N. Charman, and I.J. Murray:** Visual safety of quartz linear lamps. *Ann. Occup. Hyg. 37*:191–200 (1993).
93. **National Institute for Occupational Safety and Health:** "Health Hazard Evaluation Report Miller Thermal Technologies, Inc., Appleton, Wisconsin," by C.E. Moss and R.L. Tubbs (Rep. no. HETA-88-136-1945; NTIS no. PB89-188031). Springfield, Va.: National Technical Information Service, 1989.
94. **National Institute for Occupational Safety and Health:** "Health Hazard Evaluation Report Cone Geochemical, Inc., Lakewood, Colorado," by C.E. Moss (Rep. no. HETA 91-095-2142; NTIS no. PB92- 133214). Springfield, Va.: National Technical Information Service, 1992.
95. **National Institute for Occupational Safety and Health:** "Health Hazard Evaluation Report Ormet Corporation, Hannibal, Ohio," by C.E. Moss and R.L. Stephenson (Rep. no. HETA 88-229-1985; NTIS no. PB90-180704). Springfield, Va.: National Technical Information Service, 1988.
96. **National Institute for Occupational Safety and Health:** "Health Hazard Evaluation Report, Louie Glass Factory, Weston, West Virginia," by C.E. Moss, R.L. Tubbs, L.L. Cameron, and E. Freund, Jr. (Rep. no HETA 88-299-2028; NTIS no. PB91-115311). Springfield, Va.: National Technical Information Service, 1990.
97. **Okuno, T., H. Saito, and J. Ojima:** Evaluation of Blue-Light hazards from Various Light Sources. In *Progress in Lens and Cataract Research.* Hockwin, O., M. Kojima, N. Takahashi, and D. H. Sliney (eds.). Basel: Karger, 2002. Dev. Ophthalmol. Vol. 35, pp. 104-112.
98. **Chu, T.S., and M.J. Gans:** High speed infrared local wireless communication. *IEEE Comm. Mag. 25(8)*:4–10 (1987).
99. **Smythe, P.P., D. Wood, S. Ritchie, and S. Cassidy:** Optical wireless: New enabling transmitter technologies. *IEEE International Conference on Communications '93, Technical Program, Conference*, vol. 1, pp. 562–566. New York: IEEE, 1993.
100. **Sisto, R., I. Pinto, N. Stacchini, and F. Giuliani:** Infrared radiation exposure in traditional glass factories. *AIHAJ 61*:5–10 (2000).
101. **Lydahl, E., A. Glansholm, and M. Levin:** Ocular exposure to infrared radiation in the swedish iron and steel industry. *Health Phys. 46*:529–536 (1984).
102. **Devereux, H., and M. Smalley:** Are infrared illuminators eye safe? *Proceedings of the Institute of Electrical and Electronics Engineers 29th Annual 1995 International Carnahan Conference on Security Technology* (IEEE Cat. no. 95CH3578-8), pp. 480–481. New York: IEEE, 1995.
103. **Chou, B.R., and A.P. Cullen:** Ocular hazards of industrial spot welding. *Optom. Vis. Sci. 73*:424–427 (1996).
104. **American Conference of Governmental Industrial Hygienists (ACGIH):** *2001 TLVs® and BEIs.* Cincinnati, Ohio: ACGIH, 2001.
105. **National Institute for Occupational Safety and Health (NIOSH):** *Occupational Exposure to Ultraviolet Radiation* (HSM 73-11009). Cincinnati, Ohio: NIOSH, 1972.
106. **International Commission on Non-Ionizing Radiation Protection:** Guidelines on UV radiation exposure limits. *Health Phys. 71*:978 (1996).
107. **Sliney, D.H.:** Ultraviolet radiation exposure criteria. *Radiat. Prot. Dosim. 91*:213–222 (2000).
108. **Rea, M.S. (ed.):** *IESNA Lighting Handbook: Reference and Application*, 9th ed. New York: Illuminating Engineering Society of North America, 2000.
109. **Gies, H.P., C.R. Roy, S. Toomey, and D. Tomlinson:** The ARL solar UVR measurement network: Calibration and results. *SPIE 2282*:274–284 (1994).
110. **Klein, R.M.:** Cut-off filters for the near ultraviolet. *Photochem. Photobiol. 29*:1053–1054 (1979).
111. **Racz, M., I. Reti, and S. Ferenczi:** Measurement of UV-A and UV-B irradiance with glass filtered detectors. *SPIE 2022*:192–195 (1993).
112. **Landry, R.J., and F.A. Andersen:** Optical radiation measurements: Instrumentation and Sources of error. *J. Natl. Cancer Inst. 69*:155–161 (1982).
113. **Fanney, J.H., and C.H. Powell:** Field measurement of ultraviolet, infrared, and microwave energies. *Am. Ind. Hyg. Assoc. J. 28*:335–342 (1967).
114. **Tug, H., and E.M. Baumann:** Problems of UV-B radiation measurements in biological research: Critical remarks on current techniques and suggestions for improvements. *Geophys. Res. Lett. 21*:689–692 (1994).
115. **McKenzie, R.L., and P.V. Johnston:** Comment on "Problems of UV-B Radiation Measurements in Biological Research: Critical Remarks on Current Techniques and Suggestions for Improvements" by H. Tug and M.E.M. Baumann. *Geophys. Res. Lett. 22*:1157–1158 (1995).

116. **Rosenthal, F.S., M. Safran, and H.R. Taylor:** The ocular dose of ultraviolet radiation from sunlight exposure. *Photochem. Photobiol. 42*:163–171 (1985).
117. **Diffey, B.L.:** A comparison of dosimeters used for solar ultraviolet radiometry. *Photochem. Photobiol. 46*:55–60 (1987).
118. **Wong, C.F., S. Toomey, R.A. Fleming, and B.W. Thomas:** UV-B radiometry and dosimetry for solar measurements. *Health Phys. 68*:175–184 (1995).
119. **Sliney, D.H., F.C. Bason, and B.C. Freasier:** Instrumentation and measurement of ultraviolet, visible, and infrared radiation. *Am. Ind. Hyg. Assoc. J. 32*:415–431 (1971).
120. **Gies, H.P., and C.R. Roy:** Bilirubin phototherapy and potential UVR hazards. *Health Phys. 58*:313–320 (1990).
121. **Koller, L.R.:** *Ultraviolet Radiation*, 2d Ed. New York: John Wiley & Sons, 1965.
122. **Sliney, D.H., C.E. Moss, C.G. Miller, and J.B. Stephens:** Semitransparent curtains for control of optical radiatiion hazards. *Appl. Opt. 20*:2352–2366 (1981).
123. **Wuest, J.R., and T.A. Gossel:** Update on sunscreens: Part I. *Kentucky Pharm. 55*:185–188 (1992).
124. **Kollias, N., and A.H. Baqer:** Photoprotection by the natural pigment: Melanin. *Human Exposure to Ultraviolet Radiation: Risks and Regulations*, pp. 121–124. Amsterdam: Elsevier Publishers B.V. (Biomedical Division), 1987.
125. **Wolf, P., C.K. Donawho, and M.L. Kripke:** Effect of sunscreens on UV radiation-induced enhancement of melanoma growth in mice. *J. Nat. Cancer Inst. 86*:99–105 (1994).
126. **Armstrong, B.K., and A. Kricker:** Epidemiology of sun exposure and skin cancer. *Cancer Surveys 26*:133–153 (1996).
127. **Hersey, P., M. MacDonald, C. Burns, and S. Schibeci:** Analysis of the effect of a sunscreen agent on the suppression of natural killer cell activity induced in human subjects radiation from solarium lamps. *J. Invest. Dermatol. 88*:271–276 (1987).
128. **Wuest, J.R., and T.A. Gossel:** Update on sunscreens: Part II. *Kentucky Pharm. 55*:213–216 (1992).
129. **Sayre, R.M., N. Kollias, R.D. Ley, and A.H. Baqer:** Changing the risk spectrum of injury and the performance of sunscreen products throughout the day. *Photodermatol. Photoimmunol. Photomed. 10*:148–153 (1994).
130. **Hawk, J.L.M., A.V.J. Challoner, and L. Chaddock:** The efficacy of sunscreening agents: Protection factors and transmission spectra. *Clin. Exp. Dermatol. 7*:21–31 (1982).
131. **Koh, H.K., and R.A. Lew:** Sunscreen and melanoma: Implications for prevention. *J. Nat. Cancer Inst. 86*:78–79 (1994).
132. **Gies, H.P., C.R. Roy, C.R. Elliott, and W. Zongli:** Ultraviolet radiation protection factors for clothing. *Health Phys. 67*:131–139 (1994).
133. **Sliney, D.H., R.E. Benton, H.M. Cole, S.G. Epstein, and C.J. Morin:** Transmission of potentially hazardous actinic ultraviolet radiation through fabrics. *Appl. Ind. Hyg. 2*:36–44 (1987).
134. **Parisi, A.V., M.G. Kimlin, L.R. Meldrum, and C.M. Relf:** Field measurements on protection by stockings from solar erythemal ultraviolet radiation. *Radiat. Prot. Dosim. 86*:69–72 (1999a).
135. **Kimlin, M.G., A.V. Parisi, and L.R. Meldrum:** Effect of stretch on the ultraviolet spectral transmission of one type of commonly used clothing. Photodermatol. *Photoimmunol. Photomed. 15*:171–174 (1999).
136. **Diffey, B.L., and I. Cheeseman:** Sun protection with hats. *Br. J. Dermatol. 127*:10–12 (1992).
137. **Parrish, J.A., R.R. Anderson, F. Urbach, and D. Pitts:** *UV-A Biological Effects of Ultraviolet Radiation with Emphasis on Human Responses to Longwave Ultraviolet*. New York: Plenum Press, 1978.
138. **Sliney, D.H., and B.C. Freasier:** Evaluation of optical radiation hazards. *Appl. Opt. 12*:1–24 (1973).
139. **Tenkate, T.S.D., and M.J. Collins:** Angles of entry of ultraviolet radiation into welding helmets. *Am. Ind. Hyg. Assoc. J. 58*:54–56 (1997).
140. **Tenkate, T.S.D., and M.J. Collins:** Personal ultraviolet radiation exposure of workers in a welding environment. *Am. Ind. Hyg. Assoc. J. 58*:33–38 (1997).
141. **Moseley, H.:** Ultraviolet and visible radiation transmission properties of some types of protective eyewear. *Phys. Med. Biol. 30*:177–181 (1985).
142. **Rosenthal, F.S., A.E. Bakalian, and H.R. Taylor:** The effect of prescription eyewear on ocular exposure to ultraviolet radiation. *Am. J. Pub. Health 76*:1216–1220 (1986).
143. **Oriowo, O.M., B.R. Chou, and A.P. Cullen:** Glassblowers' ocular health and safety: Optical radiation hazards and eye protection assessment. *Ophthal. Physiol. Opt. 17*:216–224 (1997).
144. **Franks, J.K.:** Potential ocular hazards from reflective surfaces. *Proceedings of the 1992 International Laser Safety Conference*, pp. 7I-55–7I-60. Orlando, Fla.: Laser Institute of America, 1993.
145. **Puliafito, C.A., and R.F. Steinert:** Short-pulsed Nd:YAG laser microsurgery of the eye: Biophysical considerations. *IEEE J. Quantum Electon. QE-20*:1441–1448 (1984).

146. **Kochevar, I.E.:** Biological effects of excimer laser radiation. *Proc. IEEE 80*:833–837 (1992).
147. **Ham, W.T., Jr., H.A. Mueller, J.J. Ruffolo, Jr., and A.M. Clarke:** Sensitivity of the retina to radiation damage as a function of wavelength. *Photochem. Photobiol. 29*:735–743 (1979).
148. **Ham, W.T., Jr., H.A. Mueller, and D.H. Sliney:** Retinal sensitivity to damage from short wavelength light. *Nature 260*:153–155 (1976)
149. **National Institute for Occupational Safety and Health:** "Health Hazard Evaluation, University of Utah Health Sciences Center, Salt Lake City, Utah," by C.E. Moss, C. Bryant, J. Stewart, W.-Z. Whong, A. Fleeger, and B.J. Gunter (Rep. no. HETA 88-101-2008; NTIS no. PB91-107789). Springfield, Va.: National Technical Information Service, 1990.
150. **Hitchcock, T. (ed.):** *LIA Guide to Non-beam Hazards Associated with Laser Use*. Orlando, Fla.: Laser Institute of America, 1999.
151. **Kokosa, J.M.:** Hazardous chemicals produced by laser materials processing. *J. Laser Appl. 6*:195–201 (1994).
152. **Tarroni, G., C. Melandri, T. De Zaiacomo, C. Lombardi, C., and M. Formignani:** Characterization of aerosols produced in cutting steel components and concrete structures by means of a laser beam. *J. Aerosol Sci. 17*:587–591 (1986).
153. **Hardaway, G.A.:** Lasers in metalworking and electronic industries. *Arch. Environ. Health 20*:188–192 (1970).
154. **Hietanen, M., A. Honkasalo, H. Laitinen, L. Lindross, I. Welling, and P. von Nandelstadh:** Evaluation of hazards in CO_2 laser welding and related processes. *Ann. Occup. Hyg. 36*:183–188 (1992).
155. **Haferkamp, H., M. Goede, K. Engel, and J.-S. Witebecker:** Hazardous emissions: Characterization of CO_2 laser material processing. *J. Laser Appl. 7*:83–88 (1995).
156. **National Institute for Occupational Safety and Health:** *Occupational Hazards of Laser Material Processing*, by R.J. Rockwell, Jr., R.M. Wilson, S. Jander, and R. Dreffer (NTIS no. PB89-186530). Springfield, Va.: National Technical Information Service, 1976.
157. **Ball, R.D., B. Kulik, and S.L. Tan:** The assessment and control of hazardous by-products from materials processing with CO_2 lasers. In *Industrial Laser Handbook*, pp 3–13. Tulsa, Okla.: Penn Well Books, 1988.
158. **Kiefer, M., and C.E. Moss:** Laser generated air contaminants released during laser cutting of fabrics and polymers. *J. Laser Appl. 9*:7–13 (1997).
159. **Doyle, D.J.:** Spectroscopic evaluation of toxic by-products produced during industrial laser processing. In *Proceedings of the International Laser Safety Conference*, pp. 3-109–3-114. Orlando, Fla.: Laser Institute of America, 1991.
160. **Kwan, J.K.:** Tocicological characterization of chemicals produced from laser irradiation of graphite composite materials. In Proceedings of the International Laser Safety Conference, pp. 3-69–3-96. Orlando, Fla.: Laser Institute of America, 1991.
161. **Attwood, D., H.J. Sidhu, P. Rumsby, D. Thomas, and L. Vassie:** Analysis of emissions created during UV laser processing of carbon fibre reinforced composite. *Proceedings of the 2nd EUREKA Industrial Laser Safety Forum*, pp. 65–78. Bonn-Bad Godesburg, Germany: EUREKA/COST, 1993.
162. **National Institute for Occupational Safety and Health:** "Health Hazard Evaluation Report Photon Dynamics Ltd., Inc. Longwood, Florida," by C.E. Moss and A. Fleeger (Rep. no. HETA 89-331-2078; NTIS no. PB91-188946). Springfield, Va.: National Technical Information Service, 1990.
163. **Fleeger, A., and C.E. Moss:** Airborne emissions produced by the interaction of a carbon dioxide laser with glass, metals, and plastics. In *Proceedings of the International Laser Safety Conference*, pp. 3-23–3-31. Orlando, Fla.: Laser Institute of America, 1991.
164. **Engel, K., A. Hampe, D. Seebaum, I. Vinke, and J. Wittbecker:** Review of scientific research in the federal republic of germany concerning emissions in laser material processing. In *Proceedings of the International Laser Safety Conference*, pp. 5-29–5-52. Orlando, Fla.: Laser Institute of America, 1991.
165. **Kokosa, J.M., and J. Eugene:** Chemic*al Composition of Laser-Tissue Interaction Smoke Plume. J. Laser Appl. 1*(3):59–63 (1989).
166. **National Institute for Occupational Safety and Health:** "Health Hazard Evaluation, University of Utah Health Sciences Center, Salt Lake City, Utah," by C.E. Moss, C. Bryant, J. Stewart, W.-Z. Whong, A. Fleeger, and B.J. Gunter (Rep. no. HETA 88-101-2008; NTIS no. PB91-107789). Springfield, Va.: National Technical Information Service, 1990.
167. **Spleiss, M., and L. Weber:** Medium- and low-volatile organic compounds generated by laser tissue interaction. Proc. *SPIE 2923*:168–177 (1996).
168. **Waesche, W., and H.J. Albrecht:** Investigation of the distribution of aerosols and VOC in plume produced during laser treatment under OR conditions. *Proc. SPIE 2624*:270–275 (1996).
169. **Wollmer, W.:** Investigations of laser plume in medical applications. In *Proceedings of the International Laser Safety Conference*, pp. 383–392. Orlando, Fla.: Laser institute of America, 1997.

170. **Ferenczy, A., C. Bergeron, and R.M. Richart:** Human papillomavirus DNA in CO_2 laser-generated plume of smoke and its consequences to the surgeon. *Obstet. Gynecol. 75*:114–118 (1990).
171. **Matchette, L.S., T.J. Vegella, and R.W. Faaland:** Viable bacteriophage in CO_2 laser plume: Aerodynamic size distribution. *Lasers Surg. Med. 13*:18–22 (1993).
172. **Sawchuk, W.S., and R.P. Felten:** Infectious potential of aerosolized particles. *Arch. Dermatol. 125*:1689–1692 (1989).
173. **Sliney, D.H., and T.N. Clapham:** Safety with medical excimer lasers with an emphasis on compressed gases. *J. Laser Appl. 3*(3):59–62 (1991).
174. **Benoit, H., J. Clark, and W.J. Keon:** Installation of a commercial excimer laser in the operating room. *J. Laser Appl. 1*(3):45–50 (1989).
175. **Lorenz, A.K.:** Gas handling safety for laser makers and users. *J. Lasers Appl. 6*(3):69–73 (1987).
176. **Kues, H., and G. Lutty:** Dyes can be deadly. *Laser Focus 11*(4):59–60 (1975).
177. **Miller, G.:** Industrial hygiene concerns of laser dyes. In *Proceedings of the International Laser Safety Conference*, pp. 3-97–3-105. Orlando, Fla.: Laser Institute of America, Orlando, 1991.
178. **Wuebbles, B.J.Y., and J.S. Felton:** Evaluation of laser dye mutagenicity using the ames/salmonella microsome test. *Environ. Mutagen. 7*:511–522 (1985).
179. **Rockwell, R.J., Jr., and C.E. Moss:** Optical radiation hazards of laser welding processes. Part II: CO_2 laser. *Am. Ind. Hyg. Assoc. J. 50*:419–427 (1989).
180. **Hietanen, M., and P. Von Nandelstadh:** Scattered and plasma-related optical radiations associated with industrial laser processes. In *Proceedings of the International Laser Safety Conference*, pp. 3-105–3-108. Orlando, Fla.: Laser Institute of Ameica, 1991.
181. **O'Neill, F., C.E. Turcu, D. Xenakis, and M.H.R. Hutchinson:** X-ray Emission from plasmas generated by an XeCl laser picosecond pulse train. *Appl. Phys. Lett. 55*:2603–2604 (1989).
182. **Kuhnle, G., F.P. Schafer, S. Szatmari, and G.D. Tsakiris:** X-Ray production by irradiation of solid targets with sub-picosecond excimer laser pulses. *Appl. Phys B 47*:361–366 (1988).
183. **Chen, H., Y.-H. Chuang, J.A. Delettrez, S. Uchida, and D.D. Meyerhofer:** Study of X-ray emission from picosecond laser-plasma interaction. *Proc. SPIE 1413*:112–119 (1991).
184. **Seitz, T.A., and C.E. Moss:** RF-Excited Carbon Dioxide Lasers: Concerns of RF Occupational Exposures. In *Proceedings of the International Laser Safety Conference*, pp. 3-35–3-40. Orlando, Fla.: Laser Institute of Ameica, 1991.
185. **Bowman, J.D., D.H. Garabrant, E. Sobel, and J.M. Peters:** Exposures to extremely low frequency (ELF) electromagnetic fields in occupations with elevated leukemia rates. *Appl. Ind. Hyg. 3*:189–194 (1988).
186. **Bauman, N.:** Laser accidents: Why only 10% get reported. *Laser Med. Surg. News Adv.* 1-7 (1988, August).
187. **Bandle, A.M., and B. Holyoak:** Laser incidents. In *Medical Laser Safety-Report #48*, pp. 47–55. London, England: U.K. Institute of Physical Sciences, 1988.
188. **Haifeng, L., G. Guanghuang, W. Dechang, et al.:** Ocular injuries from accidental laser exposure. *Health Phys. 56*:711–716 (1989).
189. **Rathkey, A.S.:** Accidental laser burn of the macula. *Arch. Ophthal. 74*:346–348 (1965).
190. **Zweng, H.C.:** Accidental Q-switched laser lesion of human macula. *Arch. Ophthal. 78*:596–599 (1967).
191. **Curtin, T.L., and D.G. Boyden:** Reflected laser beam causing accidental burn of retina. *Am. J. Ophthal 65*:188–189 (1968).
192. **Gabel, V.-P., R. Birngruber, and B. Lorenz:** Clinical observations of six cases of laser injury to the eye. *Health Phys. 56*:705–710 (1989).
193. **Boldrey, E.E., H.L. Little, L., M. Flocks, and A. Vassiliadis:** Retinal injury to industrial laser burns. *Ophthalmol. 88*:101–107 (1981).
194. **Pleven, C.:** A description of fourteen accidents caused by lasers in a research environment. *Lasers et Normes de Protection (First International Symposium on Laser Biological Effects and Exposure Limits)*, pp. 406–417. Paris: Centre de Recherches du Service de Sante des Armees, 1986.
195. **Wolfe, J.A.:** Laser retinal injury. *Military Med. 150*:177–185 (1985).
196. **Henkes, H.E., and H. Zuidema:** Accidental laser coagulation of the central fovea. *Ophthalmologica 171*:15–25 (1975).
197. **Rockwell, R.J., Jr.:** Learning from case studies: How to avoid laser accidents. *Expert Strategies for Practical and Profitable Management*, pp. 57–66. Atlanta: American Health Consultants, 1985.
198. **Rockwell, R.J., Jr.:** Laser accidents: Are they all reported and what can be learned from them? *J. Laser Appl. 1*(4):53–57 (1989).
199. **Asano, T.:** Accidental YAG laser burn. *Am. J. Ophthalmol. 98*:116–117 (1984)
200. **Stuck, B.E., H. Zwick, J.W. Molchany, D.J. Lund, and D.A. Gagliano:** Accidental human laser retinal injuries from military laser systems. *Proc. SPIE 2674*:7–20 (1996).
201. **Laitinen, H., and T. Jarvinen:** Accident risks and the effect of performance feedback with industrial CO_2 lasers. *Opt. Laser Technol. 27*:25–30 (1995).

202. **Makhov, G.O.:** Accidents and incidents in the laser entertainment industry. In Proceedings of the 1992 International Laser Safety Conference, pp. 7I-39–7I-43. Orlando, Fla.: Laser Institute of America, 1993.
203. **Acland, K.M., and R.J. Barlow:** Lasers for the dermatologist. *Br. J. Dermatol. 143*:244–255 (2000).
204. **Armstrong, C.E.:** Eye injuries in some modern radiation environments. *J. Am. Opt. Assoc. 41*:55–62 (1970).
205. **Zamir, E., I. Kaiserman, and I. Chowers:** Laser pointer maculopathy. *Am. J. Ophthalmol. 127*:728–729 (1999).
206. **Sell, C.H., and J.S. Bryan:** Maculopathy from handheld diode laser pointer. *Arch. Ophthalmol. 117*:1557–1558 (1999).
207. **American National Standards Institute:** *American National Standard for the Safe Use of Lasers* (ANSI Z136.1-2000). Orlando, Fla.: Laser Institute of America, 2000.
208. **International Commission on Non-Ionizing Radiation Protection:** Guidelines on limits of exposure to laser radiation of wavelengths between 180 nm and 1000 μm. *Health Phys. 71*:804–819 (1996).
209. **International Commission on Non-Ionizing Radiation Protection:** Revision of guidelines on limits of exposure to laser radiation of wavelengths between 400 nm and 1.4 ?m. *Health Phys. 79*:431–440 (2000).
210. **International Electrotechnical Commission:** *Safety of Laser Products Part 1—Equipment Classification, Requirements and User's Guide* (IEC 60825-1 Ed. 1.1:1998-01 ə Am. 2 2001-01). Geneva: IEC, 1993.
211. **American National Standards Institute:** *American National Standard for Safe Use of Lasers in Health Care Facilities* (Z136.3-1996). Orlando, Fla.: Laser Institute of America, 1996.
212. **Hattin, H.C.:** Laser safety in health care facilities: A national standard of Canada. *J. Clin. Eng. 19*:218–221 (1996).
213. **American National Standards Institute:** *American National Standard for the Safe Use of Optical Fiber Communications Systems Utilizing Laser Diodes and LED Sources* (Z136.2-1997). Orlando, Fla.: Laser Institute of America, 1997.
214. **International Electrotechnical Commission (IEC):** *Safety of Laser Products Part 2—Safety of Optical Fibre Communications Systems* (IEC 60825-2). Geneva: IEC, 1993.
215. **American National Standards Institute:** *American National Standard for the Safe Use of Lasers in Educational Institutions* (Z136.5-2000). Orlando, Fla.: Laser Institute of America, 2000.
216. **American National Standards Institute:** *American National Standard for the Safe Use of Lasers Outdoors* (Z136.6-2000). Orlando, Fla.: Laser Institute of America, 2000.
217. **Curtis, R.A.:** OSHA standards related to laser safety. In *Proceedings of the International Laser Safety Conference*, pp. 1-35–1-39. Orlando, Fla.: Laser Institute of America, 1991.
218. **Rockwell, R.J., Jr., and J. Parkinson:** State and local government laser safety requirements. *J. Laser Appl. 11*:225–231 (1999).
219. **Marshall, W.J., and P.W. Conner:** Field laser hazard calculations. *Health Phys. 52*:27–37 (1987).
220. **Marshall, W.J., and W.P. Van DeMerwe:** Hazardous ranges of laser beams and their reflections from targets. *Appl. Optics 25*:605–611 (1986).
221. **Marshall, W.J.:** Laser reflections from relatively flat specular surfaces. *Health Phys. 56*:753–757 (1989).
222. **Marshall, W.J.:** Determining hazard distances from non-gaussian lasers. *Appl. Optics 30*:696–698 (1991).
223. **Marshall, W.J.:** Comparative hazard evaluation of near-infrared diode lasers. *Health Phys. 66*:532–539 (1994).
224. **Marshall, W.J.:** Understanding laser hazard evaluation. *J. Laser Appl. 7*:99–105 (1995).
225. **Marshall, W.J., R.C. Aldrich, and S.A. Zimmerman:** Laser hazard evaluation method for middle infrared laser systems. *J. Laser Appl. 8*:211–216 (1996).
226. **Lyon, T.L.:** Hazard analysis technique for multiple wavelength lasers. *Health Phys. 49*:221-226 (1985).
227. **Lyon, T.L.:** Laser measurement techniques guide for hazard evaluation (tutorial guide—part 1). *J. Laser Appl. 5*(1):53–58 (1993).
228. **Marshall, W.J.:** Focused laser beam hazard calculations. In *Proceedings of the International Laser Safety Conference*, pp. 9-33–9-39. Orlando, Fla.: Laser Institute of America, 1991.
229. **Lyon, T.L.:** Laser measurement techniques guide for hazard evaluation (tutorial guide—part 2). *J. Laser Appl. 5*(2ə3):37–42 (1993).
230. **Rockwell, R.J., Jr., and C.E. Moss:** Hazard zones and eye protection requirements for a frosted surgical probe used with an Nd:YAG laser. *Lasers Surg. Med 9*:45–49 (1989).
231. **Rockwell, R.J., Jr.:** Utilization of the nominal hazard zone in control measure selection. In *Proceedings of the International Laser Safety Conference*, pp. 7-25–7-42. Orlando, Fla.: Laser Institute of America, 1991.

232. **Labo, J.A., and M.E. Rogers:** Can Broken fiber optics produce hazardous laser beams? *Proc. SPIE 1892*:176–187 (1993).
233. **Swope, C.H.:** The eye—protection. *Arch. Environ. Health 18*:428–435 (1969).
234. **Sliney, D.H.:** Laser eye protectors. *J. Laser Appl. 2*(2):9–13 (1990).
235. **Hack, H., and N. Neuroth:** Resistance of optical and colored glasses to 3-nsec laser pulses. *Appl. Optics 21*:3239–3248 (1982).
236. **Swearengen, P.M., W.F. Vance, and D.L. Counts:** A study of burn-through times for laser protective eyewear. *Am. Ind. Hyg. Assoc. J. 49*:608–612 (1988).
237. **Tucker, R.J.:** Damage testing of polycarbonate laser protective eyewear. In *Proceedings of the International Laser Safety Conference*, pp. 9-25–9-27. Orlando, Fla.: Laser Institute of America, 1991.
238. **Lyon, T.L., and W.J. Marshall:** Nonlinear properties of optical filters—implications for laser safety. *Health Phys. 51*:95–96 (1986).
239. **Mayo, M.W., W.P. Roach, C.M. Bramlette, and M.D. Gavornik:** Nonlinear transmittance through laser protective material: Reverse photosaturation of 1-phenylazo 2-napthalenol in polymer host. *Proc. SPIE 1864*:86–95 (1993).
240. **Scott, T.R., R.J. Rockwell, Jr., and P. Batra:** Optical density measurements of laser eye protection materials. In *Proceedings of the International Laser Safety Conference*, pp. 8-7–8-16. Orlando, Fla.: Laser Institute of America, 1993.
241. **Adams, A.J., and J.E. Skipper:** Safe use of infrared viewing cards. *Health Phys. 59*:225–228 (1990).
242. **Mumford, W.W.:** Some technical aspects of microwave radiation hazards. *Proc. IRE 49*:427–447 (1961).
243. **Hitchcock, R.T., and R.M. Patterson:** *Radio-Frequency and ELF Electromagnetic Energies: A Handbook for Health Professionals*. New York: Van Nostrand Reinhold, 1995.
244. **Eriksson A., and K. Hansson Mild:** Radiofrequency electromagnetic leakage fields from plastic welding machines. *J. Microwave Power 20*:95–107 (1985).
245. **Martin, C.J., H.M. McCallum, and B. Heaton:** An evaluation of radiofrequency exposure from therapeutic diathermy equipment in the light of current recommendations. *Clin. Phys. Physiol. Meas. 11*:53–63 (1990).
246. **McKinlay, A.F., et al.:** Review of the Scientific Evidence for Limiting Exposure to Electromagnetic Fields (0-300 GHz). London: NRPB, 2004.
247. **Goldstein, L., M. Dewhirst, M. Repacholi, and L. Kheifets:** Summary, conclusions and recommendations: adverse temperature levels in the human body. *Int. J. Hyperthermia 19(3)*:373–84 (2003).
248. **Sirenko, Y., M. Stroscio, and K. Kim:** Elastic vibrations of microtubules in a fluid. *Phys. Rev. E53*:1003–10 (1996).
249. **Kotnik, T. and D. Miklaveic:** Second-order model of membrane electric field induced by alternating external electric fields. *IEEE Trans. Biomed. Eng. 47*:1074–81 (2000).
250. **Laurence, J., P. French, R. Lindner, and D. McKenzie:** Biological effects of electromagnetic fields-mechanisms for the effects of pulsed microwave radiation on protein conformation. *J. Theor. Bio. 206*:291–98 (2000).
251. **Bohr, H. and J. Bohe:** Microwave-enhanced folding and denaturation of globular proteins. *Phys. Rev. E61*:4310–14 (2000).
252. **Chiabrera, A., B. Bianco, E. Moggian, and J. Kaufman:** Zeeman stark modeling of the RF EMF interaction with ligand binding. *Bioelectromag. 21*:312–24 (2000).
253. **Schwan, H.:** EM-filed induced effects. In *Interactions Between Electromagnetic Fields and Cells*. Chiabrera, A., C. Nicolini, and H. Schwan (eds.). New York: Plenum Press, 1985. pp 371–390.
254. **Adair, R.:** Effects of weak high-frequency electromagnetic fields on biological systems, In: *Radiofrequency Standards*. Klauenberg, B., M. Grandolfo, and D. Erwin (eds.). New York: Plenum Press, 1994. pp 207–222.
255. **Woodward, J., C. Timmel, K. McLauchlan, and P. Hore:** Radiofrequency magnetic field effects on electron-hole recombination. *Phys. Rev. Letts. 87*:077602 1-4 (2001).
256. **Challis, L.J.:** Mechanisms for interaction between RF fields and biological tissue [review]. *Bio Elect. Mag. 26(S7)*:S98–S106 (2005).
257. **Kovisto, M., C. Krause, A. Revonsuo, M. Lane, and H. Hamalainen:** The effects of electromagnetic fields emitted by cellular telephones on response times in humans. *Neuroreport. 11(8)*:1641–43 (2000).
258. **Haarla, C., L. Bjornberg, M. Ek, A. Revonsuo, M. Koivisto, and H. Hamalainen:** Effect of a 9002 MHz electromagnetic field emitted by mobile phones on human cognitive function: A replication study. *Bioelectromag. 24(4)*:283–88 (2003).
259. **Frey, A.H.:** Headaches from cellular telephones: Are they real and what are the implications? *Env. Health Persp. 6(3)*:101–03 (1998).
260. **Hocking, B.:** Preliminary report: Symptoms associated with mobile phone use. *Occ. Med. 48*:357–60 (1998).
261. **Sandstrom, M. et al.:** Mobile phone use and subjective symptoms. *Occ. Med. 51*:25–35 (2001).
262. **Koivisto, M., et al.:** GSM phone signal does not produce subjective symptoms. *Bioelectromag. 22(3)*:212–15 (2001).

263. **Hietanen, M., A-.M. Hamalainen, and T. Husman:** Hypersensitivity symptoms associated with exposure to cellular telephones: No causal link. *Bioelectromag. 23*:264–70 (2002).
264. **Zwamborn, A.P.M., S.H.J.A. Vossen, B.J.A.M. van Leersum, M.A. Ouwens, and W.N. Makel:** Effects of global communication system radiofrequency fields on well being and cognitive functions of human subjects with and without subjective complaints. TNO-report FEL-03-C148, 2003.
265. **Elder, J.:** Ocular effects of radiofrequency energy. *Bioelectromag. 24*:S148–S61 (2003).
266. **Elwood, J.:** A critical review of epidemiologic studies of radiofrequency exposure and human cancers. *Env. Health Persp. 107(1)*:155–68 (1999).
267. **Independent Expert Group on Mobile Phones (IEGMP):** Mobile phones and health, report of an independent expert group on mobile phones, Chilton, U.K.: IEGMP, 2000.
268. **Inskip, P.D., R.E. Tarone, E.E. Hatch, et al.:** Cellular-telephone use and brain tumors. *New. Engl. J. Med. 344*:79–86 (2001).
269. **Muskat, J., et al.:** Handheld cellular telephone use and risk of brain cancer. *J. A. Med. Assoc. 284*:3001–07 (2001).
270. **Advisory Group on Nonionising Radiation (AGNIR):** Health effects from radiofrequency electromagnetic fields. *NRPB 14(2)*:1–177 (2003).
271. **Patterson, R.M., and R.T. Hitchcock:** Nonionizing radiation and fields. In *Health and Safety Beyond the Workplace*, pp. 143–176. New York: John Wiley & Sons, 1990.
272. **Hitchcock, R.T.:** Radio-frequency and microwave radiation. In *Patty's Toxicology*, 5th ed., vol 8, pp. 197–247. New York: John Wiley & Sons, 2001.
273. **U.S. Environmental Protection Agency:** "Biological Effects of Radiofrequency Radiation," edited by J.A. Elder and D.F. Cahill (Report no. EPA-600/8-83-026F). Springfield, Va.: National Technical Information Service, 1984.
274. **Polk, C., and E. Postow (eds.):** *Handbook of Biological Effects of Electromagnetic Fields*, 2nd ed. Boca Raton, Fla.: CRC Press, 1996.
275. **National Radiological Protection Board:** *Human Health and Exposure to Electromagnetic Radiation*, by J.A. Dennis, C.R. Muirhead and J.R. Ennis (NRPB-R241). Chilton, Didcot, Oxon, U.K.: NRPB, 1992.
276. **World Health Organization:** *Electromagnetic Fields* (300 Hz to 300 GHz) (Environmental Health Criteria 137). Geneva: WHO, 1993.
277. **Teixeira-Pinto, A.A., L.L. Nejelski, Jr., J.L. Cutler, and J.H. Heller:** The behavior of unicellular organisms in an electromagnetic field. *Exp. Cell Res. 20*:548–564 (1960).
278. **Schwan, H.P.:** Nonthermal cellular effects of electromagnetic fields: AC-field induced ponderomotoric forces. *Br. J. Cancer 45* (suppl. V):220–224 (1982).
279. **Michaelson, S.M.:** Subtle effects of radiofrequency energy absorption and their physiological implications. In *Interactions Between Electromagnetic Fields and Cells*, pp. 581–601. New York: Plenum Press, 1985.
280. **Elder, J.:** Radiofrequency radiation activities and issues: A 1986 perspective. *Health Phys. 53*:607–611 (1987).
281. **U.S. Air Force:** *Radiofrequency Radiation Dosimetry Handbook*, 2nd ed., by C.H. Durney, C.C. Johnson, P.W. Barber, et al. (School of Aerospace Medicine Report SAM-TR-78-22), pp. 31–32. Brooks Air Force Base, Tex.: U.S Air Force, 1978.
282. **D'Andrea, J., O. Gandhi, and J.L. Lords:** Behavioral and thermal effects of microwave radiation at resonant and non-resonant wavelengths. *Radio Sci. 12*(6S):251–256 (1977).
283. **de Lorge, J.O.:** The Effects of Microwave Radiation on Behavior and Temperature in Rhesus Monkeys. In Biological Effects of Electromagnetic Waves (HEW [FDA] Pub. No. 77-8010). Rockville, MD: Bureau of Radiological Health, 1976. pp. 158–174.
284. **de Lorge, J.O.:** Disruption of behavior in mammals of three different sizes exposed to microwaves: Extrapolation to larger mammals. In *Proceedings of the 1978 Symposium on Electromagnetic Fields in Biological Systems*, pp. 215–228.Edmonton, Canada: International Microwave Power Institute, 1978.
285. **de Lorge, J.O.:** The thermal basis for disruption of operant behavior by microwaves in three animal species. In *Microwaves and Thermoregulation*, pp. 379–399. New York: Academic Press, 1983.
286. **D'Andrea, J.A.:** Microwave radiation absorption: behavioral effects. *Health Phys. 61*:29–40 (1991).
287. **D'Andrea, J.A.:** Behavioral evaluation of microwave irradiation. *Bioelectromagnetics 20*:64–74 (1999).
288. **Dodge, C.H.:** *Clinical and Hygienic Aspects of Exposure to Electromagnetic Fields. In Biological Effects and Health Implications of Microwave Radiation.* Washington, D.C.: U.S. Government Printing Office, 1969.
289. **Silverman, C.:** Nervous and behavioral effects of microwave radiation in humans. *Am. J. Epidemiol. 97*:219–224 (1973).
290. **Silverman, C.:** Epidemiology of microwave radiation effects in humans. In *Epidemiology and Quantitation of Environmental Risk in Humans from Radiation and Other Agents*, pp. 433–458. New York: Plenum Press, 1985.

291. **Baranski, S., and P. Czerski:** Biological effects of microwaves. Stroudsburg, Pa.: Dowden, Hutchinson & Ross, 1976.
292. **Forman, S.A., C.K. Holmes, T.V. McManamon, and W.R. Wedding:** Psychological symptoms and intermittent hypertension following acute microwave exposure. *J. Occup. Med. 24*:932–934 (1982).
293. **Williams, R.A., and T.S. Webb:** Exposure to radio-frequency radiation from an aircraft radar unit. *Aviat. Space Environ. Med. 51*:1243–1244 (1980).
294. **Lai, H., A. Horita, C.K. Chou, and A.W. Guy:** A review of microwave irradiation and actions of psychoactive drugs. *IEEE Eng. Med. Biol. Mag. 6*(1):31–36 (1987).
295. **Frey, A.H., and L.S. Wesler:** Interaction of psychoactive drugs with exposure to electromagnetic fields. *J. Bioelect. 9*:187–196 (1990).
296. **Lary, J.M., D.L. Conover, E.D. Foley, and P.L. Hanser:** Teratogenic effects of 27.12 mhz radiofrequency radiation in rats. *Teratology 26*:299–309 (1982).
297. **Lary, J.M., D.L. Conover, P.H. Johnson, and J.R. Burg:** Teratogenicity of 27.12-MHz radiation in rats is related to duration of hyperthermic exposure. *Bioelectromagnetics 4*:249–255 (1983).
298. **Lary, J.M., D.L. Conover, P.H. Johnson, and R.W. Hornung:** Dose-response relationship and birth defects in radiofrequency-irradiated rats. *Bioelectromagnetics 7*:141–149 (1986).
299. **Berman, E., H. Carter, and D. House:** Observations of Syrian hamster fetuses after exposure to 2450-MHz microwaves. *J. Microwave Power 17*:107–112 (1982).
300. **Berman, E., H. Carter, and D. House:** Reduced weight in mice offspring after in utero exposure to 2450-MHz (CW) microwaves. *Bioelectromagnetics 3*:285–291 (1982).
301. **Cohen, B.H., A.M. Lilienfeld, S. Kramer, amd L.C. Hyman:** Parental factors in Down's syndrome: Results of the second Baltimore case-control study. In *Population Cytogenetics—Studies in Humans*, pp. 301–352. New York: Academic Press, 1977.
302. **Kallen, B., G. Malmquist, and U. Moritz:** Delivery outcome among physiotherapists in Sweden: Is non-ionizing radiation a fetal hazard? *Arch. Environ. Health 37*:81–84 (1982).
303. **Kolmodin-Hedman, B., K.H. Mild, M. Hagberg, E. Jonsson, M.-C. Andersson, and A. Eriksson:** Health problems among operators of plastic welding machines and exposure to radiofrequency electromagnetic fields. *Int. Arch. Occup. Environ. Health 60*:243–247 (1988).
304. **Taskinen, H., P. Kyyronen, and K. Hemminki:** Effects of ultrasound, shortwaves, and physical exertion on pregnancy outcome in physiotherapists. *J. Epidemiol. Comm. Health 44*:196–201 (1990).
305. **Schnorr, T.M., B.A. Grajewski, R.W. Hornung, et al.:** Video display terminals and the risk of spontaneous abortion. *New Engl. J. Med. 324*:727–733 (1991).
306. **Nielsen, C.V., and L. Brandt:** Spontaneous abortion among women using video display terminals. *Scand. J. Work Environ. Health 16*:323–328 (1990).
307. **Brandt, L., and C.V. Nielsen:** Congenital malformations among children of women working with video display terminals. *Scand. J. Work Environ. Health 16*:329–333 (1990).
308. **Larsen, A.I., J. Olsen, and O. Svane:** Gender-specific reproductive outcome and exposure to high-frequency electromagnetic radiation among physiotherapists. *Scand. J. Work Environ. Health 17*:324–329 (1991).
309. **James, W.H.:** Sex ratio of offspring of female physiotherapists exposed to low-level high-frequency electromagnetic radiation. *Scand. J. Work. Environ. Health 21*:68–69 (1995).
310. **Lancranjan, I., M. Maicanescu, E. Rafaila, I. Klepsch, and H.I. Popescu:** Gonadic function in workmen with long-term exposure to microwaves. *Health Phys. 29*:381–383 (1975).
311. **Weyandt, T.B.:** *Evaluation of Biological and Male Reproductive Function Responses to Potential Lead Exposures in 155 MM Howitzer Crewmen* (AD-A247 384). Springfield, Va.: National Technical Information Service, 1992.
312. **Schrader, S.M., R.E. Langford, T.W. Turner, et al.:** Reproductive function in relation to duty assignments among military personnel. *Reprod. Toxicol. 12*:465–469 (1998).
313. **Grajewski, B., C. Cox, S.M. Schrader, et al.:** Semen quality and hormone levels among radiofrequency heater operators. *J. Occup. Environ. Med. 42*:993–1005 (2000).
314. **Lerman, Y., R. Jacubovich, and M.S. Green:** Pregnancy outcome following exposure to shortwaves among female physiotherapists in Israel. *Am. J. Ind. Med. 39*:499–504 (2001).
315. **Larsen, A.I.:** Congenital Malformations and exposure to high-frequency electromagnetic radiation among Danish physiotherapists. *Scand. J. Work Environ. Health 17*:318–323 (1991).
316. **Ouellet-Hellstrom, R., and W.F. Stewart:** Miscarriages among female physical therapists who report using radio- and microwave-frequency electromagnetic radiation. *Am. J. Epidemiol. 138*:775–786 (1993).
317. **Kues, H.A. L.W. Hirst, G.A. Lutty, S.A. D'Anna, and G.R. Dunkelberger:** Effects of 2.45-GHz microwaves on primate corneal endothelium. *Bioelectromagnetics 6*:177–188 (1985).

318. **Kues, H.A., and S. D'Anna:** Changes in the monkey eye following pulsed 2.45-GHz microwave exposure. In *Proceedings of the Ninth Annual Conference of the IEEE Engineering in Medicine and Biology Society,* vol. 2, pp. 698–700.New York: Institute of Electrical and Electronic Engineers, 1987.
319. **Kamimura, Y., K.I. Saito, T. Saiga, and Y. Amemiya:** Experiment of 2.45 GHz microwave irradiation to monkey's eye. In *1994 International Symposium on Electromagnetic Compatibility,* pp. 429–432. New York: Institute of Electrical and Electronics Engineers, 1994.
320. **Carpenter, R., and C. Van Ummersen:** The action of microwave radiation on the eye. *J. Microwave Power 3*:3–19 (1968).
321. **Guy, A.W., J.C. Lin, P.O. Kramar, and A.F. Emery:** Effect of 2450-MHz radiation on the rabbit eye. *IEEE Trans. Microwave Theory Tech. MTT-23*:492-498 (1975).
322. **Michaelson, S.M., J.W. Howland, and W.B. Deichmann:** Response of the dog to 24,000 and 1285 MHz microwave exposure. *Ind. Med. 40*:18–23 (1971).
323. **Appleton, B., S.E. Hirsch, and P.V.K. Brown:** Investigation of single-exposure microwave ocular effects at 3000 MHz. *Ann. N.Y. Acad. Sci. 247*:125–134 (1975).
324. **Appleton, B., and G.C. McCrossan:** Microwave lens effects in humans. *Arch. Ophthalmol. 88*:259–262 (1972).
325. **Zydecki, S.:** Assessment of lens translucency in juveniles, microwave workers and age-matched groups. In *Biologic Effects and Health Hazards of Microwave Radiation,* pp. 273– 280. Warsaw, Poland: Polish Medical Publishers, 1974.
326. **Cleary, S.F., B.S. Pasternack, and G.W. Beebe:** Cataract incidence in radar workers. *Arch. Environ. Health 11*:179–182 (1965).
327. **Cleary, S.F., and B.S. Pasternack:** Lenticular changes in microwave workers. *Arch. Environ. Health 12*:23–29 (1966).
328. **Majewska, K.:** Investigations on the effect of microwaves on the eye. *Pol. Med. J. 38*:989–994 (1968).
329. **Siekierzynski, M., P. Czerski, A. Gidynski, S. Zydecki, C. Czarnecki, E. Dziuk and W. Jedrzejczak:** Health surveillance of personnel occupationally exposed to microwaves. III. Lens translucency. *Aerospace Med. 45*:1146–1148 (1974).
330. **Bonomi, L., and R. Bellucci:** Considerations of the ocular pathology in 30,000 personnel of the Italian telephone company (SIP) using VDTs. *Bollettion Di Oculistica 68*(suppl. 7):85–98 (1989).
331. **Paulsson, L.-E., Y. Hamnerius, H.-A. Hansson, and J. Sjostrand:** Retinal damage experimentally induced by microwave radiation at 55 mW/cm². *Acta Ophthalmol. 57*:183–197 (1979).
332. **Kues, H.A., and J.C. Monahan:** Microwave-induced changes to the primate eye. *Johns Hopkins APL Tech. Dig. 13*:244–254 (1992).
333. **Lu, S.-T., S.P. Mathur, B. Stuck, et al.:** Effects of high peak power microwaves on the retina of the rhesus monkey. *Bioelectromagnetics 21*:439–454 (2000).
334. **Szydzinski, A., A. Pietraszek, M. Janiak, J. Wrembel, M. Kalczak, and S. Szmigielski:** Acceleration of the development of benzopyrene-induced skin cancer in mice by microwave radiation. *Dermatol. Res. 274*:303–312 (1982).
335. **Szmigielski, S.A., A. Szudzinski, A. Pietraszek, M. Bielec, M. Janiak, and J. Wrembel:** Accelerated development of spontaneous and benzopyrene-induced skin cancer in mice exposed to 2450 MHz microwave radiation. *Bioelectromagnetics 3*:171–191 (1982).
336. **Santini, R., M. Hosni, P. Deschaux, and H. Pacheco:** B16 melanoma development in black mice exposed to low-level microwave radiation. *Bioelectromagnetics 9*:105–107 (1988).
337. **Wu R.Y., H. Chiang, B.J. Shao, N.G. Li, Y.D. Fu:** Effects of 2.45-GHz microwave radiation and phorbol ester 12-o-tetradecanoylphorbol-13-acetate on dimethylhydrazine colon cancer in mice. *Bioelectromagnetics 15*:531–538 (1994).
338. **Adey, W.R., C.V. Byus, C.D. Cain, et al.:** Spontaneous and nitrosourea-induced primary tumors of the central nervous system in fischer 344 rats chronically exposed to 836 MHz modulated microwaves. *Radiat. Res. 152*: 293–302 (1999).
339. **U.S. Air Force:** *Effects of Long-Term Low-Level Radiofrequency Radiation Exposure on Rats,* vol. 9 (Summary by A.W. Guy, C.-K. Chou, L.L. Kunz, J. Crowley, and J. Krupp; School of Aerospace Medicine Report USAF-SAM-TR-85-64), pp. 16–19. Brooks Air Force Base, Tex.: U.S. Air Force, 1985.
340. **Chou, C.-K., A.W. Guy, L.L. Kunz, R.B. Johnson, J.J. Crowley, and J.H. Krupp:** Long-term, low-level microwave irradiation of rats. *Bioelectromagnetics 13*:469–496 (1992).
341. **Elwood, J.M.:** A critical review of epidemiologic studies of radiofrequency exposure and human cancers. *Environ. Health Perspect. 107*(suppl. 1):155–168 (1999).
342. **Robinette, D., C. Silverman, and S. Jablon:** Effects upon health of occupational exposure to microwave radiation (radar). *Am. J. Epidemiol. 112*:39–53 (1980).
343. **Garland F.C., E. Shaw, E.D. Gorham, C.F. Garland, M.R. White, and P.J. Sinsheimer:** Incidence of leukemia in occupations with potential electromagnetic field exposure in United States Navy personnel. *Am. J. Epidemiol. 132*:293–303 (1990).

344. **Szmigielski, S.:** Cancer morbidity in subjects occupationally exposed to high frequency (radiofrequency and microwave) electromagnetic radiation. *Sci. Total Environ. 180*:9–17 (1996).
345. **Grayson, J.K.:** Radiation exposure, socioeconomic status, and brain tumor risk in the US Air Force: A nested case-control study. *Am. J. Epidemiol. 143*:480–486 (1996).
346. **Hill, D.G.:** *A Longitudinal Study of a Cohort with Past Exposure to Radar: The MIT Radiation Laboratory Follow-Up Study.* Ann Arbor, Mich.: University Microfilms International, 1988.
347. **Muscat, J.E., M.G. Malkin, S. Thompson, et al.:** Handheld cellular telephone use and risk of brain cancer. *J. Am. Med. Assoc. 284*:3001–3007 (2000).
348. **Morgan, R.W., M.A. Kelsh, K. Zhao, A. Exuzides, S. Heringer, and W. Negrete:** Radiofrequency exposure and mortality from cancer of the brain and lymphatic/hematopoietic systems. *Epidemiology 11*:118–127 (2000).
349. **Hardell, L., A. Nasman, A. Pahlson, A. Hallquist, and K.H. Mild:** Use of cellular telephones and the risk for brain tumours: A case-control study. *Int. J. Oncol. 15*:113–116 (1999).
350. **Finkelstein, M.:** Cancer incidence among Ontario police officers. *Am. J. Ind. Med. 34*:157–162 (1998).
351. **Dolk, H., G. Shaddick, P. Walls, et al.:** Cancer incidence near radio and television transmitters in Great Britain I. Sutton Coldfield transmitter. *Am. J. Epidemiol. 145*:1–9 (1997).
352. **Dolk, H., P. Elliott, G. Shaddick, P. Walls, and B. Thakrar:** Cancer incidence near radio and television transmitters in Great Britain I. All high power transmitters. *Am. J. Epidemiol. 145*:10–17 (1997).
353. **Hocking, B., I.R. Gordon, H.L. Grain, and G.E. Hatfield:** Cancer incidence and mortality and proximity to TV towers. *Med. J. Australia 165*:601–605 (1996).
354. **Hirsch, F.G., and J.T. Parker:** Bilateral lenticular opacities ocurring in a technician operating a microwave generator. *AMA Arch. Ind. Hyg. Occup. Med. 6*:512–517 (1952).
355. **Dougherty, J.D., J.C. Caldwell, W.M. Howe, and W.B. Clark:** Evaluation of an alleged case of radiation induced cataract at a radar site. *Aerospace Med. 36*:466–471 (1965).
356. **Rose, V.E., G.A. Gellin, C.H. Powell, and H.G. Bourne:** Evaluation and control of exposures in repairing microwave ovens. *Am. Ind. Hyg. Assoc. J. 30*:137–142 (1969).
357. **Joyner, K.H.:** Microwave cataract and litigation: A case study. *Health Phys. 57*:545–549 (1989).
358. **Lim, J.I., S.L. Fine, H.A. Kues, and M.A. Johnson:** Visual abnormalities associated with high-energy microwave exposure. *Retina 13*:230–233 (1993).
359. **Fleck, H.:** Microwave oven burn. *Bull. N.Y. Acad. Med. 59*:313–317 (1983).
360. **Dickason, W.L., and J.P. Barutt:** Investigation of an acute microwave-oven hand injury. *J. Hand Surg. 9A*:132–135 (1984).
361. **Ciano, M., J.R. Burlin, R. Pardoe, R.L. Mills, and V.R. Hentz:** High-frequency electromagnetic radiation injury to the upper extremity: local and systemic effects. *Ann. Plast. Surg. 7*:128–135 (1981).
362. **Tintinalli, J.E., G. Krause, and E. Gursel:** Microwave radiation injury. *Ann. Emerg. Med. 12*:645–647 (1983).
363. **Hocking, B., K. Joyner, and R. Fleming:** Health aspects of radio-frequency radiation accidents. Part I: Assessment of health after a radio-frequency radiation accident. *J. Microwave Power Electromag. Energy 23*:67–74 (1988).
364. **Schilling, C.J.:** Effects of acute exposure to ultrahigh radiofrequency radiation on three antenna engineers. *Occup. Environ. Med 54*:281–284 (1997).
365. **Rosenthal, D.S., and S.C. Beering:** Hypogonadoism after microwave radiation. *J. Am. Med. Assoc. 205*:105–108 (1968).
366. **Rubin, A., and W.J. Erdman:** Microwave exposure of the human female pelvis during early pregnancy and prior to conception. *Am. J. Phys. Med. 38*:219–220 (1959).
367. **Brodkin, R.H., and J. Bleiberg:** Cutaneous microwave injury. *Acta Dermatol. 53*:50–52 (1973).
368. **Heins, A.P.:** "RF Investigation Involving the Maersk Constellation." 1990. [Personal communication] U.S. Department of Labor, Health Response Team, Salt Lake City, Utah.
369. **Shepich, T.J.:** "Safety Hazard Information Bulletin on Radiofrequency Radiation-Caused Burns." Washington, D.C.: U.S. Department of Labor, Occupational Safety and Health Administration, 1990.
370. **Hocking, B., K.J. Joyner, H.N. Newman, and R.J. Allred:** Radiofrequency electric shock and burn. *Med. J. Australia 161*:683–685 (1994).
371. **McLaughlin, J.T.:** Tissue destruction and death from microwave radiation (radar). *Calif. Med. 86*:336–339 (1957).
372. **Ely, T.S.:** Microwave death. *J. Am. Med. Assoc. 6*:1394 (1971).
373. **Ely, T.S.:** Science and standards—a letter to the editor. *J. Microwave Power 20*:137 (1985).
374. **Archimbaud, E., C. Charrin, D. Guyotat, and J.-J. Viala:** Acute myelogenous leukemia following exposure to microwaves. *Br. J. Haematol. 73*:272–273 (1989).

375. **Jauchem, J.R.:** Correspondence: Leukaemia following exposure to microwaves: Analysis of a case report. *Br. J. Haematol. 76*:312 (1990).
376. **Archimbaud, E.:** Correspondence. *Br. J. Haematol. 73*:313 (1990).
377. **Hocking, B., and M. Garson:** Correspondence. *Br. J. Haematol. 76*:313–314 (1990).
378. **Budd, R.:** Burns associated with the use of microwave ovens. *J. Microwave Power Electromag. Energy 27*:160–163 (1992).
379. **Reeves, G.I.:** Review of extensive workups of 34 patients overexposed to radiofrequency radiation. *Aviat. Space Environ. Med. 71*:206–215 (2000).
380. **Feucht, B.L., A.W. Richardson, and H.M. Hines:** Effects of implanted metals on tissue hyperthermia produced by microwaves. *Arch. Phys. Med. 30*:164–169 (1949).
381. **Hepfner, S.T.:** Radio-frequency interference in cochlear implants. *New Engl. J. Med. 313*:387 (1985).
382. **Chou, C.K., J.A. McDougall, and K.W. Chan:** Absence of radiofrequency heating from auditory implants during magnetic resonance imaging. *Bioelectromagnetics 16*:307–316 (1995).
383. **Hocking, B., K.H. Joyner, and A.H.J. Fleming:** Implanted medical devices in workers exposed to radio-frequency radiation. *Scand. J. Work Environ. Health 17*:1–6 (1991).
384. **Davias, N., and D.W. Griffin:** Effect of metal-framed spectacles on microwave radiation hazards to the eyes of humans. *Med. Biol. Eng. Comput. 27*:191–197 (1989).
385. **Cook, C.F., and P.A. Huggins:** Effect of radio frequency interference on common industrial hygiene monitoring instruments. *Am. Ind. Hyg. Assoc. J. 45*:740–744 (1984).
386. **Shackford, H., and B.E. Bjarngard**: Disturbance of diode dosimetry by radiofrequency radiation. *Med. Phys. 22*:807 (1995).
387. **Carrillo, R., O. Garay, Q. Balzano, and M. Pickels:** Electromagnetic near field interference with implantable medical devices. In *IEEE International Symposium on Electromagnetic Compatibility*, pp. 1–3. New York: IEEE, 1995.
388. **Coray, R., and H. Schaer:** Immunity of cardiac pacemakers and risk potential of pacemaker patients, with special regard to high-power medium- and short-wave transmitters. In *Ninth International Conference on Electromagnetic Compatibility* (Conf. pub. no. 396), pp. 6–12. Manchester, UK: Institution of Electrical Engineers, 1994.
389. **Boivin, W.S., S.M. Boyd, J.A. Coletta, and L.M. Neunaber:** Measurement of radiofrequency electromagnetic fields in and around ambulances. *Biomed. Instrum. Technol. 31*:145–154 (1997).
390. **Kingston, H.M., P.J. Walter, W.G. Engelhart, and P.J. Parsons:** Chemical laboratory microwave safety. In *Microwave Enhanced Chemistry: Fundamentals, Sample Preparation, and Applications* (ACS Professional Reference Book Series). Washington, D.C.: American Chemical Society, 1997.
391. **Tell, R.A., and E.D. Mantiply:** Population exposure to VHF and UHF broadcast radiation in the United States. *Proc. IEEE 68*:6–12 (1980).
392. **Environmental Protection Agency:** *The Radiofrequency Radiation Environment: Environmental Exposure Levels and RF Radiation Emitting Sources*, by N.N. Hankin (EPA 520/1-85-014). Washington, D.C.: U.S. Government Printing Office, 1986.
393. **Mild, K.H., and K.G. Lovstrand:** Environmental and professionally encountered electromagnetic fields. In *Biological Effects and Medical Applications of Electromagnetic Energy*, pp. 48–74. Englewood Cliffs, N.J.: Prentice Hall, 1990.
394. **Environmental Protection Agency:** A review of radiofrequency electric and magnetic fields in the general and work environment: 10 kHz to 100 GHz, by E.D. Mantiply, S.W. Poppell, and J.A. James. In *Summary and Results of the April 26–27, 1993 Radiofrequency Radiation Conference*, vol. 2 (402-R-95-011), pp. 1–23. Washington, D.C.: U.S. Government Printing Office, 1995.
395. **National Council on Radiation Protection and Measurements:** *A Practical Guide to The Determination of Human Exposure to Radiofrequency Fields* (NCRP Report No. 119). Bethesda, Md.: NCRP, 1993.
396. **Conover, D.L., W.E. Murray, E.D. Foley, J.M. Lary and W.H. Parr:** Measurement of electric- and magnetic-field strengths from industrial radio-frequency (6-38 MHz) plastic sealers. *Proc. IEEE 68*:17–20 (1980).
397. **Stuchly, M.A., M.H. Repacholi, D. Lecuyer, and R. Mann:** Radiation survey of dielectric (RF) heaters in Canada. *J. Microwave Power 15*:113–121 (1980).
398. **Cox, C., W.E. Murray, and E.P. Foley:** Occupational exposures to radiofrequency radiation (18–31 MHz) from RF dielectric heat sealers. *Am. Ind. Hyg. Assoc. J. 43*:149–153 (1982).
399. **Gandhi, O., J.-Y. Chen, and A. Riazi:** Currents induced in human beings for plane-wave exposure conditions 0–50 MHz and for RF sealers. *IEEE Trans. Bio-Med. Eng. BME-33*:757–767 (1986).
400. **Conover, D.L., C.E. Moss, W.E. Murray, et al.:** Foot currents and ankle SARs induced by dielectric heaters. *Bioelectromagnetics 13*:103–110 (1992).

401. **Stuchly, M.A., and D.W. Lecuyer:** Induction heating and operator exposure to electromagnetic fields. *Health Phys. 49*:693–700 (1985).
402. **Desrosiers, R.:** "Radio Frequency (RF) Using Tools and Some Observations on RF Emissions." September 30, 1986. [Personal Communication] IBM Corporation, Burlington, VT 05452.
403. **Ungers, L.J., J.H. Jones, and G.J. Mihlan:** "Emission of Radio-Frequency Radiation from Plasma-Etching Operations." Paper presented at the 1985 American Industrial Hygiene Conference, Las Vegas, NV, May 19–24, 1985.
404. **Joyner, K.H., and M.J. Bangay:** Exposure survey of civilian airport radar workers in Australia. *J. Microwave Power 21*:209–219 (1986).
405. **Tell, R.A., and J.C. Nelson:** Microwave hazard measurements near various aircraft radars. *Rad. Data Rep. 15*:161–179 (1974).
406. **Tell, R.A., N.N. Hankin, and D.E. Janes:** Aircraft radar measurements in the near field. In *Operational Health Physics, Proceedings of the Ninth Midyear Topical Symposium of the Health Physics Society.* McLean, Va.: Health Physics Society, 1976.
407. **Food and Drug Administration:** *Measurement of Power Density from Marine Radar*, by D.W. Peak, D.L. Conover, W.A. Herman and R.E. Shuping [Publication no. HEW [FDA] 76-8004]. Washington, D.C.: U.S. Government Printing Office, 1975.
408. **National Institute for Occupational Safety and Health:** "Hazard Evaluation and Technical Assistance Report Technical Assistance to the Federal Employees Occupational Health Seattle, Washington," by C.E. Moss (Rep. no. HETA 89-284-L2029; NTIS no. PB91-107920). Springfield, Va.: National Technical Information Service, 1990.
409. **National Institute for Occupational Safety and Health:** "Hazard Evaluation Report United States Coast Guard Governors Island, New York," by C.E. Moss and A.T. Zimmer (Rep. no. HETA 93-002-22829; NTIS no. PB93-215051). Springfield, Va.: National Technical Information Service, 1993.
410. **Fisher, P.D.:** Microwave exposure levels encountered by police traffic radar operators. *IEEE Trans. Electromag. Compat. 35*:36–45 (1993).
411. **Ontario Ministry of Labour:** *Microwave Emissions and Operator Exposures from Traffic Radars Used in Ontario*, by M.E. Bitran, D.E. Charron, and J.M. Nishio. Weston, Ontario: Ministry of Labour, 1992.
412. **National Institute for Occupational Safety and Health:** "Health Hazard Evaluation Report Norfolk Police Department, Norfolk, Virginia," by R. Malkin (Rep. no. HETA 92-0224-2379; NTIS no. PB 94-183456). Springfield, Va.: National Technical Information Service, 1994.
413. **Fink, J.M., J.P. Wagner, J.J. Congleton, and J.C. Rock:** Microwave emissions from police radar. *Am. Ind. Hyg. Assoc. J. 60*:770–776 (1999).
414. **U.S. Air Force:** *Radio Frequency Radiation Hazard Survey 141 Tactical Control System Ramey PR*, by N.D. Montgomery (AFOEHL Rep. 90-088RC00679ERA; NTIS no. AD-A225-343). Springfield, Va.: National Technical Information Service, 1990.
415. **Curtis, R.A.:** Occupational exposures to radiofrequency radiation from FM radio and TV antennas. In *Nonionizing Radiation—Proceedings from a Topical Symposium*, pp. 211–222. Cincinnati, Ohio: American Conference of Governmental Industrial Hygienists, 1980.
416. **Tell, R.A.:** "Induced Body Currents and Hot AM Tower Climbing Assessing Human Exposure in Relation to the ANSI Radiofrequency Protection Guide" (NTIS no. PB92-125186). [Rep prep. for Federal Communications Commission] Springfield, Va.: National Technical Information Service, 1991.
417. **Joyner, K.H., and M.J. Bangay:** Exposure survey of civilian airport radar workers in Australia. *J. Microwave Power 21*:209–219 (1986).
418. **Environmental Protection Agency:** *An Evaluation of Selected Satellite Communication Systems as Sources of Environmental Microwave Radiation*, by N.N. Hankin (EPA-520/2-74-008). Washington, D.C.: EPA, 1974.
419. **Petersen, R.C., and P.A. Testagrossa:** Radiofrequency electromagnetic fields associated with cellular-radio cell-site antennas. *Bioelectromagnetics 13*:527–542 (1992).
420. **Environmental Protection Agency (EPA):** *An Investigation of Energy Densities in the Vicinity of Vehicles with Mobile Communications Equipment and Near a Hand-Held Walkie-Talkie*, by D.L. Lambdin (Report no. ORP/EAD 79-2). Las Vegas, NV: EPA, 1979.
421. **Food and Drug Administration:** *Measurements of Electromagnetic Fields in the Close Proximity of CB Antennas*, by P.S. Ruggera (Publication no. HEW [FDA] 79-8080). Washington, D.C.: Government Printing Office, 1979.
422. **Guy, A.W., and C.-K. Chou:** Specific absorption rates of energy in man models exposed to cellular UHF mobile-antenna fields. *IEEE Trans. Microwave Theory Tech. MTT-34*:671–680 (1986).

423. **Cleveland, R.F., and T.W. Athey:** Specific absorption rate (SAR) in models of the human head exposed to hand-held UHF portable radios. *Bioelectromagnetics 10*:173–186 (1989).
424. **Dimbylow, P.J., and S.M. Mann:** SAR calculations in an anatomically realistic model of the head for mobile communication transceivers at 900 MHz and 1.8 GHz. *Phys. Med. Biol. 39*:1537–1553 (1994).
425. **Kuster, N., and Q. Balzano:** Energy absorption mechanisms by biological bodies in the near field of dipole antennas. *IEEE Trans. Vehic. Technol. VT-41*:17–23 (1992).
426. **Rothman, K.J., C.-K. Chou, R. Morgan, et al.:** Assessment of cellular telephone and other radio frequency exposure for epidemiologic research. *Epidemiology 7*:291–298 (1996).
427. **Royal Society of Canada:** *A Review of the Potential Health Risks of Radiofrequency Fields from Wireless Telecommunications Devices* (RSC.ERP 99-1). Ottawa, Ontario: Royal Society of Canada, 1999.
428. **Independent Expert Group on Mobile Phones:** *Mobile Phones and Health.* Chilton, Didcot, Oxon, UK: National Radiological Protection Board, 2000.
429. **Center for Devices and Radiological Health:** *An Evaluation of Radiation Emission from Video Display Terminals* (Publication no. DHHS [FDA] 81-8153). Rockville, Md.: CDRH, 1981.
430. **Australian Radiation Laboratory:** *Electromagnetic Emissions from Video Display Terminals (VDTs)*, by K.H. Joyner, C.R. Roy, G. Elliott, M.J. Bangay, H.P. Gies and D.W. Tomlinson (ARL/TR067). Yallambie, Victoria: Australian Radiation Laboratory, 1984.
431. **National Institute for Occupational Safety and Health (NIOSH):** *Potential Health Hazards of Video Display Terminals*, by W.E Murray, C.E. Moss, W.H. Parr, et al. [Publication no. DHHS (NIOSH) 81-129]. Cincinnati, Ohio: NIOSH, 1981.
432. **Boivin, W.S.:** RF electric fields: VDTs vs. TV receivers. In *Proceedings of the International Scientific Conference: Work with Display Units*, pp. 36–39. Amsterdam: Elsevier Scientific Publishers, 1986.
433. **Food and Drug Administration:** *Measurements of Emission Levels During Microwave and Shortwave Diathermy Treatments*, by P.S. Ruggera [Publication no. DHHS (FDA) 80-8119]. Washington, D.C.: U.S. Government Printing Office, 1980.
434. **Stuchly, M.A., M.H. Repacholi, D.W. Lecuyer, and R.D. Mann:** Exposure to the operator and patient during short wave diathermy treatments. *Health Phys. 42*:341–366 (1981).
435. **Hansson Mild, K.:** Occupational exposure to radio-frequency electromagnetic fields. *Proc. IEEE 68*:12–17 (1980).
436. **Ruggera, P.S.:** Near-field measurements of RF fields. In *Symposium on Biological Effects and Measurement of Radio Frequency/ Microwaves* [Publication no. HEW (FDA) 77-8026], pp. 104–116. Washington, D.C.: Government Printing Office, 1977.
437. **Paz, J.D.:** Potential ocular damage from microwave exposure during electrosurgery dosimetric survey. *J. Occup. Med. 29*:580–583 (1987).
438. **Institute of Electrical and Electronics Engineers (IEEE):** *IEEE Standard for Safety Levels with Respect to Human Exposure to Radio Frequency Electromagnetic Fields, 3 kHz to 300 GHz* (C95.1-1999). New York: IEEE, 1999.
439. **International Commission on Non-Ionizing Radiation Protection:** Guidelines for limiting exposure to time-varying electric, magnetic, and electromagnetic fields (up to 300 GHz). *Health Phys. 74*:494–522 (1998).
440. **National Council on Radiation Protection and Measurements:** *Biological Effects and Exposure Criteria for Radiofrequency Electromagnetic Fields* (NCRP rep. no. 86). Bethesda, Md.: NCRP, 1986.
441. **Federal Communications Commission (FCC), Office of Engineering and Technology:** *Evaluating Compliance with FCC Guidelines for Human Exposure to Radiofrequency Electromagnetic Fields* (OET bull. 65). Washington, D.C.: FCC, 1997.
442. **Erdreich, L.S., and B.J. Klauenberg:** Radio frequency radiation exposure standards: Considerations for harmonization. *Health Phys. 80*:430–439 (2001).
443. **Gandhi, O.P.:** State of knowledge for electromagnetic absorbed dose in man and animals. Proc. IEEE 68:24–32 (1980).
444. **Aslan, E.:** Broad-band isotropic electromagnetic radiation monitor. *IEEE Trans. Instrum. Meas. IM-21*:421–424 (1972).
445. **Larsen, E.B., and F.X. Ries:** *Design and Calibration of the NBS Isotropic Electric-Field Monitor (EFM-5), 0.2 to 1000 MHz* (NBS tech. note 1033). Washington, D.C.: U.S. Government Printing Office, 1981.
446. **Tell, R.A.:** Instrumentation for measurement of electromagnetic fields: equipment, calibrations and selected applications. Part I—radiofrequency fields. In M. Grandolfo, S. Michaelson, and A. Rindi, editors, *Biological Effects and Dosimetry of Nonionizing Radiation Radio-frequency and Microwave Energies*, pp. 95–144. New York: Plenum Press, 1981.
447. **Aslan, E.:** A Low Frequency H-Field Radiation Monitor. In *Biological Effects of Electromagnetic Waves* [Publication no. HEW (FDA) 77-8011], pp. 229–238. Washington, D.C.: Government Printing Office, 1976.

448. **National Institute for Occupational Safety and Health (NIOSH):** *Development of Magnetic Near-Field Probes*, by F.M. Greene [Publication no. HEW (NIOSH) 75-127]. Cincinnati, Ohio: NIOSH, 1975.
449. **Institute of Electrical and Electronics Engineers (IEEE):** *IEEE Recommended Practice for the Measurement of Potentially Hazardous Electromagnetic Fields—RF and Microwave* (C95.3-1991). New York: IEEE, 1992.
450. **Conti, R.:** Instrumentation for Measurement of Power Frequency Electromagnetic Fields. In M. Grandolfo, S.M. Michaelson, and A. Rindi, editors, *Biological Effects and Dosimetry of Static and ELF Electromagnetic Fields*, pp. 187–210. New York: Plenum Press, 1985.
451. **Baron, D.:** Measuring EMF emissions from video display terminals. *Compliance Eng. Mag. 8*(5):1–5 (1991).
452. **Gandhi, O.P., I. Chatterjee, D. Wu, and Y.-G. Gu:** Likelihood of high rates of energy deposition in the human legs at the ANSI recommended 3–30 MHz RF safety levels. *Proc. IEEE 73*:1145–1147 (1985).
453. **Gandhi, O.P., J.-Y. Chen, and A. Riazzi:** Currents induced in a human being for plane-wave exposure conditions 0–50 MHz in RF sealers. *IEEE Trans. Biomed. Eng. 33*:757–767 (1986).
454. **Federal Communications Commission:** *Engineering Services for Measurement and Analysis of Radiofrequency (RF) Fields*, by Richard A. Tell (OET/RTA 95-01). Washington, D.C.: U.S. Government Printing Office, 1995.
455. **Lubinas, V., and K.H. Joyner:** *Measurement of Induced Current Flows in the Ankles of Humans Exposed to Radiofrequency Fields* (Rep. 8000). Clayton, Victoria, Australia: Telecom Research Laboratories, 1991.
456. **National Institute of Occupational Health:** *Guidelines for the Measurement of RF Welders*, by P. Williams and K.H. Mild (Undersokningsrapport 1991:8; Rapportkod: ISRN AI/UND-91-8-SE). Umea, Sweden: National Institute of Occupational Health, 1991.
457. **Beischer, D.E., and V.R. Reno:** Microwave reflection and diffraction by man. In *Biologic Effects and Health Hazards of Microwave Radiation*, pp. 254–259. Warsaw, Poland: Polish Medical Publishers, 1974.
458. **Beischer, D.E., and V.R. Reno:** Microwave energy distribution measurements in proximity to man and their practical application. *Ann. N.Y. Acad. Sci. 247*:473–479 (1975).
459. **Bassen, H., and J. Bing:** An EM radiation safety controller. *J. Microwave Power 14*:45–48 (1979).
460. **Eure, J.A., J.W. Nicolls, and R.L. Elder:** Radiation exposure from industrial microwave applications. *Am. J. Pub. Health 62*:1573–1577 (1972).
461. **Keiser, B.E.:** *Principles of Electromagnetic Compatibility*. Dedham, Mass.: Artech House, 1979.
462. **Ott, H.W.:** *Noise Reduction Techniques in Electronic Systems*. New York: John Wiley & Sons, 1976.
463. **Yasufuku, S.:** Technical progress of EMI shielding materials in Japan. *IEEE Elect. Insulat. Mag. 6*(6):21–30 (1990).
464. **Naishadham, K.:** Shielding effectiveness of conductive polymers. *IEEE Trans. Electromag. Compat. 34*:47–50 (1992).
465. **Colaneri, N.F., and L.W. Shacklett:** EMI shielding measurements of conductive polymer blends. *IEEE Trans. Instrum. Measure. 41*:291–297 (1992).
466. **Brailsford, F.:** *Magnetic Materials*, 3rd ed. New York: John Wiley & Sons, 1960.
467. **Trenkler, Y., and L.E. McBride:** Characterization of metals as EMC shields. In *IEEE Instrumentation and Measurement Conference* (86CH2271-5), pp. 65–69. New York: IEEE, 1986.
468. **Hoeft, L.O.:** Measured magnetic field reduction of copper-sprayed wood panels. In *IEEE 1985 International Symposium on Electromagnetic Compatibility* (85CH2116-2), pp. 34–37. New York: IEEE, 1985.
469. **Jonnada, R.K.R., and K.A. Peebles:** Effects of shield discontinuities on the performance of shielded enclosures. In *1965 Symposium Digest Seventh National Symposium on Electromagnetic Compatibility*. New York: Institute of Electrical and Electronics Engineers, 1965.
470. **Honig, E.M., Jr.:** Electromagnetic shielding effectiveness of steel sheets with partly welded seams. *IEEE Trans. Electromag. Compat. EMC-19*:377-382 (1977).
471. **Soltys, J.J.:** Maintaining EMI/RFI shielding integrity of equipment enclosures with conductive gasketing. In *IEEE International Symposium on Electromagnetic Compatibility* (CH1304-5), pp. 333–338. New York: IEEE, 1978.
472. **White, D.R.J., and M. Mardiguian:** Gasket types and materials: A basic selection guide. *EMC Technol. Interference Control News 8*(1):59–64 (1989).
473. **Molyneux-Child, J.W.:** Knitted gasketing for enclosure shielding. *New Elec. 19*(14):48, 51 (1986).
474. **Bereuter, W.A., and D.C. Chang:** Shielding effectiveness of metallic honeycombs. *IEEE Trans. Electromag. Compat. EMC-24*:58–61 (1982).

475. **Kunkel, G.M.:** Shielding characteristics of honeycomb filters. In *1986 IEEE International Symposium on Electromagnetic Compatibility* (86CH2294-7), pp. 299–303. New York: IEEE, 1986.
476. **Bureau of Radiological Health:** *Concepts and Approaches for Minimizing Excessive Exposure to Electromagnetic Radiation from RF Sealers*, by P.S. Ruggera and D.H. Schaubert (DHHS [FDA] 82-8192). Washington, D.C.: Government Printing Office, 1982.
477. **Hill, D.A.:** Effect of separation from ground on whole-body absorption rates. *IEEE Trans. Microwave Theory Tech. MTT-32*:772–778 (1984).
478. **National Institute for Occupational Safety and Health:** "Health Hazard Evaluation Report Dometic Corporation, La Grange, Indiana," by T.A. Seitz, C.E. Moss, and R. Shults (Publication no. HETA 90-389-2272; NTIS no. PB93-215028). Springfield, Va.: National Technical Information Service, 1992.
479. **Gandhi, O.P., and E.L. Hunt:** Corner-reflector applicators for multilateral exposure of animals in bioeffect experiments. *Proc. IEEE 68*:160–162 (1980).
480. **Gandhi, O.P., E.L. Hunt, and J.A. D'Andrea:** Deposition of electromagnetic energy in animals and in models of man with and without grounding and reflector effects. *Radio Sci. 6* (suppl.):39–47 (1977).
481. **Chen, J.-Y., and O.P. Gandhi:** Electromagnetic deposition in an anatomically based model of man for leakage fields of a parallel-plate dielectric heater. *IEEE Trans. Microwave Theory Tech. 37*:174–180 (1989).
482. **Reynolds, M.R.:** Development of a garment for protection of personnel working in high-power RF environments. In *Proceedings of the Fourth Annual Tri-Service Conference on the Biological Effects of Microwave Radiation* (vol. 1), pp. 71–81. New York: Plenum Press, 1961.
483. **Klascius, A.F.:** Microwave radiation protective suit. *Am. Ind. Hyg. Assoc. J. 32*:771–774 (1971).
484. **Chou, C.-K., A.W. Guy, and J.A. McDougall:** Shielding effectiveness of improved microwave-protective suits. *IEEE Trans. Microwave Theory Tech. MTT-35*:995–1001 (1987).
485. **Joyner, K.H., P.R. Copeland, and I.P. MacFarlane:** An evaluation of a radiofrequency protective suit and electrically conductive fabrics. *IEEE Trans. Electromag. Compat. 31*:129–137 (1989).
486. **Amato, J.A.:** Use protective clothing for safety in RF Fields. *Mobile Radio Technol. 12*(4):40, 42, 44 (1994).
487. **De Bruyne, R., and W. Van Loock:** New class of microwave shielding materials. *J. Microwave Power 12*:145–154 (1977).
488. **Heins, A.P., and R. Curtis:** "RF Shock Hazard Inspection Terminal 5, Port of Seattle." 1990. [Personal communication]. USDOL OSHA Health Response Team, Salt Lake City, Utah.
489. **Heins, A.P.:** R.F. Investigation Involving The Maersk Constellation. (Letter to M. Grueber). Salt Lake City, UT: USDOL OSHA Health Response Team, 1990.
490. **Tell, R.A.:** *RF Current Reduction Provided by Work Gloves at AM Radio Broadcast Frequencies* (FCC/OET contract report no. RTA 93-01; NTIS no. PB94-117041). Springfield, Va.: National Technical Information Service, (1993).
491. **Institute of Electrical and Electronics Engineers (IEEE):** *IEEE Standard for Radio-Frequency Energy and Current-Flow Symbols* (IEEE C95.2-1999). New York: IEEE, 1999.
492. **Tenforde, T.S., and W.T. Kaune:** Interaction of extremely low frequency electric and magnetic fields with humans. *Health Phys. 53*:585–606 (1987).
493. **Deno, D.W.:** Currents induced in the human body by high voltage transmission line electric field—measurement and calculation of distribution and dose. *IEEE Trans. Power Appar. Syst. PAS-96*:1517–1527 (1977).
494. **Kaune, W.T., and R.D. Phillips:** Comparison of the coupling of grounded humans, swine, and rats to vertical, 60-Hz electric fields. *Bioelectromagnetics 1*:117–130 (1980).
495. **Tenforde, T.S.:** Biological interactions of extremely-low-frequency electric and magnetic fields. *Biochem. Bioenergetics 25*:1–17 (1991).
496. **Bernhardt, J.H., H.J. Haubrich, G. Newi, N. Krause, and K.H. Schneider:** Limits for Electric and Magnetic Fields in DIN VDE Standards: Considerations for the Range 0 to 10 kHz. Paper presented at CIGRE, International Conference on Large High Voltage Electric Systems, Paris, August 27–September 4, 1986.
497. **Bawin, S.M., L.K. Kaczmarek, and W.R. Adey:** Effects of modulated VHF fields on the central nervous system. *Ann. N.Y. Acad. Sci. 247*:74–81 (1975).
498. **Blackman, C.F., S.G. Benane, L.S. Kinney, W.T. Joines, and D.E. House:** Effects of ELF fields on calcium-ion efflux from brain tissue in vitro. *Radiat. Res. 92*:510–520 (1982).
499. **Blackman, C.F., S.G. Benane, J.R. Rabinowitz, D.E. House, and W.T. Joines:** A role for the magnetic field in the radiation-induced efflux of calcium ions from brain tissue in vitro. *Bioelectromagnetics 6*:327–337 (1985).

500. **Blackman, C.F., L.S. Kinney, D.E. House, and W.T. Joines:** Multiple power-density windows and their possible origin. *Bioelectromagnetics 10*:115–128 (1989).
501. **Blackman, C.F., S.G. Benane, and D.E. House:** The influence of temperature during electric- and magnetic-field- induced alteration of calcium-ion release from in vitro brain tissue. *Bioelectromagnetics 12*:173–182 (1991).
502. **Murphy, J.C., D.A. Kaden, J. Warren, and A. Sivak:** Power frequency electric and magnetic fields: A review of genetic toxicology. *Mutation Res. 296*:221–240 (1993).
503. **McCann, J., F. Dietrich, C. Rafferty, and A.O. Martin:** A critical review of the genotoxic potential of electric and magnetic fields. *Mutation Res. 297*:61–95 (1993).
504. **McCann, J., F. Dietrich, and C. Rafferty:** The genotoxic potential of electric and magnetic fields: An update. *Mutation Res. 411*:45–86 (1998).
505. **Huuskonen, H., M.L. Lindbohm, and J. Juutilainen:** Teratogenic and reproductive effects of low-frequency magnetic-fields. *Mutation Res. 410*:167–183 (1998).
506. **Sikov, M.R., D.N. Rommereim, J.L. Beamer, R.L. Buschbom, W.T. Kaune, and R.D. Phillips:** Developmental studies of hanford miniature swine exposed to 60-Hz electric fields. *Bioelectromagnetics 8*:229–242 (1987).
507. **Rommereim, D.N., R.L. Rommereim, M.R. Sikov, R.L. Buschbom, and L.E. Anderson:** Reproductive, growth, and development of rats during chronic exposure to multiple field strengths of 60-Hz electric fields. *Fund. Appl. Toxicol. 14*:608–621 (1990).
508. **Berman, E., L. Chacon, D. House, et al.:** Development of chicken embryos in a pulsed magnetic field. *Bioelectromagnetics 11*:169–187 (1990).
509. **Rommereim, D.N., R.L. Rommereim, D.L. Miller, R.L. Buschbom, and L.E. Anderson:** Developmental toxicology evaluation of 60-Hz, horizontal magnetic fields in rats. *Appl. Occup. Environ. Hyg. 11*: 307–312 (1996).
510. **Ryan, B.M., E. Mallett, T.R. Johnson, J.R. Gauger, and D.L. McCormack:** Developmental toxicity study of 60 Hz (power frequency) magnetic fields in rats. *Teratology 54*:73–83 (1996).
511. **Juutilainen, J.:** Developmental effects of electromagnetic fields. *Bioelectromag. 7*:S107–S115 (2005).
512. **Shaw, G.M.:** Adverse human reproductive outcomes and electromagnetic fields: A brief summary of the epidemiologic literature. *Bioelectromagnetics 5*:S5–S18 (2001).
513. **Wilson, B.W., L.E. Anderson, D.I. Hilton, and R.D. Phillips:** Chronic exposure to 60-Hz electric fields: Effects on pineal function in the rat. *Bioelectromagnetics 2*:371–380 (1981).
514. **Wilson, B.W., E.K. Chess, and L.E. Anderson:** 60-Hz electric-field effects on pineal melatonin rhythms: Time course for onset and recovery. *Bioelectromagnetics 7*:239–242 (1986).
515. **Kato, M., K. Honma, T. Shigemitsu, and Y. Shiga:** Effects of exposure to a circularly polarized 50-Hz magnetic field on plasma and pineal melatonin levels in rats. *Bioelectromagnetics 14*:97–106 (1993).
516. **Lee, J.M., F. Stormshak, J.M. Thompson, et al.:** Melatonin secretion and puberty in female lambs exposed to environmental electric and magnetic fields. *Biol. Reprod. 49*:857–864 (1993).
517. **Lee, J.M., F. Stormshak, J.M. Thompson, D.L. Hess, and D.L. Foster:** Melatonin and puberty in female lambs exposed to EMF: A replicate study. *Bioelectromagnetics 16*:119–123 (1995).
518. **Truong, H., and S.M. Yellow:** Continuous or intermittent 60 Hz magnetic field exposure fails to affect the nighttime rise in melatonin in the adult Djungarian hamster. *Biol. Reprod. 52*:72 (1995).
519. **Levine, R.L., J.K. Dooley, and T.D. Bluni:** Magnetic-field effects on spatial discrimination and melatonin levels in mice. *Physiol. Behav. 58*:535–537 (1995).
520. **Grota, L.J., R.J. Reiter, P. Keng, and S. Michaelson:** Electric field exposure alters serum melatonin but not pineal melatonin synthesis in male rats. *Bioelectromagnetics 15*:427–438 (1994).
521. **Yaga, K.R.J. Reiter, L.C. Manchester, H. Nieves, J.H. Sun, and L.D. Chen:** Pineal sensitivity to pulsed static magnetic-fields changes during the photoperiod. *Brain Res. Bull. 30*:153–156 (1993).
522. **Selmaoui, B., and Y. Touitou:** Sinusoidal 50-Hz magnetic-fields depress rat Pineal NAT activity and serum melatonin. Role of duration and intensity of exposure. *Life Sci. 57*:1351–1358 (1995).
523. **Rogers, W.R., R.J. Reiter, L. Barlow-Walden, H.D. Smith, and J.L. Orr:** Regularly scheduled, day-time, slow onset 60 hz electric and magnetic field exposure does not depress serum melatonin concentration in nonhuman primates. *Bioelectromagnetics 3*(suppl.):111–118 (1995).
524. **Rogers, W.R., R.J. Reiter, H.D. Smith, and L. Barlow-Walden:** Rapid-onset/offset, variably scheduled 60 Hz electric and magnetic field exposure reduces nocturnal serum melatonin concentration in nonhuman primates. *Bioelectromagnetics 3*(suppl):119–122 (1995).
525. **National Institute of Environmental Health Sciences:** *Assessment of Health Effects from Exposure to Power-Line Frequency Electric and Magnetic Fields.* Research Triangle Park, N.C.: NIEHS: 1998.

526. **Noonan, C., J. Reif, M. Yost, and M. Touchstone:** Occupational exposure to magnetic fields in case-referent studies of neurogenerative diseases. *Scan. J. Work Env. Health 28(1)*:42–48 (2002).
527. **Juutilainen, J., R.G. Stevens, L.E. Anderson, et al.:** Nocturnal 6-hydroxymelatonin sulfate excretion in female workers exposed to magnetic fields. *J. Pineal Res. 28*:97–104 (2000).
528. **Hong, S.C., Y. Kurokawa, M. Kabuto, and R. Ohtsuka:** Chronic exposure to ELF magnetic fields during night sleep with electric sheets: Effects on diurnal melatonin rhythms in men. *Bioelectromagnetics 22*:138–143 (2001).
529. **Graham, C., M.R. Cook, M.M. Gerkovich, and A. Sastre:** Examination of the melatonin hypothesis in women exposed at night to EMF or bright light. *Environ. Health. Perspect. 109*:501–507 (2001a).
530. **Graham, C., M.R. Cook, M.M. Gerkovich, and A. Sastre:** Melatonin and 6-OHMS in high-intensity magnetic fields. *J. Pineal Res. 31*:85–88 (2001).
531. **Davis, S., W.T. Kaune, D.K. Mirick, C. Chen, and R.G. Stevens:** Residential magnetic fields, light-at-night, and nocturnal urinary 6-sulfatoxymelatonin concentration in women. *Am. J. Epidemiol. 154*:591–600 (2001).
532. **Burch, J.B., J.S. Reif, C.W. Noonan, and M.G. Yost:** Melatonin metabolite levels in workers exposed to 60-Hz magnetic fields: Work in substations and with 3-phase conductors. *J. Occup. Environ. Med. 42*:136–142 (2000).
533. **McCann, J., R. Kavet, and C.N. Rafferty:** Assessing the potential carcinogenic activity of magnetic fields using animal models. *Environ. Health Perspect. 108*(suppl 1):79–100 (2000).
534. **Boorman, G.A., D.L. McCormick, J.M. Ward, J.K. Haseman, and R.C. Sills:** Magnetic fields and mammary cancer in rodents: A critical review and evaluation of published literature. *Radiat. Res. 153*:617–626 (2000).
535. **Heath, C.W.:** Electromagnetic field exposure and cancer: A review of epidemiologic evidence. *Ca. Cancer J. Clin. 65*:29–44 (1996).
536. **Carstensen, E.L.:** Magnetic fields and cancer. *IEEE Eng. Med. Biol. Mag. 14*:362–369 (1995).
537. **Advisory Group on Non-Ionising Radiation:** ELF electromagnetic fields and the risk of cancer. In *Documents of the NRPB*, vol. 12, pp. 1–179. London: NRPB, 2001.
538. **International Agency for Research on Cancer (IARC):** *Static and Extremely Low Frequency Electric and Magnetic Fields.* Lyon, France: IARC, 2002.
539. **Feychting, M.:** Occupational exposure to electromagnetic fields and adult leukemia: A review of the epidemiological evidence. *Radiat. Environ. Biophys. 35*:237–242 (1996).
540. **Miller, R.D., J.S. Neuberger, and K.B. Gerald:** Brain cancer and leukemia and exposure to power-frequency (50-to 60-Hz) electric and magnetic fields. *Epidemiol. Rev. 19*:273–293 (1997).
541. **Kheifets, L.I., E.S. Gilbert, S.S. Sussman, et al.:** Comparative analyses of the studies of magnetic field and cancer in electric utility workers: Studies from France, Canada, and the United States. *Occup. Environ. Med. 56*:567–574 (1999).
542. **Kheifets, L.I., A.A. Afifi, P.A. Buffler, Z.W Zhang, and C.C. Matkin:** Occupational electric and magnetic field exposure and leukemia. *J. Occup. Environ. Med. 39*:1074–1091 (1997).
543. **Ahlbom, A., N. Day, M. Feychting, et al.:** A pooled analysis of magnetic fields and childhood leukaemia. Br. J. Cancer 83: 692–698 (2000).
544. **Greenland, S., A.R. Sheppard, W.T. Kaune, C. Poole, and M.A. Kelsh:** A pooled analysis of magnetic fields, wire codes, and childhood leukemia. *Epidemiology 11*:624–634 (2000).
545. **Wartenberg, D.:** Residential EMF exposure and childhood leukemia: Meta-analysis and population attributable risk. *Bioelectromagnetics 5*(suppl): S86–S104 (2001).
546. **Kheifets, L.I., A.A. Afifi, P.A. Buffler, and Z.W. Zhang:** Occupational electric and magnetic field exposure and brain cancer: A meta-analysis. *J. Occup. Environ. Med. 37*:1327–1341 (1995).
547. **Kheifets, L.I.:** Electric and magnetic field exposure and brain cancer: A review. *Bioelectromagnetics 5*(suppl): S120–S131 (2001).
548. **Erren, T.C.:** A meta-analysis of epidemiologic studies of electric and magnetic fields and breast cancer in women and men. *Bioelectromagnetics 5*(suppl):S105–S119 (2001).
549. **Brainard, G.C., R. Kavet, and L.I. Kheifets:** The relationship between electromagnetic field and light exposures to melatonin and breast cancer: A review of the relevant literature. *J. Pineal Res. 26*:65–100 (1999).
550. **Caplan, L.S., E.R. Schoenfeld, E.S. O'Leary, and M.C. Leske:** Breast cancer and electromagnetic fields—a review. *Ann. Epidemiol. 10*: 31–44 (2000).
551. **Kheifets, L., J. Swanson, and S. Greenland:** Childhood Leukemia, Electric and Magnetic Fields, and Temporal Trends. *Bioelectromag. 27*:545–52 (2006).
552. **Khekfets, L., A. Afifi, and R. Shimkhada:** Public health impact of extremely low-frequency electromagnetic fields. *Env. Health Persp. 114(10)*:1532–37 (2006).

553. **Sahl, J.D., M.A. Kelsh, and S. Greenland:** Cohort and nested case-control studies of hematopoietic cancers and brain cancers among electric utility workers. *Epidemiology 4*:104–14 (1993).
554. **Theriault, G., M. Goldberg, A.B. Miller, et al.:** Cancer risks associated with occupational exposure to magnetic fields among electric utility workers in Ontario and Quebec, Canada, and France: 1970–1989. *Am. J. Epidemiol. 139*:550–72 (1994).
555. **Savitz, D.A., and D. P. Loomis:** Magnetic field exposure in relation to leukemia and brain cancer mortality among electric utility workers. *Am. J. Epidemiol. 141*:123–34 (1995).
556. **International Commission for Non-Ionizing Radiation Protection, Standing Committee on Epidemiology:** Review of Epidemiologic Literature on EMF and Health. *Env. Health Persp. 109(6)*:911–33 (2001).
557. **Hitchcock, R.T., S. McMahan, and G.C. Miller:** *Extremely Low Frequency (ELF) Electric and Magnetic Fields.* Fairfax, Va.: American Industrial Hygiene Association, 1995.
558. **Grandolfo, M., and P. Vecchia:** Natural and man-made environmental exposures to static and ELF electromagnetic fields. In M. Grandolfo, S. Michaelson and A. Rindi, editors, *Biological Effects and Dosimetry of Static and ELF Electromagnetic Fields*, pp. 49–70. New York: Plenum Press, 1985.
559. **Kaune, W.T.:** Assessing human exposure to power-frequency electric and magnetic fields. *Environ. Health Perspect. 101*(suppl 4):121–133 (1993).
560. **Skotte, J.H.:** Exposure to power-frequency electromagnetic fields in Denmark. *Scand. J. Work Environ. Health 20*:132–138 (1994).
561. **Tenforde, T.S.:** Spectrum and intensity of environmental electromagnetic fields from natural and man-made sources. In *Electromagnetic Fields Biological Interactions and Mechanisms*, pp. 13–35. Washington, D.C.: American Chemical Society, 1995.
562. **Randa, J., D. Gilliland, W. Gjertson, W. Lauber, and M. McInerney:** Catalogue of electromagnetic environment measurements, 30–300 Hz. *IEEE Trans. Electromag. Compat. 37*:26–33 (1995).
563. **Maruvada, P.S.:** Characterization of power frequency magnetic fields in different environments. *IEEE Trans. Power Del. 8*:598–606 (1993).
564. **Merchant, C.J., D.C. Renew, and J. Swanson:** Exposures to power-frequency magnetic fields in the home. *J. Radiol. Prot. 14*:77–87 (1994).
565. **Friedman, D.R., E.E. Hatch, R. Tarone, et al.:** Childhood exposure to magnetic fields: Residential area measurements compared to personal dosimetry. *Epidemiology 7*:151–155 (1996).
566. **Silva, M., N. Hummon, D. Rutter, and C. Hooper:** Power frequency magnetic fields in the home. *IEEE Trans. Power Del. 4*:465–478 (1989).
567. **Kavet, R., J.M. Silva, and D. Thornton:** Magnetic field exposure assessment for adult residents of Maine who live near and far away from overhead transmission lines. *Bioelectromagnetics 13*:35–55 (1992).
568. **Hartwell, F.:** Magnetic fields from water pipes. *Elec. Const. Main. 92*(3):63–70 (1993).
569. **Florig, H.K., and J.F. Hoburg:** Power-frequency magnetic fields from electric blankets. *Health Phys. 58*:493–502 (1990).
570. **Gauger, J.R.:** Household appliance magnetic field survey. *IEEE Trans. Power Apparat. Systems PAS-104*:2436–2444 (1985).
571. **Tofani, S., P. Ossola, G. D'Amore, and O.P. Gandhi:** Electric field and current density distributions induced in an anatomically based model of the human head by magnetic fields from a hair dryer. *Health Phys. 68*:71–79 (1995).
572. **P reece, A.W., W. Kaune, P. Grainger, S. Preece, and J. Golding:** Magnetic fields from domestic applicances in the UK. *Phys. Med. Biol. 42*:67–76 (1997).
573. **Sun, W.Q., P. Heroux, T. Clifford, V. Sadilek, and F. Hamade:** Characterization of the 60-Hz magnetic fields in schools of the Carleton Board of Education. *Am. Ind. Hyg. Assoc. J. 56*:1215–1224 (1995).
574. **Breysse, P., P.S.J. Lees, M.A. McDiarmid, and B. Curbow:** ELF magnetic field exposures in an office environment. *Am. J. Ind. Med. 25*:177–185 (1994).
575. **Walsh, M.L., S.M. Harvey, R.A. Facey, and R.R. Mallette:** Hazard assessment of video display units. *Am. Ind. Hyg. Assoc. J. 52*:324–331 (1991).
576. **Kerr, L.N., W.S. Boivin, S.M. Boyd, and J.N. Coletta:** Measurement of radiated electromagnetic field levels before and after a changeover to energy-efficient lighting. Biomed. *Instrum. Technol. 35*:104–109 (2001).
577. **Tell, R.A.:** *An Investigation of Electric and Magnetic Fields and Operator Exposure Produced by VDTs: NIOSH VDT Epidemiology Study* (NTIS no. PB91-130500/XAB). Srpingfield, Va.: National Technical Information Service, 1990.
578. **Ontario Ministry of Labour:** *Background ELF Magnetic Fields in Ontario Offices*, by M. Bitran, D. Charron, and J. Nishio. Toronto, Ontario: Ministry of Labour, 1995.
579. **Phillips, K.L.:** "Characterization of Occupational Exposures to Extremely Low Frequency Magnetic Fields in a Health-Care Setting." Master's thesis, School of Public Health, University of Texas, Houston, Tex., 1993.

580. **National Institute for Occupational Safety and Health:** *Electric and Magnetic Fields in a Magnetic Resonance Imaging Facility: Measurements and Exposure Assessment Procedures*, by T.D. Bracken (NTIS no. PB94-174489). Springfield, Va.: National Technical Information Service, 1994.
581. **Paul, M., K. Hammond, and S. Abdollahzadeh:** Power frequency magnetic field exposures among nurses in a neonatal intensive care unit and a normal newborn nursery. *Bioelectromagnetics 15*:519–529 (1994).
582. **Li, C.Y., R.-S. Lin, C.-H. Wu, and F.-C. Sung:** Occupational exposures to pharmacists and pharmaceutical assistants to 60 Hz magnetic fields. *Ind. Health 38*:413–419 (2000).
583. **Minder, Ch.E., and D.F. Pfluger:** Extremely low frequency electromagnetic field measurements (ELF-EMF) in Swiss railway engines. *Radiat. Prot. Dosim. 48*:351–354 (1993).
584. **Department of Transportation:** *Safety of High Speed Guided Ground Transportation Systems. Magnetic and Electric Field Testing of the Amtrak Northeast Corridor and New Jersey Transit/North Jersey Coast Line Rail Systems*, vol. I, by F.M. Dietrich, W.E. Ferro, P.N. Papas, and G.A. Steiner (Publication no. DOT/FRA/ORD-93/01.I; NTIS no. PB93-219434). Springfield, Va.: National Technical Information Service, 1993.
585. **Department of Transportation:** *Safety of High Speed Guided Ground Transportation Systems. Magnetic and Electric Field Testing of the Amtrak Northeast Corridor and New Jersey Transit/North Jersey Coast Line Rail Systems*, vol. II, by F.M. Dietrich, D.C. Robertson, and G.A. Steiner (Publication no. DOT/FRA/ORD-93/01.II; NTIS no. PB93-219442). Springfield, Va.: National Technical Information Service, 1993.
586. **Fisher, R.B.:** Electric and magnetic fields and electric transit systems. *Trans. Res. Rec. 1503*:69–76 (1995).
587. **Yost, M.:** Alternative magnetic field exposure metrics: occupational measurements in trolley workers. *Radiat. Prot. Dosim. 83*:99–106 (1999).
588. **Silva, M., and D. Huber:** Exposure to transmission line electric fields during farming operations. *IEEE Trans. Power Apparat. Syst. PAS-104*:2632-2640 (1985).
589. **Enk, J.O., and M.M. Abromavage:** Exposure to low-level extremely low frequency electromagnetic fields near naval communications facilities. *IEEE J. Oceanic Eng. OE-9*:136-142 (1984).
590. **National Institute for Occupational Safety and Health:** "Chicago Television Stations Chicago, Illinois," by R. Malkin and C.E. Moss (Publication no. HETA 93-0424-2486; NTIS no. PB95-241121). Springfield, Va.: National Technical Information Service, 1995.
591. **Barroetavena, M.C., R. Ross, and K. Teschke:** Electric and magnetic fields at three pulp and paper mills. *Am. Ind. Hyg. Assoc. J. 55*:358–363 (1988).
592. **Vogt, D.R., and J.P. Reynders:** An experimental investigation of magnetic fields in deep level gold mines. In *Seventh International Symposium on High Voltage Engineering 1991*, pp. 63–66. Dresden, Germany: Dresden University of Technology, 1991.
593. **National Institute for Occupational Safety and Health:** "Electro-Galvanizing Company Cleveland, Ohio," by C.E. Moss and D. Mattorano (Publication no. HETA 93-1038-2432 L-S). Springfield, Va.: National Technical Information Service, 1995.
594. **Stuchly, M.A., and D.W. Lecuyer:** Exposure to electromagnetic fields in arc welding. *Health Phys. 56*:297–302 (1989).
595. **Skotte, J.H., and H.I. Hjollund:** Exposure of welders and other metal workers to ELF magnetic fields. *Bioelectromagnetics 18*:470–477 (1997).
596. **Rosenthal F.S., and S. Abdollahzadeh:** Assessment of extremely low frequency (ELF) electric and magnetic fields in microelectronics fabrication rooms. *Appl. Occup. Environ. Hyg. 6*:777–784 (1991).
597. **Lovsund P., P.A. Oberg, and S.E.G. Nilsson:** ELF magnetic fields in electrosteel and welding industries. *Radio Sci. 17*(5S):35S–38S (1982).
598. **Cartwright, C.E, P.N. Breysse, and L. Booher:** Magnetic field exposures in a petroleum refinery. *Appl. Occup. Environ. Hyg. 8*:587–592 (1993).
599. **Wenzl, T.B.:** Assessment of magnetic field exposures for a mortality study at a uranium enrichment plant. *Am. Ind. Hyg. Assoc. J. 60*:818–824 (1999).
600. **Hayashi, N., K. Isaka, and Y. Yokoi:** ELF electromagnetic environment in power substations. *Bioelectromagnetics 10*:51–64 (1989).
601. **Vinh, T., T.L. Jones, and C.H. Shih:** Magnetic fields near overhead distribution lines—measurements and estimating technique. *IEEE Trans. Power Del. 6*:912–921 (1991).
602. **Sahl, J.D., M.A. Kelsh, R.W. Smith, and D.A. Aseltine:** Exposure to 60 Hz magnetic fields in the electric utility work environment. *Bioelectromagnetics 15*:21–32 (1994).
603. **Bracken, T.D., R.F. Rankin, R.S. Senior, J.R. Alldredge, and S.S. Sussman:** Magnetic field exposure among utility workers. *Bioelectromagnetics 16*:216–226 (1995).

604. **Miller, D.A.:** Electrical and magnetic fields produced by commercial power systems. In *Biological and Clinical Effects of Low-Frequency Magnetic and Electric Fields*, pp. 62–70. Springfield, Ill.: Charles C. Thomas, 1974.
605. **Kromhout, H., D.P. Loomis, G.J. Mihlan, et al.:** Assessment and grouping of occupational magnetic field exposure in five electric utility companies. *Scand. J. Work Environ. Health 21*:43–50 (1995).
606. **Deadman, J.E., M. Camus, B.G. Armstrong, et al.:** Occupational and residential 60-Hz electromagnetic fields and high-frequency electric transients: Exposure assessment using a new dosimeter. *Am. Ind. Hyg. Assoc. J. 49*:409–19 (1988).
607. **Straum, A., A. Johnson, and G. Oftedal:** ELF-magnetic flux densities measured in a city environment in summer and winter. *Bioelectromag. 29*:20–28 (2008).
608. **Nicholas, J.S., G.C. Butler, D.T. Lackland, W.C. Hood, D.G. Hoel, and L.C. Mohr, Jr.:** Flight deck magnetic fields in commercial aircraft. *Am. J. Ind. Med. 38*:548–554 (2000).
609. **Kavet, R., W. Bailey, T. Bracken, and R. Patterson:** Recent advances in research relevant to electric and magnetic field exposure guidelines. *Bioelectromag. 29*:499–526 (2008).
610. **IEEE/ICES International Committee on Electromagnetic Safety:** IEEE Standard for Safety Levels with Respect to Human Exposure to Electromagnetic Fields, 0-3 kHz. Standard C96.6. New York: IEEE, 2002.
611. **Bailey, W.H., S.H. Su, T.D. Bracken, and R. Kavet:** Summary and evaluation of guidelines for occupational exposure to power frequency electric and magnetic fields. *Health Phys. 73*: 433–453 (1997).
612. **Environment & Society Working Group, Union of the Electricity Industry:** *Status Report Power-Frequency EMF Exposure Standards* (Ref: 2001-2650-0010). Brussels, Belgium: Eurelectric, 2001.
613. **Mathes, R.:** Response to questions and comments on ICNIRP guidelines for limiting exposure to time-varying electric, magnetic, and electromagnetic fields (up to 300 GHz). *Health Phys. 75*:438–439 (1998).
614. **IEEE Magnetic Fields Task Force:** An evaluation of instrumentation used to measure AC power system magnetic fields. *IEEE Trans. Power Del. 6*:373–383 (1991).
615. **Environmental Protection Agency:** *Final Report Laboratory Testing of Commercially Available Power Frequency Magnetic Field Survey Meters by SC&A, Inc. and Science Applications International Corporation* (EPA 400R-92-010). Washington, D.C.: EPA, 1992.
616. **Zipse, D.W.:** Electric and magnetic fields: Equipment and methodology used for obtaining measurements. IEEE Trans. Ind. Appl. 30:262–268 (1994).
617. **Bartington, G.:** Sensors for low level low frequency magnetic fields. In *Low Level Low Frequency Magnetic Fields* (Digest no. 1994/096), pp. 2/1–2/9. London, UK: Institute of Electrical Engineers, 1994.
618. **Sussman, S.S.:** Exposure assessment at extremely low frequencies: Issues, instrumentation, modeling, and data. *Radio Sci. 30*:151–159 (1995).
619. **Deno, D.W., and M. Silva:** Method of evaluating human exposure to 60 Hz electric fields. *IEEE Trans. Power Apparat. Sys. PAS-103*:1699–1705 (1984).
620. **Hayashi, N., K. Isaka, S. Yura, and Y. Yokoi:** Development of magnetic field dosimeter for exposure application. In *7th International Symposium on High Voltage Engineering*, vol. 9, pp. 83–86. Dresden, Germany: Lechnische Universitat, 1991.
621. **Dlugosz, L., K. Belanger, P. Johnson, and M.B. Bracken:** Human exposure to magnetic fields: A comparative assessment of two dosimeters. *Bioelectromagnetics 15*:593–597 (1994).
622. **Lo, C.C., T.Y. Fujita, A.B. Geyer, and T.S. Tenforde:** A wide dynamic range portable 60-Hz magnetic dosimeter with data acquisition capabilities. *IEEE Trans. Nuc. Sci 33*:643–646 (1986).
623. **Lindh, T., and L.-I. Andersson:** Comparison between two power-frequency electric-field dosimeters. *Scand. J. Work Environ. Health 14*(suppl 1):43–45 (1988).
624. **Heroux, P.:** A dosimeter for assessment of exposures to ELF fields. *Bioelectromagnetics 12*:241–257 (1991).
625. **Douglas, J.:** Taking the measure of magnetic fields. *EPRI J. 17*:16–17 (1993).
626. **Kaune, W.T., J.C. Niple, M.J. Liu, and J.M. Silva:** Small integrating meter for assessing long-term exposure to magnetic fields. *Bioelectromagnetics 13*:413–427 (1992).
627. **National Institute for Occupational Safety and Health:** Manual for Measuring Occupational Electric and Magnetic Field Exposures, by J.D. Bowman, M.A. Kelsh, and W.T. Kaune (Publication no. DHHS [NIOSH] 98-154). Cincinnati, Ohio: NIOSH, 1998.
628. **Patterson, R.M.:** Exposure assessment for electric and magnetic fields. *J. Exp. Anal. Environ. Epidemiol. 2*:159–176 (1992).
629. **Zaffanella, L.E.:** Magnetic field exposure characterization during environmental field surveys for the EMF RAPID program. In A.E. McBride, editor, *Proceedings of the American Power Conference*, vol. 58-1, pp. 263–268. Chicago, Ill.: Illinois Institute of Technology, 1996.

630. **Methner, M.M., and J.D. Bowman:** Hazard surveillance for industrial magnetic fields: I. Walkthrough survey of ambient fields and sources. *Ann. Occup. Hyg. 44*: 603–614 (2000).
631. **Bowman, J.D., and M.M. Methner:** Hazard surveillance for industrial magnetic fields: II. Field characteristics from waveform measurements. *Ann. Occup. Hyg. 44*:615–633 (2000).
632. **Chadwick, P.:** Assessment of industrial exposure to magnetic fields. *Radiat. Prot. Dosim. 83*:47–52 (1999).
633. **Institute of Electrical and Electronic Engineers (IEEE):** *IEEE Standard Procedures for Measurement of Power Frequency Electric and Magnetic Fields from AC Power Lines* (ANSI/IEEE 644-1994). New York: IEEE, 1994.
634. **IEEE Magnetic Fields Task Force:** Measurements of power frequency magnetic fields away from power lines. *IEEE Trans. Power Del. 6*:901–911 (1991).
635. **IEEE Magnetic Fields Task Force:** A protocol for spot measurements of residential power frequency magnetic fields. *IEEE Trans. Power Del. 8*:1386–1394 (1993).
636. **Yost, M.G., G. M. Lee, D. Duane, J. Fisch, and R. R. Neutra:** California protocol for measuring 60 Hz magnetic fields in residences. *Appl. Occup.Environ. Hyg. 7*:772–777 (1992).
637. **Kaune, W.T.:** Assessing human exposure to power-frequency electric and magnetic fields. *Environ. Health Perspect. 101*(suppl 4):121–133 (1993).
638. **Cotten, W.L., K.C.K. Ramsing, and C. Cai:** Design guidelines for reducing electromagnetic field effects from 60-Hz electrical power systems. *IEEE Trans. Ind. Appl. 30*:1462–1471 (1994).
639. **Feero, W.E.:** Electric and magnetic field management. *Am. Ind. Hyg. Assoc. J. 54*:205–210 (1993).
640. **Farag, A.S., M.M. Dawoud, and I.O. Habiballah:** Implementation of shielding principles for magnetic field management of power cables. *Elec. Power Sys. Res. 48*:193–209 (1999).
641. **World Health Organization (WHO):** Environmental Health Criteria 232. Static Fields. Geneva: WHO, 2006.
642. **International Commission on Non-Ionizing Radiation Protection (ICNIRP):** ICNIRP Guidelines on Limits of Exposure to Static Magnetic Fields. *Health Phys. 96(4)*:504–14 (2009).
643. **Gowland, P.:** Present and future magnetic resonance sources of exposure to static fields. *Prog. Biophys. Mol. Bio. 87*:175–83 (2005).
644. **Glaser, Z.R.:** Organization and management of a nonionizing radiation safety program. In *CRC Handbook of Management of Radiation Protection Programs*, 2nd ed., pp. 43–52. Boca Raton, Fla.: CRC Press, 1992.
645. **National Institute for Occupational Safety and Health (NIOSH):** *Radiofrequency (RF) Sealers and Heaters: Potential Health Hazards and Their Prevention* (Current Intelligence Bulletin 33, #80-107). Cincinnati, Ohio: NIOSH, 1979.
646. **U.S. Air Force:** *Exposure to Radiofrequency Radiation* (AFOSH Standard 161-9). Washington, D.C.: Department of the Air Force, 1987.
647. **U.S. Department of Defense:** *Protection of DoD Personnel from Exposure to Radiofrequency Radiation and Military Exempt Lasers* (DoD Instruction 6055.11). Washington, D.C.: Department of Defense, 1995.
648. **U.S. Department of Energy:** *Industrial Hygiene Standard for Non-Ionizing Radiation* (Draft 11/16/92). Washington, D.C.: U.S. Department of Energy, 1992.

Outcome Competencies

After completing this chapter, the reader should be able to:

1. Define underlined terms used in this chapter.
2. Describe the physics of radiation interaction with matter.
3. List categories of ionizing radiation.
4. Explain dosimetry and attenuation.
5. List radiation detection devices.
6. Recall the operating principles for radiation detection devices.
7. Summarize the sources of exposure to ionizing radiation.
8. Describe radiation production equipment.
9. Describe the biological consequences of exposure to ionizing radiation.
10. Recall agencies that regulate ionizing radiation.

Key Terms

absorption • agreement state • atomic • atomic mass • atomic number • attenuation • beta • bremsstrahlung • Compton effect • contamination • critical target • densitometer • gamma rays • Geiger counter • ionizing radiation • isotope • LD37 • LD_{50} • Naturally Occurring Radioactive Material (NORM) • neutrino • neutron • nucleon • nuclides • pair production • photoelectric effect • positrons • proportional counter • radioactivity • radionuclide • radon progeny • sensitive volume • specific activity • standard man • survey • total absorption process

Prerequisite Knowledge

Basic college physics, college chemistry, mathematics to the level of calculus.

Prior to beginning this chapter, the user should review the following chapters:

Chapter Number	Chapter Topic
4	Occupational Exposure Limits
5	Occupational Toxicology
25	Nonionizing Radiation

Key Topics

I. Introduction
II. Quantities and Units
   A. Activity
   B. Exposure
   C. Absorbed Dose
III. Interactions
   A. Ionization
   B. Interaction by particles
   C. Interaction by photons
IV. Biological Effects and Risks
   A. Cell Sensitivity
   B. Dose Response Curve
   C. Linear, No Threshold Theory
   D. Factors Affecting Biological Damage
   E. Risks in Perspective
V. Sources of Ionizing Radiation
   A. Natural
   B. Medical
   C. Consumer Products
   D. Industrial Uses
   E. Energy
VI. Measurements and Monitoring
   A. Instruments
   B. External Exposure Measurements
   C. Internal Exposure Measurements
VII. Protection Methods
   A. External
   B. Internal
   C. Emergency Response
   D. Employee Workplace Awareness
   E. Considerations in Rescue and Recovery Operations
VIII. Regulations
   A. Agencies
   B. Exposure Limits
   C. Licensing
   D. ALARA
IX. Summary

Ionizing Radiation

26

By Bill R. Thomas, CIH, CHP and Carol D. Berger, CHP

Introduction

Radiation is the emission or giving off of energy in the form of rays or particles from unstable atoms. Most people are familiar with one form of radiation, the X-ray, used for medical diagnosis and treatment. Other forms occur naturally in materials such as soil, rocks, food and air. They are the power source for electric generating plants, submarines, and can be found elsewhere in medicine, industry, the military, research, and every-day life.

Although radiation is a valuable tool in these applications, over-exposure can be harmful. Millions of people work with radioactivity and radiation-producing machines on a daily basis, and are able to take advantage of what the science has to offer. However, they depend upon radiation protection professionals, such as health physicists or industrial hygienists, to ensure their workplace is safe.

Protecting people and the environment from the potentially hazardous ramifications of radiation and radioactivity, while still permitting its peaceful and beneficial use, is the overall objective of the radiation safety professional. This chapter presents the concepts of radiation and radioactivity. Included herein is a brief introduction to the various quantities and units used in this field, as well as how ionizing radiation interacts with matter. Discussions on biological effects and risks, sources of ionizing radiation, measurement/monitoring methods, and basic protection methods are also included. Finally, the agencies that regulate the use of radiation and radioactivity are presented, along with applicable rules.

It is important to note, however, that regulations and guidance documents that pertain to ionizing radiation are based upon a set of international standards. However, there is little consistency between federal regulatory authorities on which set of standards are applicable. For example, the Occupational Safety and Health Administration bases its radiation safety rules on the 1951 recommendations of the International Commission on Radiological Protection (ICRP). The U. S. Nuclear Regulatory Commission's regulations, on the other hand, are based upon the ICRP's 1976 recommendations. The U. S. Department of Energy bases theirs on the 1981 ICRP version, and much of the international community, including Canada and Mexico, subscribe to the most recent version of the ICRP recommendations (i.e., ICRP Publication No. 103, dated 2007). Because most commercial users of radiation and radioactivity are licensed by the USNRC or an Agreement State, the basis for the information presented in this Chapter will be consistent with current USNRC rules and thus the 1976 ICRP recommendations.

Quantities and Units

The phenomenon of radioactivity is based upon nuclear instability. The number of protons and neutrons in the nucleus of an atom determines whether an atom will be stable or unstable (radioactive). If radioactive, a variety of ionizing radiations can be ejected/emitted during the process of radioactive decay, each with different properties.

Various quantities and units have evolved since radiation was discovered in

1895 (by Roentgen) and radioactivity was identified in 1896 (by Becquerel) to aid in the understanding and measurement of these nuclear emissions.

Radiation dose units are limited to ionizing radiation photons and ionizing particles (Tables 26.1, 26.2, 26.3 and 26.4, below). Typically, ionizing radiation photons are defined in terms of energy expressed in multiples of the electron volt, kiloelectron volt (keV) or megaelectron volt (MeV), rather than wavelength (λ) or frequency (Hz).

Table 26.1 — Radiation Units

Dose Unit	*SI Unit*	*Comment*
Exposure dose	C/kg	used only for X-ray machine; not SI, but quantity
Activity	becquerel	limited to radionuclides only; quantity
Absorbed dose	gray	any classification of radiation dose; quality
Dose equivalent	sievert	only for human dose monitoring; integrated quality
Linear energy transfer	LET	energy transfer per path length (keV/μm)
Absorbed dose	KERMA	dose for indirectly ionizing radiation, quality

KERMA = kinetic energy released in material

Table 26.2 — Scaling Factors for Ionizing Radiation

Relative biological effectiveness (RBE)	ratio of a standard cell effect to test effect
Quality factor (QF)	factor to convert Gy to Sv (rad to rem)
f-factor	factor to convert R to Gy (energy dependent)

Table 26.3 — Quality Factor

Type of Radiation	*QF (One Significant Figure)*
Photons, electrons, betas	11
Thermal neutrons (<10 keV)	13
Neutrons (>10 keV)	10
Protons	10
Alpha	20
Heavy recoil nuclei	20

Source: Code of Federal Regulations, Title 10, Part 835.

Table 26.4 — SI units used in radiation protection

Exposure

Roentgen R, the charge produced in air by x or gamma rays. The SI unit is in terms of coulombs per kilogram of air (C/kg).

1 R= 2.58 × 10^{-4} C/kg

1 C/kg = 3,876 R

KERMA (Kinetic Energy Released in Material)

An exposure of 1 R (2.58 × 10^{-4} C/kg corresponds to an air KERMA of about 0.87 rad (8.7 mGy) or a tissue KERMA of about 0.97 rad (9.7 mGy).

Radiation Absorbed Dose

The SI unit is the gray (Gy).

1 gray = 100 rad
1 rad = 0.01 Gy

Radiation Dose Equivalent

The SI unit is the sievert (Sv).

1 sievert (Sv) = 100 rem
1 rem = 0.01 Sv

Activity

The SI unit of activity is the becquerel (Bq).

1 becquerel (Bq) = 1 disintegration per second
1 Bq = 2.7 × 10^{-11} Curie (Ci)
1 Ci = 3.7 × 10^{10} Bq = 37 Gbq

Additional Useful Conversions

1 μCi = 37kBq
1 mCi = 37MBq
1 Bq = 27 pCi
370 MBq = 10 mCi
1 μSv = 0.1 mrem

Common Prefixes for SI Units Submultiples

10^{-3}	milli m
10^{-6}	micro μ
10^{-9}	nano n
10^{-12}	pico p

Multiples

10^{+3} kilo k
10^{+6} mega M
10^{+9} giga G
10^{+12} tera T

Source: Health Physics Society, A Guide To SI Units In Radiation Protection, Operational Radiation Safety, Volume 80, No.5, May, 2001

Source: National Council of Radiation Protection and Measurements, SI Units in Radiation Protection and Measurements, Report Number 82, 1985.

Table 26.5 — Category of Ionizing Radiation

The following table summarizes the characteristics of the major types of ionizing radiation:

Type	*Symbol*	*Composition*	*Mass (amu)*	*Charge*	*Typical Energies*	*Range (air)*	*Range (tissue)*	*Primary Hazard*
alpha particle	α	2p+2n	4	+2	4–8 Mev	few centimeters	50–70 µm	internal
beta particle	β	electron	0.00055	+ or - 1	0.018–3 MeV	few meters	few millimeters	external and internal
gamma ray	γ	electro-magnetic ray	0	0	0.01–2 MeV	indefinite	indefinite	external and internal
x-ray	x	electro-magnetic ray	0	0	0.01–150 keV	indefinite	indefinite	external and internal
neutron	n	free neutron	1	0	0.025 eV–5 MeV	indefinite	indefinite	external

Source: Cember, Herman. Introduction to health physics / Herman Cember.3rd ed. New York : McGraw-Hill, Health Professions Division, c1996.

Wavelength units typically apply to the part of the electromagnetic spectrum in the optical, infrared, and microwave region and frequency units to the lower energy portion of radio and television regions. Though physically the same in any unit, measurement in the electromagnetic spectrum historically is described in the unit in which the component can be measured. For biological measurement that compares ionizing photons with ionizing particles, measurement in energy units is required. It is appropriate to state the energy of ionizing photons in units of keV or MeV. Heretofore, the term radiation will assume ionizing radiation. The common types of radiation commonly encountered in medical and manufacturing applications are listed in Table 23.5, below.

The following are fundamental radiation quantities and units used in health physics and radiation safety. Once again, they are limited to ionizing radiation with specific applications.

Roentgen

The Roentgen, symbolized "R", is the historical (classical) unit for measuring the quantity "exposure." The unit is named after Wilhelm Roentgen who discovered x-rays in 1895 and is defined only for the amount of ionization (charge) produced in air. This applies only to gamma and x-ray radiations. It is an archaic unit that, while still widely used, has limited usefulness and is no longer officially recognized by recommending bodies (e.g., the International Commission on Radiological Protection) and is considered an outdated quantity.

Absorbed Dose

Rad

The Rad, is a conventional unit for measuring the quantity "absorbed dose". In fact the term "rad" is the acronym for "Radiation Absorbed Dose". The absorbed dose results from energy being deposited by the radiation in a mass of material (i.e., energy deposited per unit mass). Unlike the roentgen, the rad is defined for any material (air, water, tissue, etc.) and applies to all ionizing radiations. Its prime limitation is that it does not consider the potential biological effect that different radiations have on the human body. In the System International (SI) System of Units, the gray (Gy) is the unit for absorbed dose. The conversion between Gy and rad is a factor of 1000:

1 Gy = 100 rads

Dose Equivalent

Rem

The Rem is an acronym for "roentgen equivalent man". It is a conventional unit used in radiation protection for measuring the "dose equivalent", a quantity which has no precise or exact meaning. It is an administrative concept subject to change. It is perhaps, however, the most commonly used unit of radiation dose referring to the amount of biological damage produced by a particular type of radiation and a given exposure to radiation. The dose equivalent is calculated by multiplying the absorbed dose (in rads or Gy) by the quality factor (the administrative factor that is typically a conservative measure of the biological effectiveness of the radiation). See Table 26.2 and Table 26.3.

For example, one (1) rad of x-rays or gamma rays and one (1) rad of alpha particles are equivalent in terms of the absorbed dose. However, photon radiations are considered to be approximately twenty (20) times less hazardous than alpha particles. See Table 26.3. Therefore, one rad of photon radiation interacting with the body is equivalent to one (1) rem, whereas, one (1) rad of alpha radiation is equal to a dose equivalent of 20 rem In short, the rem takes into account the energy absorbed (dose) and the effectiveness of the radiation in producing biological changes in the body. The conversion between Sv and rem is a factor of 1000:

1 Sv = 100 rem

Activity (Radioactivity)

The quantity activity (radioactivity) is typically measured in terms of the number of disintegrations (decays) that the radionuclide/radioactive material undergoes in a certain period of time, otherwise known as the "decay rate". The conventional unit of activity is the Curie (Ci) which is defined as 37 billion decays occurring each second (3.7×10^{10} dps). It was defined by the International Radiological Congress in 1910 as the amount of radioactivity emitted from one gram of radium and named in honor of Pierre Curie.[1] The unit for activity in the SI System is the becquerel (Bq) which is equivalent to one (1) decay per second, respectively. The following conversions show the relationship between Ci and dps:

1 Curie (Ci) = 3.7×10^{10} dps (2.22×10^{12} dpm)

1 millicurie (mCi) = 3.7×10^{7} dps (2.22×10^{9} dpm)

1 microcurie (μCi) = 3.7×10^{4} dps (2.22×10^{6} dpm)

1 nanocurie (nCi) = 3.7×10^{1} dps (2.22×10^{3} dpm)

1 picocurie (pCi) = 2.7×10^{-2} dps (2.22 dpm)

Each of these units can be converted into another. For example, 1 Ci = 1,000,000 μCi. Another is 1 nCi = 0.001 μCi. However, please keep in mind that a curie of radioactivity is quite large. A picocurie, on the other hand, is very small and is a unit often used to characterize the levels of radioactivity found in the environment such as in the air we breathe and the water we drink.

Specific Activity

The term Specific Activity defines the decay rate per unit mass. Typical units include the Ci/g (Curie per gram) or Bq/kg (becquerel per kilogram). Specific activity is related to the half-life of the radionuclide in that as the half-life gets shorter, the specific activity becomes higher. Conversely, as the half-life increases, the specific activity decreases. The specific activity for Plutonium-239, for example, is low (6.13×10^{-2} Ci/g) because of its long half-life of 24,000 years.

Half Life

The term half-life means the length of time for half of a collection of radioactive atoms to decay to a stable state. The units for half-life are expressed in minutes, hours, years, etc. For example, the half-life of Potassium-40, a naturally occurring radionuclide, is 1.27 billion years. Over that time, one-half of the activity present at the beginning of the period will have decayed away to stable potassium.

Contamination

Radioactive contamination is typically measured in units of radioactivity, curies or becquerels. The unit, counts per minute (cpm) is defined as the number of radiation events ("counts") from a radioactive source detected by an instrument over a specified time frame. The count rate (cpm) can be converted to the disintegration rate (dpm) by using a conversion factor which takes into account the "efficiency" of the radiation instrument for the radiation type of interest. In other words, the count rate observed from a radioactive source divided by the instrument's ability to detect that radiation (detector efficiency) is a measure of the

[1] Pierre Curie was killed on the streets of Paris on April 19, 1906 by a horse drawn wagon. He was returning from a meeting to draft legal codes to prevent laboratory accidents.

actual number of radioactive atoms decaying over a certain time (i.e., disintegration rate). Please note that contamination is a quantity of radioactivity spread over an area. Thus, units of contamination will be the activity present divided by the area over which it is distributed (e.g., becquerels per square meter, disintegrations per minute per 100 square centimeters).

SI Units

Radiation measurements are provided using a system consistent with the metric system or the International System of Units (SI System). The International Commission on Radiation Units and Measurements (ICRU) published units to correspond to each type of measurement.[1,2] Table 26.4 lists each of the SI units and the corresponding conversion factor. In this text, the SI unit is provided as well as the conventional radiation units, defined before 1975. The USNRC issued a Policy Statement in 1992 requiring licensees to report surveys and dose assessments using the SI units.[3] In practice, the conventional radiation units are still used today by many health physicists in the United States.

Interactions

Ionization

Ionizing radiation is a general term that applies to both electromagnetic waves and/or particulate radiation capable of producing ions by interaction with matter. Ionization is the process of removing electrons from neutral atoms which results in the breaking up of an electrically neutral atom or molecule into charged components or ions. If enough energy is supplied to remove electrons from the atom, the remaining atom has a positive (+) charge. The positively charged atom and the negatively charged electron are called an ion pair.

Do not confuse ionization with radiation. Radiation is simply energy and/or mass in motion. As a result of its interaction and deposition of energy in matter, ionization may occur. Ions (or ion pairs) produced as a result of radiation interactions with atoms allow the detection and measurement of radiation. The four basic types of ionizing radiation that are of primary concern in the nuclear industry are alpha particles, beta particles, gamma or X-rays and neutrons. See Table 26.5.

Non-ionizing radiation is radiation that does not have a sufficient amount of energy to ionize an atom. Examples of non-ionizing radiation include ultraviolet light, ultrasound, radar waves, microwaves and visible light. Although the word "radiation" refers to both ionizing and non-ionizing radiation, it is most often used to mean ionizing radiation, which is how it will be used in this chapter.

Radioactivity is a property of the nucleus of atoms that contains an unstable configuration of protons or neutrons. Radioactive atoms emit radiation in the form of particles or energy in an attempt to achieve stability. Radioactive material is thus any material containing unstable radioactive atoms that emit radiation.

Only certain combinations of neutrons and protons result in stable atoms. If there are too many or too few neutrons for a given number of protons, the resulting nucleus will contain too much energy in it and will not be stable. The unstable atom will attempt to become stable by giving off excess energy in the form of particles or waves (radiation). The exact mode of those emissions, called radioactive decay, depends on two factors, whether the ratio of neutron to protons is either too high or too low for the specific nuclide under consideration, and on the mass to energy relationship among the parent nucleus, and the emitted particle.[7]

Interactions by Particles

A charged particle loses energy in a medium proportional to charge and mass, and inversely proportional to its velocity squared. If the particle is created by a radioactive decay process, its maximum energy is predicable. The plot of specific energy loss, which can be related to specific ionization, along the track of a charged particle is called a Bragg Curve. A typical Bragg Curve is depicted in the Figure 26.1 for an alpha particle of several MeV of initial energy; this manner of energy loss is typical of any monoenergetic charged particle. As the energy is lost to the air molecules or the medium containing the charged particle, an electron will attach to the particle, dramatically lowering the specific energy loss.

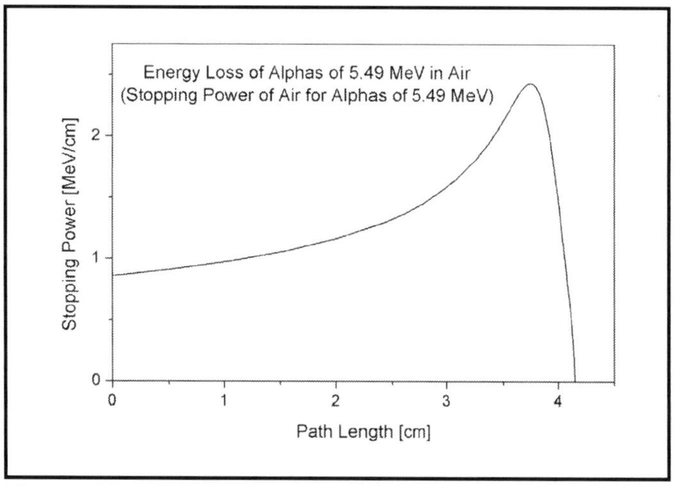

Figure 26.1 — Bragg Curve.

Alpha Radiation

The alpha particle follows this model of the Bragg Curve. An alpha particle is a highly charged helium nucleus that is emitted from the nucleus of the radioactive isotope when the neutron to proton ratio is too low. The alpha particle is positively charged, consisting of an assembly of two protons and two neutrons. See Figure 26.2. As the particle slows down and spends more time per path length, the curve increases in ionizing density and terminates at a predicable depth dependent on the density of the attenuating material and kinetic energy of the alpha particle. Because of its large mass and double positive charge, an alpha particle is limited to a very short range. The alpha particle deposits a large amount of energy in a short distance of travel. This large energy deposit limits the penetrating ability of the alpha particle to a very short distance. In air the typical 5 MeV alpha particle has a range of approximately 5 cm and in skin is attenuated by the dead or top layer of tissue. Alpha particles are primarily considered to be an internal hazard. Should an alpha emitter be inhaled or ingested, it becomes a source of internal exposure. Internally, the source of the alpha radiation is in close contact with body tissue and can deposit large amounts of energy in a small volume of body tissue. Typical sources of alpha radiation are transuranic materials such as plutonium, neptunium, and uranium, and other elements with atomic numbers greater than 82.

Beta Radiation

The negatively-charged beta, called an electron, or a positively-charged beta, called a positron, are emitted in radioactive decay with its companion neutrino, sharing the total energy. The beta particle is essentially an electron which is emitted from the nucleus instead of orbiting the atom. It has the mass of an electron and can be either negatively (-1) or positively (+1) charged. See Figure 26.3. As a result, beta particles are not emitted from the nucleus with the same energy. While the energy is not monoenergetic, the energy is statistically predictable. The kinetic energy of the beta varies between zero and a maximum value.
The neutrino, the energy of which varies between the maximum value and zero, is

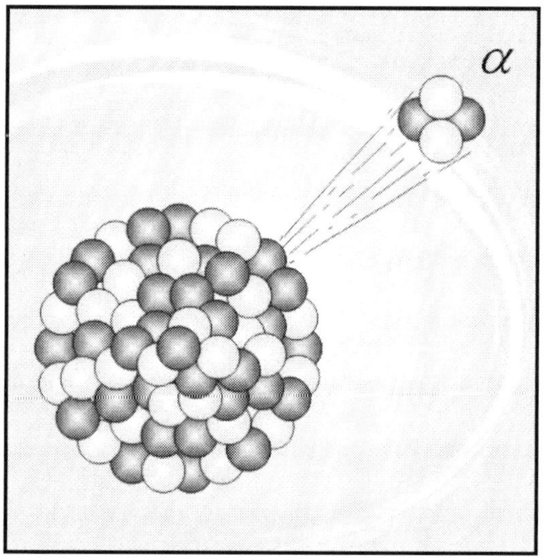

Figure 26.2 — Alpha particle.

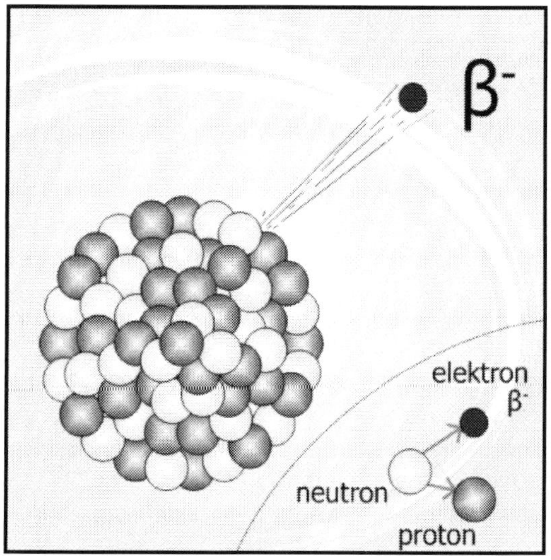

Figure 26.3 — Beta particle.

not considered interactive with matter and is ignored for radiation protection purposes. Beta particles created from radioactive decay are listed according to an average energy E_{av}, which is approximately one-third the maximum energy. Beta particles have a greater penetrating ability than alpha particles and constitute both an internal and external radiation hazard. Its typical range in air is several feet, but this is dependent upon the energy of the particle. For example, a one million electron volt (1 MeV) beta particle has a range in air of about ten (10) to twelve (12) feet. A less energetic beta particle would not travel as far in air, etc. Beta particles and free ionizing electrons deposit energy in tissue to a depth of 0.5 cm for each MeV. A 10 MeV electron (or beta) will penetrate the skin to about 5 cm. Most beta particles are completely absorbed by plastic, glass, metal foil, or safety glasses. If ingested or inhaled, a beta emitter can be an internal hazard because of the amount of energy deposited in a short range of tissue. Externally, beta particles are potentially hazardous to the skin and eyes. Sources of beta radiation include fission products such as Cesium-137 (Cs-137), Strontium-90 (Sr-90), uranium decay products, and Tritium (H-3).

Neutron Radiation

Neutrons are particles ejected from the nucleus with mass (unlike photon radiations), but no electrical charge (unlike alpha and beta radiations). With no net charge, a neutron can interact with a target nuclei by being captured by the target nucleus to create, in most cases, an unstable nuclide. This process is known as neutron activation and serves as the beginning of artificially produced radionuclides. The activated nucleus thus provides a beta/gamma emitting product as it attempts to achieve stability. If in the process of capture, a particle is ejected, the newly formed nuclide is transmuted or changed into a new element.

Neutrons have a relatively high penetrating ability and are difficult to shield against. Their range in air, like gamma rays, is indefinite. Neutron radiation is best shielded by materials with high hydrogen content, such as water or plastic. Neutrons are considered to be an external whole body hazard because of their high penetrating ability.

Neutrons may be found in nuclear facilities where fission and neutron activation are of interest. There are no pure neutron emitters; Cf-252 is a close approximation with some gamma emission. Free neutrons are considered radioactive with a half-life of about 10.4 minutes. Their interaction can be either elastic scattering (fast neutrons with energy > 100 keV) or inelastic, in which a small fraction of the neutron energy is transferred to the target, resulting in gamma ray emission (medium energy of 100 eV-100 keV; slow 0.025–100 eV). It is the thermal neutron with kinetic energy of the order of room temperature (~ 0.025 eV) that undergoes capture.

The objective in neutron radiation protection is to reduce the energy of high energy neutrons by inelastic scattering and then capture them with an appropriate absorber material. Materials that slow down or thermalize neutrons are made from low Z materials such as water, plastic, or paraffin. Neutron capture is accomplished by boron or cadmium. Protection from secondary radiation is provided by specially selected materials impregnated in the protective shielding. Neutron dosimetry is complex, and measurements involve the use of special neutron detectors.

A summary of relative attenuation for a variety of radiation types is shown in Table 26.6. The energies associated with the processes are in Table 26.7.

Interaction by Photons

Gamma/x-ray radiations are electromagnetic waves, called photons, with no electrical charge and negligible mass. Gamma rays are similar in nature to x-rays except for their place of origin. Gamma radiation originates in the nucleus; whereas x-rays originate outside the nucleus as a result of electron transitions (see Figure 26.4). In addition, as a general rule, gamma rays possess higher energies than x-rays.

Because gamma/x-ray radiations have no charge or mass, they have high penetrating power. They essentially have an indefinite range in air, and are best shielded by dense materials, such as concrete, lead or steel. Gamma/x-ray radiations are considered to be an external hazard and can result in radiation exposure to the whole body. Sources of gamma radiation include decay products of natural uranium, U-233, or

Table 26.6 — Interactions with Matter

Photon	attenuation is exponential monoenergetic gamma from radionuclides bremsstrahlung or X-rays from machines can compare energy of different photons by half value layer (HVL) radionuclides emitting gamma have specific gamma factor
Alpha particle	always monoenergetic MeV energy range displays Bragg curve of specific ionization limited range in tissue
Beta particle (positive & negative)	not monoenergetic energy of disintegration shared by positive beta and neutrino or negative beta and antineutrino average energy approximated by 1/3 maximum energy does not display Bragg curve finite range in matter (for electrons in tissue range in cm = 1/2 E in MeV) energy deposited in a medium by beta is because of inelastic collisions that are directly proportional to the Z of the medium and to the energy of the particle (to shield from beta use low Z medium to lower danger from bremsstrahlung-produced during collisions)

Note: HVL = half value layer, which is defined as that amount of a given material necessary to shield a given amount of radiation to one half of its original intensity.

Source: **Cember, H.:** *Introduction to Health Physics*, 3rd edition. New York: McGraw-Hill, Health Professions Division, 1996.

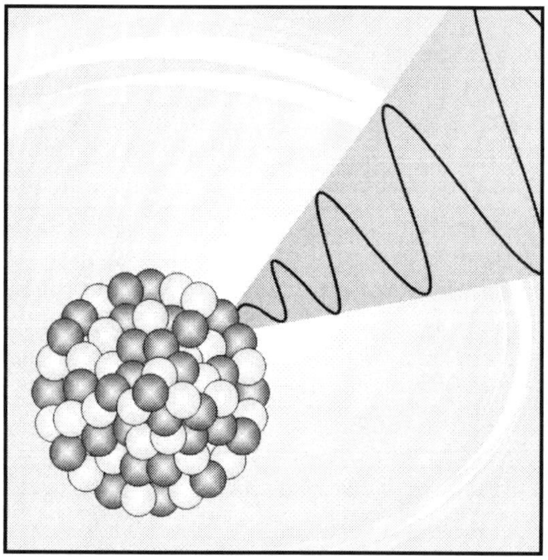

Figure 26.4 — Gamma ray.

fission products such as cesium-137 (Cs-137). The best example of an x-ray source is an x-ray machine used for radiography or medical examination. Nomenclature pertaining to electromagnetic waves refers to their origin. Photons produced from nuclear transition emissions are called gamma rays, typically with energies ranging from keV to MeV. Those photons produced from electron transitions in high atomic mass nuclides are called characteristic X- rays.

There are similarities between the attenuation of free particles and attenuation of photons in matter. Both have an associated wavelength and also characterized by energy. However, the differences are greater than the similarities. Photons are exponentially attenuated; particles deliver the energy, the dose, in a finite, short range. Particles created by cyclotrons or accelerators, of course, will have a long range. Photons carry no charge; most particles are charged. Even the uncharged neutron freed from the nucleus will decay into two charged particles.

Photons produced from free electron interactions, typically keV, are called X-rays or bremsstrahlungen. A bremsstrahlung (plural bremsstrahlungen) is an X-ray created when a high energy particle is decelerated or slowed down over a very short distance and the kinetic energy is transformed into an ionizing photon.[7] Depending on the rate of deceleration, the energy of the photon ranges between the lower limit of ionizing radiation and the maximum kinetic energy of the particle. The particle can be

Table 26.7 — Summary of Attenuation Processes

Process	*Z*	*Energy*	*Threshold*
Elastic scattering	—	1/E	entire EM spectrum
Photoelectric effect	Z^3	$1/E^3$	K binding energy of Z
Compton effect	independent	1/E	No threshold observed
Pair production	Z or Z^2	E	incident photon of 1.02 MeV
Photodisintegration			nuclear binding energy

Source: **Cember, H.:** *Introduction to Health Physics*, 3rd edition. New York: McGraw-Hill, Health Professions Division, 1996.

any charged particle such as a beta from radioactive decay, a proton in a cyclotron, or electrons in an X-ray machine. Bremsstrahlung radiation can also be created while shielding sources of beta radiation and may require additional shielding.

Photons whose origins are extraterrestrial are called cosmic electromagnetic rays. There are also cosmic particles. Characteristic X-rays, bremsstrahlungen, X-rays in general, gamma rays, and cosmic electromagnetic rays are collectively called photons, independent of origin and of energy level. Direct reference made to the energy (wavelength, frequency) of the photon or groups of photons is termed "quality" while the reference to the number of photons may be termed "quantity."

For both particles and photons the incident ray can interact elastically or inelastically. The word "scattering" is misused. In the strictest sense it applies to interactions of either photon or particle radiation in which an incident ray is changed in direction with or without an energy loss. In inelastic scattering, energy is imparted from the ray to the medium. Scattering does not apply to secondary processes such as characteristic X-ray production or annihilation radiation. Photons are attenuated exponentially; particles are attenuated to a finite depth.

The processes described below are organized into two major groups — interactions without energy deposition and interactions with energy deposition. The conservation laws of physics governing all interactions are not explicitly stated. Processes in which a reduction in intensity of a beam, particles, and/or photons is known but energy transfer is unknown is termed "<u>attenuation</u>." For those processes relating to energy transfer from the beam to the medium, then the word <u>absorption</u> can be applied. For the majority of radiation dose processes applicable to humans (the photoelectric and the Compton Effect from medical sources and background) the photon interacts with an electron within the body. It is sufficient to state that the photon must interact with an electron attached to an atom, ion, or radical and not with a free electron. A free electron is one not bound in an atomic structure and that can have energy or momentum equal to zero.

The energy of the photon after scattering is the same as before scattering. Therefore, the frequency and the wavelength remain the same. The only difference is that the direction of travel probably changes. At the atomic level, the photon is absorbed and re-emitted at the same energy. There is a chance that it can be emitted in the same general direction, called forward scatter. Elastic scattering is less probable in the ionizing range than in the nonionizing region of the electromagnetic spectrum, and its probability diminishes with an increase in photon energy. See the discussion of the Compton Effect later in this section for inelastic or modified scattering.

Photoelectric Effect

For photons (E > 10 keV) the most probable interaction in matter depends on its energy. Low energy photons are those whose energies lie between 10 and 125 keV; medium energy photons those with energies from ~100 keV to ~10 MeV; and high energy photons are those with threshold energies beginning at 1.02 MeV, but predominate at energies greater than 10 MeV.[7] The electrons released or created in these interactions deposit energy. The specific names for these interactions apply to photon interactions only and not to nuclear interactions.

For photons whose energies begin at the ionization energy to about 125 keV, the photoelectric effect is the predominant absorption process.[8][2] The <u>photoelectric effect</u>, also called a <u>total absorption process</u>, occurs when an inner shell electron of an atom absorbs the energy of an incident photon. See Figure 26.5. The energy of a photon must exceed the binding energy of the electron. The electron is ejected from its atomic shell with the kinetic energy of the initial photon minus the binding energy of the particular shell. The electron deposits its energy within a local region of where it was released. This energy is the dose deposited from the primary interaction and is specifically called the photoelectron. After the initial removal of an inner shell electron to become the photoelectron, an outer shell electron quantum

[2] This value changes depending on the materials in which the photon is being adsorbed. The photoelectric effect may extend to 125 kev when impinging on soft tissue but as high a s250 kev when striking a sodium iodide crystal during analysis.

mechanically moves to fill in the space of the ejected photoelectron. This transitional electron must release excess energy in the process of moving to a lower energy level. The release of its energy is considered a secondary process. The original atom is now an ion and will eventually collect an electron to balance the charge after a secondary process has occurred.

There can be two secondary processes from the primary photoelectric effect. These two processes statistically compete with each other depending on the atomic number of the target atom. The fluorescent yield is the fraction of secondary photons (characteristic X-ray production) compared with the secondary electrons (Auger process) created in the secondary process subsequent to the photoelectric effect.

For atoms of low atomic number Auger electron emission predominates. The Auger electron is one of the atomic electrons given the energy from the transitional electron. Statistically, the Auger electron originates from the same atomic shell as the photoelectron. Given the shell level, this energy is predictable and is considered monoenergetic. Most detectors measure photons and not electrons, and thus would not measure the energy of Auger electrons, but this secondary electron still contributes to the radiation dose.

For atoms with high atomic number, the excess energy from the transitional electron appears as a photon (or photons) equal in energy to the shell(s) of transition. In materials with a large number of protons (e.g. high Z material) such as tungsten, copper, materials used in shielding, and target material, these photons have energies in the ionizing region and are termed characteristic X-rays.

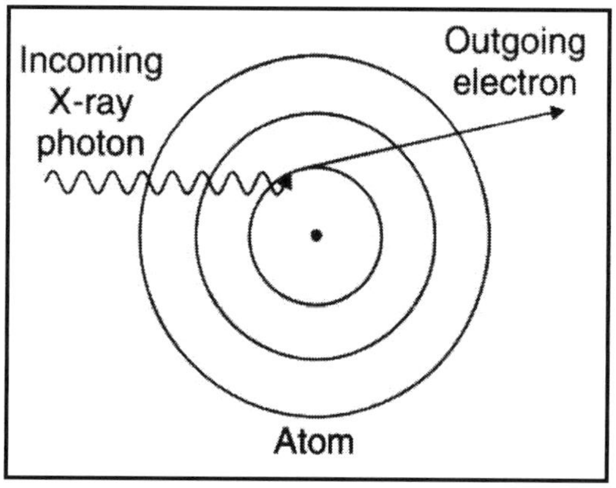

Figure 26.5 — Photoelectric effect.

They have characteristic energy of the atomic shell, and, therefore, of the element (e.g. number of protons or Z) creating them and are X-rays from creation by electrons. These X-rays are attenuated as any other ionizing photon. Any condition removing an inner shell electron from an atom will induce a similar secondary effect of characteristic X-ray(s) or the Auger electron process.

The photoelectric effect is the principle attenuating process underlying the use of diagnostic X-rays and dental films. The Z-cubed dependence of the absorbing medium for the same energy photons allows a differential absorption of incident photons. Film, tape, or other imaging media can record these photons in a way that permits fine differences between normal and abnormal medical conditions to be detected. With low energy, Z-dependent, incident photons, personnel protection includes the use of lead gloves, lead thyroid blockers for patients of dental and diagnostic x-rays, lead aprons with thyroid shields for personnel, and lead glass to absorb the incident radiation photons and ejected photoelectrons.

Compton Effect

The Compton Effect, also called inelastic scattering, predominates in attenuating photons in the energy region between 100 keV and 10 MeV. The incident photon interacts with any outer shell electron. Outer shell electrons are loosely bound at typically low electron volt (eV) binding energies. The incident photon is absorbed and re-emitted from the interaction site as a scattered photon but with less energy. The energy imparted to the electron releases the Compton electron at an angle obeying conservation laws. The scattered photon is reduced in energy but still carries a large fraction of the initial energy. The atom is now an ion. There is no secondary process for the Compton Effect. See Figure 26.6.

The Compton process is considered to be Z-independent for equal numbers of electrons, and interaction occurs with outer-shelled electrons.[9] The medical field of radiation therapy is predicated on use of the Compton Effect in which a tumor ($Z \sim 7$) can be irradiated through non-homogeneous material and through relatively high Z biological material such as bone ($Z \sim 13$). The Compton Effect is electron density dependent and is likely to be observed in materials with high electron density. Oxygenated tumors with high electron density respond best radiation therapy.

Pair Production

For photons with a minimum energy of 1.02 MeV the attenuation process of <u>pair production</u> can occur but predominates at high energies above 10 MeV. The threshold requirement of 1.02 MeV is predicated on the mass equivalent of 0.511 MeV for the mass equivalent of one electron. A high energy photon passes in the local region near the nucleus of an atom. The threshold energy of 1.02 MeV of the photon is converted into the mass of two electrons (1.02 MeV total) with the remaining energy transferred to the two created electrons as kinetic energy. To obey conservation of momentum and charge, two electrons must be created with opposite charges. See Figure 26.8. The (negative) electron continues in the medium as a high energy electron until its kinetic energy is dissipated. The positive electron, the positron, is an antiparticle, which cannot exist very long in matter. The positron loses its kinetic energy until its velocity is zero relative to a newly found electron and then necessarily undergoes the secondary process of annihilation radiation.

Somewhere in the vicinity of the positron is an electron. Opposite charges attract. On collision when kinetic energy is zero, the mass of the positron and the mass of the electron annihilate each other by changing the energy from the rest masses into photons. Rest mass means that there is no kinetic energy. These two photons have 0.511 MeV of energy each and travel in opposite (180° or p radian) directions from one another.

Any two particles with the same mass but opposite charge and angular momentum are termed antiparticles of each other. Examples include antiprotons and antineutrons. Annihilation radiation is a process that necessarily follows any particle-antiparticle annihilation process, releasing photons with the mass-equivalent energies. The most common one is the 0.511 MeV positron-electron interaction. Annihilation radiation is used in some nuclear medicine procedures. Rather than use a positron to interact with an electron, a positive beta is

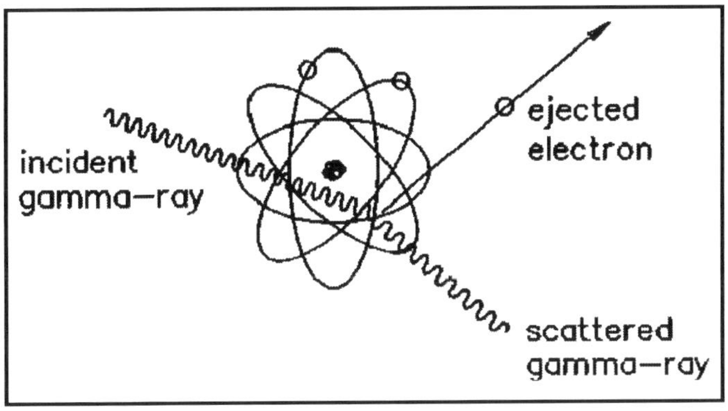

Figure 26.6 — Compton effect.

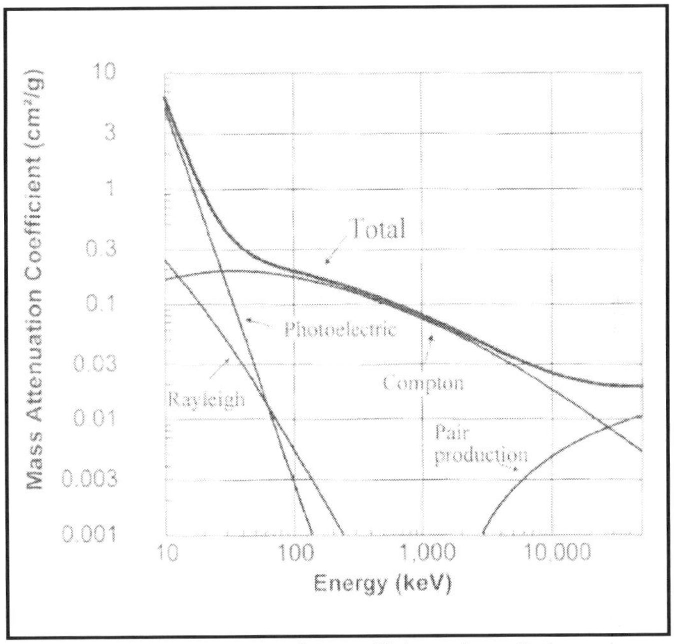

Figure 26.7 — Mass attenuation coefficients for soft tissue.

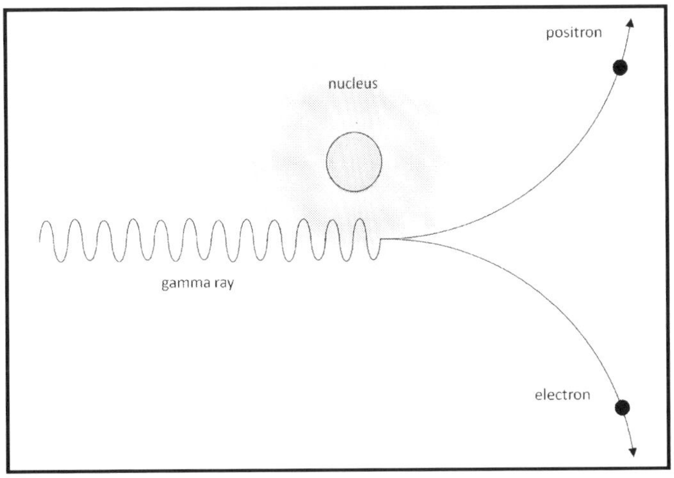

Figure 26.8 — Pair production.

created by selecting the appropriate radioactive material to yield a positive beta. Positive betas and positrons differ only in nomenclature relating to their origin. The 0.511 MeV photons are measured with coincidence counters.

Photodisintegration completes the attenuation processes for photons. An incident photon with a threshold energy approximately 8 MeV or greater interacts with the nucleus of an atom emitting a nucleon or a combination of nucleons. One exception is Be-9 with threshold energy of 1.66 MeV for a gamma-in, neutron-out reaction. With a high threshold and low probability of interaction, this process is limited to high energy machines in research applications.

Table 26.8 describes the various attenuation processes versus photon energy. Figure 26.7 provides a graphical display of the photon interactions.

Biological Effects and Risks

Of all the environmental exposures in the world, more is known about the biological effects of ionizing radiation than any of the others. Rather than just being able to base our information on animal studies, a large body of data and information regarding exposures to humans is available. There are four (4) major groups of people that have been exposed to significant levels of radiation and subsequently studied. The first involves early medical workers such as radiologists who received large doses of radiation before the biological effects were recognized. The second group is the more than 100,000 survivors of the atomic bombs that were dropped at Hiroshima and Nagasaki in 1945. These survivors received estimated doses in excess of 0.5 Sv (50,000 mrem). The third group is individuals who have been involved in radiation accidents, the most recent being the Chernobyl accident that took place in 1986. The fourth and largest groups of individuals are patients who have undergone radiation therapy for cancer and other disease treatment.

Exposure to high levels of radiation such as those cited above is rare in the nuclear industry. It is the goal of the scientific community, however, to study people exposed to these high levels of radiation, and to use the information obtained to predict the consequences of exposures that other people might receive.

Table 26.8 — Process by which ionizing radiation is absorbed in soft tissue

Energy Range	*Attenuation Process*
10–50 keV	photoelectric much more than Compton
60–90 keV	photoelectric and Compton equally
100–200 keV	Compton more than photoelectric
200 keV–2 MeV	Compton alone
2–5 MeV	Compton and some pair production
5–50 MeV	pair production begins to predominate
>50 MeV	pair production most important

Note: Water Z ~ 7.4.

Source: **Cember, H.:** *Introduction to Health Physics*, 3rd edition. New York: McGraw-Hill, Health Professions Division, 1996.

Cell Sensitivity

Radiation can cause damage to human cells through ionization of atoms in the cell. Atoms make up cells that are building blocks for the tissues and organs of the body. Any potential radiation damage to our body begins with damage to atoms that make up the cells.

A cell is made up of several components, with the nucleus acting like the brain of the cell. The nucleus controls the processes that take place within the cell. When ionizing radiation hits a cell, it may cause damage directly to the nucleus or any other part of the cell. This interaction may cause physical damage, chemical damage, or both to occur to the cell. Some cells are more sensitive to environmental factors such as viruses, toxicants and ionizing radiation. Radiation damage on the cellular level depends on how sensitive the cells are to radiation. When a cell is in the process of dividing, it is less able to repair any damage. Therefore, cells that are actively dividing are more sensitive to environmental factors such as ionizing radiation. Examples of non-specialized cells that are rapidly dividing include, blood forming cells, the cells that line the intestinal tract, hair follicles, and cells that form sperm in males. Cells that are more radioresistant are those that divide at a less rapid pace or are more specialized (such as brain cells, nerve cells, or muscle cells) are not as sensitive to damage by ionizing radiation.

Chromosome morphology and normal recombination events can be altered by radiation. This alteration can lead to death of the cell, can be carried on as a mutation, or repaired. Background radiation is of the order of 2–3 mSv (200–300 mrem) per year and is not considered a significant influence on ionizing radiation risk.

That ionizing radiation at significant doses above background radiation that can cause measurable cellular damage has been known since shortly after its discovery. The initiation of the field of what is now known as radiobiology began when Pierre Curie asked two French biologists, Bergonie and Tribondeau, around the year 1906 to study the effect of radiation on the development of frog eggs. The thesis of their work has been generalized into a law named after them, the "Law of Bergonie and Tribondeau", which states "the radiosensitivity of a tissue is directly proportional to the reproductive activity and inversely proportional to the degree of differentiation."[(10,11)] This statement applies to most mammalian cells.

The critical target for ionizing radiation damage in any cell is the deoxyribonucleic acid (DNA).[(12)] Damage is caused by an interaction or the initiation of free radicals at the point of interaction between the ionizing radiation and the target cell. These lesions, as they are called, are classified as either the result of a direct or an indirect hit. A direct hit is one in which the interaction from the ionizing radiation actually occurred on the DNA molecule. The particle or photon deposits all or part of its energy at the site and causes the immediate death of the cell. Immediate cell death is defined for the time that the cell dies during a particular part of the cycle, the time being dependent on many variables. Death of a cell is defined as the loss of reproductive integrity and not necessarily loss of viability. Cell survival is defined as the ability of a cell to produce daughter cells.

The direct radiation effect on DNA is the disruption of the DNA strand, either a single strand break or a double strand break, causing a major discontinuity in the primary structure. If a direct effect of ionizing radiation on cells causes a double strand break, the event is usually lethal to the cell within a very short time, defined as a period shorter than the cycling time of the cell. Most cells with double strand breaks do not have the capacity to repair, and therefore die. They are selectively removed from the statistical pool of those cells that are the precursors of alterations in the cell. High linear energy transfer (LET) and high relative biological effectiveness (RBE) ionizing radiation, such as alpha and low-energy beta particles, tend to cause more direct hit cell deaths; however, the few cell survivors from this type of radiation induce more chromosomal aberrations than the more plentiful survivors from low LET damage.[(12)3] Sublethal damage caused by high LET radiation is not repaired to the same extent as that from exposure to low LET radiation.

Indirect hits typically interact with a water molecule other than DNA molecules, which then releases a free radical or radicals.[(12)] Damage from the indirect effect requires more time to manifest itself in cell damage. Since cell content is mostly water, the majority of free radicals are free water radicals. The free radical then interacts with the DNA strand to cause the lesion. The amino acid bases of irradiated DNA display a relative radio sensitivity: thymine (most sensitive), cytosine, adenine, and guanine (least sensitive). The lesions may or may not end in the death of the cell but may produce altered cellular metabolism.

The majority of surviving cells from a radiation interaction can be injured with sublethal damage caused by an indirect hit. Low LET and low RBE radiation and high energy beta particles are not efficient in the production of double strand breaks and usually produce single strand breaks. The intermediaries of the free radicals in the cell cause the majority of DNA damage, but are not usually lethal to the cell due to repair. However, repair mechanisms themselves are subject to aberrations, and the cell line may be altered with repeated injury.

In the nomenclature of toxicology, the terms direct and indirect as applied to the effects of chemicals on DNA have different definitions from those used in radiation physics. The direct effect in toxicology means that the DNA has a chemical additive, an

[3] Linear energy transfer is defined as the rate at which energy is deposited per unit length of the particle track, expressed in terms of kiloelectron volts per micrometer (keV/μm) of track length in any medium, such as soft tissue. The LET of diagnostic x-rays is about 3 keV/μm, whereas the LET of 2 MeV alpha particles is 250 keV/μm.

adduct, attached to the DNA.[13] That attachment is the cause of disruption of normal functioning, which may lead to cancer. The indirect chemical effect, an epigenetic effect, requires chemical modification by a metabolic process to initiate the damage process. The activated form of the molecule is then the putative cause of a change in the DNA and lesions that can cause cancer or birth defects.

Membrane integrity is required for normal cell metabolism. Damage to the cell membrane is one of the major factors causing cell death. Membranes can be degraded in one of two ways; either by hydrolyzing phospholipids into fatty acids or by free radical attack. Free radicals are generated in normal cell metabolism, and all free radical formation is highly soluble in lipids, causing damage to the cell membrane. In particular, unsaturated lipids are susceptible to oxidation by ionizing radiation. Radiation injury, like chemical and ultraviolet radiation exposure to membranes, increases cell free radical formation and thus cellular damage.

Other chemicals can enhance or diminish cellular damage. Certain chemicals in cigarette smoke, for instance, are associated with lung cancer. In uranium mine worker epidemiological studies, the nature of the dust is important in the evaluation of lung cancer risk. If the factors influencing membrane composition are altered, as with chemical application or excessive cell regeneration (hyperplasia), the sensitivity to radiation can be modified, increased, or even decreased.

In summary, particle radiations, in comparison to photons, have higher LET and tend to kill the cells directly with double strand DNA breaks. There are relatively few survivors to this damage, but those that survive will tend to have greater chromosomal damage even after repair. Photons with a low RBE and low LET tend to kill and injure the cells indirectly by free radical attack and cause single strand DNA breaks. This type of damage occurs more frequently and can possibly be handled by cell repair mechanisms at lower dose rates.

Dose Response Curve

The dose response curve is a mathematical relationship between the severity of the radiation effect and the total dose (see Figure 26.9).[12] Dose response curves are used to characterize living systems, such as individual cells in a cell line or a complete animal such as the standard test animals used by the National Toxicology Program (NTP). Even with the standard rabbit or laboratory inbred rat lines, individual variation to a toxin necessitates the establishment of a response curve under controlled conditions to represent the median response. Epidemiology and animal studies are used to estimate the dose response of humans.

In 1949 the ICRP formulated the first "standard man," a human model to specify the masses of important critical organs and tissue to be used for radiation dose evaluation and response determination. Refinement of the model in 1959 included distribution of the elements in the total body, effective radii of organs, intake and excretion rates. The ICRP model is now called Reference Man and describes an occupational radiation worker who is a 70-kg, 1.7 m tall, 20–30 year old Caucasian male, who lives and therefore breathes in a temperate climate of 10–20°C and has Western European or North American habits.[14]

The value of the dose at the median response is called the LD_{50} (lethal dose to 50% of the population). Human population radiation doses are expressed as $LD_{50/30}$, indicating death to 50% of the population within 30 days. The overall shape of this curve is sigmoid. Deviations from the characteristic shape can provide information about hypothesized mechanisms. The slope of the linear portion from ionizing dose will depend heavily on the dose rate. In radiation studies, radiation dose rate is one of the most important variables that must remain constant throughout the experiment. For low LET radiation, the linear quadratic model for the dose response curve governs the shape.[12] A reduction in the dose rate reduces the quadratic coefficient, which changes the slope of the linear portion of the curve. If the slope rises too rapidly, a small error in the dose delivered will be reflected in a large change in cell death. Relatively high dose rates introduce a much higher rate of double strand breaks. Likewise, a shallow slope will be displayed with a large change in dose with a relatively small change in cell death, typically found at low dose rates.

At low LET, there is a finite probability that the radiation will not interact within the two strands separating the critical biological target, the DNA. Strands are separated at about 3 nanometers (nm). Radiation can cause single or double strand breaks, the double strand break being more serious. At a high spatial rate of energy deposition (high LET) the probability of interaction between the radiation and the DNA increases and approaches 1. The DNA is highly likely to receive a double strand break from the high LET radiation. The frequency of double strand breaks is associated with chromosomal aberrations. Somatic chromosome abnormalities are found at a low rate in the general population but are omnipresent in cancer cells.

Investigation of the low dose portion of the response curve and its mathematical approach to the x-axis can yield information on the occurrence of a threshold response. The ICRP adopted a univariate logistic regression linear nonhreshold model for radiation protection in 1977 based on the consensus of the scientific community. Now the existence for the possibility of a threshold is being debated. No effects have ever been observed at doses below 50 mSv (5,000 mrem) delivered over a one year period.[15] In fact, effects seen when humans are exposed whole body to 1 Gy (100,000 mrad) over a short time period are temporary and reversible. It takes a short-term whole body dose of well over 5 Gy (500,000 mrad) to cause a fatality. Assessment of the cancer risks that may be associated with low doses of radiation are projected from data available at doses larger than 10 rem (greater than 0.1 Sv).[16] For radiation protection purposes, these estimates are made using the straight line portion of the linear quadratic model (See Figure 26.10, Curve 2).[15]

The probabilities of cancer are available only for high doses, that are greater than 50 rem (0.5 Sv) (See Figure 23.10, solid line). Only in studies involving radiation doses above occupational limits are there dependable determinations of the risk of cancer, primarily because below the limits the effect is small compared to the differences in the normal cancer incidence from year to year and place to place.

The ICRP, NCRP and other standards setting organizations assume for radiation protection purposes that there is some risk, no matter how small the dose (See Figure 23.10, Curves 1 and 2). Some scientists believe that the risk drop off to zero at some low dose, the threshold effect (See Figure 23.10, Curve 3). The ICRP and NCRP endorse the linear quadratic model as a conservative means of assuring safety (See Figure 23.10, Curve 2).

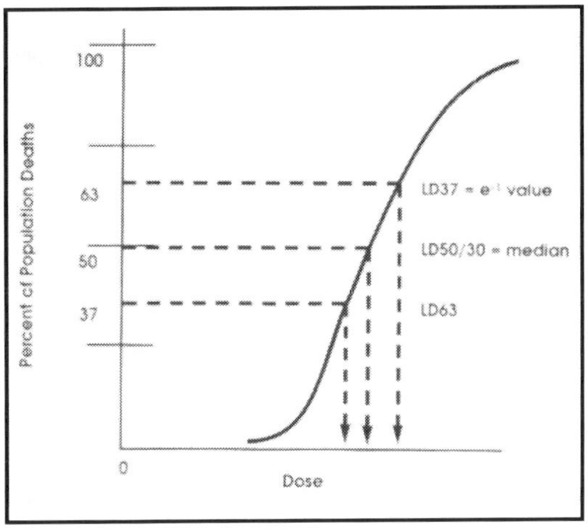

Figure 26.9 — Radiation dose response curve.

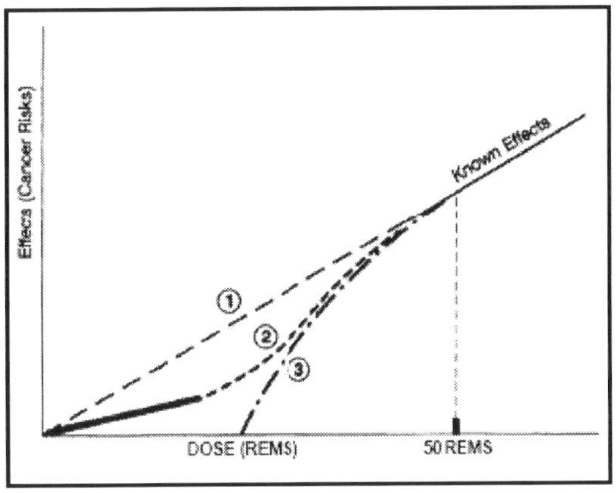

Figure 26.10 — Proposed models for how effects of radiation vary with low doses of radiation.

For regulatory purposes, the USNRC uses the straight line portion of Curve 2, which shows the number of effects decreasing linearly as the dose decreases. Because the scientific evidence does not conclusively demonstrate whether there is or is not an effect at low doses, the USNRC assumes for radiation protection purposes, that even small doses have some chance of causing cancer. Thus, a principle of radiation protection is to do more than merely meet the allowed regulatory limits. Radiation doses should be kept as low as reasonably achievable (ALARA).

Linear, No Threshold Hypothesis

The underlying basis for "Linear No Threshold" or LNT hypothesis is the worthwhile objective of controlling radiation doses in humans for the purpose of limiting the potential for effects. The hypothesis states that scientists have observed a linear relationship between radiation dose and effect at high doses. Exposure to naturally occurring radiation eliminates a truly radiation free environment to test the linear relationship at low doses (assumed to be less than 200 mSv or less than 20,000 mrem). Consequently, it is assumed, for radiation protection purposes, that the relationship is indeed linear at low doses as well.

This leads to the obvious conclusion that any dose, no matter how small, may be capable of causing some biological damage or detriment. Nonetheless, it has been considered for the past 40 years or so to adopt the philosophy that radiation exposure at any level is harmful.

There is no tested scientific evidence to support the assumption that irrepairable biological damage occurs at low doses. Therefore, it must remain a theoretical concept. Some professionals refer to the LNT as a theory rather than a hypothesis. In this discussion, the two proposed ideas will be used interchangeably to avoid the subtle distinctions between these two phrases.

The LNT hypothesis has been adopted by every national and international body that offers radiation protection recommendations or interprets scientific data. These include, but are not limited to, the National Council on Radiation Protection and Measurements (NCRP), the International Commission on Radiological Protection (ICRP), the National Academy of Sciences (NAS) Biological Effects of Ionizing Radiation (BEIR) Committees, the International Atomic Energy Agency (IAEA), and the United Nations Scientific Committee on the Effects of Atomic Radiation (UNSCEAR). In addition, the Health Physics Society (HPS), endorses the "As Low As Reasonably Achievable" (ALARA) philosophy (i.e., that there is no absolutely safe dose threshold), as a reasonable basis for radiation protection programs.[17]

These publications are recommendations by committees and organizations that were established to offer standards and guidance in the areas of radiation safety and dose control. However, regulatory agencies almost always adopt the recommendations of these organizations, in one form or another. For example, in the United States, federal and state regulatory agencies overseeing the safe use of radiation and radioactivity require the application of the ALARA principle, with its LNT basis, in licensee or contractor radiation protection programs.

Natural background doses vary greatly over the world. However, even in populations where background levels are much higher than those typical of the United States, and even much higher than radiation doses typical of occupational radiation work, no ill effects have ever been observed in the survivors. If the LNT theory were true in these dose ranges, there should be an increased incidence of radiation-related health effects. However, this increase is not observed. The philosophy "no dose, no matter how small, has some risk associated with it" is conservative and cannot be defended. In the case of natural background, there are certain areas of the world where levels of natural radioactivity are quite high relative to what is encountered in the United States. Particular examples include Ramsar, Iran, and the Kerala region in India. Even so, no adverse health effects of natural radiation have been found in either these regions (or any other areas of elevated background for that matter). In the workplace setting, no evidence of detriment to the workers occupationally exposed to radiation within the established regulatory limits has been shown.

Unlike other areas of study, such as health risks from exposure to air pollutants, where there is a great deal of direct data in the region of interest, radiation effects have been extrapolated far below the region where any meaningful data exist. This has generated no end of controversy in the radiation safety community regarding its continued applicability. Because it has not been proven, use of the LNT hypothesis requires that latent cancer fatalities be projected from accumulated exposures to very small levels of ionizing radiation. And because they are nothing more than projections, there is no assurance of their validity. In the case of cancer, quantitative estimates of "risk" are reported as the number of cancers per unit dose (e.g., Sievert or rem). If the LNT hypothesis is incorporated into the development of risk factors, the risk factors are assumed to be valid for all doses, and dose rates, even those approaching zero.

These risk factors arise from epidemiological data from the atomic bomb blasts of Hiroshima and Nagasaki. The argument can be made that these risk estimates are not relevant to "normal" radiological protection situations, where individuals are irradiated with very low doses (on the order of 1 mSv (100 mrem) delivered over an extended period (i.e., one year). In Japan, for example, a certain proportion of the population was irradiated "acutely", that is, in a fraction of a second or a few seconds with near lethal doses as high as 5 Sv (500,000 mrem). These dose rates were orders of magnitude higher than those commonly encountered in radiological protection. Extrapolating over such a vast dose-rate span is certainly grounds for arguing the scientific merits of the LNT assumption. Keep in mind that the LNT hypothesis states that even the lowest, close to zero, radiation dose is detrimental, and can produce a cancer or a hereditary effect. However, no hereditary effects have been discovered in the progeny of survivors of Hiroshima and Nagasaki irradiated with high sub-lethal doses. In fact, certain symptoms are clearly demonstrated to have a threshold of exposure, above which the effect is observed. These effects, termed non stochastic effects, are reported for skin, eyes, specific organ damage, etc.[18] Stochastic effects are defined as those without a defined threshold of exposure, including but not limited to, the onset of various cancers.

Radiation carcinogenesis is often viewed as a straightforward process. It is assumed that if the DNA in one cell in the body absorbs one photon, a cancer will inevitably result from the interaction of one particle of radiation and ultimately results in a single mutation. However, the assumption that cancer induction is caused by a single mutation in one cell is probably erroneous based on ongoing studies which describe the complexity of this process. In actuality, a cell may have to divide millions of times before a cancer is formed. If true, predicting cancer as an "outcome" of radiation exposure is not consistent with the present state of knowledge

Within error bars, the LNT has merit. However, adoption of the LNT hypothesis as the basis for radiation protection regulations means that significant sums of money are spent in the United States and in other countries around the world to remediate or clean-up residual radioactivity in soils, in buildings, on equipment, and in potentially useful feed materials, even though there is no demonstrable health effect associated with the presence of those materials. There are certainly grounds for contesting these expenditures.

Factors Affecting Biological Damage

In general, the greater the radiation dose, the greater the biological effects. Likewise, the faster the dose is delivered, the less time the cell has to repair, thus the greater the damage. The type of radiation affects the amount and type of damage, with alpha radiation being more damaging than beta or gamma radiation for the same energy deposited.

Effects are related to the area of the body exposed. The larger the area of the body that is exposed, the greater the biological impact. Because they do not contain critical organs, extremities are less sensitive to radiation than internal organs. This helps explain why the annual dose limit for extremities is higher than for a whole body exposure that irradiates the internal organs. Rapidly dividing cells are the most sensitive to radiation exposure. The developing embryo/fetus is considered to be the most sensitive because of its rapid cell division rate. Some individuals are more sensitive to environmental factors such as ionizing radiation. Children are more sensitive than adults. In general, the human body becomes less sensitive to ionizing radiation with increasing age.

Risks in Perspective

Because ionizing radiation can damage the cell's chromosomes, it is possible that through incomplete or incorrect repair, a cell could become cancerous. However, at low levels of radiation exposure, it is difficult to quantify precisely what the risks are because of inherent problems with measuring long term effects that can be directly attributed to radiation at such low exposures. It is possible to take into account results/data from known radiation exposures that led to an effect and project an estimate of risk at lower levels of radiation exposure.

No increases in cancer have been observed in individuals exposed to ionizing radiation at occupational levels, i.e., chronic doses. The possibility of cancer induction cannot be dismissed because an increase in cancers has not been observed. Risk calculations have been derived primarily from individuals who have been exposed to high levels of radiation that is greater than 0.1 Sv (> 10 rem).[19]

Acceptance of a risk is a highly personal matter and requires a good deal of informed judgment. The risks associated with occupational radiation doses are considered acceptable as compared to other occupational risks by virtually all the scientific groups who have studied them.

Biological effects on humans and associated risks from ionizing radiation received in the workplace can be better understood first through a knowledge and appreciation of the natural and man-made sources of radioactivity that the general public, are exposed to each day. These "chronic" levels of radiation interact continuously with the human body, necessitating an understanding of radiation effects on the cellular level.

While the body has mechanisms in place to repair damage caused by low-level radiation, much larger doses — known as acute doses — may overwhelm the body, preventing sufficient time for repair. Acute doses can cause various types of cancer on a probability basis, and possibly genetic effects in human offspring (though this has never been observed). Acute doses above a "threshold" dose are known to cause various somatic effects, such as the onset of cataracts and hair loss. Mothers receiving large acute doses in utero have given birth to deformed children. In rare (accident) situations, acute doses have been lethal. For these reasons, emphasis is placed in the occupational setting on understanding the biological risks from ionizing radiations and subsequently implementing measures to minimize these risks.

Table 26.9 — Radiation Exposures Received by Typical Members of the U.S. Population

1300 mrem per year for the average cigarette smoker
650 mrem per nuclear medicine examination of the brain
509 mrem per nuclear medicine examination of the thyroid
405 mrem per barium enema
245 mrem per upper gastrointestinal tract series
150 mrem per nuclear medicine examination of the lung
110 mrem per computerized tomography of the head and body
7.5 mrem per year to spouses of recipients of certain cardiac pacemakers
6 mrem per dental x-ray
5 mrem per year from foods grown on lands in which phosphate fertilizers are used.
4 mrem per year from highway and road construction materials
2 mrem per year from the use of gas mantles
1.5 mrem from each cross-country airline trip (one way)
1 to 6 mrem per year from domestic water supplies
1 mrem per year from television receivers
0.5 mrem from eating one-half pound of Brazil nuts.
0.3 mrem per year from combustible fuels, (i.e., coal, natural gas, and liquefied petroleum)
0.2 mrem from drinking a quart of Gatorade each week
0.1 mrem per year from sleeping with one's spouse (or "significant other")

Source: **National Council on Radiation Protection and Measurements:** *Radiation Exposure of the U.S. Population from Consumer Products and Miscellaneous Source.* NCRP Report No. 95. Bethesda, MD: NCRP, 1987.

Sources of Ionizing Radiation

A series of reports to advise the U.S. government on health consequences of radiation exposures are authored by the National Research Council's (NRCs) committees on the Biological Effects of Ionizing Radiation (BEIR).[12,20] The result of these reports is the analysis of the bulk of ionizing radiation data to produce a comprehensive updated review of ionizing radiation health effects. The focus of these committees is divided as follows: heritable genetic effects; cellular radiobiology and carcinogenic mechanisms; radiation carcinogenesis; radiation effects on the fetus; and radiation epidemiology and risk modeling. The radiation values are then used by EPA to set guidelines and promulgate radiation safety regulations. A listing of typical annual exposures is provided in Table 26.9.

In the early 1980's, medically-based exposure to radiation accounted for only about 15 percent of the ionizing radiation exposure of the population of the United States.[21] Background radiation made up 83 percent of the total exposure. Background is from naturally occurring radiation from rocks and soil, radioactive materials in one's body, exposure from the atmosphere, and also from radon gas seeping into buildings. Radiation exposure from industrial and research uses and occupational tasks, represented only about 0.3 percent, and consumer products accounted for only about 2 percent. In 2006, radiation from medical sources accounted 48 percent of the U.S. population's exposure.[22] See Figure 26.11. Background radiation exposure accounted for 50 percent, while occupational and industrial sources dropped to approximately 0.1 percent, and sources of consumer based radiation exposure remained around 2 percent of the total. From the early 1980s to 2006, the average effective radiation dose per individual in the U.S. from medical sources increased by approximately 6 times, from 0.53 mSv (53 millirem) to 3 mSv (300 millirem).

Background radiation, on the other hand, has not changed significantly from 3 mSv (300 millirem) in the early 1980s to 3.11 mSv (311 millirem) in 2006. Sources of occupational and industrial radiation exposures was reported to be 0.010 mSv (10 millirem) in the early 1980s, and was reported to be approximately 0.008 mSv 98 millirem) in 2006. Exposures from consumer-based products accounted from between 0.5 and 0.13 mSv (50 to 130 millirem) in the early 1980s, and approximately 0.13 mSv (130 millirem) in 2006.

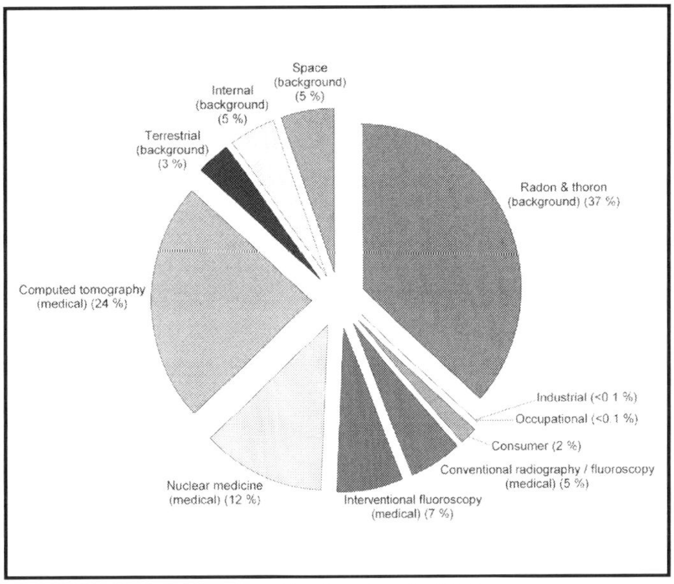

Figure 26.11 — Collective effective dose in 2006.

Natural

Some radiation received by man is natural in origin and ubiquitous.[23] Terrestrial radiation is emitted by the long-lived radionuclides in rocks and soils, some of which become incorporated into the human body through the food and water supply. See Table 26.10. Soils formed from igneous rock contain large amounts of uranium and, therefore, radon. Most soils contain some uranium, making radon omnipresent. The U.S. Environmental Protection Agency (USEPA) estimates that radon contributes two-thirds of the natural dose to the average American. Indoor radon exposure is reducible, and low concentration levels are mandated. This topic is given more consideration later in this chapter.

Cosmic radiation (photons and particles) originates in outer space and contributes to external radiation dose (around 8% of total) especially at high altitudes closer to the propagating sources without the benefit of

Table 26.10 — Natural radioactivity

Series Name	Mass	Initial N	Final N	Initial Isotope	$T_{1/2}$ years	Stable Isotope
Thorium	4n + 0	58	52	^{232}Th	10^{10}	^{208}Pb
Neptunium	4n + 1	60	52	^{237}Np	10^{6}	^{209}Bi
Uranium	4n + 2	59	51	^{238}U	10^{9}	^{206}Pb
Actinium	4n + 3	58	51	^{235}U	10^{9}	^{207}Pb
40 K		40 Ca			10^{9}	
14 C		14 N			10^{4}	

$T_{1/2}$ = physical half-life in year

Note: All nuclides with Z > 84 are naturally radioactive; some with Z < 84 are naturally radioactive. In particular, ^{40}K and ^{14}C are important. There are three naturally occurring series of radionuclide. The fourth series, the neptunium series, has a half-life so short that any naturally occurring members of the series have decayed. It can be produced in the laboratory.

Source: **United Nations Scientific Committee on the Effect of Atomic Radiation:** *Sources, Effects and Risks of Ionizing Radiation*. New York: United Nations, 1993.

air attenuation. Internal dose (about 11% of total) results from radionuclides (C-14) created in the upper atmosphere distributed by meteorological conditions. Long-lived Potassium 40 (K-40) contributes to internal dose via food consumption.[12,24]

The natural radioactivity in the environment is just about the same activity today as it was at the beginning of the Neolithic Age, more than 10,000 years ago. Human bodies harbor measurable amounts (>1x10^9 atoms) of radioactive atoms. About half of the radioactivity in the body comes from K-40, a naturally-radioactive form of potassium. Potassium is vital and is especially important for the brain and muscles. The remainder is from radioactive carbon and hydrogen. There exists about 4.4 kBq (120 nCi) of radioactivity in the human body. These naturally-occurring radioactive substances expose man to as much as 250 microSv (25 millirem per year) (mrem/yr).[21,25,26]

Most radioactive substances enter the body from food, water or air. The radioactive as well as the nonradioactive isotopes of essential elements such as iodine and sodium can be found in all foods. In a few areas of the United States, the naturally-occurring radioactivity in the drinking water can result in a dose of more than 0.01 Sv or 10 mSv (> 1,000 mrem in one year).[21]

In general, the foods contain varying concentrations of radium-226, thorium-232, potassium-40, carbon-14, and hydrogen-3, also known as tritium.[27] Examples include: Salad Oil 181 Bq/l(4,900 pCi/l); Milk 52 Bq/l (1,400 pCi/l); Whiskey 44 Bq/l (1,200 pCi/l); Beer 14 Bq/l (390 pCi/l); Tap Water 1 Bq/l (20 pCi/l); Brazil Nuts 0.5 Bq/g (14.00 pCi/g); Bananas 0.1 Bq/g (3.00 pCi/g); Tea 0.01 Bq/g (0.40 pCi/g); Flour 0.01 Bq/g (0.14 pCi/g); and Peanuts and Peanut butter 0.004 Bq/g (0.12 pCi/g). These very small but detectable levels of radioactivity are a natural consequence of life itself. People are exposed to a constant stream of radiation from the sun and outer space. Radioactivity resides in the ground, the air, the buildings, the food, the water, and the products in use.[21]

Another type of natural radiation is cosmic radiation given off by the sun and stars in outer space. Because the earth's atmosphere absorbs some of this radiation, people living at higher altitudes receive a greater dose than those at lower altitudes. In Ohio, for example, the average resident receives a dose of about 400 μSv/yr (40 mrem) in one year from cosmic radiation. In Colorado, it is about 1,800 μSv (180 mrem) in one year. Generally, for each 100-foot increase in altitude, there is an increased dose of one (1) millirem per year. Flying in an airplane increases exposure to cosmic radiation. A coast-to-coast round trip gives a dose of about 40 μSv (4 mrem).

In Ohio, radiation in soil and rocks contributes about 600 μSv (60 mrem) per year to the total annual exposure level. In Colorado, it is about 1,050 μSv (105 mrem) per year. In Kerala, India, this radioactivity from soil and rocks can result in an exposure in excess of 30 mSv (3,000 mrem) per year, and at a beach in Guarapari, Brazil, radiation levels have been measured in excess of 50 μSv (5 mrem) in a single hour. Some of the residents who use that beach receive doses approaching 10 mSv (1,000 mrem) per year. In a wooden house, the natural radioactivity in the building materials results in a dose of 300 to 500 μSv (30 to 50 mrem) per year. In a brick house, the dose is 500 to 1,000 μSv (50 to 100 mrem) per year. And, if a home is so tightly sealed that the leakage of outside air into the home is small, natural radioactive gases (radon) can be trapped for a longer period of time and thus increase dose.

There are many examples of naturally occurring radioactive materials present in consumer products beyond those already discussed. These include highway and road construction materials, mining and agricultural products (e.g., fertilizers and other phosphate products), and combustible fuels (coal, oil, natural gas, etc.). Optical lenses (eyeglasses, etc.) are noted for their thorium content (and consequently may contain elevated levels of thorium) because this element often appears as an impurity in the rare earth oxides used to produce certain types of glass.

Tobacco contains naturally occurring radioactive materials. Since tobacco is a crop grown in the soil, it will chemically bioaccumulate atoms of naturally occurring uranium and thorium series as well as potassium-40 (K-40), a ubiquitous naturally occurring beta-gamma emitter with a long half-life (1.28 × 10^9 year). Of greatest importance from a radiological perspective, tobacco contains polonium-210 (Po-210) and lead-210 (Pb-210) - radioactive progeny (daughter products) produced in the uranium series.

The presence of these radionuclides can be explained by at least plausible reasons. First, Po-210 and Pb-210 are present on tobacco leaves from the deposition and subsequent decay of airborne progeny of radon-222 (Rn-222). Secondly, the tobacco plant also has a preference for concentrating Pb-210 found naturally in soil. Lastly, phosphate fertilizers, routinely used in tobacco fields, contain measurable concentrations of Pb-210 and Po-210 (from the decay of uranium found in the phosphate).

The effects of tobacco on human health and the link to lung cancer is widely cited and discussed, but that is not the focus of this discussion. Radiologically, it has been estimated that the amount of Pb-210 and Po-210 residing in the lungs and bones of U.S. smokers is approximately four (4) times and two (2) times that of non-smokers, respectively. Lastly, the additional annual dose equivalent to a particular region of the lung - the bronchial epithelium - from smoking the daily average consumption of thirty (30) cigarettes is approximately 0.15 Sv (15,000 mrem).[24]

Radioactivity commonly found in building materials includes uranium, thorium, and potassium. Radiation exposures from these sources are not excessive especially when compared to the annual natural background. Dose estimates place the average annual whole body external dose at 70–100 μSv (7 to 11 millirem) from homes of masonry and concrete construction.[24]

Most homes are constructed on soil that also contains naturally occurring materials. Decay of uranium and thorium results in the formation of gaseous radon and daughter progeny which contributes to lung dose. In addition, naturally occurring radioactive materials can appear in well water used inside a home as a domestic water supply. Internal exposure is of greater importance, especially in poorly-ventilated or tightly-enclosed homes.[28] For this reason, the U.S. Environmental Protection Agency (USEPA) has advocated for several years that homeowners evaluate their homes for the presence of radon gas.[29]

Uranium is commonly found in colored glazes. It was used in different chemical forms as far back as the 1920s and produced brown, green, the entire spectrum from yellow to red glazes. Beginning in the 1930s, the orange color was quite popular in the production of a particular line of dinnerware known as "Fiesta-Ware™". While the current manufacturer of Fiesta-Ware™ no longer uses uranium in its manufacturing process, these dinner services can still be found in flea markets and in many homes. Emissions of primarily beta and gamma radiation can be detected from the plates. Even though alpha particles are emitted during the decay of uranium, these radiations are absorbed and contained within the glaze. The radiation emanating from Fiesta-Ware™ is detectable using any common radiation detection device such as a Geiger counter. External surface dose rates range from 5 to 200 μGy (0.5 to 20 millirad per hour), with an average dose rate from a complete Fiesta-Ware™ setting being about 30 μGy (3 mrad per hour) at a distance of one inch, the approximate distance to the hands. The dose rate to the whole body would be 10 or more times lower.[27]

In the 1970's, thorium was added to eyeglasses to produce a pink tint. Another application involved its incorporation into very high quality lenses in order to improve the transmission of light. This characteristic has been used by the military in their night sights, for example. It has also been used in older vintage 35 mm Pentax™ cameras and television cameras. The limits appear in the USNRC regulation (10 CFR 40.13). For contact lenses, eyeglasses, binoculars, etc., items in close contact with the eye, this regulation places a limit of 0.05% by weight of thorium. For lenses that are not designed for eye contact, limits up to 30% by weight are permitted. Older lenses still in use could result in non-trivial doses to the outer (germinal epithelial) layer of the cornea. For example, eyeglasses containing the maximum (0.05%) thorium limit could result in an annual dose of 40 mSv/yr (4,000 mrem/yr) to this area. Because of this potential exposure, direct exposure of the eye to lenses at a close distance for extended periods of time should be avoided. There have also been isolated cases reported where higher than permitted thorium quantities (greater than 0.05% by weight) were added to eyepieces without proper marking/labeling signifying the addition of thoriated glass.

Thorium can be found in tungsten welding rods ("thoriated tungsten") to produce easier starting, greater arc stability, and less weld metal contamination. According to the NCRP, about 300,000 people work either directly or indirectly with thorium-bearing welding rods.[27] Doses from welding rods result through their distribution, use, and disposal. However, actually using the devices is the primary source of exposure. Welding rods contribute both an external whole body dose and an internal (inhalation) dose. The latter pathway predominates, particularly during tip grinding. While doses from external exposures are estimated to be less than 10 μSv/yr (1 mrem/yr), the whole body and bone dose commitments from internal exposures varies widely depending on the relative use ("heavy", "occasional", personnel assisting the welder, etc.).[30] The highest whole body and bone dose estimates are 140 μSv (14 mrem) and 20,000 μSv (2,000 mrem), respectively.

Human activity raises the radiation background because of discharges from coal fired nuclear power plants. Radioactive discharges from nuclear power plants are limited to authorized discharge levels above environmental background. Radioactivity from coal fired plants, on the other hand, is not regulated. Population exposure from operation of a 1000-MW coal fired plant is 100 times that for a nuclear plant 4.9 person-Sv/yr (490 person-rem/yr compared to 4.8) and releases 5.2 tons of uranium and 12.8 tons of thorium to the atmosphere each year.[27,31]

Radon

Radon, a noble gas, is classified as a lung carcinogen in humans when delivered in high doses. Exposure to naturally occurring radon and its progeny is regarded as the largest contributor of radiation exposure from natural sources to humans. EPA projects that 5000–20,000 lung cancers per year are associated with radon exposure in air.[20,32] The National Academy of Sciences estimates 13,300 deaths per year are due to radon exposure.[20]

Elevated radon in drinking water poses a risk of cancer from ingested water, based on 1 L per day intake. EPA uses a 10^4 to 1 transfer coefficient of radon in water to radon in air (10,000 pCi/L of radon in water contributes 1 pCi/L of radon in air) and estimates that about 5% of radon in the home originates in drinking water. Exposure to radon in drinking water is about 20% of the risk of inhaled radon.[33,34]

The origin of the radon (Ra-222) in air and in water derives from the naturally occurring decay chain of uranium.[28] Each of the intermediate decay products in this chain has a characteristic half-life before terminating in the stable nuclide of Pb-206. There are two other isotopes of radon (Rn-219 and Rn-220) produced in natural soils from other natural decay schemes. However, uranium other than U-238 and radon other than Rn-222 are given the individual mass number and contribute trivial radiation dose to humans.

As a monatomic noble gas, radon is relatively insoluble, and after being inhaled is exhaled rather than absorbed. If it decays during residence in the lung, a particulate daughter is produced. It is the progeny of radon, not radon per se, that contribute to lung dose.

The daughter products exist as unattached ions, atoms, condensation nuclei, or attached to particles, all of which emit high energy alpha radiation that cause lung damage. The term radon daughters refers to any of the decay products of radon, however the term <u>radon progeny</u> typically applies to the first four decay products of Rn-222, Po-218, Pb-214, Bi-214, and Po-214. These four progeny have short enough half-lives to decay in the lung (and deposit energy) before being physiologically removed. They are responsible for the radiation dose delivered to the lung. The target cell in the lung from radon exposure is the bronchial epithelium, which is the site of the majority of lung cancers considered to be caused by radon. The fifth decay step is Pb-210, which has a long enough half-life (22.3 years) to be removed from the lung by physiological processes before it decays.

The radon concentration in air above typical soil depends on meteorological conditions. When confined to a defined volume, the radon progeny decay by secular equilibrium to Pb-210 in approximately 4 hours. The equilibrium fraction is the fraction of decaying daughters divided by the number of radon atoms. A fraction of 1 is the value when the number of decay products from progeny equals the number of decay products from the Ra-226. If a fraction of the radon is removed from the defined volume, the fraction of progeny decreases. The values of radon progeny outdoors are at about 70% of the equilibrium value. EPA estimates that the average outdoor concentrations are 8 Bq/m^3 or 200 pCi/L or 0.001 working level (WL) for someone working outdoors continuously.(32)

The WL (J/m^3) is a derived standard based on human epidemiological studies of working miners to relate the risk from radon exposure to the incidence of lung cancer.(35) The working level month (WLM) is defined in terms of energy deposition over a working month. The dose equivalent unit of the Sievert is not used for the evaluation of radon in air.

The progeny of radon are solid, ionized nuclei, which have a high likelihood of becoming electrostatically attached to aerosols. Because they are ionized, progeny can attach to an aerosol or remain unattached. It has a characteristically high surface area to volume ratio with a geometric diameter range between 0.001 mm–100 mm. Neutral particles adsorb on aerosols. Then, when inhaled, the aerosols deposit on the interior surfaces of the lung. The aerosol factors include the size distribution of the particle, the fraction unattached, and the equilibrium factor. Outdoors, the unattached fraction is below 10%. Unattached fractions consist of free ions, micrometer-size agglomerates with water molecules, which plate out with about 100% efficiency in the lung. Thus, the dose (per WLM) from one unit of an unattached fraction will be greater than the dose (per WLM) from the same unit of an attached fraction.(32)

Radon dosimetry becomes complex when the radon becomes attached to particles with different solubilities and particle size. This distribution of the fraction of the attached/unattached groups is critical to dose evaluation since the dose is proportional to the unattached fraction. For example, nasal breathing influences unattached radon deposition, which is cleared from the nasal passages on exhale. Particle size attachment determines in which part of the airway radon will be deposited. Radiation dose to the bronchial epithelium depends on the amount of radon, the aerosol mixture, and the physiology of the lung.

When confined to a constant volume, radon remains in equilibrium with its progeny. Measurement of radon in air requires knowing or estimating the equilibrium constant. When radon is subject to air convection currents or ventilation, the equilibrium value is reduced from a value of 1 for equilibrium conditions. When trapped indoors, the fraction of radon in equilibrium with its progeny is dependent on the ventilation rate for the structure. The equilibrium fraction used by BEIR IV and the International Commission on Radiological Protection (ICRP) for the risk evaluation from radon exposure is 0.5 for existing housing and is the fraction required for EPA evaluation.(27) The rationale of radon mitigation is that the equilibrium fraction is disrupted and reduced in value to 0.5 by venting the radon to an outside air space, where the decay process continues away from the living space. Measurement of radon in air in a dwelling is predicated on a constant 0.5 fraction and is defined as "closed house conditions."

Radon in water and radon in air in the home and public buildings in excess of a mandated level are required to be mitigated. The mandates govern public water systems, which are defined as having 15 or more service connections or regularly serving at least 25 persons for 60 or more days per year. Normally, a public water supply does not have elevated levels of radon but may have other regulated radionuclides.

Radon mitigation regulations cover indoor air and drinking water but do not account for the environmental fate of the radon in outdoor air. The U.S. Geological Survey and EPA developed the Map of Radon Zones to pinpoint communities of high radon concentration.(36) Table 26.12 lists the USEPA's action levels for indoor air, and Table 26.13 presents the instruments and methods used to measure indoor radon concentrations.

Medical

Ionizing radiation has been used for both diagnostic and therapy procedures for more than 50 years. The use of ionizing radiation requires licenses and registrations from a regulatory authority, particularly when dose will be delivered to humans. The quantity of radiation received by a single patient is

Table 26.12 — EPA action levels for indoor radon in air

Concentration (pCi/L)	*EPA Protocol*
<0.25	not practical; considered de minimis
1–4	recommend reduction
4 (0.02 WL)	action level as annual average
4–20	action required within year
20–200	action required within months
>200	action required weeks

Table 26.13 — Instrumentation approved for indoor radon measurements

Note: Outdoor radon standards are limited to uranium and phosphorus mine vents. (For more information, see www.epa.gov).

Measurement Device	*Closed House*	*Minimum Time*	*Potential Interferences*
Continuous radon monitors	Yes	48 hours	equilibrium conditions required for diffusion chamber
Alpha track detectors	No	90 days	uncertainty at low concentration
Electret™ ion chambers	No	No limit	temperature dependent ±10°F
Activated charcoal adsorption	No	2–7 days	not integrate uniformly; moisture sensitive
Charcoal liquid scintillation cells	No	2–7 days	not integrate uniformly; moisture sensitive
Grab radon sampling with pump and collapsible bag	Yes	4–24 hours	Required radon equilibrium
Unfiltered track detectors	Yes	4 hours	Uncertainty at low concentrations. Not sensitive to radiation less than 5 Mev
Continuous working level monitors	No	48 hours	radon equilibrium with daughters
Radon progeny integrating sampling units with alpha track	No	48 hours	Uncertainty at low concentrations.
Grab sample to measure working level	Yes	5 minutes	measurement of flow rate through a filter short duration

prescribed by the authorized physician according to the diagnosis and approved treatment. The radiation doses received by a patient may exceed those authorized for radiation workers and allowable occupational exposures because the benefit of the exposure significantly outweighs the risk.

A conventional X-ray machine accelerates electrons in an evaluated tube to a maximum voltage, into a target (see Figure 26.12). When the electrons slow, X-rays are produced by the conversion of kinetic energy to electromagnetic energy. The majority of X-rays produced come from a target at a back angle with a spectrum of photon energies that ranges from a minimum associated with any inherent filtration to the peak voltage energy. The energy produced is stated in terms of kVp, the "p" referring to peak voltage set on the controls. The bremsstrahlung curve is called the continuous X-ray distribution curve. The window of an X-ray machine is made of low Z material to allow penetration of the lower energy X-rays.

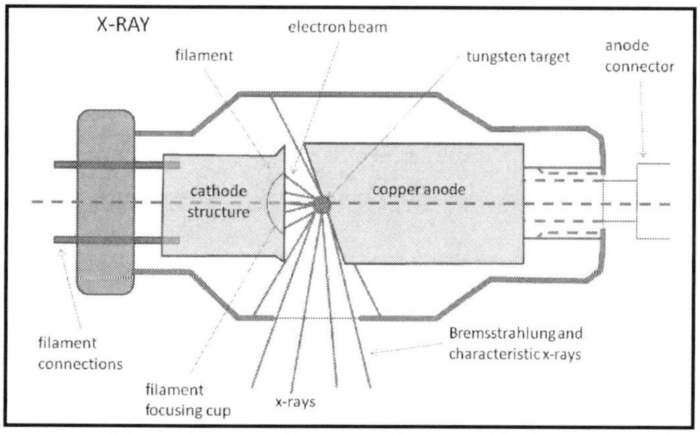

Figure 26.12 — Diagram of an X-ray tube.

The average energy of an X-ray spectrum is determined by a process called the half value layer. An output radiation rate for each machine is specified with the peak voltage value and the half value layer. All dental, diagnostic radiology and some superficial radiation therapy machines fall into this group. Research X-ray machines require personnel protection, particularly for the hands and eyes.

X-ray machines for medical use fall into special categories, and their operation and compliance requirements fall under state jurisdiction. Current applications of such machines are listed in Table 26.14.

Table 26.14 — Machines that produce ionizing radiation

Machine	Particle	Direction	Product	Use
Van De Graff	Electron	linear	Photons and electrons	Research, Radiation therapy
Cyclotron	Any charged particle	circle	Radionuclides	Radiopharmaceuticals
Betatron	electron	circle	Photons and electrons	Medical
Linac	Any charged particle	linear	Radionuclides	Research, Radiation therapy
Medical Linac	electron	linear	Photons and electrons	Medical
Xray	electron	linear	Photons	Research and medical
Reactor	neutron	any	Fission products	Energy source, free neutrons

The NCRP recently updated its 1987 publication, NCRP Report No. 93 that described sources of ionizing radiation and exposures to the general public in the U.S.[22] It examined the various sources of ionizing radiation in the U.S. as of 2006, estimated the total amount of radiation, and compared those amounts to the estimates published in 1987. Among other findings, exposures to naturally-occurring amounts of radiation changed very little. The new report, No. 160, concluded that there has been a dramatic increase in the amount of radiation from medical imaging procedures, including computed tomography (CT) and cardiac nuclear medicine examinations. The report stated that the average effective radiation dose individuals in the U.S. received in 2006 increased about 1.7-times since the early 1980s from 3.6 mSv (360 millirem) to 6.2 mSv (620 millirem).

The use of computerized tomography (CT) for medical diagnosis has increased in the last few decades as the technology has become more sophisticated, often replacing risky, invasive tests. CT and other medical imaging procedures have nearly eliminated exploratory surgery and enabled minimally invasive surgery both which have shortened or eliminated hospitalization and reduced the risk of surgery related problems like infection.[37] CT scanners have also reduced the volumes of radiation therapy fields, thereby reducing the probability of radiation harm, including second malignancies. The number of procedures per year was typically a few million per year in the 1980s while there were more than 60 million CT procedures performed in 2006.

Current CT scanners modify the radiation dose to the specific exam type and individual. Modern CT systems are equipped with automatic exposure control systems that reduce patient dose levels to the minimum necessary for the examination. Cardiac nuclear medicine studies have increased by a factor of 15 since the 1980s and deliver approximately 75 percent of the dose from nuclear medicine procedures.[38] Combined, radiation exposures from CT and nuclear medicine procedures deliver approximately 36 percent of the total population dose, equivalent to the dose from radon and thoron.

The latest NCRP report calculated the total radiation dose for all CT scans performed in 2006 and divided that by the number of people in the U.S. population for that year. It was observed that much of the U.S. population received a much smaller dose from medical imaging or participated in other imaging exams that did not use ionizing radiation, such as magnetic resonance imaging (MRI) or ultrasound procedures. The NCRP report did not attempt to quantify the associated health risks nor specify the actions that should be taken in light of their new findings.

Consumer Products

There many examples of radiation and radioactivity in products commonly used by members of the public. Examples include electronically generated radiation, radioactivity in consumer products, and radionuclides intentionally added to a product.[39] Examples of each type of radiation are provided below, including the nature of the product, the radioactivity concentrations and/or radiation levels likely to be present.

The best and most widely-used example of a consumer product that produces radiation through electronic means is the tried-and-true old-time television set. Other examples are video display terminals (VDTs), airport inspection systems and obsolete shoe-fitting fluoroscopes. The type of radiation associated with these devices is x-ray, a type of photon radiation produced when high energy electrons impact a stationary object, such as the television picture tube or a computer monitor. The x-rays are not necessary for the operation of a television set and this is just one example where the radiation is a byproduct, meaning it is incidental or extraneous to the purpose for which the consumer product was originally designed.

The operating voltage is the primary cause of x-ray emissions from old-style television sets. As the voltage is increased, which was often done in order to improve the picture, the x-ray intensity increased. The use of thick walls in picture tubes effectively shielded some of the low energy x-ray emissions, however, the highest x-ray emission levels recorded were produced in two particular years (1968 and 1969) when color television sets first became popular. These levels have since diminished markedly with technological advancements such as solid-state designs. The limits for radiation exposure from television sets and similar devices is currently enforced by the United States Food and Drug Administration (FDA).[40] All television sets must meet a limit of less than 0.5 milliRoentgen per hour (0.5 mR/hr or less than 5 μGray/hr at a distance of five (5) centimeters (cm) from any accessible point on the external surface of the set. Recent estimates place the annual radiation dose to the U.S. population at much less than 10 μSv/yr (< 1 mrem/yr) from color televisions, and even lower for black and white sets.[27] Typical radiation exposures from video display terminals, such as a computer screen, are similar to television receivers.

According to the NCRP, there has always been a mistaken assumption that VDTs constitute a source of personnel exposure worthy of attention. Studies conducted on x-ray emissions from these devices show no differences when compared to television emissions. In addition, studies conducted on possible health effects associated with the continued use of VDT's, such as cataracts, birth defects, and others, have to date found no evidence of health hazards. An annual dose of much less than 10 μSievert (1 mrem) has been estimated for VDT use as well.

Smoke detectors are one of the most commonly available consumer products. Used to signal the presence of smoke/fire, these detectors typically contain an americium-241 (Am-241) source with a small amount of radioactivity, on the order of 37 kBq (1 μCurie). When smoke particles enter the detector, they disrupt the flow of current (electrons) created by the ionization of alpha particles produced from the decay of the americium. This disruption triggers an alarm. For this reason, they are known as "ionization-type" smoke detectors. The radiation levels emitted from these devices cannot be distinguished from background levels. To further the point, it has been estimated that the annual average dose equivalent to the U.S. population from these devices is less than 0.08 μSv (< 0.008 millirem), far below the annual natural background in the U.S.[27] Most importantly, they save lives.

Radioluminescent products include radionuclides such as radon (Ra-226), promethium-147 (Pm-147), and tritium (H-3). Ra-226 is an alpha/beta/gamma emitter with a half-life of 1,600 years. Pm-147 is a beta emitter with a half-life of 2.6 years. Tritium, a radioactive isotope of hydrogen, has a relatively short half-life of 12.3 years. Zinc sulfide (ZnS) is the most commonly used scintillating material for this application. The products are simple devices. The radionuclide and the scintillator are mixed together and then plated on some kind of surface like a glass tube. When either alpha or beta radiations interact with the zinc sulfide, a small flash of light is produced. This type of product is typically found in watches and clocks. Watches and clocks employing Ra-226 have not been produced in the U.S. since 1968 and 1978, respectively, although there are a number of these old antiques still available

In the U.S., the USNRC requires the manufacturer to obtain a radioactive materials license for watches/clocks containing either Pm-147 or H-3. The USNRC also limits the amount of radioactivity that may be present in an individual timepiece. For Pm-147, there is an additional limitation on the permissible dose rate. Health concerns have been reduced by eliminating the use of radium and using the weak beta emissions of the shorter half-life tritium and the less hazardous Pm-147.

Timepieces containing tritium have been known to occasionally leak, resulting in a small whole body dose from inhalation or absorption through the skin and contamination of clothing, surfaces, etc. There is no particular concern with Pm-147, although specific dose rate limits are cited for this radionuclide at a stated distance (e.g., 1 cm, 10 cm) from the timepiece depending on its type (i.e., wrist watch, pocket watch, clock). For both H-3 and Pm-147, the estimated annual dose equivalent to an individual user is much less than 10 μSievert (1 millirem).

Tritium is also used in a variety of other applications, including self-luminous aircraft and commercial exit signs (those red things with the blue-colored light seen at the bulkheads of airplanes), luminous dials and gauges, and the production of luminous paints. Care must be taken in production and use of the products because the weak beta emission is essentially impossible to detect with conventional survey instruments.[4] Therefore, if a leak occurs in a production facility, the entire facility can become contaminated and the problem remains undiscovered for some time unless specialty instruments are used for routine surveillance. More importantly, however, is the fact that, in the last few years, there have been instances where tritium exit signs have been stolen. These devices are "generally licensed" by the USNRC and may contain up to 925 GBq (25 Ci) of tritium, thus there has been recent regulatory interest in increased controls.

Static eliminators have been used for a number of years in an industrial setting to reduce electrical charge buildup in various materials. In a more general application Po-210, an alpha emitter produced from the decay of U-238, is incorporated into so-called "static eliminators" to reduce/eliminate the static charge during the manufacture and use of photographic film and phonograph records. Those individuals familiar with phonograph records (before the advent of CD's, DVD's, etc.) may well have used a Po-210 static eliminator to reduce the amount of dust on the record surface. In brief, ionizations from the polonium alpha particles neutralize the charge on the dust particles, reducing their accumulation on the surface being cleaned.

Industrial Uses

There are wide-spread uses of radiation and radioactivity in industrial operations. Manufacturers and researchers take advantage of the following four characteristics of radiation sources for industrial uses: that radiation affects materials; that materials affect radiation exposure; that radiation traces materials; and that radiation produces heat and power in a variety of industries.[(41)] Applications such as pasteurization and sterilization of food, polymerization of organic compounds, sterilization of medical supplies, and elimination of static electricity are possible.[(5)] Likewise, the intensity of nuclear radiation is reduced by thicker or denser materials that are in the path of the radiation. This is the characteristic that is responsible for such applications as radiographs.

In the metals industry, where blast furnace operations are used, radioactivity is used to study the residence time and distribution of constituents in the various metallurgical processes. Other tracer studies compare methods of chemically cleaning copper and stainless steel parts, evaluating plating techniques, and adding knowledge about the structure of electroplated coatings. Radionuclides have also been used to evaluate the diffusion of gases into metals (causing brittleness), and they have been used to provide valuable information on the rate of tool wear.

Using radioactivity to gauge thicknesses has been well-recognized by industry.[(41)] It permits continuous control of the uniformity of the thickness of various kinds of sheets and layers to very close tolerances. Furthermore, these types of systems can be completely automated so that the response to thickness changes can be used to actuate rollers, thus providing closer control than would otherwise be possible. In addition to thickness, radioactivity can be used to measure the density of various materials. The density of liquid slurries, powders, and granular solids can be measured by having a radiation source and a detector mounted on opposite sides of the material being measured (i.e., like in a hopper or pipe line). If the detected intensity of radiation from the source increases or decreases, the density of the material has decreased or increased, respectively.

The major advantage of radiography with a radiation source versus an x-ray machine for pipe and weld inspection is portability, the absence of electrical wires and connectors, and the ability to make exposures with the source of radiation placed inside a complex shape. The use of

[4] - Tritium decays by beta radiation and emits a 18 kiloelectron volts maximum beta particle and an average beta energy of six (6) keV.

cobalt-60 (Co-60) for flaw detection in masses of metal was one of the earliest applications of radionuclide radiography.[5] Most foundry operations maintain a selection of radiation sources, including radioactive cobalt, iridium, and cesium, among others. While x-ray machines are still used, radiation sources are the preferred methodology where the shape and accessibility of the casting makes x-ray techniques less effective. Although the purchase price of a radioactivity-bearing device can be much less than the price of an x-ray machine, compliance costs for users of radioactivity tend to be much higher than for users of radiation-producing machines.

There are uses of radioactivity in the electrical industry also. One example is the use of krypton gas (Kr-85) for leak testing. This procedure involves exposing electronic components to the gas under pressure for some period of time, during which any leaky components are at least partially filled with the gas. After the exposure period, the surfaces of the components are cleaned, and the leaky components are quickly identified by detecting the residual radioactivity. For example, they are used to study adsorption and desorption of mercury by glass surfaces in mercury switches. In addition, there are studies of corrosion of silver contacts by fused salt, the development of a high-integrity compression seals, evaluation of methods for cleaning metal surfaces prior to electroplating or enameling, wear testing of bearings, determination of lubrication and seal characteristics, and improving the doping of semiconductors by investigating the mechanisms of the diffusion.

Radiation sources are also used in fire detection equipment. Certain navigational lights also contain radioactivity. In addition, there has been considerable interest in the use of radionuclides to replace batteries and related power sources. The use of radionuclides in this industry is widespread and includes many different categories. Petroleum refiners were among the first industrial operations to use radionuclides. Refineries pump large amounts of fluids, including raw materials and other in-plant inventory and products. Radiation sources are used as part of the automatic (computerized) control of the flow of these fluids.

By far the most extensive use of radionuclides in this and other chemical industries is its use as a tracer. For example, radioactive sulfur can be used to determine the efficiency of separation; radioactive gold and iodine can be used to determine the thoroughness of mixing; radioactive sodium and bromine are used for locating leaks; and radioactive cobalt and cesium are used for gauging liquid or solid levels. Other radiation sources might be used to study process stream flow patterns, locate pipe obstructions, study mass balances in refinery streams, measure flow velocities, study catalyst movement, study carbon deposits in fuel research for drug metabolism studies, determine tire wear, study diffusion in glass, eliminate static, and sterilize medical supplies.

Trace amounts of radioactivity (Ru-106 or Rh-106) are sometimes used for determining the rate of wear in floor wax.[42] It can also be used to assess laundering efficiencies of various detergents. Radioactivity has been used to determine the firmness of cigarettes, the rate of pesticide removal from surfaces, the metabolism of food additives, biosynthesis, the movement of textile layers, the control of solid and liquid levels of foods and beverages in their containers, sterilization and pasteurization of food, and even the migration of dyes in the printing business.

Energy

A nuclear reactor operates on the physical principle that uranium fissions (splits) easily using neutrons. With the absorption of the neutron, the uranium atom disintegrates into two fission nuclei as well as gamma rays and, on average, two free neutrons. A nucleus is said to be fissile if absorption of a thermal neutron will cause a split into two nuclei. Fissile material contained in a fuel rod is covered with cladding to contain the uranium fission by-products and transfer heat. Control rods such as boron or cadmium made of low Z material with a high cross section for neutrons reduce the kinetic energy of free neutrons for a capture and control of subsequent fission.

Most reactors are intended for electric power generation, but there are a few for research. Any reactor can be used as a source of neutrons for research. Often non-radioactive material is lowered through a specialized port in the reactor for exposure to neutrons. When the neutrons are captured in the material, a radioactive isotope is formed. However, a key disadvantage of neutron activation for isotope production is that the end product is a mixture of radioactive and nonradioactive isotopes. The time of irradiation can be lengthened to increase specific activity, but the radioactive component decays, prohibiting the practicality of the use of very short lived radionuclides.

Measurements and Monitoring

Instruments

Survey instruments are used to detect and/or measure the radiation dose from a field of radiation. Selection of the appropriate detector is critical in the evaluation of the radiation dose or dose rate. The sensitive volume is that part of the detector where interaction between the radiation and the detection medium actually occurs. Survey devices or equipment consist of portable, multi-scaled radiation detectors to evaluate radiation dose over a relatively short period of time (usually dose per minute).

Survey instruments can operate on batteries, be light enough for an adult to carry in one hand, and respond in multiple ways to radiation fields. Many have audio speakers in addition to multi-staged scaling factors, and some can measure particles and/or photons.

Monitoring devices or equipment may be used to evaluate a radiation field over a relatively long period of time (week or month). Personnel monitors are generally analyzed on a monthly or quarterly schedule. Personnel who require shorter time evaluation wear special monitors. Room monitoring equipment may be active continuously with threshold warning devices. Table 26.15 provides an overview of radiation detectors with health physics application; Table 26.16 gives more detail on the common survey methodologies.

The principles of ionization and excitation are the fundamental interactions that provide the basis for the operation of radiation detectors. Detectors operate in one of two modes: a) counting mode; and b) spectroscopy mode. In either case, radiation transfers energy to a detector which is connected to a high voltage power supply. The interaction of ionizing radiation with the detector produces pulses of energy which are sent to a processor (e.g., amplifier or discrimination). Once the pulses are shaped

Table 26.15 — Classification of ionizing radiation detecting equipment

Classification	*Sensitive Volume*	*Energy Range (rad)*	*Health Physics Function*
Electrical			
Ionization	Gas	All energies	Survey meter
Proportional counter	Gas	All energies	Survey meter
Geiger Mueller	Gas	0.001–100	Survey meter
Solid State material	Ge(Li) or Si(Li)	All energies	Analytical
Chemical			
Film	AgX	$0.01–10^4$	Diagnostic and personnel
Fricke	Ferrous sulfate	$5–10^8$	Calibration
Light			
Scintillation	Crystal NaI	All photon energies	Survey meter, gamma spectroscopy
Scintillation	Liquid cocktail	Not applicable	Analytical, Low energy beta
Thermoluminescence			
TLD	LiF	$0.01–10^5$	Tissue equivalent monitor
TLD	CaF_2	$0.01–10^5$	High energy photon
Heat			
Calorimeter	Thermistor	$1–10^5$	Calibration, high intensity radiation field

Note: An absolute dosimeter is one in which all the primary and secondary ionizing events are measured.
N/A=not applicable

and accepted, they are counted using either a scalar or rate meter. Rate meters, however, are commonly associated with survey and not laboratory instrumentation.

The basic distinction between counting and spectroscopy is that detectors operating strictly in the counting mode will indicate that radiation is present, but will not supply information as to the energy of the radiation or the identity of the radionuclide. Spectroscopy units, on the other hand, can analyze the height of the pulse and relate that height to the incident energy. Once that is known, the identity of the source can be determined.

Gas-Filled Detectors

There are three (3) types of gas-filled detectors. These are: Geiger counters or

Table 26.16 — Radiation detectors

Detector	*Types of radiation measured*	*Typical Units*	*Primary Use*	*Typical background*	*Advantages*	*Disadvantages*
G-M Detectors, End window, pancake	X-rays	Counts per minute (cpm), mR/hr*	Personnel surveys, contamination surveys	< 100 cpm	Inexpensive Simple, reliable Rapid response Sensitive to most contamination	Significant dead time (counts lost at high count rates) Will not detect verify low energy beta or alpha (α<4 Mev, β< 70 keV) Energy dependant
G-M detectors-side window	α, β, λ, X-rays	Counts per minute (cpm), mR/hr*	Personnel surveys, contamination surveys	< 100 cpm	Inexpensive Simple, reliable Rapid response, Easily adjusted to respond to gamma or x-rays only	Significant dead time, Will not detect alpha radiation at any energy, will not detect beat radiation less than 200 keV, Energy dependant
Proportional Counter — Gas flow	α, β	cpm	contamination surveys	Near 0 cpm	Ability to separate alpha and beta radiation , Insensitive to humidity	Relatively heavy, Flammable gas
Proportional Counter — air	α	cpm	contamination surveys	Near 0 cpm	Alpha radiation only, light weight, No special gas required	Sensitive to humidity, High maintenance
Sodium iodide scintillation detector	λ, X-rays	cpm (µR/hr)*	Area surveys for low levels of gamma and x-ray radiation	Several thousand cpm	Very sensitive, Rapid response	Detects gamma and x-ray radiation only, Relatively expensive, High background, fragile
Zinc Sulfide scintillation detector	α	cpm	Contamination surveys for alpha radiation	Near 0 cpm	Detects alpha radiation only, Light weight	Sensitive to light leaks
Ionization chamber	β, λ, x-rays	R/hr, mR/hr, µR/hr*, mrad/hr for β	Area survey for gamma and x-ray radiation, intense beta radiation	Less than 0.1 mR/hr	Directly measures mR/hr Virtually no dead time Capable to measure relatively intense levels of gamma radiation	Slow response Sensitive to temperature, pressure and humidity

Note: Appropriate calibration factor and/or instrument design required

Source: **Knoll, G.F.:** *Radiation Detection and Measurement.* New York: John Wiley and Sons, 1979.

Geiger Mueller detectors; Proportional counters; and Ionization Chambers. Each contains a central wire known as the anode which initially carries a positive (+) charge. Alpha and beta particle interactions inside the gas produce primary ion pairs. The electron component of the ion pair will be attracted to the anode. The positive member of the ion pair will be attracted to the outer wall which is initially negatively (-) charged with respect to the anode (i.e., cathode). Gamma ray interactions will more than likely occur first within the cathode wall rather than the fill gas. These interactions will eject electrons from the wall that then ionize the gas as noted above.

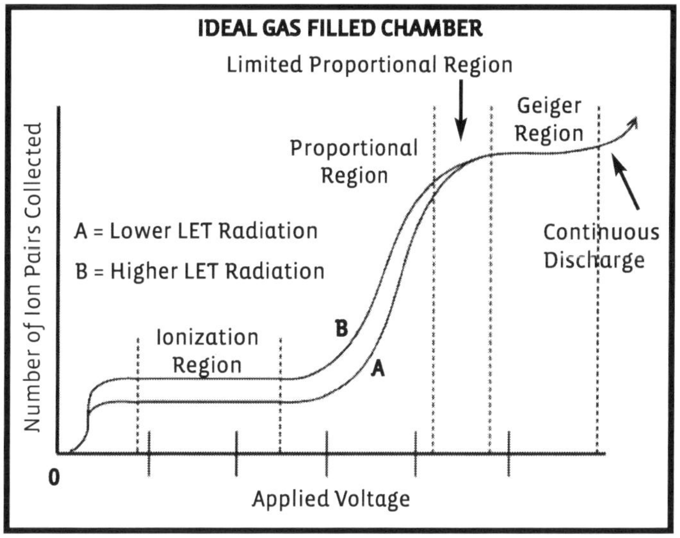

Figure 26.13 — Response of ideal gas-filled chamber to radiation.

Solid Detectors

There are three (3) basic types of solid detectors. These are: Sodium Iodide (NaI); Zinc Sulfide (ZnS); and High Purity Germanium (HPGe)

Sodium iodide detectors are crystalline solids which respond to gamma radiation by producing visible light flashes. Hence, they are known as scintillators. Zinc sulfide detectors are also crystalline solids useful for the detection of alpha radiation. They, too, rely on the scintillation process. In both cases, the light is converted into an electronic signal for recording purposes.

Detectors utilizing germanium are referred to as semiconductor or solid-state detectors. They are used exclusively for the detection of gamma radiation. Table 26.16 contains a summary of the types, uses, advantages, and disadvantages of radiation survey instruments that are commonly applied for licensed facilities.

A radiation survey is performed to measure the intensity of a radiation field; measure contamination levels, fixed or removable; and/or measure airborne radioactivity. For contamination survey instruments, one should use the "fast" response on the instrument (if available) to achieve the highest detector sensitivity. The instrument response can be switched to the "slow" setting for recording purposes. The operator should use headphones when available to detect increases in count rate by the audible meter output. This allows the surveyor to watch the probe and the surface being evaluated, rather than the meter itself.

The speed at which the detector moves should be relatively slow. Accelerated movement of the probe can result in failure to detect the radioactivity, although an experienced surveyor can often counter this problem. Typical scanning speeds are on the order of one detector width per second. Most detectors respond differently depending on the direction in which they are pointed. Typical detection limits and the variables that affect the sensitivity of the instrument were evaluated by the USNRC in 1998.[43]

Radiation survey instruments serve a wide variety of purposes and as a consequence, a wide variety of types are available. The selection of the correct instrument for the desired application requires an understanding of not only the type and form of the radiation to be measured but also the features and limitations of the specific detector. Table 26.17 describes the features that one should consider when selecting the correct instrument to characterize radiation or radioactive materials.

External Exposure Measurements

To assess each worker's external radiation exposure, special types of monitoring equipment are used and are selected based on the radiological hazards present. Personnel dosimeter measurements are considered the preferred source of information for evaluating external doses (relative to workplace monitoring programs or other personnel monitoring programs). Examples of primary personnel monitoring devices (that is, those

Table 26.17 — Instrument Use Considerations

Regardless of the instrument type, the following should be considered when using a radiation survey instrument:
Select an appropriate survey instrument for the radionuclide/radiations of interest.
Unless the instrument is being used strictly as a detection device, the instrument should be calibrated for the radionuclide and energy(ies) of interest.
Calibration sources and devices should be traceable to the National Institute for Standards and Technology (NIST).
Background and operability checks (high voltage, battery, source checks, etc.) should be performed daily (often two-three times in the same day).

Source: National Council on Radiation Protection and Measurements: Instrumentation and Monitoring Methods for Radiation Protection. Report 57. Bethesda, MD: NCRP, 1978.

typically used for the measurement of the dose equivalent received) include: thermoluminescent dosimeters (TLD's), film badges and track etch dosimeters. Direct reading pocket ionization chambers, electronic dosimeters, and audible-alarm dosimeters, are examples of supplemental dosimetry — devices often worn in addition to or located near the primary dosimeter.

The use of personnel dosimeters is an important aspect of a radiation monitoring program. These devices not only detect radiation in a qualitative manner but measure the amount of exposure in a precise manner. They permit radiation protection professionals to not only ensure personnel are not being exposed excessively, but to demonstrate that regulatory dose limits have not been exceeded. Routine monitoring is an element of the radiation protection program and the philosophy to keep one's radiation exposure as low as reasonably achievable (ALARA).

Regulatory requirements for the assessment and recording of external exposures are set forth by different federal agencies such as the Nuclear Regulatory Commission (USNRC) and the Department of Energy (DOE).[44–46] The armed services (Army, Navy, Marine Corps, Air Force, and the Coast Guard) have their own set of regulations which closely parallel those issued by the USNRC. In addition, many states have their own set of radiation protection regulations addressing this particular issue. Radiation protection requirements were developed and are periodically revised to attain consistency with radiation-related guidance that has been submitted by the Environmental Protection Agency (USEPA) to the President of the United States.[47] This guidance is based on current recommendations provided by consensus standards organizations.

External exposures usually involve a derived or inferred quantity since directly measuring the dose (or energy imparted) to every organ or tissue in the body with extreme accuracy is not realistic. There are several important elements of external monitoring programs, all of which are necessary for their successful operation.[48,49] For example, the staff that operates the program must be well-trained. In addition, the monitoring devices must be suitable for the radiations present at the facility, and their use parameters (deployment duration, position on the body, etc.) must be designed to ensure the measured result is representative of the true exposure. Finally, the records associated with the measurements and their interpretation is almost as important as the measurements themselves.

One of the most popular types of personnel monitoring devices contains small chips of a salt called "thermoluminescent dosimeters", or TLDs. Another type that contains film similar to the film used by a dentist for x-raying teeth, called a "film badge". Both of these types of monitoring devices require processing before the data are available. Primary personnel monitoring devices, that is those typically used for the official measurement of the exposure received for record-keeping purposes, include TLD and film badges. A thermoluminescent dosimeter, or TLD, can contain a variety of different materials. When these materials are exposed to radiation, the absorbed energy is "trapped" and held indefinitely. When the materials are heated at a later date in a device known as a "TLD reader" (the basis for the word "thermo"), the trapped energy is released in the form of light or luminescence. The amount of light is then related to the radiation dose. The fact that the absorbed radiation energy is trapped indefinitely is a prime advantage because the user can decide when the TLD will be read and the results reported. It is not uncommon for a period of several months to pass between the radiation exposure and the read-out of the TLD.

A typical TLD may have several salt chips or "elements" for different dose monitoring requirements. For example, the mylar window covers the shallow dose measurement area used for measuring skin/beta dose at a depth in the body of 0.007 centimeters (cm). The next area is the deep dose (whole body) section — the area is filled with Teflon™ and is thick enough to represent deep dose skin penetration — and is often rounded to detect radiation from any angle. This element is designed for detection of higher energy beta particles, x-rays, and gamma rays that penetrate at least one centimeter into the body. The third area above the deep dose rounded area or "bump" provides for x-ray detection. This area has a copper filter for x-ray discrimination.

Another advantage is that TLDs come in a variety of materials, sizes and shapes. These dosimeters are small, light, easy to handle, and can be worn comfortably by the individual. They are capable of covering a wide range of radiation exposures, from less than a few thousandths of a Sievert (millirem) to greater than 10 Sievert (> 1,000 rem). In addition, they have applicability for environmental measurements as well - a situation which is possible because certain types of TLDs are very sensitive to very low radiation exposures (the type of exposure levels found in the environment).

A TLD can only be read once, that is, once the trapped electrons have been heated, the amount of light produced, and the results recorded, the TLD cannot be re-read to confirm the results. It is also possible for a certain degree of "fading" to take place whereby some of the trapped electrons leave their excited energy states and return to the ground state prior to being read in the reader. This potentially results in a lower estimate of the individual's exposure. Many TLD materials, however, do not have this problem, and for those that do, correction factors can be applied to account for this situation. Finally, most TLD materials exhibit energy dependence, which means its response, is dependent upon the energy of the radiation that interacted with it.

X-ray film, used as a personnel dosimeter, was a common practice 20 years ago but has mostly been replaced in most facilities with more sensitive detectors. The sensitive volume is the silver ion of either silver bromide or silver iodide. The percentage of silver iodide (AgI) is about 10% to allow the atomic number of I (Z=53) to attenuate radiation by the photoelectric effect. Care must be taken to handle and store unexposed film as it is highly dependent on processing controls, pressure, humidity, storage on edge and not flat, and artifacts by air pockets. Processing of exposed film must be done using standard conditions. The use of film for external radiation exposures is not common among current licensees.

Small intense sources of radiation may expose small areas of the body in a different manner than the whole body. Fingers or skin may receive a higher dose than the whole body and must be evaluated correctly. Extremity dosimeters consist of a TLD chip encased in thin plastic and surrounded by a metallic ring. A flexible band of various sizes, each having a Velcro™ closure, is typically used for holding the dosimeter in place. As the name implies, extremity dosimeters are used to measure the external dose received at the extremities. The arms below the elbow and the legs below the knee are defined as extremities. Like the eyes, the extremities have a specific regulatory exposure limit. The limit is much higher than the limit for the whole body because there are few blood-forming organs in the extremities, thus they are less sensitive to radiation exposure. When monitoring the exposure of the extremities, dosimeters are typically placed at the most exposed portion of the body. Ring badges, wrist badges, toe badges, and ankle badges that are custom-designed to provide as little movement restriction as possible are readily available for this purpose. Their use is important in those situations where the extremities are likely to receive higher doses than the whole body. They measure the beta and gamma dose to the extremities. Typically, doses from beta radiation are the most variable by distance because they are easily shielded and their energies vary greatly. Because of this, the hands are usually in a higher dose rate field than the whole body of the whole body dosimeter.

The USNRC (or applicable Agreement State) allows the extremities to receive higher doses than the whole body. The reason for this is that the extremities contain no vital organs or extremely radiosensitive tissues. The limiting tissue is the skin. Unless otherwise directed by radiation safety personnel to wear the dosimeter in an atypical location, e.g., the ankles, the extremity dosimeters should be worn on the middle fingers with the TLD chip on the palm side of the hand, label facing the skin. The dosimeter should always be worn on the inside of gloves, if worn, in order to get an accurate measurement of the dose to the tissue itself. Extremity dosimeters should always be issued and worn in pairs and should never be worn in any area of the body other than the extremities. Extremity dosimeters are worn for a particular job. They are to be worn only while performing that job, not all of the time. When not in use, the extremity dosimeters should be placed inside of the plastic bag provided and stored according to instructions provided by the Radiation safety organization. This usually includes keeping them away from moisture and monitoring them for contamination after each use to avoid false high dose readings.

There are small instruments that function like gas-filled survey meters. These devices can be direct-reading, and provide real time information about the accumulated exposure received, or they can make noise whenever the accumulated exposure reaches a pre-determined level. Audible-alarm dosimeters and direct-reading pocket ionization chambers are examples of supplemental dosimetry devices often worn with or located near the primary dosimeter. The latter devices are not to be used as the official record of the exposure received.

An alarming dosimeter often contains a small Geiger-Mueller (G-M) detector and some electronics. Typically, the electronic circuit causes a series of "beeps" or "chirps" when the G-M detector responds to radiation. If calibrated properly, the number of "chirps" can be made equivalent to a known amount of radiation exposure. For example, if the device is set to "chirp" every time the G-M counter is exposed to 1 milliroentgen, a dosimeter that "chirps" five times during the next hour reflects an exposure of 5 milliroentgens.

When these devices are used in industry, their primary purpose is to make noise when a pre-set exposure or exposure rate has been exceeded. As such, it serves as a warning device rather than as a true dosimeter to measure the exposure received.

It is most important that the device be checked for functionality before work in a radiation field occurs. At that time, the device is typically pre-set to a specific alarm set point. However, it is equally important that the device be calibrated periodically to ensure the set points correspond to true radiation exposures. These dosimeters can create a false sense of security for workers as they can malfunction. A dosimeter that has been dropped, or that has low batteries, or that is worn such that the G-M detector inside cannot detect the radiation exposure, serves little purpose. An alarming dosimeter should never be used as a substitute for a radiation survey instrument, for job pre-planning, or for basic common sense.

A direct-reading dosimeter, also called a "pocket meter" or "pocket ionization chamber", is a small air-filled instrument, typically the size of a short, fat pen. It operates on the principle of radiation ionizing air, and it is capable of responding, primarily, to photon radiation (i.e., gamma rays, x-rays) and sometimes high-energy beta radiation. Specially-modified direct-reading dosimeters can also be used to measure neutron radiation. A direct-reading dosimeter contains both a "fixed" and a "movable" quartz fiber. When first put into use, an electrical charge is placed on both fibers. Because of their similar charge, the two fibers "repel" each other. As radiation enters the chamber and ionizes the air that is inside, the charge on the fibers is neutralized, and they begin to move closer together. The degree of movement, which is proportional to the amount of exposure received, can be seen by observing one of the fibers through an eyepiece that is on the end of the device. And this is perhaps the greatest advantage of using a direct-reading dosimeter. A user can determine his/her exposure at any time by holding the pocket dosimeter up to a light source and directly reading the value off a numerical scale. This allows workers to keep track of the amount of radiation exposure received over each day's work. The greatest disadvantage associated with these devices is that they are fragile. Simply dropping one of them can cause the two fibers to "discharge". In addition, they can "leak" some of their charge, meaning the fibers inside the dosimeter move even though there is no radiation exposure occurring. Finally, if the user forgets to "charge" the dosimeter before use, the device serves no purpose. It is for these reasons that a film badge or TLD is almost always used in conjunction with a direct-reading dosimeter.

Personnel monitoring programs are designed and conducted at nuclear facilities for several reasons. Among these are: protecting the health of personnel; identifying poor work practices; detecting changes in radiological conditions; verifying the effectiveness of engineering and process controls; meeting ALARA (reducing ones radiation exposure to "as low as is reasonably achievable") considerations; demonstrating compliance with regulatory requirements; and keeping adequate records. From a regulatory standpoint, personnel monitoring is required when an individual has the potential to receive 10% of the regulatory exposure limit from occupational exposure (i.e., as part of his or her work).[44] For facilities licensed by the nuclear regulatory commission, adult occupational workers must be monitored if they have the potential to receive a dose greater than 5 mSv (>500 millirem). For minors and declared pregnant women, however, monitoring is required when the individual is likely to receive more than 0.5 mSv(>50 millirem).

The USNRC has developed a comprehensive safety program for the industrial radiography industry.[50] These individuals typically use MBecquerel (multi-Curie) sealed sources of radiation to "radiograph", "image," or take x-ray pictures of pipes, to examine the adequacy of welds and to perform related activities. For a variety of reasons, these intense radiation sources can and have caused exposures in excess of regulatory limits. In some cases, very serious overexposures that resulted in observable health effects occurred.

The USNRC has issued specific regulations that impose additional external monitoring requirements for radiographers.[51] These regulations require radiographers and their assistants to wear a direct reading pocket dosimeter and either a film badge or TLD. An alarming device is also required except for permanent radiography facilities where alarming/warning devices are in routine use. Records documenting external exposures received by workers are required by federal and state agencies. These records must be maintained to document compliance, and they must be retained until their disposition is authorized by the overseeing agency. Examples of required records include those related to results of individual external exposure measurements; documentation of occupational exposures received during both current and prior years; data necessary to allow future verification or reassessment of recorded exposures; results of surveys, measurements, and calculations used to determine individual occupational exposures; results of maintenance and calibration performed on personnel monitoring devices; training records; results of internal audits; and declarations of pregnancy. Reports are required which include, but are not limited to, radiation exposure data for monitored individuals; and records of exposure for terminating employees. In addition, an annual radiation dose report (NRC Form 5) must be provided in writing to each individual who was monitored over the past year.

Several of the federal radiation protection regulations (e.g. 10 CFR Part 20 and 10 CFR Part 835) do not mandate where personnel monitoring devices should be located on the worker. However, assistance in this regard can be found in other radiation-related guidance documents. To determine the whole body exposure, dosimeters should be placed on the trunk of the body (between the neck and the waist) and positioned so that the front of the badge holder is facing the source of the radiation.[52] The dosimeter should be attached to the anterior portion of the torso. Dosimeters should not be attached to loose-fitting clothing, lapels, or worn on neck chains. Exposure to the lens of the eye is one concern for radiation protection professionals, and there is a separate regulatory limit for the eyes. For uniform exposures, a measurement at the surface of the torso is usually assumed to be equivalent to the exposure in the location of the eye. Non-uniform exposures, however, which include localized beams of radiation, x-ray machines, or beta sources, would require the placement of a dosimeter somewhere near the eyes. Typically, a dosimeter is mounted on the side of the head or on the forehead, such that it is located adjacent to the eye. Another circumstance is estimating the radiation exposure to the embryo/fetus of a pregnant worker. Again, wearing a conventional whole body personnel dosimeter (e.g., TLD or film badge) between the neck and the waist typically provides an adequate result. However, in the case of non- uniform fields or when exposures begin to approach the applicable exposure limit, an additional dosimeter is mounted near the mother's waist area or abdomen.

The National Voluntary Laboratory Accreditation Program, abbreviated "NVLAP", provides accreditation for testing and calibration laboratories, including those that provide personnel radiation dosimetry programs.[53] The NVLAP accreditation process is designed to assess how precise and how accurate the devices are, and how competent the processor is in providing the service. Competence, as used here, requires not only that the dosimeters perform adequately, but also that the processor demonstrates it has the staff, facilities and equipment, procedures, records and reports, and a quality assurance program to ensure reliable results. Any facility that provides personnel monitoring services is afforded the opportunity to attain accreditation. Once received, NVLAP accreditation is valid for a period of one year. After this period, re-accreditation is required. Concerns about personnel dosimetry performance date back to the 1950s. Efforts to implement dosimetry performance standards have been attempted several times but were always unsuccessful, primarily because only the performance of the dosimeter and not the dosimetry processor was addressed. The goal of the NVLAP remains the satisfactory performance of personnel dosimeters, and of equal import, that of the processor.

Internal Exposure Measurements

Potential sources of internal exposures can be placed into two categories. One category is natural radioactivity in food, water, air, and medical procedures that use radioactive materials. The other category is accidental or inadvertent internal uptake of radioactive material (internal contamination) that can cause additional dose to the whole body or individual organs. Internal exposure results from the inhalation, ingestion, injection, or absorption of uncontained radioactive material. Sensitive instruments and discrete samples collected from individuals are used to directly or indirectly measure the amount of radioactive material present inside the body, whether from naturally occurring or inadvertent uptakes. Indirect bioassay is the measurement of radioactivity in urine, feces, secretions, and other body samples, such as blood and other tissues. Direct bioassay is the measurement of the radiation emitted from the body using an external detector. Bioassay programs are established whenever there is a potential for internal exposures. These programs exist for radiological workers, declared pregnant workers, and minors, students, visitors, and members of the public depending on the dose potential. Bioassay programs are designed to assess baseline radioactivity, routine monitoring, diagnostic (or special) evaluation, termination evaluations, confirmatory monitoring, and operational monitoring.

The primary internal dosimetry techniques are lung and whole body counting measurements (direct bioassay) and urine/fecal sampling (indirect bioassay). The following sections describe these methodologies in greater detail.

The purpose of lung counting is to measure the amount of photon-emitting (gamma and low-energy X-ray) radioactive material present in the lungs. The lung counter utilizes sensitive gamma detectors placed above and beneath the lungs and is used routinely for those with a potential for internal exposure if any unsuspected activity shows up in bioassay samples, whole body scans, or during screening for baseline data. The measurement time is usually 20 to 40 minutes.

Whole body counting is a colloquial term for the measurement of the penetrating radiations emitted from radioactive materials that are contained in the human body, emitted through the body, and detected externally. The whole body counter utilizes a set of gamma detectors that moves or scans over the whole body while the individual being monitored lies on a bed. The scan time can vary from as short as 10 minutes or as long as an hour. The results can be used to screen large numbers of personnel or establish pre-exposure baseline data.

The purpose of the bioassay program involves the indirect measurement of a body elimination product, such as urine, to determine the amount of activity contributing to an internal exposure over a period of time. This program is particularly useful for alpha and beta emitters which cannot be measured by detectors external to the body.

Urinalysis is a useful measurement tool for soluble radionuclides that either distribute themselves uniformly throughout the body into the body fluids, or are taken up by a target organ and then slowly released into the body fluids. Either way, the contaminant is filtered by the kidneys and passed out in the urine. This bioassay method can be used to determine the amount of radioactivity present in the body at the time of measurement but cannot directly determine the amount that was present at some previous time.[49] That quantity must be inferred from the measured body content of the specific radioactive material, followed by application of mathematical models which describe the behavior of that material in the body.

Indirect bioassay, or excretion analyses, refers to identifying and quantifying radioactive materials that are excreted or removed from the body. Indirect bioassay procedures are used routinely in radiation protection work to monitor personnel for possible accidental intakes of radioactive materials.[54]

After an intake has occurred by inhalation or ingestion, a portion of the radioactive material will be absorbed into the bloodstream and deposited in various body organs or tissues or excreted from the body. Therefore, by analyzing an individual's excreta, an indication of whether an intake has occurred can be accessed. Examples of excreta that can be used for indirect bioassay include urine, feces, tissue, blood, fingernails, hair, teeth, saliva, sweat, and exhaled breath. However, for most routine internal radiation monitoring programs, urine bioassay, or urinalysis, is the methodology of choice.[55,56] As time passes and the body begins to excrete radioactive materials retained by various organs, standard indirect bioassay procedures can detect the presence of smaller amounts of radionuclides than is possible by standard whole body counting techniques. This difference in detection capability becomes even greater when insoluble radioactive materials are involved. The actual procedures are specific for the type and form of radioactivity being used in the work place. In general, however, one or more samples of urine are collected into a sterile bottle, the bottle is sealed, and the sample is shipped to a laboratory that performs radionuclide analysis. The actual analysis procedure is specific for the radioactivity in question. One common method is to place the sample directly over a radiation detector that is connected to a computer-based analyzer. This simple method is actually quite sensitive and requires no sample preparation other than to measure the total volume of the sample. Other methods generally require the sample to be dissolved into a solution, mixed with certain chemicals, and then poured through a device that is designed to extract the radionuclide in question.

Air sampling and monitoring programs, which are one means of assessing internal radiation exposures, can detect the presence of radioactive material in the air; and quantify the amount for dose assessment purposes. Air sampling devices are designed to collect particulates such as dusts, mists or fumes, etc. and gases (e.g., radon, radioiodine, tritium, etc.) The radioactivity of the sampled material is quantified at a later time. These devices are useful in identifying the amount and type of airborne radiation to which an individual has been exposed. Some air monitoring devices incorporate a direct reading detector and sound an alarm when a specified limit is exceeded. These monitors are generally not suitable for monitoring individual exposures. However, they do provide an immediate indication of airborne radiation in the work area.

Continuous monitoring or sampling for airborne radioactivity should be implemented whenever there is a significant potential for airborne exposure.[57,58] Breathing zone (BZ) sampling may performed for short-term periods at low flow rates with the intent of collecting a sample representative of what the worker is breathing. The use of these lapel monitors may be hampered by the low air sample volumes and consequently an unacceptable high detection limit when compared to the derived air concentration. A fixed air sample may be required in order to collect a much larger air sample volume and achieve the desired detection limit. When collecting air samples, information regarding sample number, equipment, sampling parameters and worker/workplace data is recorded on an appropriate data sheet. During sampling, the system is checked periodically to assure that the desired sampling rate is being maintained. Flow rate adjustments or changes are performed as necessary. Air is drawn through the collection media for the duration described in the work or project plan or until field conditions (e.g., excessive dust loading on a filter) necessitate the termination of sample collection. The pump is turned off at the predetermined time and the ending sample time and flow rate recorded.

The average flow rate is determined and recorded on the appropriate data sheet. However, the data sheet is checked for completeness upon termination of the air sampling activity. Sample collection media are transferred to appropriate envelopes/containers and labeled. Equipment is cleaned and operability checks performed before initiating further sampling.

Calculated radiation doses from bioassay measurements, breathing zone sampling, personnel monitoring devices, etc., are assessed on a planned and periodic basis by the radiation safety organization. All results are maintained in the worker's dosimetry records file. Under the provisions of the licensees radiation protection program plan, occupational workers who are monitored by the personnel dosimetry program may be provided an annual report of their total dose, external and internal. Upon request, a current radiation dose record must be provided to the employee. Terminating employees are provided a report within 90 days of the last day of employment which summarizes the radiation dose received for the total period of employment at the reporting facility. Upon request, a written estimate, based upon available information, may be provided upon termination. The results of both external and internal radiation exposures comprise a workers total radiation exposure history.

Protection Methods

External

There are several ways to protect oneself from external sources of radiation. However, the three most important ones are the concepts of "time", "distance", and "shielding." The time spent in a radiation field is the first major method for limiting exposure to an external radiation source. To apply this method, it is important to realize that the amount of radiation one receives is directly proportional to the time spent in the radiation field. For example, that a radiation detection instrument, held in a particular room, gives a reading of 50 microRoentgens per hour (50 uR/hr). If a worker stands in that location for one hour, a total exposure of 50 μR is reached. However, if the person remains in that location for two hours, the exposure will increase to 100 μR. On the other hand, if one half hour is the total time, the exposure will decrease to 25 μR. There-fore, to minimize the amount of radiation received, the time spent in the radiation field should be kept as short as possible.

Increasing the distance from the source of radiation is another major exposure-reducing method. In essence, for gamma emitters, such as a sealed source, the exposure drops by the "inverse square" of the distance from the radiation source. If the exposure is 50 μR at one (1) foot from a radiation source, the exposure at four (4) feet from that same source drops by a factor of one over four squared, or one sixteenth, or 3 μR. The distance between a radiation source and a person has an even greater influence over the total exposure than the amount of time one stands in the radiation field. While the exposure-time relationship follows a direct dependence (i.e., reducing the time spent in a radiation field by one-half reduces the exposure to the worker by one-half), doubling the distance from a source reduces the exposure by a factor of four. It is important to note here that inverse square law only is observed when the shape and size of the radiation source is a point source, rather than a line or a cylinder shape. However, generally speaking, the farther one moves away from a radiation source, the lower one's exposure will be. The inverse square law is calculated:

$$I_1 = I_2(D_2/D_1)^2$$

Where:

I_1 = is the intensity at a distance, D_1
I_2 = is the intensity at a distance, D_2.

This formula applies to effective point sources but fails when the distances are too close to the source of radiation, where particle radiation may be included for radioactive sources. Remember that particles have a finite range in air. Since sources are labeled with activity and date of that activity for that particular radionuclide, the exposure rate for gamma emitters can be calculated at any distance by use of the specific gamma constant defined as follows. Examples of gamma constants for selected isotopes are listed in Table 26.18.

Exposure rate (R/hr) = G A/d^2

Where:

G = specific gamma ray constant listed in texts in units of R m^2/Ci hour
A = activity of radionuclide in Curies, and
d = distance from a point source of radioactivity in meters.

Gamma constants can be found in any standard text or requested from the gamma emitter manufacturer. Diagnostic and therapeutic X-ray machines are calibrated with dose rate exposures at a given distance and field size and in some cases filtration thickness.

Different types of non-photon radiations can be stopped or "blocked" by using shields constructed of a variety of materials. Alpha particles typically have energies on the order of four (4) to eight (8) million electron volts (MeV). However, they quickly lose this energy through the ionization process. Hence, the range of an alpha particle in a particular type of material is quite short. In fact, a single sheet of paper can be used to completely eliminate the exposure from most alpha radiations. Beta particles lose their energy just like alpha particles — through the ionization process — but they do not ionize to the same ionization density in the absorbing medium as alpha radiation. Therefore, for the same energy particle they have a greater range than an alpha particle in various types of matter. Nonetheless, it is still fairly easy to shield or "block out" beta radiation. For average beta energies of less than 1 MeV, a few inches of wood or a few tenths of an inch of aluminum will effectively eliminate the exposure.

Because they are uncharged and electromagnetic in nature, gamma radiation is more difficult to shield than particles like alphas and betas. Exponential attenuation of gammas implies that there will be some radiation that penetrates the barrier. The basic approach to gamma ray shielding is to optimize the thickness and density of the shield such that the intensity of the beam is reduced to an acceptable level, most likely background. In other words, a very thin layer of lead or steel may be just as effective of a shield as a much thicker layer of concrete or wood. Neutron shielding is based on "moderating" or slowing down neutrons until their energy is low enough to permit them to be "captured" by a near-by atom. A wide range of shielding materials are used for these purposes, with some of the most common being water or cement.

Charged particle radiations like alphas and betas travel fixed distances in different materials, with the actual distance dependent upon their energies (in MeV). The greater the energy, the greater the distance the radiation will travel, and the thicker the shield for a given density must be to stop it. However, shielding for gamma rays and neutrons is more complex. In reality, the range for these radiations is indefinite. It is possible for these radiations to travel for miles before being stopped.

The quantity (amount) of radioactive material [activity measured in Becquerel (Bq) or Curie (Ci)] in the source also influences the exposure received. If one source has only half the amount of radioactivity in it as another equivalent source, only half of the radiations will be emitted. Therefore, the exposure rate at a given location away from the small source will be only half that of the larger source, not accounting for absorption in the air.

In general, radiation sources are designed to achieve a given purpose. Therefore, reducing the radioactivity in them may not be practical. However, if radiation sources are no longer necessary nor

Table 26.18 — Examples of gamma constants

Units of rem/hr @ 1 m from a 1 Ci point source	
Cesium 137	0.3818
Cobalt 60	1.3701
Iodine 131	0.2829
Radium 226	0.0121
Uranium 238	0.0652

Source: **Oak Ridge National Laboratory, Radiation Safety Information Computational Center:** Specific Gamma-Ray Dose Constants for Nuclides Important to Dosimetry and Radiological Assessment, ORNL/RSIC-45, May, 1982.

needed, it is a good idea to reduce the inventory. Likewise, when residual radioactivity in the form of "contamination" is present, it is clearly prudent to reduce its amount to the greatest extent practical so that the exposure rate from it will likewise be reduced. Therefore, good housekeeping is just as important in the business of radiation and radioactivity as it is anywhere else.

Internal

The purpose of a contamination control program is a structured program designed to reduce internal as well as external radiation exposures that result from the presence of contamination on surfaces of buildings, equipment and other areas. The goal of a contamination control program is not necessarily to eliminate contamination but to control its spread. An effective contamination control program contains several components including procedural requirements, worker training, the ALARA philosophy, and a Quality Assurance (QA) plan to assure verification.[59]

One key element to minimize internal exposures is the correct classification of an area that contains radioactive contamination and whether it is "fixed" or "removable".[60] As the words imply, "fixed" contamination means radioactive materials adhere onto the surface such that typical handling and touching of that surface does not dislodge the radioactivity. On the other hand, "removable" contamination is radioactivity that can be easily dislodged or transferred. Areas are often classified according to their contamination levels. The level of contamination control practiced in that area is dependent on the type and amount of contamination present.

Typical designations include "controlled area", "contaminated area", "highly contaminated area", "airborne radioactivity area", and "radioactive materials" area.[60,61] Areas having (or likely to have) loose, i.e., removable or transferable surface contamination in excess of specified limits, should be posted as noted above or in another appropriate fashion. Barriers and signs should also be placed at entrances and perimeters around the area to warn personnel of any inherent hazards. The requirements for entering the area should also be posted. Proper posting, followed by training all workers in the meaning of the signs and entrance requirements, serves to limit the spread of contamination and reduces personnel exposures to radiation. See Figure 26.14.

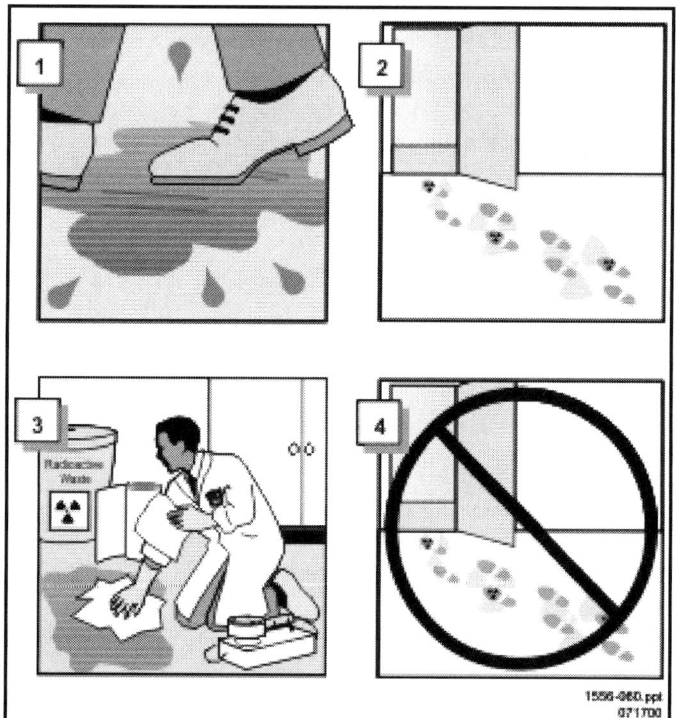

Figure26.14 — Tracking removable contamination.

One way to minimize the spread of contamination is to employ covering techniques. Contamination of clean areas can be minimized by covering those areas with materials such as plastic, paper or strippable coatings. Slightly contaminated areas can be prevented from becoming highly contaminated areas through the use of protective coverings. Safety hazards are often a factor when selecting a particular type of covering. Polyethylene materials, for example, become very slippery when moisture is present. Flammability is an issue with cloth and polyethylene materials. Coverings placed in high traffic areas can promote slipping if not securely fastened to the floor. Consideration must be given to all the safety hazards associated with these covering techniques to reduce the need for excessive decontamination while at the same time minimizing cost, time and excessive exposures. The amount of preparation required to protect an area can vary greatly. Consideration of the type of work and degree of contamination present will determine the appropriate type of covering and the number of layers required. Covering techniques, however, should be balanced against the volume and cost of radioactive waste generated, i.e., the use of unnecessary amounts of plastic, paper, etc., leading to waste disposal problems.

Control of internal exposures is a prime objective at sites that use radiation and radioactivity for several reasons. For one, assessing internal exposures is a much more difficult process than assessing external exposures. In addition, the analysis and interpretation of the results is time consuming, especially because of regulatory requirements and a relatively new dose reporting system where both internal and external exposures are summed and reported as one value. Each of these considerations should serve to encourage both worker and line management to minimize internal exposures by controlling the amount and spread of contamination.

There are specific contamination control methods that will minimize internal exposures. To reduce the possibility of internal contamination, eating, chewing, application of make-up, drinking and/or smoking should be allowed only in designated areas.[60] Such areas include uncontrolled areas or designated clean areas (permanent/temporary) within controlled areas. Basic contamination control practices dictate that before any individual eats, drinks or smokes, he or she must (1) remove all protective clothing, (2) perform a personal contamination survey and initiate decontamination efforts if necessary, and (3) follow common personal hygiene practices (e.g. washing hands).

The design of a facility, with consideration for proper engineering controls, contributes toward controlling contamination and reducing internal exposures. Engineering controls are those that are built into the design of the facility. These include things like ventilation systems with associated filters for trapping particulates and gases. Fume hoods and glove boxes, remote handling devices, and shielding may also be employed as confinement and containment devices. When these fail on occasion or become ineffective, respiratory protection may be required. Of course restricting entry to contaminated areas only to those that need to be there, and posting these areas appropriately, reduces the probability of contamination and personnel dose. In addition, detection and alarm systems can alert people to changes in the levels of airborne radioactivity, signifying possible loss of contamination control. Contamination on surfaces such as floors, tools and equipment can be tracked to different locations, spreading the contamination and increasing the possibility of worker exposure. In certain instances, transferable contamination on floors can become airborne through re-suspension (the contamination is removed from the floor surface by friction, such as "kicking" or simply walking on the floor, and becomes airborne.

Hot particles may be encountered in some facilities and may create a problem to limit the spread of radioactive materials. Hot particles are microscopic particles formed from degraded nuclear reactor fuel (i.e., fuel "fleas") or bits of metal that are made radioactive when they are carried by water into the core of a nuclear reactor.[59] Their origin indicates that they pose the greatest concern for operating nuclear reactors. Their small size and high radioactivity demands special contamination controls because they are difficult to detect, yet effective in delivering radiation exposure when they contact the skin. Control of hot particles in the workplace includes both specific procedures tailored to this particular type of contaminant, and significant job preplanning before doing any work in areas where hot particles are known to exist. In addition, special monitoring devices and survey techniques are used to identify and retrieve particles. Controlling their spread by restricting movement of personnel and equipment into hot particle areas is also important. In addition, optimum use of special filters, vacuuming, and wet towel wiping of internal valves and floor surfaces are all effective in reducing the number of hot particles. Typically, only the exposure to a small area on the anterior region of the body is evaluated as a measure of the whole body exposure. The possibility exists that other, more localized areas could have been highly exposed. If an overexposure occurs, it may be necessary to reconstruct the exposure situation (never the preferred method).

Contamination control points are special areas at nuclear facilities that are equipped with personal clothing racks or lockers, bins stocked with protective clothing, tape, benches, barrels for contaminated trash and protective clothing, step-off-pads, and personnel survey stations (friskers) or personnel contamination monitors. A properly located and equipped control point is necessary for contamination control. The control point is typically positioned in such a manner to provide a clear view of the entire work area and positive control of all activities within the area.[60] In addition, the location is chosen so that the flow of personnel and equipment entering or exiting a contamination area can be easily monitored and regulated. Step-off-pads provide an effective method of contamination control by serving as the boundary between the contaminated area and the contamination control point. Generally, step-off-pads are considered clean (uncontaminated). They should not be located in areas where a safety hazard may result, such as in stairwells or elevators.

Equipment used in or removed from contaminated areas should be prepared to minimize the spread of contamination. One or more of the following methods may be used: (1) adhesive tape applied to small items such as flashlights or wheels of a hand cart; (2) sheet material such as plastic or paper to cover large or bulky items; (3) sleeves for hoses and cables; (4) plastic bags to enclose portable instruments or other equipment that do not provide a remote display; (5) strippable coatings to apply to large flat surfaces; or (6) sealing exposed surfaces with paint or other durable coverings. Before removal from a contaminated area, items that are potentially contaminated must be surveyed for the presence of radioactive contamination.

During the operation of any facility where loose radioactive material is used, contamination is likely to be encountered and decontamination efforts must be applied. Each technique must be evaluated and modified as necessary, to accommodate the task or item being decontaminated.[7] Decontamination of contaminated tools, equipment and/or surfaces must be completed before work commences. This approach reduces the likelihood that the contamination will be spread to other uncontrolled areas and also reduces the potential exposure to the employees assigned to the area. A typical scenario includes: Surveying the item or surface with an acceptable radiation survey instrument; determining whether the contamination is "fixed" or "loose" by smear techniques; and applying detergents or other agents to the area of interest using a brush or tool to scrub the surface.[41,48,60] If the effort is successful, the tools and equipment can be released to the "uncontrolled" area, and the postings and barriers surrounding the controlled area may be removed. If unsuccessful, the tools and equipment can either be discards as radioactive waste or placed in a specific area with the appropriate controls and postings. Any liquids or material used to decontaminate the equipment or surface should be tested to determine the correct disposal option. In many situations, it is discarded as radioactive waste. Liquids must be absorbed in porous solids before radioactive disposal; mixing with Portland™ cement is a common treatment method in proportions that no free standing liquid remains.

In cases of personnel decontamination, the method should be selected based on the effectiveness of removing the contamination, but also on the effect the method will have on the individual.[62] There are three primary objectives of personnel decontamination, including reducing radiation exposure, minimizing the absorption of radionuclides into the body and prevent localized contamination from spreading to clean, uncontaminated areas. The following steps should be followed when personnel decontamination is required:

Survey the individual over the skin, hair, clothing, etc., using an appropriate instrument. See Figure 26.15. If the contamination is widespread, the individual should shower with soap and water and then dry off. The survey should be repeated, to verify that the contamination has been reduced to a localized portion of the body. Superficial contamination should always be removed by first washing the affected area with lukewarm water and mild soap. Scrubbing with soft bristle brushes should be done only when absolutely necessary. Hard bristle brushes should not be used because excessive irritation can lead to a loss of integrity of the skin barrier. Hot water which opens pores such that contamination can enter or cold water which closes pores around contamination should be avoided if possible. In addition, when showering, care should be taken to prevent contaminating body orifices with contaminated runoff.[62] Localized areas can often be decontaminated by taping a surgeon's glove, plastic bag, etc. over the affected area. The contamination is removed by sweating through the skin.

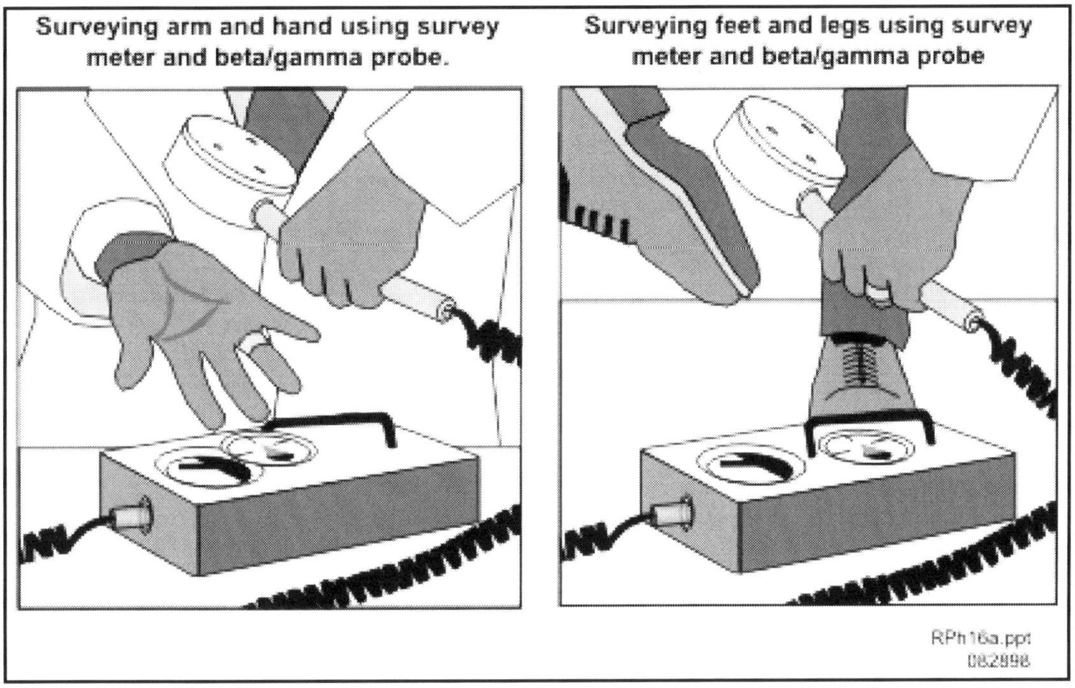

Figure 26.15 — Method for personnel radiation survey.

Contamination present in the eyes, mouth and wounds should be handled by flushing the areas with copious amounts of water (sterile water for eyes) and relying on trained medical personnel for further decontamination efforts. Potential evidence of internal contamination can be determined by taking nasal swipes with cotton swabs and counting each swab in a G-M counter. Based on the preliminary findings, the individual may be asked to blow his/her nose repeatedly; additional nose swabs are then taken and recounted.

Decontamination efforts should be repeated several times for a given procedure. If after up to four attempts, the contamination levels are not being reduced significantly, additional measures should be employed. These include applying mixtures of corn starch or cornmeal with detergent to the affected area. Only if these physical methods fail should the use of chemical agents be considered.

Detailed records should be maintained which include the initial level and extent of contamination, removal methods, skin condition, and final contamination levels. Protective clothing is worn by people working or entering contaminated areas to prevent contamination on their clothes or skin. It provides personnel with an easily removed outer layer, so that if contamination is present on the clothing, the wearer is no longer exposed after the clothing is removed. In addition, protective clothing may provide some shielding for beta radiation. The amount of protection gained by wearing protective clothing depends to a large degree on how the clothing is worn and used by personnel.

Several types of protective clothing are used depending on the work activity, associated levels of contamination, and whether the contamination is in a dry or wet state. These include lab coats, coveralls (e.g., cotton or Tyvek™), plastic suits, gloves, shoe covers (ranging from cotton to plastic to rubber overshoes), and head gear (e.g., surgeon's caps and hoods). Instructions should be provided to document the requirements for personal protective equipment and may change depending on conditions encountered in the controlled area.

Protective clothing must be selected to assure that it will fit properly. Clothing that is too large for the wearer makes work more difficult and may drag along the floor spreading contamination. Clothing which is too small for the wearer does not give adequate protection, because as the wearer moves, the joints where the clothing meets (i.e., points where coverall sleeves meet gloves) can separate, exposing skin to possible contamination. Protective clothing should be comfortable and provide sufficient mobility for the wearer. An improper fit reduces worker efficiency and could result in increased exposure from increased stay times. Prior to donning, each article of protective clothing should be inspected for contamination, holes, torn seams, missing buttons, broken zippers, etc. If defects are found, the item should be marked for repair or discarded, and another article selected. When using rubber gloves, check for small holes to ensure that the glove will not leak. Inflate the glove (not by mouth blowing) to check for air leaks. When selecting gloves, be sure the style used is suitable for the type of work being performed. For example, if "finger tip" type work is to be performed, surgeon's gloves would be the logical choice. Rubber gloves, which are large and bulky, would not be suitable.

Emergency Response

Working in a radiological environment requires more precautionary measures than performing the same job in a non-radiological setting. This premise holds true if an emergency arises during radiological work. The approach to limit the extent of an emergency is dependent on the nature of the emergency.

For minor injuries in radiological areas, one should leave the immediate work area following normal radiation safety organization procedures, if possible, and notify radiation safety organization personnel. Radiation safety organization personnel will survey the injury and direct personnel to the medical department or other designated area for treatment.

Appropriate first aid and other immediate medical needs of injured individuals should not be neglected, delayed, or ignored because of suspected contamination.[63] The name and telephone number of the Radiation Safety Officer (RSO) or an alternate person(s) should be posted conspicuously in areas of use, so that they are readily available to workers in case of emergencies. The licensee should have emergency equipment readily available for handling spills. Spill kits should include personal protective equipment such as disposable gloves, housekeeping gloves, disposable lab coats, disposable head coverings, disposable shoe covers, roll of absorbent paper with plastic backing, masking tape, plastic trash bags with twist ties, "Radioactive Material" labeling tape, marking pen, "Radioactive Material" labeling tags, instructions for "Emergency Procedures," and appropriate calibrated survey instruments including batteries (for survey meters).

For serious injuries in radiological areas, the major consideration is the immediate health of the individual rather than routine radiation safety organization procedures, such as removing protective clothing and monitoring. If a person needs immediate attention, a typical procedure is to contact the emergency response staff by performing a series of actions in a preferred order; (1) Dialing previously specified site-specific telephone numbers; or (2) Using an Emergency Pull Box, or (3) Utilizing a site radio system. Immediate first aid procedures should be provided only for which the responder is trained and emergency personnel should not move the injured person unless the location of the person could be considered life-threatening. There are additional situations that might require immediate exit from a radiologically-controlled area, such as a lost or damaged TLD; an off-scale direct-reading dosimeter (or one that reads 75% of full-scale); torn protective clothing; indications that radiological conditions in the area have changed; an area radiation or CAM alarm; or when directed to do so by radiation safety organization personnel.

Survey all personnel who could possibly have been contaminated. Decontaminate personnel by removing contaminated clothing and flushing contaminated skin with lukewarm water and then washing with a mild soap. Allow no one to return to work in the area unless approved by the RSO. Persons involved in the incident should cooperate with RSO or designated RSO staff so that a thorough investigation of root cause can be completed and bioassay samples can be submitted, if required. Those persons involved should follow the instructions of the RSO or designated RSO staff regarding decontamination techniques, surveys, provision of bioassay samples or requested documentation. The RSO should confirm decontamination of personnel. If decontamination of personnel was not fully successful, consider inducing perspiration by covering the area with plastic. Then wash the affected area again to remove any contamination that was released by the perspiration. The RSO should supervise decontamination activities and document the results. The documentation should include location of surveys and decontamination results. The cause and needed corrective actions should be determined and the need for bioassays should be evaluated if licensed material may have been ingested, inhaled, and/or absorbed through the skin.

In the event of a spill of radioactive material, certain actions should be initiated

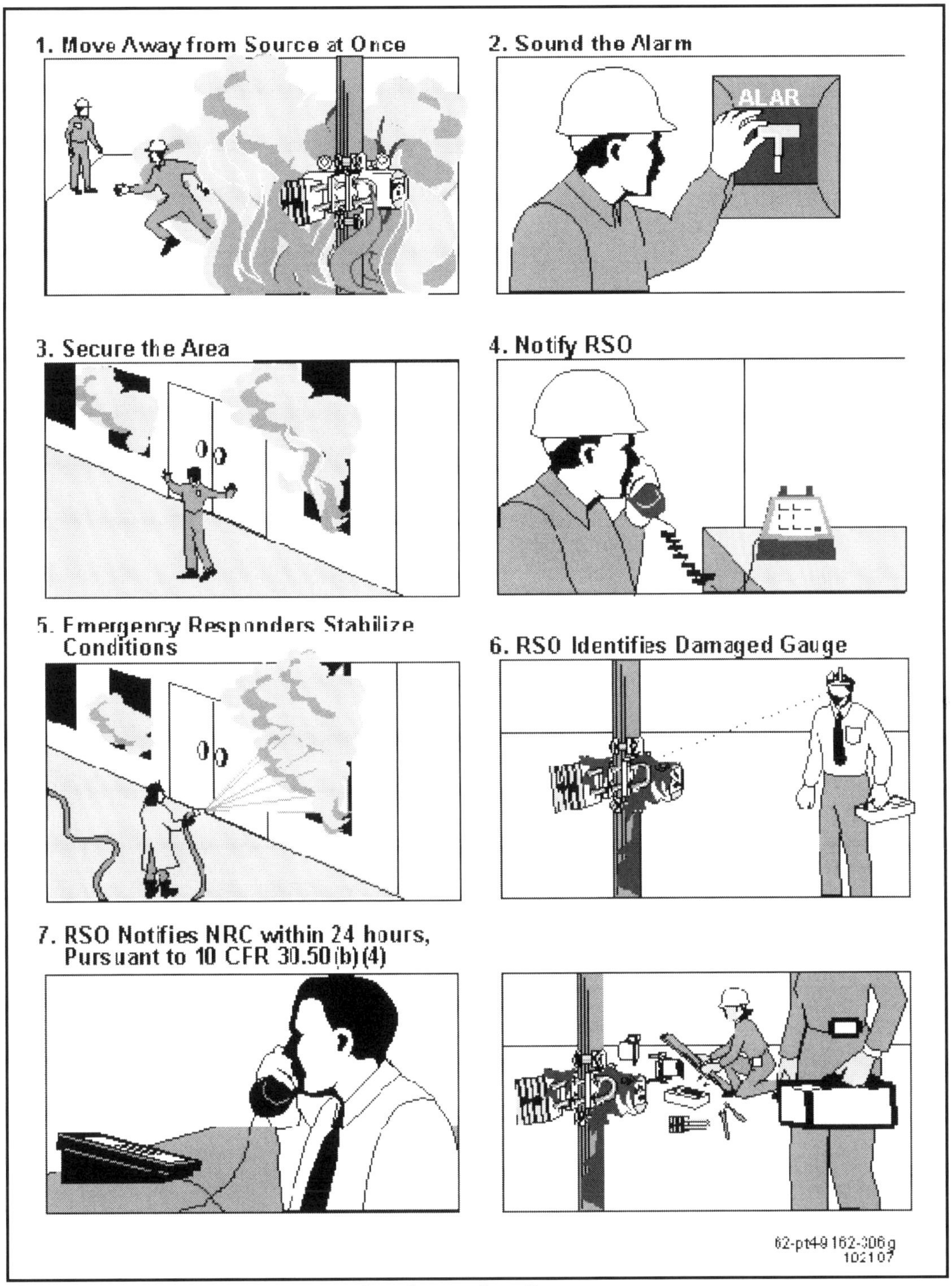
1. Move Away from Source at Once
2. Sound the Alarm
ALAR
3. Secure the Area
4. Notify RSO
5. Emergency Responders Stabilize Conditions
6. RSO Identifies Damaged Gauge
7. RSO Notifies NRC within 24 hours, Pursuant to 10 CFR 30.50(b)(4)
62-pt49 162-306g
102107

Figure 26.16 — Emergency response actions for a radioactive source.

immediately after the situation is identified (e.g., an uncontrolled leak from a radioactive system, an overturned sample bottle containing a radioactive liquid, etc.). If the spill is from a system that may have more material to leak out (i.e., an overturned container or process pipe), promptly stop the leak if possible. Do not collect the liquid (for purposes of criticality control where applicable). If the spill is of a minor nature, (e.g., a few milliliters of water spilled on a smooth surface), immediately cover the spill with an absorbent material such as rags. Warn other personnel who may become contaminated by the spill or who may be able to control it. Staying at the site while sending others for assistance can help to prevent accidental contamination of other personnel and prevents the spread of contamination to other previously uncontaminated areas.
Isolating the area will minimize the spread of contamination and will also assist the clean-up personnel in knowing the extent of the spill. Personnel, rope or tape placed at the entry points may be used to isolate the area and keep unnecessary personnel away. Ones radiation exposure can be minimized by Standing upwind and move toward the edge of the spill; Using protective clothing if available; not touching areas suspected of being contaminated; prevent tracking contamination to other areas; Securing unfiltered ventilation; Performing this task, as appropriate, to prevent airborne activity from entering unfiltered ventilation pathways. In any event, radiation safety personnel and supervision should be notified. Table 26.19 summarizes the sequence of events recommended to reduce the severity of a spill.

After the spill is secured and the event is complete, survey the area with an appropriate low-range radiation detector survey meter or other appropriate technique.[63]

Table 26.19 — SWIMS

The acronym SWIMS can be used to remember the initial responses to a spill:

STOP the spill
WARN other personnel
ISOLATE the area
MINIMIZE your own exposure
SECURE unfiltered ventilation

Source: Lawrence Berkeley National Laboratory, Emergency Preparedness Guide, 2008.

Check the area around the spill for contamination. Also check hands, clothing, and shoes for contamination. Report the incident to the RSO promptly. Allow no one to return to work in the area unless approved by the RSO.

In the event of a fires, explosions, or major emergencies, all personnel should be instructed to leave the area immediately and report to the designated emergency areas. The RSO and other facility safety personnel should ensure that injured personnel receive medical attention. Upon arrival of firefighters, inform them where radioactive materials are stored or where radionuclides were being used; inform them of the present location of the licensed material and the best possible entrance route to the radiation area, as well as any precautions to avoid exposure or risk of creating radioactive contamination by use of high pressure water. Allow no one to return to work in the area unless approved by the RSO. Notify emergency medical personnel of any injured individuals who may be contaminated. Provide radiation safety assistance (e.g., monitoring) as needed or requested. The RSO should coordinate activities with local fire department or other emergency personnel. Set up a controlled area in concert with firefighting personnel or other emergency personnel where personnel can be surveyed for contamination of their protective clothing and equipment after the fire is extinguished. Once the fire is extinguished, provide assistance to firefighters or other emergency personnel who may need to re-enter restricted areas to determine the extent of the damage to the licensed material use and storage areas. To the extent practical, assist firefighters and emergency personnel in maintaining their exposures ALARA if the fire resulted in a significant release of radioactive material or loss of shielding capability, such that excessive radiation levels (> 100 mrems/hr) are created. The RSO should perform thorough contamination surveys of firefighters and emergency personnel and their equipment before they leave the controlled area, and decontaminate if necessary. The RSO should supervise decontamination activities of both emergency response personnel and persons in the contaminated areas. The RSO should consider bioassays if licensed material may have been ingested or inhaled.

Employee Workplace Awareness

All employees must be aware of conditions, hazards, and potential emergencies in their workplace. Some thought should be given to what actions one would take in the event of an incident before it occurs. At a minimum, each employee should know the location of emergency exits; the location of nearest fire extinguisher and emergency pull box; the location of other emergency equipment (first aid kits, eye wash stations, etc.); the location of nearest telephone; and the location of applicable assembly station

Consideration in Rescue and Recovery Operations

In extremely rare cases, emergency exposure to high levels of radiation may be necessary to rescue personnel or protect major property. Rescue and recovery operations that involve radiological hazards can be a very complex issue with regard to the control of personnel exposure. The type of response to these operations is generally left up to the officials in charge of the emergency situation. The official's judgment is guided by many variables which include determining the risk versus the benefit of the action, as well as how to involve other personnel in the operation. Since these situations often involve a substantial personnel risk, volunteers are used. The use of volunteers is based on their age, experience, and previous exposure. Suggested emergency total effective dose equivalent limits for rescue and recovery of personnel are summarized in Table 26.20.

Table 26.20 — Recommended radiation dose limits for emergency rescue

• For protecting major property (only on a volunteer basis where the lower dose limit of five (5) rem is not practicable) — less than 10 rem.
• For lifesaving or protection of large populations (only on a volunteer basis where the lower dose limit is not practicable) — less than 25 rem
• For lifesaving or protection of large populations (only on a voluntary basis to personnel fully aware of the risks involved) — greater than 25 rem.

Source: **U.S. Department of Energy:** Radiological Control Manual, DOE/EH-0256T, Revision 1, Chapter 2, Appendix A, April, 1994.

Regulations

Agencies

The U.S. Nuclear Regulatory Commission (USNRC) is an independent agency established by the U.S. Congress under the Energy Reorganization Act of 1974 to ensure adequate protection of the public health and safety, the common defense and security, and the environment in the use of radioactive materials in the United States.[64–66] Licensing and related regulatory functions were transferred to the USNRC. The USNRC's scope of responsibility includes regulation of commercial nuclear power reactors; nonpower research, test, and training reactors fuel cycle facilities; medical, academic, and industrial uses of nuclear materials the transport, storage, and disposal of nuclear materials and waste. The Commission consists of five commissioners; the Chairman is appointed by the U.S. President. Each commissioner must be confirmed by the U.S. Senate.

The licensing and regulation of radionuclides in the United States are shared by the USNRC, the U.S. Environmental Protection Agency (USEPA), and many State governments. The USEPA is also responsible for, among other things, setting air emission and drinking water standards for radionuclides. The States regulate radioactive substances that occur naturally or are produced by machines, such as linear accelerators or cyclotrons. The Food and Drug Administration (FDA) regulates the manufacture and use of linear accelerators; the States regulate their operation.

The USNRC is the federal agency given the task of protecting public health and safety and the environment with regard to the safe use of nuclear materials. Among its many responsibilities, the USNRC regulates medical, academic, and industrial uses of nuclear materials generated by or from a nuclear reactor. Through a comprehensive inspection and enforcement program, the USNRC ensures that these facilities operate in compliance with strict safety standards.

Regulations established by the USNRC are published in the Federal Register and become incorporated into the Code of Federal Regulations. In addition to regulations, the USNRC publishes Regulatory Guides, Branch Technical Position Papers and NUREG reports which provide supporting information.

The USNRC has relinquished its authority to regulate certain radioactive materials, including some radionuclides. As of 2008, thirty five states had completed the process to regulate and license the use of radioactive materials in their specific state. These States, which have entered into an agreement assuming this regulatory authority from the USNRC, are called Agreement States.[67] Agreement States, like the USNRC, regulate reactor produced radionuclides within their borders and must provide at least as much health and safety protection as under the USNRC.

The Office of Federal and State Materials and Environmental Management Programs is responsible for establishing and maintaining effective communications and working relationship between the USNRC and States, local government, other Federal agencies and Native American Tribal Governments, serving as the primary contact for policy matters between USNRC and these external groups.[67] It keeps the external groups informed on USNRC activities, keeps the Agency appraised of these groups' activities as they may affect USNRC, and conveys to USNRC management these groups' views toward USNRC policies, plans, and activities as well as administers the Agreement State Program.

As of 2008, the USNRC maintained approximately 3,770 licenses for the use of radioactive materials, and the Agreement States maintained approximately 18,482 materials licenses.[68] Every license specifies the type, quantity, and location of radioactive material that may be possessed and used. When radioactive material is transported, special packaging and labeling are required. Also specified in each license are the training and qualification of workers using the materials, specific procedures for using the materials, and any special safety precautions required. Every licensee is inspected periodically either by the USNRC or the Agreement State to ensure that radioactive materials are being used and transported safely. Violators of regulatory requirements are subject to fines and other enforcement actions, including loss of license.

When used properly, radionuclides are a productive part of today's world. The USNRC and the Agreement States remain committed to protecting public health and safety in the use of these nuclear materials by inspecting medical, academic, and industrial applications carefully, and monitoring users to ensure safe work practices.

The use of radioactive materials is governed by a license issued by the USNRC or an Agreement State. The licensee not only must satisfy the requirements of the applicable federal or state regulations, but must also implement a site specific program to minimize the potential for radiation exposures.[69] The USNRC recognizes that effective radiation safety program management is vital to achieving safe and compliant operations. USNRC believes that consistent compliance with its regulations provides reasonable assurance that licensed activities will be conducted safely. USNRC also believes that effective management will result in increased safety and compliance. The licensee is responsible for Radiation safety, security and control of radioactive materials, and compliance with regulations. The licensee must implement the elements defined in the license and application as well as comply with current USNRC and Department of Transportation (DOT) regulations. The licensee must establish operating and emergency procedures. The licensee must make a commitment to provide adequate resources (including space, equipment, personnel, time, and, if needed, contractors) to the radiation protection program to ensure that the public and workers are protected from radiation hazards and meticulous compliance with regulations is maintained. The company must select and assign a qualified individual to serve as the Radiation Safety Officer (RSO) with responsibility for the overall radiation safety program.

The licensee must establish appropriate administrative procedures to assure the control of procurement and use of byproduct material. Some licenses are specific and authorize the licensee to perform only certain tasks in a specific manner. On other licenses, termed broad scope licenses, the licensee may use larger quantities of radioactive materials in a variety of applications. In this case, the licensee may be required to complete safety evaluations of proposed uses that consider the adequacy of facilities and equipment, training and experience of the user, and operating and handling procedures.[63] As applicable the licensee must review and approve the safety evaluations of proposed uses. Broad scope licensees must specify the duties and responsibilities of management, the Radiation Safety Committee (RSC) as well as the duties of the RSO. See Figure 26.17. These organizations must review and approve program and procedural changes before the changes are implemented. The RSO must complete periodic audits of licensed operations to determine compliance with the license and applicable regulations. All three functions, Management, RSC and the RSO, must take appropriate actions when noncompliance is identified. The licensee is expected to complete an analysis of the cause, corrective actions, and actions to prevent recurrence. Program changes are authorized, through use of the license conditions, as long as the program change or revised procedures are reviewed and approved by the RSC prior to implementation. Any change must satisfy regulatory requirements and may not change existing license conditions. The changes must not decrease the effectiveness of the Radiation Safety Program.

A licensee must be familiar with the regulations promulgated by the USNRC, including but not limited to:

10 CFR Part 2, "Rules of Practice for Domestic Licensing Proceedings and Issuance of Orders"

10 CFR Part 19, "Notices, Instructions and Reports to Workers: Inspection and Investigations"

10 CFR Part 20, "Standards for Protection Against Radiation"

10 CFR Part 21, "Reporting of Defects and Noncompliance"

10 CFR Part 30, "Rules of General Applicability to Domestic Licensing of Byproduct Material"

10 CFR Part 31, "General Domestic Licenses for Byproduct Material"

10 CFR Part 32, "Specific Domestic Licenses to Manufacture or Transfer Certain Items Containing Byproduct Material"

10 CFR Part 51, "Environmental Protection Regulations for Domestic Licensing and Related Regulatory Functions"

10 CFR Part 71, "Packaging and Transportation of Radioactive Material". Part 71 requires that licensees or applicants who transport licensed material or who may offer such material to a carrier for transport must comply with the applicable requirements of the United States Department of Transportation (DOT) that are found in 49 CFR Parts 170 through 189.

10 CFR Part 170, "Fees for Facilities, Materials, Import and Export Licenses and Other Regulatory Services Under the Atomic Energy Act of 1954, as Amended"

10 CFR Part 171, "Annual Fees for Reactor Operating Licenses, and Fuel Cycle Licenses and Materials Licenses, Including Holders of Certificates of Compliance, Registrations, and Quality Assurance Program Approvals and Government Agencies Licensed by USNRC".

Each agreement state has equivalent regulations which may be identical or more stringent than the requirements established by the USNRC. Each licensee is responsible to determine which regulations apply to their operation and implement those elements into their specific program.

Exposure Limits

To minimize the potential risks of biological effects associated with radiation, dose limits and administrative control levels are established and implemented at all licensed facilities. The radiation dose limits that established for occupational workers are based on guidance from the USEPA; the National Council on Radiation Protection and Measurements (NCRP); and the International Commission on Radiological Protection (ICRP). These limits are also consistent with the "Radiation Protection Guidance to Federal Agencies for Occupational Exposures" signed by the President. USNRC (or Agreement State) dose limits are established based on extensive scientific study. They are designed to allow activities which might result in radiation exposure, while protecting individuals, their offspring and the general population.

Before discussing the various limits and control levels, it is important to understand what portion of the body where limits and controls are applied. Dose limits are based on the risk of exposure to various organs and tissues in the body. The area of the body which contains the vital organs (whole body) will have lower allowable doses than those areas of the body containing no vital organs (extremities). For purposes of external exposures, the USNRC defines the whole body as the head, trunk (including male gonads), arms above and including the elbow, and legs above and including the knee.[70] These are the location of most of the blood-producing and vital organs. See Figure 26.18.

External exposure results from a radiation source outside the body. Internal exposure is a result of radioactive material being inhaled, ingested, or absorbed through the skin or wound. The USNRC dose limits are based on the sum of internal and external exposure.

Committed and Effective Dose Equivalents

The USNRC dose limit involves the combination of internal and external exposures. The process of combining the two involves the Committed Dose Equivalent and the Effective Dose Equivalent.

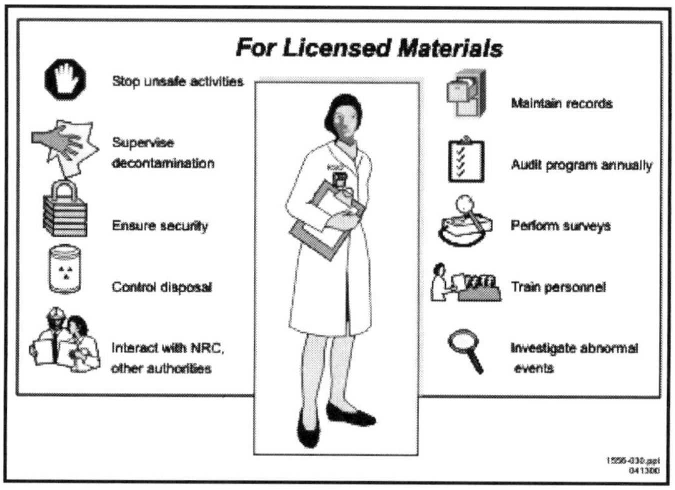

Figure 26.17 — Typical duties and responsibilities to RSOs.

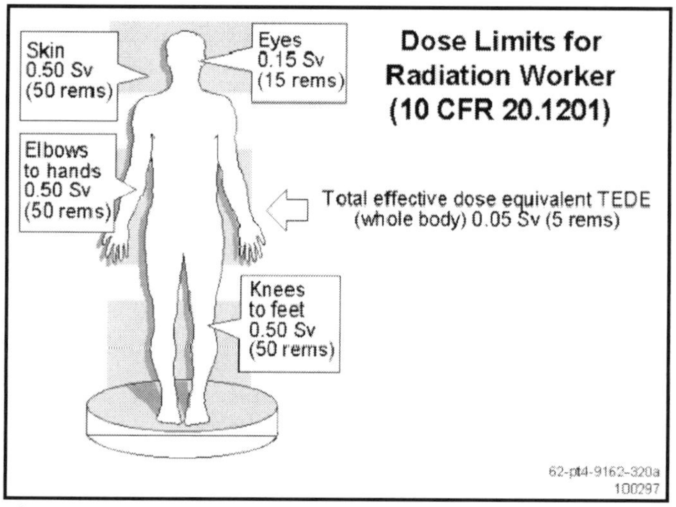

Figure 26.18 — Dose limits for radiation workers.

Committed Dose Equivalent

The Committed Dose Equivalent is the dose to some specific organ or tissue that is received from an intake of radioactive material by an individual during the 50-year period following the intake (see 10 CFR Part 20.1003). It is possible to calculate the radiation dose to individual organs after incorporating specific radionuclides into the organ or near the organ of concern.[71] Radioactivity travels to individual organs (depending on its chemical nature) and resides in the organs for a period of time. At some point, the body begins to remove the radioactivity in the organ, and eventually eliminates it.

While the radioactivity is contained in the organs, it is depositing radiation dose in them. The dose equivalent to the organs is committed over the period of time that the body is eliminating the radioactivity. The total dose equivalent associated with an intake of radioactivity is represented by a single value for each organ exposed to the radiation. This total dose equivalent is called the committed dose equivalent.

Effective Dose Equivalent

When a human is exposed to radiation from outside of the body, the resulting dose equivalent is typically associated with the whole body. When radioactivity is absorbed into the body, however, the dose equivalent is limited to one or more organs. It is not possible to compare these dose equivalents directly because of the different parts of the body exposed.

To combine these dose equivalents, the USNRC has adopted a series of weighting factors for the different organs. These weighting factors convert the dose equivalent received by an organ into a comparable dose equivalent to the whole body. This is an effective dose equivalent.

When adjusted to the comparable whole body dose, the internal exposure becomes a committed effective dose equivalent, which can be added to the external exposure that the body has received. When the external dose equivalent and the committed effective dose equivalent are combined, the total measure of the amount of radiation that has been absorbed can be determined. This measure is called the total effective dose equivalent.

Current occupational dose limits for adults may be found in 10 CFR 20.1201 and are shown in Table 26.21. The 50 rem limit to the skin is designed to prevent nonstochastic (i.e., direct) effects. Planned special exposures and emergency exposures are considered separately from the above limits. Radiation dose limits are not restricted simply to radiation workers. Limits for other situations also exist. For example, visitors and members of the public are allowed 0.1 rem (100 mrem) in a year from the sum of internal and external radiation sources.

A female radiological worker is encouraged to voluntarily notify her employer, in writing, when she is pregnant. The employer must provide the option of a mutually agreeable assignment of work tasks — with no loss of pay or promotional opportunity — such that further occupational radiation exposure is unlikely. For a declared pregnant worker who chooses to continue working as a radiological worker, the dose limit for the embryo/fetus (during the entire gestation period) is 500 mrem. Measures shall be taken to avoid substantial variation above the uniform exposure rate necessary to meet the 500 mrem limit for the gestation period. Efforts should be made to avoid exceeding 0.05 rem/month (50 mrem/month) to the declared pregnant worker.

If the dose to the embryo/fetus is determined to have already exceeded 0.5 rem (500 mrem) when a worker notifies her employer of her pregnancy, the worker shall not be assigned to tasks where additional occupational radiation exposure is likely during the remainder of the pregnancy.

The USNRC recommends that licensees use implementing procedures in order to satisfy the requirements of 10 CFR 20. Women should report in writing any suspected pregnancy as soon as possible to the appropriate department and their immediate supervisor, although this is not mandatory. A workplace evaluation should be conducted by the appropriate department once the pregnancy is declared. Declared pregnant females will be removed from work areas where the dose equivalent could exceed 0.5 rem (500 mrem) for the entire pregnancy. Declared pregnant females should be informed of the risks from radiation exposure to the unborn child through consultations with radiation safety personnel. Monthly control goals should be established so that the limiting value will not be exceeded. An upper value of 50 mrem/month, for example, (equivalent to approximately 0.25 mrem/hr) is an acceptable goal. Declared pregnant females are encouraged to report any changes in work duties or workplace assignments to the appropriate department/individuals to determine if additional workplace evaluations are necessary. Declared pregnant females should be allowed to withdraw their declaration of pregnancy at any time, thus terminating any work restrictions, but she must do so in writing. It is the licensee's legal responsibility to remove such restrictions. All aspects of the withdrawal of the declaration of pregnancy must be maintained as confidential and private.

Table 26.21 — Occupational dose limits

Description Limit	*Annual Limit*
Total Effective Dose Equivalent (TEDE)	5 rem (.05 Sv)
Deep Dose Equivalent and Committed Dose Equivalent (Summation)	50 rem (0.5 Sv)
Eye Dose Equivalent	15 rem (0.15 Sv)
Shallow Dose Equivalent to the Skin or Extremities	50 rem (0.5 Sv)

Notes

The 50 rem limit to the skin is designed to prevent nonstochastic effects. Planned special exposures and emergency exposures are considered separately from the above limits.

Radiation dose limits are not restricted simply to radiation workers. Limits for other situations also exist. For example, visitors and members of the public are allowed 0.1 rem (100 mrem) in a year from the sum of internal and external radiation sources.

Extremity means hand, elbow, arm below the elbow, foot, knee, or leg below the knee. Monitoring badges must include the whole body. Higher limits such as a finger dose require separate monitoring.

Source: U.S. Nuclear Regulatory Commission, Title 10 Code of Federal Regulations Part 20.1201

Licensing

The USNRC recognizes that effective radiation safety program management is vital to achieving safe and compliant operations.[72] USNRC also believes that consistent compliance with its regulations provides reasonable assurance that licensed activities will be conducted safely. USNRC also believes that effective management will result in increased safety and compliance. "Management" refers to the processes for conduct and control of a radiation safety program and to the individuals who are responsible for those processes and who have authority to provide necessary resources to achieve regulatory compliance. To ensure adequate management involvement, a duly authorized management representative must sign the submitted application acknowledging management's commitments and responsibility for the radiation safety, security and control of radioactive materials, and compliance with regulations; completeness and accuracy of the radiation safety records and all information provided to USNRC (10 CFR 30.9); knowledge about the contents of the license and application; and compliance with current USNRC and Department of Transportation (DOT) regulations and the licensee's operating and emergency procedures. The licensee must provide a commitment to provide adequate resources (including space, equipment, personnel, time, and, if needed, contractors) to the radiation protection program to ensure that public and workers are protected from radiation hazards and meticulous compliance with regulations is maintained. Management must select and assign a qualified individual to serve as the Radiation Safety Officer (RSO) for their licensed activities and prohibit discrimination of employees engaged in protected activities.[73] The licensee must obtain the USNRC's prior written consent before transferring control of the license and notify the appropriate USNRC regional administrator in writing, immediately following filing of petition for voluntary or involuntary bankruptcy.

Licensees should develop written procedures for use of different unsealed radionuclides so that users know the types of shielding, protective clothing, survey instruments, surveys, and decontamination activities that are required.[63] Examples of such procedures are included below.

Example 1:

If using more than 37 MBq (1 mCi) of iodine-123 or iodine-131, special safety instructions should be provided to users, including provisions for the following: A mandatory radiation survey and wipe test for radioactive contamination after each use, Bioassay procedures for individuals working with mCi quantities of radioiodine, The use of vented hoods for iodination and for the storage of mCi quantities of radioiodine, A dry run prior to the performance of unfamiliar procedures, in order to preclude unexpected complications. In addition, it is recommended that the RSO be present during new procedures and those for measuring the concentration of radioiodine effluents from the hoods.

Example 2:

If using more than 37 MBq (1 mCi) of fluorine-18, special safety instructions should be provided to users, including provisions for the following: The use of high-density materials (e.g., lead, tungsten) in order to keep radiation exposure to a minimum, A daily radiation survey and wipe test for radioactive contamination should be performed, The use of extremity monitors for procedures that involve one mCi or more, and A dry run prior to the performance of unfamiliar procedures in order to preclude unexpected complications. In addition, it is recommended that the RSO be present during new procedures.

When using a sealed radioactive source, the licensee must provide the source manufacturer's or distributor's name and model number for each requested sealed source and device. Licensees are authorized to possess and use only those sealed sources and devices specifically approved or registered by USNRC or an Agreement State.

The USNRC or an Agreement State performs a safety evaluation of fixed gauges before authorizing a manufacturer or distributor to distribute the gauges to specific licensees. The safety evaluation is documented in a Sealed Source and Device (SSD) Registration Certificate. The license should consult with the proposed source manufacturer or distributor to verify that requested sources and devices are compatible and conform to the sealed source and device designations registered with USNRC or an Agreement State. Licensees may not make any changes to the sealed source, device, or source/device combination that would alter the description or specifications from those indicated in the respective registration certificates, without obtaining USNRC's prior permission in a license amendment. Such changes may necessitate a custom registration review, increasing the time needed to process a licensing action. SSD Registration Certificates contain sections on "Conditions of Normal Use" and "Limitation and Other Considerations of Use." These sections may include limitations derived from conditions imposed by the manufacturer or distributor, by particular conditions of use that would reduce radiation safety of the device, or by circumstances unique to the sealed source or device. For example, working life of the device or appropriate temperature and other environmental conditions may be specified. Except as specifically approved by the USNRC, licensees are required to use gauges according to their respective SSD Registration Certificates. Accordingly, applicants may want to obtain a copy of the certificate and review it with the manufacturer or distributor or with NRC or the issuing Agreement State to ensure that it correctly reflects the radiation safety properties of the source or device.

There are many different uses of radioactive materials and accordingly there are a variety of licenses and associated conditions that may be employed by the licensee. The USNRC has provided detailed guidance about the minimum requirements for each type of license, entitled NUREG 1556. More than 20 volumes have been published to date which provide the requirements for licensing and model procedures that are considered to be acceptable to the USNRC. Agreement States have adopted many of the procedures and guidance documents related to licensing and applicable radiation safety programs.

ALARA

As described in previous sections of this chapter, a basic radiation protection concept or philosophy in current radiation protection programs is to maintain employee exposure to radiation to ALARA.(74) Being consistent with the purpose for which the licensed activity is undertaken, taking into account the state of technology, the cost of improvements in relation to state of technology, the cost of improvements in relation to benefits to the public health and safety, and other societal and socioeconomic considerations. These means are in relation to utilization of nuclear energy and licensed materials in the public interest.[5]

The element of ALARA is considered to be the continuation of good radiation protection programs and practices. This approach has been effective in keeping the average and individual exposures for monitored workers well below the limits.(75) The application of ALARA clearly includes the specification that economic and social factors be considered. Thus, the application of ALARA will inherently be different, not necessarily standardized across different sources or facilities. The application of ALARA is founded in the professional judgment of radiation-safety managers and personnel and is not, therefore, able to be used as a measure as to whether or not a particular radiation-safety program is adequate in comparison with other programs. Additionally, the ALARA concept does not provide a numerical limit below which the ALARA concept is achieved.

Reducing radiation exposures to levels that are "as low as reasonably achievable" has long been a goal of radiation safety programs.(76) The concern over possible genetic effects (effects that can be passed from adults to their children) in the 1960s led the Atomic Energy Commission (AEC), the predecessor to the Nuclear Regulatory Commission (USNRC) and the Department of Energy (DOE), — two federal regulatory authorities in the U.S. — to require that human exposures be kept "as low as practicable" (the "ALAP" philosophy). Additional emphasis on the ALARA philosophy heightened in the 1970s when scientists studying Japanese survivors of the atomic bomb blasts noticed an increased incidence of solid tumors (i.e., tumors other than leukemia). Similar increases were also observed in patients undergoing medical treatments. These increases were associated with very large radiation doses and high dose rates. Unfortunately, the scientists were not able to evaluate whether the same

[5] HPS definition of ALARA: http://www.hps.org/publicinformation/radterms/radfact1.html

results occur at small doses. However, ALARA is not a dose limit, but rather a goal. It exemplifies a mind set to achieve radiation exposures which are as far below the applicable limits as is reasonably achievable.

There are three guiding principles that must govern all work activities with the potential for exposure to radiation or radioactive materials in order to implement an effective ALARA program. Specifically, no activity or operation will be conducted unless its performance will produce a net positive benefit; all radiation exposures will be kept ALARA considering economic and societal costs; and no individual will receive radiation doses in excess of the federal limits.

ALARA principles can be utilized in an infinite number of situations. For example, the proper design of a nuclear facility may be modified depending on ALARA considerations. The cost of additional shielding may be justified for an area routinely occupied by members of the public and the corresponding decrease in potential exposure.[77] In addition, designing an X-ray facility for medical applications requires consideration of the amount of shielding needed to ensure that individuals located near the facility (e.g., on the other side of the wall from the x-ray unit) do not receive any more dose than is really necessary during operation of the x-ray device. It is important reasonable to place emphasis on the physical design features at a nuclear facility rather than on administrative controls such as procedures, or personal practices. The design of a nuclear facility is important in the eventual success of an effective ALARA program. If designed satisfactorily, worker doses and releases of radioactivity to the environment can not only be controlled but reduced substantially. An improperly designed facility, on the other hand, may require subsequent modifications, often at considerable expense to reach the desired dose rates and with a corresponding impact on existing operations.

A successful ALARA program requires an appreciation, understanding, and acceptance from each individual involved in work with radioactivity and radiation-producing machines. More specifically, an ALARA program must have some (preferably all) of the following: a strong commitment from facility management at all levels and throughout the entire organization, dedicated staff, an ALARA program manual or approved program procedures, education and training programs, a well-defined ALARA organization with established responsibilities, a Radiological Safety Committee which reports to upper management on ALARA issues, and routine internal and external audits of the effectiveness of the dose reduction program. Each person involved in radiological work is expected to demonstrate responsibility and accountability through an informed, disciplined and cautious attitude toward radiation and radioactivity. Each radiological worker is responsible for maintaining his or her own exposure to radiation or radioactive material ALARA. In addition, each worker should promptly identify any radiological control deficiencies and concerns and be involved in their resolution. Maintaining a good work environment by establishing excellent housekeeping and cleaning up after the task has been concluded is essential. Finally, each worker should understand that proper radiological control is an integral part of their daily duties and that they are held accountable for their radiological control performance.

Implementing the ALARA concept involves six general categories. These are: 1) eliminating or reducing the source of radiation; 2) containing the source; 3) minimizing the time spent in a radiation field; 4) maximizing the distance from a radiation source; 5) using radiation shielding; and 6) using optimization analyses.[77] Eliminating the source of radiation can be accomplished by substituting other appropriate technologies or materials. For example, using an ultrasound exam (sonogram) in prenatal examinations, rather than an X-ray exam, is a much preferred practice because of the type of radiation received by the fetus. The control of contamination on building surfaces, equipment, etc. is an important ALARA consideration in source reduction. Removing/reducing the source of contamination will in turn eliminate (or at least reduce) the likelihood of worker contamination and dose. Radioactivity be controlled and contained is a subset of the first source reduction principle and involves containment, ventilation, and filtration. Containment involves using leak-tight or controlled-opening enclosures to prevent radioactive materials from migrating to other areas. Containment may be used temporarily and then removed after the job is complete, or be a permanent component (as, for example, from a structural standpoint). See the section related to contamination control. Proper ventilation is the flow of air and other gases in a certain direction and rate such that radioactive airborne particles and gases are captured and directed to collection filters, followed by release to the atmosphere once appropriate release limits have been met. A well-designed ventilation system will limit the potential for intakes of radioactive material. For example, designing the flow of air containing small amounts of radioactive materials away from people will help to ensure unnecessary exposure. To meet ALARA objectives in a radiation protection program, it may be necessary to use some or all of the following items: ventilated fume hoods, glove boxes (used to handle radioactive materials), exhaust systems, water filtration and processing systems, ventilation cleanup systems, and double-walled pipes and tanks, leak-tight valves, etc.

Minimizing time spent in a radiation field can be considered the third principle. Simply put, the less time spent in a radiation field, the lower the dose. To meet ALARA goals, no more time should be spent in a radiation field than is necessary to perform the required tasks. There are several design factors which can be utilized in a nuclear facility to promote this principle. For example, personnel who have to work in the vicinity of radioactive sources often conduct rehearsals in low dose areas to ensure that they keep their time in the area to a minimum and that they have all the tools they need, etc.

In the case of distance, the farther away from a radiation source, the lower the dose. This is especially true for "point" sources of radiation which follow the inverse-square law. As with time, several design factors are available to aid in maximizing the distance from radioactive sources. Shielding a radiation source involves the use of different materials placed between the worker and the source to absorb the radiation. The choice of shielding depends on the type of radiation and may either be temporary or permanent. As with time and distance, several design factors are available to reduce worker dose.

Finally, optimization requires that cost-benefit analyses are performed to balance economic considerations with the expected benefits. Optimization is used to demonstrate that any expenses involved — in terms of money, time spent by personnel, dose received, etc. — are justified in terms of the benefit received.[60,77] Thus, reducing radiation exposures can be weighed against competing conflicts (technical considerations, social, operational, and economic).

Working in an area containing radiation and/or radioactive materials requires pre-job planning (the extent of which depends on the complexity of the job), implementation of pre-established ALARA controls and tracking of worker doses, and a post-job review to evaluate the "lessons learned". These steps allow the application of ALARA principles before the job is started, ensure that the principles are being applied correctly, and assist in improving performance on future jobs.

Summary

Human exposure to ionizing radiation is part of the natural coexistence with the planet. Background radiation includes exposure from long-lived radioactive nuclides in the earth, water, and air. With the advent of modern medicine, exposure from dental and medical X-rays, nuclear medicine studies, and radiation therapy add to the accumulated exposure for both the patient and the occupational worker. Industrial and consumer products add to the body burden. Radiation limitation levels are set for the occupational worker, with more limited measures taken for the general public reduced by a factor of 10 or more. The accumulated knowledge of the biological effects of radiation, the collection of which spans more than a century, is reviewed by government agencies and is eventually translated into radiation protection for the worker and the general public.

References

1. **Health Physics Society:** *A Guide to SI Units in Radiation Protection, Operational Radiation Safety.* Volume 80, No.5. McLean, VA: Health Physics Society, May, 2001.
2. **International Commission on Radiation Units and Measurements (ICRU):** *Quantities and Units in Radiation Protection Dosimetry.* Report 51. Bethesda, MD: ICRU, 1993.

3. **U.S. Nuclear Regulatory Commission:** Commission's Policy on Conversion to Metric System, Volume 57. Federal Register, page 46202. October 7, 1992.
4. **Turner, J. E.:** *Atoms, Radiation, and Radiation Protection*, 2nd edition. New York: Wiley, 1995.
5. **Shapiro, J.:** *Radiation Protection: A Guide For Scientists and Physicians,* 4th edition. Cambridge, MA: Harvard University Press, 2002.
6. **Thompson, M.A., et al.:** *Principles of Imaging Science and Protection*. Philadelphia, PA: Saunders, 1994.
7. **Cember, H.:** *Introduction to Health Physics,* 3rd edition. New York: McGraw-Hill, Health Professions Division, 1996.
8. **Lapp, R. and H. Andrews:** *Nuclear Radiation Physics,* 4th edition, Upper Saddle River, NJ: Prentice-Hall, 1972.
9. **Chandra, R.:** *Nuclear Medicine Physics: The Basics*, 5th edition. Baltimore, MD: Williams & Wilkins, 1998.
10. **Bergonie, J. and L. Tribondeau:** De quelques resultats de la Radiotherapie, et esaie de fixation d'une technique rationelle, Comptes Rendu des Seances de l'Academie des Sciences. Volume 143. Comptes-Rendus des Séances de l'Académie des Sciences, 1906. pp. 983–985.
11. **Bergonie, J. and L. Tribondeau:** Interpretation of some results of radiotherapy and an attempt at determining a logical technique of treatment. *Radiat. Res. 11*:587 (1959).
12. **National Academy of Sciences:** *Health Effects of Exposure to Low Levels of Ionizing Radiation.* Biological Effects of Ionizing Radiation Report V, BEIR V. Washington, D.C.: National Academy Press, 1990.
13. **U.S. Department of Health and Human Services, Public Health Service (PHS):** Seventh Annual Report on Carcinogens. Summary 1994. Research Triangle Park, NC: PHS, 1994.
14. **International Commission on Radiological Protection:** Report of the Task Group on Reference Man. Report 23. Ottawa, Ontario: ICRP, 1975.
15. **U.S. Nuclear Regulatory Commission:** Instruction Concerning Risks from Occupational Radiation Exposure. Regulatory Guide 8.29, Revision 1. Rockville, MD: U.S. Nuclear Regulatory Commission, February 1996.
16. **International Commission on Radiological Protection:** Annuals of the ICRP, Risks Associated with Ionising Radiation, Volume 22, Number 1. Oxford, U.K.: Pergammon Press, 1991.
17. **Health Physics Society:** *Ionizing Radiation — Safety Standards for the General Public,* Position Statement PS-005. McLean, VA: Health Physics Society. September, 1992, reaffirmed February, 2009.
18. **International Commission on Radiological Protection (ICRP):** *Nonstochastic Effects of Ionizing Radiation.* (ICRP pub. 41). Oxford, U.K.: Pergamon Press, 1984.
19. **Health Physics Society:** *Radiation Risk in Perspective,* Position Statement PS-010-1. McLean, VA: Health Physics Society, August, 2004.
20. **National Academy of Sciences:** *Health Effects of Exposure to Radon, Biological Effects of Ionizing Radiation.* Report VI, BEIR VI. Washington, D.C.: National Academy Press, 1999.
21. **National Council of Radiation Protection and Measurements:** *Ionizing Radiation Exposure of the Population of the United States.* Bethesda, MD: NCRP, 1987.
22. **National Council of Radiation Protection and Measurements:** *Ionizing Radiation Exposure of the Population of the United States.* Bethesda, MD: NCRP, 2009.
23. **U.S. Environmental Protection Agency, Office of Radiation Programs (EPA):** Risk Assessments Methodology. Environmental Impact Statement. NESHAPS for Radionuclides. Background Information Document, vol. 2 (EPA 520/1-89-006-2). Washington, DC: EPA, 1989.
24. **United Nations Scientific Committee on the Effect of Atomic Radiation:** *Sources and Effects of Ionizing Radiation,* Volume I. New York: United Nations, 2000.
25. **National Commission on Radiation Protection:** *Use of Bioassay Procedures for Assessment of Internal Radionuclide Deposition.* NCRP Report No. 87. Bethesda, MD: National Commission on Radiation Protection and Measurements, 1987.
26. **National Council on Radiation Protection and Measurements:** *Exposure of the U.S. Population from Natural Background Radiation.* NCRP Report No. 94. Bethesda, MD: National Council on Radiation Protection and Measurements, 1987.
27. **National Council on Radiation Protection and Measurements:** *Radiation Exposure of the U.S. Population from Consumer Products and Miscellaneous Sources.* NCRP Report No. 95. Bethesda, MD: National Council on Radiation Protection and Measurements, 1987.
28. **National Council on Radiation Protection and Measurements:** *Exposures from the Uranium Series with Emphasis on Radon and Its Daughters.* NCRP Report No. 77. Bethesda, MD: NCRP, 1984.

29. **U.S. Environmental Protection Agency, Office of Radiation Programs (EPA):** *Radon Reference Manual* (EPA 520/1-87-20). Washington, DC: EPA, 1987.
30. **U.S. Nuclear Regulatory Commission:** *Estimated Radiation Doses from Thorium and Daughters Contained in Thoriated Welding Electrodes.* NUREG/CR-1039. Rockville, MD: U.S. Nuclear Regulatory Commission, December, 1979.
31. **National Council on Radiation Protection and Measurements:** *Public Radiation Exposure from Nuclear Power Generation in the United States.* NCRP Report 92. Bethesda, MD: National Council on Radiation Protection and Measurements, 1987.
32. **U.S. Environmental Protection Agency, Office of Radiation Programs (EPA):** *Indoor Radon and Radon Decay Product Measurement Protocols.* (EPA 520/1-86-04). Washington, DC: EPA, 1989.
33. **U.S. Environmental Protection Agency (EPA):** *Protocols for Radon and Radon Decay Product Measurements in Homes.* (EPA 402-R-92-003). Washington, DC: EPA, 1992.
34. **United Nations Scientific Committee on the Effect of Atomic Radiation. Sources:** *Effects and Risks of Ionizing Radiation.* New York: United Nations, 1993.
35. **National Academy of Sciences:** *Health Effects of Radon and Other Internally Deposited Alpha-Emitters, Biological Effects of Ionizing Radiation.* Report IV. National Academy Press, 1988.
36. **U.S. Environmental Protection Agency (EPA):** EPA Map of Radon Zones. http://www.epa.gov/radon/zonemap.html, [Accessed on July 29, 2011].
37. **American Association of Physicists in Medicine:** *The Measurement, Reporting and Management of Radiation Dose in CT.* Report of AAPM Task Force 23. Report Number 96. College Park, MD: AAPM, January, 2008.
38. **National Council on Radiation Protection and Measurements:** *Ionizing Radiation Exposure of the Population of the United States.* Report 160. Bethesda, MD: National Council on Radiation Protection and Measurements, 2006.
39. **U.S. Nuclear Regulatory Commission:** The Regulation and Use of Radioisotopes in Today's World. NUREG/BR-0217, Revision 1. Rockville, MD: U.S. Nuclear Regulatory Commission, April, 2000.
40. **U.S. Food and Drug Administration (FDA):** *Performance Standards for Ionizing Radiation Emitting Products.* Title 21, Code of Federal Regulations, Part 1020. Silver Spring, MD: FDA, 2010.
41. **Gollnick, D.A.:** *Basic Radiation Protection Philosophy,* 2nd edition. Altadena, CA: Pacific Radiation Corporation, 1988.
42. **Chemical Rubber Company:** *Handbook or Radioactive Nuclides.* Wang, Y. (ed.). Boca Raton, FL: Chemical Rubber Co., 1969.
43. **U.S. Nuclear Regulatory Commission:** *Minimum Detectable Concentrations with Typical Radiation Survey Instruments for Various Contaminants and Field Conditions.* NURG 1507. Rockville, MD: U.S. Nuclear Regulatory Commission, June 1998.
44. 10 CFR Part 20.1502. *Conditions Requiring Individual Monitoring of External and Internal Occupational Dose.* Rockville, MD: U.S. Nuclear Regulatory Commission, 1998.
45. 10 CFR Part 835. *Occupational Radiation Protection.* Washington, D.C.: U.S. Department of Energy, 1993.
46. **National Council on Radiation Protection and Measurements:** *Recommendations on Limits for Exposure to Ionizing Radiation.* NCRP 91. Bethesda, MD: National Council on Radiation Protection and Measurements, 1987.
47. **U.S. Environmental Protection Agency (EPA):** *Radiation Protection Guidance to Federal Agency for Occupational Exposure.* Volume 52, Federal Register. January 27, 1987. p. 2822.
48. **U.S. Department of Energy (DOE):** U.S. *Department of Energy Radiological Control Manual.* DOE/EH-0256T (Revision 1). Washington, D.C.: U.S. Department of Energy, April, 1994.
49. **Toohey, R.E., et al.:** Current Status of Whole Body Counting as a Means to Detect and Quantify Previous Exposures to Radioactive Materials. *Health Physics 60(Sup. 1)*:7–42 (1991).
50. **U.S. Nuclear Regulatory Commission:** Program-Specific Guidance about Industrial Radiography Licenses. NUREG-1556, Volume 2. Rockville, MD: U.S. Nuclear Regulatory Commission, August, 1998.
51. Code of Federal Regulations, Title 10, Part 34, Licenses for Industrial Radiography And Radiation Safety Requirements For Industrial Radiographic Operations.
52. **U.S. Nuclear Regulatory Commission:** Monitoring Criteria and Methods to Calculate Occupational Radiation Doses. Regulatory Guide 8.34. Rockville, MD: U.S. Nuclear Regulatory Commission, July, 1992.
53. **National Institute of Standards and Technology (NIST):** *National Voluntary Laboratory Accreditation Program, Procedures and General Requirements.* NIST Handbook 150. Gaithersburg, MD: NIST, 2006.

54. **U.S. Environmental Protection Agency, Office of Radiation Programs (EPA):** *Indoor Radon and Radon Decay Product Measurement Protocols.* (EPA 520/1-86-04). Washington, D.C.: EPA, 1989.
55. **American National Standards Institute (ANSI):** *Performance Criteria for Radiobioassay.* Report No. ANSI-N13.30. New York: ANSI, 1987.
56. **National Commission on Radiation Protection and Measurements:** Use of Bioassay Procedures for Assessment of Internal Radionuclide Deposition. , NCRP Report No. 87. Bethesda, MD: National Commission on Radiation Protection and Measurements, 1987.
57. Code of Federal Regulations. Title 10, Part 20.1502. Conditions requiring individual monitoring of external and internal occupational dose.
58. **U.S. Nuclear Regulatory Commission:** *Air Sampling in the Workplace.* NUREG 1400. Rockville, MD: U.S. Nuclear Regulatory Commission, September 1993.
59. **National Council on Radiation Protection and Measurements:** Limit for Exposure to "Hot Particles" on the Skin. NCRP 106. Bethesda, MD: National Council on Radiation Protection and Measurements, 1989.
60. **Pacific Northwest Laboratory:** Health Physics Manual of Good Practices for Reducing Radiation Exposure to Levels that are As Low As Reasonably Achievable. PNL-6577. Prepared for the U.S. Department of Energy, June 1988.
61. Code of Federal Regulations. Title 10, Code of Federal Regulations, Part 20, Section 1101, Radiation protection programs. U.S. Nuclear Regulatory Commission.
62. **National Council on Radiation Protection and Measurements:** *Management of Persons Accidentally Contaminated with Radionuclides.* NCRP Report No. 65. Bethesda, MD: National Council on Radiation Protection and Measurements, 1980.
63. **U.S. Nuclear Regulatory Commission:** Program-Specific Guidance about Licenses of Broad Scope — Final Report. NUREG-1556, Volume 11, Appendix R. Rockville, MD: U.S. Nuclear Regulatory Commission, April, 1999.
64. **U.S. Nuclear Regulatory Commission:** The U.S. Nuclear Regulatory Commission and How It Works. NUREG 0256. Rockville, MD: U.S. Nuclear Regulatory Commission, August, 2000.
65. **U.S. Nuclear Regulatory Commission:** Citizen's Guide to U.S. Nuclear Regulatory Commission Information. (NUREG/BR-0010, Rev 3). Rockville, MD: U.S. Nuclear Regulatory Commission, 1998.
66. **U.S. Nuclear Regulatory Commission:** A Short History of Nuclear Regulation, 1946-1999. NUREG/BR-0175 Rev. 1. Rockville, MD: U.S. Nuclear Regulatory Commission, November, 2000.
67. **U.S. Nuclear Regulatory Commission:** The USNRC Agreement State Program. http://www.USNRC.gov/about-USNRC/state-tribal/agreement-states.html. [Accessed July 29, 2011.]
68. **U.S. Nuclear Regulatory Commission:** Information Digest 2008–2009. NUREG 1350, Volume 20. Rockville, MD: U.S. Nuclear Regulatory Commission, August, 2008.
69. **U.S. Nuclear Regulatory Commission:** *Consolidated Guidance about Materials Licenses.* NUREG 1556. Rockville, MD: U.S. Nuclear Regulatory Commission, May, 1997.
70. Code of Federal Regulations. Title 10, Part 20. Standards for Protection against Radiation. Rockville, MD: U.S. Nuclear Regulatory Commission.
71. **Medical Internal Radiation Dose Committee (MIRD):** *Primer for Absorbed Dose Calculations,* rev. edition. Maryland Heights, MO: Mathews Medical Book Co., 1991.
72. **U.S. Nuclear Regulatory Commission:** Program-Specific Guidance about Fixed Gauge Licenses. NUREG 1556, Volume 4. Rockville, MD: U.S. Nuclear Regulatory Commission, October, 1998.
73. Title 10, Code of Federal Regulations, Part 30.7,
74. **U. S. Nuclear Regulatory Commission:** *Operating Philosophy for Maintaining Occupational Radiation Exposures As Low As Is Reasonably Achievable.* Regulatory Guide 8.10. Rockville, MD: U.S. Nuclear Regulatory Commission, 1977.
75. **National Council on Radiation Protection and Measurements:** *Limitations of Exposure to Ionizing Radiation.* NCRP Report No. 116. Bethesda, MD: National Council on Radiation Protection and Measurements, 1993.
76. **International Commission on Radiological Protection:** *Implications of Commission Recommendations that Doses be Kept as Low As Reasonably Achievable.* ICRP 22. New York: Pergamon Press, 1973.
77. **International Commission on Radiological Protection:** *Cost Benefit Analysis in the Optimization of Radiation Protection.* ICRP 37. New York: Pergamon Press, 1982.

Outcome Competencies

After completing this chapter, the reader should be able to:

1. Define underlined terms used in this chapter.
2. Evaluate the role of major physiological systems relating to heat strain.
3. Evaluate thermal injuries and prescribe first aid treatment.
4. Evaluate the role of cold in cumulative trauma disorders.
5. Evaluate environments that may precipitate heat/cold stress problems.
6. Analyze heat/cold stress problems to identify the most effective and practical solutions.
7. Describe administrative, engineering, and job controls for protecting against heat/cold stress.
8. Develop appropriate mechanisms to identify heat/cold problems arising from new work situations.
9. Develop appropriate mechanisms to prevent new heat/cold problems.
10. Describe the major physiological systems that respond to heat and cold stress.
11. Evaluate the worker qualitatively with respect to potential heat/cold strain problems.

Key Terms

acclimatization • air temperature • conduction • convection • dry bulb temperature • electrolytes • evaporation • frostbite • heat strain • heat stress • heat stroke • hyponatremia • hypothermia • hypotonic • metabolic heat • microenvironment • radiation • relative humidity • shock • thermal balance • water intoxication

Prerequisite Knowledge

Basic biology, basic chemistry, and basic physics.

Key Topics

I. Worker Responses in Hot and Cold Environments
  A. Introduction
  B. Personal Protective Clothing & Equipment
  C. Thermal Strain Disorders
  D. Heat Stroke
  E. First Aid for Heat Stroke
  F. Heat Exhaustion and Cramps
  G. Heat Syncope, Heat Rash and Other Problems
  H. Cold Strain Disorders
  I. Heat and Cold Injuries

II. Mechanisms of Thermal Exchange
  A. Heat Production
  B. Evaporation
  C. Convection
  D. Radiation

III. Environmental and Microenvironmental Strain
  A. Hypothalmic Regulation of Temperature and Cerebral Blood Flow
  B. Stress from the Microenvironment
  C. Assessing Environmental and Microenvironmental Strain
  D. Measuring Deep Body Temperature of Workers

IV. Factors Affecting Thermal Strain
  A. Controllable Factors Affecting Strain
  B. Uncontrollable Factors Affecting Strain

V. Controlling Thermal Exposure
  A. Administrative Controls
  B. Engineering Controls
  C. Environmental Controls
  D. Microenvironmental Control
  E. Microclimate Cooling

VI. Prediction of Thermal Work Tolerance
  A. Generalized Prediction of Thermal Tolerance
  B. Individualized Prediction of Thermal Tolerance

VII. Summary

Applied Physiology of Thermoregulation and Exposure Control

27

By Michael D. Larrañaga, PhD, CIH, CSP, PE

Worker Responses in Hot and Cold Environments

Introduction

The purpose of this chapter is to provide the necessary background information to permit evaluation of the thermal characteristics of the working environment, determine the need for intervention, and devise appropriate, practical intervention methods. Hot and cold environments are thermal stressors, and workers experience a physiological stress as a result. It would be impossible to anticipate every possible situation that could arise and every potential solution that could be implemented. Therefore, the approach of this chapter is to elucidate the basic principles necessary to enable industrial hygienists to solve the specific problems in their workplaces.

For example, an industrial hygienist might be called on to participate in the planning of a new industrial facility, a new expansion of production or space, or a new process. Anticipating potential worker heat stress (external stress from hot conditions) in the planning phase can improve safety and permit relatively low-cost improvements in environmental control systems that may preclude later health and productivity problems. In another scenario, the hygienist may need to plan for fieldwork involving encapsulating protective clothing. The biophysics of the microenvironment, that space between the skin and the outer clothing, may greatly affect manpower needs or work-hour requirements. Understanding the microenvironment may save your company money and, more importantly, may prevent an injury or death. A hygienist also may be called upon to help with an emergency in extremely hot or cold conditions. A basic knowledge of the biophysics of the thermal environment and how to minimize the dangers to workers while maximizing productivity is essential in all of these situations. Similarly, knowledge of the advantages and disadvantages of different thermal remediation techniques may lead to more rapid and efficient solutions.

Essentially, hot and cold environments may reduce both safety and productivity. Besides the obvious dangers from frostbite or heatstroke, even a milder thermal strain can be problematic. Environments do not have to be life threatening to cause problems. A cold environment, for example, may increase the risk of cumulative trauma disorders.[1,2]

Worker performance deteriorates during cold stress before physiological limits have been reached.[3] Even if the deep body is warm, hand dexterity begins to decrease when skin temperatures fall to 15–20°C (59–68°F)[3–5], and muscle strength declines when muscle temperature falls below 28°C (82°F).[6] Likewise, a warm environment can compromise the concentration, steadiness, or vigilance of workers.[7] Even moderately warm environments may require interruption of work with extensive rest breaks, especially when protective clothing is worn.

Across most of the United States, and in many other places in the world, the outdoor environment can pose problems for workers. For example, the average wet-bulb globe temperature (WBGT) in July for much of North and South America, Europe, and Asia, is above 29°C (84°F).[8] Even cooler temperatures can cause problems for workers. In the

U.S., for example, the first moderately warm days of spring tend to result in more heat-stress medical emergencies than the hotter days of summer, because of the lack of heat acclimatization. Likewise, cold exposure problems can be a serious threat to utility employees responding to an ice storm even if temperatures are not extremely cold.

Some potential hot work areas are easily anticipated, such as foundry operations. Many occupational and protective clothing environments result in WBGTs as high as 43°C (109°F).[9] The heat stress is less obvious in other occupations and becomes apparent only through experience. For example, heating and air conditioning contractors working in the attic of a residence can encounter dry bulb temperatures higher than 49°C (120°F), even when the weather is moderate. The situation is more complex when a worker must greatly vary his or her work rate while wearing semi-permeable chemical protective clothing. During the periods of heavy work in cold environments, the worker may become overheated; yet during periods of very light work, the wetness accruing from previous sweating can result in hypothermia.

Personal Protective Clothing and Equipment

Protective clothing and equipment of all types may compound thermal problems for workers. Welders, for example, may suffer from the heat in warm environments and from the cold in cool environments because their protective clothing retains heat in the summer, but the design of welding masks and gloves hampers adding adequate insulation in winter. Chemical protective clothing can create a microenvironment under the clothing that may be uncomfortably warm or hot during work, even when ambient temperatures are comfortable.

Thermal Strain Disorders

Human deep-body temperature is maintained within a few degrees of 37°C (98.6°F). Extreme variations from this deep body temperature can adversely affect important chemical reactions and the structure and function of proteins. The most common thermo-physiological threats to worker safety and productivity in industry are heat stress disorders. Heat stress disorders range from simple heat syncope (fainting) to life-threatening heatstroke. These disorders are interrelated and seldom occur as discrete entities. Of these, the most serious risk is heatstroke. If heatstroke continues unchecked, it will result in blood clots, tissue death, cerebral (brain) damage, general central nervous system dysfunction, and finally death.[10] Death from heat strain (the body's response to heat stress) occurs when deep body temperature approaches 43°C (109°F). Likewise, hypothermia, or low deep body temperature, can be dangerous. If the body temperature begins to drop, shivering will commence at 34°C (93°F), at 26.5°C (80°F) workers can become unresponsive, and death due to cold occurs rapidly at a rectal temperature of about 25°C (77°F).

Heat Stroke

Unacclimatized workers exposed to moderately warm temperatures or acclimatized workers exposed to hot temperatures should be continuously monitored to detect signs of potential heat injury. Typically, workers in the early stages of heatstroke evidence hot, dry skin; however, in exertional heatstroke, the skin can also be wet. The skin is typically red but may be mottled or pale blue-gray (indicating very low oxygen delivery), and deep body temperature will be very high.[11] The victim may evidence mental confusion or lose consciousness. Confusion is a key symptom. Breathing may be faster and deeper than normal. All workers who may be exposed to heat stress, or who supervise others exposed to heat stress, should be reminded periodically of these symptoms and first aid procedures. Heat stroke is a life-threatening medical emergency, and trained medical help should be summoned immediately, even if the diagnosis is uncertain.

First Aid for Heat Stroke

While waiting for medical help or while transporting potential heatstroke victims, first aid should be initiated. For all heat injuries, remove the victim from the heat source. Stricken workers should be cooled as rapidly as possible, as danger increases the longer cooling is delayed. Cooling is best accomplished by maximizing airflow across the body by fanning, removing clothing, and cooling by whatever additional means are available. Supplement this by applying the coldest water available including whole-body ice or cold-water immersion. The American Red Cross recommends the use of ice packs on the victim's wrists, ankles, groin, each armpit, and the neck. In either case, cooling must be stopped once the victim's temperature is lowered to about 39°C (102°F) to prevent hypothermia. Conscious victims can be given half a glass (4 ounces) of water every 15 minutes (drinking too fast can cause vomiting).[12] Anyone giving first aid should observe universal precautions against blood borne pathogens (i.e., avoid direct contact with body fluids.

Victims of heat injury can go into shock, or circulatory collapse, which can be life-threatening itself. Rapid breathing and a rapid, irregular pulse characterize shock. It should be treated by placing the victim in a comfortable horizontal position. If shock is present, and there are no head, neck, or back injuries, elevate the feet[12] and continue cooling the person, but do everything possible to secure immediate medical treatment. Administration of intravenous fluids by qualified personnel is usually needed, and getting the victim to medical care should not be delayed even if the person regains consciousness. Death typically occurs when deep body temperature exceeds 43°C (109°F) and is a result of cardiovascular failure, although brain damage can occur earlier in the process.[13]

Heat Exhaustion and Cramps

Less dangerous but more common than heat stroke are heat exhaustion and heat cramps. Although these disorders do not put life at risk, they may be intermediate steps on the way to heatstroke. Workers who experience undue fatigue or muscle cramps while working in the heat are likely to be suffering from heat exhaustion and should be required to sit or lie down in a cooler environment. Heat exhaustion victims often have a headache and may feel nauseous as well. Their skin is usually pale, and they may feel faint. They should be kept well hydrated and observed closely. If sweating stops suddenly, or the worker loses consciousness or becomes disoriented, he or she should be treated as a heatstroke victim and medical help should be summoned immediately. If heat cramps persist, an intravenous infusion, and hence skilled medical care, will be required. Any worker who has experienced a previous heat injury is more susceptible to a subsequent injury and should be afforded more protection, such as reduced heat exposure, more frequent or longer rest periods, etc.[14]

Since it may be difficult to distinguish between heat exhaustion and heatstroke, it is wise to observe all heat exhaustion victims very closely. If they show any confusion, bizarre behavior, or loss of consciousness, they should be treated as heatstroke victims, and emergency medical assistance should be called immediately.

Heat Syncope, Heat Rash and Other Problems

Heat syncope presents as fainting while a person stands erect or immobile in the heat. The underlying physiological cause is pooling of the blood in dilated vessels of the skin and lower parts of the body. A predisposing factor is lack of acclimatization and treatment involves moving to a cooler area. Recovery is typically prompt and complete unless the person was injured during fainting. The onset of heat syncope can be prevented effectively with intermittent physical activity to assist venous return to the heart.[15]

The final common form of heat injury is heat-related rashes. Kerslake[16], in his classic text on heat strain, provides a detailed explanation of how sweat glands can become clogged. Sweat glands often become infected, causing discomfort that may reduce worker productivity. If large areas of skin become affected, sweat production can be compromised, reducing heat tolerance. Professional medical treatment will be required.

Other complications of work in hot situations include sweat in the eyes and dripping sweat, which may damage sensitive equipment and cause electrical hazards. In impermeable clothing, considerable quantities of sweat can collect in boots and gloves. Thermal stress can distract workers, reduce concentration, and lead to early fatigue, all of which are likely to reduce worker safety. Ramsey and Kwon[17] have reported deterioration of other performance variables during heat stress situations.

Cold Strain Disorders

Cold strain injuries are also potentially dangerous. The most dangerous cold threat is hypothermia (abnormally low deep body temperature), which fortunately is rare in industry. However, anyone who could be exposed to near-freezing temperatures for prolonged periods should be trained in the prevention and treatment of hypothermia. This could include workers such as highway maintenance personnel and search and rescue personnel (including volunteers) working in cold climates.

Extremely low temperatures can interfere with vital biochemical processes. The best data suggest that humans with deep body temperatures near 25°C (77°F) or lower would be expected to die. Symptoms of hypothermia include uncontrollable shivering and intense feelings of cold, falling blood pressure, and irregular heartbeat. Victims become incoherent and disoriented and may be very drowsy. Once hypothermia begins, the blood vessels near the skin may dilate, causing further heat loss[11], which may result in further reduction in deep body temperature and cause death even after a person is moved to a warmer environment. Any person who cannot be warmed at the first onset of hypothermia symptoms should receive medical treatment as soon as possible. First aid consists of warming the person as rapidly as possible and protecting against shock by keeping the feet elevated and the trunk warm. Care should be taken to gently warm hypothermia victims to prevent cardiovascular complications. Since circulatory and ventilatory function may be compromised in hypothermia, cardiopulmonary resuscitation may be needed. The victim's pulse and breathing should be checked periodically. Victims of hypothermia are in grave danger and in need of expert medical assistance.

Frostbite is more common than hypothermia. Frostbite is a result of freezing the extracellular fluid in the skin, which can permanently damage the tissue. It usually occurs on the extremities, such as the tips of the fingers, ears, and nose and manifests itself with initial pain at the afflicted site, which subsides as nerves are damaged. The tissue becomes white or grayish. Since the face is often less protected than other body parts, the victim may be unaware of the first signs of frostbite on the nose and ears because he or she cannot see the discoloration. Though not life-threatening, frostbite damage can be severe and permanent, so prompt medical attention is required.

Rapid heat transfer by conduction can occur if a body part comes in contact with a very cold object, even if the ambient air temperature is mild. Workers should be trained to avoid contact with cold metal or cryogenic fluids, and liquids of low vapor pressure such as alcohol or cleaning fluids, all of which can increase the possibility of frostbite.[3] Workers should try to avoid direct contact with metallic surfaces below 0°C (32°F).[5] Workers exposed to extreme cold or moderate cold with high wind (25 mph or greater), are in danger of frostbite and hypothermia. However, frostbite can occur in even warmer temperatures if workers are not properly clothed.[11]

Problems can arise before serious cold injury occurs. Cold exposure can reduce dexterity and strength.[3] For example, even if the deep body temperature is normal, dexterity begins to decline when hand skin temperature falls to 15–20°C (59–68°F), which is a very common temperature for work in cold environments.

Heat and Cold Injuries

Protecting against heat strain disorders is primarily a matter of anticipating problems and trying to prevent even mild disorders from developing. Gradually acclimatizing workers, keeping them well-hydrated (discussed in more detail later), and detecting symptoms early, are the most important defensive measures. Workers showing initial signs of any heat or cold disorder should be removed from exposure and given fluids for rehydration. It is especially important to note that the use of encapsulating protective clothing may hamper both the worker's temperature control and rehydration. It is difficult to evaluate problems when workers are entirely clad in coveralls, respiratory protective masks, and other equipment. For workers in hazardous environments, the need for respirator removal and decontamination before drinking may greatly hamper adequate hydration.

Self-monitoring is often difficult, hence it is imperative that both workers and work site supervisors appreciate the importance of the symptoms the worker may display.

Workers should be paired with others for work in hot or cold environments, with instructions to watch for signs of thermal strain in each other.[5] It is also important for workers and supervisors to realize that there is tremendous variability among workers in thermal tolerance; what one worker may find merely uncomfortable could result in a dangerous level of heat strain for other workers doing the same work in the same environment. Often it is the most industrious "get-the-job-done" employees who place themselves at greatest risk for heat or cold injury.

Mechanisms of Thermal Exchange

Workers' body temperatures are a function of the heat balance equation:

Metabolic heat production minus evaporative cooling ± heat gain or loss due to convection ± heat gain or loss due to conduction ± heat gain or loss due to radiation = ± heat stored or lost which determines body temperature. For a detailed description of the body's thermal balance equation, see Chapter 28 "Thermal Standards and Measurement Techniques". The industrial hygienist, at times, must adjust the factors in the equation to ensure that workers' body temperatures are maintained within the narrow limits that are required for the preservation of human health. The following sections provide qualitative descriptions of each of the factors of heat balance.

Heat Production

When the body uses food for energy, about 70–80% of the energy available is released as heat.[18] This heat energy always moves from hotter to cooler locations, and in a closed ideal system would achieve equilibrium, or uniform distribution of heat energy.

Muscles represent the largest single group of tissues in the body, typically accounting for about 45% of body weight. At rest, the muscles account for about 20 to 25% of the total metabolic heat production. The heat produced by the muscles during exercise or work can be many times higher than at rest, and most of the energy released in the body during work is released in the muscles and will manifest itself as heat. As heat is produced, muscle temperature rises, and heat transfer occurs from the muscle to the cooler blood. As body core temperature increases, there is an increase in skin blood flow. This raises skin temperature to facilitate losses (or reduced gains) by convection and radiation. With the onset of sweating, the heat is also dissipated by evaporative cooling. The circulation to the skin is matched to deliver to the skin surface the amount of excess heat necessary to maintain thermal equilibrium, if it can be maintained. During heat strain, heat generated in the muscles is carried to the inactive tissues and to the skin, which in most cases is much cooler than the blood. For simplicity then, in terms of thermal strain, the worker's body should be thought of as having two principal components: a deep body consisting of the brain and viscera and the outer shell comprised of the skin and muscles. The temperature in the shell may vary considerably, whereas ideally the deep body temperature is maintained within about 3°C (5°F) of its mean temperature (37°C, 98.6°F).

The amount of heat produced is determined by the rate of muscular activity. A person resting quietly produces about 44 W/m^2 (1.1 kcal/min) depending on body size (standard man is 1.8 m^2). In general, the bigger the person, the higher the resting metabolic heat production will be. Some normal bodily functions, such as food digestion, increase heat production even further.

During work, metabolic heat production increases. Among very physically fit workers, the metabolic rate can be sustained as high as 700 W (600 kcal/hour) for 4 or more hours. Actual energy requirements for a given task will vary according to the mechanical efficiency of the task and the worker (efficiency tends to increase to an upper limit as task experience increases), body or limb weight, loads carried, speed of activity, and clothing worn.

Evaporation

In humans the primary means for heat dissipation is the evaporation of sweat. Sweating occurs over a wide range of thermal exposure in amounts sufficient to achieve enough evaporative cooling to offset the total heat load represented by metabolic heat production, and heat gained through radiation, convection, and conduction. Sweat, a hypotonic fluid (i.e., more

Table 27.1 — Approximate Metabolic Requirements of Some Representative Work Activities

Activity	*kcal/hour*
Keyboarding, quiet standing	108
Seated writing	120
Driving tractor	150
Sewing with a machine	190
Cooking	198
Machining	198
Sheet metal work	198
Carpet sweeping, wallpapering	200
General carpentry	210
Lathe operation	210
Welding	210
Raking	222
Electrical Work	234
Mopping floors	252
Scraping and painting	260
Vacuuming, feeding animals	264
Tapping and drilling	265
Laundry	270
Planting seedlings	288
Chain saw work	305
Plastering	320
Walking—smooth road	325
Shoveling grain	348
Erecting mine supports	360
Forestry hoeing	372
Tipping molds	378
Drilling coal, rock	384
Walking at 4 mph	396
Steel Forging	408
Shoveling coal	438
Mowing	456
Tending steel mill furnace	516
Trimming trees	528
Felling trees	540
Barn cleaning	552
Rapid marching	582
Digging trenches	594
Fast ax chopping	1212

Note: Adapted from Mcardle et al.[18] These approximations are based on 68 kg body weight. Adjust by proportionate body weight (e.g., a worker weighing one-third more will use roughly one-third more energy). See text for additional considerations.

dilute than most body fluids), is secreted from thousands of glands per square inch all across the body. The evaporation of sweat under optimal conditions requires the absorption of about 0.58 kcal/mL at normal body temperature. Sustained sweat rates as high as 10 mL/min for almost 8 hours and short-term sweat rates as high as 1 L/hour have been reported[19] and even higher rates have been reported for very short durations.[16,20,21] Thus, if 1 L of sweat were totally evaporated from the skin in 1 hour, 580 kcal/hour of heat would be lost, which, under ideal conditions, would be adequate for most work activities. For maximal effectiveness, evaporation must occur from the skin, not from the clothing, although evaporation from the clothing may provide some cooling.[22] However, in many industrial situations, although 1 L of sweat may be produced in an hour, seldom can this much sweat be evaporated from the skin.

Thus, the body has a tremendous capability to dissipate heat under normal circumstances. With regard to heat balance, it is important to realize that in many industrial situations, the primary means for workers to dissipate heat is by evaporation of sweat. Therefore, during heat stress, any time sweat evaporation is hampered, the potential for overheating becomes very serious.

Heat loss through sweat evaporation can be restricted in many industrial situations. Sweat evaporation becomes critically reduced when the relative humidity level nears 100%, and ambient temperature is near skin temperature. Humidity alone, which is a function of air temperature, is not the controlling factor in evaporation, but rather the gradient between the vapor pressure at skin temperature and the water vapor pressure of the air.[23] Evaporation ceases when the ambient water vapor pressure equals that of the skin. This is more likely to occur under protective clothing and equipment such as welding aprons, firefighting garments, or encapsulating chemical protective coveralls. Under encapsulating clothing the microenvironment (i.e., the environment lying between clothing and skin) may become saturated by evaporated sweat and approach 100% relative humidity after only a few minutes of work.[24]

Similarly, any failure to produce adequate sweat will result in rapid overheating. Lack of sweat can occur due to extreme dehydration and in heatstroke when the sweat glands simply shut down.

Convection

The transfer of heat by the flow of some liquid or gas is termed convection and is vital to thermoregulation in the body. Convection results in heat loss by two avenues: (1) within the body by blood circulation, and (2) by movement of water or air across the skin. This process controls the heat flow between the shell and deep body through the movement of blood.

In most cases, the skin is cooler than the blood because the body takes steps to ensure this. In fact, the skin and surface muscles act dynamically to protect the stability of the deep body where most vital organs lie. In hot situations some amount of heat can be stored in this shell (periphery) before the deep body temperature starts to rise. Likewise, this shell tissue can cool significantly before the deep body temperature begins to drop.[25] Since convective heat flow between the deep body and the skin can be controlled by adjusting blood flow, and since blood flow is typically well-controlled, a good system exists for controlling deep body temperature.

The motion of cooler air across the skin also transfers heat. Convective heat loss can be experienced as the dangerous windchill in cold environments, or the pleasant cool breeze in warm environments. The importance of convective heat loss is that equilibrium will occur eventually in any situation. When the air next to the skin is still, and there is no air convection, the air nearest the skin will achieve temperature equilibrium by conduction and also may become saturated with water vapor from the skin. When thermal equilibrium occurs, effective heat transfer by convection or by evaporation of sweat ceases. This illustrates the need for air movement, especially if humidity is relatively high. If heat loss is desired, increasing the movement of even humid air across the skin will help to increase the evaporation rate.

In the cold, convective loss of heat is usually undesirable. If cool air is continuously brought into contact with the skin, that air will continue to absorb heat as it tries to reach equilibrium, and heat will be continuously lost. Thus, when trying to protect from the cold, a layer of dead (nonconvective) air is needed to prevent continuous convective heat loss.

Conduction

Heat transfer by conduction occurs when there is direct contact between a hotter and a colder substance. In most industrial situations conduction of heat to substances other than air is not usually important because there is relatively little contact between the skin and other materials. However, when workers are required to handle cold materials, particularly those with high thermal conductivity, conduction can lead to localized frostbite, which can be very serious. When large areas of the body are in contact with a surface of high conductivity (e.g., workers in prone postures lying on metal plating), the gain or loss of heat can be significant. Likewise, heat conduction through machinery and equipment and through tools can lead to serious burns if there is a substantial heat source and good conductivity.

The best conductors of heat are very dense materials, such as metals. Conversely the worst conductors of heat, and hence the best insulators, are of low density, such as an expanded foam insulation or motionless (nonconvective) air. Even the warmth of fur is primarily attributed to the air it traps.[16]

One can keep warm in a cold environment by layering insulative clothing to trap nonmoving air between the multiple layers (and removing layers to prevent wetting from sweat). If, however, the outer layer is snug because of the bulk of clothing underneath, the clothing may actually lose dead air space (loft) and become a conductor itself. For example, wearing three or four pairs of socks underneath boots that were intended to fit well with only a single pair, probably will result in a situation wherein the insulating layer of air is displaced by the sock, and the sock fabric forms a conductive link between the foot and the outside environment. Blood flow to the foot may be reduced as well. Similarly, wearing a heavy coat over a down vest will compress the down and reduce the vest's insulating capability.

Conduction is also an important factor in wet clothing, in which the water will displace air. Water is denser than air, and is 23 times more conductive[13], which will result in a rapid loss of heat.

Radiation

Radiation is the electromagnetic transfer of heat energy without direct contact. Radiant heating from the sun provides the best illustration. Passing through the vacuum of space, sunlight strikes the earth's surface (and other objects) and only then is it both absorbed and reflected, producing heat.

Workers in hot environments exposed to high radiant loads will benefit from shielding from radiant heat. This, of course, explains the appeal of shade to those laboring in the sun. It is important to recognize that all objects radiate to other objects, thus the total thermal radiation to which a worker is exposed is the sum of all direct and indirect (reflected) radiation, minus the worker's radiation to cooler objects. For simplicity, when the mean radiant temperature of local objects and material is above about 35°C (95°F) (a common mean skin temperature during work in warm environments), the body will gain heat, whereas below 35–36°C (95–97°F), the body loses heat through radiation to cooler surroundings. Again, both the macro- and the micro- environments must be taken into account.

Environmental and Microenvironmental Strain

Humans are homeotherms and must maintain an internal body temperature within a narrow range near 37°C. Humans' inherent thermal homeostasis provides temperature regulation within suitable limits by the involuntary control of blood flow from sites of metabolic heat production (muscles and deep tissues) to the cooler body surface (skin). Heat loss takes place through the mechanisms of radiation, convection and evaporation.[26]

Hypothalamic Regulation of Temperature and Cerebral Blood Flow

The temperature regulating center for humans lies in a region at the base of the brain known as the hypothalamus. Under normothermic conditions, the hypothalamus responds to changes in its own temperature as well as to incoming nerve impulses from temperature receptors in the skin. It activates heat loss or gain by altering blood flow to the skin. Such physiological reactivity leads to interaction with the thermal environment so as to offset the increase or decrease in body temperature, thus maintaining body temperature within an acceptable range.[26]

Cerebral blood flow delivers substrates necessary for cell function to the brain and also serves to remove heat from the brain while at rest and during activity. The brain is especially vulnerable to the effects of heat stress[27], and during periods of hyperthermia, neural activity in the brain and cerebral blood flow circulation are reduced. The decreased cerebral blood flow results in the storage of heat in the brain and is an inevitable consequence of hyperthermia. Therefore, the subjective feelings of central fatigue (reduced central nervous drive to the muscles); a decreased arousal, motivation, or drive to continue working or complete a task; and/or the reduced ability to sustain motor activity in response to hyperthermia should be considered warning signs of reaching high core and brain temperatures.[28]

Stress from the Microenvironment

The integration of all the biophysical factors determines the physiological status of the worker. Figure 27.1 illustrates the composite problem. At the onset of work, blood temperature increases due to metabolic heat production from the working muscles. The hypothalamus, the brain's thermostat, integrates the signals from the body's deep sensors plus those from thermal sensors in the skin. The central processor signals appropriate responses at the skin level. If the clothing characteristics, the skin temperature, and the metabolic rate are such to cause an increase in deep body, or core, temperature, the response is to try to cool the body to the normal deep body temperature (assuming no fever). To dissipate more heat, the body will dilate the skin blood vessels to permit convective heat transfer to the skin. Skin temperature will rise, allowing convective heat loss if there is air movement, and conductive heat loss if there is contact with cooler materials. In addition, the skin will radiate to surrounding cooler objects. Heart rate will increase to provide this needed extra blood flow to the skin for cooling. Sweat glands will be signaled to start releasing sweat to the skin surface where it can be evaporated. Sweat rate will increase to a maximal level depending on the individual and the degree of heat acclimatization. If the sweat is not evaporated, physiological feedback will reduce the sweat rate.

All of this will occur in the microenvironment between the clothing and the skin. Since the volume of air in the microenvironment is relatively small, the air will be greatly affected by the heat and moisture delivered to it by the body. If it is relatively tightly sealed and the ambient environment is cool, the microenvironment may become very different from the ambient macroenvironment. However, if the microenvironment has good exchange with the external environment (clothing is porous, highly permeable to water vapor, loose fitting, with generous openings at the cuffs and neck), the two environments will be more similar.

Once heat dissipation equals heat production, a new deep body temperature equilibrium will be established. In hot jobs, once metabolic rate or the ambient heat stress is decreased, the heat dissipation mechanisms will slowly return toward that individual's normal deep body temperature of approximately 37°C (98.6°F).

If the worker's metabolic rate and clothing are such that deep body temperature begins to fall, shivering and voluntary movements will commence to generate more metabolic heat to try to maintain deep body temperature. If possible, the worker will add more clothing or seek a warmer, less drafty (less convective), work location.

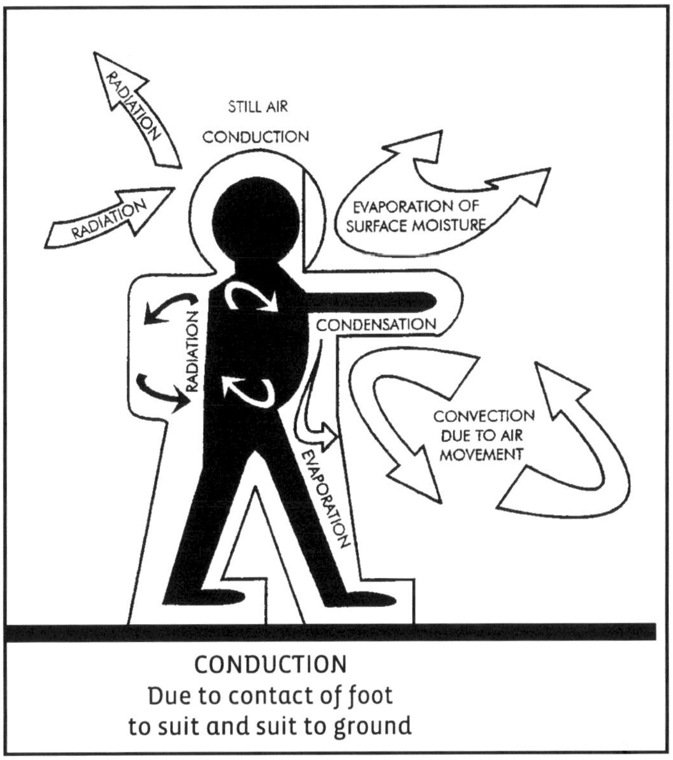

Figure 27.1 — Thermal factors affecting workers in Class A totally encapsulating protective clothing. Heat is produced by the working muscles and metabolic processes. It is carried to the skin through blood flow (convection). From the skin it may be lost (or in some cases gained) by radiation, evaporation, conduction, and convection depending upon the condition inside the suit (the micro-environment). The worker plus suit also reacts with the external (macro-) environment to gain or lose heat depending upon the conditions. The integration of both the micro- and macro- heat exchanges will determine whether the worker's average body temperature continuously rises or establishes equilibrium at some higher temperature. (Drawing by John Kelly).

Assessing Environmental and Microenvironmental Strain

The first and simplest step in assessing the thermal environment is to recognize that many jobs are inherently thermally stressful. High temperatures are frequently encountered in fire fighting, smelting, boiler cleaning or maintenance, plastics extrusion or molding, and asphalt paving or roofing in the summer, , among others. Very low-temperature jobs include emergency work in inclement weather (including unseasonable but otherwise mildly cool weather), and any task in which workers may become wet in cold environments.

Since work involves the production of energy through metabolism, workers are constantly producing heat. The higher the work rate is, the higher the rate of heat production will be. Whether a worker is cooling off or heating up depends on the balance of heat production through metabolism combined with heat gains or losses caused by interaction with the environment (see Chapter 28). This is typically illustrated in the heat balance equation discussed earlier. The body uses metabolic production to help control body temperature. Hence, shivering is an involuntary mechanism that causes the muscles to raise their metabolic rate to produce more heat. Lethargy reduces the metabolic rate and results in less heat production.

Since at any given moment, different parts of the body are individually generating various amounts of heat and experiencing different interactions with the external environments, the heat balance equation is very complex. This partly explains why simple equations cannot be used to accurately predict how workers will respond to a given environment. However, understanding the heat balance equation is very useful in predicting thermal problems for workers and in devising solutions.

A qualitative assessment of the heat balance equation can be very useful in assessing the potential for heat or cold problems. Consider the example of an unacclimatized worker laboring at an accident site with a hazardous chemical spill on an interstate highway on a warm sunny spring day. If the air temperature is 18°C (64°F), the humidity level is 50%, the wind is still, the sun is out, and the worker is performing moderately hard work in Class A protective clothing (i.e., totally enclosed suit with a self-contained breathing system that offers the greatest protection from chemical hazards), the suit's microenvironment creates a very good potential for heat problems despite the relatively mild temperatures. The microenvironment relative humidity will quickly rise, thereby reducing evaporative cooling. The suit also prevents convective cooling by outside air. The radiant energy from the sun will also result in heat gain. If the metabolic heat production is high, the lack of evaporative and convective cooling can lead to considerable heat strain.

Although a quantitative approach to evaluating thermal strain is useful, sole reliance on quantitative evaluation is usually ill-advised. Accurately predicting any individual worker's response to a given thermal environment is very difficult, and there is much data to support great variability among workers in response to the environment.[20,29,30] Exactly what causes this variability is not fully understood. Undoubtedly, there are many differences among workers in size, state of acclimatization, amount and distribution of fat (which is insulative), and function of the cardiovascular and sweat production systems. Theoretically, a given quantity of heat will raise the temperature of a smaller worker more rapidly than that of a larger worker. However, this simple observation is complicated by the fact that cardiovascular fitness may vary, and the surface area-to-mass ratio is higher in smaller workers than in bigger workers. More will be said about the contribution of individual factors later in this section.

Since humans are so highly variable, the only way to determine the true thermal strain is to measure the individual's response. In hot environments, deep body temperature should be monitored as the best single gauge of heat strain; but in the cold, skin temperature is also important, because frostbite can easily occur while deep body temperature is normal.

Accurate prediction of the heat strain experienced by workers through modeling is extremely difficult.[31] At present, the simplest approach to controlling heat stress is to monitor environmental conditions and take appropriate precautions in hot or cold situations. It must be kept in mind that some workers may experience heat intolerance problems even in very mild warm conditions. Ideally, in warm to hot environments, every worker's deep body temperature would be monitored, and protective and rehabilitative procedures would be instituted whenever deep body temperatures reached a certain predetermined threshold. Unfortunately, that is not practical at present. Recently there have been some attempts to measure skin or ear canal temperature to predict deep body temperature, but these procedures have not been found to be valid.[32–34]

The Occupational Safety and Health Guidance Manual for Hazardous Waste Site Activities[14] says workers should be monitored when ambient work temperature is above 21°C (70°F). Monitoring workers consists of measuring heart rate, oral temperature, and body weight (which reflects sweat losses). If heart rate exceeds 110 beats/min or oral temperature exceeds 37.6°C (99.7°F), work periods must be shortened and rest periods lengthened to reduce the physiological strain. The assumption here is that oral temperature monitoring will be an accurate reflection of deep-body temperature, and that has not been established.

In addition, this guide[35] recommends that, in temperatures of 32°C (90°F) (with no sun) or higher, when workers are wearing impermeable clothing, physiological monitoring of acclimatized workers be repeated every 15 minutes. Konz also recommends[3] multiple measures rather than a single measure of heat strain. This is to preclude a dangerous assumption based on a single faulty measurement. Multiple measures might include heart rate plus temperature, when practical. Since 2001, the American Conference of Government Industrial Hygienists recommendations[33] call for rational heat stress analysis (only applicable when encapsulating clothing is NOT used) or physiological monitoring (only option when encapsulating protective clothing is used) as the best approach to monitoring heat stress and strain for workers. Whereas this is a good theoretical approach, there are no practical, worker-acceptable, accurate means for individual monitoring while working, and a heat stress analysis is of little help in planning manpower requirements for hot jobs requiring encapsulating clothing.

Obviously, for workers in toxic environments, monitoring oral temperature, heart rate, or body weight (hydration status) will in many cases prove impractical. However, this does highlight the need for constant vigilance and extreme caution when workers wearing protective clothing are exposed to warm temperatures.

Measuring Deep Body Temperatures of Workers

The deep body temperature is the temperature of the body's internal organs. Deep body temperature is considered to be the best single measure of heat strain. Unfortunately, this measure is very difficult to obtain and can only be accurately measured during physical work by inserting a thermometer to make contact with the body's central deep internal tissue. This can be done in the following three ways: (1) inserting a thermometer 8–12 cm into the rectum, (2) inserting a wire thermometer through the nose or mouth and down the esophagus to approximately heart level, or (3) having the subject swallow a radiotelethermometer that can transmit temperature data to the outside. Understandably, most workers are not enthusiastic about any of these options.

Several alternatives have been suggested to overcome the difficulties of inserting thermometers deep into the body. Socially acceptable measures of core temperature in the workplace are not currently available.[26] As such, surrogate measures are the most frequently used in the field. Of the surrogate measures, oral temperature has the longest history. It is best measured at least 15 minutes after the last drink and with the mouth closed. The rule of thumb is to add 0.5°C to the measured value. Oral temperature and axillary (armpit) temperature are used clinically to measure pyrogenic (fever) changes in body temperature.

Likewise attempts have been made to use skin temperature and tympanic (ear drum) temperature. Ear canal temperature (as opposed to tympanic temperature, which is not recommended for safety and comfort reasons) provides some insight to core temperature. It, however, is easily influenced by environmental conditions, but in a protective fashion. That is, hot environments tend to raise ear canal temperature more than expected from an increase in core temperature.

Passive infrared devices are available for measuring tympanic temperature in a less intrusive manner are available. They have been designed for application in a climate-controlled environment and can be affected by sweat in the ear. On some devices, the offset for rectal temperature may have been selected based on data for infants. Care must be taken to use them in a workplace, although they may produce protective results due to the influence of hotter ambient conditions.

Although research has shown that the alternative methods are not sufficiently accurate to replace the less-appealing methods for measuring core temperature[34,36], in most cases, these surrogate methods are the only measurement option.

Factors Affecting Thermal Strain

Thermal stress is the external heat load placed on the body due to the characteristics of the environment, and thermal strain is the body's response. Workers will show a large variation in heat strain, even though all may be working at the same work rate in the same thermal environment. This is because many controllable and uncontrollable factors affect heat strain, as summarized in Table 27.2.

Controllable Factors Affecting Strain

Clothing

In protecting against cold, clothing insulating values are measured in clo units. One clo equals the insulating value needed for someone to be comfortable sitting in a typical office environment of 21°C (70°F), 50% relative humidity, and air speed of 10 cm/sec (20 ft/min). The clo needed is a function of the metabolic heat production. Figure 27.2 is an illustration of the relationship between activity, temperature, and clothing needed.

Clothing keeps people warm because it creates a microenvironment that results in a comfortable balance between heat production and heat loss. In other words, properly chosen clothing reduces or enhances conduction, convection, evaporation, and radiation

Table 27.2 — Summary of Variables That May Influence Work in Thermally Stressful Environments

Variable	*Impact*
Controllable Variables	
Work Task	
Rate	Metabolic rate influences heat storage rate
Type	Mobility influences ability and type of cooling possible; Psychomotor function may be affected
Workers (may be controlled through selection/training)	
Physical Fitness	Improved fitness increases thermal tolerance
Training	Increases safety
Acclimatization	Increases tolerance; with impermeable clothing, sweat effects may be mitigated
Size	Both mass/area and absolute mass may influence tolerance
Body fat content	Theoretically may influence heat loss
Hydration	Dehydration increase heat injury risk; repeated workdays may affect prework hydration and electrolytes
Electrolyte Levels	Will influence rehydration and physiological function
Health	Fever, other illness, or medication may affect tolerance
Genetics	Large interindividual variability
Gender	Generally unstudied; thermoregulation shows a sex difference, but not in overall response, except that females may be less cold-tolerant
Age	Does not affect thermal tolerance except tp the degree it affects physical fitness
Clothing (including protective clothing) required	
Insulating Value	As insulation increase, potential heat loss decreases
Permeability	As permeability decreases, less opportunity for sweat evaporation; this may retard cooling or increase clothing wetness
Weight	Increases in weight increase metabolic requirements
Stiffness	Increases in stiffness raise metabolic costs of movement
Glove/Mitten	Effects dexterity and hand/arm type fatigue
Gas MaskReduces field of vision, may fog, impedes communication, raises metabolic costs	
Uncontrollable Factors	
Work Task	
Type	Mobility will influence ability and type of cooling possible; psychomotor function may be affected
Workers	
Size	Both mass/area and absolute mass may influence tolerance
Body Fat Content	Theoretically may influence heat loss
Genetics	Large interindividual variability
Gender	Thermoregulation shows particular sex differences, but not in overall response
Age	Does not affect thermal tolerance except to the degree it affects physical fitness
Environment	
Temperature	Increases in temperature increase heat storage
Humidity	Major impact on heat tolerance, but in protective clothing the role of humidity is less
Radiant load	Can be a major heat source
Wind Velocity	Can play a major role in heat loss, in both hot and cold environments.

in such a way that the metabolic heat production will maintain deep body temperature and skin temperature. The introduction of a strong draft (i.e., convective heat loss) will alter the clo level needed for comfort, as will an increase in metabolic rate.

Minimizing sweat production and evaporation is important in cold exposures to minimize condensation that would wet the clothing (undesirable in cold), reduce clo, and increase conductive heat loss. For this reason, removing clothing to avoid excess sweating during cold exposure is very important. The ratio of clo to the impermeability-to-water-vapor is an important characteristic of clothing, known as the im/clo ratio. The higher the clo, the warmer the clothing. The higher the im/clo ratio, the greater the problems in evaporating sweat.

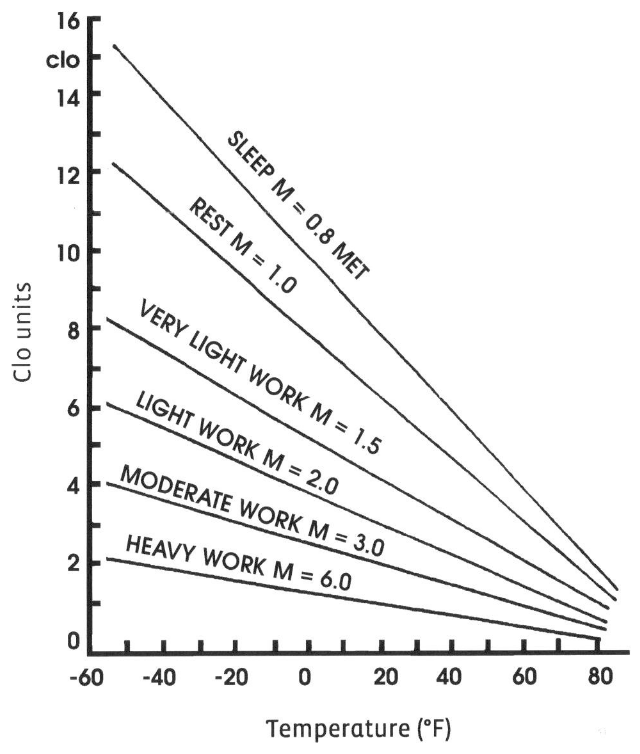

Figure 27.2 — Amount of clothing insulation (in Clo units) required at different work rates to maintain comfort. M= one MET which is the resting metabolic rate of 100 W (oxygen consumption of 3.6 mL/Kg). (From Burton & Edholm[37] with permission.)

Acclimatization

Among controllable factors, the most important is acclimatization. Acclimatization refers to a set of adaptive physiological and psychological adjustments that occur when an individual accustomed to working in a temperate environment undertakes work in a hot or cold environment. These progressive adjustments occur over periods of increasing duration and reduce the strain experienced on initial exposure. This enhanced tolerance allows a person to work effectively under conditions that might have been unendurable before acclimatization.

When workers are exposed to hot environments, particularly when they perform physical labor in hot environments, their bodies gradually adapt in several ways.

Heat acclimatization. When workers are initially exposed to hot work environments, they can show signs of distress and discomfort; develop increased core temperatures and heart rates; complain of headache, giddiness, or nausea; and present other symptoms of incipient heat exhaustion. In heat acclimatization, the human body adaptations include

- Increase in the amount of sweat, which increases evaporative cooling potential
- Earlier onset of sweating, which reduces heat storage prior to activation of evaporative cooling
- More dilute sweat (lower salt concentration), which reduces electrolyte (chiefly sodium and chloride) losses
- Increased skin blood flow, which provides greater convective heat transfer between deep body and skin
- Reduction in heart rate at any given work rate, which lowers cardiovascular strain and the oxygen requirements of the heart
- Greater use of fat as fuel during heavy work, which conserves carbohydrates that are useful when very high rates of energy production are needed.
- Reduction in skin and deep body temperature at any given work rate, which maintains a larger heat storage reserve and permits the worker to work at a higher rate.[18]

These adaptations work together to reduce the deep body and skin temperatures (i.e., heat strain) for a given amount of work, providing a greater reserve for emergency or prolonged work requirements.

Heat acclimatization occurs very rapidly, with substantial adaptation apparent

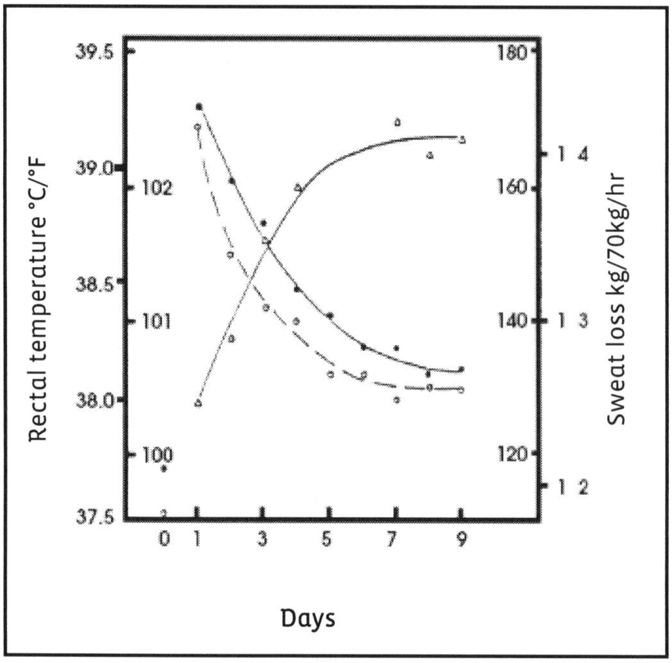

Figure 27.3 — Typical average rectal temperatures(•), pulse rates (°), and sweat loss (Δ) of a group of men during the development of acclimatization to heat. On Day 0, the men worked for 100 min at an energy expenditure of 349 W (300 kcal/hour) in a cool climate; the exposure was repeated on Days 1 to 9, but in a hot climate with dry- and wet-bulb temperatures of 48.9 and 26.7°C (120 and 80°F). (Used with permission from C.S. Leithead and A.R. Lind, *Heat Stress and Heat Disorders*, 1964).[38]

Table 27.3 — Guidelines for Acclimatization and Reacclimatization as a Percent of Effort[a]

Acclimatization Guidelines

Day	Activity (percent of full work assignment) Experienced	New
1st	50%	20%
2nd	60%	40%
3rd	80%	60%
4th	100%	80%
5th		100%

Re-Acclimatization Guidelines

Days Away from Heat-related Jobs Routine		Exposure Sequence (percent of full work assignment)			
Absence	Illness	1st	2nd	3rd	4th
<4	–	100%			
4–5	1–3	R/E[b]	100%		
6–12	4–5	80%	100%		
12–20	6–8	60%	80%	100%	
>20	>8	50%	60%	80%	100%

[a]Ref 39.
[b]Reduced Expectations by the worker and supervision.

after only 2 hours of heat exposure per day for 8 consecutive days.[19] Figure 27.3 illustrates the change in heart rate and rectal temperature during a 9-day exposure. Guidance for acclimatization to heat stress exposures is provided in Table 27.3.[39] The schedule for a new employee is more gradual than for an experienced employee based on the assumption that a new employee must also learn about the job and its related hazards.[40] Additional acclimatization will continue to occur with continuing exposure. If seasonal changes are gradual, people working outside will make a natural adaptation to either heat or cold. However, sudden weather changes may result in dangerous levels of stress, particularly of heat stress. Workers just beginning to work in high heat-stress jobs may not have a natural acclimatization, so provisions for adequate time for acclimatization are essential. Acclimatization to one heat level may only partially acclimatize the individual to higher heat exposures. Likewise, acclimatization may be temporarily lost after a long weekend or a vacation. The more time an individual spends away from the heat, the longer time is required for re-adaptation.[26] Table 27.3 provides some guidance on re-acclimatization for different periods away from heat exposures whether due to routine reasons such as reassignment, vacation or injury or for illness.[39]

Despite a high degree of acclimatization, when environmental conditions are extreme, productivity will likely decrease, and this reduced productivity should be anticipated. When workers wear impermeable encapsulating chemical protective clothing, some of the value of acclimatization may be reduced. The increased sweat rate under impermeable clothing may actually hasten dehydration without providing proportionate cooling (due to vapor saturation of the micro-environment). The other changes would be positive, and heat acclimatization most likely enhances work tolerance and certainly reduces cardiovascular strain in the heat in protective clothing.

Cold Acclimatization

Cold acclimatization, which is much less profound than heat acclimatization, produces a lowered deep body temperature and an increased blood flow through the exposed extremities.[18] These changes help conserve heat by reducing the heat loss gradient.

One physiological aspect of cold tolerance that is not part of acclimatization is the hunter or Lewis reflex. When extremities are very cold, the blood vessels will vasoconstrict (become smaller in diameter, which reduces blood flow) to conserve heat for internal body organs. When the hunter reflex occurs, the finger tips, palms, toes, sole of the foot, ear lobe, and parts of the face react to the cold exposure by occasional vasodilation (increases in the vessel diameter, which increases blood flow) that periodically rewarms peripheral tissues without the loss of excess heat that would occur if higher temperatures were maintained constantly in these areas.[13] This periodic rewarming delays frostbite and minimizes heat loss from the internal body. This reflex is seen to varying degrees in humans, being well developed in some and virtually absent in others.

Physical Fitness

Physically fit persons have distinct advantages with respect to heat tolerance, but physical fitness alone does not ensure superior acclimatization.[9,18,41] In general, the greater the physical fitness level of the worker, the quicker the worker will adapt to, and tolerate, both the heat and the cold. Physical fitness leads to better thermal tolerance mainly because fitness leads to increased blood volume and cardiovascular capabilities. Aerobic fitness is known to increase blood volume, cardiac stroke volume, maximal cardiac output, and increased capillarization of the muscles. The increase in the number of capillary blood vessels relative to muscle mass provides a larger interface between blood and muscle for the exchange of oxygen and waste products. Furthermore, the increased tone of small veins from nonmuscle tissue reduces their volumetric capacity during exertion and thus increases pressure on large, central veins returning blood to the heart. This increase in venous return causes cardiac output to increase during work with less need to accelerate the heart. Therefore a physically conditioned person, by virtue of having a higher maximum cardiovascular capacity, has a wider margin of safety in coping with the added circulatory strain of working under heat stress. These changes would lower the cardiovascular strain for any given work rate, as well as increase the physiological reserves. The resultant increased blood volume, for example, becomes important when blood must simultaneously supply the muscles with oxygen at the same time it must transport heat to the skin for dissipation.[26]

Hydration and Electrolyte Balance

The most easily controlled factor in heat tolerance is the hydration level of workers. Research by Coyle and Montain[42] has shown that fluid replacement lowers body temperature and cardiovascular strain during work in the heat, both of which are linked to heatstroke probability. Providing copious amounts of different appealing beverages to workers is considered to be one of the most important precautions that can be taken to maintain the highest blood volume.[43] Fluids with a high sugar content and caffeine should be avoided, as sugar intake can increase metabolic heat production and caffeine can have a diuretic effect.

Sweat is a mixture of water, electrolytes, and lactic acid. Electrolytes essentially are minerals that play a vital role in maintaining homeostasis within the body. Electrolytes help to regulate myocardial and neurological function, fluid balance, oxygen delivery, acid-base balance and other biological functions. Sweat of acclimatized workers contains 1–4 g/L of electrolytes, and the sweat of unacclimatized workers contains even more. During heavy sweating, it may be very difficult to maintain the body's electrolyte levels.

Armstrong et al.[44] showed that the losses of sodium and calcium resulting from 6 hours of work can exceed the normal daily intake. This suggests that workers exposed to repeated days of profuse sweating may incur electrolyte deficits that can pose a serious health risk. Nadel et al.[45] argue that rehydration cannot be complete until all the electrolytes lost in sweat are restored such that all the body fluid compartments are returned to pre-exposure status. They also point out that the thirst drive is reduced too quickly by drinking low-concentrate (over-diluted with water as a cost saving measure) electrolyte-replenishing beverages and recommend that the drinks not be diluted.

A typical American diet (10 to 15 g/day of salt) supplies the needs of an acclimatized worker producing 6 to 8 kg of sweat during a single shift, for whom 1 kg of sweat contains 1 to 2 g of salt. During acclimatization, however, workers require additional salt. Although maximal sweating rates in un-acclimatized persons are lower, salt concentrations are higher than after acclimatization. Thus an unacclimatized person may lose 18 to 30 g of salt per day, resulting in a negative salt balance. Salt supplements in the form of tablets should never be used. A preferable practice is to consume small portions of salty snacks (salted nuts or crackers) and potassium-rich foods such as bananas, oranges, cantaloupe, or strawberries, and drink electrolyte replenishing fluids throughout the day. Consuming caffeine and drinks high in sugar content(including juice and fruit drinks) should be avoided. In view of the high incidence of elevated blood pressure in the U.S. population and the relatively high salt content of the typical U.S. diet, recommending increasing the amount of salt intake during meals is probably not warranted.[40]

Water lost from sweating of 1 kg (1.4% of body weight in a 70-kg person) can be tolerated without serious effects. Water deficits of 1.5 kg or more during work in the heat reduce the volume of circulating blood, resulting in signs and symptoms of increasing heat strain, including elevated heart rate and body temperature, thirst, and severe heat discomfort. At water deficits of 2 to 4 kg (3 to 6% of body weight), work performance is impaired; continued work under such conditions leads to heat exhaustion.[40,41] Therefore, sweating workers should drink at frequent intervals, at least two or three times per hour, to assure adequate fluid replacement. Coyle and Montain[42] suggest workers try to drink enough to make up for about 80% of the working sweat loss. For example, if workers lose 1 kg (2.2 lbs) of sweat, they need to replace the lost sweat with 800 mL of fluid intake. Between shifts, the remaining deficit should be recovered so that workers start each shift fully hydrated.

Workers chronically exposed to hot environments or conducting heavy work in encapsulating personal protective equipment or firefighting garments should have their body weights monitored routinely. NIOSH[14] suggests that body weight loss in a workday should not exceed 1.5%. It is important to recognize that it takes a great deal of effort for workers to maintain body weight within 1.5% over the course of a work shift when engaged in heavy work resulting in heavy sweating. Regardless, complete rehydration should be achieved before the start of the next shift. Hydration guidelines that may be helpful are included in Table 27.4.

Table 27.4 — Fluid Replacement Guidelines

- Workers should be careful to consume a well-balanced diet and drink plenty of nonalcoholic beverages in the day preceding severe heat exposure.
- Workers should avoid diuretic drinks immediately prior to work and drink as much as a half liter prior to commencement of work.
- During work, workers should try to drink as much and as frequently as possible.
- Workers should be provided cool drinks that appeal to them. Fluids can contain 40–80 g/L of sugar and 0.5 to 0.7 g/L of sodium.
- Workers should be encouraged to drink as much as possible and consume foods rich in electrolytes between work shifts and during breaks.
- Body weight should be monitored at the start and end of each shift to ensure that progressive dehydration is not occurring.

Note: These guidelines were adapted, in part, from McArdle, et al.[18]

When hydration is maintained, workers seem to be able to undergo several successive days of intense heat exposure without obvious cumulative adverse effects. Solomon et al.[21] measured the stability of tolerance for protective clothing within subjects across days. Subjects varied somewhat from day to day in work tolerance, work/rest ratio, sweat production, and perception of effort, but there were no clear trends in the data suggesting a cumulative increase or decrease in work tolerance.

It must be recognized that in the American culture, most workers tend to be reluctant to sacrifice convenience for safety. It is best if the employer maximizes the availability of appealing fluids.[43] This may take some extra planning in situations requiring respirator use, since the respirator greatly inconveniences drinking.

If workers replace water losses without adequate salt intake, a progressive dehydration occurs because thermoregulatory controls in the human body are geared to maintain a balance between electrolyte concentration in tissue fluids and body cells.

Deficient salt intake with continued intake of water dilutes the tissue fluid, which in turn suppresses the release of antidiuretic hormone (ADH) by the pituitary gland. The kidney then fails to reabsorb water and excretes dilute urine containing little salt. Under these conditions, homeostasis maintains the electrolyte concentration of body fluids but at the cost of depleting body fluids and ensuing dehydration. Under continued heat stress, the symptoms of heat exhaustion (elevated heart rate and body temperature plus severe discomfort) develop similarly to those resulting from water restriction, but signs of circulatory insufficiency are more severe and there is notably little thirst. An excellent diagnostic tool for salt deficiency is the presence of a very low level of chloride (less than 3 g/L) in the urine.[26,41]

In extreme cases, water intoxication, or hyponatremia (low blood sodium levels), can result from uncompensated electrolyte loss combined with ingestion of large quantities of water. In this situation, body electrolytes fall so low that coma can ensue. Regardless, workers should be encouraged to drink as often and as much as they can tolerate. Those who sweat a great deal should be encouraged to eat foods high in electrolytes (e.g., cantaloupe, bananas) as well as drink electrolyte replacement drinks low in sugar content. Conversely, workers with diagnosed electrolyte problems or who are on sodium-restricted diets should not work in the heat.[26]

Confounding Factors

Alcohol and Drug Use (Including Medication)

Many therapeutic and social drugs can have an impact on a worker's tolerance for heat or cold tolerance. Alcohol has been identified as a contributing factor in the occurrence of heatstroke.[38] Excessive social drinking of alcoholic beverages can leave a worker dangerously dehydrated. Alcohol also interferes with central and peripheral nervous function and is associated with dehydration by suppressing ADH production. Notwithstanding the potential hazards from central nervous system (CNS) depression, the ingestion of alcohol before or during work in the heat should not be permitted, because it reduces heat tolerance and increases the risk of heat-related illnesses.

Many prescription and over-the-counter drugs prescribed or taken for therapeutic purposes can interfere with thermoregulation.[46] Almost any drug that affects CNS activity, cardiovascular reserve, or body hydration could potentially affect heat or cold tolerance. Some therapeutic drugs, such as heart-rate controlling (beta-blocking) drugs, will compromise work ability in jobs with high heart strain, such as moderate or hard labor in hot conditions. Vasoactive (affecting blood vessel size) drugs can influence heat loss and blood supply and thereby contribute to hypothermia or frostbite. The Physician's Desk Reference Guide to Drug Interactions, Side Effects and Indications lists medications that may affect heat tolerance and many more that affect hydration levels in some manner.[47] Any worker who is taking any medication should receive medical clearance before being exposed to hot or cold conditions.

It is difficult to separate the heat- or cold-disorder implications of drugs used therapeutically from those which are used socially. Nevertheless, there are many drugs other than alcohol that are used on social occasions. Some of these have been implicated in cases of heat disorder, sometimes leading to death.

Uncontrollable Factors Affecting Strain

Body Size and Fatness

Two uncontrollable factors that influence heat and cold tolerance are body size and fatness. The larger the person, the greater the energy required to perform work (and hence the higher the metabolic heat production), particularly for weight-supported activities such as walking or lifting. Also, the bigger the person, the lower the surface area-to-mass ratio, which reduces the person's ability to dissipate heat, and it takes longer for the person to cool off once exposure to heat ceases. In the cold, large size is generally an advantage because typically more heat is generated in the body, and the reduced surface area-to-mass ratio keeps the worker warmer.[26]

It is well established that obesity is a risk factor for heat disorders.[38] The acquisition of fat means that additional weight must be carried, resulting in a greater expenditure of energy to perform a given task and the use of a greater proportion of the aerobic capacity. In addition, the body surface to body weight ratio becomes less favorable for heat dissipation. Probably more important is the lower levels of physical fitness and decreased maximum work and cardiovascular capacities associated with obesity.

Fat is a good insulator, which means that the fatter the person is, the less heat tolerant and more cold tolerant they should be. However, the extra weight raises the energy costs and metabolism for workers who must support and transport their body weight as part of the job (e.g., if the worker must squat and rise repeatedly). There is much individual variation in the influence of size and fatness on heat and cold tolerance.

Age

Older, healthy workers perform well in hot jobs if allowed to proceed at a self-regulated pace. Under demands for sustained work output in heat, an older worker is at a disadvantage compared with the younger worker. First, the older worker has less cardiocirculatory reserve. Second, under levels of heat stress above the prescriptive zone, an older worker compensates for heat loads less effectively than do younger persons, as indicated by higher core temperature and peripheral blood flow for the same work output. This occurs because of a delay in the onset of sweating and a lower sweat-rate capacity with age, thus resulting in greater heat storage during work and longer time required for heat recovery.

Aging leads to a more sluggish response of the sweat glands, resulting in less effective control of body temperature. Aging also results in a greater level of skin blood flow associated with exposure to heat.[40] When two groups of male coal miners of average age 47 and 27 years worked in several comfortable or cool environments, they showed little difference in their responses to heat near the REL with light work. In hotter environments, however, the older men showed substantially greater thermoregulatory strain than their younger counterparts. The older men also had lower aerobic work capacities.[18] In analyzing the distribution of 5 years' accumulation of data on heatstroke in South African gold mines, Strydom[48] found a marked increase in heatstroke with increasing age of the workers. Thus men over 40 years of age represented less than 10% of the mining population, but they accounted for 50% of the fatal and 25% of the nonfatal cases of heatstroke. The incidence of cases per 100,000 workers was 10 or more times greater for men over 40 years than for men under 25 years of age. In all the experimental and epidemiologic studies described above, the workers had been medically examined and were considered free of disease. Total body water decreases with age, which may be a factor in the observed higher incidence of fatal and nonfatal heatstroke in the older group.[40]

Worker Health

Sick workers, especially those with a fever, are at special risk in stressful work environments since body temperature will be regulated to a higher temperature than normal. This means that the same amount of work will produce the same heat storage, but at a higher, more dangerous temperature. A worker who ordinarily tolerates the heat well will thus be impaired.

Any disease that may influence cardiovascular or kidney function or hydration state (e.g., diarrhea results in dehydration) may impact heat tolerance. Generally speaking, it is dangerous for the ill to work in hot environments.[49] Workers and supervisors should be trained to screen themselves and each other to avoid unsafe heat and cold exposures.

Heat Stress and Reproduction

The effects on reproduction of acute and chronic exposure to physical labor in combination with heat are not well known. The effects on pregnant women are potentially very serious. Exposure of pregnant women to high deep body temperatures during the first trimester (3 months) of pregnancy may result in fetus malformation.[3,18] This is vital information for workers, since it is possible that a female worker might not realize she is pregnant until well into the first trimester. It is well known that intense work can elevate rectal temperature as high as 40°C (104°F) even in moderate environments. Female workers who might be pregnant should be protected from heat exposure. Any work to be conducted in heat exposure by a pregnant female should first be reviewed and approved by a licensed physician.

In men, the potential impact of heat on reproduction would be chiefly manifest in terms of its effects on fertility. Based on the available research, it does not appear that heat exposure has a major effect on reproduction in men, but further research may lead to other conclusions.

Gender Differences in Thermal Tolerance

Studies that matched the cardiorespiratory fitness levels and size of male and female subjects found that women's heat tolerance was at least as good and occasionally better than that of men.[50–54] Additionally, when working at similar proportions of their maximum aerobic capacity, women perform similarly or only slightly less well than men.[9] However, due to lower aerobic capacities, the average woman or small man is at a disadvantage when performing the same hot job as the average-sized man. Although all aspects of heat tolerance in women have not been fully examined, gender-related differences in thermoregulatory capacities have been reviewed extensively. Lower sweat rates for females are widely reported in the literature, and related differences in physiological response by males and females are well established.[9]

In contrast, it appears that for very low work rates, such as inspection or supervision tasks, gender differences in cold tolerance should be considered and female worker offered additional protection. For work rates eliciting substantial amounts of metabolic heat production, gender responses are somewhat different, but the net effect is a similar overall response, regardless of gender. For work tasks requiring more than minimal energy expenditure, considerations other than gender, such as size, acclimation state, and physical work capacity, should be used in assigning workers to tasks involving thermal tolerance. Additionally, individual differences in response to heat loads in particular tend to be very great.[30,55–57]

Controlling Thermal Exposure

Administrative Controls

Administrative control methods minimize employee exposures by altering work practices, limiting exposure times, increasing the number and duration of rest periods, reducing or sharing workloads, and allowing workers to self-limit exposure on the basis of the signs and symptoms of heat strain. The key to effective administrative control of heat stress is effective training and the provisions for hydration with potable water and electrolyte replenishing fluids. Fluids with a high sugar content and caffeine should be avoided. Untrained workers may not recognize the importance of preventative measures or the onset of heat stress and may misinterpret the onset of the protective mechanisms of central fatigue, exhaustion, and a decreased drive to continue work.

Worker Selection

There are several ways of controlling the physical strains of hot and cold environments. As always, administrative controls can be used to advantage. One obvious, though complex, administrative approach is worker selection, which raises ethical and moral issues. For example, excluding women from some hot jobs may be unethical and illegal sex discrimination, but exposing known pregnant women to jobs that threaten heat strain is certainly unethical. Keeping workers with heart conditions from performing certain jobs may be highly ethical in some situations and unethical in others, depending on the circumstances. Ethical issues must be considered on a case-by-case basis.

Workers may be selected based on the nature of the work and a number of other criteria. Selecting workers based on obvious factors seems reasonable. For example, an acclimatized, fit, lean worker generally would be expected to tolerate greater heat stress than a fat, unfit, unacclimatized worker. Although this is generally true, the only way to determine worker tolerance is to observe workers over a period of time to see who is most tolerant of a given work load and environmental combination. Measuring deep-body temperature response to work would be desirable but is generally impractical.

Worker Training

Appropriate training includes ensuring that workers understand the signs and symptoms of heat strain, principles of prevention and hydration, management of personal factors (acclimatization, alcohol usage, medications, diet, fitness and health status, age, etc.) and the interaction of these in avoiding heat-related illnesses. Proactive and paced fluid replacement rather than reactive response to the thirst is critical to the prevention of heat-related illness.[58] The California Occupational Safety and Health Administration investigated 46 medically confirmed heat-related illnesses in 2005 and 2006, and 96% of the cases showed medical evidence of dehydration; Drinking water was available on site in 90% of the cases but consumption was not adequate to remain hydrated.[59] Routine recording of worker body weight can be utilized to monitor fluid replacement levels and identify employees requiring hydration. The support of management is critical to the successful use of administrative controls for the management of heat stress. All employees including supervisors and managers should be trained to recognize the signs and symptoms of heat strain and should permit workers to interrupt their work if they exhibit or self-report symptoms of heat strain.[26,60] Individual workers should be afforded as much control as possible over the pace of the work and the ability to take recovery breaks.[5]

Teaching workers to recognize potential hot/cold problems and training them to deal with these should improve both safety and productivity. For example, training workers to maintain good levels of hydration, even in the cold, and to select protective clothing that provides the maximum protection with the minimum heat or cold strain improves safety and productivity. Research has shown that if workers select impermeable protective coveralls when only a regular (uncoated) fabric needed, the heat strain is much higher than necessary, and worker productivity and safety are reduced.[57] Workers and supervisors should be taught that therapeutic and recreational drugs may alter hot/cold tolerance, and that workers who report a fever should be protected from heat exposure.

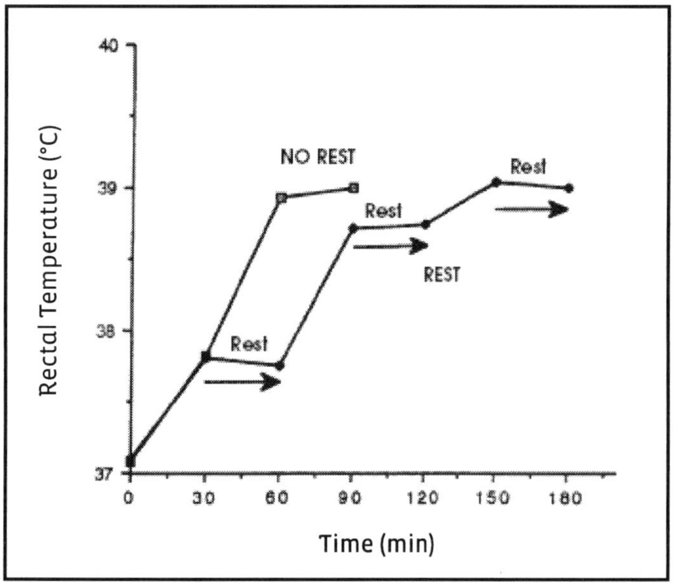

Figure 27.3 — Mean rectal temperature for intermittent work in protective clothing with and without rest. Adapted with permission from Bishop et al.[61]

Scheduling

Most industries do not have a great degree of scheduling flexibility, but annual planning and careful scheduling to minimize stressful exposure to heat or cold when possible would improve safety and increase productivity. Factors to be considered in scheduling include time of day, season, and locale. Time of day, especially for hot outside work, can have a major impact on heat stress. When possible, work in very hot outdoor environments should be scheduled for night, or for early and late in the day. Outside work requiring protective clothing should, when practical, be scheduled for the coolest months.

Work-Rest Intervals

Work-rest intervals have been used to control the environmental exposure of workers. As heat strain increases, the ratio of work-to-rest must fall.[15] Safe and wise scheduling of work and rest is not as simple as it might at first appear. For example, it was discovered that in protective clothing in very hot environments when rest must occur while wearing the clothing, it was preferable to have workers work continuously rather than work and rest, because they were unable to cool off during rest.[61] See Figure 27.3.

Resting in the protective clothing in this situation would only result in a longer duration of heat exposure without an increase in productivity. The balance between work and rest must consider both safety and the thermal physiology, because workers resting in protective clothing may not cool much; however, doffing and donning protective clothing would increase worker risk of toxic chemical exposure. There is useful information on work-rest intervals in other sources.

Engineering Controls

Engineering controls can also be employed to improve safety and productivity in hot and cold environments. For example, improving seals and insulation and/or painting hot surfaces such as kilns, ovens, or boilers with aluminum paint (thereby decreasing the emissivity of the hot surface) can decrease the heat energy transferred into a workspace. These controls offer several advantages: less heat transfers to workers nearby, protecting workers; and heat is conserved inside the units resulting in decreased energy costs.[64] Installing radiant heat shields may be very cost effective in many situations because of the resulting increase in worker productivity. Job redesign may be necessary to lower worker metabolic rates (i.e., lower metabolic heat production) to reduce heat strain, which can increase productivity.

Hot Environments

Eastman Kodak[4,5] lists several steps that can be taken to minimize thermal stress in hot environments. These include engineering and administrative controls and the use of personal protective equipment:

- Macro cooling (i.e., cooling the general work environment)
- Reducing ambient humidity to increase rate of evaporative cooling and the efficiency of evaporation (usually accomplished through mechanical cooling of the work space or spot cooling of cool, dehumidified air)
- Increasing air velocity in cases where the ambient temperature is equal to or less than the skin temperature
- Lowering metabolic rate by implementation of slower work rate or provision of mechanical assistance
- Adjusting clothing to decrease evaporative resistance
- Adding microenvironmental cooling
- Providing radiant shielding or isolation of hot surfaces using insulation or lowering the emissivity of hot surfaces
- Providing a cool location, or at least spot-cooling, for rest breaks
- Providing plenty of palatable fluids of the workers' preference for rehydration

Cold Environments

For cold environments, they recommend[4,5]:

- Provide cold stress training for work in temperatures below 5°C (41°F).
- Provide proper clothing. Choose fabrics that inherently trap air (e.g., wool) and stop air penetration (e.g., windbreakers).
- Allow for self-limiting of work exposure to cold.
- Reducing air velocity and minimizing drafts (e.g., windbreaks).
- Balancing work rate so that periods of intense work are not followed by low work rates.
- Increasing the clothing insulation.
- Using windproof clothing as appropriate.
- Provide hand warming for fine work below 16°C (61°F).
- Providing opportunities and equipment to dry clothing that is wet or damp.
- Increasing radiant heat with micro- or spot heaters.
- Providing general or spot heating and warming shelters.
- Minimize conductive cooling of the hands and other body surfaces from cold surfaces .
- Avoiding long periods of inactivity.
- Provide for the use of the buddy system.
- Allow for productivity reductions due to the use of personal protective equipment.
- Schedule work/recovery cycles.
- Use active warming systems (microenvironmental heating).
- For work below 2°C (36°F), replace clothing immediately if it becomes wet.
- Provide hydration with warm, sweet, non-caffeinated drinks.
- Encourage a balanced diet.

Environmental Controls

Macroenvironmental change to reduce thermal problems is the most obvious but sometimes the least practical change. When the macroenvironments cannot be changed, the microenvironments can sometimes be improved. One simple and well-studied example is the microenvironment inside protective clothing. As previously discussed, this microenvironment can quickly become very warm and humid. Such a microenvironment can be cooled in a variety of ways.

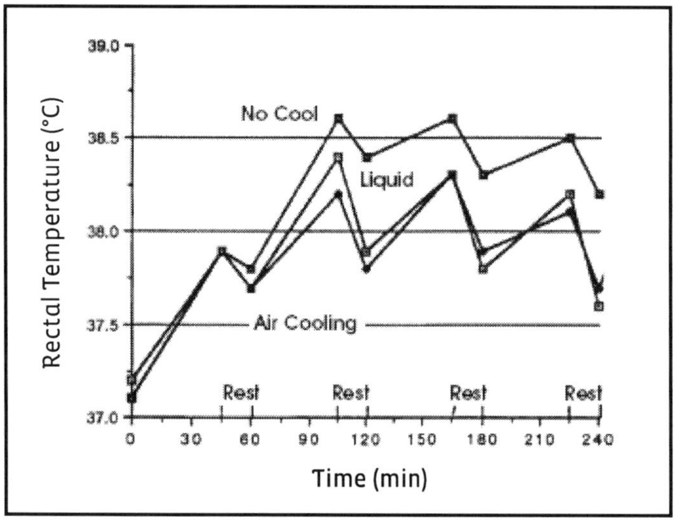

Figure 27.4 — Mean rectal temperatures for intermittent work in protective clothing (metabolic rate of 430 W or 370 kcal/hr) at WBGT = 25°C (77°F) with no cooling (n=14), air and liquid cooling (n=13)during rest. Number of subjects completing 240 min was: no cool = 5, liquid cool = 6, air cool = 11. Adapted with permission from Bishop et al.[61]

Microenvironmental Control

The simplest means of controlling the microenvironment is to control the clothing worn. In hot jobs, adjust clothing to protect against radiant loads, but maximize air movement and evaporation of sweat. Sometimes this can be accomplished simply by minimizing clothing. If protective clothing must be worn, use a fabric or design that maximizes sweat evaporation and air movement.[61]

In cold conditions, microenvironmental control means using outer clothing that minimizes airflow across the skin and maximizes the insulating, or clo, value. There is a practical limit to how much clo can be raised, because of both the bulk and the increase in surface area. Increase in clo is negated, at some point, by the increase in surface area. This is why mittens are superior to gloves in keeping hands warm. The microclimate of the head is also especially important, since at -4°C (25°F), the heat loss from the head on average is about 50% of resting metabolism. Adding 2.4 clo units of insulation to the head reduces heat loss equivalent to adding 4 clo to the rest of the body.[3]

Microclimate Cooling

As illustrated in Figure 27.4, all micro-cooling is most effective in hot temperatures and declines in impact as the temperature falls. Good results have been observed in some situations by cooling workers only during rest. For example, a worker in protective clothing who must be mobile on a hazardous waste site might spend 30–60 minutes working and plan to finish near a support site, where he or she could be attached to either a clean liquid or air cooling system for a rest break. It should also be recognized that the worker's subjective comfort may be as important, and sometimes more important, than physiologic benefits.

There are basically three options for micro-environmental cooling. Phase change vests are passive cooling devices with limited cooling capacity but are relatively cheap.[65] Liquid cooling systems come in both mobile and tethered forms and are more expensive, but provide greater cooling power.[20] Air cooling systems are mostly tethered systems which provide more comfort than the others because of evaporative cooling (and drying), but are limited by the air-supply tether.[20]

Microenvironmental Heating

Conversely, in cold situations the use of space heaters, heated boots, socks, or gloves may alter the microenvironments to improve safety and cost-effectiveness. However, improperly used heaters can be dangerous due to fire and burn potential and carbon monoxide production. Since heat generation requires a lot of energy, the monetary cost of low productivity must be balanced against heating costs. Phase change, solid and liquid fuel, circulating fluid, and thermoelectric heating have been used to provide microenvironmental heating, but the physiological and cost-effectiveness of these methods have not been reported.

Prediction of Thermal Work Tolerance

Generalized Prediction of Thermal Tolerance

Because hot environments (micro- and macro-) particularly limit work tolerance and pose a significant health and safety threat, there is a strong need for accurate prediction of worker tolerance in hot and cold environments. Prediction generally takes two forms: (1) a generalized prediction equation that attempts to predict for groups of people, and (2) an individualized approach that tries to use individual information to predict for a single worker.[31] Because of the great variability among workers in their heat/cold responses, one of the greatest needs in the prevention of heat strain is a practical means of monitoring or predicting heat strain within individuals rather than generally. There are no accurate and practical personal monitors at present.

Individualized Prediction of Thermal Tolerance

Previous attempts to predict individual responses have not been accurate for a broad range of workers in a broad range of situations. Some type of personalized prediction is likely to be more accurate for individual workers than a generic prediction in which one tolerance time is predicted for all workers in a given situation. Presently, these individual predictions are not sufficiently accurate to provide adequate worker safety. Worker monitoring seems the most practical near-term solution to protecting workers in very hot conditions, and innovative effective approaches to this task would be very valuable.

Summary

Protecting the worker against the stresses of the thermal environment requires recognition of potential problems, minimization of heat or cold strain, and determination of the most practical and effective solutions. This can best be achieved by helping workers and supervisors to understand the fundamentals of worker thermoregulation and exposure control. Undoubtedly, there will be major advances in materials, equipment, and techniques in the future. Evaluating and selecting the most appropriate innovations in individual situations is again a function of grasping the underlying principles.

Work in protective clothing, in hot or warm environments, shortens work tolerance even for the most hardy workers, and work-rest scheduling may not extend work time effectively in hot, hazardous environments.[66] In previous military studies, workers in protective clothing have suffered from physical and heat exhaustion after relatively short work duration and even in cool temperatures (WBGT = 9°C, 48°F), which emphasizes the need for constant efforts to ensure worker safety when protective clothing is used even in cool ambient conditions. Worker safety in protective clothing is not strictly an issue of work rates. Workers in some military studies have performed relatively light duty tasks in protective clothing, such as patient medical care, and consequently suffered heat problems.[67]

Microenvironmental cooling effectively increases work tolerance and worker comfort. Liquid, air, and phase-change cooling have all proved effective. Phase-change vest cooling presently appears the most feasible for short-term cooling of mobile workers.

In addition to the serious diminution of physical work capacity, work in winter clothing and chemical protective clothing can also result in possible loss of dexterity, strength, work capacity, and perceptual motor performance. This loss results in a higher safety risk as well as decreased productivity.

The reduction of work capacity in hot and cold conditions presents occupational hygienists and ergonomists with a very challenging problem. Currently, guidance for employers of personnel in hot environments is very restrictive of productivity and is thus problematic for industry. Continued research and cooperation is needed to maximize productivity while simultaneously minimizing health risks for workers in extremely hot and cold environments. A checklist to help improve worker safety and productivity in extreme environments is included in Tables Table 27.5 and Table 27.6.

Table 27.5 — Checklist for Heat Exposures

- ❑ Are adequate supplies of a variety of appealing cool drinks available?
- ❑ What is the major source of heat stress and how can it be mitigated (e.g., protective clothing requires particular strategies)?
- ❑ If radiant shielding (including shade) is possible, is it in the most strategic location?
- ❑ Is temperature-monitoring equipment available at the work site?
- ❑ Are work guidelines that are appropriate to the situation available to workers and supervisors?
- ❑ Are first aid supplies available that are appropriate to heat/cold emergencies?

- ❑ Has an appropriate work rate and work-rate schedule been determined, and is there sufficient manpower to stay on schedule despite a slower work pace?
- ❑ Have supervisors been instructed to remove workers at the first sign of problems?
- ❑ Have workers been properly and thoroughly acclimatized (or reacclimatized after time away from the stressing environment)?
- ❑ Is a cool recovery/rest area available?
- ❑ Are workers and supervisors trained in recognizing the symptoms of, and providing first-aid treatment for heat injury?
- ❑ Is there a means of calling emergency medical support? Do workers know how and where to call emergency medical support?
- ❑ Is the clothing appropriate (minimal obstruction of sweat evaporation and maximal protection from radiant heat; i.e., use the lightest, most permeable clothing that provides adequate safety)?
- ❑ Is air velocity as high as practical?
- ❑ Are workers well hydrated at the beginning of work?
- ❑ Is spot cooling available?
- ❑ Is microclimate cooling available as needed?
- ❑ Have workers who might be pregnant, or those with cardiovascular problems, previous heat injuries, on problematic medications, and who have fever, been protected from elevated deep body temperatures?
- ❑ Have workers been reminded of appropriate safety precautions?

Table 27.6 — Checklist for Cold Exposures

- ❑ Are workers and supervisors trained in recognizing the symptoms of and providing first-aid treatment for frostbite and hypothermia?
- ❑ Is there a means of calling emergency medical support? Do workers know how and where to call emergency medical support?
- ❑ Are appropriate clothing and replacements for wet items available?
- ❑ Is emergency warming available?
- ❑ Are there facilities available for drying clothing items that become damp or wet?
- ❑ Are windbreaks erected in the most beneficial locations?
- ❑ Is a windchill chart available?
- ❑ Have supervisors been instructed to remove workers at the first sign of problems?
- ❑ Are hand/foot warmers available?
- ❑ Has the work rate been modified as much as possible to avoid following very high work rates with very low ones (i.e., avoid causing workers to sweat, followed by very low work rates that might cause them to become hypothermic)?
- ❑ Is spot warming available?
- ❑ Are drinks available? (Avoid drinks high in caffeine since caffeine is a vasodilator.[3])

Nomenclature

°C = degrees Celsius
°F = degrees Fahrenheit
°K = degrees Kelvin
C = convective heat
E = evaporative heat
E_{max} = maximum evaporative capacity of the climate
E_{req} = evaporative heat required
h_c = the convective heat transfer coefficient
h_r = the linear radiation exchange coefficient
H_{res} = respiratory heat loss (convective and evaporative)
I_{cl} = insulation, clothing
K = conductive heat
M = metabolic heat
R = radiant heat
S = heat storage
t_a = air temperature
t_{ch} = equivalent chill temperature
t_{cl} = dry heat loss from clothing to environment
T_g = globe temperature
T_r = the mean radiant temperature
t_{sk} = heat conducted from the skin
v = air velocity
v_{ar} = relative air velocity, m/sec
w = the skin wetness
W = external work rate
WCI = windchill index

References

1. **Kroemer, K.H.:** Avoiding cumulative trauma disorders in shops and offices. *Am. Ind. Hyg. Assoc. J. 53*:594–604 (1992).
2. **Frederick, L.J.:** Cumulative trauma disorders an overview. *Am. Assoc. Occup. Health Nurses J. 40(3)*:113–16 (1992).
3. **Konz, S.:** *Work Design*, 4th edition. Scottsdale, AZ: Publishing Horizons, 1995. pp. 378, 381-383, 389, 390.
4. **Eastman Kodak Company:** *Ergonomic Design for People at Work*, Vol. 1. Rodgers, S.H. (ed.). Lifetime Learning Publications: London, 1983. pp. 253, 267, 271.
5. **Eastman Kodak Company:** Kodak's *Ergonomic Design for People at Work*, 2nd edition. Chengalur, S.N., S.H. Rodgers, and T.E. Bernard (eds.). 2004, Wiley: Hoboken, NJ. xxvii, 704 p.
6. **Simonson, E. and A.R. Lind,(eds.):** *Fatigue in static effort. In Physiology of Work Capacity and Fatigue*. Simonson, E. (ed.). Springfield, IL: C.C. Thomas Publishing, 1971.
7. **Robinson, M.D. and P.A. Bishop:** Influence of thermal stress and cooling on fine motor and decoding skills. *Int. J. Sports Med. 9*:148 (1988).
8. **Sawka, M.N., C.B. Wenger, and K.B. Pandolf:** Thermoregulatory responses to acute exercise-heat stress and heat acclimation. In *Handbook of Physiology*. Fregly, M.J. and C.M. Blatteis, (eds.). New York: Oxford University Press, 1996. pp. 157–161.
9. **Pandolf, K.B., M.N. Sawka, and R.R. Gonzalez (eds.):** *Human Performance Physioloy and Environmental Medicine at Terrestrial Extremes*. Carmel, IN: Cooper Publishing Group, 1986.
10. **Werner, J.:** Temperature regulation during exercise. In *Perspectives in Exercise Science and Sports Medicine*. Gisolfi, C.V., D.R. Lamb, and E.R. Nadel (eds.). Dubuque, IA: Brown and Benchmark, 1993. pp. 63–38.
11. **Alpaugh, E.L.:** Temperature extremes, in *Fundamentals of Industrial Hygiene*, B.A. Plog, B.A. (ed.). Washington, D.C.: National Safety Coucil, 1988.
12. **American Red Cross:** *Community First Aid and Safety*. St. Louis, MO: American Red Cross, 1993. pp. 146, 147, 221.
13. **Folk, G.E.:** *Textbook of Environmental Physiology*. Philadelphia, PA: Lea & Febiger, 1974. p. 105, 154-55, 244.
14. **National Institute for Occupational Safety and Health (NIOSH);** Occupational Safety **and Health Administration (OSHA); U.S. Coast Guard; and the U.S. Environmental Protection Agency:** Occupational Safety and Health Guidance Manual for Hazardous Waste Site Activities (DHHS [NIOSH] pub. 85-115). 1985, Washington, D.C.: U.S. Government Printing Office, 1985. pp. 8–21.
15. **Ramsey, J.D. and T.E. Bernard:** Heat Stress. In *Patty's Industrial Hygiene*, 5th edition. Harris, R. (ed.). New York: Wiley-Interscience, 2000. p. 925-984.
16. **Kerslake, D.M.:** *The Stress of Hot Environments*. Cambridge, U.K.: Cambridge University Press, 1972. p. pp. 95, 96, 134, 147, 238.
17. **Ramsey, J. and Y.G. Kwon:** Recommended alert limits for perceptual motor loss in hot environments. *Int. J. Ind. Ergon. 9*:245–57 (1992).
18. **McArdle, W.D., F.I. Katch, and V.L. Katch, (eds.):** *Excercise Physiology*, 4th edition. Baltimore, MD: Williams & Wilkins, 1996. pp. 157-158, 169, 512, 521.
19. **Brief, R.S.:** *Basic Industrial Hygiene, A Training Manual*. New York: Exxon Corp., 1975. pp. 189, 191, 192.
20. **Bishop, P.A., S.A. Nunneley, and S.H. Constable:** Comparisons of air and liquid personal cooling for intermittent heavy work in moderate temperatures. *Am. Ind. Hyg. Assoc. J. 52*:393–97 (1991).
21. **Solomon, J., et al.:** Responses to repeated days of light work at moderate temperature in protective clothing. *Am. Ind. Hyg. Assoc. J. 55*:16–19 (1994).
22. **Robinson, S., S.D. Gerking, and L.H. Newburgh:** Interim Report #27 to the CMR, Jul 1945. Cited in *The Physiology of Heat Regulation and the Science of Clothing*. Newburgh, L.H. (ed.). Philadelphia, PA: W.B. Saunders Co., 1949. p. 351.
23. **Goldman, R.F.:** Prediction of human heat tolerance. In *Environmental Stress: Individual Adaptations*. Folinsbee, L.F., et al., (eds.). New York: Academic Press, 1978, p. 57.
24. **Bishop, P., D. Gu, and A. Clapp:** Climate under impermeable protective clothing. *Int. J. Ind. Ergon. 25(3)*:233–38 (2000).
25. **Bazett, H.C.:** The regulation of body temperatures. In *The Physiology of Heat Regulation and the Science of Clothing*. Newburgh, L.H. (ed.). Philadelphia, PA: W.B. Saunders Co., 1949. p. 110.
26. **Larrañaga, M.D. and T.E. Bernard:** Heat Stress. In *Patty's Industrial Hygiene*. Rose, V. and B. Cohrssen (eds.). In Press, Wiley-Interscience.
27. **Brinnel, H., M. Cabanac, and J. Hales:** Critical upper levels of body temperature, tissue thermosensitivity and selective brain cooling in hyperthermia. In *Heat Stress: Physical Exertion and Environment*. Hales, J. and D. Richards (eds.). Amsterdam: Excerpta Medica, 1987. p. 363–403.
28. **Nielsen, B. and L. Nybo:** Cerebral Changes During Exercise in the Heat. *Sports Med. 33(1)*:1–11 (2003).

29. **Bishop, P.A., et al.:** Limitation to heavy work at 21°C of personnel wearing the U.S. military chemical defense ensemble. *Aviat. Space Env. Med. 62(3)*:216–20 (1991).
30. **Mar'yanovich, A.T., et al.:** Individual features of responses to a combination of heat and physical exertion. Hum. Physiol., 1984. 10: p. 49–55 (1984).
31. **Bishop, P.A.:** A new approach to predicting response to work in hot environments. In *Advances in Ergonomics and Safety II*. Das, B. (ed.). New York: Taylor & Francis, 1990. p. 913-918.
32. **Morgans, L.F., S.A. Nunneley, and R.F. Stribley:** Influence of ambient and core temperatures on auditory canal temperature. *Aviat. Space Environ Med. 52(5)*:291–93 (1981).
33. **American Conference of Governmental Industrial Hygienists (ACGIH®):** *2001 TLVs and BEIs: Threshold Limit Values for Chemical Substances and Physical Agents and Biological Exposure Indices*. Cincinnati. OH: ACGIH®, 2001.
34. **Green, J.M., A.J. Clapp, D.L. Gu, and P.A. Bishop:** Prediction of rectal temperature by the Questemp II Personal Heat Strain Monitor under low and moderate heat stress. *Am. Ind. Hyg. Assoc. J. 60*:801–06 (1999).
35. **National Institute for Occupational Safety and Health (NIOSH):** *The Industrial Environment — Its Evaluation and Control*. Washington, D.C.: U.S. Government Printing Office, 1973.
36. **Reneau, P.D. and P.A. Bishop:** Validation of a Personal Heat Stress Monitor. *Am. Ind. Hyg. Assoc. J. 57*:650–57 (1996).
37. **Burton, A.C. and O.G. Edholm:** *Man in a Cold Environment*. London: Edward Arnold Publishing, 1955.
38. **Leithead, C.S. and A.R. Lind:** *Heat Stress and Heat Disorders*. Philadelphia, PA: F.A. Davis, 1964.
39. **Bernard, T.E.:** Thermal Stress. In *Fundamentals of Industrial Hygiene*. Plog, B. (ed.). Chicago, IL: National Safety Council, 2001.
40. **National Institute for Occupational Safety and Health (NIOSH):** Criteria for a Recommended Standard-Occupational Exposure to Hot Environments Revised Criteria. Washington, D.C.: U.S. Department of Health Education and Welfare, 1986.
41. **Minard, D.:** Physiology of Heat Stress. In *The Industrial Environment — Its Evaluation and Control*. Washington, D.C.: NIOSH, 1973.
42. **Coyle, E.F.a.S.J.M.:** Thermal and cardiovascular responses to fluid replacement during exercise. In *Perspectives in Exercise Science and Sports Medicine*. Gisolfi, C.V., D.R. Lamb, and E.R. Nadel (eds.). Dubuque, IA: Brown and Benchmark, 1993. pp. 183–187.
43. **Clapp, A.J., et al.:** Palatability ratings of different beverages of heat exposed workers in a simulated HOT industrial environment. *Int. J. Ind. Erg. 26*:57–66 (2000).
44. **Armstrong, L.E., et al.:** Fluid electrolyte losses in uniforms during prolonged exercise at 30°C. *Aviat. Space Environ. Med. 63*:351–55 (1992).
45. **Nadel, E.R., G.W. Mack, and A. Takamata:** Thermoregulation, exercise, and thirst: interrelationships in humans. In *Perspectives in Exercise Science and Sports Medicine*. Gisolfi, C.V. D.R. Lamb, and E.R. Nadel (eds.). Dubuque, IA: Brown and Benchmark, 1993. p. 248.
46. **Nadel, E. and M.R. Cullen:** Thermal Stressor. In *Textbook of Clinical Occupational and Environmental Medicine*. Rosenstock, L. and M.R. Cullen (eds.). Philadelphia, PA: W.B. Saunders Co., 1992.
47. **Thomson Healthcare:** *Physicians' Desk Reference, PDR Guide to Drug Interactions, Side Effects, and Indications*. Vol. 63. New York: Thomson Healthcare., 2009. p. 2235.
48. **Strydom, N.B.:** Age as a Casual Factor in Heat Stroke. *J. S. Afr. Inst. Mining Metall. 72*:112–14 (1971).
49. **MacPherson, R.K.:** The effect of fever on body temperature regulation in man. *Clin. Sci. 18*:281–87 (1959).
50. **Frye, A.J. and E. Kamon:** Responses to dry heat of men and women with similar aerobic capacities. *J. Appl. Physiol. 50*:65–70 (1981).
51. **Avellini, B.A., E. Kamon, and J.T. Krajewski:** Physiological responses of physically fit men and women to acclimation to humid heat. *J. Appl. Physiol. 44*:254–61 (1980).
52. **Kamon, E., B.A. Avellini, and J. Krajewski:** Physiological and biophysical limits to work in the heat for clothed men and women. *J. Appl. Physiol. 41*:71–76 (1976).
53. **Paolone, A.M., C.L. Wells, and G.T. Kelly:** Sexual variations in thermoregulation during heat stress. *Aviat. Space Environ. Med. 49*:715–19 (1978).
54. **Drinkwater, B.L., et al.:** Thermoregulatory responses of women to intermittent work in the heat. *J. Appl. Physiol. 41*:57–61 (1976).
55. **Wyndham, C.H., et al.:** Relation between VO2 max and body temperature in hot humid air conditions. *J. Appl. Physiol. 29*:45–50 (1970).
56. **Wyndham, C.H., et al.:** *Studies on the Effects off Heat on Performance of Work, in Applied Physiology Laboratory Reports*. South Africa: Transvaal and Orange Free State Chamber of Mines, 1959.
57. **Reneau, P. and P. Bishop:** A comparison of two vapor barrier suits across two thermal environments. *Am. Ind. Hyg. Assoc. J. 58(9)*:646–49 (1997).

58. **Brake, D. and G. Bates:** Fluid losses and hydration status of industrial workers under thermal stress working extended shifts. *Occup. Env. Med. 60*:90–96 (2003).
59. **Neidhart, A. and J.C. Prudhomme:** Cal/OSHA's Investigations of 2005 Heat Illness Cases. 2006; Available from: http://www.cal-osha.com/Resources.aspx#heat.
60. **Helgerman McKinnon, S. and R.L. Utley:** Heat Stress. *Professional Safety April*:41–47 (2005).
61. **Bishop, P., P. Ray, and P. Reneau:** A review of the ergonomics of work in the U.S. military chemical protective clothing. *Int. J. Ind. Ergon. 15*:278–83 (1995).
62. **Electrical Power Research Institute (EPRI):** Heat Stress Management Program for Nuclear Power Plants (NP-4453). Palo Alto, CA, EPRI, 1986.
63. **Bureau of Medicine and Surgery:** N.D. Manual of Naval Preventative Medicine (NAVMED-P-5010-3). Palo Alto, CA: Research Reports Center, 1988.
64. **American Industrial Hygiene Association (AIHA):** *Heating and Cooling for Man in Industry* 2nd edition. Akron, OH: AIHA, 1975.
65. **Muir, H.I., P. Bishop, and P. Ray:** Effects of novel ice-cooling technique on work in protective clothing at 28, 23 and 18oC WBGT. *Am. Ind. Hyg. Assoc. J. 60*:96–104 (1999).
66. **Carter, B.J. and M. Cammermeyer:** Biopsychological responses of medical unit personnel wearing chemical defense ensemble in a simulated chemical warfare environment. *Mil. Med. 150(5)*:239–49 (1985).
67. **Carter, B.J. and M. Cammermeyer:** Emergence of real casualties during simulated chemical warfare training under high heat conditions. *Mil. Med. 150(12)*:657–63 (1985).

Outcome Competencies

After completing this chapter, the reader should be able to:

1. Define underlined terms used in this chapter.
2. Recognize instruments and methods for measuring environments.
3. Evaluate heat and cold exposure limits.
4. Demonstrate the process for making decisions concerning thermal environments.

Prerequisite Knowledge

Basic chemistry, physics, and general occupational hygiene background.

Prior to beginning this chapter, the user should review the following chapters:

Chapter Number	Chapter Topic
1	History of Industrial Hygiene
4	Occupational Exposure Limits
27	Applied Physiology of Thermoregulation and Exposure Control

Key Terms

dew point temperature • dry bulb temperature • globe thermometer • globe temperature • hygrometer • mean radiant temperature • natural wet bulb temperature • permissible exposure limit (PEL) • psychrometer •psychrometric chart • psychrometric wet bulb • radiometer • relative humidity • thermometer • vapor pressure

Key Topics

I. Measuring Thermal Environments
   A. Thermal Components
   B. Psychrometric Chart
   C. Instruments and Methods for Measuring Thermal Components

II. Heat Stress Indices
   A. Thermal Balance Equation
   B. Metabolic Heat Estimation
   C. Heat Stress Index (HSI)
   D. Effective Temperature (ET) and Corrected Effective Temperature (CET)
   E. Wet Bulb Globe Temperature (WBGT)
   F. Thermal Stress and the Required Sweat Rate
   G. Other Heat Indices

III. Heat Exposure Limits
   A. WBGT Recommendations
   B. NIOSH Recommendations
   C. ACGIH® Threshold Limit Values®
   D. ISO
   E. Effects of Clothing on WBGT Calculations
   F. Comparison of WBGT Recommendations

IV. Cold Exposure Limits
   A. Windchill Index
   B. ACGIH® Recommendations
   C. Required Clothing Insulation

V. Thermal Effects on Performance and Safety
   A. Effects of Heat
   B. Effects of Cold
   C. Effects on Safety Incident (Accident) and Safety Behavior

VI. Evaluating the Hot Workplace: An Example

VII. Evaluating the Cold Workplace: An Example

Thermal Standards and Measurement Techniques

28

By Michael D. Larrañaga, PhD, CIH, CSP, PE

Introduction

This chapter covers the standards and measurement techniques for natural and artificial thermal environments, including measurement of thermal environments, heat stress indices, heat and cold exposure limits, and examples to demonstrate the use of this information to make decisions concerning environmental exposures. The units and symbols used in this chapter are those proposed by the International Organization for Standardization (ISO), i.e., units of the System International (SI units).[1]

Measuring Thermal Environments

The thermal environment can be assessed by measuring its thermal components: dry bulb (air) temperature, psychrometric wet bulb temperature, natural wet bulb temperature, relative humidity, vapor pressure, dew point temperature, air velocity, globe temperature, and mean radiant temperature.

The dry bulb temperature is measured with a thermometer, commonly a liquid-in-glass thermometer. Temperature units are expressed in degrees Celsius (°C), Kelvin (K) (K = Celsius + 273), or degrees Fahrenheit (°F) (F = 9/5 Celsius + 32). Celsius (often called Centigrade) and Kelvin units are used for temperature in SI units.[1] The term air temperature is synonymous with dry bulb temperature.

The psychrometric wet bulb temperature, commonly called wet bulb temperature, is measured by a thermometer on which the sensor is covered by a wetted cotton wick that is exposed to forced movement of the air. A clean wick, distilled water, and proper shielding to prevent radiant heat gain are needed to produce accurate wet bulb temperature measurements. The natural wet bulb temperature is the temperature measured when the wetted wick covering the sensor is exposed only to naturally occurring air movements.

The percentage value of the ratio of the actual amount of moisture in the air to the amount of moisture that the air could hold if saturated at a given temperature is used to define the relative humidity.

The water vapor pressure is the pressure at which a vapor can accumulate above its liquid (water) if the vapor is confined over the liquid and the temperature is held constant. Normal units for vapor pressure are mm Hg, torr, or kPa, where 1 mm Hg = 1 torr, and 7.5 torr = 1 kPa.

The dew point temperature is the temperature, at a given state of humidity and pressure, at which condensation of water vapor in a space begins as the temperature is reduced. There is a unique dew point temperature associated with each combination of dry and wet bulb temperatures.

The globe temperature is a measure of radiant heat. It is obtained by placing the sensor of a thermometer in the center of a hollow copper sphere, usually 15 cm (6 in) in diameter and painted a matte black to absorb the incident infrared radiation. Globe temperature can also be obtained from electronic instruments that use black spheres with diameters about 5 cm (2 in.).

The mean radiant temperature is the temperature of an imaginary black enclosure, of uniform wall temperature, that provides the same radiant heat loss or gain as the environment measured. It can be approximated from readings of globe temperature, dry bulb temperature, and air velocity. The velocity of the air movement is also called wind speed. Units for air velocity are meters per second (m/sec), feet per min (ft/min), or miles per hour (mph).

A comprehensive discussion of the instruments and methods for measuring the components of thermal environments can be found in ISO 7726.(2)

Psychrometric Chart

The psychrometric chart (Figure 28.1) is the graphic representation of the relationship between the dry bulb temperature, wet bulb temperature, relative humidity, vapor pressure, and dew point temperature.(3,4) If any two of these thermal components of the environment are known, the other three can be obtained from the chart. For example, if the dry bulb temperature and wet bulb temperature of an environment are 43 and 24°C, respectively, it can be determined from Figure 28.1 that the relative humidity, vapor pressure, and dew point temperature of this environment are 20%, 13 mm Hg, and 15°C, respectively. Note that at 100% relative humidity, dry bulb temperature = wet bulb temperature = dew point temperature.

Instruments and Methods for Measuring Thermal Components

Temperature Measurements

Any instrument that measures temperature is called a thermometer. The term is most commonly used, however, for liquid-in-glass thermometers. Thermometers can be classified according to the nature, properties, characteristics, and materials of the sensing element. The main types are liquid-in-glass, bimetallic, and resistance thermometers, and thermocouples. Depending on the methods and setup used for taking the measurements, the same type of thermometer can be used to measure dry bulb, psychrometric wet bulb, natural wet bulb, or globe temperature. Following are some tips for obtaining accurate temperature measurements:

- The time allowed for measurement must be longer than the time required for thermometer stabilization.
- The measured temperature must be within range of the thermometer.
- Under radiant conditions (i.e., when temperatures of the surrounding surfaces are different from the air temperature), the accuracy of air temperature measurement can be improved either by shielding the sensing element or by

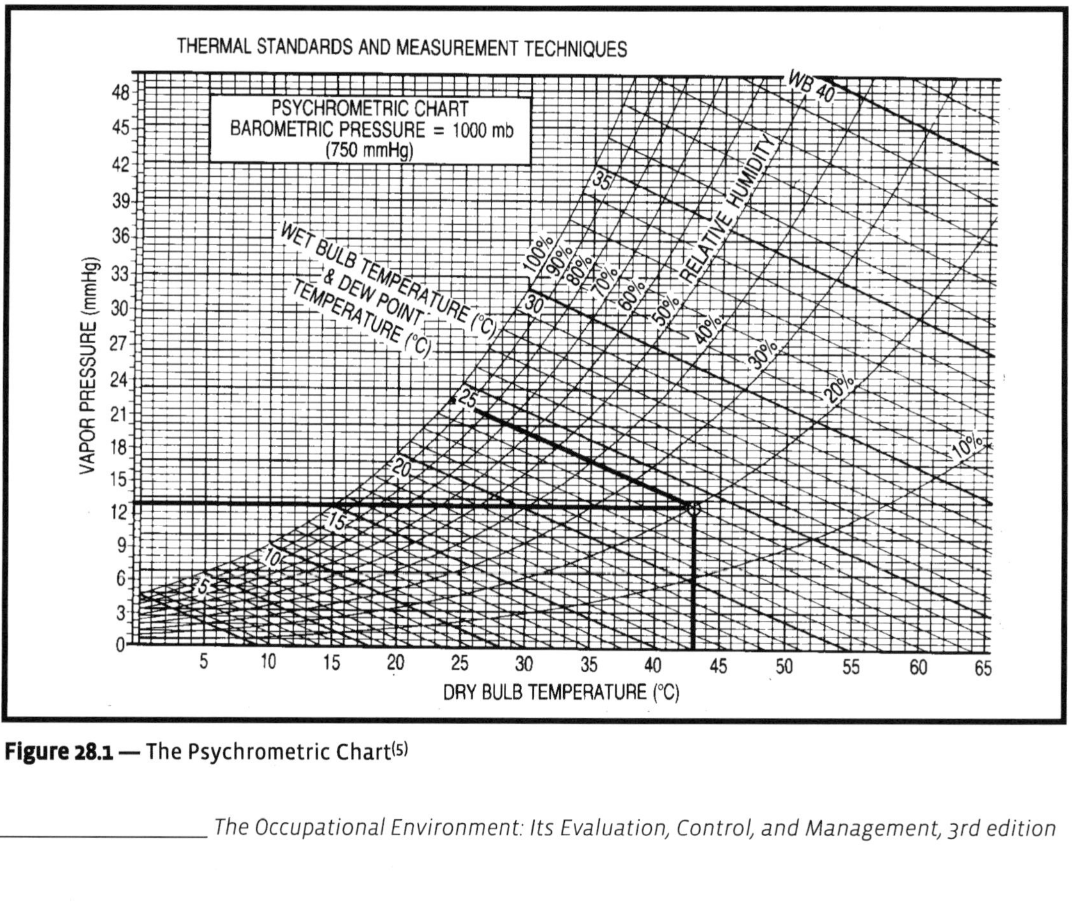

Figure 28.1 — The Psychrometric Chart(5)

accelerating the movement of the air. Under high radiant conditions, both shielding the sensor and accelerating the air may be required.
- The sensing element must be in contact with, or as close as possible to, the area of interest.

Liquid-in-Glass Thermometers

The liquid-in-glass thermometer, first developed in 1706, is the most widely used and familiar type of thermometer. The most commonly used liquids are mercury and alcohol. Mercury-in-glass thermometers have wider application, but one exception is the measurement of extreme cold, since the freezing point of alcohol (-114°C) is considerably lower than that of mercury (-40°C).

The liquid-in-glass thermometer consists of a bulb and a stem of glass. The bulb serves as the liquid container; the stem has a capillary tube into which the liquid will expand when heated. The length of the liquid in the capillary tube depends on the temperature to which the thermometer is exposed. The calibration of the temperature scale on the thermometer stem depends on the coefficient of expansion of both the glass and the liquid.

Two major types of liquid-in-glass thermometers are available. The total immersion thermometer is calibrated by immersing the whole thermometer in a thermostatically controlled medium. It should be used when the whole thermometer is exposed to the measured temperature, such as when measuring the air temperature. The partial immersion thermometer is calibrated by immersing only the bulb of the thermometer in a thermostatically controlled medium. It should be used when only the sensing element (the bulb) is exposed to the measured temperature (as in measuring wet bulb and globe temperatures).

Bimetallic Thermometers

A bimetallic thermometer consists of two strips of different metals of equal length welded or soldered together on one end, with the free ends connected to an indicator. This thermometer operates on the principle that each metal has a specific linear coefficient of expansion. When the thermometer is exposed to a certain temperature, the two strips change length according to their coefficients of expansion, which produces calibrated movement of the indicator.

Bimetallic thermometers are usually in a dial form. The temperature range and the sensitivity of the thermometer can be altered by changing the material and length of the metallic strips. A longer the strip provides a more sensitive response.

Resistance Thermometers

The resistance thermometer functions based on the principle that a changing temperature creates a change in electric resistance. A resistance thermometer consists of a resistor (the sensing element) and a wheatstone bridge, galvanometer, or other means for measuring the change in resistance that results from the temperature change. The thermometer may be calibrated to give a direct temperature reading. The resistor is either a metal wire or a semiconductor. The resistance increases as the temperature increases for the metal wire, whereas the resistance decreases as the temperature increases for the semiconductor. When a semiconductor is used as a sensor, the resistance thermometer is called a thermistor.

Thermocouples

The thermocouple thermometer uses the principle that when a junction of two wires of dissimilar metals is formed, an electromotive force is generated. A thermocouple is simply a junction of two wires of different metals, formed by soldering, welding, or merely twisting the two wires together. A thermocouple circuit is formed when the free ends of the wires are also joined together. If one junction is kept at a constant reference temperature, the temperature of the second junction can be determined by measuring the existing electromotive force or the induced electric current with a potentiometer or a millivoltmeter. The temperature of the second junction is determined from an appropriate calibration table or curve.

Humidity Measurements

Humidity is the amount of water vapor within a given space. It is commonly measured as the relative humidity. It has an important effect on human thermal exchange with the environment: A lower humidity level allows faster sweat evaporation from the skin and larger amounts of heat removal from the body. Two types of instruments are used for measuring relative humidity. A psychrometer gives an indirect measurement of the relative humidity, and a hygrometer gives a direct measurement.

Psychrometers

A psychrometer consists of two mercury-in-glass thermometers. One thermometer measures dry bulb temperature, and the other measures wet bulb temperature; in the latter case, the bulb is covered with a cotton wick wetted with distilled water. The thermometers are mounted parallel to each other on the frame of the psychrometer. The relative humidity and water vapor pressure can be determined from the dry and wet bulb values, using a psychrometric chart as shown in Figure 28.1.

Often this is presented as a table or nomogram drawn on the psychrometer frame. The wet bulb thermometer must be read only after the application of forced air movement. Forced air movements can be obtained manually with a sling psychrometer or mechanically with a motor-driven or an aspirated psychrometer.

The sling psychrometer is usually whirled by a handle for approximately one minute. Accurate measurement is obtained when both thermometers stabilize (i.e., no temperature changes between repeat readings). On the aspirated psychrometer, a battery or spring-operated fan blows air across the wick. To ensure appropriate fan speed, the battery must be checked before using the psychrometer. Air blown across the wet wick must not pass over the dry bulb thermometer or errors in air temperature readings may result. The sensors of both the sling psychrometer and the aspirated psychrometer must be shielded from radiant heat. Sling psychrometers are simple to use and easily calibrated in the field utilizing ice water at 0°C and lukewarm water (temperature varies). The psychrometer is correctly calibrated if both thermometers read the same temperature in both the cold and lukewarm water.

Hygrometers

Any instrument that measures humidity is a hygrometer; however, the term is commonly used for instruments that provide a direct reading of the relative humidity. Organic hygrometers do not provide a high degree of accuracy, but because of their low cost they are widely used. Organic hygrometers operate on the principle that organic materials change their length according to their moisture content, which depends on the humidity of the ambient air. The change in length of the organic material can be transferred as a direct readout of relative humidity on a percentage scale.

Other types of hygrometers for laboratory and more precise applications include dew point, electrolytic, electronic, and chemical hygrometers. Dew point hygrometers measure the dew point temperature, and the relative humidity is determined from a conversion chart. The principle of electrolytic hygrometers is that the electric resistance of a salt film depends on the humidity of the exposed atmosphere. On electronic hygrometers, a sulfonated polystyrene strip is the sensing element whose conductance varies as it absorbs water vapor. Chemical hygrometers (e.g., lithium chloride) measure the humidity directly by extracting and weighing the water vapor from a known sample.

Air Velocity Measurements

The movement of air affects the mechanism of exchange of convective and evaporative heat between the human body and the environment. In a warm, dry environment, an increase in air velocity reduces the effects of the environment on the body because the resultant heat loss through evaporation is greater than the heat gain from convective heat. However, in a hot, humid environment, in which air temperature exceeds skin temperature and the water vapor pressure of ambient air exceeds the water vapor pressure of the skin, an increase in air velocity increases the heat-loading effects of the environment on the body. In any cold environment, an increase in air velocity increases the rate of heat loss by convection.

Any instrument that measures air velocity or wind speed is an anemometer. Typical types of anemometers include the vane anemometer (velometer) and the thermal anemometer (thermoanemometer). Accurate determination of an air velocity contour map in a work area is very difficult, or often impossible, due to the variability in air movement in both time and space. Also, most of the available anemometers are insensitive to low air velocity.

If an anemometer is not available for accurate indoor air velocity measurement, air velocity (v) in meters per second can be estimated as follows:

- No sensation of air movement (closed room with no air source): $v < 0.2$ m/sec
- Sensing light breezes (perception of slight air movement): $0.2 \le v \le 1.0$ m/sec
- Sensing moderate breezes (at a few meters from a fan, definite perception of air movement, causing tousling of hair and movement of paper): $1.0 < v \le 1.5$ m/ sec
- Sensing heavy breezes (located close to a fan, air causes marked movement of clothing): $v > 1.5$ m/sec

Sensitivity to air movement is increased when the skin is wet and/or when body movements generate air flow across the skin.

Vane Anemometers

Measuring air velocity with vane (or cup) anemometers involves measuring either the rotation of a fan (rotating vane anemometer) or the deflection of an internal vane (velometer) by placing the anemometer in the airstream. The vane anemometer usually has an air inlet and an air outlet. The vane or fan is placed in the pathway perpendicular to the direction of the air movement, so that air causes vane deflection or causes the fan wheel to rotate, producing a direct reading of air velocity.

Thermal Anemometers

The basic concept of the thermal anemometer is to determine air velocity by measuring the cooling effects of air movements on an electrically heated thermometer. Two types of thermal anemometers are commonly used: hot-wire anemometers which use resistance thermometers, and heated thermocouple anemometers.

One technique for measuring the cooling effects of air movement is to heat the wire by applying an electric current of specified value and then determine the air velocity from a calibration chart based on air velocity and the resultant wire resistance (hot-wire) or the resultant electromotive force (heated thermocouple). A second technique is to bring the resistance, or the electromotive force, to a specified level and then measure the current required to maintain this level. The air velocity is obtained from a calibration chart relating air velocity to the required electric current. In both cases a correction is made for air temperature.

Radiant Heat Measurement

Determining radiant heat exchanges is necessary to define the thermal environment. A variety of radiometers have been used to measure radiant flux in surface pyrometry and meteorological applications.[6] The net radiometer has been used to measure the radiant energy balance of human subjects.[7] A radiometer with a sensor consisting of a reflective polished disk and a black absorbent disk can also be used. These laboratory and special purpose instruments, however, are not commonly used in occupational heat measurements.

In the occupational environment, the Vernon globe thermometer[8] is the most commonly used device for estimating radiant heat. The thermometer recommended by the National Institute for Occupational Health and Safety (NIOSH)[9] and described above under the definition of globe temperature, has an emissivity of 0.95. The globe temperature is an integrated measure that has a time lag, but it does provide a means for approximating the mean radiant temperature (T_r) from air temperature (T_a), globe temperature (T_g), and air velocity (v), according to the following equation.

$$T_r = T_g + (1.8v^{0.8})(T_g - T_a)°C \qquad (28.1)$$

The globe thermometer exchanges heat with the environment by radiation, convection, and conduction. It stabilizes when the heat exchange by radiation is equivalent to that by convection and conduction: normally 15 to 20 min is required for a globe that is 15 cm in diameter. It has been demonstrated that the globe diameter affects heat exchange and stabilization time, but that appropriate conversion equations can be applied so that black globes of different diameters will yield functionally equivalent results. There are small globe thermometers (4.2 cm) that reduce the response time to one-quarter that required for the standard Vernon globe thermometer.[10]

The precise evaluation of mean radiant temperature for use in research or critical occupational applications is discussed elsewhere.[2]

Heat Stress Indices

As noted in Chapter 27, heat stress is the aggregate of environmental and physical work factors that constitute the total heat load imposed on the body. The environmental components of heat stress are air temperature, water vapor pressure, radiant heat, and air movement. Physical work contributes to total heat stress by producing metabolic heat in the body in proportion to the work intensity.

A heat stress index is a composite measure used for the quantitative assessment of heat stress. Over the years, various indices have been developed to integrate the components of thermal environment and/or the physical and personal factors that influence heat transfer between the person and the environment into a single number. Heat indices can be classified as those based on physical factors of the thermal environment, thermal comfort assessment, rational heat balance equations, and physiological strain.[11]

Thermal Balance

A major criterion for evaluating the usefulness of a heat stress index is its correlation with the changes that occur in human physiological response to heat strain. The major, readily measured physiological responses to heat stress are increases in body temperature, which are measured by oral, tympanic, esophageal, or rectal temperature; heart rate; and sweat production.[12,13] Oxygen consumption is affected less by heat exposure than by the physical work load.

In addition to the environmental and physical factors mentioned above, age, physical fitness, health status, clothing, and acclimatization are also major factors contributing to heat strain. Unfortunately, an index that integrates all these parameters and correlates them precisely to one or more physiological responses has not yet been developed.[14,15] However, there are several indices for measuring heat stress, each with special advantages that make it more suitable for use in a particular environment.

Several thermal indices use the basic construct of thermal balance or heat exchange between the human body and the environment, as represented by the following equation.

$$M \pm R \pm C \pm K - E = \pm S \qquad (28.2)$$

Where:

M = metabolic heat
R = radiant heat
C = convective heat
K = conductive heat
E = evaporative heat
S = heat storage

Equation 28.2 represents the basis for understanding thermal stress both qualitatively and quantitatively. For a quantitative analysis, measurements or reliable estimates of metabolic heat production, air temperature, air water vapor pressure (humidity), air velocity, and mean radiant temperature are necessary. In this equation, heat storage equals zero if the body is in heat balance. The metabolic heat is positive as a heat gain, while the evaporative heat is negative as a heat loss. Other components may be positive or negative based on their influence in the thermal exchange. The conductive heat is very small and is usually neglected. Heat production resulting from external work is sometimes identified separately from metabolic heat. Similarly, respiratory heat loss by evaporation and convection may be considered separate components in the heat balance equation.[14] These components have a relatively small impact on heat balance and normally are neglected unless metabolic heat is to be accurately measured. Heat exchange is measured in terms of the watt or kilocalories per hour (kcal/hour), where one watt equals 0.8606 kcal/hour.

Metabolic Heat Estimation

The metabolic heat generated by work or activity represents a major component in human heat balance and is more difficult to measure than are the environmental components. Metabolic heat can be measured directly or estimated indirectly from physiological measurements such as oxygen consumption. In the evaluation of occupational environments, however, metabolic heat is usually estimated by means of tabulated descriptions of energy cost for typical work activity, as shown in Table 28.1[15], or from tables that specify incremental metabolic heat resulting from activity or movement of different body parts, such as arm work, leg work, standing, and walking.[16] The metabolic heat can then be estimated by summing the component metabolic heat values based on the actual body movements of the worker. In cases where it is necessary to determine oxygen uptake or pulmonary ventilation requirements for certain tasks based on work output or metabolic rate.[17–18]

ISO has recommended determining the metabolic rate analytically by adding values of basal metabolic rate, metabolic rate from body position or body motion, metabolic rate from type of work, and metabolic rate related to work rate. The basal metabolic rate is a function of age, body weight, and height and equals 44 watts/m^2 for a standard man. Metabolic rate values for body position, body motion, and type of work are specified in Table 28.2. For example, the metabolic rate estimate for a standard man sitting and performing average handwork is 84 watts/m^2; (44 watts/m^2 basal, 10 watts/m^2 sitting, 30 watts/m^2 average handwork). Assuming a surface area of 1.8 m^2 (standard man) results in an estimated metabolic rate of 1.8 m^2 × 84 watts/m^2 = 151 watts. Tables for assessing metabolic rate related to work speed are also presented in the ISO standard.[19]

Several tables, charts, and equations relating to metabolic rate determination have been summarized in a procedure for systematic work load estimation.[20] Figure 28.2 shows this system, which can be used with an activity log to determine metabolic heat as a function of stationary, walking, or extra effort work for one hand, two hands, or whole body work. The numbers assigned to each row represent the range of intensity for the activity, with the lower numbers indicating slow or light activity and the higher numbers indicating fast or heavy activity. For example, a worker standing and doing heavy two-arm work would be coded S-9, which shows a metabolic heat around 280 to 330 watts.

Heat Stress Index (HSI) and Predicted Heat Strain

Belding and Hatch developed the heat stress index (HSI) to express thermal stress of a hot climate as the ratio of the evaporative heat required (Ereq) to maintain the body in thermal equilibrium to the maximum evaporative capacity of the climate (Emax).[21] Therefore:

$$HSI = \frac{E_{req}}{E_{max}} \times 100 \qquad (28.3)$$

This index assumes individuals of average build (weight, 70 kg; height, 1.7 m; body

Table 28.1 — Some Selected Types of Work Classes According to Work Load Level[15]

Work Load	*Energy Expenditure Range (M)*
Level 1, resting	Less than 117 watts (100 kcal/hr)
Level 2, light	117–232 watts (100–199 kcal/hr)
Sitting at ease: light handwork (writing, typing, drafting, sewing, bookkeeping); hand and arm work (small bench tools, inspecting, assembly or sorting of light materials); arm and leg work (driving car under average conditions, operating foot switch or pedal). Standing: drill press (small parts); milling machine (small parts); coil taping; small armature winding; machining with light power tools; casual walking (up to 0.9 m/sec, i.e., 2 mph). Lifting: 4.5 kg (10 lb) < 8 lifts/min; 11 kg (25 lb) < 4 lifts/min	
Level 3, moderate	233–348 watts (200-299 kcal/hr)
Hand and arm work (nailing, filing); arm and leg work (off-road operation of trucks, tractors, or construction equipment); arm and trunk work (air hammer operation, tractor assembly, plastering, intermittent handling of moderately heavy materials, weeding, hoeing, picking fruits or vegetables); pushing or pulling lightweight carts or wheelbarrows; walking 0.9–1.3 m/sec (2–3 mph). Lifting: 4.5 kg (10 lb), 10 lifts/min; 11 kg (25 lb), 6 lifts/min	
Level 4, heavy	349–465 watts (300-400 kcal/hr)
Heavy arm and trunk work; transferring heavy materials, shoveling; sledge hammer work; sawing, planting, or chiseling hardwood; hand mowing, digging, walking 1.8 m/sec (4 mph), pushing or pulling loaded hand carts or wheelbarrows; chipping castings; concrete block laying. Lifting: 4.5 kg (10 lb), 14 lifts/min; 11 kg (25 lb), 10 lifts/min	
Level 5, very heavy	above 465 watts (400 kcal/hr)
Heavy activity at fast to maximum pace; ax work; heavy shoveling or digging; climbing stairs, ramps, or ladders; jogging, running, or walking faster than 1.8 m/sec (4 mph). Lifting: 4.5 kg (10 lb) > 18 lifts/min; 11 kg (25 lb) > 13 lifts/min	

Table 28.2 — Metabolic Rate for Body Posture, Type of Work, and Body Motion Related to Work Speed[19]

Body Posture	*Metabolic Rate (watts/m²)*
Sitting	10
Kneeling	20
Crouching	20
Standing	25
Standing stooped	30
Type of Work	*Mean (Range)*
Handwork	
Light	15 (<20)
Average	30 (25–35)
Heavy	40 (>35)
One-arm work	
Light	35 (<45)
Average	55 (45–65)
Heavy	75 (>65)
Two-arm work	
Light	65 (<75)
Average	85 (75–95)
Heavy	105 (>95)
Trunk work	
Light	125 (<155)
Average	190 (155–230)
Heavy	280 (230–330)
Very heavy	390 (>330)
Work Speed Related to Distance	
Walking, 2 to 5 km/hr	110
Walking uphill, 2 to 5 km/hr	
Inclination, 5°	210
Inclination, 10°	360
Walking downhill, 5 km/hr	
Declination, 5°	60
Declination, 10°	50
Walking with load on back, 4 km/h	
10 kg load	125
30 kg load	185
50 kg load	285
Walking upstairs	1725
Walking downstairs	480
Mounting inclined ladder	
Without load	1660
10 kg load	1870
50 kg load	3320
Mounting vertical ladder	
Without load	2030
10 kg load	2335
50 kg load	4750

Note: Values exclude basal metabolism (44 watts/m²)

surface area, 1.8 m²), dressed in shorts and gym shoes, with a skin temperature of 35°C (95°F), and uniformly wetted with sweat. It should be noted that other investigators have concluded that 36°C is a more accurate estimate of mean skin temperature for use in heat transfer equations.[22,23] The HSI further assumes that there is no storage of heat in the body at the beginning of heat exposure, and thermal exchanges by conduction and respiration can be ignored. From the equation of heat exchange above:

$$E_{req} = M + R + C \qquad (28.4)$$

where M = metabolic heat, R = radiant heat, and C = convective heat. The equations and coefficients needed to compute the values of R, C, E_{max}, E_{req}, and HSI for various combinations of clothing are available.[11]

The approximations and assumptions introduced in the HSI construction, mainly for simplicity and practicality, have resulted in areas of reduced accuracy. For example, the HSI does not correctly differentiate between heat stress resulting from a hot, dry climate and that resulting from a warm, humid climate. Similarly, a work change that results in a 100-watt increase in metabolic heat would have a greater physiological impact than an environmental change that results in a 100-watt increase in radiant or convective heat, even though in the HSI, the effect of the environment (R + C) has the same weighting as the value of metabolic heat. Approximations and limitations notwithstanding, the HSI has been used widely and successfully as a tool for evaluating and understanding the components of hot work environments. Nomograms are also available as an aid to determining E_{req} and E_{max}.[24]

The predicted heat strain analysis recommended by the ISO[14] is a third generation rational approach, which evolved from the concepts contained in the HSI. Equations listed in Table 28.3 are the methods for estimating convective (C) and radiant (R) heat exchange. The use of predicted heat strain as a means to evaluate heat stress is described in the ISO standard[14] and elsewhere.[21,25,26]

A distinct advantage of the HSI and PHS in practice is that the components offer an excellent starting point for specifying corrective measures when heat exposure is excessive.

The relative values of the convective exchange C, radiant exchange R, and evaporative capacity E_{max} not only provide a rigorous way to estimate heat stress, but also offer a basis for a rational approach to the evaluation of alternative corrective engineering measures.

Effective Temperature (ET) and Corrected Effective Temperature (CET)

The effective temperature (ET) scale was developed by Houghten and Yaglou in

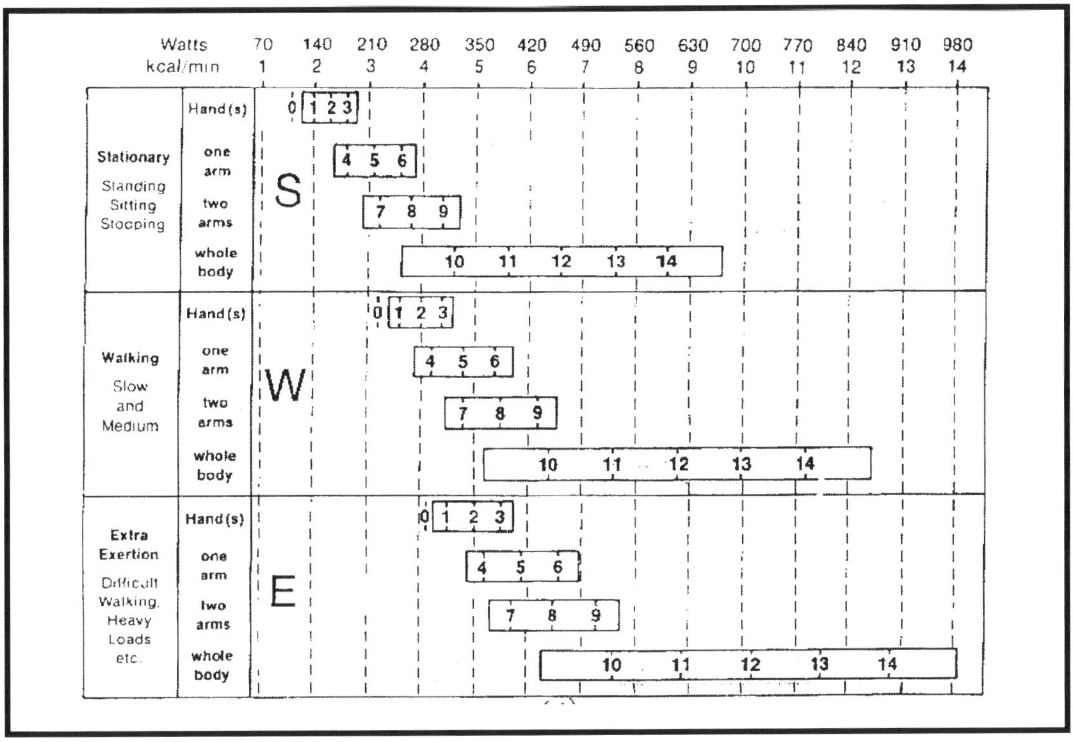

Figure 28.2 — Systematic work load estimation (SWE) schema.[20]

Table 28.3 — Components of Thermal Balance[14]

E_{req} = Evaporation rate required (watts/m²) for the maintenance of the thermal equilibrium = M – C – R

M = Heat flow by metabolism (watts/m²)

C = Heat flow by convection at the skin surface (watts/m²) = $h_c \times F_{cl} (\bar{t}_{sk} - \bar{t}_a)$

R = Heat flow by radiation at the skin surface (watts/m²) = $H_r \times F_{cl} (\bar{t}_{sk} - \bar{t}_r)$

E_{MAX} = Maximum evaporation rate (watts/m²) if skin is completely wetted = $(P_{sk,s} - p_a)/R_T$

w_{req} = Required skin wetness (dimensionless) = E_{req}/E_{max}

SW_{req} = Required sweat rate (SW_{req}, watts/m²) = E_{req}/r_{req}

where:

- h_c = the convective heat transfer coefficient, watts/m² K
- F_{cl} = the reduction factor for sensible heat exchange due to the wearing of clothes (dimensionless)
- $\bar{t}_{sk}$ = the mean skin temperature, °C
- $\bar{t}_a$ = the air temperature, °C
- h_r = the radiative heat transfer coefficient, watts/m², K
- r = the mean radiant temperature, °C
- $P_{sk,s}$ = the saturated vapor pressure at the skin temperature, kilopascals (kPa)
- p_a = the partial water vapor pressure in the working environment, kPa
- R_T = the total evaporative resistance of the limiting layer of air and clothing, m² kPa/watt
- r_{req} = the evaporative efficiency of sweating (dimensionless), which corresponds to the required skin wetness

1923.[27] It was the first heat index and, in revised form, is still one of the widely used indices for evaluating thermal environments. The scale was based on equivalent subjective estimates of the thermal environments with different combinations of air temperature, air velocity, and humidity.

Two environmental chambers were used. Subjects moved between a reference chamber and a second chamber while adjustments were made until the subjects felt they had equivalent thermal sensations. All conditions that had the same effects were grouped together under the same ET as the still, saturated conditions of the reference chamber.

Two ET scales were developed: the normal scale for men wearing ordinary, indoor summer clothing and the basic scale for men stripped to the waist. Measuring the ET of a room requires dry bulb temperature, wet bulb temperature, and air velocity values. An example of ET, using the normal scale, can be obtained from the nomogram in Figure 28.3. If the dry and wet bulb temperatures and the air velocity of an environment are 30°C, 20°C, and 2 m/sec, respectively, the corresponding ET value for this environment is 23°C. This means that the standard man wearing ordinary, summer clothing will sense a thermal environment of 30°C dry bulb temperature, 20°C wet bulb temperature, and 2 m/sec air velocity as equivalent to a 23°C dry bulb temperature environment of still, saturated air (i.e., zero air velocity and 100% relative humidity).

Because radiant heat measuring devices were not available, the radiant parameter was not included in the ET scale. Later, after the introduction of the Vernon globe temperature[8], Bedford (1946)[28] amended the ET scale to include allowances for radiant heat. This scale, called corrected effective temperature (CET), uses the globe temperature instead of the dry bulb temperature. CET can also be determined from Figure 28.3.

Although the ET and CET scales have been widely used, they make limited

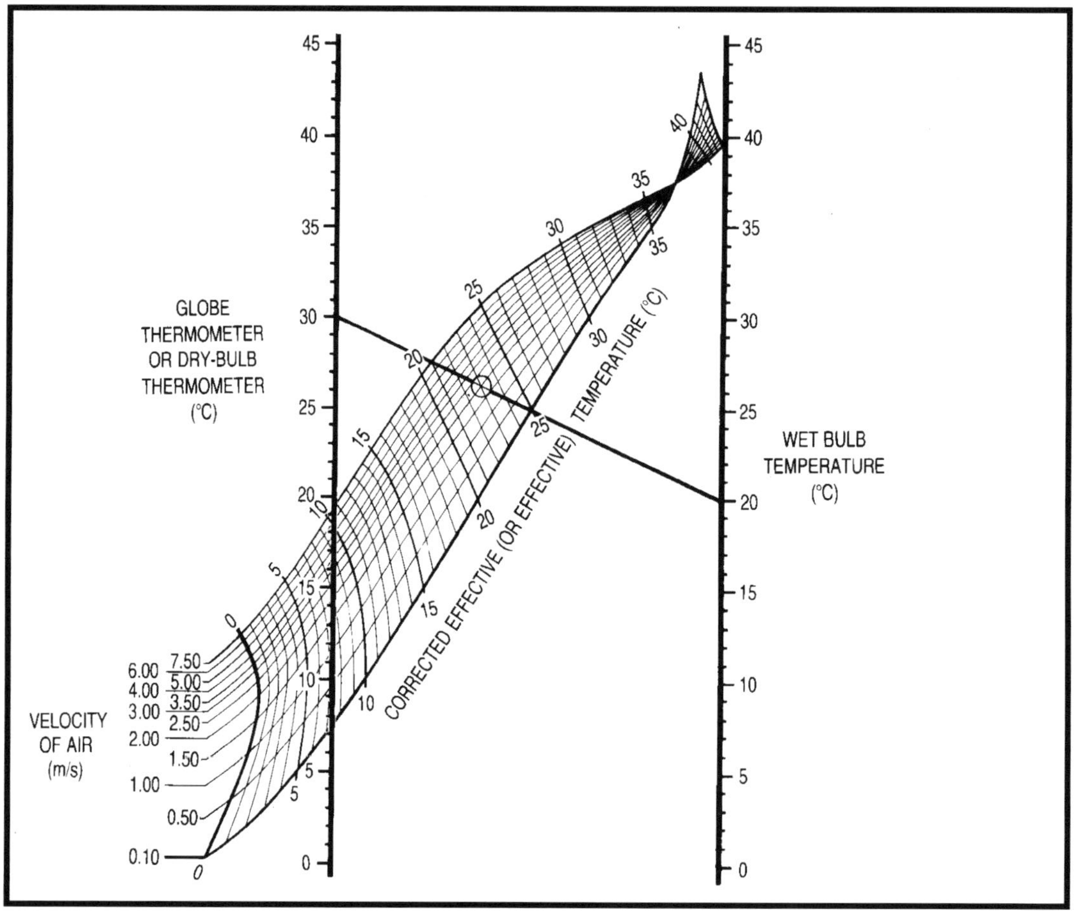

Figure 28.3 — Nomogram for the CET, or ET, normal scale.[5]

allowance for the effects of clothing worn and no allowance for the level of physical activity. Under severe conditions approaching the limits of tolerance, wet bulb temperature becomes the major determinate of heat strain, and the ET scale may underestimate the severity of these conditions.[29]

Wet Bulb Globe Temperature (WBGT)

The wet bulb globe temperature (WBGT) developed by Yaglou and Minard[30] was not based on analysis of a new set of prime data. Rather, it was derived from, and was a means for estimating, the CET. It was originally developed for use in controlling heat casualties at military training centers.[30]

The WBGT combines the effect of the four main thermal components affecting heat stress: air temperature, humidity, air velocity, and radiant heat, as measured by the dry bulb (T_{db}), natural wet bulb (T_{nwb}), and globe (T_g) temperatures. For indoor conditions (or outdoors without solar load, e.g., cloudy or shaded), WBGT values can be determined from the following equation:

$$WBGT = 0.7T_{nwb} + 0.3T_g \qquad (28.5)$$

For conditions with solar radiation, the equation becomes

$$WBGT = 0.7T_{nwb} + 0.2T_g + 0.1T_{ab} \qquad (28.6)$$

Different forms of these equations have been proposed to define WBGT estimates under different conditions, but these two are the most widely used and accepted.

In 1969, a panel of international experts from the World Health Organization (WHO) reviewed several thermal indices including CET and HSI. The panel determined that none of the indices specifically predicted the physiological strain to be expected from exposure to heat.[31]

NIOSH later established five principal criteria for a standard heat stress index for industrial use.[9] Based on these criteria it recommended the WBGT index as the standard heat stress index. The Occupational Safety and Health Administration (OSHA) Advisory Committee[32], American Conference of Governmental Industrial Hygienists (ACGIH®)[16], and ISO[33] have also recommended the WBGT as the primary heat stress index.

NIOSH (1972)[9] suggested the use of a tripod with thermometers measuring air, natural wet bulb, and globe temperature as the standard means for determining the WBGT. Integrated electronic instruments for measuring WBGT, such as those shown in Figure 28.4, are also commercially available. Such instruments provide a direct or digital readout of WBGT and, in some models, air velocity, dry bulb, wet bulb, and globe temperatures. The stabilization time required for the WBGT standard tree is at least 20 min, since it includes a globe thermometer that is 15 cm (6 in.) in diameter. The stabilization time required for the integrated electronic instruments is usually about 5 min, since all the sensors are resistance thermometers, and the globe has a small diameter of approximately 4 cm (< 2 inches).

Electronic instruments for personal heat stress monitoring are also available to register

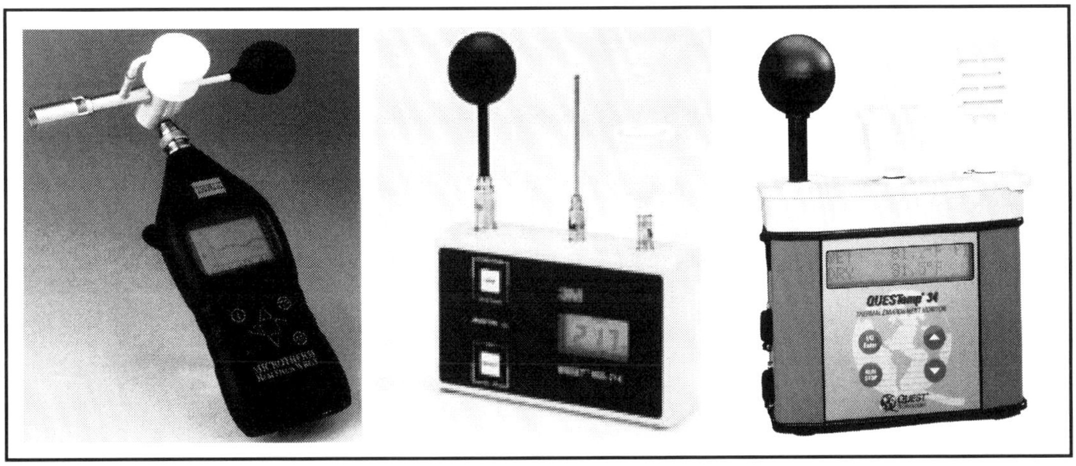

Figure 28.4 — Typical Electronic Instruments for Evaluating Heat Stress.

heart rate and/or body temperature via wrist, ear, or chest-placed sensors but correlation to body core temperature has shown to be inconsistent. Therefore, data gathered using these instruments should be analyzed carefully. Many attempts have been made to develop a single-reading heat stress instrument for assessing and integrating the environmental factors of air temperature, air speed, humidity, and radiant temperature. Among the instruments that have been proposed are the globe thermometer[34], the heated globe thermometer[35], the wet Kata thermometer[36], the eupathescope, the thermointegrator[37], and the wet globe thermometer.[38] Several of these instruments have been largely abandoned, and the search continues for improved single-reading instruments.

Typically, however, if the work allows it, a worker trained to recognize heat illness can recognize limiting conditions and make the necessary changes in his/her location duration or work intensity. Prediction of thermal work tolerance is discussed in Chapter 27.

Thermal Stress and the Required Sweat Rate

The international standard ISO 7933 incorporates the latest scientific information for computation and interpretation of thermal balance and the sweat rate required to maintain this balance, i.e., the required sweat rate.[14] This rational approach to assessing hot environments requires measurements of the thermal environment as well as a determination of the metabolic heat production and the clothing being worn. This approach is not valid for the worker wearing protective clothing. These data serve as input to the previously discussed basic heat balance equation, and calculations of each heat balance component are made using the equations shown in Table 28.3. Although this standard includes equations for respiratory heat loss and mechanized power, these are excluded here since they typically have less effect on thermal balance than is represented by the imprecision in determining metabolic heat.

Comparison of the required sweat rate and skin wetness with the maximum limiting values for skin wetness and sweat rate provides an indication of thermal severity of the work and heat. The resulting limits are expressed for both acclimatized and unacclimatized workers. Heat storage and the resulting increases in body temperature occur when thermal equilibrium is exceeded. Two levels of heat limits (warning and danger) are presented in terms of heat storage and maximum water loss. These limiting values for thermal stress and strain are shown in Table 28.4.

Allowable exposure time, or duration of limiting exposure, can also be calculated when thermal balance is not achieved. These thermal balance relationships are based on a 36°C body temperature associated with the onset of sweating. They also assume no impermeable protective clothing is being worn.

This ISO document also includes a BASIC language computer program for calculating all parameters used in the standard. This rational method provides useful information for engineering controls in the workplace, since the contribution of each thermal component is individually determined.

Other Heat Indices

Other indices that have been reported in the literature include predicted 4-hour sweat rate[39]; new effective temperature[40]; wet kata cooling power of air[41]; wet bulb-dry bulb index[42]; wet globe index[38]; temperature humidity index[43]; index of physiological effect[44]; index of thermal stress[45]; relative strain index[46]; reference index[47]; and others.[11]

The potential severity of heat stress is determined largely by weather conditions, even in the hot industries. The prevailing meteorological conditions, the onset of hot weather, and heat wave episodes can have a significant effect on the heat stress experienced by workers, and the public. Since 1985, the U.S. National Weather Service (NWS) has been using an abbreviated apparent temperature (called a heat index) as an index of heat discomfort during the summer months. This index includes the amplifying effect of increasing humidity on the discomfort level and is frequently reported by the news media to complement the report of daily summertime air temperatures. As shown in Table 28.5, an air temperature of 38°C/100°F and a 50% relative humidity "feels like" a temperature of 49°C/120°F. Apparent temperature ranges associated with different heat syndromes/ risks are also presented. The original apparent temperature model was reported in the field of meteorology.[48]

The U.S. and most countries around the world maintain details on environmental measurements that can be a useful supplement to the climatic factors measured at a work site. The NWS data include daily observations at 1 and 3-hr intervals for air temperature, wet bulb temperature, dew point temperature, relative humidity, wind velocity, sky cover, ceiling, and visibility. A summary of daily environmental measurements includes maximum, minimum and average temperatures as well as wind velocity (direction and speed), extent of sunshine and sky cover. These data can be used for an approximate assessment of the worksite environmental heat load for outdoor jobs or for some indoor jobs where air conditioning is not in use.

Table 28.4 — Reference Values for the Different Criteria of Thermal Stress and Strain[14]

	Nonacclimatized Subjects		*Acclimatized Subjects*	
Criteria	*Warning*	*Danger*	*Warning*	*Danger*
Maximum skin wetness (wmax)	0.85	0.85	1.0	1.0
Maximum sweat rate:				
Rest: (M < 65 watts/m²)[A]				
SW_{max}, watts/m²	100	150	200	300
SW_{max}, g/hr	260	390	520	780
Work: (M > 65 watts/m²)[A]				
SW_{max}, watts/m²	200	250	300	400
SW_{max}, g/hr	520	650	780	1040
Maximum heat storage				
Q_{max}, watts hr/m²	50	60	50	60
Maximum water loss				
D_{max}, watts hr/m²	1000	1250	1500	2000
D_{max}, g	2600	3250	3900	5200

[A]M = metabolic heat

Table 28.5 — Apparent Temperatures, °C/°F, and Heat Syndromes (adapted from National Oceanic and Atmospheric Administration)[48]

Air Temp. (°C / °F)	Apparent Temperatures[A]									
	10%	20%	30%	40%	50%	60%	70%	80%	90%	100%
52/125	51/123	61/141								
49/120	47/116	54/130	64/148							
46/115	44/111	49/120	57/135	66/151						
43/110	40/105	44/112	51/123	58/137	66/150					
40/105	38/100	40/105	45/113	51/123	57/135	65/149				
38/100	35/95	37/99	40/104	43/110	49/120	56/132	62/144			
35/95	32/90	34/93	36/96	38/101	42/107	45/114	51/124	58/136		
32/90	29/85	31/87	32/90	34/93	36/96	38/100	41/106	45/113	50/122	
29/85			29/84	30/86	31/88	32/90	34/93	36/97	39/102	42/108
27/80				26/79	27/81	28/82	29/85	30/86	31/88	33/91
24/75					24/75	24/76	25/77	26/78	26/79	27/80

Percent Humidity

[A]130°F or more (extremely hot), heatstroke or sunstroke is imminent; 105–130°F (very hot), sunstroke, heat cramps, and heat exhaustion likely, and heatstroke possible with prolonged exposure and physical activity; 90–105°F (hot), sunstroke, heat cramps, and heat exhaustion possible with prolonged exposure and physical activity; 80–90°F (very warm), fatigue possible with prolonged exposure and physical activity.

In 2000, the NWS instituted a Heat Index Program with Alert Procedures when the heat index is expected to exceed 105° to 110°F (depending on local climate) for at least two consecutive days.[49] The NWS heat index is based on the shady and light wind conditions and considers dry bulb temperature (>80°F and relative humidity from 40 to 100 percent in the determination of the heat index. The NWS issues advisories or warnings to the public when the heat index is expected to have a significant impact on public safety. At-risk populations are identified as the elderly, children, chronic invalids, those on certain medications or drugs, persons exercising or working outdoors, and persons with weight and alcohol problems. Heat Wave/Heat Index advisories and warnings include the extent of the hazard including heat index values, at risk populations, and recommendations for reducing risk. The NWS system utilizes a tabulated value from a Heat Index Chart to determine the risk associated with the expected conditions. The tabulated value is applied to the information in Table 28.6 for interpretation.[49]

Complicating factors such as the use of personal protective equipment, exposure to full sun, exposure to dry and hot wind, work other than light work limit somewhat the usefulness of the NWS Heat Index Program in the workplace. In 2006, 84% of the medically confirmed heat-related illnesses in the state of California occurred during a 12 day heat wave.[50] Therefore, the NWS Heat Index Program predictions can provide useful information about the conditions expected for outdoor work and allow time for assessment and implementation of controls. Heat stress monitoring of workers is suggested when a NWS Heat Index Program alert is issued.[51]

Heat Exposure Limits

The heat stress indices incorporate important thermal variables into a single number or scale with different degrees of success. The major application for a single index number is to define limits for exposure to hot occupational environments. Such limits may correspond to the upper, midrange, or lower levels of physiological impact and risk. Threshold values of thermal indices represent exposures above which a worker will be at some risk to heat illness. Upper, tolerance, or ceiling limits represent absolute maximum exposures above which work should not continue because the risk of heat illness is high. The term permissible exposure limit has been used in the literature alternately to represent threshold and ceiling limits as well as the range in between, and this has generated confusion at times.

Heat exposure limit values are typically based on some set of assumed physiological, personal, and/or environmental conditions. A number of factors, however, create variability and imprecision in the application of such limits: individual differences, worker populations, age, acclimatization, and health status, or errors in measuring or estimating metabolic work load or the environment.[52–55]

Since threshold limits are not associated with the high risk of heat illness, they may be defined in terms of levels at which nearly all, or some specific percentile of workers (e.g., 95%) may be repeatedly exposed without adverse effects. Upper or tolerance limits, however, are commonly based on a selected individual worker or a select work group in a hot environment rather than on the general population of workers.

Table 28.6 — National Weather Service Heat Index Advisory and Warning Interpretations.

Descriptive Zone	*Heat Index (°F)*	*Possible Heat Disorders for Higher Risk Groups*
Extreme Danger	130° or Higher	Heatstroke highly likely with continued exposure
Danger	105°– 130°	Heat cramps or heat exhaustion likely, and heatstroke possible with prolonged exposure and/or physical activity
Extreme Caution	90°–105°	Heat cramps or heat exhaustion likely, and heatstroke possible with prolonged exposure and/or physical activity
Caution	80° – 90°	Fatigue possible with prolonged exposure and/or physical activity

WBGT Recommendations

The most commonly used index for expressing limiting thermal exposure levels in occupational environments is the WBGT. The WBGT index has proved to be very successful in monitoring heat stress and minimizing heat casualties in the United States and has been widely adopted. The WBGT index provides a quick, convenient method to assess conditions that pose threats of thermal strain, with a minimum of operator skills. Because of its simplicity and close correlation with CET, it was adopted in 1971 (and has prevailed) as the principal index for the TLV® for heat stress established by the ACGIH®.[56]

One fundamental assumption used in threshold heat stress limits is that a worker's deep body temperature should not exceed 38°C. This was recommended by a WHO panel of physiologists[31] and is similar to the strain criteria of the Belding and Hatch HSI[21], which suggest that deep body temperature should not increase by more than 1°C.

Another major support for both the WHO recommendation and the development of the WBGT limits are Lind's prescriptive zone studies.[41,57] To use these studies to develop WBGT threshold limits, it was necessary to account for the effects of metabolic heat gain caused by work and to convert studies reported in ET into WBGT units. Lind's studies used ET measures with subjects who were unacclimatized and wore only shorts, whereas an industrial worker normally would be acclimatized and wear some form of worker uniform. The effect of clothing, which lowers the limits, and the effect of acclimatization, which raises them, were assumed to be approximately equal in magnitude and opposite in direction, and thus would cancel each other with no further modification. Lind's data using the basic ET scale for partially clothed men was first converted to the normal ET scale for clothed men and then to WBGT, using the relationships suggested by Minard.[58] This resulted in the development of a threshold permissible exposure limit (PEL). The PEL was designed to represent a work temperature and WBGT combination that protected 95% of the workers from exceeding an average deep body temperature of 38°C.The 38°C limit is widely accepted as an average limit for prolonged daily exposure to heavy work; however, it is considered conservative as a limit for many individuals and for short exposure periods. Persons who are medically screened and under experimental surveillance commonly exceed 39°C without noticeable ill effects.[59] One way to circumvent debate on the 38°C/39°C limits is to reference rate of changes in deep body temperature to specific physiological heat tolerance and exposure limits.[60]

Although the WBGT index is convenient and simple to use, the WBGT is not a perfect predictor of physiological strain. Ramanathan and Belding, among others, have shown that environmental combinations yielding the same WBGT levels can result in different physiological strains.[61] This suggests that WBGT has limitations as a heat stress index, especially at high levels of severity. In addition, when impermeable clothing is worn, the WBGT will not be a relevant index, because evaporative cooling (wet bulb temperature) will be limited. Nevertheless, WBGT has become the index most frequently used and recommended for use throughout the world.[62]

Time-Weighted Average

Because any workday or work period can consist of varying levels of both thermal exposure (WBGT) and metabolic heat (M), it is necessary to calculate time-weighted average (TWA) values to determine the total heat or work impact. To calculate the time-weighted average of the variable x.

$$TWA(x) = \frac{(x_1t_1 + x_2t_2 + \dots + x_nt_n)}{(t_1 + t_2 + \dots + t_n)} \qquad (28.7)$$

where:

x = value of WBGT or M
x_n = value during period n of WBGT or M
t_n = time in minutes of period n

NIOSH Recommendations

A criteria document for a recommended standard concerning occupational exposure to hot environments was developed by NIOSH.[9] This document recommended that one or more work practices be instituted when "exposure of an employee is continuous for one hour or intermittent for a period of two hours at a time-weighted average WBGT that exceeds 79°F (26.1°C) for men or 76°F (24.4°C) for women." The suggested limits represent the point of WBGT intersection with 400 kcal/hour (465 watts) workload on the WBGT chart (Figure 28.5). This workload is the maximum anticipated as an hourly TWA in American industry. The lower value for women was intended to compensate for differences from men. Subsequent research concerning male/female differences has established that such differences more commonly represent differences in physical work capacity or heat acclimatization, and that different limits would be better based on these factors than on gender.[59]

A revised criteria document was issued in 1986 that changed exposure limit calculations to a 1-hour TWA and also removed the differential related to gender.[63] Also included in this revision were recommended alert limits (RAL) for unacclimatized workers, recommended exposure limits (REL) for acclimatized workers, and ceiling limits (CL) beyond which appropriate and adequate heat protective clothing and equipment should be required. A summary of the recommended limits for acclimatized workers (REL) is shown in Figure 28.6. The RAL values for unacclimatized workers are lower than the REL by 2°C for light work, 2.5°C for moderate work and 3°C for heavy work. These limits were based on a "standard worker" of 70 kg body weight and 1.8 m² body surface.

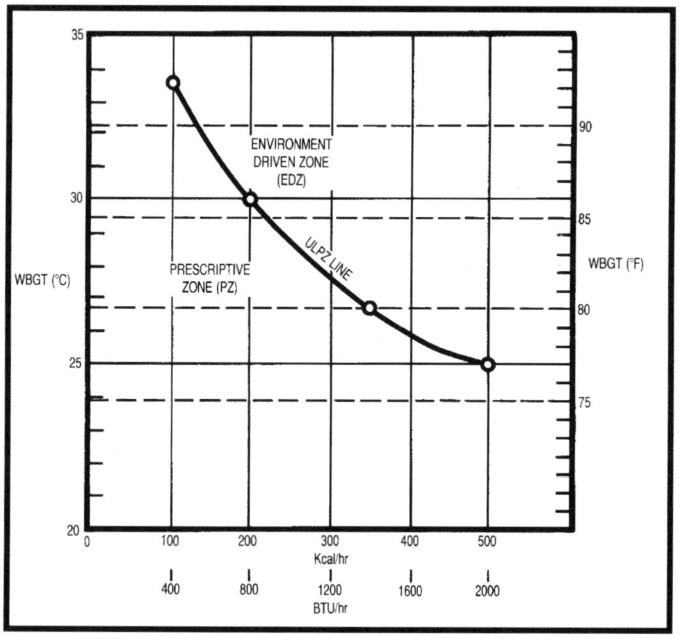

Figure 28.5 — Permissible exposure limit chart.[14]

Bernard has developed a set of equations for estimating the NIOSH recommended limits shown in Figure 28.6.[64] These limits are depicted in Figure 28.6 and can be calculated as follows:

$$REL = 56.7 - 11.5 \log_{10} M \quad (28.8)$$

$$RAL = 60.0 - 14.1 \log_{10} M \quad (28.9)$$

$$CL = 70.0 - 13.5 \log_{10} M \quad (28.10)$$

where:

REL = Recommended Exposure Limit (°C WBGT)
RAL = Recommended Alert Limit (°C WBGT)
CL = Ceiling Limit (°C WBGT)
M = Metabolic Rate (W)

ACGIH® Threshold Limit Values®

The permissible heat exposure Threshold Limit Values® (TLVs®) developed by ACGIH® served as a basis for the original NIOSH criteria document recommendations.[9] For many years the TLVs®[65] for acclimatized and unacclimatized workers have been basically the same, except for name changes, as in the 1986 NIOSH REL and RAL, respectively.[5] The 2001 TLVs® and BEIs® edition published by ACGIH®, however, departed from earlier editions in its approach to heat stress and heat strain.[66]

The 1999 Notice of Intended Change to the ACGIH® TLVs® proposed a change of title from "Heat Stress" to "Heat Stress and Heat Strain," and important changes in content and format continued through several iterations until a final version was approved in 2007.[62,67] ACGIH® identifies the formerly titled "Permissible heat exposure TLVs®" as "Screening Criteria for Heat Exposure". If screening values are exceeded a detailed analysis would be conducted following rational models of heat stress such as those found in ISO 7933[14] to determine if there is excessive heat stress. If detailed rational analysis shows excessive heat stress, physiological monitoring of the individual worker heat strain would be indicated. Since most WBGT-based heat exposure assessment was developed for traditional work uniforms, physiological monitoring was also recommended for evaluating heat strain of workers in impermeable clothing. The 2001 edition[66] also removed the details of determining metabolic workload, and it refers the reader to documentation in other industrial hygiene and safety sources. As shown in Table 28.7, TLV® screening values for acclimatized workers working 50–75% of the time with light, moderate, and heavy work demands are 31.0°C, 29.0°C, and 27.5, respectively. For unacclimatized workers the values are 28.5°C, 26.0°C, and 24.0°C, respectively. Note that the TLVs® are based on allocation of work in a cycle of work and recovery (rest) and must be adjusted accordingly. Additionally, screening criteria values for heavy (up to 25% rest) and very heavy work (up to 50% rest) are not provided because the physiological strain associated with these levels of work among less fit workers are not recommended and detailed analysis and/or physiological monitoring should be used.[16] Table 27.3 provides some guidance on re-acclimatization for different periods away from heat exposures whether due to routine reasons such as reassignment, vacation or injury or for illness.[64]

Although both NIOSH and ACGIH® originally used the same basic relationships between environmental heat (WBGT) and metabolic heat (M) to determine the threshold exposure limits, the TLVs® included the information in tabular format as well as the graphic form depicted in Figure 28.6.[63] The table extracted from this graph in the past, however, was represented in its most conservative interpretation in that WBGT TLVs® were associated with the maximum metabolic rate in the range. This meant for example the TLV® of 25°C for all heavy work (between 400 W and 580 W) was selected at an M of 580 W, a level which probably never occurs as an hourly time-weighted average in a work-place in the U.S.

The table format for expressing a WBGT limit for different proportions of work was retained, but it should be emphasized that the table represents screening criteria and not the TLV® because of the approximations that are required.

The WBGT values have been increased for each proportion of metabolic rate from previous values because a mid-range value for metabolic rate was used rather than the high end value of past practice. This provides a rational and appropriate, but less conservative screening criterion.

The TLV® also provides information such as the measurement and calculation of WBGT, correction factors for different clothing ensembles, methods for assessment of work load, water and salt supplementation, acclimatization, and adverse health effects. A flow chart provides a simplified format for evaluation process, which starts with the screening criteria, to a more detailed WBGT evaluations and rational heat stress assessments as well as physiological criteria for heat-stressed workers, which better addresses the protection of those wearing impermeable clothing.

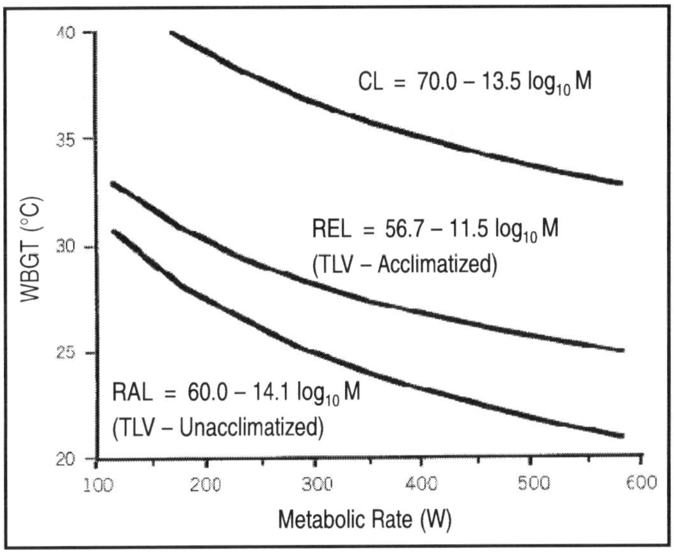

Figure 28.6 — NIOSH recommended heat stress alert limits (RAL) and recommended exposure limits (REL) as well as the ceiling limit (CL). (Note: The ACGIH® Action Limit is equivalent to the RAL and is called the TLV® for unacclimatized workers in the figure, and the TLV® is the same as the REL and was called the TLV® for acclimatized workers.). (This figure is provided courtesy of the National Safety Council, Itasca, Illinois.).[64]

Table 28.7 — Current ACGIH® Screening Criteria for Heat Stress Exposure where WBGT Criterion Values for Work Rate Categories are Based on Acclimatization State and Percent of Work in a One to Two Hour Cycle.[16]

% Work	*Acclimatized*			
	Light	*Moderate*	*Heavy*	*Very Heavy*
100% to 75%	31.0	28.0	—	—
75% to 50%	31.0	29.0	27.5	—
50% to 25%	32.0	30.0	29.0	28.0
<25%	32.5	31.5	30.5	30.0
% Work	*Unacclimatized (Action Limit)*			
	Light	*Moderate*	*Heavy*	*Very Heavy*
100% to 75%	28.0	25.0	—	—
75% to 50%	28.5	26.0	24.0	—
50% to 25%	29.05	27.0	25.5	24.5
<25%	30.0	29.0	28.0	27.0

ISO Recommendations

ISO[33] has also adopted a heat stress standard based on the WBGT index. Limits are based on 1-hour time-weighted WBGT values for workers who are normally clothed, physically fit, of standard size with surface area of 1.8 m^2, and in good health. Included are five metabolic rate classes that range from resting to a very high metabolic rate and an adjustment for acclimatization. Limits for most unacclimatized workers are 1 to 3°C lower than for acclimatized workers. In the case of heavy and very heavy metabolic work load, a different WBGT is indicated where there is sensible air movement compared with no sensible air movement. These limits are shown in the summary information of Table 28.9. When limits are exceeded ISO 7243 recommends rational methods described in ISO 7933[14] be used to better evaluate worker heat exposure.

Effects of Clothing on WBGT Calculations

The principal purpose of clothing in a work environment is to provide a barrier against hazardous chemical, physical, and biological agents. But clothing also alters the rate of heat exchange between the skin and the ambient air by convection, radiation and evaporation; and this effect can be significant. When estimating worker-environment heat exchange, correction factors must be used to reflect the type, amount and characteristics of the clothing being worn. The recent TLVs® include some basic guidelines for adjusting WBGT calculations depending on the type of clothing utilized.[67]

Table 28.8 — Clothing Adjustment Factors (CAF) Reported by the ACGIH® and Others.[26,67–70]

Clothing	*CAF [°C]*
Work Clothes	0
Cloth Coveralls	0
FR Cloth Clothing	0
Two-Layer Cloth Clothing	3
SMS Polypropylene Coveralls Over Modesty Clothing	0.5
Tyvek® Coveralls Over Modesty Clothing	1
Polyolefin coveralls	1
Limited-use Vapor Barrier Coveralls Over Modesty Clothing	10
Hood Configuration with Above	+1

Adjustments to the measured WBGT for clothing ensembles other than ordinary work clothes can be made. Some of these are provided in Table 28.8.[16,26,67–70]

Comparison of WBGT Recommendations

Table 28.9 summarizes and compares several of the proposed Screening Criteria for the TLV® where work load levels have been specified to correspond to certain WBGT values. When the different metabolic heat assumptions are considered and criteria are compared, a strong pattern of consistency is observed: resting, 33°C; light, 30–31°C; moderate, 28°C; heavy, 25–26°C; and very heavy, 23–25°C. Given the imprecision attendant on estimating metabolic work load and the variability of metabolic costs during the day and from day to day, the WBGT threshold values in Table 28.9 are all basically equivalent.

Limited Exposure Times

There are times when an exposure to heat stress is not sustained for long periods (over two hours). In these cases, the job risk factors are the traditional environment, work demands, clothing, and time. Short exposure times at heat stress conditions above the WBGT-based occupational exposure limits (e.g., REL and TLV®) remain to be safe. The U.S. Navy in their Physiological Heat Exposure Limit (PHEL) curves and the Electric Power Research Institute (EPRI) Action Times recognize the time factor. The following is guidance may be an aide in setting safe exposure times above the TLV®.[71] It applies to times between 10 and 120 minutes.

$$\text{Time Limit [min]} = 22{,}000/(WBGT_{adj}[°C] - TLV_M[W]^3) + 10 \qquad (28.11)$$

$$TLV_M[W] = 57.6 - 11.5 \log_{10} M[W] \qquad (28.12)$$

$$WBGT_{adj}[°C] = WBGT_{measured} + CAF - 0.02(380 - M[W]) \qquad (28.13)$$

Cold Exposure Limits

Limits for exposure to cold environments are difficult to specify since the amount of clothing and its insulating characteristics have such a dominant effect on the extent of cold exposure. The effects of exposure to cold environments also vary dramatically based on the amount of metabolic heat being generated by any work being performed. A sleeping bag can provide enough insulation to withstand extreme cold conditions, even though the contribution of metabolic heat is low. The worker dressed in heavy clothing may be comfortable at light work, sweating inside these clothes during heavy work periods, then very cold during a subsequent rest break with the damp clothing and low metabolic heat. Thus, the worker can go through zones of comfort, heat stress, and cold stress with the same clothing and thermal exposure.

Table 28.9 — A Comparison of Proposed WBGT Threshold Values for Acclimatized Workers

Work Load	*ACGIH®(16)*	*ISO(33)*	*NIOSH[63]*
Resting		33°C <100 kcal/hr (<117 watts)	
Light	31°C 100–200 kcal/hr (117-233 watts)	30°C 100–201 kcal/hr (117–234 watts)	30°C <200 kcal/hr (<233 watts)
Moderate	28°C 201–300 kcal/hr (234–349 watts)	28°C 201–310 kcal/hr (234–360 watts)	28°C 201–300 kcal/hr (234–349 watts)
Heavy		25°CA, 26°CB 310–403 kcal/hr (360–468 watts)	26°C 301–400 kcal/hr (350–465 watts)
Very Heavy		23°CA, 25°CB >403 kcal/hr (>468 watts)	25°C 401–500 kcal/hr (466-580 watts)

[A]Low air velocity (no sensible air movement)
[B]High air velocity (sensible air movement)

Windchill Index

In 2001, the NWS implemented an updated Windchill Temperature Index (WCI) in collaboration with the Meteorological Service of Canada so that there would be one WCI for all of North America.(72) The change improves upon the former WCI Index used by the NWS and the Meteorological Service of Canada, which was based on the 1945 Siple and Passel Index. The original Siple and Passel Index was developed using the freezing rate of a plastic container of water, while the updated WCI utilized human subjects and is based on the human face model.(73)

The WCI represents the most universally accepted scale for describing the combined cooling effects of air temperature and wind velocity. This index provides a more accurate description of cold thermal conditions than air temperature alone since, at constant temperature, the risk of tissue freezing increases with air movement (convection). The current formula uses advances in science, technology, and computer modeling to provide a more accurate, understandable, and useful formula for calculating the dangers from winter winds and freezing temperatures. The WCI provides a useful means of estimating those combinations of temperature and wind speed likely to freeze non-wetted exposed human flesh.(25,73) The NWS does not provide the updated WCI in metric units, but the Meteorological Services of Canada published an equivalent equation to calculate the WCI in metric units.(72) The new WCI formulas are:

$$WCI_{new}[°F] = 35.74 + 0.6215T_a - 35.75(V_{ar}^{0.16}) + 0.4275(V_{ar}^{0.16}) \quad (28.14)$$

$$WCI_{new}[°C] = 13.12 + 0.6215T_a - 11.37(V_{ar}^{0.16}) + 0.3965(V_{ar}^{0.16}) \quad (28.15)$$

where:

WCI = windchill index, °C (metric), °F (US)
V_{ar} = relative air velocity, km/hr (metric), miles/hr (US)
T_a = air temperature, °C (metric), °F (US)

For the first time, the new Wind Chill Chart includes a frostbite indicator, showing the points where temperature, wind speed and exposure time will produce frostbite on exposed human flesh. Table 28.10 includes three shaded areas of frostbite danger. Each shaded area shows how long (30, 10, and 5 minutes) bare skin can be exposed before frostbite develops.(18) Although the WCT is expressed on a temperature scale (°C or °F), it is *not* a temperature: it expresses the human sensation of the cooling power of wind.(72) For example, a temperature of 0°F and a wind speed of 15 mph will produce a wind chill temperature of -28.6°C (-19.5°F). Under these conditions, exposed skin can freeze in 30 minutes.(73) Special precautions to protect bare skin against the cold must be taken when the wind chill is less than -27°C (-17°F).(18)

The WCI does not recognize the amount of clothing being worn, but relates instead to bare skin such as the face and hands. It does provide a comparative scale for cooling power, but exaggerates the importance of wind for the person dressed in heavy clothing and having face/hand protection.[25] This overstatement of freezing power results in WCI values that are conservative and, thus, safe to use. Environment Canada's protective recommendations based on the WCI are summarized in Table 28.11.

ACGIH® Recommendations

Windchill reflects the cooling power of wind on exposed flesh and is commonly expressed by a related index called equivalent temperature. When equivalent temperature is below freezing, cold injury can occur. The ACGIH® TLV's® for cold stress are expressed in terms of equivalent temperature. The higher the wind speed and the lower the temperature in the work area, the greater the insulation value of the protective clothing required. The 2009 ACGIH® TLV's® for cold stress provide recommendations and provisions for protection from the cold, protective clothing, and work-warming regimens for working in the cold (in dry clothing). Workers who become wet should not work in the cold and should seek warm shelter immediately. The equivalent chill temperature should be utilized when estimating the combined cooling effect of wind and low air temperatures on skin or when determining clothing insulation requirements to maintain the body's core temperature.[16] The cooling power of wind on exposed flesh is shown in Table 28.12.

Adequate insulating dry clothing and provisions for total body protection must be provided to workers if work is performed below 4°C (39.2°F). This represents a body temperature above the point of intense shivering and more serious health effects. The uncontrollable physiological response of shivering provides a good warning signal to the worker that the combined exposure effects of temperature, clothing, and metabolic heat are going beyond discomfort and into potential health-related problems. See the ACGIH® TLVs® and BEIs®[16] for more detailed information and to determine work-warming regimens.

Required Clothing Insulation (IREQ)

An index of required clothing insulation (IREQ) is presented in ISO/TR 11079.[75] This index uses the same general concepts of thermal equilibrium as previously discussed for hot environments. Originally proposed by Holmér[76,77] IREQ assumes a minimal cold tolerance level for skin temperature of 30°C and skin wetness of 0.06 in a stationary standing man. With these assumptions the amount of

Table 28.10 — Updated Wind Chill Temperature Index (°C) as a combination of temperature and wind speed (calculated using Environment Canada formula).[72]

Wind Speed		Temperature (°F)														
		25	20	15	10	5	0	-5	-10	-15	-20	-25	-30	-35	-40	-45
mph	km/h	Temperature (°C)														
Calm	Calm	-4	-7	-9	-12	-15	-18	-21	-23	-26	-29	-32	-34	-37	-40	-43
5	8	-7.3	-10.6	-13.9	-17.1	-20.4	-23.6	-26.9	-30.2	-33.4	-36.7	-40.0	-43.2	-46.5	-49.8	-53.0
10	16	-9.4	-12.9	-16.3	-19.8	-23.2	-26.7	-30.1	-33.5	-37.0	-40.4	-43.9	-47.3	-50.8	-54.2	-57.7
15	24	-10.8	-14.3	-17.9	-21.5	-25.0	-28.6	-32.1	-35.7	-39.3	-42.8	-46.4	-49.9	-53.5	-57.1	-60.6
20	32	-11.8	-15.4	-19.1	-22.7	-26.4	-30.0	-33.7	-37.3	-41.0	-44.6	-48.3	-51.9	-55.5	-59.2	-62.8
25	40	-12.6	-16.3	-20.0	-23.8	-27.5	-31.2	-34.9	-38.6	-42.3	-46.1	-49.8	-53.5	-57.2	-60.9	-64.6
30	48	-13.3	-17.1	-20.9	-24.6	-28.4	-32.2	-36.0	-39.7	-43.5	-47.3	-51.1	-54.8	-58.6	-62.4	-66.1
35	56	-13.9	-17.7	-21.6	-25.4	-29.2	-33.0	-36.9	-40.7	-44.5	-48.3	-52.2	-56.0	-59.8	-63.6	-67.5
40	64	-14.4	-18.3	-22.2	-26.1	-29.9	-33.8	-37.7	-41.5	-45.4	-49.3	-53.1	-57.0	-60.9	-64.8	-68.6
45	72	-14.9	-18.8	-22.7	-26.7	-30.6	-34.5	-38.4	-42.3	-46.2	-50.1	-54.0	-57.9	-61.9	-65.8	-69.7
50	80	-15.4	-19.3	-23.2	-27.2	-31.1	-35.1	-39.0	-43.0	-46.9	-50.9	-54.8	-58.8	-62.7	-66.7	-70.6
55	89	-15.8	-19.7	-23.7	-27.7	-31.7	-35.7	-39.7	-43.6	-47.6	-51.6	-55.6	-59.6	-63.5	-67.5	-71.5
60	97	-16.1	-20.1	-24.2	-28.2	-32.2	-36.2	-40.2	-44.2	-48.2	-52.3	-56.3	-60.3	-64.3	-68.3	-72.3
Time to Frostbite:					30 minutes		10 minutes		5 minutes							

Table 28.11 — Adapted from the Meteorological Service of Canada's Wind Chill Hazards and Recommendations for Protection against the cold for a person who is dry.[72]

Wind Chill	*Temperature Description*	*Concern Level (Health Concerns)*	*Recommendations*
0 to -9	Low	Caution (Slight increase in discomfort.)	Dress warmly, with the outside temperature in mind.
-10 to -24	Moderate	Caution (Uncomfortable. Exposed skin feels cold. Risk of hypothermia if outside for long periods without adequate protection.)	Dress in layers of warm clothing, with an outer layer that is wind resistant. Wear a hat, mittens and scarf, and appropriate footwear. Keep active.
-25 to -44	Cold	Extreme Caution (Risk of skin freezing (frostbite). Risk of hypothermia if outside for long periods without adequate protection.)	In addition to the recommendations above for moderate: • Wear a neck tube and/or face mask. • Cover all exposed skin, particularly your face and hands. • Check face, fingers, toes, ears and nose for numbness or whiteness. • Be observant and careful.
-45 to -59	Extreme	DANGER (Exposed skin may freeze in minutes. Serious risk of hypothermia if outside for long periods.)	In addition to the recommendations above for cold: • Be prepared to shorten or cancel outdoor activities. • Be observant and very careful.
≤ -60	Extreme	EXTREME DANGER (Outdoor conditions are dangerous. Exposed skin may freeze in less than 2 minutes.)	Stay indoors. Cancel all non-emergency activities.

Table 28.12 — Cooling Power of Wind on Exposed Flesh Expressed as Equivalent Temperature. Adapted from (74) to include the ACGIH® TLV® recommendations for additional dry clothing.[16]

Equivalent Chill Temperature

Estimated Wind Speed		Actual Temperature Reading															
		(°F)								(°C)							
mph	km/hr	50	40	20	10	0	-10	-30	-50	10	4.4	-6.7	-12	-18	-23	-34	-45.6
calm	calm	50	40	20	10	0	-10	-30	-50	10	4.4	-6.7	-12	-18	-23	-34	-45.6
5	8	48	37	16	6	-5	-15	-36	-57	8.9	2.8	-8.9	-14	-21	-26	-38	-49.4
10	16	40	28	4	-9	-24	-33	-58	-83	4.4	-2.2	-16	-23	-31	-36	-50	-63.9
15	25	36	22	-5	-18	-32	-45	-72	-99	2.2	5.6	-21	-28	-36	-43	-63	-72.8
20	32	32	18	-10	-25	-39	-53	-82	-99	0	-7.8	-23	-32	-39	-47	-63	-72.8
30	48	28	13	-18	-33	-48	-63	-94	-125	-2.2	-11	-28	-36	-44	-53	-70	-87.2
40	64	26	10	-21	-37	-53	-69	-100	-132	-3.3	-12	-29	-38	-47	-56	-73	-91.1
Winds above 40 mph (64 km/h) have little additional effect.		LITTLE DANGER (1)			INCREASING DANGER (2)			GREAT DANGER (3)		LITTLE DANGER (1)			INCREASING DANGER (2)			GREAT DANGER (3)	

Freeze Danger

(1) Little Danger from freezing (< 1 hr exposure with dry skin). Max. danger of false sense of security.

(2) Increasing Danger from freezing of exposed flesh w/in one minute.

(3) Great Danger from freezing of Exposed flesh may freeze w/in 30 seconds.

Note: Trenchfoot and immersion foot may occur at any point on this chart.

[shaded] Equivalent chill temperature requiring dry clothing to maintain core body temperature above 36°C (96.8°F) per cold stress TLV.

insulation required to obtain thermal balance can be calculated. Equilibrium in the cold occurs when the heat conducted from the skin (t_{sk}) to the clothing surface equals the dry heat loss from the clothing surface to the environment (t_{cl}). Thus, IREQ can be expressed as

$$IREQ = \frac{t_{sk} - t_{cl}}{M} - W - H_{res} - E \qquad (28.16)$$

where:

$$M - W - H_{res} - E = R + C(17)$$

and

t_{sk} = heat conducted from the skin
t_{cl} = dry heat loss from clothing to environment
M = metabolic rate
W = external work rate
H_{res} = respiratory heat loss (convective and evaporative)
E = evaporative heat loss
R = radiative heat loss
C = convective heat loss

Calculation of IREQ requires an iterative procedure since t_{cl} is not a measured value. Computer programs are available for this and related calculations.[78]

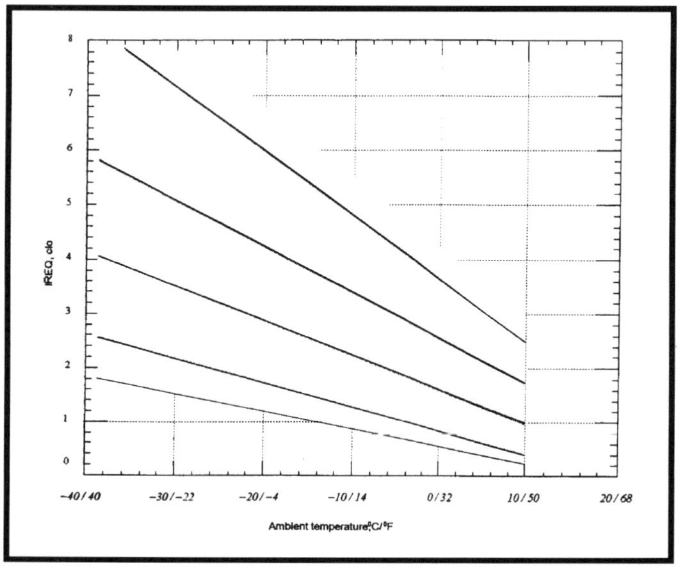

Figure 28.6 — Required Clothing Insulation (IREQ) for Different Classes of Activity.[77]

The low skin temperature (30°C) and wetness (0.06) relate to uncomfortably cool conditions that will not produce sweating and the interference from moisture absorbing into the clothing, refreezing, and producing complications in determining the insulation requirements. Figure 28.6 depicts typical relationships of IREQ and metabolic rate, where increased metabolic rate allows reduction in insulating requirements at any given temperature.

To determine IREQ for a specific environment requires a measurement of the various temperatures, air velocity, and an estimate of metabolic activity using methods or tables previously discussed. Then the basic thermal balance equations are used to determine the IREQ, which is not exactly the same as the clothing insulation (clo) value normally cited with standard clothing. In most cases a higher clothing insulation value should be selected since differences in motion and wind penetration affect heat loss and reduce the effectiveness of the clothing. These factors are included in the IREQ.

Thermal Effects on Performance and Safety

Effects of Heat

Effects on Physical Performance

The effects of hot environments on physical work output and on manual task performance are reasonably well understood and documented.[79,80] Physical work in a hot environment generates physiological responses that are readily measurable and physical fatigue that is readily noticeable.

Thermal exposure of such intensity and duration that it contributes to localized or general fatigue will negatively affect physical work capacity. Loss of performance capacity during physical activity in the heat can be measured in reduced production output, speed, quality, or repetitions per unit time. Deterioration in work output due to heat, as measured by military marching rates, has been observed.[78] It has been concluded that hot environments significantly reduce the work load of manual handling tasks. A temperature increase from 17 to 27°C WBGT has reduced workload by 20% for lifting, 16% for pushing, and 11% for carrying tasks.[81] Scheduling interim rest cycles during physical work under hot, ambient conditions has been suggested as a means to increase work efficiency by reducing physiological cost.[82]

Effects on Perceptual-Motor Performance

Although decreases in physical work capacity in the heat are relatively predictable, human performance is much more unpredictable when it involves sedentary work, low metabolic costs, perceptual-motor skills, or mental activities. Research concerning the effect of heat on perceptual-motor performance has been extensive and often contradictory.

Many studies have attempted to isolate the effects of heat on a sedentary or standing person performing light work-load tasks involving perceptual motor and mental tasks. Several authors have summarized or generalized from these individual investigations.[83–87] The data summarized by Wing[83] became the basis for the upper limits of exposure for unimpaired mental performance suggested by NIOSH.[63] However, these recommendations were omitted from the revised criteria document.[63]

Continuing research has indicated that the degree of performance decrement on such work tasks in the heat is dominated by the type of task being performed. Heat appears to have a very small effect on mental or very simple tasks and, indeed, brief exposures to the heat may even enhance task performance. This does not imply that work on a simple task will not deteriorate in performance over time, but simply that it will not deteriorate differently based on the presence of heat. Other perceptual motor tasks such as tracking, vigilance, eye-hand coordination, and combinations of these tasks do tend to show losses in performance due to heat. These tasks depict a pattern of onset of performance decrement in the 30–33°C (86–91°F) WBGT temperature range, and the decrement appears to be relatively independent of exposure time.[88] This is the same temperature range that is associated with the onset of physiological heat stress for the worker performing sedentary or light work, as shown in the REL for Figure 28.6.

In summary, performance on specific task, under a specific set of thermal conditions, is difficult to predict precisely due to the wide range of individual personal characteristics that relate to the handling of thermal loads and to the person's skill in performing the specific task. General relationships that may be useful, however, in designing work tasks in hot environments include the following:[87]

- Performance in a hot environment and for exposure periods that yield general fatigue will also yield general performance decrements.
- Acclimatization will aid physiological adjustment and reduce the strain of a task. With perceptual-motor tasks, the effect is less pronounced, although there is evidence that acclimatization reduces performance variability and improves performance.
- Performing mental or simple perceptual-motor tasks during brief exposure to high temperature levels results in only minor decrement, or even enhancement of performance because of the arousal effects of the heat. Most other tasks, however, show onset of performance decrement around 30–33°C (86–91°F) WBGT.
- Hot temperatures seem to affect skilled or trained persons differently, depending on the level of mental or physical load at non-heat levels. If the work task does not load the operator, the addition of heat causes an arousal effect that enhances or minimally affects the performances. If the work task has already created an overload, the addition of heat will tend to degrade performance.
- Perceptual-motor performance within the comfort zone is generally best at the cooler end of the zone.
- A commonly reported relationship between performance of perceptual-motor tasks and the thermal conditions is the inverted U, where performance is highest at midrange temperatures and decreases with positive or negative changes in temperature.

Effects of Cold

The most significant effect of cold exposure is on manual dexterity. Many studies of performance in cold have emphasized the effects of cold on the skillful use of the hands. An individual required to work in the cold normally has protective, insulating layers of clothing consistent with the severity of the cold. Thus, the internal microclimate of the body may be relatively stable under normal cold conditions. Adequately protecting the hands, however, is difficult because manual dexterity and general handwork are adversely affected by increased thermal insulation and protection. Dusek[89] reported that at finger temperatures below 15.6°C (60°F), significant decrease in manual performance occurred. Below 10°C (50°F), there is onset of pain and extensive loss of manual abilities. Below 4.4°C (40°F), tactual discrimination is lost, as is the ability to perform fine manipulative movements. Significant correlations were observed between manual task performance and the skin temperatures of the hand, the finger, and the upper arm, mean skin temperature and mean body temperature during cold exposure.[90] The skin temperature of the hand and the mean skin temperature showed highest correlations with performance. After a 1-hour exposure to cold, manual performance of subjects wearing cold-protective clothing with cotton work gloves showed continuing deterioration as the environmental temperature level lowered to -20°C (-4°F).[90]

Motor skill loss in the cold occurs more rapidly for fine motor skills than for gross motor skills. The National Association of Building Contractors considers guidelines for reduction in motor skills as 10%, 20%, and 25%, for gross motor skills and 60%, 80%, and 90% for fine motor skills at -18°C (0°F), -23°C (-10°F), -29°C (-20°F) ET, respectively. These guidelines assume that the worker has the proper clothing to provide protection. The consensus is that loss of perceptual-motor performance in the cold is primarily a deterioration of motor capabilities rather than mental deterioration. The opportunity to warm the hands or remove them from cold exposure periodically can help reduce the loss of manipulative motor skills. Hand protection is recommended, if manual dexterity is not critical, for temperatures below 16°C (60.8°F) for sedentary work or below -7°C (19.4°F) for moderate work.[65] Mittens offer more protection than gloves since air does not have contact with each finger. A layered ensemble of gloves covered with mittens offers the highest degree of cold protection. Performance losses as a function of lower body temperature have also been reported.

Cognitive mental tasks are much less affected by the cold than are motor tasks. However, it is often difficult to separate these effects because results of mental activity are generally manifested in some motor movement that is more likely to be affected by cold. Cold exposure affects visual acuity as a result of ocular discomfort, including tearing and sensations of dryness accompanies by frequent blinking.[91] The general psychological responses to prolonged work in the cold can be significant. Elements of isolation and confinement due to cold work locations as well as discomfort from the cold have been noted to result in behavioral responses. These include changes in arousal, perception, mood, personality, apathy, etc.[25]

Prolonged contact with surfaces having temperatures be3low 15°C (59°F), may impact dexterity; below 7°C (45°F) may induce numbness; and below -0°C (32°F) may induce frost nip or frostbite.(77) When surfaces are below -7°C (19.4°F), warnings should be given to prevent inadvertent contact by bare skin, and hand protection should be provided if air temperature is below -17.5°C (0°F).[65]

Effects on Safety Incident (Accident) and Safety Behavior

There have been only a few extensive studies of thermal effects on safety. One report describes a study of over 2000 accidents in four types of industrial workshops[92], air temperature had a significant effect on accidents in two of the observed plants; the observed temperatures were in the 15–24°C (59–75°F) range and higher accident rates occurred at the lower temperatures. In the third plant, there were no temperature effects on accidents. The fourth plant was analyzed differently because of the small number of accidents.

As previously mentioned, NIOSH recommendations for upper limits of thermal exposure for unimpaired mental performance imply that a thermal environment that impairs mental performance may also negatively affect safety and incident frequency. Results of a 4-year study of accidents in a steel mill show that peak accident rates occur during peak air and dew point temperatures.[93]

Surry[94] states that “the conditions for thermal comfort are essentially the same for peak work efficiency and for minimum accident rates,” and other studies have confirmed similar relationships. A summary of over 30 independent studies on thermal comfort reports that the preferred air temperature in these studies to be between 17°C (63°F) and 26°C (79°F)[95], with the highest preference being between 23–25°C.[96] Studies included data for both males and females, from offices, schools, laboratories, and light industry. It was further noted that as the monthly mean outdoor temperatures increase, the preferred temperature for comfort tends to increase.

Comfort is also affected by metabolic work load and clothing. In general, the higher the metabolic work load and/or the clothing insulation, the lower the temperature required for comfort. By the addition or removal of clothing, the individual can establish his or her comfort temperature.[5]

Thermal effects on safety behavior have been reported in a 14-month study conducted in a metal products manufacturing plant and a foundry. A wide variety of industrial work tasks and workstations were observed.[97] Conclusions from this investigation support the relationship between unsafe work behavior and ambient temperatures as a U-shaped curve, with the minimum unsafe behavior rate occurring in the preferred temperature zone of 17°C (63°F) to 23°C (73°F) WBGT, and with the unsafe behavior rate increasing when the ambient temperatures increase or decrease from this range. Grouping work tasks according to metabolic work load and different job risk groups, but the basic U-shaped relationship was consistently portrayed. A generalized curve demonstrating this relationship between unsafe behavior rate and temperature is shown in Figure 28.7.[97]

Evaluating the Hot Workplace: An Example

The potentially hot workplace will usually become apparent; it will be obvious, or the workers will make the hot conditions known. The important objective, however, is to determine if the workplace is excessively hot according to heat stress standards or heat illness criteria. Such a determination can be made using the steps described below. Example calculations in this section will use SI units, i.e., °C, watts, and m/sec. Other practitioner guidelines for evaluation of hot working environments are also available and may be of assistance.[18,78,98]

(1) Preliminary Review. The hot work site should be observed as to the nature of the work, the thermal characteristics, type of clothing worn, and other relevant job and worker information. Records of prior heat-related injury or illness should be reviewed. This information will be helpful in deciding what kind of heat stress assessment is to be made. Worksheets for both quantitative and qualitative analysis of workplace heat exposure are provided in Kodak.[18]

(2) Select a Heat Index. A heat stress index should be selected that best represents the hot work in question. Rational indices based on calculations of thermal balance have been discussed. For most applications, the WBGT is preferred for initial evaluation. It is relatively easy to measure and to interpret the results, and it is also the most widely used and accepted index. Rational analysis methods require a measure of professional sophistication and instrumentation and cannot be covered in this simple example. Please refer to earlier discussions of thermal stress and the required sweat rate.[14]

(3) Select Instruments. WBGT can be calculated after measuring the thermal components of globe temperature, air temperature, and natural wet bulb temperature. Or, WBGT can be obtained directly using electronic instruments (Figure 28.4).

(4) Measure the Thermal Environment. Measurement of the thermal environment requires care. The instruments should be placed in the actual working

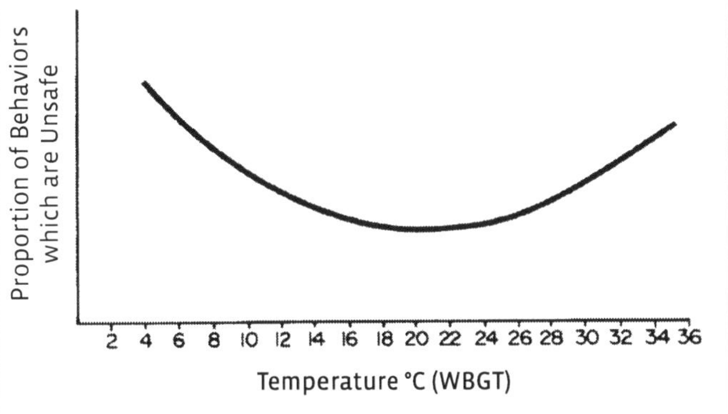

Figure 28.7 — Effects of workplace thermal conditions on safe work behavior.[97]

locations to ensure the readings are representative of the heat exposure. Instruments should be allowed time to stabilize to the environment, dry bulb and wet bulb thermometers should be shielded from sun or radiant sources, and wicks on the wet bulb thermometers should be clean and fully wetted. Repeated readings may be desirable if conditions can change during the period for which a TWA is to be calculated. The temperatures and the amount of time spent at each location (work or rest) must be determined.

(5) Calculate the WBGT. If direct reading instruments are not used, the WBGT can be easily calculated using equations 28.5 or 28.6. For example, assume the temperature readings obtained at an indoor workplace were: T_{db} = 35°C; T_{nwb} = 30°C; and T_g = 39°C.

The WBGT is calculated as:

$$WBGT = 0.7(30°C) + 0.3(39°C) = 32.7°C$$

(6) Calculate TWA for WBGT. Frequently the worker's thermal exposure varies during the hottest hour of the day due to working at different locations or due to changing thermal conditions. If so, it will be necessary to calculate a WBGTTWA. Assume the measurements at the work site show a 30 minute exposure at 30°C WBGT, a 20 minute exposure at 28°C WBGT, and a 10 minute exposure at 38°C WBGT.

Then using Equation 28.7:

$$WBGT_{TWA} = \frac{30\text{ min}(30°C) + 20\text{ min}(28°C) + 10\text{ min}(38°C)}{60\text{ min}}$$

$$WBGT_{TWA} = \frac{900 + 560 + 380}{60} = 30.7°C$$

(7) Estimate Metabolic Heat. The work effort and intensity required by the job being performed in the heat must be well understood, since it makes such a major contribution to total heat load on the worker. Thermal balance during the work hour is affected by the cumulative heat load so it is necessary to consider all tasks and rest periods in the assessment of metabolic heat. Table 28.1, Table 28.2, and Figure 28.2 represent some of the common approaches to relating the work to its energy cost, or metabolic heat. For example, assume the worker is carrying and stacking boxes, which appears from Figure 28.2 to represent a W-8 work load (i.e., 390 watts). If the heaviness of this work requires a 15 min. rest break (S-0 workload, or 115 watts) after each 45 min of work, the best estimate of metabolic heat would again be the hourly TWA calculated using Equation 28.7:

$$M_{TWA} = \frac{45\text{ min}(390W) + 15\text{ min}(115W)}{60\text{ min}}$$

$$M_{TWA} = \frac{17550 + 1725}{60} = 321W$$

(8) Evaluate Recommended Threshold Limits. Various proposals for heat stress thresholds are available and reasonable, but most are very similar. Those presented by ACGIH®[16] or NIOSH[63] are most commonly recommended. From the above calculated example, metabolic heat = 321 watts, and using the RELs from Figure 28.6, a WBGT limit of 27°F is indicated. The calculated WBGT was 30.7°F, which is above the REL and below the ceiling limit of 37°F. The REL represents a threshold value of heat stress and the onset of increased risk of heat illness.

(9) Determine Thermal Components. Although WBGT provides a good composite index of heat load on the body, knowledge of the specific thermal components can provide diagnostic information concerning control of the heat. High globe temperature readings support the use of radiant shielding, low velocity speaks for increased ventilation, and high natural wet bulb temperature relates to high moisture and the

call for moisture control or refrigeration. The use of the equations of Table 28.3 and measurement of the individual thermal components can provide quantification of the convective, radiant, and evaporative heat flow useful in making engineering modifications at the workplace.

(10) Modify the Hot Work Exposure. When a job or work site has been identified as above the REL, a broad array of practices can be considered for protecting the worker. Actions related to the worker can involve acclimatization, clothing, personal protection, fluid replacement, health issues, and self-determination during exposure. It is especially important that individual workers are knowledgeable about the symptoms and control of heat illness. Many engineering controls are also available and can be selected based on the specific thermal components in a work environment. These include ventilation, spot cooling, refrigeration, fans, radiant shielding, moisture reduction, and isolation. Relevant administrative practices for consideration are training about heat stress, reducing metabolic heat through mechanization or work scheduling, providing rest breaks, and use of a buddy system. Thermal environment controls are discussed more extensively in Chapter 27.

(11) Re-evaluate Heat Limits. After modifications of the hot work have been made, the work should be re-evaluated using the previously described methods. Note that these threshold limits do not represent upper limits for work in the heat. They imply that risk for heat stress is increasing, and appropriate work practices and other controls must be implemented. As with most occupational hygiene controls, the use of engineering modifications provides a more complete and permanent solution. However, in the case of heat stress, humans have their own built-in sensors of heat strain, so the understanding and use of all practices should be a requirement for anyone who works in the heat. Rational methods for heat stress evaluation[14,40,99,100] or personal physiological monitoring of workers should be used in those situations where heat stress is considered to be excessive and to present an unacceptable risk.

Evaluating the Cold Workplace: An Example

Occupational exposure to the cold can occur indoors or outdoors. Indoor cold work in refrigerated areas is typically easier to evaluate and control since the conditions of temperature, wind speed, and total working environment are more consistent. Also, indoor thermal conditions can often be modified (e.g., changing wind speed) and the work clothing and work schedule can be finally selected for the environment. The larger variability in temperature and wind found with outdoor cold work or with "indoor" work sites dominated by outdoor temperatures, makes it more difficult to establish a safe and healthful workplace.

There are considerably fewer guidelines concerning cold work from standards, recommendations, and even the research literature than are found for hot work. The steps in evaluation of a cold outdoor work site are discussed in the example below. Again, the example will be presented in SI units.

(1) Preliminary Review. The cold work site should be observed to determine the nature of the work, the characteristics of both the work and warm-up areas, clothing worn, and other relevant job and worker information. Climatic records and injury/illness records may also be useful in determining the type of analysis to be made.

(2) Decide Type of Analysis. An initial decision involves selecting either a simple and general analysis or a more detailed, rational analysis. The general approach involves less measurement, more estimates, and the use of tables for decision making. The basic equations of thermal balance can be used along with additional measurements to evaluate rationally the effects of environment, work, and clothing parameters. A general analysis is recommended as appropriate for most cold work decisions.

(3) Measure the Thermal Environment. The primary measurements are air temperature (t_a) and wind speed (v). If air velocity instruments are not available, wind

speed can be estimated: 2 m/sec (5 mph)-light flag moves; 4 m/sec (10 mph)-light flag fully extended; 7 m/sec (15 mph)-raises newspaper sheet; 9 m/sec (20 mph)-blowing and drifting snow.[65] It may be proper in some instances to use temperature information from the National Weather Service as a substitute for actual readings. Assume in this example T_a = -18°C and v = 7 m/sec.

If rational analysis is to be used, measures of mean radiant temperature and humidity must also be obtained.

Surface temperatures should be measured when bare skin/hands can contact cold surfaces. Assume a surface temperature of -9°C (16°F) is measured using a surface thermistor. This surface would be considered uncomfortably cold and hand protection would be recommended.

(4) Determine Windchill Index. The WCI could be calculated directly and converted to an equivalent chill temperature or this information could be obtained from tables, if available. For this example, air temperature = -18°C and air velocity = 7 m/sec, an equivalent chill temperature of -36°C would be determined. This represents a condition where exposed skin should be covered, since flesh is likely to freeze within a few minutes.

(5) Estimate Metabolic Heat. The metabolic heat can be estimated using the information found in Table 28.1, Table 28.2, and Figure 28.2. For example, assuming the work involves arm and trunk work of intermittent handling of boxes, Table 28.1 would suggest this to be moderate work.

(6) Determine Insulation Required. The IREQ of clothing adequate for thermal balance in an environment can be calculated if all variables have been measured. Generally an adequate approximation of clothing requirements can be obtained from Figure 28.6. For the example air temperature = -18°C and moderate work, Figure 28.6 shows an IREQ between 1.7 clo and 2.7 clo, where 1 clo = 0.155 meter square °C per watt. Clothing for this work and temperature combination should provide insulation of this level.

(7) Modify the Cold Work Exposure. There are a large number of practices that may be useful in alleviation of cold stress. Of major importance is assurance that the worker is adequately educated and trained concerning all aspects of controlling and responding to cold environments. The selection and use of clothing and of personal protection for the head and extremities is critical. Engineering controls may also be applicable including the proper selection of tools, equipment, and machinery; the use of shielding or heated enclosures, local or personal heaters; mechanization of the work to reduce human exposures, etc. Administrative controls should also be considered as they relate to careful planning and preparation for the work, work scheduling, work sharing, work breaks, and the use of buddy systems. An extensive discussion of cold stress preventive measures can be found in Holmér[77], Environment Canada[72] and ACGIH®.[16] If modifications of the work or environment are substantial, it may be useful to re-evaluate the situation using the previously described methods.

Evaluating the Thermal Workplace: Summary

Adverse thermal environments represent a commonly encountered occupational exposure, and the risks to humans are real and recognizable.

The hot and cold workplace examples cited above demonstrate some of the methods and procedures discussed in this chapter, and they provide guidance on evaluating and making decisions for hot and cold occupational exposures where conditions are simple and straightforward. Most often, however, the making of thermal environment decisions in the real workplace involves knowledge and application of the broader principles covered throughout this chapter.

References

1. **Ellis, F.P., F.E. Smith, and J.D. Walters:** Measurement of environmental warmth in SI units. *Br. J. Ind. Med. 29*:361–377 (1972).

2. **International Organization for Standardization (ISO):** *ISO 7726:1998: Ergonomics of the thermal environment-Instruments for Measuring Physical Quantities.* Geneva: International Organization for Standardization, 1998.
3. **Minard, D.:** Physiology of Heat Stress. In *The Industrial Environment—Its Evaluation and Control,* Washington, D.C.: Department of Health Education and Welfare, 1973.
4. **National Institute for Occupational Safety and Health (NIOSH):** *The Industrial Environment — Its Evaluation and Control.* Washington, D.C.: U.S. Government Printing Office, 1973.
5. **Fanger, P.O.:** *Thermal Comfort, Analyses and Applications in Environmental Engineering.* Copenhagen, Denmark: Danish Technical Press, 1970.
6. **Gagge, A.P.:** Effective radiant flux, an independent variable that describes thermal radiation on man. In *Physiological and Behavioral Temperature Regulation.* Hardy, J.D., A.P. Gagge, and J.A.J. Stolwijk (eds.). Springfield, IL: Charles C. Thomas, 1970.
7. **Cena, K. and J.A. Clark:** Physics, Physiology, and Psychology. In *Bioengineering, Thermal Physiology, and Comfort.* Cena, K. and J.A. Clark (eds.). New York: Elsevier Publishing Co.: 1981.
8. **Vernon, H.:** The measurement of radiant heat in relation to human comfort. *J. Ind. Hyg. 14*:95 (1932).
9. **National Institute for Occupational Safety and Health (NIOSH):** *Criteria for a Recommended Standard-Occupational Exposure to Hot Environments: HSM-72-10269, in U.S. Department of Health Education and Welfare.* Washington, D.C.: U.S. Department of Health Education and Welfare, HSM-72-10269, 1972.
10. **Keuhn, L.A. and L.E. Machattie:** A fast responding and direct-reading WBGT index meter. *Am. Ind. Hyg. Assoc. J. 36*:325–331 (1975).
11. **Witherspoon, J.M. and R.F. Goldman:** Indices of thermal stress. *ASHRAE Bull. LO-73-8*:5-13 (1974).
12. **Belding, H.S.:** *Strains of exposure to heat. Standards for Occupational Exposure to Hot Environments, in Standards for Occupational Exposure to Hot Environments, Proceedings of Symposium,* S.M. Horvath and R.C. Jensen (eds.). U.S. Government Printing Office: Washington, D.C.: U.S. Government Printing Office, 1976.
13. **Wyndham, C.H. and A.J. Heyns:** The Accuracy of the Prediction of human strain from heat stress indices. *Arch. Sci. Physiol. 27*:295–301 (1973).
14. **International Organization for Standardization (ISO):** *ISO 7933:2004: Hot Environments-Analytical Determination and Interpretation of Thermal Stress Using Calculation of the Predicted Heat Strain.* 2004, Geneva, Switzerland: International Organization for Standardization.
15. **Smith, J.L. and J.D. Ramsey:** Designing physically demanding tasks to minimize levels of worker stress. *Ind. Eng. 14*:44–50 (1982).
16. **American Conference of Governmental Industrial Hygienists (ACGIH®):** *Threshold Limit Values and Biological Exposure Indicies for Chemical Substances and Physical Agents.* Cincinnati, OH: ACGIH®: 2009.
17. **Konz, S.:** *Work Design*, 4th edition. Scottsdale, AZ: Publishing Horizons, 1995. pp. 378, 381–383, 389, 390.
18. **Eastman Kodak Co.:** *Kodak's Ergonomic Design for People at Work*, 2nd edition. S.N. Chengalur, S.H. Rodgers, and T.E. Bernard (eds.). Hoboken, NJ: Wiley, 2004. p. xxvii, 704.
19. **International Organization for Standardization (ISO):** *ISO 8996:2004: Ergonomics of the thermal environment-Determination of Metabolic Rate.* Geneva, Switzerland: International Organization for Standardization. 2004.
20. **Tayyari, R., C.L. Burford, and J.D. Ramsey:** Guidelines for the Use of Systematic Workload Estimation. *Internatl. J. Ind. Ergo. 4*:61–65 (1989).
21. **Belding, H.S. and T.F. Hatch:** Index for Evaluating Heat Stress in Terms of Resulting Physiological Strain. *Heat, Pip. Air Cond. 27*:129–135 (1955).
22. **Gagge, A.P. and R.R. Gonzalez:** Physiological bases of warm discomfort for sedentary man. *Arch. Sci. Physiol. 27*:409 (1973).
23. **Vogt, J.J., V. Candas, and J.P. Libert:** Graphical determination of heat tolerance limits. *Ergo. 25*:285–294 (1982).
24. **McKarns, J.S. and R.S. Brief:** Nomographs give refined estimate of heat stress index. *Heat./Piping/Air Cond. 38*:113–116 (1966).
25. **Parsons, K.C.:** *Human Thermal Environments: The Effects of Hot, Moderate, and Cold Environments on Human Health, Comfort, and Performance*, 2nd edition. London: Taylor and Frances, LTD., 2003. pp. xxiv, 527.
26. **Malchaire, J., et al.:** Development and validation of the predicted heat strain model. *Ann. Occup. Hyg. 45(2)*:123–135 (2001).
27. **Houghton, F.C. and C.P. Yaglou:** Determining Lines of Equal Comfort. *J. Am. Soc. Heat & Vent. Engrs. 29*:165–176 (1923).
28. **Bedford, T.:** *Environmental Warmth and its Measurement. Medical Research Council War Memo No. 17.* 1946: London.

29. **MacPherson, R.K.:** *Physiological Responses to Hot Environments. Med. Res. Coun. Special Report Serial No. 298.* London: His Majesty's Safety Office, 1960.
30. **Yaglou, C.P. and D. Minard:** Control of Heat Casualties at Military Training Camps. *Arch. Ind. Health 16*:302–316 (1957).
31. **World Health Organization (WHO):** *Health Factors Involved in Working Under Conditions of Heat Stress.* In *Who Technical Report Series 412.* Geneva, Switzerland: WHO, 1969.
32. **Ramsey, J.D.:** Heat Stress Standard: OSHA's advisory committee recommendations. *Natl. Safety News 68*:89–95 (1975).
33. **International Organization for Standardization (ISO):** *ISO 7243-1989: Hot Environments-Estimation of Heat Stress on Working Man Based on the WBGT Index (Wet Bulb Globe Temperature).* Geneva, Switzerland: ISO, 1989.
34. **Vernon, H.M.:** *The Measurement of Radiant Heat in Relation to Human Comfort.* Journal of Physiology—Proceedings of the Physiological Society, 1930. p. xv-xvii.
35. **Yaglou, C.P.:** Heated Globe Thermometer for Evaluating Environmental Conditions for Comfort and For Studying Radiation-Convections Effects. *J. Ind. Hyg. 17(9)*: 185–198 (1935).
36. **Hill, L.:** *Medical Research Council Special Report No. 32, Part I.* London, 1919.
37. **Winslow, C.E.A. and L. Greenburg:** *Am. Soc. Heat. Vent. Eng. Trans. 41*:149 (1935).
38. **Bostford, J.H.:** A Wet Globe Thermometer for Environmental Heat Measurement. *Am. Ind. Hyg. Assoc. J. 32*:1–10 (1971).
39. **McCardle, B., et al.:** *The prediction of the physiological effects of warm and hot environments: The P4SR index, in R.N.P. Report 47:391.* London: Medical Research Council, 1947.
40. **Gagge, A.P.:** *Rational temperature indices of thermal comfort, in Bioengineering, Thermal Physiology and Comfort.* Clark, K.C. and J.A. Clark (eds.). New York: Elsevier Scientific Publishing Co., 1981.
41. **Young, P.A., W.L. W.L. Potts, and A.C. Mandal:** Kata thermometry in relation to the specific cooling power of a mine environment. *J. Mine Vent. Soc. S. Afr. 31*:136–137 (1978).
42. **Lind, A.R.:** *Tolerable limits for prolonged and intermittent exposures to heat,* in *Temperature: Its Measurement and Control in Science and Industry.* Hardy, J.D. (ed.). New York: Van Nostrand Reinhold, 1963.
43. **Thom, E.C.:** A new concept for cooling degree-days. *Air Cond. Heat. Vent. 54(6)*:73–80 (1957).
44. **Robinson, S., E.S. Turrell, and S.D. Gerking:** Physiologically equivalent conditions of air temperature and humidity. *Am. J. Physiol. 143*:21–32 (1945).
45. **Givoni, B.:** *The influence of work and environmental conditions on the physiological responses and thermal equilibrium of man, in Proceedings of a UNESCO Symposium on Arid Zone Physiology and Psychology.* 1962, UNESCO: Lucknow, India.
46. **Lee, D.H. and A.H. Henschel:** *Evaluation of Thermal Environment in Shelters (Public Health Service pub. TR-8).* Washington, D.C.: U.S. Department of Health, Education, and Welfare, 1963.
47. **Pulket, C., et al.:** A comparison of heat stress indices in a hot- humid environment. *Am. Ind. Hyg. Assoc. J. 41*:442–444 (1980).
48. **Steadman, R.G.:** The assessment of sultriness, part I: A temperature humidity index based on human physiology and clothing science. *J. Climate Appl. Meteorol. 18*:861–873 (1979).
49. **National Weather Service:** *National Weather Service: Heat Wave, Heat Index, NWS Alert Procedures, in Document NOAA/PA 85001.* 2000, National Oceanic and Atmospheric Administration.
50. **Neidhart, A. and J.C. Prudhomme:** *Cal/OSHA's Investigations of 2005 Heat Illness Cases. 2006* [cited; Available from: http://www.cal-osha.com/Resources.aspx#heat].
51. **Helgerman McKinnon, S. and R.L. Utley:** Heat Stress. *Professional Safety April*:41–47 (2005).
52. Physicians' Desk Reference, *PDR Guide to Drug Interactions, Side Effects, and Indications.* Vol. 63. Thomson Healthcare, 2009.
53. **Seales, D.R.:** *Influence of aging on autonomic-circulatory control at rest and during exercise in humans.* in *Perspectives in Exercise Science and Sports Medicine.* Gisolfi, C.V. D.R. Lamb, and E.R. Nadel (eds.). Dubuque, IA: Brown and Benchmark, 1993. pp. 291–293.
54. **MacPherson, R.K.:** The effect of fever on body temperature regulation in man. *Clin. Sci. 18*:281–287 (1959).
55. **Frye, A.J. and E. Kamon:** Responses to dry heat of men and women with similar aerobic capacities. *J. Appl. Physiol. 50*:65–70 (1981).
56. **American Conference of Governmental Industrial Hygienists (ACGIH®):** *Threshold Limit Values® for Chemical Substances and Physical Agents in the Workroom Environment with Intended Changes for 1971.* Cincinnati, OH: ACGIH®, 1971.
57. **Lind, A.R.:** A Physiological Criterion for Setting Thermal Environmental Limits for Everyday Work. *J. Appl. Physiol. 18*:51–56 (1963).
58. **Minard, D.:** *Effective Temperature Scale and its Modifications (NMRI research rep. 6).* 1964, Naval Medical Research Institute: Bethesda, MD.

59. **Goldman, R.A.:** *Prediction of heat strain, revisited 1979–1980*, in *Proceedings of a NIOSH Workshop on Recommended Heat Stress Standards (DHHS [NIOSH] pub. 81-108)*. Dukes-Dobos, F.N. and A. Henschel (eds.). Washington, D.C.: U.S. Government Printing Office, 1980.
60. **Dasler, A.R.:** *Heat Stress, Work Function and Physiological Heat Exposure Limits in Man (special pub. 491)*. Washington, D.C.: National Bureau of Standards, Commerce Department, 1977. p. 65-92.
61. **Ramanathan, N.L. and H.S. Bedling:** Physiologic Evaluation of the WBGT Index for Occupational Heat Stress. *Am. Ind. Hyg. Assoc. J. 34(9)*:375–383. (1973)
62. **Larrañaga, M.D. and T.E. Bernard:** Heat Stress. In *Patty's Industrial Hygiene*, 6th edtion. Rose, V. and B. Cohrssen (eds.). Hoboken, NJ: Wiley-Interscience, 2010.
63. **National Institute for Occupational Safety and Health (NIOSH):** *Criteria for a Recommended Standard-Occupational Exposure to Hot Environments Revised Criteria, in U.S. Department of Health Education and Welfare*. Cincinnati, OH: NIOSH, 1986.
64. **Bernard, T.E.:** *Thermal Stress, in Fundamentals of Industrial Hygiene*, B. Plog, Editor. 2001, National Safety Council: Chicago. Chapter 12.
65. **American Conference of Governmental Industrial Hygienists (ACGIH®):** *1998 TLVs® and BEIs®: Threshold Limit Values® for Chemical Substances and Physical Agents and Biological Exposure Indices®*. Cincinnati, OH: ACGIH®, 1998.
66. **American Conference of Governmental Industrial Hygienists (ACGIH®):** *2001 TLVs® and BEIs®: Threshold Limit Values® for Chemical Substances and Physical Agents and Biological Exposure Indices®*. Cincinnati, OH: ACGIH®, 2001.
67. **American Conference of Governmental Industrial Hygienists (ACGIH®):** *Threshold Limit Values® and Biological Exposure Indices® for Chemical Substances and Physical Agents*. Cincinnati, OH: ACGIH®, 2007.
68. **O'Connor, D.J. and T.E. Bernard:** Continuing the search for WBGT clothing adjustment factors. *Appl. Occup. Env. Hyg. 14*:119–125 (1999).
69. **Bernard, T.E., et al.:** WBGT clothing adjustment factors for four clothing ensembles and the effects of metabolic demands. *J. Occup. Env. Hyg. 5*: 1–5 (2008).
70. **Ashley, C.D. and T.E. Bernard:** Effects of hoods and flame retardant fabrics on WBGT clothing adjustment factors. *J. Occup. Env. Hyg. 5*:59–62 (2008).
71. **Bernard, T.E. and C.D. Ashley:** *Short-term heat stress exposure limits based on WBGT and adjusted for clothing*. in *International Conference on Environmental Ergonomics*. 2007. Piran Slovenia.
72. **Meteorological Service of Canada:** *Wind chill and Environment Canada's new program*. Environment Canada, 2003.
73. **National Weather Service:** *Wind Chill Temperature Index for Winter 2001–2002*. Washington, D.C.: National Oceanic and Atmospheric Administration-United States Department of Commerce, 2001.
74. **U.S. Army Research Institute of Environmental Medicine:** *Cold Injury (TG No. 172)*. Aberdeen Proving Ground, MD: U.S. Army Environmental Hygiene Agency, 1989.
75. **International Organization for Standardization (ISO):** *ISO/TR 11079:2007: Evaluation of Cold Environments-Determination of Required Clothing Insulation (IREC)*. Geneva, Switzerland: ISO, 2007.
76. **Holmér, I.:** Required clothing insulation (IREQ) as an analytical index of cold stress. *ASHRAE Trans. 90*:1116–1128 (1984).
77. **Holmér, I.:** Cold stress: part I-Guidelines for the practitioner. *Int. J. Ind. Ergonom. 14*:139–149 (1994).
78. **Ramsey, J.D., T.E. Bernard, and F.N. Dukes-Dobos:** Evaluation and control of hot working environments: part I-guidelines for the practitioner. *Int. J. Ind. Ergonom. 14*:119–127 (1994).
79. **Mackworth, N.H.:** High incentives versus hto and humid atmospheres in a physical work task. *Br. J. Psychol. 38*:90–102 (1947).
80. **Pepler, R.D.:** *Performance and Well-Being in Heat*, in *Temperature-Its Measurement and Control in Science in Industry Vol. 3, Part 3*. Hardy, J.D. (ed.). New York: Van Nostrand Reinhold, 1963.
81. **Snook, S.H. and V.M. Ciriello:** The effects of heat stress on manual handling tasks. *Am. Ind. Hyg. Assoc. J. 35*:681–685 (1974).
82. **Kamon, E., J. Benson, and K. Soto:** Scheduling work and rest for the hot ambient conditions with radiant heat source. *Ergo. 26*:181–192 (1983).
83. **Wing, J.E.:** *A Review of the Effects of High Ambient Temperature on Mental Performance (AMRL-TR-65-102)*. Wright Patterson Air Force Base, OH: U.S. Department of the Air Force, Aerospace Medical Research Laboratory, 1965.
84. **Grether, W.F.:** Human performance at elevated environmental temperatures. *Aerosp. Med. 44*:747–755 (1973).
85. **Ramsey, J.D. and S.J. Morrissey:** Isodecrement curves for task performance in hot environments. *Ergo. 9*:66–72 (1978).

86. **Kobrick, J.L. and B.J. Fine:** *Climate and Human Performance.* In *The Physical Environment at Work.* Osborne, D.J. and M.M. Gruneberg (eds.). Chichester, U.K.: John Wiley & Sons, 1983. pp. 69-107.
87. **Ramsey, J.D.:** Task performance in heat: a review. *Ergo. 38*:154–163 (1995).
88. **Ramsey, J. and Y.G. Kwon:** Recommended alert limits for perceptual motor loss in hot environments. *Int. J. Ind. Ergon. 9*:245–257 (1992).
89. **Dusek, E.R.:** *Effect of Temperature on Mental Performance. Protection and Functioning of the Hand in Cold Climates.* Washington, D.C.: National Academic Science, Natural Resource Council, 1957.
90. **Tanaka, M., et al.:** Thermal reaction and manual performance during cold exposure while wearing cold-protective clothing. *Ergo. 26*:141–150 (1983).
91. **Kobrick, J.L.:** Effects of exposure to low ambient temperature and wind on visual acuity. *J. Eng. Psychol. 4*:92–98 (1965).
92. **Powell, P.I., et al.:** *"2000 Accidents, A shop Floor Study of Their Causes." (Rep. 21).* London: National Institute of Industrial Psychology, 1971.
93. **Belding, H.S., et al.:** Recent Developments in Understanding of Effects of Exposure to Heat. In *International Congress of Occupational Health.* New York: 1960.
94. **Surry, J.:** *Industrial Accident Research: A Human Engineering Approach.* Toronto, Canada: University of Toronto, Department of Industrial Engineering, 1968.
95. **Humphreys, M.A.:** The Dependence of Comfortable Temperatures Upon Indoor and Outdoor Climates. In *Bioengineering, Thermal Physiology and Comfort.* Cena, K. and J.A. Clark (eds.). New York: Elsiever Scientific Publishing Co., 1981.
96. **Reddy, S.P. and J.D. Ramsey:** Thermostat variations and sedentary job performance. *ASHRAE J. 18*:32–36 (1976).
97. **Ramsey, J.D., et al.:** Effects of workplace thermal conditions on safe work behavior. *J. Safety Res. 14*:105–114 (1983).
98. **Ramsey, J.D.:** Abbreviated guidelines for heat stress exposure. *Am. Ind. Hyg. Assoc. J. 39*:491–495 (1978).
99. **Dukes-Dobos, F.N.:** Rationale and provisions of the work practices standard for work in hot environments as recommended by NIOSH. In *Standards for Occupational Exposure to Hot Environments, Proceedings of Symposium.* Horvath, S.M. and R.C. Jensen (eds.). Washington, D.C.: U.S. Government Printing Office (DHEW/NIOSH pub.), 1976. pp. 76–100.
100. **Parsons, K.C.:** International standards for the assessment of the risk of thermal strain on clothed workers in hot environments. *Ann. Occup. Hyg. 43(5)*:297–308 (1999).

Outcome Competencies

After completing this chapter, the reader should be able to:

1. Define underlined terms used in this chapter.
2. Calculate the pressure at any habitable depth under water or altitude above sea level.
3. Calculate the molar fraction or partial pressure of oxygen, nitrogen, carbon dioxide, etc., in air at any of the above pressures.
4. Anticipate the effects and estimate the incidence of hypoxia and benign acute mountain sickness.
5. Propose some potential control schemes for hypoxia and benign acute mountain sickness.
6. Anticipate the effects of nitrogen narcosis, oxygen and carbon dioxide toxicities and the conditions at which they might occur.
7. Explain the principles behind changing the composition of the air used in NITROX and saturation diving.
8. Calculate the change in trapped gas volume resulting from a change in depth or altitude.
9. Anticipate the magnitude of change associated with barotrauma.
10. Discuss the cause and forms of decompression sicknesses and describe the control approaches used to mitigate decompression sickness.

Key Terms

acclimatization • airtight caisson • barotrauma • benign acute mountain sickness • bottom time • Boyle's law • carbon dioxide toxicity • Dalton's law • decompression schedule • decompression sicknesses • dysbaric osteonecrosis • dysbarism • hematocrit • hemoglobin • Henry's law • high altitude cerebral edema • high altitude pulmonary edema • high pressure nervous syndrome • hyperbaric • hypobaric • hypoxia • NITROX • oxygen toxicity • partial pressure • pressure • saturation diving • solubility coefficient • time of useful consciousness • Valsalva maneuver

Prerequisite Knowledge

Prior to beginning this chapter, the reader should review the following chapters:

Chapter Number	Chapter Topic
2	Environmental and Occupational Toxicology
13	Principles and Instrumentation for Calibrating Air Sampling Equipment

In addition, a college-level knowledge of physics, chemistry, and mathematics is helpful.

Key Topics

I. Physical Principles
   A. Boyle's Law
   B. Dalton's Law
   C. Henry's Law

II. Hypobaric Hazards
   A. Recognition of Hypobaric Hazards
   B. Control of Hypobaric Hazards

III. Hyperbaric Hazards
   A. Recognition of Hyperbaric Hazards
   B. Control of Hyperbaric Hazards

IV. Changing Pressure Effects
   A. Recognition of Changing Pressure Hazards
   B. Control of Pressure Changes

Barometric Hazards

29

William Popendorf, PhD, CIH

Introduction

Although hygienists should be able to contribute to improving the control of barometric hazards, there are currently no Occupational Safety and Health Administration (OSHA) regulations governing work at altitude, and hygienists seem to have had little direct influence on managing diving hazards. Similarly, although several books and numerous book chapters are available on health hazards associated with abnormal atmospheric pressure, the focus of most of these references is more on the physiological and medical responses to pressure, rather than on the environmental elements and work practices that hygienists might be trying to control. This chapter begins with the basic science needed to anticipate and recognize the physical conditions constituting a barometric hazard, and discusses the health effects associated with each type of hazard, but tries to put an emphasis on the management and control of barometric hazards in some of industry's more novel workplaces.

From an occupational hygiene perspective, barometric hazards can be categorized as (1) hypobaric (low pressure) hazards, (2) hyperbaric (high pressure) hazards, and (3) hazards from changes in pressure (predominantly, but not exclusively, decreases from high to low pressure). This chapter is organized to follow these three categories.

Hypobaric conditions produce adverse health effects due to a lack of oxygen, specifically the low absolute partial pressure of oxygen (PO_2 in mmHg). Health effects include both direct symptoms of hypoxia and groups of indirect symptoms including benign acute mountain sickness (AMS) and the more life-threatening high-altitude pulmonary edema (HAPE) and high-altitude cerebral edema (HACE). In normal air (20.9% oxygen) these effects do not begin to be detectable until at least 2000 m (6000 ft) above sea level (ASL); however, the same range of effects can occur at or near sea level if the fraction of oxygen is reduced as might be present in a confined space.

Hyperbaric conditions can produce narcotic-like effects from high inert gas pressure (especially nitrogen, although high-pressure helium also can have neurologic effects) and toxic effects from high oxygen or carbon dioxide pressure. Nitrogen and helium are also responsible for adverse health effects following a rapid decrease in total pressure during ascent after an extended period of pressurization.

Changes in pressure can cause adverse health effects via at least two mechanisms: (1) pain or traumatic injury from the expansion or contraction of trapped gas as the pressure changes, and (2) the formation of inert gas bubbles within supersaturated tissues that can produce a range of decompression sicknesses (DCSs). A combination of the two mechanisms can produce a potentially fatal arterial gas embolism. DCS most commonly arises following a rapid decrease from a "hyperbaric" pressure to normal pressure (typical of diving, underwater construction, and work in pressurized caissons or tunnels); however, DCS can also occur following a rapid decrease from near sea level pressure to a hypobaric pressure (typical of flight crews).

The following sections of this chapter first discuss the physical principles and

Table 29.1 — Common Units of Pressure Equivalent to One Standard Atmosphere

14.696 pounds per square inch (psi)	101325 Newtons per square meter (N/m^2)
29.920 inches of mercury (in Hg)	101.325 kiloPascals (kPa)
760 millimeters of mercury (mm Hg)	1.01325 bars (B)

physiological mechanisms underlying all of these barometric hazards, then discuss each of the categories of hazards individually. The general sequence covers conditions defining each hazard, the nature of its health effects, and viable controls for these hazards. This chapter does not stress medical diagnosis, treatment, or the toxicological mechanisms underlying these hazards; the interested reader is directed toward the extensive bibliography cited throughout.

Physical Principles

Dysbarism is a generic term applicable to any adverse health effect due to a difference between ambient pressure and the total gas pressure in tissues, fluids, or cavities of the body. To understand the physical and physiological effects of pressure, an occupational hygienist should have a thorough understanding of three physical gas laws: Boyle's law, Dalton's law, and Henry's law, which are discussed in subsequent sections. These three laws underlie most of the hazards associated with dysbarisms. All three of these laws relate to ambient pressure that changes with altitude above sea level and with depth below the surface of water. Pressure is the force per unit surface area exerted by the molecules of a fluid in contact with a body. Barometric hazards to humans are most easily referenced to differences from the normal living environment of one standard atmosphere, which can be expressed in several common units, as listed in Table 29.1. Pressure measured relative to the local atmosphere is sometimes called "gauge pressure" with units such as "psig," in which "g" is for gauge. Hypobaric and diving conditions are reported in the literature as absolute pressure, but conditions in compressed air construction work is usually stated in gauge pressure.

Boyle's Law

Boyle's law (postulated in 1662) states that the volume of a gas at constant temperature is inversely proportional to its pressure. As a historical footnote, Robert Boyle hired a then young Robert Hooke to make an air pump with which he not only studied the physical behavior of gases but also observed animal responses to pressure. Boyle's law can be formulated as Equation 29-1 or as the more general universal (or ideal) gas law, Equation 29-2.

$$P \times V = \text{constant} \tag{29-1}$$

$$P \times V = n \times R \times T \tag{29-2}$$

where:

P = total pressure, atmospheres
V = gas volume, L
n = moles of gas; its mass in g divided by its molecular weight.
R = universal gas constant, 0.08205 L × atm /K/mole
T = absolute temperature in degrees Kelvin, K = °C + 273.15

Boyle's law applies to the expansion and contraction of gases within the body due to changes in external pressure. Expanding gas trapped within the lung, middle ear, sinuses, or stomach (gastrointestinal [GI] tract) can cause pain, and rapidly expanding gas can actually cause traumatic injury, called a barotrauma. One use of the universal gas law familiar to occupational hygienists is to find the molar volume of any gas at normal temperature (T=25°C = 298.15 K) and pressure (P=1 atm):

$$\frac{V}{n} = \frac{RT}{P} = \frac{0.08205 \text{ L} \times \text{atm/K/mole} \times 298.15 \text{ K}}{1 \text{ atm}}$$

$$= 24.45 \text{ L/mole} \tag{29-3}$$

Another useful application is finding the density (ρ) of a known gas. For instance, the density of air can be found knowing its molecular weight (MW) is 28.96 g/mole (see Table 29.2):

$$\rho = \frac{mass}{V} = \frac{n\,MW}{V} = \frac{(28.96\text{ g/mole})}{24.45\text{ L/mole}} = 1.184\text{ g/L} \quad (29\text{-}4)$$

The pressure created by a fluid depends on the height and density of the fluid above it. Thus, pressure decreases with altitude above sea level and increases with depth below the surface of water. Changes in absolute pressure with depth are easy to anticipate because water is practically incompressible. Thus, pressure increases linearly with depth. However, water density does differ between fresh water at 1 kg/L (62.4 lb/ft;) and sea water 1.026 kg/L (64.0 lb/ft;). And it is important to remember that the pressure at the water's surface is always 1 local atmosphere (and at sea level the local atmosphere is approximately 1 standard atmosphere). Thus, the pressure in absolute total atmospheres (ATA) at any depth in terms of either feet or meters may be found using Equation 29-5:

$$P_{underwater} = P_{local} + (depth/\kappa) \approx 1\text{ atm.} + (depth/\kappa) \quad (29\text{-}5)$$

where P_{local} = either 1 atm or a lower air pressure if above sea level (see Equation 29-6) and κ= chosen from Table 29.3 based on the density of the water and units of depth.

Example 1. Find the total pressure while repairing an oil rig at a depth of 185 feet under the Gulf of Mexico. Use κ = 33 in Equation 29-5 to find the total pressure at a depth in sea water given in feet (denoted as fsw for feet of sea water). Because the surface is at sea level, $P_{underwater}$ = 1 atm + 185/33.1 = 1 atm + 5.6 = 6.6 ATA.

Changes in pressure with altitude are slightly more complex because air is compressible. Its density varies according to Boyle's law inversely with pressure, which itself varies with the height of the atmosphere above it. If the air temperature were constant, this change in pressure with altitude would be an exact exponential relationship of the form in Equation 29-6.

Table 29.2 — Chemical Composition of Standard Dry Air

Chemical Component	*Molecular Weight*	$MW_i \times Y_i$	Y_i (%)
Nitrogen (N^2)	28.0134	78.084	21.8740
Oxygen (O^2)	31.9988	20.948	6.7031
Argon (A)	39.948	0.934	0.3731
Carbon dioxide (CO^2)	44.0099	0.0314	0.0138
Neon (Ne)	20.183	0.00182	0.0004
Helium (He)	4.0026	0.00052	0.00000
Sum of molar fractions =		99.9997	
Molecular weight via Equation 29-9 =			28.96440

Source: Reference 1

Table 29.3 — Values of κ for Use in Equation 29.5 with Depth Below the Surface of Water

	Depth in Feet	*Depth in Meters*
Fresh Water	33.8	10.3
Sea Water	33.1	10.1

Table 29.4 — Values of κ for Use in Equation 29-6 (or Power of 2) to Anticipate the Normal Pressure at Altitudes Above Sea Level (ASL)

	≤ 20,000 ft	*≤ 6100 m*
For Equation 29-6	25,970	7915
For Power of 2	18,000	5500

$$P_{ASL} = P_{at\ sea\ level} \times e^{(-altitude/\kappa)} \quad (29\text{-}6)$$

where κ is chosen from Table 29.4 based on the units of altitude ASL.

Although air temperature does change with altitude,[1] it turns out that this change is sufficiently uniform that atmospheric pressure can still be approximated by an exponential formula.(1) The coefficients in Table 29.4 were optimized to predict P to within ±1% for most terrestrially accessible altitudes (up to 20,000 ft or 6100 m), but they will overestimate P by >10% above 35,000 ft. Table 29.4 also includes coefficients for powers of two, which some readers may find more intuitive (similar to a half-life). Thus, the atmospheric pressure at an altitude of 18,000 ft or 5500 m is approximately one-half that at sea level.

[1] Under normal conditions, temperature drops about 2°C per 1000 ft in altitude. This is called an "adiabatic lapse rate," which in the NOAA standard atmosphere is 1.9803EC = 3.5645EF) up to 36,000 feet (~11,000 m) where the constant temperature stratosphere begins.

Example 2. Find the local barometric pressure at Logan, Utah (altitude 4455 ft or 1358 m ASL), on a normal day.

$P_{at\ sea\ level}$ = normal pressure = 1 atm = 760 mm Hg

$P_{at\ Logan} = 760 \times e^{(-1358/7915)} = 760 \times 0.842 = 640$ mm Hg

$P_{at\ Logan} = 760 \times 2^{(-4455/18,000)} = 760 \times 0.842 = 640$ mm Hg

This example predicts that normal atmospheric pressure at that location measured by a barometer will be 640 mm Hg. Note, however, that weather bureaus and airports always adjust their readings for their local altitude and would still "report" a pressure of 760 mm Hg or 29.92 inches Hg on a normal day. Changes in the equivalent sea level pressure caused by weather fronts are normally within ±25 mm Hg (or ±1 inch Hg). Thus, a hygienist could specify a nonstandard local pressure either by inserting the pressure reported by a local weather bureau or airport into Equation 29-6 with errors within ±1%, by assuming the day is standard and insert 760 or 29.92 into Equation 29-6 with errors of ±3% (25/760 or 1/29.92), or by finding a working barometer (although the pressure may still easily change ±1% during a day).

Dalton's Law

Dalton's law involves a term called "partial pressure." The partial pressure of substance i (abbreviated P_i) is simply the force per unit surface area exerted by molecules of one specific chemical in contact with a body. John Dalton conducted extensive research in physical chemistry and formulated the modern atomic theory (for which the unit of atomic mass was given his name). Dalton's law (1801), sometimes called the law of partial pressures, states that the total pressure (P) of a mixture of gases is equal to the sum of its independent partial pressures, Equation 29-7.

$$P_{ATA} = \Sigma P_i = \Sigma[Y_i \times P_{ATA}] = (Y_1 + Y_2 + \ldots + Y_n) \times P_{ATA} \qquad (29\text{-}7)$$

where Y_i = the molar fraction of gas i in the total mixture = $P_{i/PATA}$.

Table 29.5 — Solubility Parameters (Henry's Constants) of Some Gases of Physiologic Interest

Gas	*S in Water (cc/mL/atm)*	*S in Lipid (cc/mL/atm)*	*S Lipid / S Water*
Cyclopropane	.204	11.2	55.0
Argon	.0262	.1395	5.3
Nitrogen	.01206	.0609	5.0
Oxygen	.0238	.112	4.7
Nitrous oxide	.435	1.4	3.2
Helium	.0087	.0148	1.7
Carbon dioxide	.5797	.88	1.5
Ethyl ether	15.6	15.2	1.0

The partial pressure exerted by each component is proportional to its molecular concentration in the mixture. Thus, partial pressure (P_i) is but one measure of airborne concentration. Equation 29-8 relates Pi to the more familiar occupational hygiene concentration term of parts per million (ppm), or molecules of a contaminant per million molecules of air.

$$ppm_i = \frac{P_i \times 10^6}{P_{ATA}} = Y_i \times 10^6 \qquad (29\text{-}8)$$

Dalton's law can be used to determine how much oxygen is available in the ambient air, in the lung, or in the alveoli either at altitude when the total P is low or when high concentrations of other gases displace oxygen even at sea level. The molecular composition of air is quite constant with altitude. Table 29.2 lists the U.S. and internationally agreed standard composition applicable to all humanly habitable altitudes.[2] This table also calculates the molecular weight (MW) of standard dry air using Equation 29-9[(1)]; humidity can reduce the molecular weight of air by 0.1 to 0.2 g.

$$MW_{mixture} = \frac{\Sigma(Y_i \times MW_i)}{\Sigma(Y_i)} \qquad (29\text{-}9)$$

Henry's Law

Henry's law (proposed by William Henry in 1803) states that the equilibrium concentration of a gas dissolved into a liquid will

[2] The U.S. standard atmosphere is identical to those adopted by the ISO and ICAO (International Civil Aviation Organization) through 11 km.

equal the product of the partial pressure of the gas times its solubility in the liquid. The gas solubility in a given liquid (shown in Equation 29-10 as S_i) is usually called Henry's constant.

$$C_{i\ in\ solution} = S_i \times P_i \tag{29-10a}$$

$$V_{i\ in\ solution} = V_{liquid} \times C_i \tag{29-10b}$$

where

- C_i = concentration of gas i dissolved in solution, cm^3/mL = cc/mL
- P_i = partial pressure of gas i, atm
- S_i = solubility coefficient of gas i in a given solute, cc/mL/atm
- V_i = volume in either cc of dissolved gas i or mL of liquid

Henry's law has been successfully used outside the body to relate a contaminant's concentration in water (or other solvent) to its vapor pressure and, therefore, to its rate of evaporation from or absorption into that media.[2–5] Physiologically, Henry's law can predict the body's absorption of most gases from the alveoli of the lung, its rate of transport via the blood, and the amount of gas that can be stored in tissue where it can eventually have an adverse effect. It is important to realize that because blood is mostly water, the rates of gas absorption, transportation to tissues, and eventual desorption from tissues are all primarily dependent on the gas's water solubility (with the exception of oxygen because of hemoglobin). However, the mass of gases stored in lipid tissues, such as myelinated neurons and collagen at joints, is determined by the gas's lipid solubility. Henry's law predicts that the greater the ratio of a gas's lipid to water solubility, the more slowly these gases can be carried back out of lipid tissues after leaving high pressure, which is especially a problem for poorly perfused tissues like collagen within joints. It also turns out that the anesthetic quality of a gas is highly correlated to its lipid or oil solubility (related to the lipid nature of myeline). Values of Henry's constants for some physiologically important gases are listed in Table 29.5, rank ordered by their lipid/water solubility ratios.

Example 3. Assuming that a carbonated beverage is initially bottled in equilibrium with carbon dioxide at 1 atm (i.e., 100% CO_2), how much CO_2 gas is dissolved in a 12 oz (0.355 L) bottle? Use Equation 29-10 to find the concentration of gas in the bottled liquid, then the volume of gas trapped in the bottle.

$$CCO_2 = 1\text{ atm} \times .5797\text{ cc/mL/atm} = 580\text{ cc/L}$$
(analogous to 58% CO_2)

$$VCO_2 = Vliquid \times CCO_2 = 355\text{ mL} \times .580\text{ cc/mL} = 206\text{ cc.}$$

The same method can be used to find that only about 0.06 cc of CO_2 will be in the bottle if it is left open until it comes into equilibrium with normal air that contains only about 314 ppm according to Table 29.2. Thus, one can see that when that bottle is first opened, there is 3185 times more CO_2 in the beverage than there will be when it comes back into equilibrium with ambient air.

$$\frac{CO_2\text{ in a fresh beverage}}{CO_2\text{ in an old beverage}} = \frac{1{,}000{,}000\text{ ppm}}{314\text{ ppm}} = 3185$$

This "supersaturated" ratio is sufficient to cause bubbles to form rapidly within the beverage when it is opened, bubbles that can comprise as much as 58% of its liquid volume. Only if the pressure is released slowly and the evolved gas can dissipate, is it possible for such a beverage to lose its fizz without forming bubbles.

Hypobaric Hazards

Occupational examples of hypobaric conditions include high-altitude construction or mining, and aviation (especially aircrews or passengers under rapid loss of pressurization conditions). The number of hygienists actively involved in these settings is probably less than warranted by the range of hazards and number of people exposed. Effects of hypobaric health hazards include the following.

(1) Hypoxia due to insufficient oxygen produces symptoms that range from barely detectable to completely disabling depending on the severity of the cellular oxygen depletion. Normal increases

in respiratory ventilation cannot prevent some decrease in a person's ability to perform extended strenuous work. In cases of rapid decompression or removal of supplemental oxygen, one's ability to perform lifesaving responses can be limited to a potentially very short time of useful consciousness.

(2) Benign AMS (also referred to as simple AMS or mild/moderate AMS) is a constellation of symptoms highlighted by frontal headaches that can range from discomforting to incapacitating. Benign AMS is precipitated by a rapid ascent, has no objective diagnostic criteria, but will generally resolve spontaneously within 3 to 5 days.

(3) High altitude cerebral edema (HACE, also termed cerebral AMS) is believed to be the endpoint of progressive benign AMS. High altitude pulmonary edema (HAPE, also termed pulmonary AMS), may or may not be preceded by benign AMS. HACE and HAPE both reveal definitive objective findings, and their symptoms can progress rapidly to become life threatening if not treated by a prompt descent to a lower altitude. For this reason HACE and HAPE are categorized by some to be malignant AMS in contrast to less serious benign AMS.[6]

(4) Chronic mountain sickness (CMS or Monge's disease) can affect long-term mountain residents. CMS is a loss in pulmonary acclimatization that results in alveolar hypoventilation and ensuing cyanosis, low arterial saturation, increased erythrocytosis with increased hematocrit, pulmonary hypertension, and right heart enlargement. Affected individuals have varied neuropsychological symptoms. Because the time of response of CMS is so delayed relative to industrial personnel transfers, it is considered herein to be outside the occupational hygienist's realm (if that is possible). The interested reader is referred to Heath and Williams[6] or Ward et al.[7]

(5) DCS can occur at high altitude with symptoms identical to but usually less severe than those following underwater diving. A full discussion of DCS is deferred to the Changing Pressure Effects section.

Recognition of Hypobaric Hazards

As previously discussed, the ambient total pressure at any practical altitude can be predicted using Equation 29-6. If total pressure decreases but the mixture of gases stays the same, the partial pressures of oxygen and nitrogen decrease in parallel with the total pressure. Thus, a quantitative prediction of these ambient partial pressures at any altitude can be made by applying the molar composition YN_2 and YO_2 from Table 29.2 and the change in total pressure from Equation 29-6:

$$P_{\text{ambient N2}} = 0.78084 \times 760 \times 2^{(\text{feet}/18,000)} \qquad (29\text{-}11a)$$

$$P_{\text{ambient O2}} = 0.20948 \times 760 \times 2^{(\text{feet}/18,000)} \qquad (29\text{-}11b)$$

As long as there are no local sources of emission, absorption, or consumption of either gas, the molar ratio of 78.084% nitrogen to 20.948% oxygen in ambient air will always be about 3.73 to 1. Now, using Dalton's law (Equation 29-7) and adjusting for the presence of other natural inert gases:

$$0.99032\ P_{ATA} = PN_2 + PO_2 = 3.73\ PO_2 + PO_2$$

$$= 4.73\ PO_2 \qquad (29\text{-}11c)$$

Therefore, in ambient air, $PO_2 \approx P_{ATA}/4.78$. Physiologically, the situation becomes a little more complicated. The composition of gases changes as air enters the respiratory tract, as summarized in Table 29.6.[8,9] One of the first changes to occur is the complete humidification of the air before reaching the alveoli. The lung's concentration of water vapor is nominally always 47 mm Hg, equal to the vapor pressure of water at the body's core temperature of 37.2°C (or 99°F). This constant PH_2O of 47 mm Hg is a small molar fraction when the total P is 760 mm Hg at sea level, but it becomes an increasing fraction as the total pressure drops with altitude. The body can easily exhale 1 to 2 L of water per day, continually humidifying typically dry mountain air and contributing an additional risk of dehydration at altitude.[7]

The next change is the simultaneous absorption of oxygen and release of carbon dioxide within the alveoli. Alveolar PO_2 is less than lung PO_2 because some oxygen is

Table 29.6—Physiological Partial Pressures (mmHg) when Breathing Normal Air

Altitude (ft ASL)	*Ambient Air total P*	*PO_2*	*Physiological Pressures[A,B] PH_2O*	*PCO_2*	*ΔPO_2*	*Alveolar[B] PO_2*
0	760	159	47	40 (40)	−38 (−38)	104 (104)
10,000	523	110	47	36 (23)	−26 (−19)	67 (77)
20,000	349	73	47	24 (10)	−19 (−9)	40 (53)
30,000	226	47	47	24 (7)	−15 (−6)	18 (30)
40,000	141	29	47	not humanly tolerable		
50,000	87	18	47	not humanly tolerable		
62,800	47	10	47	water at body temperature boils		

[A]The partial pressures (mmHg) of alveolar CO_2 exhaled and O_2 absorbed decreases at higher altitudes due to increasing respiratory minute volume.
[B]The first set of PO_2 are unacclimatized values; the second are for acclimatized persons.[8,9]

absorbed into the blood for distribution to the body. This absorbed oxygen (listed in Table 29.6 as ΔPO_2) is ~38 mm Hg at sea level and decreases with altitude in a nonlinear fashion in response to both the decreasing oxygen initially within the alveoli and the increasing respiratory minute volume (the latter varies with the degree of acclimatization). Increased respiration decreases the amount of oxygen absorbed per breath (ΔPO_2), thereby increasing the average alveolar oxygen and helping to maintain the oxygen saturation within the blood. Meanwhile, the PCO_2 released from blood into the alveoli is about 40 mm Hg at sea level and decreases at higher altitudes to a plateau of about 24 mm Hg at 24,000 feet (7300 m). The normal ambient PCO_2 is so much smaller than physiologic levels at any altitude in Table 29.6 that it may be disregarded.[3]

Dalton's law can be used again to approximate the physiological dynamics of respiration at increased altitudes shown in Table 29.6. The effect of a potential inert gas is inserted here for completeness because the same hypoxic effects caused by a low total pressure of air at altitude can also occur at sea level if an inert gas displaces air. Inert gas concentrations are normally negligible except in confined spaces (discussed in Chapter 46). Applying Equation 29-7 similar to its use in Equation 29-11c:

$$P_{\text{ambient total}} = SP_i = PN_2 + PO_2 + (P_{\text{inert gas}}) \quad (29\text{-}12a)$$

$$P_{\text{ambient total}} = 4.78PO_2 + (P_{\text{inert gas}}) \quad (29\text{-}12b)$$

$$PO_2 = \frac{P_{\text{ambient total}} - P_{\text{inert gas}}}{4.78} \quad (29\text{-}12c)$$

Accounting for the presence of water vapor in the lung and for the liberation of physiologic PCO_2 yields a new distribution of gases, and in particular a reduced concentration of oxygen reaching the lung:

$$P_{\text{lung total}} = 4.78PO_2 \text{ in lung} + PH_2O + PCO_2 + (P_{\text{inert gas}}) \quad (13a)$$

$$PO_2 \text{ in lung} = [P_{\text{lung total}} - PH_2O - PCO_2 - (P_{\text{inert gas}})] / 4.78 \quad (29\text{-}13b)$$

From this oxygen initially reaching the lungs, an experimentally predictable amount of oxygen will be absorbed into the alveoli (ΔPO_2) to yield Equation 29-14:

$$PO_2 \text{ in alveoli} = [\text{Pambient total} - PH_2O - PCO_2 - (\text{Pinert gas})] / 4.78 - \ PO_2 \quad (29\text{-}14)$$

Example 4. Find the alveolar oxygen partial pressure in an unacclimatized person at 30,000 feet, the approximate height of Mount Everest. Equations 29-6 and 29-12–29-14 can be used in sequence:

$$P_{\text{ambient total}} = 760\ e^{(30{,}000/24{,}540)} = 224 \text{ mm Hg}$$
(versus 226 from NOAA[1])

[3] Because ambient YCO2 is only about 315 ppm (Table 29.2), ambient PCO_2 found using Equation 7 is only 0.2 mm Hg at sea level and decreases with altitude (similar to Equation 11).

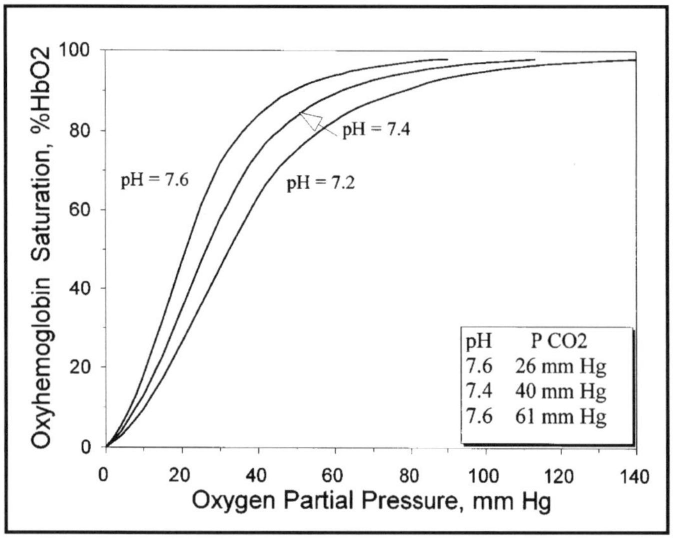

Figure 29.1—The oxyhemoglobin dissociation curves for human blood at 37°C and pH of 7.6, 7.4 (normal), and 7.2.[10]

alveolar PH_2O = 47 mm Hg (at body core temperature)

alveolar PCO_2 = 24 mm Hg (known by experiment)

ΔPO_2 = 15 mm Hg (also known by experiment)

alveolar PO_2 = (224 – 47 – 24) / 4.78 – 15 = 17 mm Hg (versus 18 mm Hg from Table 25.6).

Hemoglobin's affinity for oxygen is a major contributor of physiological tolerance to hypobaric conditions. Hemoglobin in red blood cells carries about 50 times more oxygen than is dissolved in blood plasma. One can calculate using Dalton's law, Henry's law, and sea level data from Tables 29.5 and 29.6, that only about 0.2 cc O_2 can be dissolved into 100 mL of blood plasma acting as water versus about 20 cc O_2/100 mL (often called "20 volume percent") contained in normally oxygenated blood with hemoglobin. Moreover, rather than a linear relationship with the partial pressure of oxygen predicted by Henry's law, hemoglobin binds with oxygen in a beneficially nonlinear way. As shown by the center line in Figure 29.1, which depicts hemoglobin at a normal blood pH of 7.4 (corresponding to an alveolar PCO_2 of 40 mm Hg), blood is at least 95% oxygen saturated at an alveolar oxygen partial pressure as low as 85 mm Hg. The body's response to less oxygen in the blood is to increase its respiration rate, driving off CO_2, increasing the blood's pH, and further increasing the carrying capacity of hemoglobin.[9] Thus, hemoglobin gives the body a very robust tolerance to modest altitudes, as summarized in Table 29.7.

One of the first physiological symptoms of hypoxia is shortness of breath on exertion. The unacclimatized person's initial physiologic response of increasing respiration will be somewhat thwarted by the secondary effect of hyperventilation to decrease the blood's carbon dioxide concentration (see PCO_2 in Table 29.7), which increases its pH and tends to lower respiration. The body will partially acclimatize to altitude in 2–5 days, facilitating hyperventilation (see further discussion in Control of

Table 29.7 — Summary of Direct Physiological Responses to Hypobaric Pressures[11–14]

Altitude (ft)	*Ambient PO_2 mmHg*	*Alveoli PO_2 mmHg*	*Blood O_2 % sat.*	*Health Effects*	*YO_2*	*Eqv. Sea Level Y_{inert}*
< 6000	>127	>82	>95	none except on maximum exertion	17%	21%
12,000	101	65	90-95	decreased night vision and AMS symptoms	13%	37%
18,000	79	44	75-85	euphoria, loss of coordination	10%	51%
>18,000 limited by the time of useful consciousness (TUC)						
20,000	73	40	74-82	TUC = 10-20 minutes	9.6%	55%
25,000	59	25	45-55	TUC = 3-5 minutes	8%	63%
30,000	47	21	30-40	TUC = 1-2 minutesA	6%	71%
35,000	37	12	15-20	TUC = 30-60 secondsA	5%	77%
40,000	29	12	10-15	TUC = 15-20 secondsA	4%	82%

Note: The concentrations of inert gas sufficient to create the equivalent levels of hypoxia at sea level were calculated from ambient PO_2 using Equation 29-12.

AComplete loss of consciousness will result above 30,000 feet.

Hypobaric Hazards section). The combined benefits of hemoglobin's natural affinity for oxygen, an initial increase in cardiac output, and even modest increases in respiration are so effective that very little physiologic effects of altitude can be detected below 6000 feet (1800 m) except that an oxygen debt can develop more rapidly if near maximum exertion. This was perhaps most vividly demonstrated in the 1968 Summer Olympics in Mexico City (2300 m; 7546 ft) in which no world records were established in events lasting longer than 2.5 minutes.[14] Mental performance is also not affected below a PO_2 equivalent to 6000 ft.[11]

Regarding inert gases in confined spaces, it can be noted in Table 29.7 that 6000 feet is equivalent to 17% oxygen at sea level. Figure 29.1 shows that the oxyhemoglobin will still be >95% saturated under this condition. This observation implies that the OSHA requirement to ventilate any time the oxygen content is less than 19.5% [29 CFR 1910.94(d)(9)(vi)] has no real basis in health. The American Conference of Governmental Industrial Hygienists' threshold limit value recommendation of a YO_2 the molar fraction of oxygen, of 18% or an equivalent PO_2 of 135 mm Hg is a similarly conservative health hazard at sea level that if applied literally (using Equation 29-11) would ban all work over 3750 feet above sea level. Such guidance might best be described as a good practice standard. Given that providing fresh air to a workplace is generally cheap (although perhaps time-consuming), abundant oxygen should be available unless it is consumed, an unreasonable amount of some other gas or vapor is allowed in the workplace air (that is likely to be toxic or explosive well before it creates an oxygen deficient health hazard), or ventilation is marginal. However, more severe displacements of oxygen at sea level (shown on the right side of Table 29.7) are capable of causing the full range of hypoxic symptoms.

The decrease in night vision acuity among the next group of symptoms in Table 29.7 manifests itself in lower sensitivity to stimuli and decreased peripheral vision and contrast discrimination.[10,12] The percentage increase in the light intensity necessary to maintain an equivalent retinal response may be estimated using Equation 29-15, determined by regressing the data summarized by Gagge and Shaw.[8]

$$\frac{\%\ \text{increase in}}{\text{light intensity}} = 80 \times \ln(1 - \text{altitude in feet}/19{,}400) \qquad (29\text{-}15)$$

This effect suggests that special precautions should be taken to avoid working in poor lighting conditions at high altitude work sites. A discussion of the cluster of the less direct and slightly delayed symptoms collectively called AMS that can occur about 12,000 feet will be postponed briefly.

Except for the aviation industry and recreation, work above 18,000 is quite rare. High altitude hazard recognition training for pilots and flight crews includes their exposure to the early symptoms of hypoxia (lightheadedness and peripheral tingling) that usually precedes euphoria, incoordination, and the loss of the ability to take corrective steps to ensure ones own survival. The special case of responding to rapid decompression at altitudes above 20,000 ft emphasizes the limited time of useful consciousness[8] sometimes also called the effective performance time.[10] It is incumbent on the flight crew (and beneficial to passengers) to don masks providing 100% oxygen within the sometimes very short times listed in Table 29.7.

In contrast to the direct effects of hypoxia described previously, two clinically important, related, yet distinct groups of indirect and slightly delayed responses to altitude have been identified. What was initially called AMS has now been subdivided into benign AMS and what at least some call malignant AMS.[15]

Benign AMS constitutes an array of symptoms that may begin to develop in travelers from near sea level within 6–12 hours after arriving at altitudes above 8000 ft (2500 m), especially when travel is rapid as by air or car. Symptoms include headache (very common and nearly always in the frontal region), difficulty sleeping (the next most common symptom), lightheadedness or dizziness, nausea or vomiting, and fatigue or weakness. Symptom severity ranges from mild (discomforting) to severe (incapacitating). Physical examination of those with symptoms has revealed that about 25% exhibited chest crackles or peripheral pulmonary edema.[16] Symptoms beyond a headache normally increase gradually, peak on the second or third day, and resolve

Table 29.8 — Reported Incidence of Benign AMS

Altitude (ft)	Altitude (meters)	Incidence	Data Source
6200-9600	1900-2940	25%	17
9350	2850	9%	18
10,000	3050	13%	18
11,975	3650	34%	18
14,250	4343	43%A	16
13,910	4240	53%	19

AIf the person is flown to 9186 ft, 60% incidence; 31% if hiking from 3940 ft.

themselves by the fourth or fifth day. Thus, the term "benign" was adopted to differentiate this pattern from the more life-threatening manifestations of AMS.[6,7] The incidence of benign AMS can be anticipated from prior studies as summarized in Table 29.8, although the subjective nature of benign AMS makes its diagnosis a variable.[6,7]

Symptoms of benign AMS subside spontaneously (without treatment) and will not necessarily affect the same traveler repeatedly or with the same severity. Treatment of symptoms with ibuprofen may be better at relieving symptoms of headache than aspirin, but Ward et al.[7] advocates voluntary hyperventilation, which also promotes acclimatization. Acetazolamide (Diamox®, 250 mg twice daily) may be used either as a prophylaxis beginning 24 to 48 hours before ascending or to relieve symptoms.[7] Dexamethasone has been found to be equally effective for treatment.[20] Prevention by avoiding rapid ascents is widely touted,[6,7] but the recommended schedule of 1 to 2 days per 1000 feet above 9000 feet is not compatible with the fast pace of most non-recreational temporary assignments.

It is important to be able to differentiate benign AMS symptoms from the less common but more severe and life-threatening forms of AMS that may develop. Dickinson[15] proposed the term "malignant AMS" to encompass HAPE and HACE, although this categorization is not as widely accepted as benign AMS.[6] The edema in HAPE is characterized by the release of large quantities of a high protein fluid into the lung. Differential symptoms (often denied by the patient) include severe breathlessness (in 84% of cases) and chest pain (in 66%), with or without the above symptoms of benign AMS. Symptoms of patients with HAPE rapidly progress to a dry cough, production of a foamy pink sputum, audible bubbling and gurgling sounds during breathing, and cyanosis of the lips and extremities. Early recognition of these acute symptoms, conservative field diagnosis, and prompt action is essential to prevent further progression into a coma followed by death within 12 hours. The patient should be given oxygen, restricted in activity, and taken immediately to a lower altitude. If oxygen or descent is not possible, oral nifedipine should be administered.[20] Recovery without complications is normally quite rapid. Although the recovered patient should be cautious, he or she may later return to high altitude without further trouble.[6,7]

The incidence of HAPE is uncertain. One study reported rates of 0.9% in residents returning to 10,000 feet ASL after short visits to a lower altitude.[21] Heath and Williams summarized the incidence among studies of mixed populations at altitudes between 10,000 and 20,000 ft (2800–6195 m) as 0.5 to 1.5%.[6] They also cited studies reporting rates of subclinical pulmonary edema diagnosed radiologically ranging from 12 to 66%. HAPE is slightly more prevalent among the young, apparently healthy, and therefore probably more active segments of a population. The mechanism(s) of HAPE is unclear. It may or may not be related to the mechanisms causing benign AMS, but the most prevalent theory imputes pulmonary vasoconstriction due to the accumulation of water in extravascular spaces. Preventive guidelines are broadly similar to those for benign AMS with the added caution against overexertion the first few days after rapidly traveling or returning to altitudes above 9000 ft (2700 m). Nifedipine can be taken as prophylaxis in people with a history of HAPE.[20] Acetazolamide (Diamox) is not protective against HAPE.[7]

HACE is even less understood than HAPE. Ward et al.[7] and Hackett et al.[20] believe that HACE is a direct progression of benign AMS to include cerebral edema, whereas Heath and Williams[6] believe that thrombosis also plays a part. The symptoms of HACE include many benign AMS symptoms but are differentiated by disturbed consciousness (irrationality, disorientation, and even hallucinations), abnormal reflex and muscle control (ataxia, bladder dysfunction, and even convulsions), and/or papilloedema (swelling of the optic disc). HACE is rarer than HAPE, although symptoms of mixed HACE and HAPE frequently occur. As with HAPE, early recognition and action are essential to prevent a fatal HACE outcome. Fortunately, both conditions require the same treatment with oxygen and evacuation to a lower altitude. If medication is feasible, dexamethasone should be administered immediately, and acetazolimide should be given if descent is delayed.[20] Knowledge of HAPE and HACE is a vital component of a hazard communication program for supervisors and workers at high altitude.

Control of Hypobaric Hazards

The full paradigm of occupational hygiene controls is applicable to the hypobaric workplace. The classically preferred option of source control is only practical in aircraft where the total pressure inside a pressurized cockpit or cabin can be increased. Modern commercial, turbine powered aircraft maintain a maximum interior-to-exterior pressure differential of about 8.6 psi, which will maintain a cabin altitude of no more than 8000 feet. General aviation operations are restricted to cabin altitudes of 12,500 ASL without personal protection.

Various forms of personal protective equipment similar to supplied-air respirators are available to increase the YO_2 in the breathing air. The maximum option of providing 100% oxygen extends the no-effect zone to about 35,000 feet.[9,11] An annoying, sometimes painful, but usually resolvable result of breathing 100% oxygen is the tendency for the body to absorb the high concentrations of oxygen from the middle ear overnight.[22] If the Eustachian tube does not open spontaneously to relieve the resulting pressure difference, the Valsalva maneuver described in the Changing Pressure Effects section should be performed. Supplemental oxygen is generally limited to short-term use in aircraft systems or Himalayan expeditions. However, Ward et al.[7] suggests adding 5% oxygen indoors via the use of electrically powered oxygen concentrators to relieve symptoms of hypoxia.

Acclimatization is a remarkably effective long-term control for habitable high altitudes. Acclimatization changes the balance between two respiratory control mechanisms. After initial exposure to low oxygen, the reaction of peripheral chemoreceptors (PO_2 sensors in the carotid and aortic bodies) is to increase the respiratory minute volume; however, increased respiration decreases the blood PCO_2 and increases its pH, which decreases the stimulation of the respiratory center within the brain. This natural balance initially limits the body's ability to increase respiration in response to a feeling of breathlessness. For example, the work capacity of a new arrival at 17,000 feet would be expected to be reduced by 50%.[9] This would be aggravated if the work required a respirator.

The first adaptation to altitude is a reduction over 2 to 5 days in the blood's bicarbonate ion concentration (HCO_3), decreasing the negative sensitivity of the respiratory center to increased ventilation. Thereafter, the peripheral chemoreceptors can more easily increase respiratory minute volumes four- to fivefold, increasing one's work capacity back toward normal. This is also the time period over which symptoms of benign AMS (should they occur) generally subside. The length of a corresponding administrative restriction to the intensity of a new arrival's work schedule is shorter than but roughly analogous to the 1 week often recommended for heat stress acclimatization.

For more extended stays at altitude, longer term physiologic changes further benefit one's working capacity. After a period of 2–3 weeks, the body's hematocrit[4] and blood volume begin to increase up to 50 to 90% above normal, and the initial increase in cardiac output begins to return toward normal. Following the initial drop to 50% of one's sea level capacity at 17,000 feet, these changes can be expected to raise one's work capacity to about 70% within 2 to 3 months.[9] Other changes in cardiovascular circulation occur even more slowly but are most pronounced in persons born and raised at high altitude.

Selection criteria for temporary work at high altitude are not particularly restrictive. Among the factors not considered detrimental

[4] Hematocrit is the percentage of cellular matter in a volume of whole blood, normally 42% (15 g Hb/100 mL) for men and 38% (13.5 g Hb/100 mL) for women.[9]

to high altitude are increased age, postmyocardial infarction if symptom-free for several months, controlled hypertension, asthma, and well-controlled diabetes.[6] Travel to high altitudes is not recommended for those with effort angina, a recent myocardial infarction, chronic bronchitis, emphysema, and interstitial lung disease.[6] Hard data on reproductive hazards to pregnant women have not been developed, but high altitude travel while pregnant is generally not advised due to fetal oxygen requirements.[6,7]

Hyperbaric Hazards

The most common occupation associated with hyperbaric conditions is underwater diving.[23] Occupational diving is expanding into new frontiers like fish farming.[24]

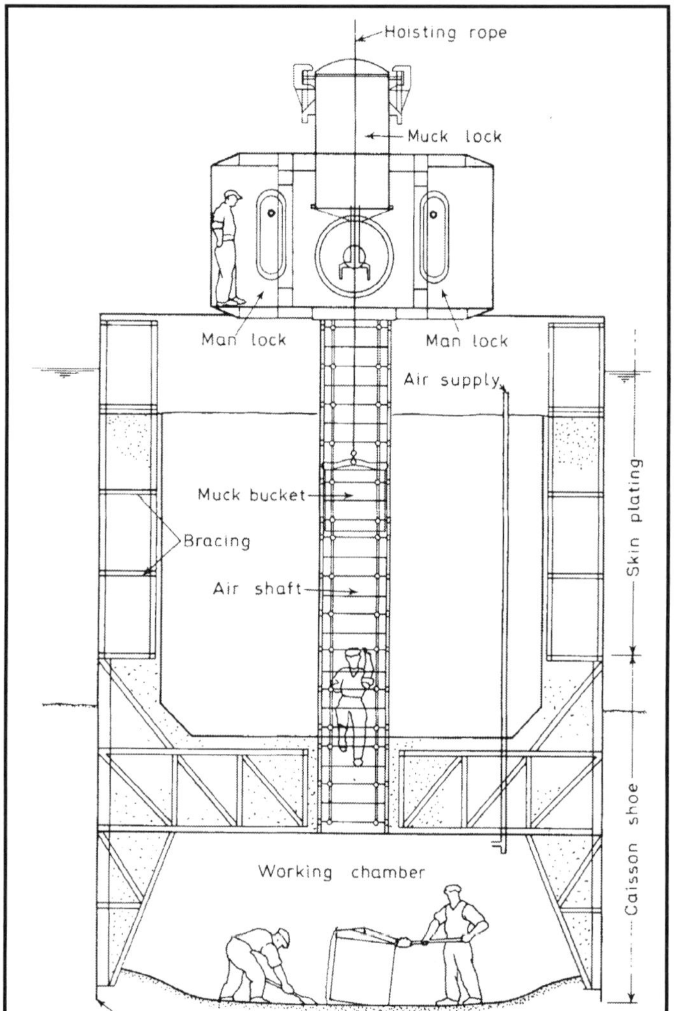

Figure 29.2—A compressed air caisson with separate air locks for personnel and bottom muck.[25]

Compressed air work in construction is a less common occupation. Pressure supplied to an airtight caisson used to be a common technique to reduce the infusion of water or mud while digging bridge pilings (see Figure 29.2). As workers removed the undersurface mud and sand, the caisson would settle until reaching a stratum where a stable structural foundation could be formed. Air pressure has also been applied in tunnels and mines to control water intrusion during construction. A 1975 National Institute for Occupational Safety and Health document estimated there were about 5000 professional divers and caisson workers in the United States exposed to hyperbaric hazards.[26] OSHA limits compressed air workers' maximum pressures to the equivalent of 112 fsw to protect them not only from the direct hazards of hyperbaric conditions described in this section, but also from the indirect hazards resulting after return to normal pressures (described in the Changing Pressure Effects section). Hygienists are often involved in construction projects but rarely have direct responsibilities for diving operations. The material covered in this section and the Changing Pressure Effects section should provide the technical bases to enhance hygienists' support functions to specialized and highly trained supervisory staff.

Three major health hazards (among a wide array of all hazards) associated with hyperbaric conditions are discussed here.

(1) Gas narcosis caused by nitrogen in normal air during dives of more than 120 feet (35 m); helium, substituted for nitrogen in "mixed gas diving," can cause a contrasting effect called high pressure nervous syndrome beyond 500 fsw.
(2) Gas toxicity caused by oxygen and carbon dioxide; the damage of oxygen to the lung and brain (central nervous system [CNS]) varies with the time of exposure and depth. Although a carbon dioxide partial pressure of 15–40 mmHg will stimulate the central respiratory sensor, concentrations >80 mmHg suppress respiration.
(3) Another group of effects can occur after leaving hyperbaric conditions too rapidly. Because they do not occur during residence in one barometric condition, DCS and dysbaric osteonecrosis

are discussed in the Changing Pressure Effects section.

Divers and (more commonly) compressed air workers can face other nonbarometric risks including microbes and parasites,[27–31] noise,[27,28,32–34] silica,[35] radon,[36] fire,[23,28,37] and toxic chemicals during underwater cleanup operations.[28] Thus, the recognized acute and chronic barometric effects covered herein are only a portion of the total health risks faced by these workers. Some novel effects from high pressure have also be reported on typical occupational hygiene evaluation equipment, such as a negative indication of oxygen sensors in response to sudden changes in pressure.[38] Other long-term hyperbaric effects, such as those summarized by Farmer and Moon[39] are neither well established nor otherwise discussed herein.

Recognition of Hyperbaric Hazards

The first of these hazards is the result of the narcotic effect of any gas absorbed into neural tissues. The potential of a gas to produce a narcotic effect is proportional to its solubility in the lipid layers surrounding neural tissue (the Meyer Overton rule for anesthetic gases). Thus, the narcotic effect of a gas increases with its oil solubility and with its partial pressure in accordance with Henry's law (Equation 29-10). Henry's constants for selected anesthetic gases (cyclopropane, nitrous oxide, and ethyl ether) are provided in Table 29.5 as useful points of reference. Pressure increases with depth underwater, as described by Equation 29-5. Each component of the breathing air maintains its own constant molar fraction of the increasing total pressure in accordance with Dalton's law (Equation 29-7). Thus, the partial pressure and potential lipid concentration of each gas can be predicted at any depth (or pressure created by other means).

Example 5. Find the N_2 partial pressure in air and the potential concentration of nitrogen in saturated tissues for a worker repairing an oil rig 185 feet under the Gulf of Mexico.

Starting with a total pressure of 6.6 ATA from Example 1, Dalton's law as expressed in Equation 29-7 can be used to find the fraction of the total pressure contributed by nitrogen:

Table 29.9 — Severity of Nitrogen Narcosis Symptoms with Depth in Feet and Pressure in ATA

Depth (ft)	P_{ATA} (atm)	PN_2 (atm)	Symptoms
100	4.0	3.1	reasoning measurably slowed.
150	5.5	4.3	joviality; reflexes slowed; idea fixation.
200	7.0	5.5	euphoria; impaired concentration; drowsiness.
250	8.6	6.7	mental confusion; inaccurate observations.
300	10.1	7.9	stupefaction; loss of perceptual faculties.

Sources: References 9, 22, 28

$$PN_2 = YN_2 \times P^{ATA} = 0.7808 \times 6.6 = 5.2 \text{ atm.}$$

The concentration of nitrogen in solution can then be determined from Henry's law as expressed in Equation 29-10 and data from Table 29.5:

$$CN_2 \text{ in water} = SN_2 \text{ in water} \times PN_2 =$$
$$0.01206 \text{ cc/mL/atm} \times 5.2 \text{ atm} = 0.062 \text{ cc/mL}$$

$$CN_2 \text{ in lipid} = SN_2 \text{ in lipid} \times PN_2 =$$
$$0.0609 \text{ cc/mL/atm} \times 5.2 \text{ atm} = 0.314 \text{ cc/mL}$$

One can see that the concentration of N_2 in lipid tissues at saturation is much more than in the blood. Although it takes time for sufficient nitrogen to be transported by the blood to saturate the whole body, neurologic tissue is so perfused by blood that symptoms of nitrogen narcosis can be quite rapid. Because the severity of symptoms listed in Table 29.9 depends on the gas concentration in neural lipids, severity depends primarily on depth and not on time at depth; however, severity also depends strongly on personal susceptibility, experience, training, rate of descent, and level of exertion.[22,27,28,40]

The second group of hyperbaric hazards is due to the toxicity of common air constituents such as oxygen and carbon dioxide at high pressures. The hazards of oxygen were first explored as a result of World War II attempts to dive with pure oxygen to avoid nitrogen hazards and creating bubbles of exhaled air by using a closed circuit self-contained breathing apparatus (called a rebreather).[22,28,41,42] Most symptoms of oxygen toxicity can be categorized as either pulmonary (coughing,

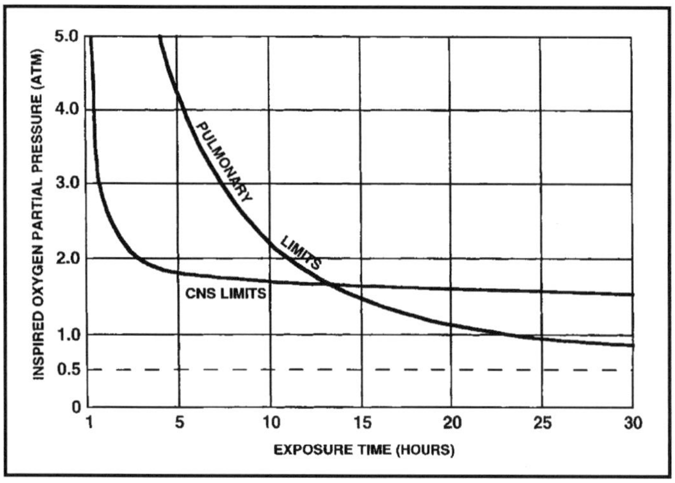

Figure 29.3—Recommended limits of exposure to inspired oxygen.[28]

substernal soreness, and pulmonary edema) or CNS (including body soreness, nausea, muscular twitching, and convulsions).[27,40,45] The toxic mechanism is believed to be related to the increase in oxygen free radicals.[9,43,44] Both symptoms and severity vary inversely with pressure and time of exposure, as shown in Figure 29.3.[27,40,42,45,46] CNS hazards predominate for exposures in the time frame of a working day, whereas pulmonary effects are more of a concern after longer times, such as during saturation diving or recompression therapy for DCS. The pulmonary curve in Figure 29.3 corresponds to about a 12% change in vital capacity.[46] The CNS curve is more judgmental. Although the CNS curve implies an asymptote near 1.5 ATA,[22,45] a plan should be in place to deal with convulsions any time the oxygen partial pressure exceeds 1.0 atm.[27] It is notable that the onset of life-threatening convulsions is not necessarily preceded by the less severe symptoms.[22,41]

Carbon dioxide becomes toxic when it suppresses respiration. Normally an increase in PCO_2 decreases blood pH, which acts to increase the respiratory minute volume. However, at PCO_2 >80 mmHg (about twice the IDLH value), the respiratory control center becomes depressed and soon ceases to function.[47] Thus, carbon dioxide is not toxic at exhaled air concentrations at sea level (40 mmHg in Table 29.6). Nor is it toxic if normal ambient air (314 ppm CO_2 in Table 29.2) is compressed over 90 times to 3000 fsw, yielding PCO_2 = 24 mmHg. However, the combination of the accumulation of exhaled carbon dioxide at increased pressure (either in the breathing system's dead space or due to a malfunction) can rapidly cause toxic effects.[48] Using Henry's law and Table 29.5, the concentration of carbon dioxide in lipids at 80 mmHg is less than half that of nitrogen at 3.6 ATA, supporting the suggestion that the toxic effect of carbon dioxide may be due to a different mechanism than that of oxygen and nitrogen.[49] On the other hand, there is likely to be an interaction between the early response to carbon dioxide causing an increase in respiration and an episode of CNS oxygen toxicity.[22,28]

Control of Hyperbaric Hazards

The options available to control hyperbaric hazards get progressively more complex. Prevention of carbon dioxide toxicity is simply a matter of good system design and maintenance. OSHA regulations for commercial diving operations (29 CFR 1910.430 and 1926.1090) limit CO_2 to 1000 ppm in supply air and to 0.02 ATA within the mask, usually by assuring that the flow of surface supplied air to masks and helmets is at least 4.5 actual cubic feet per minute at any depth at which they are operated. The 0.02 ATA is equivalent to 1000 ppm at 20 atm (or 627 fsw).

Most oxygen toxicity can be prevented by keeping oxygen's partial pressure below 1 atm, and when that is not possible, by limiting the diver's time of exposure above 1 atm. Dalton's law indicates how the partial pressure of oxygen can be controlled by reducing its molar fraction (YO_2) in the breathing air.[22,28] In fact, dives to depths of over 1000 ft (300 m) use only around 1% oxygen to keep PO_2 to less than 0.5 ATA.[39] The U.S. Navy Diving Manual recommends keeping the oxygen partial pressure during routine saturation diving at 0.21 ATA (equivalent to normal air at sea level), to between 0.44 and 0.48 ATA during depth changes, and to a maximum of 1.25 ATA for short intervals.[22] The NOAA Diving Manual time limits when diving with pure oxygen (which NOAA admits are conservative) are superimposed on Figure 29.3.[28]

Administratively limiting depth is a simple but only marginally effective control for nitrogen narcosis. For instance, the deepest routine air supplied dive recommended in the U.S. Navy Diving Manual is 190 fsw.[22] The 5.3 atm of N_2 is well into the range of nitrogen narcosis symptoms described in Table 29.9, and the 1.4 atm of O_2 is approaching the time limited range of oxygen toxicity in Figure 29.3. Reducing or removing nitrogen within the source of breathing air can be a cost-effective control in certain conditions. Reducing the nitrogen/oxygen ratio by using enriched oxygen mixtures (called NITROX) can speed the ascent rate, thus decreasing the total diving time, but NITROX is limited to a shallower depth than air diving because of oxygen's own toxicity at pressures of more than 1 atm. A separate published decompression schedule limits diving with 68% N_2 32% O_2 NITROX to a depth of 130 fsw.[22,28]

Substituting helium for all or most of the nitrogen (called "mixed gas diving") is a cost-effective control for deeper dives. Helium's major advantage is its lower lipid solubility, allowing deeper dives than with normal air. Its higher molecular diffusivity and lower lipid/water solubility ratio than nitrogen also allow it to reach and depart from equilibrium with the body's tissues more quickly during a dive. Unfortunately, helium is less stable in solution, requiring its decompression schedule to have more stops and take longer than nitrogen to prevent bubbles from forming in tissues, that is, supersaturation is limited to 1.7× ambient, compared with 2 to 3× for nitrogen. Schedules for surface supplied He/O_2 dives to 380 fsw are available.[22,28] Deeper dives are only practical by keeping the diver under pressure for several days (called "saturation diving"). A slow rate of compression is necessary to avoid symptoms of high pressure nervous syndrome such as nausea, fine tremors, and incoordination that can begin to appear at about 500 fsw.[22,28] Dives deeper than 1000 fsw have been made using a trimix of nitrogen, helium, and oxygen; physiological research has found that the narcotic potential of a small amount of nitrogen can be used to balance the stimulatory effect of helium at high pressure. Helium presents other problems. Its high thermal diffusivity combined with the high gas density and specific heat at depth cause more rapid heat exchange rates requiring careful protection from hypothermia in the typically cold underwater temperatures.[22,27,50,51] Helium's low molecular weight causes a high-pitched distortion of human speech (a "Donald Duck" effect) that eventually requires electronic processing to become intelligible.[22,52]

Changing Pressure Effects

The recognized adverse health effects of changing pressure include two acute symptoms and one chronic symptom. The following effects can occur in changing either from normal to hypobaric conditions or from hyperbaric to normal or hypobaric conditions.

(1) Expanding or contracting trapped gases can cause pain, potentially leading to barotrauma. This acute symptom and potential damage can occur during either ascent or descent but are potentially most severe when gases are expanding. Barotrauma to the lungs (pulmonary barotrauma) can result in a fatal arterial gas embolism.
(2) DCS due to the evolution of inert gas bubbles inside the body. Acute symptoms of DCS can occur during a decrease in pressure, but most commonly occur soon after an ascent has been completed.
(3) Dysbaric osteonecrosis causes detectable bone lesions most commonly on the body's long bones. Although its etiology is unknown, this chronic disease is likely to be related to the evolution of gas bubbles that may be too small to cause symptoms diagnosed as DCS.

Recognition of Changing Pressure Hazards

Pain and barotrauma from expanding or contracting gases while transiting between pressure zones are direct effects predictable from Boyle's law. The most common sites of pain from trapped gases are teeth, the GI tract, sinuses, middle ear, and lungs (the latter particularly during ascent).[53–55] In addition, compression of trapped gases between the individual and his or her equipment can also cause trauma. For example, if the airspace between diver and mask is not regularly equalized, a diver could end up with small blood vessel hemorrhage of the eyes. A tight fitting wet-suit hood against the ear could cause an external ear barotrauma. The expansion of trapped gas caused by dental decay can actually cause a tooth to crack or a dental filling to become dislodged during ascent; good dental care will prevent this problem. Divers and flyers should anticipate and not attempt to suppress the release of natural gases of digestion that expand during ascent.

The sinuses are hollow, membrane-lined spaces within the skull bones connected to the nasal cavity by narrow passages. Blockage of these passages due to nasal congestion or a head cold can cause pain during either ascent or descent. Sinus pain during descent is called "sinus squeeze." Divers should be trained to detect blocked sinuses and not dive with a cold or an allergic inflammation.

The most common source of pain on descent is from the contraction of air in the middle ear if the Eustachian tubes are inflamed or blocked. The Eustachian tubes normally relieve outwardly (during ascent) at a small pressure difference (ΔP) of only a couple of mmHg. However, it usually requires at least 15 mmHg to relieve inwardly (during descent). If not relieved, pain can begin to occur at 50–100 mmHg, and the eardrum will rupture at 100–500 mmHg. Equation 29-5 can be used to find the change in depth for any pressure. Some examples are given in Table 29.10. However, because pressure is not linear with altitude above sea level, the change in altitude to achieve a similar fixed ΔP varies with the starting altitude above sea level and the direction (ascending or descending), as given by Equation 29-6. To achieve an air pressure difference of 500 mmHg is rare, because it requires, for instance, a descent to sea level starting at a pressure altitude of at least 27,000 feet ASL (8200 m).

$$\Delta\text{altitude descending} = \kappa \times \ln\left[1 - (\Delta P/P)\right] \quad (29\text{-}16a)$$

$$\Delta\text{altitude ascending} = \kappa \times \ln\left[(\Delta P/P) + 1\right] \quad (29\text{-}16b)$$

Table 29.10 — Change in Seawater Depth Corresponding to a Selected Change in Absolute Pressure (ΔP)

ΔP		*Δdepth*	
mm Hg	*atm*	*fsw*	*m*
15	0.020	0.662	0.202
50	0.066	2.18	0.667
100	0.132	4.37	1.33
500	0.658	21.78	6.65

where κ = the altitude coefficient for Equation 29-6 taken from Table 25.4; ΔP = the change in pressure in the same units as P, following; P = the initial pressure found using Equation 29-6.

For most people, opening the Eustachian tubes during descent requires some conscious action like yawning or swallowing. The Valsalva maneuver is a more active technique used by flyers and some divers to force air up their Eustachian tubes by closing their mouth, holding their nose, and trying to exhale. This technique may also clear slightly blocked sinuses. However, external forces on the Eustachian tube at a ΔP of 90 mmHg usually prevent it from opening, even with the help of the Valsalva maneuver.[54] Thus, Farmer and Moon[39] recommend that divers clear their ears every 2 ft (corresponding to 50 mmHg in Table 25.10). Should a blockage occur, divers should be trained to stop and rise back up a few feet before attempting to clear and proceed.[22]

The most severe outcome of expanding gases is pulmonary barotrauma. An increase in gas volume of 20 to 30% can cause an initially full lung to rupture. A trapped gas volume expands in proportion to the change in relative pressure, as predicted by Boyle's law. In contrast with changes in absolute pressure as described previously, changes in relative pressure are not constant with depth. Equation 29-17 (derived from Equation 29-5) can be used to find the change in depth necessary to create a given relative change in pressure.

$$\Delta\text{depth} = -\left([\text{initial depth}] + \kappa\right) \times \left[1 - \frac{V_{\text{initial}}}{V_{\text{final}}}\right] \quad (29\text{-}17)$$

where κ = coefficient from Table 29.3 depending on the water density and units of depth; V = the gas volumes before and after the change in depth.

During ascent, Δdepth is negative, gases expand, and the initial volume is smaller than the final (larger) volume. This ratio is also the final (lower) pressure to the initial (higher) pressure. Example 6 uses Equation 17 to show that equal relative changes in pressure and volume occur over smaller distances at shallow depths than when starting from deeper depths. This implies an important lesson to be conveyed in training: the risk of pulmonary barotrauma is actually greater for a given ascent starting from a shallow depth than ascending the same distance starting a greater depth. In fact, pulmonary barotrauma has actually been documented in a breath-hold ascent to the surface from a depth of 1 m (3 ft).[56] Pulmonary barotrauma can lead to a pneumothorax (air escaping into the pleural space), interstitial emphysema (air escaping into the surrounding pulmonary tissue), and/or an arterial gas embolism of the heart or brain (air escaping into the arterial circulation). Arterial gas embolism is second to drowning as a cause of death in sport divers.[57] Divers and compressed air workers must be trained not to hold their breath during normal ascent and to consciously exhale during a rapid or emergency ascent.

Example 6. Find the change in depth necessary for a gas volume to expand by 25% starting at initial depths of 10, 100, and 500 feet of sea water.

From Table 29.3 for feet of sea water, κ = 33.1, and for this problem, Vinitial/Vfinal = 1/1.25 = 0.80. Using Equation 29-17 for the three initial depths given:

Initially at 10 feet:
depth = (10 + 33.1) × (0.80 – 1) = -8.6 feet.

Initially at 100 feet:
depth = (100 + 33.1) × (0.80 – 1) = -27 feet.

Initially at 500 feet:
depth = (500 + 33.1) × (0.80 – 1) = -107 feet.

DCS is the most commonly known of the many dysbarisms. It is sometimes referred to as "evolved gas dysbarism," "compressed air sickness," "caisson worker's syndrome," or various common names listed in Table 29.11. DCS is completely different from the preceding direct effects of expanding gases. DCS is caused indirectly by the formation of inert gas bubbles at one or more locations within the body.

Example 5 can be extended to a human analogy of the "pop bottle" in Example 3. The nominal distribution of a 70 kg human body is 58% water (or 40.6 L), 20% fats, lipids, and oils (or ~14 L), and 22% solids (mainly bone). Thus, the volumes of gas (V) in each compartment at 185 fsw can be determined using Equation 29-10:

VN_2 in body water =
0.062 cc/mL × 40.6 L = 2.5 L N_2 in water

VN_2 in body lipid =
0.314 cc/mL × 14 L = 4.4 L N_2 in lipids

A total volume of 7 L nitrogen is about the size of a basketball.

As pointed out in the Physical Principles section, when discussing high lipid-to-water solubility ratios, the rate at which inert gases such as N_2 are transported by blood is slow compared to the capacity of lipid tissue to absorb them. This difference creates a beneficial time lag for gas absorption that allows ascents from short dives to be made without any constraints on decompression. But the slow gas desorption rate creates a hazard during ascent from longer dives. Due to either desire or necessity, divers can easily decompress to lower pressures at rates much faster than the stored gases can be resorbed back into the blood and exhaled out of the body. The desorption rate from any location in the body is determined by

Table 29.11 — Distribution of Initial DCS Symptoms Reported Among Divers and Tunnel Workers

				Relative Incidence (%)		
Location of Bubbles	*Symptom(s)*	*DCS Type*	*Common Term*	*Professional Divers[58]*	*Tunnel Workers[58]*	*Recreational Divers[39,59]*
Joints	pain on flexure	I	bends	70–90%	55–90%	41%
Skin	altered skin sensation, itching, or rash	I	1–15%	0–10%	20%	
Brain-spine	dizziness, headache, loss of coordination, weakness	II	staggers	10–35%	8–25%	35%
Chest	cough, dyspnea, pain on breathing	II	chokes	2–8%	1–7%	3%

(1) the difference between tissue and blood gas concentrations, which depends on the dive's depth and "bottom time," and
(2) the perfusion of tissue(s) by blood into which the inert gas must dissolve (in general, skeletal lipid tissues are perfused less thoroughly than are muscle, CNS, or other organs).

Note that the tissue has to have a higher partial pressure compared with the blood for gas to be removed from the tissue (a ratio of the gas concentration within tissue or a liquid to its equilibrium concentration in its surrounding fluid that is greater than unity is called "supersaturation"). However, if the pressure ratio is too large, bubble formation and DCS occur.

Symptoms of DCS can range from irritating to severe. The common names given to DCS depend on its symptoms, and its symptoms in turn depend on the location of the gas bubbles (Table 29.11). The location of the bubbles largely determines the seriousness of the sickness. Beyond the descriptors in Table 29.11, a simple medical classification of DCS has evolved. Type I DCS symptoms involve only skin, lymphatic, or joint pain. Type II DCS involves respiratory symptoms, neurologic or auditory-vestibular symptoms, and symptoms of shock or barotrauma. Type II DCS is potentially life threatening. Of course, nothing is completely simple. For instance, Arthur and Margulies(60) pointed out that skin marbling (from intradermal bubbles) is indicative of impending systemic involvement and should be treated as Type II DCS. Elliott and Moon(59) reported that recreational divers suffering DCS are initially more likely to have Type I symptoms, but most eventually progress to Type II.

The incidence of DCS is largely unknown for various reasons. Literally thousands of cases of DCS have been reported among divers,(39,58,61) but the frequency of diving or even the number of divers from which rates could be assessed is unknown. The distribution of symptoms in Table 29.11 is only among those cases reported to the respective databases. The incidences following three sets of hyperbaric chamber dives are summarized in Table 29.12. Farmer and Moon(39) cited reports of DCS risk of 0.1 to 0.2% in commercial diving operations, whereas another report claims 31% of divers have experienced DCS at least once.(61) These two rates would be statistically compatible after 370 to 185 dives, respectively, if the probability of an incident were distributed randomly. The incidence of DCS among compressed air workers has been reported to be about 0.5% in two large groups(62,63) and 0.07% in another.(64) Differences in rates may be due to differences in the decompression schedules used (both between and within divers and compressed air workers), in the lack of adherence to those schedules (a function of training and supervision), or in the detection and reporting protocols (such as day-to-day versus periodic medical supervision and working almost individually versus in large groups).

Table 29.12 — Incidence of DCS Among Chamber Dive Trials in the United States and Canada

Number of Dives	*Depth Mean (range) Meters*	*Bottom Time Mean (range) Minutes*	*Breathing Gas*	*DCS Incidence*
1041	45 (15–88)	22 (5–120)	air	3.0%
647	66 (36–100)	32 (10–100)	He-O_2	4.2%
261	92 (43–123)	33 (15–90)	He-O_2	12.%

Source: Reference 65

The same DCS phenomenon can occur in hypobaric chamber trainers, in flight crews in unpressurized aircraft, in someone flown from near sea level to a high mountain facility, and in someone who flies soon after diving. Incidence rates among hypobaric chamber technicians have been reported to be as low as 0.25%(66) to about 0.35%(67,68) and as high as 0.62%(69) while hypoxia orientation training was conducted at pressure altitudes ranging from 25,000 to 30,000 ft (7500–9,000 m); however, incident rates can exceed 10% at simulated altitudes above 30,000.(70,71) Both physiological and epidemiological studies show that DCS is likely to occur at about a 15% incidence rate when underwater diving is followed by flying, that is, going from hyperbaric to hypobaric conditions.(72) The *U.S. Navy Diving Manual* Table 9-5 specifies wait times of up to 24 hours prior to flying following air dives to various depths and times (commercial airline cabin pressure is maintained at an altitude equivalent to 8000 ft ASL).

Dysbaric osteonecrosis is perhaps the least known barometric pressure hazard, both technically and publicly. Although it was first recognized among caisson workers early in the 20th century by Bornstein and

Plate[73] and is now known to also affect divers,[26,39,59,74] many believe that it is still not widely recognized, adequately researched, or effectively controlled by current practices.[26,75,76] Dysbaric osteonecrosis (also called aseptic bone necrosis) manifests itself as regions of bone and marrow necrosis, especially of the humerus, femur, or tibia (the "long bones"). The lesions are indistinguishable histologically from necrosis from other causes. The condition is generally asymptomatic, with detection relying on differential diagnosis of high quality radiographs and by excluding other causes.[75-77] In two British studies the prevalence of detectable bone lesions was reported as 24% among compressed air workers[77] and 6.2% among divers.[61] Most of these lesions were in the head, neck, or shaft of the long bones, where they are generally benign. However, 3.7% of compressed air workers had lesions adjacent to articulating surfaces, where they can cause degenerative changes.[77] "Juxtaarticular" lesions were found in 1.2% of divers, with at least 15% of these divers (0.2% overall) actually experiencing joint damage (in shoulders of divers and in shoulders and hips of compressed air workers).[61] There are strong positive associations between lesions and length of diving experience (but not age), the maximum depth dived (none were found in those who had never dived below 30 m [100 ft]), and a history of at least one prior DCS (although lesions can also occur without any known prior acute DCS symptoms).[61]

There is no direct evidence for any clear etiology to osteonecrosis. Microbubbles can be detected electronically before symptoms are detected.[78-80] In the absence of other pathological etiologies, it is plausible that these asymptomatic bubbles could account for the prevalence of osteonecrosis in divers without a history of DCS.[61] The prevalence of dysbaric osteonecrosis is significant and perhaps still being underestimated by the occupational health establishment.

Control of Pressure Changes

The risk of DCS is controlled by administratively limiting the pressure ratio during ascent (the inverse of the volume ratio used in Equation 29-17). Early experimental research by J.S. Haldane recommended a maximum ratio of 2:1 for saturated tissues, the "Haldane rule."[81] However, the majority of the recommended initial standard air decompression ratios are close to but exceed this ratio, as denoted by the gray area of Figure 29.4. Only a small portion of the long dives to depths between 35 and 60 ft complies with this 2:1 guidance.[22] It is important to understand that existing decompression schedules have been defined and refined based on symptoms rather than on preventing bubbles per se or by using good epidemiologic health surveillance.[27] The background level of DCS even when decompression guidelines are followed, the ragged pattern of the exceedance zone, and the detection of bubbles in blood by Eckenhoff et al.[79] and Ikeda et al.[80] after saturation dives to depths of only 25 ft suggest the limited degree of control afforded by these guidelines.

The substitution of helium for nitrogen (discussed in the Hyperbaric Hazards section) changes the dynamics of gas absorption and desorption but does not remove the bubble hazard. The use of one-atmosphere suits is a recent development that has some promise if issues of functional flexibility can be overcome.[39] However, the high costs and low availability of new technologies cause the vast majority of divers to continue to use conventional administrative controls that rely on decompression schedules.

Along with guidance for dives that do not require decompression, the U.S. Navy Diving Manual has four basic decompression

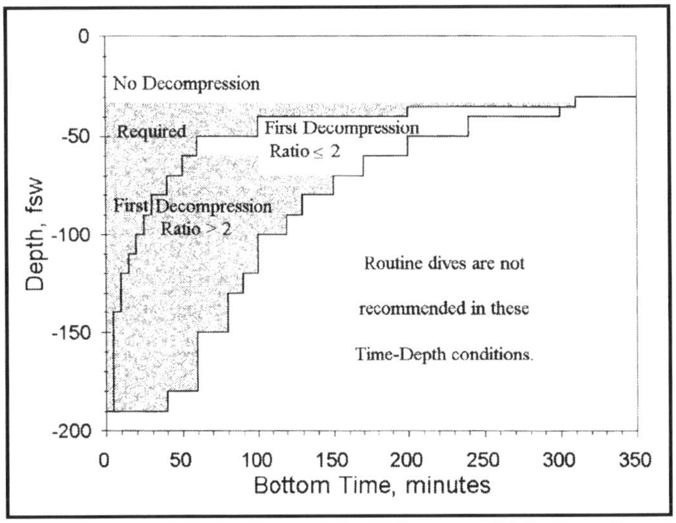

Figure 29.4—Diving conditions above the top solid line require no decompression. Conditions below the bottom solid line require exceptional approval. The first decompression stop for conditions in gray is at a pressure ratio greater than 2.[22]

schedules, each with various options, exemptions, and response contingencies.[22] These schedules are constructed to limit depth on the basis of narcosis, to limit bottom time on the basis of oxygen toxicity, and to limit ascent time on the basis of DCS and include "a practical consideration of working time versus decompression time."[22]

(1) The Standard Air Decompression schedule (see Example 7) is applicable to either scuba or surface-supplied divers breathing air, who completely decompress either in the water or in a diving bell or chamber before reaching surface pressures. The maximum recommended air dive is 190 ft for 40 minutes with emergency dives allowed to 300 ft for 180 minutes.

Example 7. The U.S. Navy schedule for in-water ("standard") decompression from a depth of 100 fsw (30.4 m; 4 ATA) and a bottom time of 120 minutes requires a total decompression time (with time for ascent at about 30 ft/min) of 134 minutes.

Stop, ft (m)	*Stop Time*	*Total Stop Time*
30 (9.1)	12	12
20 (6)	41	53
10 (3)	78	131 = 2:11 hours

(2) Surface Decompression allows ascents with minimal or no stops but requires the diver to transfer to a recompression chamber within 5 minutes of reaching the surface. Surface decompression provides more convenient and often safer conditions than in the water. Recompression with air extends the entire decompression time (see Example 8), but the faster nitrogen wash-out rate from breathing oxygen in the chamber allows a shorter decompression schedule (see Example 9). The maximum recommended dive is still 190 feet.

Example 8. The U.S. Navy schedule for surface decompression using air from the same dive as in Example 7 allows an ascent time of just over 56 minutes but requires an additional surface decompression time of 119 minutes.

Stop, feet (m)	*Stop Time*	*Chamber Time*	*Total Hold Time*
30 (9.1)	12	12	
20 (6)	41	53	
20 foot equiv.	41		94
10 foot equiv.	78		172 = 2:52 hours

Example 9. The U.S. Navy schedule for surface decompression using oxygen for the same dive to 100 ft for 120 minutes as in Example 7 allows both a shorter ascent time of 6 minutes and a reduced surface decompression time breathing oxygen of only 53 minutes.

Stop, feet (m)	*Stop Time*	*Chamber Time*	*Total Hold Time*
30 (9.1)	3		3
40 foot equiv.		53	56 = 0:56 hours

(3) Surface Supplied Helium-Oxygen Decompression procedures have undergone significant revisions since 1991. The new decompression schedule (see Example 10) can involve stops breathing the bottom-supplied mixture below 90 fsw, a 50% oxygen mixture between 90 and 40 fsw, and pure oxygen at stops of 30 and 20 fsw. The normal operating limit on this schedule is 300 feet for 30 minutes.

Example 10. U.S. Navy surface-supplied helium oxygen decompression schedule for the same dive to 100 ft for 120 minutes as in Example 7 would require a total of three stops.

Stop, feet (m)	*Stop Time on 50% O_2*	*Stop Time on 100% O_2*	*Total Hold Time*
40 (12.2)	10		10
30 (9.1)		32	42
20 (6)		58	100 = 1:40 hours

(4) To prevent decompression from Helium-Oxygen Saturation Diving the U.S. Navy Diving Manual specifies a series of ascent rates of feet per hour. For example, an ascent from saturation diving at 340 ft would require 72 hours (or 3 days). However, saturation diving allows more working time per day

(greatly reducing the total time for long jobs) and avoids the hazards of multiple compressions and decompressions.

One important exception is short dives that may be made with no decompression time. These limits for air dives are depicted as the times above the top heavy line in Figure 25.4. For deeper and/or longer dives, decompression time requirements are a cost burden on employers and a potentially boring time for employees, an inviting incentive for both parties to cut corners, resulting in a higher incidence of DCS and potentially of osteonecrosis.[58] Motivational training and close supervision are essential components of a successful diving management program.

In the United States, OSHA regulates compressed air work, diving that does not qualify as "scientific diving,"[28] and diving from vessels not subject to Coast Guard inspection (46 CFR 197.200-488). OSHA regulations may be found in either General Industry Standards Subpart T (29 CFR 1910.401-441) or Construction Standards Subpart Y. Construction Standards also include 29 CFR 1926.801 governing caissons, 29 CFR 1926.803 governing compressed air work, and 29 CFR 1926.804 that contains definitions applicable to all of Subpart S. Tables 29.13 and 29.14 provide a quick overview of these OSHA work practice standards that frequently refer to a diving manual and to other requirements that parallel the principles and mechanisms outlined here and the schedules and guidelines contained within the Navy diving manual.[22]

Table 29.13 — An Overview of OSHA 29 CFR 1910.401-441, Subpart T: Commercial Diving Operations

1910.401 -	Scope and application
1910.402 -	Definitions (a glossary of terms)
1910.410 -	Qualifications of dive team (covers training requirements)
1910.420 -	Safe practices manual (a written procedures manual shall be developed and maintained)
1910.421 -	Predive procedures (covers emergency planning)
1910.422 -	Procedures during dive (covers communication, decompression tables, and the dive depth-time record to be maintained)
1910.423 -	Postdive procedures (covers instructions to diver, provision of recompression chamber (required to be on-site if the dive is outside the "no-decompression limits" and deeper than 100 fsw), and recompression requirements if needed)
1910.424 -	Scuba diving (limited to ≤ 130 fsw and specifies certain procedures)
1910.425 -	Surface-supplied air diving (limited to 190 fsw (with 30 min to 220 fsw excepted) and specifies certain procedures)
1910.426 -	Mixed gas diving (specifies certain constraints and procedures)
1910.427 -	Lifeboating (puts certain constraints on air supplied or mixed gas diving while the support vessel is underway)
1910.430 -	Equipment (various specifications including supplied-air quality limits of 20 ppm CO and 1000 ppm CO_2, hoses, lines, masks, helmets, decompression chamber, etc)
1910.440 -	Record-keeping requirements (retention of most records by employer for 5 years except records of nonincident dives for only 1 year, and all 5-year records to be forwarded to NIOSH)

Note: Parallels 29 CFR 1926.1071-1092, Subpart Y: Construction Diving

Table 29.14 — Overview of OSHA 29 CFR 1926.800-804, Subpart S: Underground Construction, Caissons, Cofferdams, and Compressed Air

1926.800 -	Underground construction (defines general program requirements such as air quality monitoring by a "competent person")
1926.801 -	Caissons (specifies certain fall safety and pressure testing requirements)
1926.802 -	Cofferdams (e.g., specifies escape provisions in case of flooding)
1926.803 -	Compressed air (describes on-site supervision; annual medical certification of each employee; provision of a "medical lock" [decompression chamber]; medical emergency identification badges such as bracelets for all compressed air workers; posting of decompression schedules; a maximum working pressure of 50 psig; air supply ventilation; sanitation; and fire prevention requirements)
1926.804 -	Definitions (e.g., "decanting" when a person is rapidly brought to atmospheric pressure then recompressed immediately [to be undertaken only under medical direction])
Appendix A to Subpart S -	Decompression tables that differ from diving table schedules. These decompression schedules cover much longer working times (more than 8 hours at ≤ 46 psig, equivalent to ~100 fsw), continuous slow decompression (versus stops at multiple stages), and somewhat longer times than the Navy Diving Manual.[22]

A variety of sources of further emergency and routine information are available electronically. The Divers Alert Network (DAN) is the largest nonprofit medical and research organization dedicated to the safety and health of recreational scuba divers (www.diversalertnetwork.org/). An array of international organizations [IDAN] has been organized to provide expert emergency medical and referral services "24/7" to regional diving communities including central and south America, Europe, Japan, South East Asia Pacific, and Southern Africa.

Information on diving and hyperbaric medicine and physiology may also be obtained from the Undersea and Hyperbaric Medical Society, an international nonprofit organization comprised of diving or hyperbaric scientists, physicians, and technical specialists.

The National Board of Diving and Hyperbaric Medical Technology is a source of information on approved courses for becoming certified in hyperbaric technology, exams and testing schedules, training facilities, and other helpful information.

The NOAA Diving Program maintains a strong training program in support of their own and other governmental research and service missions.

Conclusion

Despite hygienists' notable absence from the extensive barometric hazard literature, hygienists have much to contribute to improving the control of hazards in each of these environments. The broad intent of this chapter was to provide both the incentive and the basic tools needed to anticipate, recognize, and control barometric hazards. The physical laws developed by Boyle, Dalton, and Henry underlie and help to quantify the following barometric hazards and adverse outcomes discussed herein.

Hypobaric hazards include hypoxia, benign AMS, and the two more life threatening forms of AMS, HAPE and HACE. Although DCS can result from rapid changes from normal to low pressure (as in decompression at high altitude), symptoms in this circumstance are less severe than those subsequent to underwater diving or compressed air work. Engineering, personal protection, and administrative controls may all be beneficially applied to hypobaric hazards.

Hyperbaric hazards include barotrauma from contracting or expanding gas, toxic effects from oxygen above 1 atm or carbon dioxide above 80 mmHg, narcosis from a PN_2 above 3 to 4 atm, and high pressure nervous syndrome from PHe above about 15 atm. Administrative control of depth to not more than 190 fsw is recommended for air diving; decreasing the nitrogen content of air (such as in NITROX) can shorten the decompression time for shallow dives, and replacing nitrogen with helium allows dives in excess of 1000 fsw.

Leaving a hyperbaric condition so rapidly that inert gas bubbles are generated within the body can cause DCS and probably leads to osteonecrosis. DCS and especially osteonecrosis remain a lingering problem with all decompression schedules.

This information should allow hygienists to be better prepared to contribute to improving the health of workers facing barometric hazards.

Additional Sources

W.N. Rom: High altitude environments. In *Environmental and Occupational Medicine*, 3rd ed., pp. 1359–1387. Philadelphia: Lippencott-Raven, 1998.

E.P. Kindwall: Medical aspects of commercial diving and compressed-air work. In C. Zenz, et al., editors, *Occupational Medicine*, 2nd ed., pp. 343–383. St. Louis: Mosby-Year Book, 1994.

References

1. **National Oceanic and Atmospheric Administration (NOAA):** *U.S. Standard Atmosphere, 1976* (NOAA-S/T 76-1562). Washington, DC: NOAA, 1976.
2. **Mackay, D., and A.T.K. Yeun:** Mass transfer coefficient correlations for volatilization of organic solutes from water. *Environ. Sci. Technol. 17*:211–217 (1983).
3. **Stiver, W., and D. Mackay:** Evaporation rate of spills of hydrocarbons and petroleum mixtures. *Environ. Sci. Technol. 18*:834–840 (1984).
4. **Fthenakis, V.M., and V. Zakkay:** A theoretical study of absorption of toxic gases by spraying. *J. Loss Prev. Process Ind. 3*:197–206 (1990).
5. **Altschuh, J., R. Bruggemann, H. Santl, G. Eichinger, and O.G. Piringer:** Henry's law constants for a diverse set of organic chemicals: experimental determination and comparison of estimation methods. *Chemosphere 39*:1871–1887 (1999).

6. **Heath, D., and D.R. Williams:** *High Altitude Medicine and Pathology*. Oxford: Oxford University Press, 1995.
7. **Ward, M.P., J.S. Milledge, and J.B. West:** *High Altitude Medicine and Physiology*, 2nd ed. London: Chapman & Hall, 1995.
8. **Gagge, A.P., and R.S. Shaw:** Aviation medicine. In O. Glasser, editor, *Medical Physics*. Chicago: Year Book Publishing, 1985.
9. **Guyton, A.C.:** Aviation, high altitude, and space physiology. In *Textbook of Medical Physiology*, 8th ed., pp. 464–470. Philadelphia: Saunders, 1991.
10. **Sheffield, P.J., and R.D. Heimbach:** Respiratory physiology. In R.L DeHart, editor, *Fundamentals of Aerospace Medicine*, pp. 72–109. Philadelphia: Lea and Febiger, 1985.
11. **Knight, D.R., C.L. Schlichting, C.S. Fulco, and A. Cymerman:** Mental performance during submaximal exercise in 13 and 17% oxygen. *Undersea Biomed. Res. 17*:223–230 (1990).
12. **McFarland, R.A., and J.N. Evans:** Alterations in dark adaptations under reduced oxygen tensions. *Am. J. Physiol. 127*:37–50 (1939).
13. **Henderson, Y., and H.W. Haggard:** *Noxious Gases*. New York: Van Nostrand Reinhold, 1943.
14. **McArdle, W.D., F.I. Katch, and V.L. Katch:** *Exercise Physiology: Energy, Nutrition, and Human Performance*. Philadelphia: Lea and Febiger, 1991.
15. **Dickinson, J.G.:** Terminology and classification of acute mountain sickness. *Brit. Med. J. 285*:720–721 (1982).
16. **Hackett, P.H., and D. Rennie:** Rales, peripheral edema, retinal hemorrhage and acute mountain sickness. *Am. J. Med. 67*:214–218 (1979).
17. **Honigman, B., M.K. Thesis, J. Koziol-McLain, et al.:** Acute mountain sickness in a general tourist population at moderate altitude. *Ann. Intern. Med. 118*:587–592 (1993).
18. **Maggiorini, M., B. Buhler, M. Walter, and O. Oelz:** Prevalence of acute mountain sickness in the Swiss Alps. *Brit. Med. J. 301*:853–855 (1990).
19. **Hackett, P.H., D. Rennie, and H.D. Levine:** The incidence, importance, and prophylaxis of acute mountain sickness. *Lancet II*:1149–1154 (1976).
20. **Hackett, P.H., and R.C. Roach:** High altitude illness. *N. Engl. J. Med. 345*:107–114 (2001).
21. **Scoggin, C.H., T.M. Hyers, J.T. Reeves, and R.F. Grover:** High-altitude pulmonary edema in the children and young adults of Leadville, Colorado. *N. Engl. J. Med. 297*:1269–1272 (1977).
22. **U.S. Navy:** *Diving Manual*, rev. 4 (NAVSEA 0910-LP-708-8001). Washington, D.C.: U.S. Navy, 1999 (Change A dated 1 March 2001). Available on-line at www.vnh.org/DivingManual/DiveManualRev4ChangeA.pdf.
23. **Elliott, D., and A.M. Grieve:** The offshore oil and gas industry. In J.M. Harrington, editor, *Recent Advances in Occupational Health*, pp. 21–36. Edinburgh: Churchill Livingstone, 1987.
24. **Douglas, J.D.M., and A.H. Milne:** Decompression sickness in fish farm workers: A new occupational hazard. *Brit. Med. J. 302*:1244–1245 (1991).
25. **Blake, L.S. (ed.):** *Civil Engineering Reference Book*, 3rd ed. London: Butterworth & Co., 1985. pp. 16–29 to 16-31.
26. **Gillen, H.W.:** Proposal for an osteonecrosis registry in the United States. In E. L. Beckman and D. H. Elliott, editors, *Proceedings of a Symposium on Dysbaric Osteonecrosis* (HEW [NIOSH] #75-153) pp. 221–226. Cincinnati, Ohio: National Institute for Occupational Safety and Health, 1974.
27. **Thalmann, E.D.:** Diving hazards. In R.L. Langley, R.L. McLymore, W.J. Meggs, and G.T. Roberson, editors, *Safety and Health in Agriculture, Forestry, and Fisheries*, pp. 617–641. Rockville, Md.: Government Institutes, 1997.
28. **National Oceanic and Atmospheric Administration (NOAA):** *NOAA Diving Manual*, 4th ed. Flagstaff, Ariz.: Best Publishing, 2001.
29. Divers' ear. *Brit. Med. J. 2*:1104–1105 (1977).
30. **Schane, W.:** Prevention of skin problems in saturation diving. *Undersea Biomed. Res. 18*:205–207 (1991).
31. **Victorov, A.N., V.K. Ilyin, N.A. Policarpov, et al.:** Microbiologic hazards for inhabitants of deep diving hyperbaric complexes. *Undersea Biomed. Res. 19*:209–213 (1992).
32. **Summitt, J.K., and S.D. Reimers:** Noise-a hazard to divers and hyperbaric chamber personnel. *Aerospace Med. 42*:1173–1177 (1971).
33. **Brady, J.I., Jr., J.K. Summitt, and T.E. Berghage:** An audiometric survey of navy divers. *Undersea Biomed. Res. 3*:41–47 (1976).
34. **Tobias, J.V.:** Effects of underwater noise on human hearing. *Polish J. Occup. Med. Environ. Health 5*:153–157 (1992).
35. **Ng, T.P., K.H. Yeung, and F.J. O'Kelly:** Silica hazard of caisson construction in Hong Kong. *J. Soc. Occup. Med. 37(2)*:62–65 (1987).
36. **Lam, W.K., T.W. Tsin, and T.P. Ng:** Radon hazard from caisson and tunnel construction in Hong Kong. *Ann. Occup. Hygiene 32*:317–323 (1988).
37. **Dorr, V.A.:** Fire studies in oxygen-enriched atmospheres. *J. Fire Flammability 1*:91–106 (1970).
38. **Dabill, D.W., J.A. Groves, and D.R. Lamont:** The effect of pressure on portable gas monitoring equipment during compressed air tunneling. *Ann. Occup. Hyg. 40*:11–28 (1996).

39. **Farmer, J.C., and R. Moon:** Occupational injuries of divers and compressed air workers. In T.N. Herington and L.H. Morse, editors, *Occupational Injuries: Evaluation, Management, and Prevention*, pp. 423–445. St. Louis: Mosby — Year Book, 1995.
40. **Bennett, P.B., and D.H. Elliott:** The *Physiology and Medicine of Diving*, 4th ed. London: W.B. Saunders, 1993.
41. **Donald, K.W.:** Oxygen poisoning in man. *Brit. Med. J. 1*:712–717 (1947).
42. **Clark, J.M., and C.J. Lambertsen:** Pulmonary oxygen toxicity: a review. *Pharmacol. Rev. 23(4)*:37–133 (1971).
43. **Jacobson, J.M., J.R. Michael, R.A. Meyers, et al.:** Hyperbaric oxygen toxicity: Role of thromboxane. *J. Appl. Physiol. 72*:416–422 (1992).
44. **Piantadosi, C.A.:** Physiologic effects of altered barometric pressure. In *Patty's Industrial Hygiene and Toxicology*, 5th ed., vol. 2, pp. 985–1014. New York: Wiley & Sons, 2000.
45. **Lipsett, M., D. Shusterman, and R.R. Beard:** Inorganic compounds of oxygen, nitrogen and carbon. In *Patty's Industrial Hygiene and Toxicology*, 4th Ed., vol. IIF, pp. 4523–4643; 4597-4621. New York: Wiley & Sons, 1994.
46. **Harabin, A.L., L.D. Homer, P.K. Weathersby, and E.T. Flynn:** An analysis of decrements in vital capacity as an index of pulmonary toxicity. *J. Appl. Physiol. 63*:1130–1135 (1987).
47. **Case, E.M., and J.B.S. Haldane:** Human physiology under high pressure I: Effects of nitrogen, carbon dioxide, and cold. *J. Hyg. 41*:225–249 (1941).
48. **Warkander, D.E., W.T. Norfleet, G.K. Nagasawa, and C.E.G. Lundgren:** CO_2 retention with minimal symptoms but severe dysfunction during wet simulated dives to 6.8 atm abs. *Undersea Biomed. Res. 17*:515–523 (1990).
49. **Hesser, C.M., L. Fagraeus, and J. Adolfson:** Roles of nitrogen, oxygen, and carbon dioxide in compressed-air narcosis. *Undersea Biomed. Res. 5*:391–400 (1978).
50. **Keatinge, W.R., M.G. Hayward, and N.K.I. McIver:** Hypothermia during saturation diving in the North Sea. *Brit. Med. J. 290*:291 (1980).
51. **Timbal, J., H. Vieillefond, H. Guenard, and P. Varene:** Metabolism and heat losses of resting man in a hyperbaric helium atmosphere. *J. Appl. Physiol. 36*:444–448 (1974).
52. **Maitland, G., and A. Findling:** Structural analysis of hyperbaric speech under three gases. *Aerospace Med. 45*:380–385 (1974).
53. **Garges, L.M.:** Maxillary sinus barotrauma-case report and review. *Aviat. Space Environ. Med. 56*:796–802 (1985).
54. **Melamed, Y., A. Shupak, and H. Bitterman:** Medical problems associated with underwater diving. *N. Eng. J. Med. 326*:30–35 (1992).
55. **Molenat, F.A., and A.H. Boussuges:** Rupture of the stomach complicating diving accidents. *Undersea Hyperbaric Med. 22(1)*:87–96 (1995).
56. **Benton, P.J., J.D. Woodfine, and P.R. Westwood:** Arterial gas embolism following a 1-meter ascent during helicopter training: A case report. *Aviat. Space Environ. Med. 67*:63–64 (1996).
57. **Bove, A.A.:** *Diving Medicine*, 3rd ed. Philadelphia: W.B. Saunders, 1997.
58. **Rivera, J.C.:** Decompression sickness among divers: an analysis of 935 cases. *Mil. Med. 129*:314–334 (1964).
59. **Elliott, D.H., and R.E. Moon:** Manifestations of the decompression disorders. In The *Physiology and Medicine of Diving*, pp. 481–505. London: W.B. Saunders, 1993.
60. **Arthur, D.C., and R.A. Margulies:** The pathophysiology, presentation, and triage of altitude-related decompression sickness associated with hypobaric chamber operation. *Aviat. Space Environ. Med. 53*:489–494 (1982).
61. Decompression sickness central registry and radiological panel: Asceptic bone necrosis in commercial divers. *Lancet II*:384–388 (1981).
62. **Golding, F.C., P. Griffiths, H.V. Hempleman, et al.:** Decompression sickness during construction of the Dartford Tunnel. *Brit. J. Ind. Med. 17*:167–180 (1960).
63. **Lo, W.K., and F.J. O'Kelly:** Health experience of compressed air workers during construction of the mass transit railway in Hong Kong. *J. Soc. Occup. Med. 37(2)*:48–51 (1987).
64. **Lee, H.S., O.Y. Chan, and W.H. Phoon:** Occupational health experience in the construction of phase I of the mass rapid transit system in Singapore. *J. Soc. Occup. Med. 38(1–2)*:3–8 (1988).
65. **Tikuisis, P., P.K. Weathersby, and R.Y. Nishi:** Maximum likelihood analysis of air and HeO_2 dives. *Aviat. Space Environ. Med. 62*:425–431 (1991).
66. **Bason, R., and D. Yacavone:** Decompression sickness: U.S. Navy altitude chamber experience 1 October 1981–30 September 1988. *Aviat. Space Environ. Med. 62*:1180–1184 (1991).
67. **Bason, R., H. Pheeny, and F. Dully:** Incidence of decompression sickness in Navy low pressure chambers. *Aviat. Space Environ. Med. 47*:995–997 (1976).
68. **Crowell, L.B.:** A five-year survey of hypobaric chamber physiological incidents in the Canadian forces. *Aviat. Space Environ. Med. 54*:1034–1036 (1983).

69. **Piwinski, S., R. Cassingham, J. Mills, et al.:** Decompression sickness incidence over 63 months of hypobaric chamber operation. *Aviat. Space Environ. Med. 57*:1097–1101 (1986).
70. **Ryles, M.T., and Pilmanis, A.A.:** The initial signs and symptoms of altitude decompression sickness. *Aviat. Space Environ. Med. 67*:983–989 (1996).
71. **Webb, J.T., K.M. Krause, A.A. Pilmanis, M.D. Fischer, and N. Kannan:** Effect of exposure to 35,000 ft on incidence of altitude decompression sickness. *Aviat. Space Environ. Med. 72*:509–512 (2001).
72. **Conkin, J., and H.D. Van Liew:** Failure of the straight-line DCS boundary when extrapolated to the hypobaric realm. *Aviat. Space Environ. Med. 63*:965–970 (1992).
73. **Bornstein, A., and E. Plate:** Uber chronische Gelekveranderungen Enstanden Durch Presslugter-krankung. *Fortchr. Feb. Roetgen-strahlem. 18*:197–206 (1911-1912).
74. **Harrison, J.A.B.:** Aseptic bone necrosis in naval clearance divers: radiographic findings. *Proc. Roy. Soc. Med. 64*:1276–1278 (1971).
75. **Lee, T.C., and K. Neville:** Barometric medicine. In W.N. Rom, editor, *Environmental and Occupational Medicine*, 2nd ed., pp. 1133–1142. Boston: Little, Brown, 1992.
76. **Downs, G.J., and E.P. Kindwall:** Aseptic necrosis in caisson workers: A new set of decompression tables. *Aviat. Space Environ. Med. 57*:569–574 (1986).
77. **Gregg, P.J., and D.N. Walder:** Caisson disease of bone. *Clin. Orthop. 210(5)*:43–54 (1986).
78. **Spencer, M.P.:** Decompression limits for compressed air determined by ultrasonically detected blood bubbles. *J. Appl. Physiol. 40*:229–235 (1976).
79. **Eckenhoff, R.G., S.F. Osborne, J.W. Parker, and K.R. Bondi:** Direct ascent from shallow air saturation exposures. *Undersea Biomed. Res. 13*:305–316 (1986).
80. **Ikeda, T., Y. Okamoto, and A. Hashimoto:** Bubble formation and decompression sickness on direct ascent from shallow air saturation diving. *Aviat. Space Environ. Med. 64*:121–125 (1993).
81. **Boycott, A.E., G.C.C. Damant, and J.S. Haldane:** The prevention of compressed-air illness. *J. Hyg. 8*:342–443 (1908).

Outcome Competencies

After completing this chapter, the reader should be able to:

1. Define underlined terms used in this chapter.
2. Understand the role ergonomics plays in overall worker health and safety.
3. Identify common work-related musculoskeletal disorders (WMSDs) and cumulative trauma disorders.
4. Identify risk factors associated with WMSDs.
5. Select controls that mitigate or eliminate work-related health and safety risks.
6. Apply anthropometric solutions to work environments to best fit the needs of workers.
7. Perform a work analysis using either the work-methods study technique or checklists.
8. Understand the basic elements of an ergonomic control program.

Prerequisite Knowledge

College-level biology and chemistry

Prior to beginning this chapter, the user should review the following chapters:

Chapter Number	Chapter Topic
1	History of Industrial Hygiene
3	Legal Aspects of Industrial Hygiene
6	Occupational Epidemiology
31	Musculoskeletal Disorders, Job Evaluation and Design Principles
32	Upper Extremities
33	Occupational Health Psychology
41	Program Management
43	Hazard Communication
45	Risk Communication

Key Terms

abduction • anthropometry • carpal tunnel • center of gravity • checklists • cumulative trauma disorders • epicondylitis • ergonomics • flexion • ligaments • methods study • physical work capacity • popliteal • pronation • supination • tendinitis • tenosynovitis • work • work-related musculoskeletal disorders

Key Topics

I. Epidemiologic Evidence of the WMSDs

II. Brief History of the Scientific Application of Ergonomics

III. Point of Connection between Occupational Hygiene and Ergonomics

IV. Work-Related Musculoskeletal Disorders (WMSDs)
   A. Why Are WMSDs a Problem?
   B. Occupational Risk Factors Associated with the Upper Extremities
   C. Occupational Risk Factors Associated with the Lower Back

V. Work Methods Evaluation
   A. Analyzing Jobs
   B. Risk Factor Assessment Techniques
   C. Psychophysical
   D. Anthropometry: Designing the Workplace to Fit the Worker

VI. Putting It All Together: Case Study Using Ergonomic Principles and Applications
   A. Ergonomics Evaluation of a Flywheel Milling Department at a Motorcycle Manufacturing Plant: An Intervention Study
   B. Methods
   C. Results
   D. Musculoskeletal Disorders
   E. Discussion

VII. Basic Elements of an Ergonomic Control Program

Ergonomics

30

By James D. McGlothlin, PhD, CPE

Introduction

Ergonomics is the science of fitting workplace conditions and job demands to the capabilities of the working population. Effective and successful "fits" assure high productivity, avoidance of illness and injury risks, and increased satisfaction among the work force. Although the scope of ergonomics is much broader, the term in this chapter refers to assessing those work-related factors that may pose a risk of musculoskeletal disorders and recommendations to alleviate them.(1)

The American Industrial Hygiene Association® (AIHA®) Ergonomics Committee defines ergonomics as

> a multidisciplinary science that applies principles based on the physical and psychological capabilities of people to the design or modification of jobs, equipment, products, and workplaces. The goals of ergonomics are to decrease risk of injuries and illnesses (especially those related to the musculoskeletal system), to improve worker performance, to decrease worker discomfort and to improve the quality of work life. The benefits of well-designed jobs, equipment, products, work methods and workplaces include: enhanced safety and health performance; improved quality and productivity; reductions in errors; heightened employee morale; reduced compensation and operating costs; and accommodation of diverse populations, including those with disabilities. Although ergonomics is an evolving science, proper application of its principles can achieve benefits that are significant and immediate.
>
> Industrial hygienists are concerned with the anticipation, recognition, evaluation, and control of all hazards in the work environment, including hazards related to musculoskeletal disorders. Ergonomics principles should be utilized by industrial hygienists to ensure that the physical and psychological demands of jobs match workers' capabilities. Appropriately trained industrial hygienists should apply the science of ergonomics to ensure that the workplace is as free of recognized hazards as possible.(2)

The National Institute for Occupational Safety and Health (NIOSH) draws a distinction between ergonomics and musculoskeletal disorders. On the NIOSH website for ergonomics, it is defined as "the science of fitting workplace conditions and job demands to the capabilities of the working population. Ergonomics is an approach or solution to deal with a number of problems—among them are work-related musculoskeletal disorders."

Musculoskeletal disorders include a group of conditions that involve the nerves, tendons, muscles, and supporting structures, including intervertebral discs. They represent a wide range of disorders, which can differ in severity from mild periodic conditions to those that are severe, chronic, and debilitating. Some musculoskeletal disorders have specific diagnostic criteria and pathological mechanisms (hand-arm vibration syndrome). Others are defined primarily by the location of pain and have a more variable or less clearly defined pathophysiology (back disorders). Examples of musculoskeletal disorders of the upper extremities include carpal tunnel syndrome, wrist tendonitis, epicondylitis, and rotator cuff tendonitis. Both nonoccupational and occupational factors contribute to the development and exacerbation of these disorders.

The International Ergonomics Association discusses on its website the domains of specialization within the discipline of ergonomics—physical ergonomics, cognitive ergonomics, and organizational ergonomics. Physical ergonomics is concerned with human anatomical, anthropometric, physiological, and biological characteristics related to physical activity. Topics that are relevant to physical ergonomics are working postures; material handling; repetitive movements; work-related musculoskeletal disorders; workplace layout; and safety and health. Cognitive ergonomics is concerned with mental processes such as perception, memory, reasoning, and motor response. Relevant topics are mental workload; decision-making; skilled performance; human-computer interaction; reliability; work stress; and training as related to human-system design. Organizational ergonomics is concerned with optimizing sociotechnical systems. This includes organizational structures, policies, and processes. Topics relevant to this specialization include communication; crew resource management; work design; teamwork; participatory design; community ergonomics; cooperative work; new work paradigms; organizations; telework; and quality management.

This chapter outlines the approach most commonly recommended for identifying and correcting work-related musculoskeletal disorders and offers practical information for applying ergonomic applications in workplaces. Additional information about the techniques, instruments, and methods mentioned in this chapter, along with references to other resources, can be found in the appendices. This chapter is focused toward health professionals, and especially occupational hygienists, who need to apply ergonomics solutions (especially in the physical domain) to the workplace to ensure safe and healthful work conditions.

As shown in Table 30.1, principles of ergonomics that are used to accomplish the broad goals of making work safe and humane, increasing human efficiency, and promoting human well-being have their origins in several scientific disciplines.[3] Specialists involved in solving ergonomic problems include psychologists; cognitive scientists; physiologists; biomechanicists; applied physical anthropologists; occupational hygienists; safety specialists; and occupational and systems engineers. The approach used by these professionals could range from the application of ergonomic principles in designing a simple tool to evaluating complex technological systems. This chapter focuses on ergonomics using a much simpler and narrower platform—anticipation, recognition, evaluation, and control of work-related musculoskeletal disorders (WMSDs) of the upper extremities and back. The reader is encouraged to seek additional information from the ergonomics journals and publications listed in the Appendices at the end of this chapter regarding the many applications of ergonomics, including the cognitive aspects.

Table 30.1 — Origins and Applications of Ergonomics and Human Factors

	Ergonomics	
Anatomy ———›	Anthropometry	Industrial engineering
Orthopedics —›	Biomechanics	Bioengineering
Physiology——›	Work physiology	Systems engineering
Medicine———›	Occupational hygiene	Safety engineering
Physiology——›	Management	Military engineering
Sociology ——›	Labor relations	Computer-aided design
	Human Factors	

Source: Adapted from reference 3, p. 347.

Epidemiologic Evidence of WMSDs

The question of whether musculoskeletal disorders are work-related was addressed in a NIOSH study titled, *Musculoskeletal Disorders and Workplace Factors: A Critical Review of Epidemiologic Evidence for Work-Related Musculoskeletal Disorders of the Neck, Upper Extremity, and Low Back.*[4] Although musculoskeletal disorders were recognized as having occupational etiologic factors as early as the 18th century, it was not until the 1970s that occupational factors were examined in a systematic way using epidemiologic methods to associate the work-relatedness of these conditions. In this document NIOSH concluded that "a large body of credible epidemiological research exists that shows a consistent relationship between MSDs and certain physical factors, especially at higher exposure levels ... and in particular when workers are exposed to several risk factors simultaneously."[4] These relationships are summarized in Table 30.2.

The National Academy of Sciences (NAS) also has weighed in on the science of ergonomics. It estimated that the cost of lost workdays and the compensation related to musculoskeletal disorders (including back discomfort and cumulative trauma disorders) ranged from 13 to 20 billion dollars annually. NAS confirmed NIOSH findings that there were causal links between musculoskeletal disorders and workplace risk factors.[5] Because the link between musculoskeletal disorders and work risk factors has been more clearly established through this body of work, logic would dictate that reducing and preventing such risk factors from occurring in the work setting should reduce the incidence and severity of such disorders as well. Ergonomic control programs may be one of the more effective mechanisms to achieve this end. In addition to the NIOSH document mentioned previously, a companion document, *Elements of Ergonomics Programs: A Primer Based on Workplace Evaluations of Musculoskeletal Disorders*[1], was developed to guide industry and labor representatives in methods to systematically evaluate, reduce, and eliminate work risk factors that may cause musculoskeletal disorders. The basic elements are outlined at the end of this chapter.

Table 30.2 — Evidence for Causal Relationship Between Physical Work Factors and MSDs

Body Part Risk Factor	*Strong Evidence (+++)*	*Evidence (++)*	*Insufficient Evidence (+/0)*
Neck and Neck/Shoulder			
Repetition		X	
Force		X	
Posture	X		
Vibration			X
Shoulder			
Posture		X	
Force			X
Repetition		X	
Vibration			X
Elbow			
Repetition			X
Force		X	
Posture			X
Combination	X		
Hand/Wrist			
Carpal tunnel syndrome			
Repetition		X	
Force		X	
Posture			X
Vibration		X	
Combination	X		
Tendinitis			
Repetition		X	
Force		X	
Posture		X	
Combination	X		
Hand-arm vibration syndrome			
Vibration	X		
Back			
Lifting/forceful movement	X		
Awkward posture		X	
Heavy physical work			X
Whole body vibration	X		
Static work posture			X

Brief History of the Scientific Application of Ergonomics

The term ergonomics is derived from the Greek roots *ergon*, meaning work, and *nomos*, meaning law. Therefore, literally translated, "ergonomics" means "the laws of work." The term "ergonomics" was first coined in 1950 by scientists in the United Kingdom to describe the interdisciplinary efforts to design equipment and work tasks to fit the person. These scientists were from the physical, biological, and psychological disciplines. Ergonomics is also known by the term "human factors engineering." Although both "ergonomics" and "human factors" are the same in meaning, the difference is that the term "human factors" has an American origin, whereas "ergonomics" has a European origin. In 1957, American engineers, behavioral scientists, and anthropometrists who performed similar work formed the Human Factors Society, and in 1992 renamed the organization the Human Factors and Ergonomics Society.

Even though the word "ergonomics" originated in 1950, the observation that musculoskeletal disorders were an occupational hazard dates back to the 1700s when the physician Ramazzini stated the following: "Manifold is the harvest of diseases reaped by craftsman... As the...cause I assign certain violent and irregular motions and unnatural postures... by which... the natural structure of the living machine is so impaired that serious diseases gradually develop therefrom."[6] Not much attention was paid to human musculoskeletal injury and illness because it was generally theorized that during the industrial revolution manual labor was plentiful and inexpensive. If someone experienced an occupational injury or illness, he or she was replaced. Indeed, it was not until the 1970s, when the Occupational Safety and Health Act was created, that musculoskeletal injuries and illnesses were identified under the General Duty Clause as problems to be prevented. This was further supported by one of the first successful cases filed by an employee against a company in a court of law. The court determined that "An injury which develops gradually over time as a result of the performance of the injured worker's job-related duties is compensable."[7] Following this historic case, industry had an economic incentive to consider ergonomics.

Point of Connection between Occupational Hygiene and Ergonomics

The scope of occupational hygiene includes a broad range of chemical, biological, and physical hazards. The application of ergonomics to solve WMSDs has become more prominent because of the loss of productivity, workers' compensation costs, and human suffering. As a result, some of the responsibilities for controlling musculoskeletal injuries and illnesses have fallen on the shoulders of the occupational hygienist. However, not all occupational hygienists have adequate training in ergonomics. Part of the reason is that there are only a handful of universities in the United States that formally teach ergonomics as part of the occupational hygiene curriculum. For example, graduate programs based in environmental and occupational health in schools of public health traditionally teach programs that focus on controlling airborne contaminants in the workplace, while graduate programs based in occupational engineering focus on ergonomic applications to control work-related physical stressors, such as repetition, force, posture, and lack of recovery time. Fortunately, the same basic skills taught in occupational engineering for ergonomic applications can be also transferred to the occupational hygiene curriculum to expand the its scope. The occupational hygienist can also apply these skills to simultaneously reduce chemical, biological, and physical hazards. For example, walk-through evaluations of the workplace by occupational hygienists enable them to see firsthand the hazards in the workplace, conduct informal interviews with workers, take measurements, and make recommendations through engineering and administrative controls. The expanded role of occupational hygienists allows them to use the same measurement techniques for musculoskeletal as well as chemical hazard controls. The key is to apply the principles of job analysis where work can be broken into its fundamental elements and then to link those elements to work risk factors. Finally, the role of the occupational hygienist is expanding to include ergonomics as part of the job responsibility. By evaluating the workplace from the perspective of reducing job-related musculoskeletal injuries and illnesses, occupational hygienists can be more comprehensive in applying their skills to workplace controls.

WMSDs

According to NIOSH, the general term "musculoskeletal disorders" describes the following: (1) disorders of the muscles, nerves, tendons, ligaments, joints, cartilage, or spinal discs; (2) disorders that are not typically the result of any instantaneous or acute event, such as a slip, trip, or fall, but reflect a more gradual or chronic development; (3) disorders diagnosed by a medical history, physical examination, or other medical tests that can range in severity from mild and intermittent to debilitating and chronic; and (4) disorders with several distinct features, such as carpal tunnel syndrome, as well as disorders defined primarily by the location of the pain (i.e., low back pain).[1]

However, the specific term "work-related musculoskeletal disorders" refers to (1) musculoskeletal disorders to which the work environment and the performance of work contribute significantly, or (2) musculoskeletal disorders that are made worse or longer lasting by work conditions. These workplace risk factors, along with personal characteristics (e.g., physical limitations or existing health problems) and societal factors, are thought to contribute to the development of WMSDs.[8] They also reduce productivity or cause dissatisfaction. Common examples are jobs requiring repetitive, forceful, or prolonged exertions of the hands; frequent or heavy lifting, pushing, pulling, or carrying of heavy objects; and prolonged awkward postures. Vibration and cold may add risk to these work conditions. Jobs or working conditions presenting multiple risk factors will have a higher probability of causing a musculoskeletal problem. The level of risk depends on the intensity, frequency, and duration of the exposure to these conditions and the individual's capacity to meet the force or other job demands that might be involved. These conditions are more correctly called "ergonomic risk factors for musculoskeletal disorders" rather than "ergonomic hazards" or "ergonomic problems." But like the term "safety hazard," these terms have become popular.

Why Are WMSDs a Problem?

Many reasons exist for considering WMSDs a problem, including: (1) WMSDs are among the most prevalent lost-time injuries and illnesses in almost every industry[9–11]; (2) WMSDs, specifically those involving the back, are among the most costly occupational problems[10–14]; (3) job activities that may cause WMSDs span diverse workplaces and job operations (see Table 32.3)[3]; (3) WMSDs may cause a great deal of pain and suffering among afflicted workers; and (4) WMSDs may decrease productivity and the quality of products and services. Workers experiencing aches and pains on the job may not be able to do good quality work.

Because musculoskeletal disorders can be associated with non-work activities (e.g., sports) and medical conditions (e.g., renal disease, rheumatoid arthritis), it is difficult to determine the proportion due solely to occupation. For example, in the general population, nonoccupational causes of low-back pain are probably more common than workplace causes.[15] However, even in these cases the musculoskeletal disorders may be aggravated by workplace factors.

WMSDs of the Upper Extremities

Musculoskeletal disorders of the upper extremities, such as carpal tunnel syndrome and rotator cuff tendonitis, resulting from work factors are common and occur in nearly all sectors of the economy. More than $2 billion in workers' compensation costs are spent annually on these work-related problems.[16] Workers' compensation costs undoubtedly underestimate the actual magnitude of these disorders. Scientific research has provided important insights into the etiology and prevention of these disorders.

Musculoskeletal disorders of the neck and upper extremities resulting from work factors affect employees in every type of workplace, including such diverse workers as food processors, automobile and electronics assemblers; carpenters; office data entry workers; grocery store cashiers; and garment workers. The highest rates of these disorders occur in the industries with a substantial amount of repetitive, forceful work. Musculoskeletal disorders affect the soft tissues of the neck; shoulder; elbow; hand; wrist; and fingers. These include the nerves (e.g., carpal tunnel syndrome), tendons (e.g., tenosynovitis, peritendinitis, epicondylitis), and muscles (e.g., tension neck syndrome).[16]

The number of nonfatal occupational injuries and illnesses as reported by the Bureau of Labor Statistics (BLS) requiring days away from work in private industry has trended downward recently. Data issued in March 2009 showed 1,158,870 total cases of nonfatal occupational injuries and illnesses involving days away from work. However, the BLS reported that the median days away from work increased to 8 days in 2008 versus 7 days in from 2004–2007. The increase in severity rates may indicate a trend where fewer workers are being exposed to more and longer duration MSD risk factors. Such employment schemes, (i.e., fewer workers doing more work), tend to occur during recessions, of which the U.S. had through 2008 and is recently recovering. (http://www.bls.gov/news.release/archives/osh2_11202008.htm)

Table 30.3 — List of Common Cumulative Trauma Disorders of the Upper Extremities

Disorder[A]	*Description*	*Typical Job Activities*
Carpal tunnel syndrome (writer's cramp, neuritis, median neuritis) (N)	Results from compression of the median nerve in the carpal tunnel of the wrist. This tunnel is an opening under the carpal ligament on the palmar side of the carpal bones, through which pass the median nerve, finger flexor tendons, and blood vessels. Swelling of the tendon sheaths reducesthe size of the tunnel opening and pinches the median nerve and possibly blood vessels. The tunnel opening is also reduced if the wrist is flexed or extended or ulnarly or radially pivoted.	buffing; grinding; polishing; sanding; assembly work; typing; keying; cashiering; playing musical instruments; surgery; packing; housekeeping; cooking; butchering; hand washing; scrubbing; hammering
Cubital tunnel syndrome (N)	Compression of the ulnar nerve below the notch of the elbow. Tingling, numbness, or pain radiating into ring or little fingers.	resting forearm near elbow on a hard surface or sharp edge or reaching over obstruction
deQuervain's syndrome (or disease) (T)	A special case of tendosynovitis that occurs in the abductor and extensor tendons of the thumb where they share a common sheath. Often results from combined forceful gripping and hand twisting, as in wringing cloth.	buffing; grinding; polishing; sanding; pushing; pressing; sawing; cutting; surgery; butchering; use of pliers; "turning" control such as on motorcycle; inserting screws in holes; forceful hand wringing.
Epicondylitis ("tennis elbow") (T)	Tendons attaching to the epicondyle (the lateral protrusion at the distal end of the humerus bone) become irritated. Often the result of impacting or jerky throwing motions, repeated supination and pronation of the forearm, and forceful wrist extension movements. Well-known among tennis players, pitchers, bowlers, and people hammering. Similar irritation of the tendon attachments on the inside of the elbow is called medical epicondylitis, also known as "golfer's elbow."	turning screws; small parts assembly; hammering; meat cutting; playing musical instruments; playing tennis; pitching; bowling
Ganglion (T)	A tendon sheath swelling that is filled with synovial fluid, or cystic tumor at the tendon sheath or a joint membrane. Affected area swells, causing a bump under the skin, often on the dorsal or radial side of the wrist. (Because it was in the past occasionally smashed by striking with a Bible or heavy book, it was also called a "Bible bump.")	buffing; grinding; polishing; sanding; pushing; pressing; sawing; cutting; surgery; butchering; use of pliers; "turning" control such as on motorcycle; inserting screws in holes; forceful hand wringing
Neck tension syndrome (M)	An irritation of the levator scapulae and trapezius group of muscles of the neck, commonly occurring after repeated or sustained overhead work.	belt conveyor assembly, typing, keying, small parts assembly, packing, load carrying in hand or on shoulder
Pronator (teres) syndrome (N)	Result of compression of the median nerve in the distal third of the forearm, often where it passes through the two heads of the pronator teres muscle in the forearm; common with strenuous flexion of elbow and wrist.	soldering, buffing, grinding, polishing, sanding

Table 30.3 — List of Common Cumulative Trauma Disorders of the Upper Extremities (cont.)

Disorder	*Description*	*Typical Job Activities*
Shoulder tendinitis (rotator cuff syndrome or tendinitis, supraspinatus tendinitis, subacromial bursitis, subdeltoid bursitis, partial tear of the rotator cuff) (T)	A shoulder disorder of the rotator cuff. The cuff consists of four tendons that fuse over the shoulder joint, where they pronate and supinate the arm and help to abduct it. The rotator cuff tendons must pass through a small bony passage between the humerus and the acromion, with a bursa as cushion. Irritation and swelling of the tendon or of the bursa are often caused by continuous muscle and tendon effort to keep the arm elevated.	Punch press operations, overhead assembly, overhead welding; overhead painting; overhead auto repair; belt conveyor assembly work; packing; storing; construction work; postal letter carrying; reaching; lifting; carrying load on shoulder
Tendinitis (tendinitis) (T)	An inflammation of a tendon. Often associated with repeated tension, motion, bending, being in contact with a hard surface, vibration. The tendon becomes thickened, bumpy, and irregular in its surface. Tendon fibers may be frayed or torn apart. In tendons without sheaths, such as within elbow and shoulder, the injured area may calcify.	punch press operation; assembly work; wiring; packaging; core making; use of pliers
Tendosynovitis (tenosynovitis, tendovaginitis) (T)	Disorder of tendons inside synovial sheaths. The sheath swells, so movement of the tendon with the sheath is impeded and painful. Tendon surfaces can become irritated, rough, and bumpy. If the inflamed sheath presses progressively onto the tendon, the condition is called stenosing tendosynovitis. DeQuervain's syndrome is a special case occurring in the thumb, and the trigger finger condition occurs in flexors of the fingers.	buffing; grinding; polishing; sanding; punch press operation; sawing; cutting; surgery; butchering; use of pliers; "turning" control such as on a motorcycle; inserting screws in holes; forceful hand wringing
Thoracic outlet syndrome (neurovascular compression syndrome, cervicobrachial disorder, brachial plexus neuritis, costoclavicular syndrome, hyperabduction syndrome) (V, N)	Results from compression of nerves and blood vessels between clavicle and first and second ribs at the brachial plexus. If this neurovascular bundle is compressed by the pectoralis minor muscle, blood flow to and from the arm is reduced. This ischemic condition makes the arm numb and limits muscular activities.	buffing; grinding; polishing; sanding; overhead assembly; overhead welding; overhead painting; overhead auto repair; typing; keying; cashiering; wiring; playing musical instruments; surgery; truck driving; stacking; material handling; postal letter carrying; carrying heavy loads with extended arms
Trigger finger (or thumb) (T)	Special type of tendosynovitis in which the tendon becomes nearly locked, so that its forced movement is not smooth but snaps or jerks. This is a special case of stenosing tendosynovitis crepitans, a condition usually found with digit flexors at the A1 ligament.	operating finger trigger; using hand tools that have sharp edges pressing into the tissue or whose handles are too far apart for the user's hand so that the end segments of the fingers are flexed while the middle segments are straight
Ulnar artery aneurysm (V, N)	Weakening of a section of the wall of the ulnar artery as it passes through the Guyon tunnel in the wrist; often from pounding or pushing with heel of the hand. The resulting "bubble" presses on the ulnar nerve in the Guyon tunnel.	assembly work

(continued on the next page.)

Table 30.3 — List of Common Cumulative Trauma Disorders of the Upper Extremities (cont.)

Disorder	*Description*	*Typical Job Activities*
SUlnar nerve entrapment (Guyon tunnel syndrome) (N)	Results from entrapment of the ulnar nerve as it passes through the Guyon tunnel in the wrist. Can occur from prolonged flexion and extension of the wrist and repeated pressure on the hypothenar eminence of the palm.	playing musical instruments; carpentering; bricklaying; use of pliers; soldering; hammering
White finger ("dead finger," Raynaud's syndrome, vibration syndrome) (V)	Stems from insufficient blood supply, bringing about noticeable blanching. Finger turns cold, numb, tingles, and sensation and control of finger movement may be lost. The condition is due to closure of the digit's arteries caused by vasospasm triggered by vibrations. A common cause is continued forceful gripping of vibrating tools, particularly in a cold environment.	chain sawing; jack hammering; use of vibrating tool that is too small for the hand, often in a cold environment

[A]N=nerve disorder; T= tendon disorder; M=muscle disorder; V= vessel disorder.

At the beginning of the second decade of the new millennium, a new picture of the U.S. economy is emerging with regard to the epidemiology of musculoskeletal disorders. The key changes, as summarized by the BLS, are presented below:

- Total musculoskeletal disorder (MSD) cases continue to decline for the 6th year in a row to 317,440 cases. Yet, the percentage of MSD cases (out of total cases) has not varied since 2005, holding steady at 29%.
- While there were overall decreases in injury and illness cases, there were increases in following categories:
  - — For workers 55 to 64 years old and workers 65 and older, injury and illness cases increased 3 percent and 13 percent, respectively
  - — For Hispanic or Latino workers in transportation and material moving occupations the number of injury and illness cases increased 10 percent to 27,770 cases.

When the BLS evaluated trends in specific occupations they reported that:

- In 2008, the top 10 occupations that had more than 18,000 injuries and illnesses. These included: 1) Laborers and freight, stock, and material movers, hand (79,590); 2) Truck drivers, heavy and tractor-trailer (57,700); 3) Nursing aides, orderlies, and attendants (44,610); 5) Construction laborers (31,310) 4) Retail salespersons (28,900); 6) Janitors and cleaners, except maids and housekeeping cleaners (28,110); 7) Truck drivers, light or delivery services (28,040); 8) Maintenance and repair workers, general (20,800); 9 Registered nurses (19,070); 10) Maids and housekeeping cleaners (18,650). This has been a trend since 2003. These top 10 occupations made up more than 33 percent of all injuries and illnesses with days away from work.
- The top occupation (Laborers and freight, stock, and material movers) experienced the an increase in the median days away from work to 8 days, an increase of one day from 2007 data.
- Tractor-trailer drivers of heavy trucks had 57,700 cases with days away from work; with 17 median days away from work (a measure of severity), up 2 days from 2007 data. This represented a 4% increase from 2007 data.
- Carpenters days away from work decreased by nearly 25% from 2007 levels and fell below the top ten occupations with less than 20,000 injuries and illnesses, a first since 2003. This drop may be more reflective of the economy than anything else.

There were 7 occupations that had days-away-from-work injury and illness rates that were three times greater than the average rate for all workers of 113 cases per 10,000 full time workers.

- Nursing aides, orderlies, and attendants showed a rate of 449 per 10,000 full time workers and decreased by 4 percent. However, the number of cases did not change significantly from 2007. Also, interesting was the severity rate showing that nursing aides, orderlies and attendants had a median of 5 days to recover from injuries and illnesses. This is 3 days fewer than for all occupations.
- The severity rate for reservation and transportation ticket agents and travel clerks increased 16 percent for days away from work.
- The severity rate for emergency medical technicians and paramedics increased by 11 percent.

One of the more interesting statistics reported by the BLS, in terms of severity of musculoskeletal injuries and illnesses, was that four sectors in industry accounted for 75 percent of the days away from work. These were: 1) trade, transportation and utilities (30 percent); 2) education and health services (17 percent); 3) manufacturing (15 percent); and 4) construction (11 percent).

The BLS report on worker characteristics for injury and illness rates were in some instances predictable and in others surprising. For example, younger workers tended to be absent from work the least number of days, while older workers (i.e., 65 years and older) had the most number of days away from work. Males were absent from work nearly twice (64%) as often compared to females. It is suggested that males are exposed to more physically demanding jobs where MSD risk factors are more prevalent and this could account for the rate differences in gender. The BLS reported that injuries and illnesses decreased for white, black and Hispanic or Latino workers. Yet, there was an increase in transportation and the material moving occupations among Hispanic and Latino workers. Again, this may have been a function of the economy more than anything else.

Case characteristics as defined by the BLS

In order to understand the events and circumstances of workplace injuries and illnesses requiring one or more days away from work it is important to include the: 1) nature, 2) part of body, 3) source, 4) event or exposure, and 5) the type of musculoskeletal disorders.

- Sixty five percent of the events or exposures for total injuries and illnesses requiring days away from work reported by the BLS were: 1) contact with objects and equipment; 2) overexertion; and 3) fall on same level.
- The most frequent events associated with injuries to laborers, freight,, stock, and material movers and construction laborers were contact with objects and equipment. Of these, 31% were reported by the BLS as cuts, lacerations, or punctures; 17% were bruises or contusions; and 12% were fractures.
- Nearly half (48%) of the injuries and illnesses occurred to nursing aides, orderlies and attendants, despite a decrease of 9% from cases in 2007.
- Cumulative Trauma Disorders (called Repetitive motion by the BLS) had the highest median days away from work at 18 days for all private industries with 18 days. This was two fewer days than what was reported in 2007.
- Overexertion and falls on the same level increased by one day between 2007 to 2008 from 9 to 10 median days, while falls to lower level required an average of 15 days away from work to recover.

Strains and Sprains:

- Nearly 4 out of 10 injury or illness showed that sprain or strain injuries required days away from work. The number of sprain or strain injuries accounted for 416,620 cases, a 7% decrease from 2007.
- Soreness and pain, including the back, accounted for 11 percent of total cases. There was no significant change from the number of cases reported between 2007 and 2008.
- Overexertion accounted for forty-five percent of sprains or strains. Bending, reaching, twisting, or slipping without falling, accounted for another 22 percent. Eleven percent of the sprains and strains were the result of falls on the same level.
- Back injury was reported in 40% of the sprain and strain cases.
- The lower extremity (including the knee and ankle) reported 1 in 4 of these were associated with sprains and strains.

- Service occupations reported 23% of the sprains and strains, a decrease of 4 percent from 2007 BLS data. In addition, production workers had a decrease of 15% in reported sprains or strains cases, down to 43,970 in 2008. Again, this may have been a function of decreased activity in the U.S. economy than anything else.
- Carpal Tunnel Syndrome (CTS) and fractures reported among workers required a median of 28 days to recover. An interesting statistic to compare this with is that amputation injuries required fewer days to recover, 26 days in 2008.

Musculoskeletal disorders (MSDs).

MSDs accounted for nearly 1 in 3 (29%) of all workplace injuries and illnesses requiring time away from work, no change from 2007. There are many definitions for musculoskeletal disorders (MSDs), the definition that BLS uses can be found on their website. The BLS reported the following for MDS for 2008:

- MSDs required a average of 10 days away from work, 2 days more than the average for all days away from work. The total number of cases reported in 2008 was 317,440. This represented a decline in the number of reported cases of nearly 5% from 2007, and a total of 11% from the 2008 total cases in 2006. There was a 2% drop in the rate of MSD injury cases from 35% to 33% cases per 10,000 full time workers, from 2007 to 2008.
- The highest number of MSD cases reported to the BLS was Transportation and material moving occupations with 66,240 in 2008. While shoulder injuries and illness would be expected for the shoulder, 10,870, cases, there were also over 4,000 MSDs reported for the knee. It took workers in this group an average of 30 days to recover.
- Occupations that had healthcare support had an average of 29,640 MSD cases.
- For the year 2008, MSD rates across several industries decreased significantly from 2007. For example, the MSD incidence rate for professional and business services decreased 3% from 17% to 14 cases per 10,000 workers; for retail trade a decrease of 10% to a rate of 38 cases per 10,000 workers; and health care and social assistance decreased 5% to a rate of 53 cases per 10,000 workers.

WMSDs of the Low Back

Low-back musculoskeletal disorders are common and costly. Although the causes of low back disorders are complex, substantial scientific evidence identifies some work activities and awkward postures that significantly contribute to the problem. In the United States back disorders account for 27% of all nonfatal occupational injuries and illnesses involving days away from work.(16) Prevention activities should be undertaken based on current knowledge, but important new research efforts are needed to assure that work-related low-back disorders are successfully prevented and treated. For some occupations and tasks there is a pressing need for more information about safe levels of exposure and for further validation of promising intervention approaches, such as mechanical lifting devices for nursing aids.

The economic costs of low-back disorders are staggering. In a recent study, the average costs of workers' compensation claim for low-back disorder was $8,300, which was more than twice the average cost of $4,075 for all compensable claims combined. Estimates of the total costs of low-back pain to society were between $50 and $100 billion per year, with a significant share (about $11 billion) borne by the workers' compensation system. Moreover, as many as 30% of American workers are employed in jobs that routinely require them to perform activities that may increase their risk of developing low back disorders.(16)

Despite the overwhelming statistics showing the magnitude of the problem, more complete information is needed to assess how changes implemented to reduce the physical demands of jobs will affect workplace safety and productivity in the future. Because a significant number of occupationally related low-back disorders are associated with certain high-risk activities, a tremendous opportunity exists for prevention efforts to reduce the prevalence and costs of low back disorders. For example, female nursing aids and licensed practical nurses were about 2.5 times more likely to experience a work-related low-back disorder than all other female workers. Male construction laborers, carpenters, and truck and tractor operators were nearly twice as likely to experience a low-back disorder than all other male workers.

Occupational Risk Factors Associated with the Upper Extremities

Several work-related risk factors associated with musculoskeletal injuries and disorders and the associated risk reduction actions have been identified.[17–23] The work risk problems and solutions are briefly summarized below.

Repetition

Controls: Work enrichment; increase rest allowances; worker rotation. Repetition, a series of motions having little variation and performed every few seconds, may produce fatigue and muscle-tendon strain. If adequate recovery time is not allowed for these effects to diminish, or if the motions also involve awkward postures or forceful exertions, the risk of actual tissue damage and other musculoskeletal problems will increase. A task cycle time of less than 30 seconds has been considered as "repetitive."

Estimates vary as to repetition rates that may pose a hazard, because other factors such as force and posture also affect these determinations. One proposal for defining high-risk repetition rates for different body parts is shown in Table 30.4.[24]

Work repetition and its relationship to carpal tunnel syndrome has been shown in studies of workers in a frozen food processing plant[25], in automotive plants[26], in a pork processing plant[27], and among supermarket workers.[28] It should be noted that in the context of evaluating jobs for work risk factors one of the first aspects of the job to be analyzed is to characterize it by the content of the job and how long it takes to do the job. As a result, cycle time, which can be a measure of job repetition, is one of the most commonly cited job risk factors in the literature. Measurement of risk factors related to posture and force are usually cited less frequently because of the nature of the job and by the degree of difficulty in analysis (i.e., it is harder and less precise to quantify posture and force issues from video analysis). Work repetition alone can be a significant risk factor, but these others risk factors can be just as significant.

Repetition can be reduced by increasing the variety of tasks performed and by a corresponding increase in cycle time or worker rotation. Additional tasks must be compatible with the original task but should not involve the same types of work stresses as the original job.[29] The feasibility of worker rotation depends on the level of skill required to perform a given job and on the existence and detail of labor contracts.

Force

Controls: Reduce weight of tools and part; handle smaller quantities; control balance of objects; use quality control program to maintain fit tolerances; use or develop mechanical aids. Changes in weight, size, shape, and balance of handheld objects can reduce the force of the exertion required to perform a task. In its simplest application, workers can pick up fewer objects at a time or lift with two hands instead of one to reduce weight-induced stresses. They need less strength to grasp an object with a power grip (fingers wrapped around the object), than with a pinch grip (finger tips supporting the load).[30,31] Grasping an object at its center of gravity is easier than elsewhere because, when balanced, the weight of the object does not tend to twist it out of the worker's hands. If the worker cannot change hand location easily, reducing, shifting, or adding weight in order of preference will shift the center of gravity. For example, attachment of an air line to a tool at a right angle can reduce the torque caused by the air line. Another factor adding to the force is the torque required to hold the tool. External torque control devices and different kinds of connectors are effective in

Table 30.4 — High-Risk Repetition Rates by Different Body Parts

Body Part	*Repetitions Per Minute*
Shoulder	more than 2.5
Upper Arm/elbow	more than 10
Forearm/wrist	more than 10
Finger	more than 200

Source: Reference 24.

controlling torque; many times these same devices can serve an additional purpose of retracting and holding the tool when it is not in use, thereby reducing the time for getting the tool.

Although there have been many studies investigating the association between force and musculoskeletal injuries and illnesses, only a few have quantitative assessments.[19,21,23] Based on these studies, it was concluded that grip force should not exceed 40–50% of the maximum grip strength. Hand tools should not weigh more than 5 lb; preferably, the weight should be under 4 lb. Forceful pinch grips, where the object is held between the thumb and finger tips, should be avoided because they require up to five times more force than power grips. To reduce force the following tool design characteristics are recommended: the tool handle should be 50–60 mm thick for power grip, and 8–13 mm thick for precision grip; the tool length should be 120 mm long for power grip, and 100 mm for precision grip (125 mm when wearing gloves).[32]

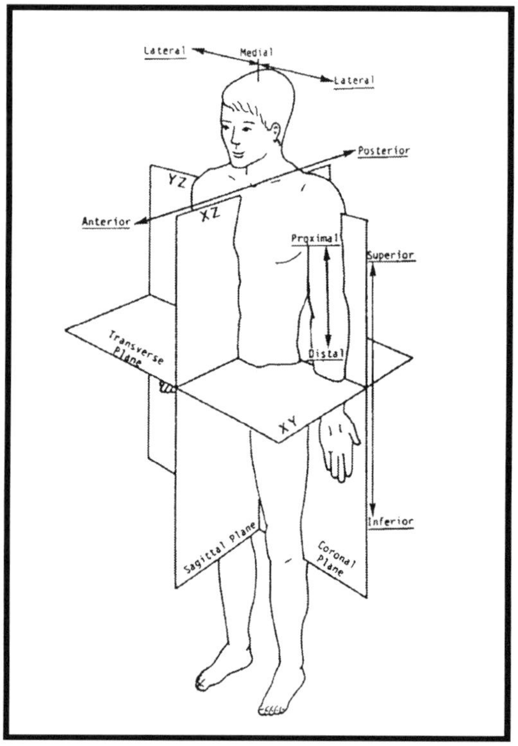

Figure 30.1 — Terminology used to define position and location on the body. (Reprinted with permission from J. Annis and J. McConville, "Anthropometry," in A. Bhattaharya and J.D. McGlothlin, editors, Occupational Ergonomic: Theory and Applications [New York: Marcel Dekker, 1996], p. 3.

Posture

Controls: Work location; work orientation; tool design. Work posture is a function of the location and orientation of the work and the design of tools used when performing the work. Posture affects the ability of workers to reach, hold, and use equipment and influences how long they can perform their jobs without adverse health effects.[33] Posture can be controlled through the location of work and design of the tool.[31,34] The controls range from the obvious to the obscure: for example, it is easier to reach a case stacked at chest height. Without stock and storage problems, the solution is apparent and simple. As the movements become more precise, the approach becomes more sophisticated. For example, if a jig can be adjusted to minimize ulnar deviation, it may not be necessary to investigate alternative tool design.

Extreme postures can lead to discomfort and joint stresses; reduced blood flow; high muscle forces; fatigue; reduced endurance time; acute shoulder and neck pain; shoulder tendonitis; and carpal tunnel syndrome. Figure 30.1 shows the standard anatomical position with classical terminology for major body movements.[7] Figure 30.2 shows the various body positions and corresponding terminology.[35]

Figure 30.3 shows the hand and wrist postures and corresponding terminology.[19] Figure 30.4 shows the various types of hand grip postures and corresponding terminology.[19] Figure 30.5 shows the postures commonly associated with cumulative trauma disorders.[36] Figure 30.6 shows grip strength as a function of degree of wrist deviation as measured in the neutral position.[19] These figures show that to reduce awkward postures, the hands should not work above mid-chest height, the shoulders should not be elevated, shoulder abduction should not be more than 30°, and that shoulder flexion, overhead reaches, elbow/forearm pronation and supination, and wrist flexion/extension should be minimized.[32]

Static Loads

Controls: Change posture; bring load closer to body; use mechanical jigs. A static load occurs when manual work is performed and muscles are isometrically contracted, but no readily observable motion occurs. During

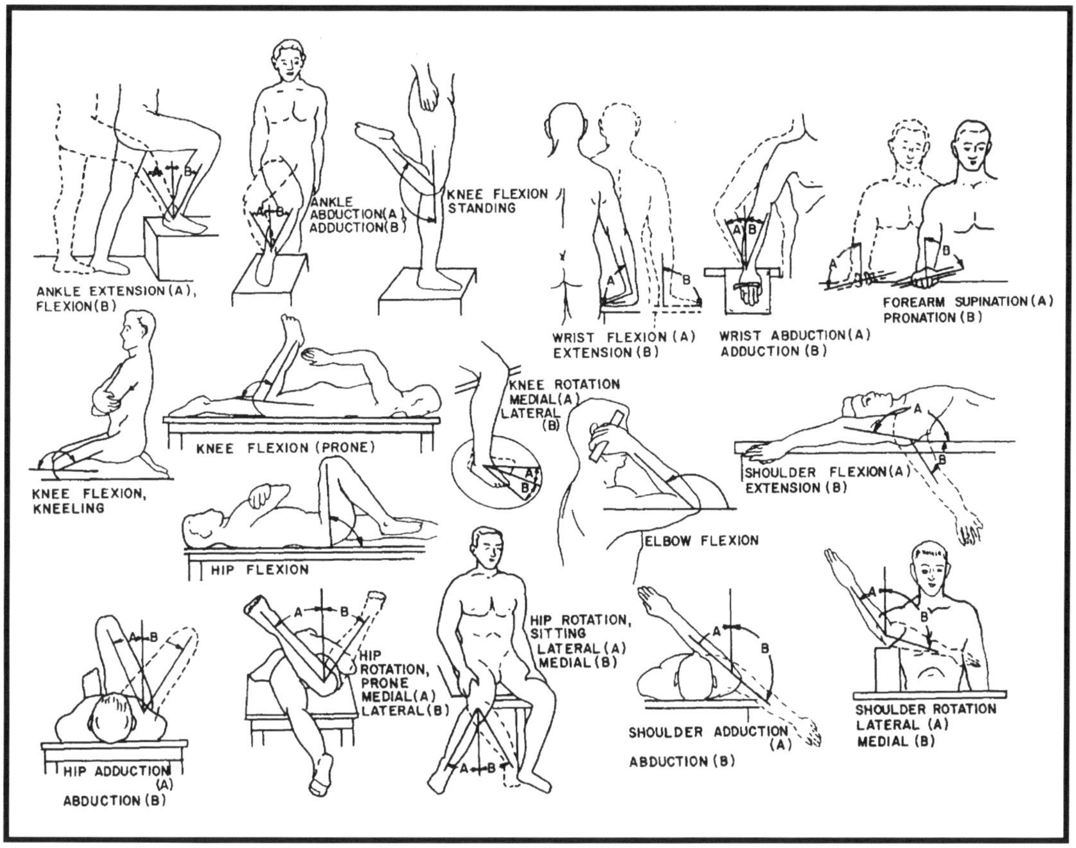

Figure 30.2 — Various body postures and corresponding terminology. (reprinted with permission from D.B. Chaffin and G.B.J. Anderson, Occupational Biomechanics, Joint Motion — Methods and Data [New York: John Wiley & Sons, 1984], p. 86.)

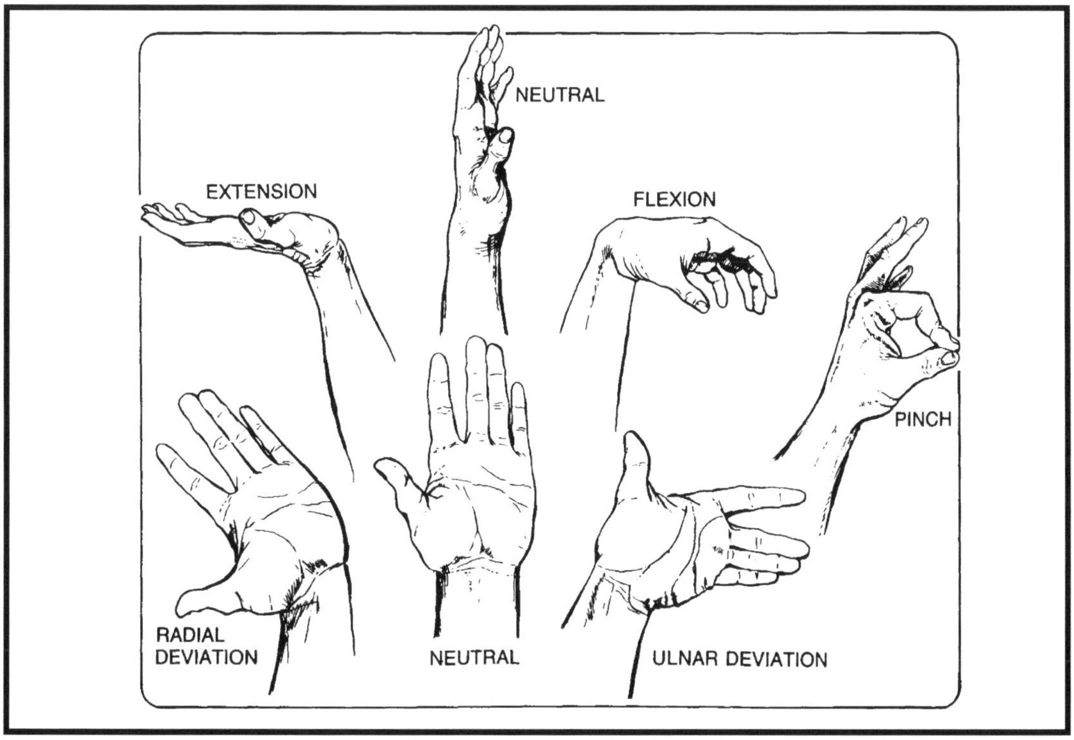

Figure 30.3 — Hand and wrist postures and corresponding terminology. (Reprinted with permission from V. Putz-Anderson (ed.), *Cumulative Trauma Disorders: A Manual for Musculoskeletal Diseases of the Upper Limbs* [Philadelphia: Taylor and Francis, 1988, p. 54).

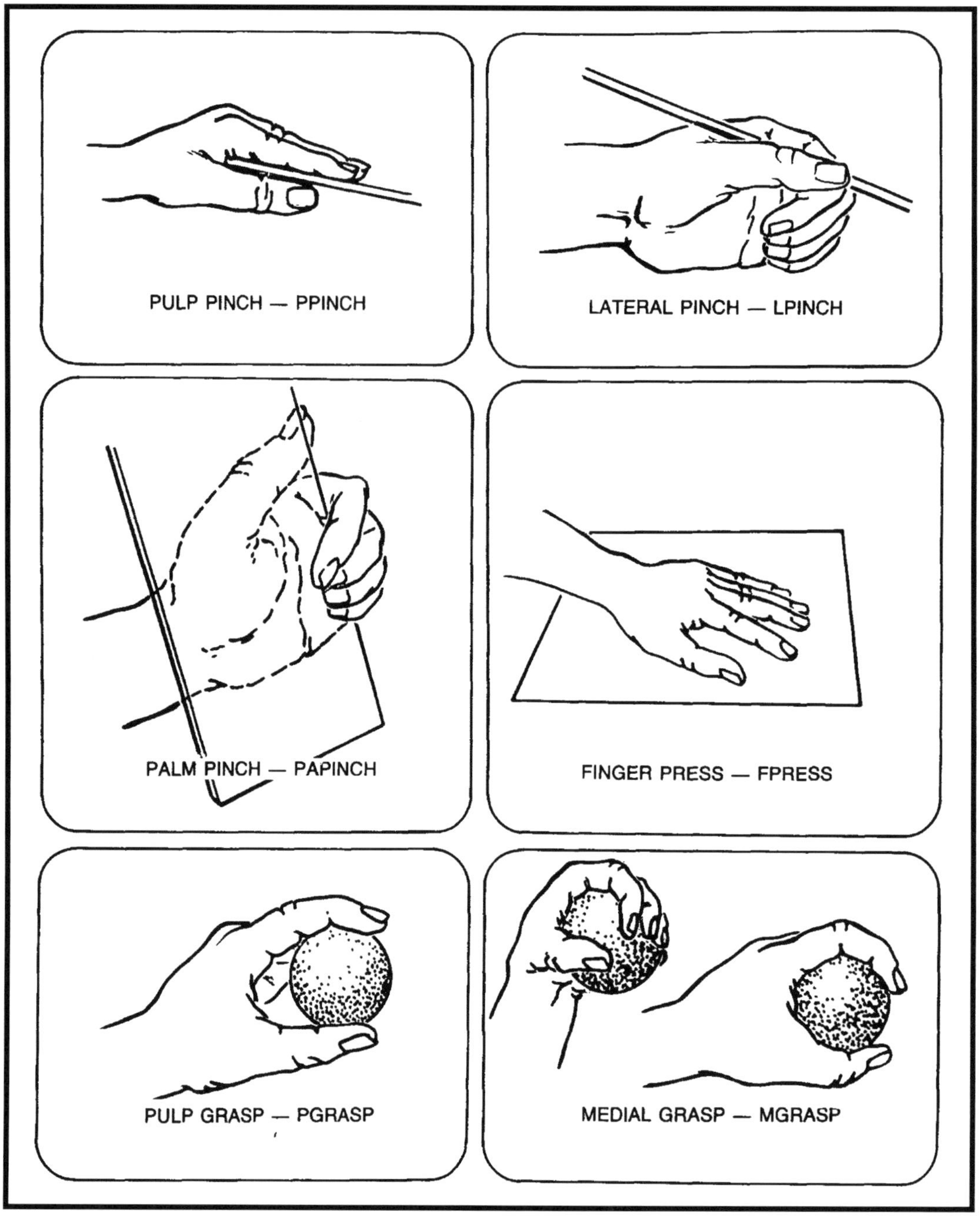

Figure 30.4 — Various types of hand grip postures and corresponding terminology. (Reprinted with permission from V. Putz-Anderson (ed.), *Cumulative Trauma Disorders: A Manual for Musculoskeletal Diseases of the Upper Limbs* [Philadelphia: Taylor and Francis, 1988], p. 56.

static loading of the muscles the body is in the same posture for an extended period of time, the metabolic energy requirements are high, and blood circulation is low. Therefore, the muscles do not receive the needed oxygen and easily become fatigued.[37] To avoid this, design the job so that the body does not remain in a fixed position for prolonged periods of time. Have a place to set the hand tool after performing a task instead of having the worker hold it to begin another piece; fashion a mechanical jig to hold parts rather than using one hand as a "bioclamp" while the other holds a tool.

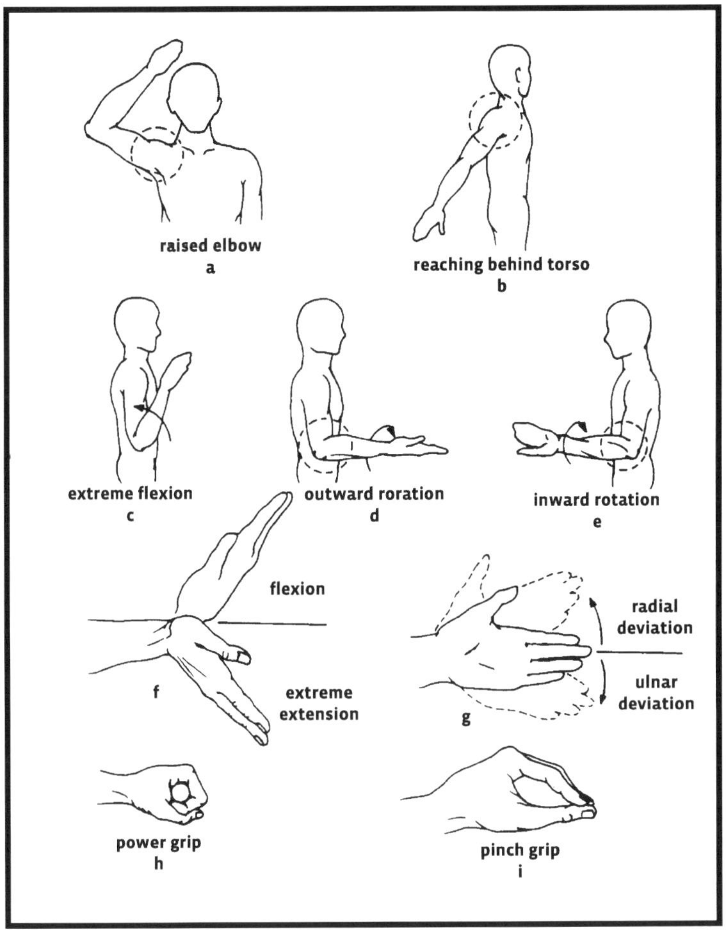

Figure 30.5 — Postures commonly associated with cumulative trauma disorders. (Reprinted with permission from T.J. Armstrong, "Upper-Extremity Posture: Definition, Measurement, and Control." In N. Corlett, J. Wilson, and I. Manenica (eds), Proceedings of the 1st International Ergonomics Symposium, Zada, Yugoslavia, April 1985 [Philadelphia: Taylor & Francis, 1985], p. 61)

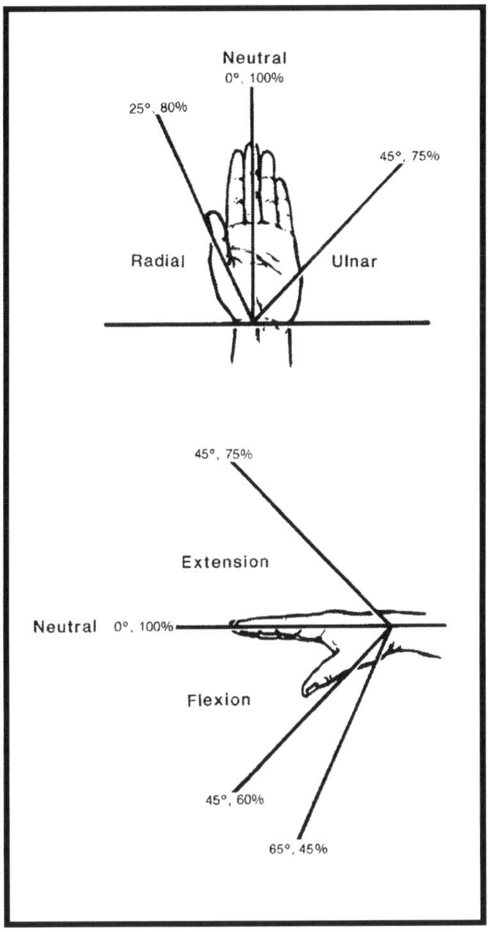

Figure 30.6 — Grip strength as a function of the wrist deviation expressed as a percentage of power grip as measured in the neutral position. (Reprinted with permission from V. Putz-Anderson (ed.), *Cumulative Trauma Disorders: A Manual for Musculoskeletal Diseases of the Upper Limbs* [Philadelphia: Taylor and Francis, 1988], p. 57.)

Mechanical Stress

Controls: Handle size; handle shape; handle materials. The average male can exert 100 to 130 pounds (444.8 to 578.3 N) of hand grip force; the average female can exert 60 to 70 pounds (266.9 to 311.4 N) of grip force.(38) Repeated exertion of these forces results in reaction stresses transmitted through the hand to the underlying tendons. For example, handheld industrial scissors used to cut fabric for clothing can cause stenosing tenosynovitis crepetans. Commonly known as "trigger finger," stenosing tenosynovitis crepetans is often associated with tools that have hard or sharp edges on their handles.(39,40) To decrease the potential for mechanical stress-related disorders, handles should have well-rounded corners, and their diameters should be at least 1.5 inches. Pliant rubber or plastic should cover metal handles. Ideally, the small joints of the hand should be near mid-flexion when applying power to tools to provide a combination of tool retention and partially stretched muscles. This is especially useful when using such tools as wirecutters and pliers.

Also, local contact stresses that are pressure concentration points, resulting from manipulating external objects (pressure caused by uneven surface projections), can cause injury to nerves, blood vessels, and skin. To avoid or reduce contact stresses, it is suggested that the contact surface area be enlarged, and the pressure on the elbows, wrists, and hands be reduced by not leaning on them.

Low Temperatures

Controls: Personal protective equipment; material temperature; environmental temperature; adjust direction of air exhausts. Workers' hands often encounter temperatures below 65°F. Cold environment exposures can occur in meat packing plants, near air exhaust systems of power tools, or from the handling of cold objects (e.g., metal hand tools). Obviously, in unheated work or storage environments the problem can be more severe in the winter. Chronic exposure to low-temperature environments or low-temperature objects can contribute to numbness, decreased blood flow, and diminished sensory feedback.(41) As a result, workers may unconsciously exert grip forces that are much greater than needed, causing unnecessary strain on tendons and possible injury. Environmental air temperatures should not be less than 20°C for a prolonged period of time if a worker's hands are in contact with tools and materials.(42–45) As before, safeguards are conceptually simple: Keep the body warm and use comfortable gloves; minimize localized cold air supplies with attachments that direct the air away from the worker; provide rubber- or plastic-handled tools to add insulation to the stress relief benefit discussed earlier. Working in cold climates can either cause or exacerbate work-related cumulative trauma disorders. Cold temperatures reduce blood flow to the upper extremities, especially the hands, affecting an abundance of motor and sensory nerves. The cold weather may reduce the sensory feedback from the hands and cause workers to have greater exertion of force to perform their jobs. Wearing gloves may also alter sensory feedback and cause the worker to grip the tool more than needed.

Vibration

Controls: Change process; change tool; change operating parameters. Workers exposed to vibration of the upper limbs often complain of numbness of fingers, wrist pain, sensitivity to cold, and circulatory disturbances in the fingers.(46) There are many factors to consider in examining vibration exposure, including frequency and magnitude of vibration, duration of exposure, temporal exposure pattern and work method, posture of hand, and type of tool. Vibration induced vascular diseases can result from frequencies between 20–1000 Hz, the range of most power hand tools.(29,47) Minimizing vibrations decreases the potential for vibration-related disorders. When the process cannot be changed, change the tool. There are many hand tools available with effective vibration dampening devices. Routine maintenance of a power tool, including basic lubrication, retards the development of wear-induced vibration. In some cases rubber and/or foam sleeves placed between the tool and hand minimize vibration.

Epidemiological studies have shown that workers who are exposed to hand-arm vibration have a greater risk of injury and musculoskeletal disorders than those who are not. Vibration causes overgripping of the tool and leads to higher forearm muscle activation and higher muscle loads. When this is combined with repetitive work, the vibration may exacerbate musculoskeletal disorders. Generally, it is recommended that segmental vibration entering the hands be avoided below 1000 Hz, specifically hand-arm vibrations in the 2–200 Hz range.(48)

Gloves

Controls: Process change; variable size gloves; glove replacement. Gloves protect the hands from environmental temperature extremes, chemical contaminants, and mechanical insult. They also enhance friction and in some tasks reduce strength requirements.(49) When a process cannot be changed, gloves are one of the most logical and cost-effective control measures to protect the hands. In manual-intensive industries the primary benefit from using gloves is to diminish mechanical insult from repetitive job tasks. A drawback is that gloves can interfere with movements of the hand and may attenuate strength by up to 30% depending on glove material and fit.(50–52) Also, task completion time may be delayed by up to 37% with certain types of gloves, which may impede performance in emergency situations such as hazardous chemical releases.(53) Getting the proper glove fit is difficult because of the variations in hand size and management's tendency to purchase only a few sizes creates problems for the workers. If gloves are needed, the best solution is to ensure that a variety of sizes is available, and that access to new, well-fitting gloves is easy and encouraged.

Fit and Reach

Controls: Adjustable workstation; assortment of hand tool sizes; bring work closer to body. The ability of individuals to fit in the workplace, to reach objects and hand tools, and to see without obstruction can force them to adopt awkward postures and have static loads that can cause musculoskeletal injuries or aggravate existing disorders. The solution is that work should accommodate the work population, from 5% females to 95% males.[7] The work, objects, and tools should be located so that the worker does not have to lean forward and flex the back, neck, shoulder, or extend arms and hands beyond their "functional" reach (approximately 12 inches from the front of the torso). Figure 30.7 shows examples of reach envelopes for a seated male and female.

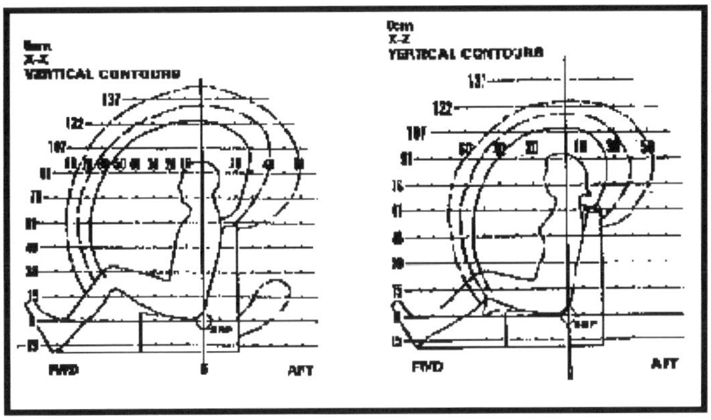

Figure 30.7 — Examples of reach envelopes for a seated male and female. Source A. Bhattaharya and J.D. McGlothlin (eds.), Occupational Ergonomics: Theory and Applications (New York: Marcel Dekker, 1996).

Work Organization

Controls: Balance work between workers; adjust line speed so workers do not "chase" parts; allow adequate recovery time between tasks. Machine pacing can cause problems because workers cannot control work pace or task frequency. Also, the type of job workers are doing may not allow them to recover from the previous task. Self-pacing versus machine pacing is preferable because it allows workers to control the frequency of the work being performed and allows them to recover from previous tasks.[20]

Multiple Risk Factor Exposures

Controls: Systems analysis of work; mechanize; worker and management input for work changes. Though each of the risk factors mentioned previously can lead to work-related cumulative trauma disorder, multiple risk factors may be more problematic not only in terms of increasing risk but also in terms of deriving solutions. For example, repetitive jobs may also have some forceful motions and awkward postures associated with them. If the job is machine paced as well, there is the additional risk factor of minimal recovery time. The combination of repetition, force, awkward postures, and insufficient recovery time may lead to an increased incidence and severity of work-related cumulative trauma disorders above that resulting from an individual exposure to one of these risk factors. Therefore, the most effective solution is to reduce risk factors by carefully examining what is being done, and then determine which solution will most benefit the worker and company.[4]

Personal Protective Equipment

Wrist Splints. Wrist splints or braces used to keep the wrist straight during work are not recommended, unless prescribed by a physician for rehabilitation. Keeping the wrist straight during work helps to optimize the biomechanical leverage of the individual to perform work. However, using a splint to achieve the same end may cause more harm than good because the work orientation may require workers to bend their wrists. If workers are wearing wrist splints, they may have to use more force to work against the brace or change the posture of the elbows or shoulders to accommodate the straight wrist. This is not only inefficient, but also may actually increase the pressure in the carpal tunnel area, causing more damage to the hand and wrist.[54] A remedy for this situation is to orient the workpiece or adjust the workstation so that the worker can perform in a neutral posture with optimum biomechanical leverage.

Occupational Risk Factors Associated with the Lower Back

Low-back pain and injuries attributed to manual lifting activities continue as one of the leading occupational health and safety issues facing the workplace today. As such, several work risk factors have been identified as leading to overexertion and musculoskeletal injuries during manual material handling. Some of these risk factors are outlined in following sections.

Posture

Controls: Avoid extreme range of motion when lifting; keep loads to be lifted between knee and heart height; avoid twisting when lifting loads; keep loads close to body when lifting. Body posture changes force requirements and may cause work to become very strenuous. Often the activity forces the body to assume different postures. For example, stoop postures can be advantageous when the load is lifted repeatedly. The squat posture is desirable when the load can fit between the knees and must be lifted occasionally. Loads that cannot fit between the knees and must be lifted repetitively should be handled by two individuals or must be moved with the help of a mechanical device.

Generally, to reduce back injury risk during manual material handling, one should avoid an extreme range of movements; moving loads from the floor; turning and twisting; "jerking motions"; fixed postures; lifting loads above heart height; and pushing or pulling heavy loads. Manual material handling should be done between knee and heart height. Use caution during material handling when the size of the load is too large to fit between the knees and a stooped lift is needed. The key words to remember, especially when lifting, are "posture" and "load"—the greater the load, the more good posture plays a role in back injury prevention. Pushing force should be exerted in an erect posture, and the load should have handles. For heavy and awkward loads, the load should be lifted by using the squat posture, the weight of the load should be less than the sum of the capacities of the individuals, and the workers engaged in lifting (i.e., buddy lift) should be similar in height. However, when the width of the load is too wide to fit between the knees, a squat lift may be inappropriate. In this case the focus of the lift should be on getting the load as close to the body as possible, thereby reducing the likelihood for back injury.

Specific recommendations for load stability include the following: The load should be rigid and symmetrical in shape; the weight should be distributed uniformly or the heavier end should be closer to the body; the center of gravity for the load should be along the line joining the two hands; the load dimension in the sagittal plane should not exceed 50 cm; the load dimension between the hands should be minimized. The load height should be determined by practical considerations, such as body size and ability to clearly view obstructions in the path. The maximum load should not exceed 51 lb., based on the NIOSH lifting guidelines.[55] More details about the NIOSH guidelines are presented in Chapter 31 Musculoskeletal Disorders, Job Evaluation and Design Principles. However, additional aspects for manual material handling are outlined in following sections.

Frequency/Repetitive Handling

Controls: Mechanize task; use "buddy" system; reduce line speed. Material handling activities that require frequent handling either should be redesigned to reduce the frequency or should depend on mechanical equipment to aid material handling. The revised NIOSH guidelines do not recommend load handling frequencies of more than 10 lifts per minute if the work is done for 8 hours. The handling frequency can increase to 12 lifts per minutes if the working duration is reduced to 2 hours. Therefore, if higher frequencies are encountered, the work time should be reduced.[32]

Static Work

Controls: Redesign work station/work area to allow freedom of movement; have adjustable workstation to allow changes in posture; remove physical barriers so worker can stand closer to work. Nearly all activities involving materials handling contain both a static and dynamic component. Tasks such as repetitive lifting have a dominant dynamic component; tasks such as load holding have a dominant static component. The static work effort is characterized by contraction of muscles over extended periods of time (e.g., adopting a posture for extended periods of time).[4]

Static work should be avoided as much as possible. Static work has high metabolic demand; however, the blood supply is reduced because of restricted circulation. Consequently, little oxygen gets to the starved muscles and fatigue quickly sets in. Therefore, it is better to design jobs so that they allow the workers to freely move their bodies during manual material handling tasks.

Handles/Couplings

Controls: All manual material handling containers should have handles; material handled should be slip resistant; handles should be designed for "power grip" handling. Good handles or couplings are essential to provide load and postural stability during materials handling. Cut-out handles should be 4.5 inches (115 mm) long, 1.0–1.5 inches (25–38 mm) wide (or diameter in the case of cylindrical handles). Cylindrical handles should have 1.2–2.0 inches (30–50 mm) clearance all around. In addition, handles should have a pivot angle of 70° from the horizontal axis of the box, and should be located at diagonally opposite ends to provide both vertical and horizontal stability for the load. According to the NIOSH lifting model, a reduction in weight of up to 10% should be made if the containers or objects being handled do not have handles.(32)

Asymmetrical Handling

Controls: Use hoists where possible to lift loads; avoid twisting when lifting loads asymmetrically; balance the load when carrying. Asymmetric handling of loads is common in industry. However, when this is done it leads to reduced load handling capabilities and strength, increased intraabdominal and intradiscal (shear) pressures, and increased muscle activity of the lower back muscles. The materials handler is advised not to keep his or her feet in a locked position, because when the worker pivots the feet in the direction of the load, the task is less stressful. The reduction in load lifting capability in such cases is expected to be no more than 15% for a 90° turn. For example, if a person can lift 50 lb (23 kg) without twisting, that person can lift approximately 42.5 lb (19 kg) when turning 90°.(32)

Space Confinement

Controls: Clear path or work area before manual material handling; use overhead hoists for manual materials handling; avoid putting materials on ground or above heart height. Performing load handling activities in small spaces is common in manual material handling tasks in industry. For loads that are to be placed on shelves, the shelf opening clearance for inserting boxes by hands should be approximately 1.2 inches (30 mm). If the workplace layout does not allow erect posture (e.g., because of limited height to stand) the load should be reduced significantly from the 51 lb (23 kg) maximum load during trunk flexion.

Personal Protective Equipment

Personal protective equipment—including shoes; gloves; vests; trousers; goggles; respirators; aprons; overalls; and masks—should permit free movement, be easily removable, and allow for personal cooling to prevent body metabolic heat build-up. Gloves should fit and be appropriate for the task to allow maintained dexterity. Shoes should be nonslip, comfortable, and water resistant.

Back Belts. The use of back belts to prevent back injury has not been shown to be a preventative measure according to a NIOSH study.(56) Specifically, the NIOSH Back Belt working group concluded the following.

- There are insufficient data indicating that typical industrial back belts significantly reduce the biomechanical loading of the trunk during manual lifting.
- There is insufficient scientific evidence to conclude that wearing back belts reduces risk of injury to the back based on changes in intra-abdominal pressure and trunk muscle electromyography.
- The use of back belts may produce temporary strain on the cardiovascular system.
- There are insufficient data to demonstrate a relationship between the prevalence of back injury in healthy workers and the discontinuation of back belt use.

The NIOSH working group recommended the following.

- The results of studies that evaluated the effects of belt use on predictions of biomechanical loading of the spine should be interpreted cautiously.
- The results of epidemiological studies related to back belt use should be used only to develop better designed epidemiological research.
- Future research should be designed to evaluate the efficacy of wearing back belts to prevent work-related back injury

Work Methods Evaluation

Analyzing Jobs

Finding out as much about the job as possible is a critical element in the recognition, evaluation, and control of musculoskeletal disorders. This procedure, known as job analysis, is one of the most tedious aspects of mastering ergonomics. Basically, there are two ways to perform a job analysis: (1) by conducting a methods study, which is a common technique used by occupational engineers; and (2) by using checklists. Both methods are briefly described in the following sections.[57–60]

Table 30.5 — Table of Work Elements Developed by the Gilbreths

Element	*Description*
Search	looking for something with the eyes or hand
Select	locating one object (that is) mixed with others
Grasp	touching or gripping an object with the hand
Reach	moving of the hand to some object or location
Move	movement of some object from one location to another
Hold	exerting force to hold an object on a fixed location
Position	moving an object in a desired orientation
Inspect	examining an object by sight, sound, touch, etc.
Assemble	joining together two or more objects
Disassemble	separating two or more objects
Use	manipulating a tool or device with the hand
Unavoidable delay	interrupting work activity because of some factor beyond the worker's control
Avoidable delay	interrupting work activity because of some factor under the worker's control
Plan	performing mental process that precedes movement
Rest to overcome fatigue	interrupting work activity to overcome the effects of repeated exertions or movements

Work-Methods Study

Work-methods study is the systematic recording and critical examination of existing and proposed ways of doing work. It is a means of developing and applying safe, easy, and effective solutions and reducing overall job costs. This method can be applied at two levels: (1) recording work sequence using a flow process chart and (2) recording work sequence using the techniques of the micromotion study. The second method of recording workplace movements is commonly used for very short cycle jobs and requires filming the job. See Appendix A for tips on properly videotaping jobs for analyses.

Jobs that have a very short cycle time, usually in seconds, and are repeated hundreds of times per day, such as in assembly jobs, are subjected to micromotion study. This is a process in which all job elements are divided into fundamental motions known as "therbligs." Therbligs were named after Frank and Lilian Gilbreth ("therbligs" is "Gilbreths" spelled backwards), who were known in the early 20th century for their research on work efficiency.[20] There are 18 fundamental motions in therblig analysis. Table 30.5 shows the basic work elements developed by the Gilbreths. Such detail can be obtained by analyzing film or videotape in slow motion and stop action. Such detail, however, can yield much information about the job and solutions to control musculoskeletal disorders.

Describing the job as a series of elements can help the researcher determine which ones may be job risk factors for musculoskeletal disorders. Elements can be grouped into tasks that are usually performed in a similar sequence. Each task should be timed by a stop watch or by calculating the elapsed time on a videotape (it is good practice to verify the timing element on the recording with a stop watch). Examples of a task include reaching for a part, grasping the part, moving the part to an assembly line, positioning the part on a jig, etc. Table 30.6 shows how such work tasks can be defined for the right and left hand for an assembly job. After this breakdown of tasks, the job can be analyzed for risk factors that can cause musculoskeletal disorders. Elements that can increase the probability of a musculoskeletal disorder are extracted from the previous table and shown in Table 30.7 with recommended solutions. Such information can be useful when complex jobs are broken down into defined units of work activity. It is also useful when trying to establish an ergonomics control program, because this approach not only documents specific exposure problems but also lists solutions. The solutions can be used in ergonomics task force meetings, where the pros and cons of the solution can be fleshed out and action can be taken.

As the Tables 30.6 and 30.7 show, breaking the job into its parts can be time-consuming and involved. However, this systematic approach yields highly specific results in terms of identifying aspects of the job that may cause musculoskeletal disorders. Additionally, it gives the evaluator a mechanism for thinking about specific ergonomic solutions.[20] With practice the evaluator can become proficient in this method. The key point here is that several job risk factors can be identified that may seem small risks, but when several of these risk factors are reduced or eliminated by ergonomic solutions, there can be a large reduction in the overall physical stressors of the job. This alleviation of physical stressors may lead, in turn, to a reduction in work-related musculoskeletal disorders.

Table 30.6 — Tasks for One Job Cycle for an Automotive Assembler

Left Hand	*Right Hand*
1. Reach to get dashboard	1. Reach to get dashboard
2. Grasp dashboard	2. Grasp dashboard
3. Move dashboard to line	3. Move dashboard to line
4. Pre-position dashboard on line	4. Pre-position dashboard on line
5. Position dashboard on line	5. Position dashboard on line
6. Release dashboard on jig	6. Release dashboard on jig
7. Reach to dashboard support	7. Idle (hand at rest)
8. Grasp dashboard support	8. Idle (hand at rest)
9. Move support to dashboard	9. Reach for tool
10. Position support on dashboard	10. Grasp screwdriver
11. Hold support on dashboard	11. Move screwdriver to dashboard
12. Hold support on dashboard	12. Position screwdriver on dashboard
13. Hold support on dashboard	13. Use screwdriver on dashboard
14. Move to load screwdriver	14. Move screwdriver to dashboard
15. Position screw on screwdriver	15. Move screwdriver to dashboard
16. Hold dashboard	16. Use screwdriver on dashboard
17. Idle (hand at rest)	17. Move screwdriver to bench
18. Idle (hand at rest)	18. Position screwdriver on bench
19. Idle (hand at rest)	19. Release screwdriver on bench
20. Idle (hand at rest)	20. Release jig posts
21. Idle (hand at rest)	21. Grasp jig posts
22. Idle (hand at rest)	22. Move (turn) jig posts
23. Idle (hand at rest)	23. Release jig posts
24. Idle (hand at rest)	24. Idle (hand at rest)
25. Idle (hand at rest)	25. Reaching for jig posts
26. Idle (hand at rest)	26. Grasp jig posts
27. Idle (hand at rest)	27. Move (turn) jig posts
28. Idle (hand at rest)	28. Release jig posts

Table 30.7 — Summary of Risk Factors and Recommendations for Automotive Assembler

Work Element	*Work Risk Factor*	*Recommendation*
5–6 10–23	Sharp edges from work bench cause uncomfortable contact pressure on operator's waist.	Pad front of bench with rounded 2-inch rubberized strip with foam core.
Right hand 12,13	Pistol-grip screwdriver used to drive screw in vertical position causes high wrist flexion	Provide in-line screwdriver to drive screw to keep wrist posture neutral.
1–27	Use of thick work gloves may decrease tactile sensitivity of the hands during work.	Use flexible lightweight gloves that fit the worker's hands to aid in sensory feedback.
Left hand 7,8	Worker reaches back (arm abduction) to get dashboard part from bin.	Move dashboard support cart next to workbench so worker does not have to reach back for the part.
Right hand 21	Grasping jig posts requires repetitive finger pinch, with high finger forces.	Provide larger grip for jig handle to improve biomechanical leverage by using the entire hand.

Checklists

Checklists provide an alternative approach to methods study. On the plus side, a checklist is easy to use because it is a qualitative method that quickly evaluates job risk factors. Depending on how checklists are structured, they can offer a "relative ranking" of jobs, from those with the highest number of job risk factors to those with the least. On the negative side, checklists are not quantitative and in some instances may identify the real risk factors. Perhaps that is why there are as many checklists as there are industries. Checklists vary from simple one-page lists with yes/no responses, to multiple page lists that try to semiquantify various risk factors. Two frequently used check lists are shown in Figures 30.8 and 30.9. The first was developed by the University of Michigan's Center for Ergonomics to evaluate risk factors for upper extremities; the other checklist was developed by NIOSH to qualitatively assess lifting hazards. A third checklist (see Figure 30.10), developed by Rogers attempts to quantify and categorize such jobs by assessing a raw score, then totaling the score for each job evaluated. Again, the objective is to rank-order each job. The advantage of Rogers' checklist is its inherent attempt to look at the synergistic nature of job risk factors—that is, to evaluate the job risk factors of repetition, force, posture, and recovery time as one value.

When using or developing checklists, one should use caution to make sure the questions are relevant, as the collection and analysis of the data can be time-consuming. More important, when working within the framework of a checklist, evaluators need to validate the checklist to ensure that it will provide enough detail to derive effective solutions. Yes/no checklists are useful for

Risk Factors	no	yes
1. Physical Stress		
1.1 Can the job be done without hand/wrist contact with sharp edges?	______	______
1.2 Is the tool operating without vibration?	______	______
1.3 Are the worker's hands exposed to temperature > 21C (70F)	______	______
1.4 Can the job be done without using gloves?	______	______
2. Force		
2.1 Does the job require exerting less than 4.5 Kg (10 lbs) of force?	______	______
2.2 Can the job be done without using finger pinch grip?	______	______
3. Posture		
3.1 Can the job be done without flexion or extension of the wrist?	______	______
3.2 Can the tool be used without flexion or extension of the wrist?	______	______
3.3 Can the job be done without deviating the wrist from side to side?	______	______
3.4 Can the tool be used without deviating the wrist from side to side?	______	______
3.5 Can the worker be seated while performing the job?	______	______
3.6 Can the job be done without "clothes wringing" motion?	______	______
4. Workstation hardware		
4.1 Can the orientation of the work surface be adjusted?	______	______
4.2 Can the height of the work surface be adjusted?	______	______
4.3 Can the location of the tool be adjusted?	______	______
5. Repetitiveness		
5.1 Is the cycle time longer than 30 seconds?	______	______
6. Tool Design		
6.1 Are the thumb and finger slightly overlapped in a closed grip?	______	______
6.2 Is the span of the tool's handle between 5 and 7 cm (2-2 3/4")?	______	______
6.3 Is the handle of the tool made from material other than metal?	______	______
6.4 Is the weight of the tool below 4 kg (9 lbs)?	______	______
6.5 Is the tool suspended?	______	______

Figure 30.8 — Michigan's checklist for upper extremity cumulative trauma disorders (Source: Lifshitz, Y. and T.J. Armstrong, "A Design Checklist for Control and Prediction of Cumulative Trauma Disorder in Intensive Manual Jobs." In Proceedings of the Human Factors Society 30th Annual Meeting, Dayton, PH, September 29-October 3, 1986, vol. 2, pp. 837-841 (Santa Monica, CA: Human Factors Society, 1986).

Risk Factors	yes	no
General		
1.1 Does the load handled exceed 50 lb?	______	______
1.2 Is the object difficult to bring close to the body because of its size, bulk, or shape?	______	______
1.3 Is the load hard to handle because it lacks handles or cutouts for handles, or does it have slippery surfaces or sharp edges?	______	______
1.4 Is the footing unsafe? For example, are the floors slippery, inclined, or uneven?	______	______
1.5 Does the task require fast movement, such as throwing, swinging, or rapid walking?	______	______
1.6 Does the task require stressful body postures, such as stooping to the floor, twisting, reaching overhead, or excessive lateral bending?	______	______
1.7 Is most of the load handled by only one hand, arm, or shoulder?	______	______
1.8 Does the task require working in environmental hazards, such as extreme temperatures, noise, vibration, lighting, or airborne contaminants?	______	______
1.9 Does the task require working in a confined area?	______	______
Specific		
2.1 Does lifting frequency exceed 5 lifts per minute?	______	______
2.2 Does the vertical lifting distance exceed 3 feet?	______	______
2.3 Do carries last longer than 1 minute?	______	______
2.4 Do tasks which require large sustained pushing or pulling forces exceed 30 seconds duration?	______	______
2.5 Do extended reach static holding tasks exceed 1 minute?	______	______

Figure 30.9 — Hazard evaluation checklist for lifting, carrying, pushing, or pulling. (Source: Waters, T., A Checklist for Manual materials Handling (Cincinnati, OH: NIOSH, Division of Biomedical and Behavioral Sciences, 1989).

walk-through surveys and can be used to rank-order jobs into high, medium, and low risk based o the number of yes or no responses for each job. Additional examples of simple yes/no proactive checklists are shown in Appendix B.

Risk Factor Assessment Techniques

The techniques to assess risk factors associated with musculoskeletal injuries and illnesses are broadly classified as (1) biomechanical, (2) physiological, and (3) psychophysical. These techniques can be qualitative or quantitative. Listed in following sections are a few examples of the techniques that can be used for risk factor assessment.

Biomechanical

Spinal stresses. Spinal stresses (compressive and shear) provide an indication of the hazard the body can be subjected to during manual material handling. Several biomechanical models have been developed to assess these stresses. Some perform static and two-dimensional analysis, whereas

Body Part		Effort Level	Continuous Effort Time	Efforts/ Minute	Priority
Neck/Shoulders	R	___	___	___	___
	L	___	___	___	___
Back		___	___	___	___
Arms/Elbows	R	___	___	___	___
	L	___	___	___	___
Wrists/Hands/	R	___	___	___	___
Fingers	L	___	___	___	___
Legs/Knees	R	___	___	___	___
	L	___	___	___	___
Ankles/Feet/	R	___	___	___	___
Toes	L	___	___	___	___

Effort Categories
1 = Light
2 = Moderate
3 = Heavy

Continuous Effort Time Categories
1 = < 6 secs
2 = 6 to 20 secs
3 = > 20 secs

Efforts/Minute Categories
1 = < 1/min
2 = 1 to 5/min
3 = > 5 -15/min

Priority for Change

Moderate = 123, 132, 213, 222, 231, 232, 312
High = 223, 313, 321, 322
Very High = 323, 331, 332

JobTitle: ______________
Specific Task: ______________
Job Number: ______________
Department: ______________
Location: ______________
Contact Person(s): ______________
Phone: ______________
Analyst: ______________
Phone: ______________
Date of Analysis: ________

Figure 30.10 — Ergonomic job analysis (Source: Rodgers, S.H., "A Functional Job Analysis Technique." In J.S. Moore and A. Gary (eds)., Occupational Medicine: State of the Art Reviews (Philadelphia, PA: Hanley and Belfuss, 1992).

others perform dynamic and three-dimensional analysis. Even though several biomechanical models are available, most are complex and not user friendly.

Before using a model, it is essential to understand the limitations of these and other existing biomechanical models. Static models consider the motion of the human body as a series of static postures and perform static analysis in each posture to determine musculoskeletal stresses. Dynamic models are more complex and can account for inertial effects of the body segments and the loading because of acceleration. However, although the static model is easy to use, some quantitative data are lost. The dynamic model gives more quantitative data and more accurate risk assessment for back injury, but the data collection and analysis are much more complex and time-consuming. As with checklists, the utility of biomechanical models is greater for comparative task analysis than for standalone task analysis to determine absolute load values. Table 30.8 shows the relationship between static versus dynamic model evaluation parameters.[61]

The static biomechanical model (two-dimensional or three-dimensional) is available from the University of Michigan's Center for Ergonomics. These static strength models predict populations capable of performing each task from a variety of inputs: body posture, object, force needed to oppose the object (average, maximum), and location of the hands.[62]

Along the same lines as the static biomechanical model is the development of several software programs that calculate the 1991 revised NIOSH lifting. These programs simply take the input data from the lifting equation and automatically calculate the NIOSH recommended weight limit (RWL) and the lifting index (LI). The LI is the ratio of the weight lifted (by the worker), divided by the RWL. For example, if the worker lifts a box weighing 75 lb (34 kg), and the RWL is 25 lb (11 kg), then, the LI is 3.0. The LI may be used to establish priorities for evaluating jobs. Details of the NIOSH Lifting Equation can be found in the NIOSH publication titled *Applications Manual for the Revised NIOSH Lifting Equation*.[63]

In recent years more research has been done using dynamic biomechanical models because static lifting models may underpredict spinal loading during dynamic lifting exertions.[7] Also, dynamic biomechanical models address muscle coactivity, which is important because of the complex loading of

Table 30.8 — Dependent and Independent Variables in the Measurement of Muscle Strength

	Isometric (Static)		*Isovelocity (Dynamic)*		*Isoacceleration (Dynamic)*		*Isojerk (Dynamic)*		*Isoforce (Static or Dynamic)*		*Isoinertia (Static or Dynamic)*		*Free Dynamic*	
Variables	*Ind.*	*Dep.*	*Ind.*	*Dep.*	*Ind.*	*Dep.*	*Ind.*	*Dep.*	*Ind.*	*Dep.*	*Ind.*	*Dep.*	*Ind.*	*Dep.*
Displacement, linear/angular	Constant[A] (zero)		C or X		C or X		C or X		C or X		C or X		C or X	
Velocity, linear/angular	o		Constant[A] (zero)		C or X		C or X		C or X		C or X			X
Acceleration, linear/angular	o		o		Constant[A] (zero)		C or X		C or X		C or X			X
Jerk, linear/angular	o		o		o		Constant[A] (zero)		C or X		C or X			X
Force, torque	C		C or X		C or X		C or X		Constant[A] (zero)		C or X			X
Mass, moment of inertia	C		C or X		C		C		C or X		Constant[A] (zero)			X
Repetition	C		C or X		C or X		C or X		C or X		C or X		Constant[A] (zero)	

Abbreviations: Ind.=independent; Dep.=dependent; C=variable can be controlled; o=variable is not present (zero); X=can be dependent variable; the boxed constant variable provides the descriptive name.
[A]Set to zero
Source: Reference 3, p. 363.

the spine. Such models are very complex, because they evaluate the compression, shear, and torsional forces on the spine. A device called a lumbar motion monitor, developed by researchers at Ohio State University, can be used to simulate spinal loading during unconstrained, free-dynamic coupled motion. Like the University of Michigan's two-dimensional and three-dimensional static strength prediction model software, the lumbar motion monitor is available on the open market and can be used by safety and health professionals to address the complex issues of back overexertion injuries during manual material handling.

Physiological Techniques

Physiological techniques are useful for repetitive and whole-body work, such as manual materials handling. The two human body responses that indicate the extent of hazard and respond to various risk factors are oxygen consumption and heart rate. These two methods are briefly described below.

Oxygen Consumption. Oxygen consumed by an individual is influenced by the intensity of the task he or she performs. Oxygen consumption is compared with the physical work capacity (PWC), also known as aerobic capacity, maximum aerobic power, and maximum oxygen uptake ($V0_2$ max). PWC is the maximum amount of oxygen that an individual can consume per minute. The higher the percentage of PWC a task requires, the higher the resulting physical stress, fatigue, and possibility of injury.

PWC can be measured by maximal or submaximal methods.[64] In the maximal method the worker is stressed to the maximum, and oxygen consumption at that level is recorded. This method is not recommended for occupational practitioners. In submaximal methods, individuals are required to perform at least three workloads on either a bicycle ergometer or treadmill, or for a specific task such as arm strength, an arm crank ergometer. The treadmill is recommended when trying to assess maximal aerobic capacity. The technique is to increase the treadmill pace from 3 mph (1.3 m/sec), 4 mph (1.8 m/sec), and 5 mph (2.2 m/sec) at a 10% slope. When the heart rate and oxygen consumption have stabilized, the values are recorded. These values are plotted on a x-y graph (e.g., heart rate on x-axis, and oxygen uptake on y-axis) and a straight line is drawn through the plotted points. The value of the maximum heart rate for the individual is determined and plotted in the x-axis. One of the more accurate formulas for an individual's maximum heart rate is:

$$\text{Maximum heart rate} = 214 - 0.71 \times \text{age in years}$$

A vertical line is projected from the maximum heart rate point. A horizontal line is projected from the point of intersection between this vertical line and the straight line joining the three plotted points. The value given by the intersection of the horizontal line and the y-axis is the PWC of the individual.

When the PWC is determined and compared with the steady state oxygen consumption of a worker on a job, an indication of the physical stress of the job is obtained. If a job requires more than 21–23% of PWC for 8-hour shifts, it is likely to lead to overexertion and, possibly, musculoskeletal disorders.[65]

Measurement of the volume of oxygen consumed can provide an overall index of energy consumption and show the energy demands of work. For example, use of 1 L of oxygen yields approximately 5 kcal. The kilocalories can be added to determine metabolic energy expenditure for several activities as shown in Table 30.11.[66] For example, an "average" man in his 20s has an average maximal capacity of 3–3.5 L/min., whereas the "average" woman of the same age has an average capacity of 2.3–2.8 L/min. This translates to approximately 1020 kcal/hour for the man, and 750 kcal/hour for the woman. It must be kept in mind that oxygen capacity diminishes with age. For example, for a 60-year-old man the average maximal capacity is 2.2–2.5 L/min, and the 60-year-old woman has a 1.8–2.0 L/min maximal capacity.

Oxygen consumption can be measured by several commercially available devices, such as the MRM-1 Oxygen Consumption Computer (Waters Instruments, Rochester, Minn.) and the Morgan Oxylog (Ambulatory Monitoring, Ardsley, N.Y.). These devices require the worker to put on a mask, breathe room air, and exhale into the mask. The exhaled air is analyzed for oxygen content and compared with oxygen content in the room's air to determine average minute oxygen uptake. The 0_2 measurements should be taken when the worker has achieved a steady-state when sampling.

Table 30.11 — Metabolic Energy Costs of Several Activities

Activity	*Kcal/hour*
Resting, prone	80–90
Resting, seated	95–100
Standing, at ease	100–110
Drafting	105
Light assembly (bench work)	105
Medium assembly	160
Driving automobile	170
Walking, casual	175–225
Sheet metal work	180
Machining	185
Rock drilling	225–550
Mixing cement	275
Walking on job	290–400
Pushing wheelbarrow	300–400
Shoveling	235–525
Chopping with axe	400–1400
Climbing stairs	450–775
Slag removal	630–750

Note: Values are for male worker of 70 kg (154 lb).
Source: Reprinted with permission from "Ergonomics Guide to Assessment of Metabolic and Cardiac Costs of Physical Work" (*Am. Ind. Hyg. Assoc. J. 32*:560-564 [1971].)

Heart Rate. Heart rate is a frequently measured indicator of physical stress. The easiest direct method is to take the pulse of the worker once steady-state has been reached. The pulse rate should be recorded for a full minute to avoid the effect of sinus arrhythmia. If the pulse rate is being recorded at the end of the work period, a 15-sec reading is sufficient; readings of longer duration tend to carry into the recovery period. A 3-min average at the steady-state should be recorded. The maximum working heart rate should not exceed 130 beats/min.

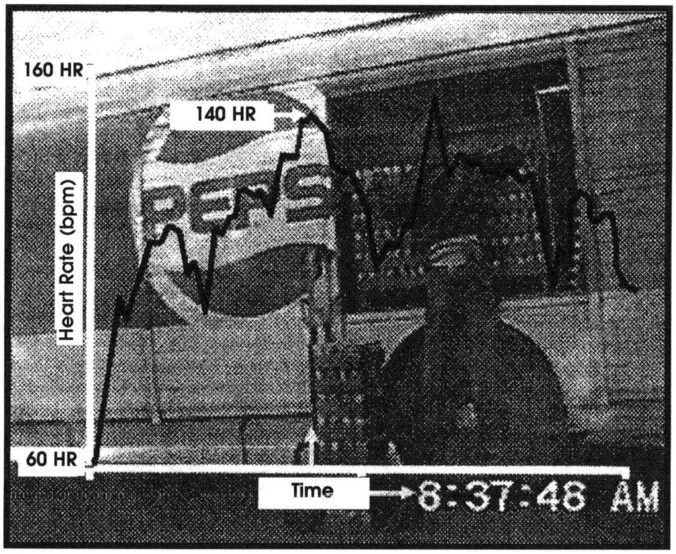

Figure 30.13 — Hear rate overlay (chart) on videograph of worker getting soft drinks from top shelf in truck. Arrow points to driver-sales-worker's current heart rate. Source: J.D. McGlothlin, *Ergonomic Inventions for the Soft Drink beverage Delivery Industry* (Cincinnati, OH: NIOSH, 1996), p. 36.

The other method for recording heart rate uses active and passive electrodes, similar to recording electrocardiogram (EKG) readings. Two electrodes are placed on the rib cage about 10 inches apart, and the ground is placed on a bony landmark. The skin is lightly abraded to get better conduction if passive electrodes are used; such electrodes are covered with an adhesive collar filled with electrode gel.

Heart rate recording devices vary from simple and relatively inexpensive ones that provide a rate only, to physiographs and data graphs that can be used to record EKGs. Physiographs and data graphs can be relatively expensive and may not be necessary for occupational use. Figure 30.13 shows the application of the heart rate monitor on a beverage delivery person, with the heart rate data are overlayed on a video monitor to show cardiovascular demands as a function of task demands.[67] Real-time monitoring of cardiovascular demands while work is videotaped can be useful when determining the job demands, as well as the impact of engineering controls and work practices to lower such demands. Table 30.12 shows the relationship between heart rate, oxygen uptake, and total energy expenditure.[64]

Psychophysical

Psychophysical techniques are suitable for repetitive as well as nonrepetitive or infrequently performed tasks. These techniques are also inexpensive, because little or no equipment is needed. The techniques described in this section can be used for both lower back and upper extremities and include measurements of postural discomfort, static and dynamic work (perceived exertion), and fatigue.

Postural Discomfort. Extreme postures or postures that are maintained for prolonged periods of time can be uncomfortable and lead to fatigue and pain. It has been determined that the level of discomfort is linearly related to the force exertion time. Maintaining the same posture is physiologically equivalent to applying a force. A body map and a 5-point scale are used to determine the body part discomfort.[68] Figure 30.14 shows both the body map and the scale.[68] The worker experiencing discomfort in the task being evaluated specifies the location of discomfort on the chart and rates it using the scale. The worker rates body parts at regular intervals ranging from 30 min to 3 hours. Some ergonomists suggest that the discomfort rating be taken just before a break to get more reliable readings.

Rating of Perceived Exertion. There is a curvilinear relationship between the intensity of a range of stimuli and workers' perception of their intensity. These perceived exertions can be rated on a Borg scale as shown in Figure 30.15.[69]

Figure 30.16(A) shows the Borg RPE for physical tasks. Note that in addition to the overall perception of exertion, these ratings are influenced by previous experience and motivation. In general, highly motivated subjects tend to underestimate their exertion.

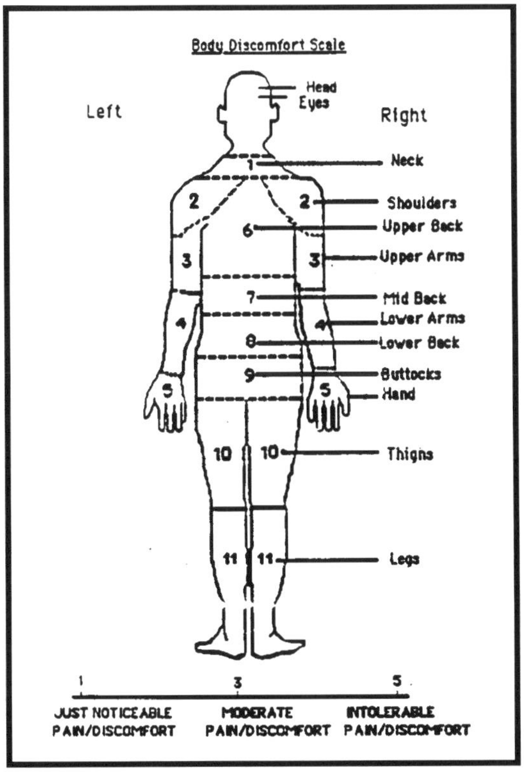

Figure 30.14 — Body part discomfort form and rating scale. (Reprinted with permission from E.N. Corlett and R.P. Bishop, "A Technique for Assessing Postural Discomfort" [*Ergo.* *19*:175–182 (1986)].

Table 30.12 — Relationship Between Heart Rate, Oxygen Uptake, and Total Energy Expenditure

Classification	*Heart Rate (beats/min)*	*Oxygen Uptake (L/min)*	*Total Energy Expenditure (Kcal/min)*
Light work (e.g., typing)	90 or fewer	up to 0.5	2.5
Medium work	100	0.5–1.0	5.0
Heavy Work	120	1.0–1.5	7.5
Very heavy work	140	1.5–2.0	10.0
Extremely heavy work (e.g., ditch digging)	160	over 2.0	15.0

Source: Adapted from reference 64, p. 502.

The scale in Figure 30.15(B) is valid only for large muscle groups and should not be used for work performed by fingers and hands. As shown in this figure, each scale has a point value. Scores for all statements are added to determine the worker's opinion.

Figure 30.16 shows the questionnaire data shown on a computer screen and filled out by a worker in the field using a light pen. This technology proved useful in a recent NIOSH study of beverage delivery workers in terms of efficient data management and analysis.[67]

6	NO EXERTION AT ALL	0	NOTHING AT ALL
7			
	EXTREMELY LIGHT	0.5	EXTREMELY WEAK
8		1	VERY WEAK
9	VERY LIGHT	2	WEAK
10		3	MODERATE
11	VERY LIGHT	4	SOMEWHAT STRONG
12		5	STRONG (HEAVY)
13	SOMEWHAT HARD	6	
14		7	VERY STRONG
15	HARD (HEAVY)	8	
16		9	
17	VERY HARD	10	EXTREMELY STRONG (ALMOST MAX)
18			
19	EXTREMELY HARD		
20	MAXIMAL EXERTION		
	A		**B**

Figure 30.15 — (A) Borg's RPE scale of physical tasks; (B) Borg's RPE scale for large muscles. (Reprinted with permission from G. Borg, An Introduction to Borg's RPE-Scale (Ithaca, NY: Movement Publications, 1985).

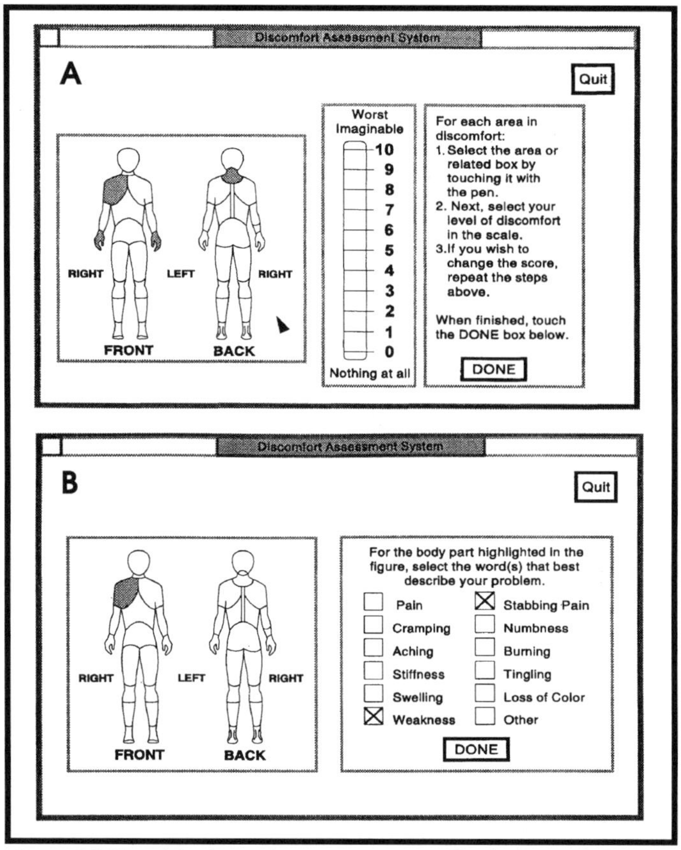

Figure 30.16 — (A) Discomfort scores screen (body figures) shown on computer and activated by light pen. (B) Discomfort descriptions screen shown on computer and activated by light pen. (From J.D. McGlothlin Ergonomic Interventions for the Soft Drink Beverage Delivery Industry [Cincinnati, OH: NIOSH], p. 36. Note: Software developed by Norka Saldana, PhD, University of Michigan, Center for Ergonomics.)

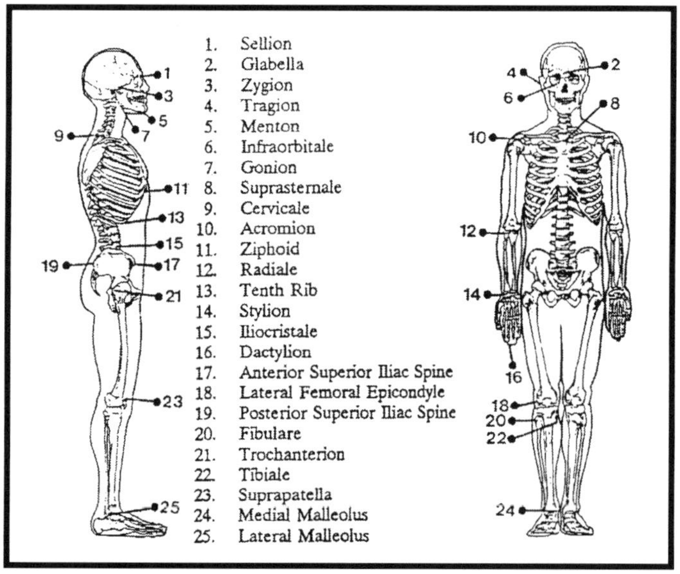

Figure 30.17 — Selected skeletal landmarks used to define traditional anthropometric measurements. (Reprinted with permission from J. Annis and J. McConville, "Ahtropometry," in A. Bhattaharya and J.D. McGlothlin, eds., Occupational Ergonomics: Theory and Applications [New York: Marcel Dekker, 1996], p. 4.

Anthropometry: Designing the Workplace to Fit the Worker

Anthropometry literately translated means "measuring the human," primarily for body size and shape. The systematic measurement of physical properties of the human body is the application of anthropometry. Measurement of humans has been done for hundreds of years, such as fitting soldiers with battle dress, but only within the last 50 years have the human dimensions been used to improve the design and sizing of everyday things.(7) It is when anthropometry is applied to the design and construction of things, from personal protective equipment to modern office furniture, that this discipline enters the realm of ergonomics. The purpose is to improve the effectiveness and efficiency of the person wearing and/or using the equipment.

Figure 30.17 shows the selected skeletal landmarks used to define traditional anthropometric measurements.(7) These landmarks are traditional dimensional descriptors of body size. The measurements provide the distance between two points obtained under static conditions. The basic categories of static dimensions include lengths, depths, breadths, and distances for body size.

This information can be useful when applied to equipment purchases, such as office furniture. For example, if the occupational hygienist was given the task of buying ergonomic office chairs, the knowledge and application of anthropometry might be useful. Table 30.13 shows body dimensions of a U.S. civilian adult sampling.(3) If the task were to purchase chairs to fit a population range from the 5th percentile woman to the 95th percentile man, the occupational hygienist would want to select chairs that could be height adjusted from 35.1 inches (89.2 cm)to 42.9 inches (109.0 cm). This is the sitting popliteal height (the distance from the floor to the joint in back of the knee) for the 5th percentile female to 95th percentile male. Therefore, when the chair can be adjusted for this range, the small woman or large man can sit in a comfortable position with the upper and lower leg approximately 90° to each. Although the example above seems deceptively simple, the applications can become very complex, and the occupational hygienist is encouraged to seek the advice from experts in this field when designing workplaces.

Hand Tools

Proper hand tool design, selection, installation, and use are crucial to the prevention of cumulative trauma disorders of the upper extremities. The physical stressors associated with hand tool operation include awkward postures, forceful exertions, repetitive motion, contact stress, and vibration. The high incidence of musculoskeletal injuries in manufacturing has prompted concern that workers be protected from excess physical stress. It has been recognized by

Table 30.13 — Body Dimensions of U.S. Civilian Adults (Women/Men in Centimeters)

Dimensions	Percentile 5th	50th	95th	Standard Deviation
Heights, Standing				
Stature ("height")	152.8/164.7	162.94/175.58	173.7/186.6	6.36/6.68
Eye	141.5/152.8	151.61/163.39	162.1/174.3	6.25/6.57
Shoulder (acromion)	124.1/134.2	133.36/144.25	143.2/154.6	5.79/6.20
Elbow	92.6/99.5	99.79/107.25	107.4/115.3	4.48/4.81
Wrist	72.8/77.8	79.03/84.65	85.5/91.5	3.86/4.15
Crotch	70.0/76.4	77.14/83.72	84.6/91.6	4.41/4.62
Overhead fingertip reach (on toes)	200.6/216.7	215.34/32.80	231.3/249.4	9.50/9.99
Heights, Sitting				
Sitting height	79.5/85.5	85.20/91.39	91.0/97.2	3.49/3.56
Eye	68.5/73.5	73.87/79.02	79.4/84.8	3.32/3.42
Shoulder (acromion)	50.9/54.9	55.55/59.78	60.4/64.6	2.86/2.96
Elbow rest	17.6/18.4	22.05/23.06	27.1/27.4	2.68/2.72
Knee	47.4/51.4	51.54/55.88	56.0/60.6	2.63/2.79
Popliteal	35.1/39.5	38.94/43.41	42.9/47.6	2.37/2.49
Thigh clearance	14.0/14.9	15.89/16.82	18.0/19.0	1.21/1.26
Depths				
Chest	20.9/21.0	23.94/24.32	27.8/28.0	2.11/2.15
Elbow–fingertip	40.6/44.8	44.35/48.40	48.3/52.5	2.36/2.33
Buttock–knee sitting	54.2/56.9	58.89/61.64	64.0/66.7	2.96/2.99
Buttock–popliteal sitting	44.0/45.8	48.17/50.04	52.8/54.6	2.66/2.66
Thumbtip reach	67.7/73.9	73.46/80.08	79.7/86.7	3.64/3.92
Breadths				
Forearm–forearm	41.5/47.7	46.85/54.61	52.8/62.1	3.47/4.36
Hip, sitting	34.3/32.9	38.45/36.68	43.2/41.2	2.72/2.52
Head Dimensions				
Length	17.6/18.5	18.72/19.71	19.8/20.9	0.64/0.71
Breadth	13.7/14.3	14.44/15.17	15.3/16.1	0.49/0.54
Circumference	52.3/54.3	54.62/56.77	57.1/59.4	1.46/1.54
Interpupillary breadth	5.7/5.9	6.23/6.47	6.9/7.1	0.36/0.37
Hand Dimensions				
Wrist circumference	14.1/16.2	15.14/17.43	16.3/18.8	0.69/0.82
Length, stylion to tip 3	16.5/17.09	18.07/19.41	19.8/21.1	0.98/0.99
Breadth, metacarpal	7.4/8.4	7.95/9.04	8.6/9.8	0.38/0.42
Circumference, metacarpal	17.3/19.8	18.65/21.39	20.1/23.1	0.86/0.98
Digit 1: breadth, distal joint	1.9/2.2	2.06/2.40	2.3/2.6	0.13/0.13
Length	5.6/6.2	6.35/6.97	7.2/7.8	0.48/0.48
Digit 2: breadth, distal joint	1.5/1.8	1.73/2.01	1.9/2.3	0.12/0.15
Length	6.2/6.7	6.96/7.53	7.7/8.4	0.46/0.49
Digit 3: breadth, distal joint	1.5/1.7	1.71/1.98	1.9/2.2	0.11/0.14
Length	6.9/7.5	7.72/8.38	8.6/9.3	0.51/0.54
Digit 4: breadth, distal joint	1.4/1.6	1.58/1.85	1.8/2.1	0.11/0.14
Length	6.4/7.1	7.22/7.92	8.1/8.8	0.50/0.52
Digit 5: breadth, distal joint	1.3/1.5	1.47/1.74	1.7/2.0	0.11/0.13
Length	5.1/5.7	5.83/6.47	6.6/7.3	0.46/0.49
Foot Dimensions				
Length	22.4/24.9	24.44/26.97	26.5/29.2	1.22/1.31
Breadth	8.2/9.2	8.97/10.06	9.8/11.0	0.49/0.53
Lateral malleolus height	5.2/5.8	6.06/6.71	7.0/7.6	0.53/0.55
Weight (kg) U.S. Army	49.6/61.6	62.01/78.49	77.0/98.1	8.35/11.10
Weight (kg) civilians*	39/58*	62.0/78.5*	85/99*	13.8/12.6*

* Estimated (from Kroemer, 1981).

Note that all values (except for civilians' weight) are based on measured, not estimated, data that may be slightly different from values calculated from average plus or minus 1.65 standard deviation.

(Excerpted from Gordon, Churchill, Clauser, et al., 1989; Greiner, 1991.)

Note: All values (except for civilians' weight) are based on measured, not estimated, data that may be slightly different from values calculated from average plus or minus 1.64 standard deviation.
Source: References 3, 66.

management and labor that the interface between the human operator and the tools frequently used for repetitive manual work can affect a large number of jobs. Consequently, manufacturers of both non-powered and powered hand tools are being challenged by customer demands for products that minimize physical stress. The physical stress associated hand tools use in manufacturing may seem small in magnitude during any single occurrence, but repeated exposure over time may lead to work-related cumulative trauma disorders. The objective when selecting installing, and using hand tools is to minimize exposures to each of the physical stress factors. The principal physical factors to consider when using tools include posture, force, repetitiveness, contact stresses, vibration, exposure time, and temperature.(70)

Tool Selection

Tool selection should be made within the context of the job. By considering the ergonomic aspect of tool application for a specific job, the adverse effects of using the wrong tool can be prevented. The appropriate hand tool for the job should (1) maximize work performance, (2) enhance work quality, (3) minimize worker stress, and (4) prevent the onset of fatigue. Also, there are process engineering requirements for tools that need to be addressed. For example, power hand tools must be capable of performing specific tasks in terms of speed; dimensions; torque; feed force; power; weight; trigger activation; spindle and chuck diameter; noise level; air pressure; precision and tolerance; bits; blades; abrasives; and power source. More important is the consideration of workers and how they will use the tools. For example, when a hand tool is selected, the worker characteristics to be considered are strength, anthropometry, manual dexterity, and motor capabilities.

Worker strength is affected by body position, the direction of exerted force relative to the body, the type of grip used to hold the tool, and the handle size. Grip strength depends on the type of grip used. The power grip is preferred because of the large muscles recruited to perform the job. To optimize grip strength, handle shape is important. It is important to know handle span and handle circumference as well as handle shape. The thumb, index, and middle fingers are the strongest fingers and should be used for producing the most grip force. By increasing the surface area of contact between the handle and the hand, the amount of torque can be increased. However, grip strength has been shown to decrease when handles with diameters greater than 50 mm are used.(71)

Worker anthropometry can affect the posture a worker assumes when operating a hand tool. The location, orientation, and tool design should all be considered together along with the stature of the worker.(29) When the work location and orientation cannot be adjusted, it may be possible to select another tool or to change the location or orientation of work.

A tool that is too large may be difficult to use for performance or precision work. The type of grip suitable for a manual tool operation is often limited by the size of the tool. For example, a power grip can provide greater strength than a pinch grip; however, a pinch grip provides greater control of precision movements. As a result, tool selection should optimize the proportion of strength that an operator must exert with the ability to make necessary movements with speed and precision. There is a tradeoff between the increased mechanical advantage provided by a long tool, versus its weight and size, and the ability for an operator to manipulate and handle it.(52)

Workstation and Task Factors

The main power hand tool characteristics and operational requirements may include the following: (1) tool weight and load distribution; (2) triggers; (3) feed and reaction force; (4) handles; (5) work location and orientation; (6) tool accessories; (7) vibration; and (8) noise. Table 32.14 shows the power hand tool mechanical properties affected by certain tool parameters.(70)

Engineering Control and Design Consideration

When controls for WMSDs are being implemented the following areas must be included in the consideration and analysis: posture; exertion/force; contact pressure; handle friction; gloves; center of gravity; tool location; tool activation and throttle; reaction torque; balancer and suspension;

and vibration. Table 30.15 shows examples of specific tool properties that are affected through design.[70]

The proper design and selection of hand tools is a complex process that must include analyzing the work station, materials, and methods; account for worker characteristics; and consider all the variations that may result from the process or the individual. To accomplish this, it is necessary to identify and understand the interrelationship of most of the process variables. This information must be integrated to critically evaluate the physical characteristics of the tool and the location of its application.

Table 30.14 — Tool Properties and Tool Parameters Affecting Tool Properties

Tool Properties	*Tool Parameters Affecting Tool Properties*
Load	center of gravity location tool mass use of counterbalance or articulating arm power line installation
Handle size	type of grip needed (power, pinch)
Handle shape	type of grip needed (power, pinch)
Handle orientation	type of grip needed (power, pinch) distribution of load work location
Feed force	type of fastener head type of fastener tip or drill bit work material
Sound level	tool speed power work material tool location
Reaction torque	spindle torque tool and handle length stiffness of joint torque reaction bar
Vibration	tool weight work material abrasive material tool speed tool power handle location moment of inertia

Table 30.15 — Physical Factors for Hand Tools and Design Objectives

Physical Factor	*Design Objectives*
Tool load	use of lightweight and composite materials optimum load distribution optimum handle location
Handle size/shape	optimum size handle optimum handle shape adjustable handle size
Handle orientation	optimum angle adjustable orientation
Work location	optimum location for tool load, handle size, and handle orientation
Sound level	motor housing and suspension mufflers
Fasteners	fastener head design
Torque	shutoff mechanism
Vibration	motor mounting tool balance and load distribution

Putting It All Together: Case Study Using Ergonomic Principles and Applications

This case study shows one of the many methods of evaluating WMSDs in the workplace, and how to evaluate the effectiveness of the interventions.

Case Study: An Ergonomics Evaluation of a Flywheel Milling Department at a Motorcycle Manufacturing Plant; An Intervention Study[72]

Background. NIOSH researchers received a joint request to evaluate musculoskeletal disorders of the upper limbs and back from the union and management of a vehicle-manufacturing facility employing approximately 650 workers. Particular concern was expressed about the flywheel milling areas.

The NIOSH request was prompted by an increase in worker's compensation costs because of a growing number of injuries. This company had experienced an economic decline during the 1970s and early 1980s resulting in worker layoffs. In the mid-1980s, after an economic recovery, experienced workers on layoff were recalled to work. Eventually, as the recovery continued, the company began hiring new employees. At about the same time, the company hired a new nurse for the health unit, who has subsequently become the safety director. She began to rigorously maintain the OSHA Log and Summary of Occupational Injuries and Illnesses and to educate workers and management concerning WMSDs. Because of a combination of these two factors the company experienced a large increase in workers' compensation cases.

Based in part on the initial NIOSH report[73], several ergonomic interventions were developed and implemented by the company, which resulted in a reduction in the number of reported musculoskeletal injuries in this department. This reduction was documented in three follow-up visits, which were conducted by NIOSH researchers. These visits resulted in information and recommendations that provided guidance to the company to help improve medical surveillance of musculoskeletal injuries.

Work Force and Physical Plant

Pre-intervention Evaluation. Approximately 253 motorcycle engines and 170 motorcycle transmissions were fabricated and assembled each day at this facility. Production was 24 hours per day, and two to three employees worked in the flywheel milling area per 8-hour shift. The flywheels came in the following two sizes: large (FL) (approximately 19 lb premilled), and small (XL) (approximately 16 lb premilled). In another area in this department there were five full-time employees assembling, truing, and balancing the flywheels. Employees rotated through the truing task every 2 to 4 hours. Occasionally, these employees would work 10- to 12-hour days to keep pace with production demands. There were 38 full-time workers in this department.

Post-intervention Evaluation. Approximately 340 motorcycle engines and 254 motorcycle transmissions were fabricated and assembled each day at this facility. Production was 24 hours per day, and two to three employees worked in the flywheel milling area per 8-hour shift. The flywheels came in the following sizes: large (FL) (approximately 17.5 lb [7.9 kg] premilled), and small (XL) (approximately 13.5 lb [6.1 kg] premilled). In another area in this department, there were seven full-time employees assembling, truing, and balancing flywheels. Because of the changes to the truing area, employees did not need to be rotated as mentioned above. Also, improved forging specifications (discussed in detail later) of the FL and XL flywheels reduced the premilled weight. There were 50 full-time employees in this department.

Process Description

The NIOSH evaluation of this motorcycle manufacturing plant focused on the flywheel milling and assembly department, where milling, assembly and truing, and balancing flywheels were done.

Milling of the flywheels consisted of a series of steps to complete the job cycle. The basic steps were manually getting the forged flywheel from a supply cart; drilling and machine milling it; grinding off metal burrs; and inspecting, measuring, and placing the finished flywheel in a receiving cart. Each milling "cell" contained three to four milling machines, a drill press, and two to three worktables. Approximately 2–3 lb of metal were cut from each flywheel during the milling process.

After milling, the flywheel unit was assembled. The unit consisted of the gear and sprocket side of the flywheel, two connecting rods, bearings, and a crank pen. These components were assembled and put together by a "marriage press." After this, the unit was taken to the truing area for straightening and centering.

Truing of the flywheel was done by manually mounting it on a fixture on top of a table, and manually rotating the flywheel to determine misalignment (a centering gauge was viewed by the operator to determine misalignment). In the initial NIOSH evaluation, when the misalignment area was found, a 5-lb (2.3 kg) brass-head hammer, which was held by the employee, was repeatedly struck against the flywheel to straighten and center (true) the unit. In the follow-up evaluations a 40-ton (36,287.4 kg) press performed the truing operation, and the hammers were eliminated. After the flywheel unit was trued, it was manually lifted and placed onto a cart, which was moved to the balancing area.

A flywheel unit was balanced by picking it up from a cart and placing it in a cradle in the balancing machine. The flywheel connecting rods were attached to balancing arms that rotated the unit at high speeds. A computer determined where holes were to be drilled to provide balance when the flywheel unit was operating at high speeds. Following this procedure, the flywheel was manually moved from the balancing machine to a cart. The weights of fully assembled postmilled flywheels (sprocket and gear) and their components (bearings, crank pin, and two connecting rods) were large, (FL) 32.5 lb (14.7 kg) (34 lb [15.4 kg] maximum weight); and small, (XL) 25.6 lb (11.6 kg) (26 lb [11.8 kg] maximum weight). The finished flywheel units were then moved from this department to the engine assembly department.

Methods

The evaluation of the flywheel milling department consisted of a walk-through survey of motorcycle engine fabrication and assembly, a review of the OSHA logs and company medical compensation data, informal interviews with employees, and an ergonomic evaluation of jobs in the flywheel milling area.

Ergonomic Evaluation

NIOSH Initial Evaluation. An in-depth ergonomic evaluation of the flywheel milling area was conducted during the initial survey; follow-up surveys consisted of assessing ergonomic changes in the flywheel milling jobs, as recommended in the in-depth report sent to the company.

The initial ergonomic evaluation consisted of (1) discussions with flywheel milling employees regarding musculoskeletal hazards associated with their job; (2) videotape of the flywheel milling process; (3) a biomechanical evaluation of musculoskeletal stress during manual handling of the flywheels; and (4) a recording of workstation dimensions. Two flywheel milling cells were evaluated.

Videotapes of the jobs were analyzed at regular speed to determine job cycle time, at slow-motion to determine musculoskeletal hazards of the upper limbs during manual material handling tasks, and using stop-action to sequence job steps and perform biomechanical evaluations of working postures. All video analysis procedures were used to document potential musculoskeletal hazards in performing the job.

Time and motion study techniques were used for the first phase of job analysis. Work methods analysis was used to determine the work content of the job. The second phase of job analysis was to review the job for recognized occupational risk factors for WMSDs. These WMSD risk factors included repetition, force, posture, contact stress, low temperature, and vibration. A biomechanical evaluation also was made of forces that were exerted on the upper limbs, back, and lower limbs of the worker while the task was performed. This two-phase approach for job analysis and quantification of forces that act on the body during materials handling formed the basis for proposed engineering and administrative control procedures aimed at reducing the risk for musculoskeletal stress and injury.

After receipt of the initial NIOSH report the company conducted several meetings over a 1- to 2-year period to engineer out specific job hazards in the flywheel milling and assembly department. The meetings led to the systematic selection of equipment based on more than 20 performance criteria. Some of these criteria were reduction or elimination of the specific hazard (vibration from hand tools); user friendly controls; noise reduction; easy access for maintenance personnel; parts availability; cycle time; machine guarding; and machine durability.

NIOSH Follow-Up Evaluations. Three follow-up evaluations were conducted.. During these evaluations NIOSH researchers spoke with the safety director, and the operators, managers, and engineers involved in the redesign of the work processes in the flywheel department. An evaluation was also done on the changes made since the initial evaluation. Specific NIOSH activities during these follow-up evaluations included (1) discussions with employees regarding changes in their job for musculoskeletal hazards; (2) videotaping the flywheel milling, truing, and balancing process; (3) reviewing company ergonomic committee activities on reducing job hazards in this department; (4) presenting education and training sessions on ergonomics to plant supervisors, engineers, and workers; and (5) reviewing OSHA logs. Recommendations were made on site during these follow-back evaluations to encourage continuous improvement of jobs to reduce musculoskeletal disorders.

Rates of Musculoskeletal Disorders. OSHA logs were obtained and coded. All musculoskeletal problems, including such conditions as sprains, strains, tendonitis, and carpal tunnel syndrome involving the upper extremities and back, were included in the analysis. It is extremely difficult to determine from the OSHA logs whether a musculoskeletal sprain or strain is due to acute or chronic trauma; therefore, all of these events were included. Musculoskeletal contusions, which are likely to be more acute events, were not included. Information on the number of employees for each year was obtained and used to develop incidence rates. Although the change in the truing machine was completed early in the evaluation, many of the other changes in the flywheel department were not in place until approximately 2 years later. Therefore, these data may not show the full effect of all the design changes.

Results

Table 32.16 summarizes the initial ergonomic recommendations for the flywheel milling area made by NIOSH researchers and the actions completed by the company on the last follow-up evaluation. This table shows that several actions were taken to address concerns about musculoskeletal injuries in the flywheel milling cell. Pre- and post-ergonomic intervention activities for the milling, assembly and truing, and balancing area are summarized in the following paragraphs.

Milling

Pre-intervention Evaluation. Milling of the FL flywheel (average weight 19.0 lbs [8.6 kg]) and the XL flywheel (average weight 16.0 lbs [7.3 kg]) consisted of 37 steps for the FL flywheel and 25 steps for the XL flywheel. It was estimated that 28,175 lbs (12,780.0 kg) of flywheels were manually handled for the FL flywheel and 18,980 lbs (9,062.8 kg) for the XL flywheel per 8-hour day. These total weights were derived by multiplying the average weight of the milled flywheel (17.5 lb [7.9 kg] FL, and 14.5 lb [6.6 kg] XL) times the average number of times the flywheel was picked up (23 and 17, respectively), times the average number of flywheels milled per day.(65)

Post-intervention Evaluation. Milling of flywheels was divided into two jobs. Instead of two flywheel castings for the left and right half (gear and sprocket sides), there was one master cast flywheel, weighing 17.5 lb (7.9 kg) for the FL flywheel, and 13.5 lb (6.1 kg) for the XL flywheel. In the first modified flywheel milling job, 13 steps were required to complete the work cycle. Approximately 84 flywheels were milled per 8-hour day; this represents 17,472 lbs (7925.2 kg) handled per day for the FL flywheel and 13,759 lbs (6241.0 kg) for the XL flywheel. In the second flywheel milling job 9 steps were needed to complete the work cycle. Approximately 84 flywheels were milled per day, representing 10,202 lbs (4627.6 kg) for the FL and 9526 lbs (4320.9 kg) for the XL flywheel handled per day. Because of the short cycle time, the worker on this job also worked on the flywheel balancing job. Table 30.17 summarizes the material handling results of the flywheel milling job before and after ergonomic interventions.

Pre-intervention Hand–Arm Vibration Exposure. In addition to the potential overexertion injuries for manual handling of the flywheels in the milling cells, another concern was excess hand–arm vibration exposure from a handheld grinder that removed metal burrs from the flywheel. It was determined that approximately 20% of the job cycle was used for removing metal burrs. As noted in Table 30.16, recommendations were provided to reduce vibration exposure and improve job efficiency.

Postintervention Hand–Arm Vibration Exposure. Vibration exposure was virtually eliminated with the purchase of a customized metal deburring machine. This machine was designed according to specifications from engineers and workers performing the job and automatically removed burrs using grinding stones inside the unit. The installation of this unit in the flywheel milling cell resulted in a more than 90% reduction in handheld grinders and a reduction from 20% of the work cycle to less than 1% (occasional touch-up) for handheld grinding operations. The deburring machine allowed the worker to move on to other work elements while this job was done, thus making the job more efficient and reducing potential hazardous vibration exposure.

The cost of the deburring machine was more than $200,000. To justify the costs over handheld grinding, the company established an evaluation program that incorporated the goal of sound engineering and production principles with ergonomic design. Table 30.18 lists the steps in which decisions and actions of plant personnel accomplished their goal as applied to the deburring machine.

Truing (Assembly and Centering)

Pre-intervention Truing Evaluation. After milling, the flywheels were assembled together with connecting rods, bearings,

Table 30.16 — Ergonomic Changes

Engineering Controls	
Initial Recommendation (January 1990)	*Result (September 1993)*
Reduce the weight of the flywheels by improving forging specifications. This will reduce milling time and the amount of weight handled over the workday.	Weight of fly wheels were reduced by improving forging specifications by nearly 2 lbs. In addition, only one type of flywheel forging (for the gear and sprocket sides) is shipped to plant and is milled to specifications. This simplifies the milling process, reduces waste and multiple handling of flywheels.
Reduce or eliminate exposure to vibration from powered hand grinder. Twenty percent of the work cycle time consists of vibration exposure from this tool.	Customized metal deburring machines were purchased to eliminate more than 90% of the exposure from the hand grinding operations. The hand grinder is used less than 1% of the work cycle time (for minor touchup of fly wheel).
Layout of the flywheel milling job is inefficient from production and material handling perspectives. Consider movable flywheel carts and/or gravity conveyors between milling work stations to reduce musculoskeletal stress.	The flywheel milling cell was reorganized into 2 work cells, reducing the number of machines per cell and the amount of material handled per worker. For the FL flywheel, this resulted in a 38% reduction in material handling from 28,175 lbs to 17,472 per shift, and a 43% reduction in the number of times the operator needed to handle the flywheel during the milling process. Similar results were documented for the XL flywheel milling process.
Reduce the size of the metal pan that is built around the base of the indexing machine and round the corners to reduce the reach distance to attach the flywheels to the machine.	The indexing machine has been eliminated and replaced by a more efficient machine. Physical barriers were designed out of this machine before it was put into operation.
Install durable rubberized floor matting around flywheel milling cells to reduce lower limb fatigue of workers.	Several types of rubberized floor matting were evaluated for durability, slip-resistance, and comfort by the operators in this department. A selection of rubberized mats was made available for the operators.
Remove all physical barriers that may cause workers to overreach, such as limited toe and leg space where the worker has to reach over barriers to manually position flywheels for processing.	Most physical barriers were eliminated because the worker was part of the workstation redesign process. Toe and leg space were considered when the work cells were redesigned. Machines such as the drill press were adjusted up to chest height of worker. This reduced stooping to position the flywheels in the machines.
Recommend workers use the "power grip" rather than the "pinch grip" when handling the flywheel. The "pinch grip" requires handling of the flywheel by the fingertips and thumb, resulting in high musculoskeletal forces and fatigue. Use of two hands was also recommended when handling parts to reduce asymmetric biomechanical loading of the limbs and back.	All workers in this department received ergonomics training on material handling techniques. When the flywheels were handled at the wheel end, both hands were used, especially when positioning flywheels in or out of the milling machines.
Wheel carts taken into the flywheel milling cell should be brought in with the cart bumper facing away from the traffic area to avoid contact with the worker's shins.	Wheel cart bumpers were retrofitted with tubular steel to reduce mechanical contact with the worker's shins. Several of the wheel carts were also fitted with hinged bumpers that can be manually rotated in the vertical position and out of the worker's way. Workers position the wheel carts close to their work area to reduce distance and material handling.
Operators should avoid overreaching while handling flywheels during milling. Overreaching may result in excess musculoskeletal stress and possibly injury, especially later in the work shift when the worker may become fatigued.	On-site training of workers about biomechanical aspects of work may have increased their awareness of overreaching while performing their job. Redesign of the workstation also helped reduce overreaching by providing leg and toe clearance and adjusting the height of the workstations to fit the workers.

Table 30.17 — Comparison of Pre- and Postinterventions of Manual Handling of Flywheel Milling

Preintervention (January 1990)	*FL Flywheel*	*XL Flywheel*
Premilled flywheel weight	19.0	16.0
Average weight	17.5	14.5
Average cycle time	5 min	4 min
No. flywheels/8-hour day	70	75
No. steps moving flywheel	23	17
No. pounds moved/8-hour shift	28,175	18,980
Postintervention First Flywheel Cell[A] (September 1993)		
Premilled flywheel weight	17.5	13.5
Average flywheel weight	16.0	12.6
Average cycle time	4 min	4 min
No. flywheels/8-hour day	84	84
No. steps moving flywheel	13	13
No. pounds moved/8-hour shift	17,472	13,759
Postintervention Second Flywheel Cell[B]		
Average weight flywheel	16.0	12.6
Average cycle time	1.5 min	1.5 min
No. flywheels/8-hour day	84[C]	84
No. steps moving flywheel	9	9
Average weight/8-hour day	12,096	9526

[A]Flywheel milling completed by another worker in adjacent cell.
[B]Second flywheel cell completes the milling process.
[C]Up to 280 flywheels can be milled per 8-hour day. However, this worker also does flywheel balancing job and only keeps pace with the first flywheel milling cell.

and a crank pen. A marriage press was used to sandwich the parts into one unit. The flywheel unit was then trued. After mounting the flywheel on a fixture, the flywheel unit was manually rotated, using a centering gauge to detect misalignment. The unit was struck, using a 5 lb brass-head hammer held by the worker. Depending on the amount of straightening necessary, the initial impact of the brass-head hammer could be as high as 92,000 pounds (41,730.5 kg). Impact forces were reduced as the flywheel was straightened to specifications. The repeated forces needed to straighten the unit were somewhat traumatizing to the workers, and they needed to be rotated from this job every 2 to 4 hours. Engineers and workers were developing ways to reduce exposure to this job when NIOSH researchers arrived for the initial visit. NIOSH researchers agreed that the job needed to be changed to reduce the impact force stressors to the upper limbs.

Post-intervention Truing Evaluation. Recommendations to reduce exposure on this job (called the "hammer slammer" job by workers) resulted in the use of a 40-ton press that was modified, based on plant ergonomic committee input, for truing the flywheels. The press completely eliminated the need for the brass hammers, thus eliminating mechanical trauma to the upper limbs from this task.

Balancing

Pre-intervention Balancing Evaluation. After the flywheel unit was trued, the next step was balancing. This process involved manually picking up the flywheel from a cart and placing it in a cradle in the balancing machine. The flywheel connecting rods were attached to balancing arms, which rotated the flywheel at high speeds. Balance sensors relayed a profile of the unit's balance characteristics to a computer, which determined where the holes were to be drilled. After the holes were drilled, the flywheel unit was rotated once more for a final balance check. The flywheel was manually picked up from the balancing machine and placed in a cart. The process was then repeated. Using the revised NIOSH Lifting Equation, it was determined that workers performing this job were occasionally at risk for back injury when manually handling the FL flywheel unit. It was determined that when the flywheel unit was picked up, a safe weight was approximately 30 lb (13.6 kg), and when it was placed in the balancing cradle, the safe weight was approximately 21 lb (9.5 kg). The difference in safe lifting weights is mainly attributable to the location of the load from the body when it was placed in the balancing cradle. Figure 30.18 summarizes the information used to determine the NIOSH Recommended Weight Limit (RWL) of 30 and 21 lb.

Post-intervention Balancing Evaluation. A similar procedure for balancing the flywheels was performed using the sensors and computer. However, because the flywheel unit was heavy, an overhead hoist mounted on an x-y trolley (gantry hoist) was used to lift the unit and place it in the balancing unit cradle. Balancing was performed by the computer, and the gantry hoist was used once more to put the finished part back in the cart. The hoist was an excellent engineering control to address this material handling problem.

Musculoskeletal Disorders

Table 30.19 shows the yearly rates of musculoskeletal disorders for the entire production facility, as well as specific rates for the most commonly affected body parts: shoulder, hand/arm, and back.

Table 30.19 also shows a breakdown of the disorders into those affecting the upper extremities and back injuries during that 5-year period for the flywheel department. Upper extremity disorders steadily decreased after the intervention program began, whereas back injuries decreased in a more erratic pattern. Because many of the interventions that would have decreased the amount of manual material handling were implemented about half way through the study, the more modest decrease in back injuries is not surprising.

Table 30.20 shows the rate of musculoskeletal disorders for the flywheel department and for all other departments combined. This table shows that the rate of injuries increased dramatically in the flywheel department and subsequently decreased. In the other departments there has been a modest but continued increase over the same period.

Figure 30.19 shows a graph of the incidence rates as well as the change in employment over the seven year period covered by the evaluation. This graph illustrates the effects of the economic recovery described at the beginning of this case study. After an

Table 30.18 — Steps in the Metal Deburring Machine Purchase

Steps	*Activity*	*Comments*
1.	NIOSH report (January, 1990), observes potential problem from hand-arm vibration exposure to handheld grinder	Recommends several options to reduce exposure, including a metal finishing machine to remove burrs.
2.	Problem-solving team formed by the company	Team participants: 1 manufacturing engineer, 2 operators, 1 maintenance machine repairman, 1 supervisor, 1 tool designer, 1 medical, 1 purchasing, and 1 facility
3.	Mission statement formed	"Deburr flywheels and connecting rods in a manner to decrease musculoskeletal injuries from hand grinders, while improving quality and reducing variability."
4.	Overview of method	(1) Three vendors quoted project; (2) team ran trials with all three and rated results on a matrix; (3) one vendor received highest quality matrix rating plus received a consensus favorable rating from the team.
5.	Definition of priorities	(1) "What the customer wants" (safety, quality, ergonomics); (2) how the company can meet these requirements: (a) reduce hand grinding >90%, (b) machine construction, (c) ease of load and unload.
6.	Analysis methods	(1) Trials and analysis; (2) interview of vendors; (3) discussion and review of machine and process details
7.	Justification	(1) Safety: (a) eliminate flywheel grinding by 90%, (b) estimated savings from prevented lost-time accidents $53,679 (1987-1991) (2) Quality, same or improved; no loose burrs, reduced variability, complexity, increase throughput (3) Ergonomic: (a) easy to load and unload, (b) no forward bending, especially with weight out in front of body, (c) both hands available to handle flywheels (4) Housekeeping and environmental: (a) noise cover, (b) eliminates flying metal
8.	Delivery and payback impacts	(a) headcount: meets planned requirements for future layout and schedule production increases; (b) meets capacity effect with less increased manual time; (c) cycle time less than 2 min/flywheel, 20 sec to load and unload; (d) labor cost savings: none except cost increase avoidance savings with increases in schedule; (e) flexibility: increased; (f) setup less than 10 min; (g) in-process inventory; (h) floor space: more than hand grinders, same for alternatives; (i) overhead: increased; annual usage cost saved (grinders and bits $1730, new process annual costs $7848)
9.	Employee modification recommendations	(a) insulation covers (noise reduction); (b) load arms presented to operator (to reduce bending over); (c) rinse cycles.
10.	Costs	$229,616
11.	Timetable	Delivery (12-23-92), installation (1-11-93), implementation (6-14-93)

Table 30.19 — Entire Production Facility Incidence Rates of Musculoskeletal Disorders from OSHA 200 Logs

Year	Total Rate (% of workers)	Shoulder Rate (% of workers)	Hand/Arm Rate (% of workers)	Back Rate (% of workers)
1987	9	3	2	3
1988	10	1	4	4
1989	14	1	5	6
1990	17	5	5	7
1991	17	4	3	7
1992	16	3	4	6
1993	13	3	3	4

initial period of increasing production, during which experienced workers were recalled to work, new and inexperienced workers were hired. This rapidly increasing rate of production, combined with the hiring of a new nurse and safety coordinator who increased awareness of work-related musculoskeletal disorders, resulting in the initial increase in rates.

Discussion

The goal of any effective ergonomic intervention effort is to eliminate the job hazards and to use reduced morbidity as a measure of success. When the process follows a systematic procedure that benefits the workers and the company, then it can be effectively repeated with high probability of success. This case study presents a process in which there was commitment from top management to provide resources to manufacture flywheels better, from company engineers to select the most cost-effective equipment available, and from workers to be involved in every aspect of the equipment from selection to custom design. The goal is a better product, made in a cost-effective manner by a healthy work force.

In this motorcycle manufacturing plant there was a strong commitment by both the management and workers to improve the ergonomic design of their equipment. Although there was a downward trend in musculoskeletal injuries particularly affecting the upper extremities, the full effect has only begun to be seen, because many design changes were implemented only recently.

The problem-solving approach used by this company was effective because it used a team of employees, engineers, managers, and medical personnel. This resulted in a participation approach in which all parties in the flywheel milling and assembly department contributed their knowledge and experience. It was noteworthy that after the committee selected this press, management supported the committee's decision. This fostered productive meetings and timely approval of other purchases to reduce and eliminate job hazards associated with musculoskeletal injuries on the job. The examples given in following paragraphs highlight these points.

A committee was formed to resolve the problem of high morbidity from the flywheel truing job. The committee included two supervisors, two truing operators, and six engineers. They first established the four most important criteria for the new process and then identified two potential vendors with machines that could meet these criteria. The selection was a 40-ton press. The next step was to send a sampling of flywheels to

Table 30.20 — Flywheel Department: Trends in WMSDs 1987–1993

	WMSD[A] Incidence Rate (% of Workers)			Lost/Restricted Workdays	
Year	Workers	Total	Lost/Restricted Workday Cases	Number of 100 Workers	Median No. per Case[B]
1987	34	17.6	11.8	110	10
1988	34	11.8	8.9	130	13
1989	36	38.9	27.6	610	13
1990	44	20.5	11.5	390	33
1991	43	27.9	18.7	480	21
1992	45	17.8	13.4	560	12
1993	48	20.8	12.5	190	11

[A]Includes all neck, upper extremity, and back cases
[B]This includes only those cases that had some lost or restricted workdays.

the press manufacturer for truing by the manufacturer's personnel. Subsequent evaluation by engineers and workers in the company's flywheel department was performed. When the quality issues were satisfied, workers from the flywheel department were sent to the press manufacturing plant to test the machine. Based on employee input, the equipment was modified prior to purchase. The new equipment was phased in as the old equipment was phased out over a 2-month period. Although some workers had reservations about the new press because they were highly skilled in their jobs, the department supervisor worked with them to allow a phase-in period during which they performed their jobs 6 hours a day using the brass hammers and 2 hours using the new press. The workers were encouraged to comment on the press and how it could be improved. Gradually the workers gave up the hammer job and used the press.

The new press cost the facility about $58,000, whereas the annual costs of brass hammers had been $40,000. Also, during the previous 6 years there had been 10 injuries from the old truing process. These injuries cost more than $20,000 in medical costs alone, plus additional expenses from lost work time.

A similar change was made for the flywheel balancing job. Using the revised NIOSH lifting equation, analysis of this task showed that manually lifting the flywheel unit from the cart, twisting the body, and placing the flywheel in the cradle of the balancing machine could pose a musculoskeletal hazard. Initially, an articulating arm having a base pod was used to perform this job. This was done without input from the committee. When the unit was installed, it proved to be too cumbersome and took too much time. The unit was soon pushed to the side, and the workers performed the job as usual. When the committee, including the worker who performed this job, thought about how to achieve the goals of reducing material handling, saving time, and keeping the unit out of the way during the balancing process, they conceived of a gantry hoist system that would do the job. The result was a suspended gantry hoist, which was easily controlled by the worker in three directions.

As these examples show, the company and its employees learned several lessons about what it takes to sustain a successful

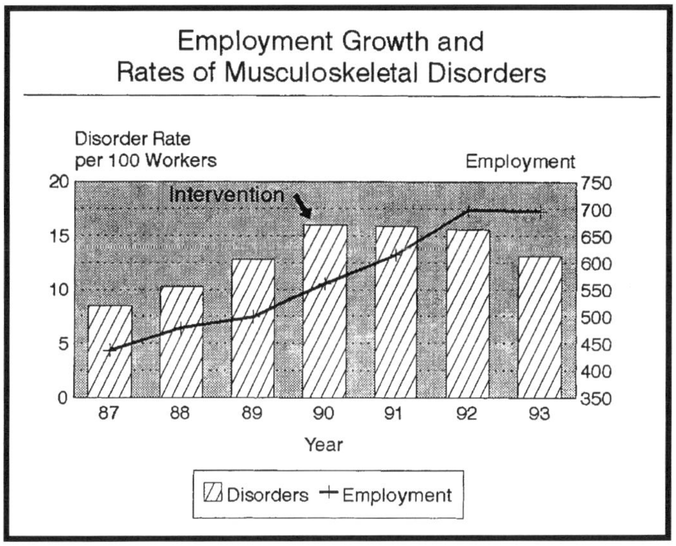

Figure 30.19 — Case study. Results of employment growth and rates of musculoskeletal disorders at a motorcycle manufacturing plant.

ergonomics program. The first lesson was that problem solving usually includes a series of steps rather than one leap from the problem to a solution. Depending on the training and resources of the company, this process can be immediate or take months. Also, resources needed to do the job can be nominal or very costly. Examples of the two extremes in this study were raising the drill press to eliminate stooping while loading flywheels into its fixture and purchasing a customized spindle deburring machine.

Another lesson is that successful ergonomic programs need to be sustained because of the dynamic nature of today's business and production environment. A variety of approaches can be used to achieve this, however, providing stimulation to the process by hiring competent outside experts can enhance the ergonomic changes. Often management may become complacent and react to problems as they arise, rather than forming a plan to engineer ergonomics into the machines and processes they control. The outside expert can assist with planning, so that ergonomic factors can be engineered into the machines and processes prior to operation.

Finally, the importance of the front-line supervisor who serves as the communicator between management and the production worker is very important. The frontline supervisor can make or break an ergonomics program. The supervisor provides a supportive environment for workers' ideas, developing their concepts into practical applications that use sound engineering principles. The frontline supervisor also needs to communicate effectively with upper management, to present needs in a systematic way, and to secure resources to get the job done right. Ergonomics training for the frontline supervisor is important, but just as important is skillful communication of the needs of the workers and the goals of the company.

Basic Elements of an Ergonomic Control Program

The first step in forming an ergonomics team is to make sure all personnel resources in the plant are represented, including management, labor, engineering, medical, and safety personnel. The team establishes a training schedule in which an outside expert, familiar with the plant operations, teaches ergonomics principles to management and workers.

Over time, medical surveillance is used to determine the effectiveness of the ergonomic interventions. Medical surveillance can be active or passive. Active surveillance is usually conducted by administering standardized questionnaires to workers in problem and non-problem jobs. Passive surveillance is conducted by examining medical injury or illness records, such as OSHA logs, workers' compensation reports, and attendance records for absenteeism. Analysis is done on both approaches to identify patterns and changes over time.

Decreases in the incidence and severity of musculoskeletal disease and injury serve as one measure of success. Increases in productivity and product quality serve as another. In many instances workers' awareness of their musculoskeletal disease and injuries show an increase in incidence rates early in the ergonomics program. However, as the program matures, both incidence and severity usually decrease. The length of time required to observe such effects can be a function of the company resources, worker participation, company size, corporate culture, and type of product produced. On average, it takes two to three years before "real" effects are seen. Two important lessons can be learned from successful ergonomics programs. First, the program should not be created as an entity separate from the mission of the plant. Rather it should be woven into existing programs, such as safety and medical programs. Second, the ergonomics program must be sustained, as it is an iterative process that incorporates the philosophy of continuous improvement, transfer of technologies from one department to another, and documentation of ergonomic success and failures.

Elements of Ergonomics Programs: A Primer Based on Workplace Evaluations of Musculoskeletal Disorders spells out seven basic training elements for developing an in-house ergonomics program.[1]

(1) Determine whether training is needed: If the evidence gathered from checking health records and results of the job analysis indicates a need to control ergonomic risk factors, then employees must be provided with the training necessary for them to gain the knowledge to implement control measures.
(2) Identify training needs: Different categories of employees require different kinds of ergonomics instruction.
(3) Identify goals and objectives: Define the objectives of training in clear, directly observable, action-oriented terms.
(4) Develop learning activities: Whatever the mode of training—live lectures, demonstrations, interactive video programs, or varied instructional aids—learning activities should be developed that will help employees demonstrate that they have acquired the desired knowledge or skill.
(5) Conduct training: Training should take into account the language and educational level of the employees involved. Trainees should be encouraged to ask questions that address their particular job concerns, and hands-on learning opportunities should be encouraged.
(6) Evaluate training effectiveness: A common tool for training evaluations is to ask questions about whether workers found the instruction interesting and useful to their jobs and whether they would recommend it to others. More important, however, are measures of the knowledge gained or improvements in skills, as may be specified in the course objectives. Knowledge

quizzes, performance tests, and behavioral observations are also evaluation tools. One exercise recommended here is that the class propose improvements in workplace conditions, based on information learned in class, and that they present these to management for their review. This relates to another level of evaluation, which is whether the training produces some overall change at the workplace. The latter measure is complicated by the time required before results are apparent, and the training may have been only one of several factors responsible for such results.

(7) Improving the program: If the evaluations indicate that the objectives of the training were not achieved, a review of the training plan elements would be in order, and revisions should be made to correct shortcomings.

Although these steps can help employers develop ergonomics training activities without having to hire outside help, much depends on the existing capabilities of the staff. If in-house expertise in ergonomics is limited, start-up activities could necessitate the use of consultants or outside special training for those employees who would ultimately assume responsibility for ergonomic activities within the workplace.

For more information on ergonomics and its applications refer to Appendix C which lists (1) journals that commonly contain articles related to ergonomics, (2) electronic sources of information, and (3) a glossary of terms. In addition, several recent publications on ergonomics and human factors have expanded the scope and depth of this discipline. One recent publication is the first edition of the *International Encyclopedia of Ergonomics and Human Factors*.[74] This three-volume ergonomics and human factors resource is divided into 12 parts: general ergonomics; human characteristics; performance related factors; information presentation and communication; display and control design; workplace and equipment design; environment; system characteristics; work design and organization; health and safety; social and economic impact of the system; and methods and techniques. The information contained in this collection may serve the safety and health professional well, especially the practicing occupational hygienist.

Acknowledgments

Thanks are extended to Robert Radwin, PhD, of the University of Wisconsin for his contribution to the section on hand tools; to Anil Mital, PhD, of the University of Cincinnati for his contribution to the section on Risk Factor Assessment Techniques; to Alex Cohen, PhD, consultant, and to Karl H.E. Kroemer, PhD, from Virginia Tech, Don Chaffin, PhD, from the University of Michigan, and Jim Annis and John McConville of Anthropology Research Project, Yellow Springs, Ohio, for their consent to use selected tables and figures. Thanks also to Sue Rogers, PhD, and Dave Ridyard for their contributions to the section on checklists. Also, thanks go to Fan Xu, my doctoral student at Purdue University, for her research assistance.

References

1. **National Institute for Occupational Safety and Health (NIOSH):** *Elements of Ergonomics Programs. A Primer Based on Workplace Evaluations of Musculoskeletal Disorders* (Publication no. 97-117). Cincinnati, Ohio: NIOSH, 1997.
2. **American Industrial Hygiene Association (AIHA®) Ergonomics Committee:** *Position Statement on Ergonomics.* Fairfax, VA: AIHA®, 2010.
3. **National Safety Council (NSC):** *Fundamentals of Industrial Hygiene*, 5th ed. Chapter 13, Recognition of Hazards: Ergonomics. Plog, B.A., J. Niland, and P.J. Quinlan (eds.). Chicago, IL: NSC, 2001. p. 357.
4. **National Institute for Occupational Safety and Health (NIOSH):** *Musculoskeletal Disorders and Workplace Factors: A Critical Review of Epidemiologic Evidence for Work-Related Musculoskeletal Disorders of the Neck, Upper Extremity, and Low Back*, edited by B. Bernard (Publication no. 97-141) Cincinnati, Ohio: NIOSH, 1997.
5. **National Academy of Sciences (NAS):** *Work-Related Musculoskeletal Disorders: Report, Workshop Summary, and Workshop Papers.* Washington, D.C.: NAS, 1999.
6. **Tichauer, E.:** *The Biomechanical Basis of Ergonomics.* New York: John Wiley & Sons, 1978.
7. **Bhattaharya, A., and James D. McGlothlin (eds.):** *Occupational Ergonomics: Theory and Applications.* New York: Marcel Dekker, Inc., 1996.

8. **Armstrong, T.J., P. Buckle, L.J. Fine, et al.:** A conceptual model for work-related neck and upper-limb musculoskeletal disorders. *Scand. J. Work Environ. Health 19*:73–84 (1993).
9. **Bureau of Labor Statistics:** *Occupational Injuries and Illnesses By Selected Characteristics for State and Local Government.* Washington, DC: U.S. Department of Labor, Bureau of Labor Statistics, (http://www.bls.gov/news.release/osh2.toc.htm 2010.
10. **Bureau of Labor Statistics:** *Characteristics of Injuries and Illnesses Resulting in Absences from Work.* Washington, DC: U.S. Department of Labor, Bureau of Labor Statistics, http://www.bls.gov/iif/osh_nwrl.htm#cases 2010.
11. **Tanaka, S., et al.:** Prevalence and work-relatedness of self-reported carpal tunnel syndrome among U.S. workers: Analysis of the occupational health supplement data to the 1988 National Health Interview Survey. *Am. J. Ind. Med. 27*:451–70 (1995).
12. **Morlock R. Mandel S:** Cost of Care for Workers' Compensation Patients with Low Back Pain Treated at a Multi-Specialty Group Practice. *Acad. Health Serv. Res. Health Policy, 18*:28. 2001
13. **Guo, H., S. Tanaka, L. Cameron, et al.:** Back pain among workers in the United States: National estimates and workers at high risks. *Am. J. Ind. Med. 28*:591–602 (1995).
14. **Frymoyer, J.W., and W.L. Cats-Baril:** An overview of the incidence and costs of low back pain. *Ortho. Clin. N. Am. 22*:262–271 (1991).
15. **Liira, J.P., H.S. Shannon, L.W. Chambers, and T.A. Haines:** Long-term back problems and physical work exposures in the 1990 Ontario health survey. *Am. J. Pub. Health 86*:382–387 (1996).
16. **National Institute for Occupational Safety and Health (NIOSH):** *National Occupational Research Agenda* Cincinnati, Ohio: NIOSH, http://www.cdc.gov/niosh/nora/ 2009.
17. **Tichauer, E.R., and H. Gage:** Ergonomic principles basic to hand tool design. *Am. Ind. Hyg. Assoc. J. 38*:622–634 (1977).
18. **Armstrong, T.J.:** *An Ergonomic Guide to Carpal Tunnel Syndrome.* Akron, Ohio: American Industrial Hygiene Association, 1983.
19. **Putz-Anderson, V. (ed.):** *Cumulative Trauma Disorders: A Manual for Musculoskeletal Diseases of the Upper Limbs.* London: Taylor & Francis, 1988.
20. **McGlothlin, J.D.:** "An Ergonomic Program to Control Work-Related Cumulative Trauma Disorders of the Upper Extremities." PhD dissertation. University of Michigan, Ann Arbor, Mich., 1988.
21. **Mital, A., and A. Kilbom:** Design, selection, and use of hand tools to alleviate cumulative trauma of the upper extremities: Parts I and II—Guidelines for the practitioner. *Int. J. Ind. Ergonom. 10(1–2)*:1–6 (1992).
22. **Westgaard, R.H., C. Jensen, and K. Hansen:** Individual and work-related risk factors associated with symptoms of musculoskeletal complaints. *Int. Arch. Occup. Environ. Health 64*:405–413 (1993).
23. **Kuorinka, I., and F. Forcier (eds.):** *Work Related Musculoskeletal Disorders (WMSDs): A Reference Book for Prevention.* London: Taylor & Francis, 1995.
24. **Kilbom, A.:** Repetitive work of the upper extremity: Part II — The scientific basis (knowledge base) for the guide. *Int. J. Ind. Ergo. 14(1–2)*:59–86 (1994).
25. **Chiang, H, Y. Ko, S. Chen, et al.:** Prevalence of shoulder and upper-limb disorders among workers in the fish-processing industry. *Scand. J. Work Environ. Health 19*:126–131 (1993).
26. **Silverstein, B.A.:** "The Prevalence of Upper Extremity Cumulative Trauma Disorders in Industry." PhD dissertation, University of Michigan, Ann Arbor, Mich., 1985.
27. **Moore, J.S., and A. Garg:** Determination of the operational characteristics of ergonomic exposure assessments for prediction of disorders of the upper extremities and back. In *Proceedings of the 11th Congress of the International Ergonomics Association,* pp. 144–146. London: Taylor & Francis, 1991.
28. **Osorio, A.M., R.G. Ames, J. Jones, et al.:** Carpal tunnel syndrome among grocery store workers. *Am. J. Ind. Med. 25*:229–45 (1994).
29. **Armstrong, T.J., et al.:** A conceptual model for work- related neck and upper-limb musculoskeletal disorders. *Scand. J. Work Environ. Health 19*:73–84 (1993).
30. **Swansen, A., I. Matev, and G. Groot:** The strength of the hand. *Bull. Prosthet. Res. 10–14*:145–153 (1970).
31. **Armstrong, T.J., J. Foulke, J. Bradley, and S. Goldstein:** Investigation of cumulative trauma disorders in a poultry processing plant. *Am. Ind. Hyg. Assoc. J. 43*:103–16 (1982).
32. **Mital, A.:** "Recognition of Musculoskeletal Injury Hazards for the Upper Extremity and Lower Back" (Final report, contract no. CDC-94071VID). Cincinnati, Ohio: National Institute for Occupational Safety and Health, 1996.
33. **Marras, W., and R.W. Schoenmarklin:** Wrist motions in industry. *Ergonomics 36*:341–51 (1993).
34. **Tichauer, E.R.:** *Occupational Biomechanics. An Introduction to the Anatomy of Function of Man at Work.* New York: Institute of Rehabilitation Medicine, New York University Medical Center, 1975.

35. **Chaffin, D.B., and G.B.J. Andersson:** *Occupational Biomechanics*, 2nd ed. New York: Wiley Interscience, 1991.
36. **Westgaard, R.H., M. Watersted, and T. Jansen:** Muscle load and illness associated with constrained body postures. In *The Ergonomics of Working Postures*. Corlett, N. and J. Wilson (eds.). London: Taylor & Francis, Ltd., 1986. Pp. 5–18.
37. **Sommerich, C.M., J.D. McGlothlin, and W.S. Marras:** Occupational risk factors associated with soft tissue disorders of the shoulder: A review of recent investigations in the literature. *Ergonomics 36*:697–717 (1993).
38. **Armstrong, T., and D. Chaffin:** Carpal tunnel syndrome and selected personal attributes. *J. Occup. Med. 21*:481–86 (1979).
39. **Tichauer, E.R.:** Biomechanics sustains occupational safety and health. *Ind. Eng. 8*:46–56 (1976).
40. **Boiano, J., A. Watanabe, and D. Habes:** *Armco Composites* (DHHS/NIOSH pub. no. HETA 81-143-1041). Cincinnati, Ohio: National Institute for Occupational Safety and Health, 1982.
41. **Schiefer, R.E., R. Kok, M.I. Lewis, and G.B. Meese:** Finger skin temperature and manual dexterity 0—some inter-group differences. *Appl. Ergon. 15*:135–41 (1984).
42. **Fox, W.F.:** Human performance in the cold. *Hum. Factors 9*:203–20 (1967).
43. **Pelmear, P.L., D. Leong, I. Taraschuk, and L. Wong:** Hand-arm vibration syndrome in foundrymen and hard rock miners. *J. Low Freq. Noise Vib. 5*:163–67 (1986).
44. **Olsen, N., S.L. Nielsen, and P. Voss:** Cold response of digital arteries in chain saw operators. *Br. J. Ind. Med. 38*:82–88 (1981).
45. **Williamson, D.K., F.A. Chrenko, and E.J. Hamley:** A study of exposure to cold in cold stores. *Appl. Ergon. 15*:25–30 (1984).
46. **Taylor, W., and P.L. Pelmear (eds.):** *Vibration White Finger in Industry*. New York: Academic Press, 1975.
47. **Brammer, A.J., W. Taylor, and J.E. Piercy:** Assessing the severity of the neurological component of the hand-arm vibration syndrome. *Scand. J. Work Environ. Health 12*:428–431 (1986).
48. **National Institute for Occupational Safety and Health (NIOSH):** *Criteria for a Recommended Standard: Occupational Exposure to Hand-Arm Vibration* (DHHS/NIOSH Publication no. 89-106). Cincinnati, Ohio: NIOSH, 1989.
49. **Riley, M.W., D.J. Cochran, and C.A. Schanbacher:** Force capability differences due to gloves. *Ergonomics 28*:441–447 (1985).
50. **Hertzberg, H.T.E.:** Some contributions of applied physical anthropology to human engineering. *Ann. NY Acad. Sci. 63*:616–629 (1995).
51. **Lyman, J.:** The effects of equipment design on manual performance in protection and functioning of the hands in cold climates. In *Production and Functioning of the Hands in Cold Climates*. Fisher, R.R. (ed.). Washington, D.C.: National Academy of Sciences, National Research Council, 1957. pp. 86–101.
52. **Sperling, L., R. Kadefors, and A. Kilbom:** Tools and hand function: The cube model—a method for analysis of the handling of tools. In *Designing for Everyone*. Queinnec, Y. and F. Daniellou (eds.). London: Taylor & Francis, 1991. pp. 176–178.
53. **Plummer, R., et al.:** Manual dexterity evaluation of gloves used in handling hazardous materials. In *Proceedings of the Human Factors Society, 29th Annual Meeting*, Santa Monica, Calif.: Human Factors Society, 1985. pp. 819–823.
54. **National Institute for Occupational Safety and Health (NIOSH):** *Investigation of Occupational Wrist Injuries in Women. Terminal Progress Report*. Cincinnati, OH: NIOSH, 1991.
55. **Waters, T.R., V. Putz-Anderson, A. Garg, and L.J. Fine:** Revised lifting equation for the design and evaluation of lifting tasks. *Ergonomics 36*:749–76 (1993).
56. **National Institute for Occupational Safety and Health (NIOSH):** *Workplace Use of Back Belts; Review and Recommendations* (Publications no. 94-127). Cincinnati, OH: NIOSH, 1994.
57. **Barnes, R.M.:** Motion and time study. Design and Measurement of Work, 7th ed. Chapter 6. Work Methods Design-Developing a Better Method. New York: John Wiley & Sons, 1980. pp. 50-60.
58. **Karger, D., and W. Hancock:** *Advanced Work Measurement*. New York: Industrial Press, 1982.
59. **Niebel, B.W.:** *Motion and Time Study*, 8th edition. Homewood, IL: Irwin, 1988.
60. **Konz, S.:** *Work Design: Industrial Ergonomics*, 3rd edition. Worthington, OH: Publishing Horizons, 1990.
61. **Marras, W.S., et al.:** *Dynamic Measures of Low Back Performance, An Ergonomics Guide*. Akron, Ohio: American Industrial Hygiene Association, 1993.
62. **Chaffin, D.B. and G.B.J. Andersson:** *Occupational Biomechanics*. New York: John Wiley & Sons, 1984.
63. **National Institute for Occupational Safety and Health (NIOSH):** Applications Manual for the *Revised NIOSH Lifting Equation*. Cincinnati, Ohio: Robert A. Taft Laboratories, Department of Health and Human Services/NIOSH DHHS (NIOSH) Pub. No. 94-110, 1994.

64. **Astrand, P.O. and K. Rodhal:** *Textbook of Work Physiology*, 3rd edition. New York: McGraw-Hill, 1986.
65. **Mital, A., et al.:** Status in human strength research and application. *Trans. Inst. Ind. Eng. 25(6)*:57–69 (1993).
66. **Gordon, C.C., et al.:** *Anthropometric Survey of U.S. Army Personnel* (TR-89-027). Natick, MA: U.S. Army Natick Research, Development, and Engineering Center, 1989.
67. **McGlothlin, J.D.:** *Ergonomic Inventions for the Soft Drink Beverage Delivery Industry* (Cincinnati, Ohio: National Institute for Occupational Safety and Health, DHHS (NIOSH) Pub No 96-109, 1996.
68. **Corlett, E.N., and R.P. Bishop:** A technique for assessing postural discomfort. *Ergonomics 19*:175–182 (1976).
69. **Borg, G.A.V.:** Psychophysical bases of perceived exertion. *Med. Sci. Sports Exerc. 14*:377–381 (1982).
70. **National Institute for Occupational Safety and Health (NIOSH):** *Proceedings of a NIOSH Workshop: A Strategy for Industrial Power Hand Tool Ergonomic Research-Design, Selection, Installation, and Use in Automotive Manufacturing* (DHHS/NIOSH Publication no. 95-114). Cincinnati, OH: NIOSH, 1995.
71. **Pheasant, S. and D. O'Neil:** Performance in gripping and turning-A study in hand/handle effectiveness. *Appl. Ergo. 6(4)*:205–208 (1975).
72. **McGlothlin, J.D., and S. Baron:** *Harley-Davidson Incorporated, Milwaukee, Wisconsin* (DHHS/NIOSH Publication no. HETA 91-0208-2422). Cincinnati, OH: NIOSH, 1994.
73. **McGlothlin, J.D., R.A. Rinsky, and L.J. Fine:** *Harley-Davidson Incorporated, Milwaukee, Wisconsin* (DHHS/NIOSH Publication no. HETA 90-134-2064). Cincinnati, OH: NIOSH, 1990.
74. **Karwowski, W. (ed.):** *International Encyclopedia of Ergonomics and Human Factors*. London: Taylor & Francis, 2001.

Chapter 31

Outcome Competencies

After completing this chapter, the reader should be able to:

1. Define the underlined terms used in this chapter.
2. Describe the anatomy and physiology of the spine.
3. Describe basic biomechanical criteria and the lever systems in the human body.
4. Utilize physiological measurements and criteria to evaluate the potential for localized muscle fatigue and whole body fatigue.
5. Identify and describe the various risk factors associated with the development of work-related lower back pain.
6. Use multiple ergonomic job analysis biomechanical models to evaluate material handling tasks and to determine the potential for the development of work-related illnesses and injuries.
7. Apply techniques used to evaluate lifting and other manual material handling tasks.
8. Understand the basic issues related to whole body vibration exposures.

Key Terms

asymmetric angle • case-control studies • cohort studies • compressive force • couplings • creep • cross-sectional studies • duration of continous lifting • duration of lifting • energy expenditure • frequency • horizontal distance • load weight • localized muscle fatigue • low back disorders • lumbar motion monitor • maximum aerobic power • maximum heart rate • odds ratio • relative risk • shear force • travel distance • vertical location

Prerequisite Knowledge

Basic anatomy and physiology

Chapter Number	Chapter Topic
30	Ergonomics
32	Upper Extremities

Key Topics

I. Introduction

II. Spine Anatomy

III. Biomechanical Criteria
   A. Compression Force Tolerance Limits
   B. Relationship Between Back Pain and Compressive Force
   C. Creep
   D. Shear Force

IV. Physiological Criteria
   A. Energy Expenditure
   B. Heart Rate
   C. Localized Muscle Fatigue

V. Epidemiological Criteria

VI. Risk Factors for LBD

VII. Ergonomic Job Analysis
   A. Biomechanical Models
   B. Revised NIOSH Lifting Equation
   C. Lifting Guidelines
   D. Pushing/Pulling

VIII. Workstation Design Recommendations
   A. Benefits of Ergonomic Job Design

IX. Whole Body Vibration
   A. Measurement and Limits
   B. Control and Prevention

X. References

Musculoskeletal Disorders, Job Evaluation, and Design Principles

31

By Arun Garg, PhD, Naira Campbell-Kyureghyan, PhD, Jay Kapellusch, PhD and Sai Vikas Yalla, PhD

Introduction

Most of the low back disorders (LBD) found in the workplace are related to manual material handling (MMH) and in particular to lifting of loads.[1,2] Work-related back injuries due to repetitive lifting are especially troublesome due to the relative severity of the injuries. Although this type of injury makes up only 14% of all injuries, they are responsible for 28% of disabling injuries, 63% of lost work time, and 58% of expenses.[3] The mean cost per case for back injuries is close to $7,000,[4] and the median lost time for repetitive motion injuries is 17 days.[5] One point worth mentioning is that prevalence has shown[6] an increasing trend in the last two decades for which there is no simple explanation due to the multifactorial nature of LBDs.

There is distinction between low back pain (LBP), impairment, and disability. LBP is chronic or acute pain in the lumbosacral, buttock, or upper leg region. Sciatic pain originates in the low back and radiates down one or both legs. Impairment is the loss of ability to perform physical activities, while disability is either time off work or placement on restricted activities.

Spine Anatomy

The human spine is a complex multijoint anatomical structure. The spine provides a framework for support of the internal organs and is the load-bearing structure for the torso and upper body. As such, the spine must have high strength and also be flexible enough to allow for a large range of motion. To provide these functions, the spine is a segmental structure. There are 24 pre-sacral vertebrae in the human spine: 7 cervical, 12 thoracic, and 5 lumbar (Figure 31.1). The vertebrae are separated by the intervertebral discs and connected by ligaments. Together, these components provide the required strength and flexibility to allow the spine to perform its functions.

The vertebrae are named according to their location in the spinal column from top to bottom (e.g., L_3 for the 3rd lumbar vertebrae). The outer shell of the vertebrae is made up of cortical bone, which is denser, stronger, and stiffer than the interior cancellous bone.

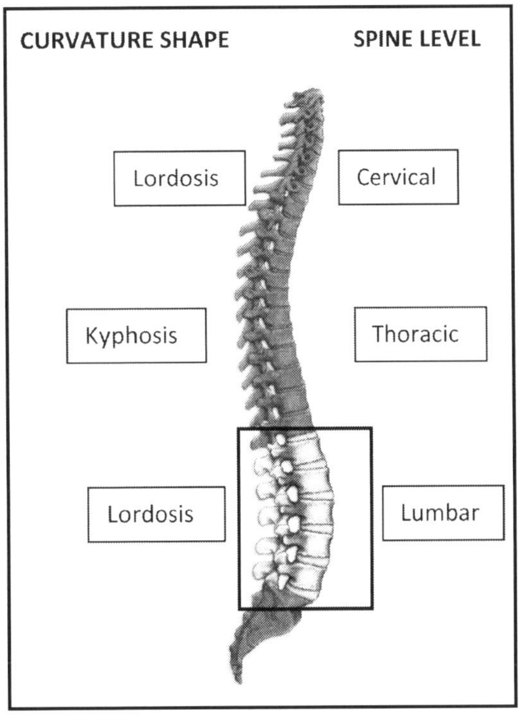

Figure 31.1 — Vertebrae and curvatures of the human spine (Adapted from The Human Spine: Vertebrae and Curvatures.[7]

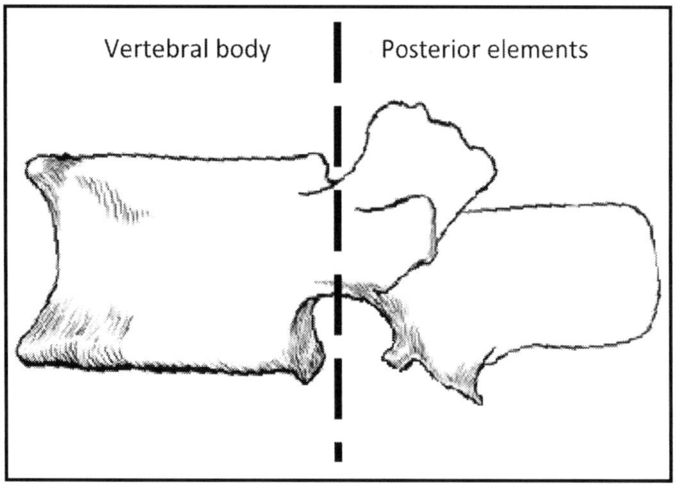

Figure 31.2 — Schematic representation of the human vertebrae.[8]

The geometry of a vertebra consists of a body and posterior elements (Figure 31.2). The body is the main load-bearing component. The posterior elements provide (1) an anchor for muscle attachment, (2) additional support for load bearing when the spine is in flexion or extension, and (3) partially bear shear forces on intervertebral discs. Since bone is a relatively stiff material, the vertebrae are able to carry large loads in both compression and shear with little deformation. Damage to the vertebrae is typically in the form of fractures caused by an acute injury, such as an accident or excessive compressive stress.

Two adjacent pre-sacral vertebrae are separated by an intervertebral disc, and the combination is called a motion segment. Intervertebral discs consist of a gel-like nucleus and a collagenous annulus fibrosis (Figure 31.3). Compressive forces (forces acting parallel to the spine) are resisted mainly by the nucleus, which acts as a nearly incompressible material and bulges laterally to compensate for compressive deformation. The annulus fibrosis provides support to the nucleus and prevents excessive bulging under load. In addition, the alternate orientation of the annulus fibrosis layers provides the shear resistance for the disc. Under external force application the disc initially deforms, and when the force is removed, the disc returns to its original shape. However, if the load is maintained (static) or repetitive, the disc exhibit viscous deformation, also known as "creep", which is characterized by a reduction of the disc height to egress of fluid. This shrinkage of the disc is typical and usually occurs as a result of the forces applied to the spine throughout daily activities. After sufficient rest, the disc recovers to its original shape.

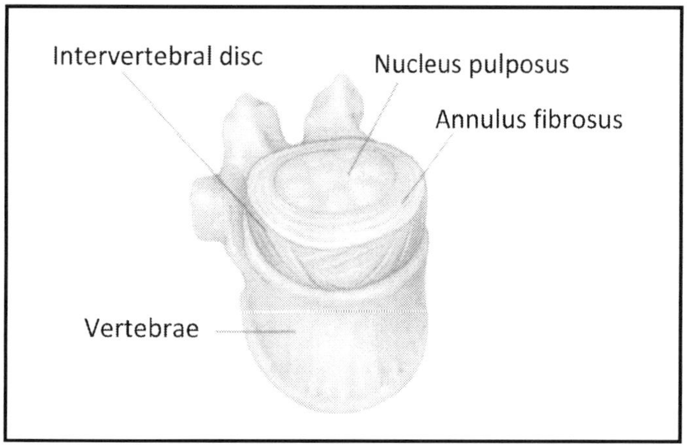

Figure 31.3 — Cross-sectional view of the intervertebral disc along with the vertebrae.[9]

Each vertebra is joined to its superior or inferior counterpart by ligaments and muscles that provide stability to the joints. Muscles are contractile tissue that produces force and motion and provide stability. Additionally, the endplate, a thin layer of cartilage, separates the disc from the vertebrae. The overall shape of the spine, viewed laterally, is lordosis, a curvature facing the posterior direction, for the lumbar and cervical spine, and kyphosis, curvature facing the anterior direction, for the thoracic spine (Figure 31.1).

Biomechanical Criteria

From a mechanical standpoint the human body can be considered as a system of levers. Body weight and external forces are resisted by muscle (and ligament) forces and compression in the skeletal system. Muscle forces can be determined by considering the moment that external forces and body weight exert on the joints. Muscle moment arms about the joints are much smaller than the moment arms for the external forces. Hence, significant muscle forces and, subsequently, compression in the skeleton are developed for even small external loads.

Consider the system shown in Figure 31.4. A 20-kg load is held at a horizontal distance of 50 cm from the L_5/S_1 intervertebral disc. Assume an upper body weight (BW) of 30 kg above the L_5/S_1 disc, centered a horizontal distance of 30 cm from the L_5/S_1 disc, and a moment arm for the muscle force of 5 cm.

Static equilibrium requires that the sum of the moments about the L_5/S_1 joint be zero, and the horizontal and vertical forces also sum to zero. From these equilibrium equations the muscle force (F_m) can be calculated. The moment for each force is the force multiplied by the distance to the center of moment, in this case, the L_5/S_1 disc in a direction perpendicular to the force. For weights this is always equal to the horizontal distance, as gravity acts vertically downward. The muscle force, however, is assumed to be parallel to the spine, and the moment arm must be the distance from the muscle perpendicular to the spine axis. The equilibrium equations for the example problem are

$$\sum M = (20kg)(9.8m/s^2)(50cm) - F_m(5cm) + (30kg)(9.8m/s^2)(30cm) = 0 \quad (31\text{-}1)$$

$$\sum F_{vertical} = (20kg)(9.8m/s^2) + (30kg)(9.8m/s^2) + F_m \sin(\theta) - C\sin(\theta) + V\cos(\theta) = 0 \quad (31\text{-}2)$$

$$\sum F_{horizontal} = F_m \cos(\theta) - V\sin(\theta) - C\cos(\theta) = 0 \quad (31\text{-}3)$$

where C is the compressive force in the spine at L_5/S_1, V is the shear force at L_5/S_1, and θ is the angle of the spine axis with horizontal (Figure 31.5). If the spine is vertical (θ = 90°), the resulting forces are

F_m = 3724 N
C = 4214 N (430 kg)
V = 0

If the spine is bent over so that the orientation is at 45° from the horizontal, the resulting forces are

F_m = 3724 N (assuming no change in moment arms)
C = 4071 N (415 kg)
V = 347 N (35 kg)

Several observations regarding spinal forces can be made.

1. Lifting even small loads can generate substantial compression and shear forces in the low back joints.
2. The simple example shown includes only an equivalent single muscle force. In reality, multiple muscles (and ligaments) are often involved, making a direct calculation of the spinal forces extremely complex.

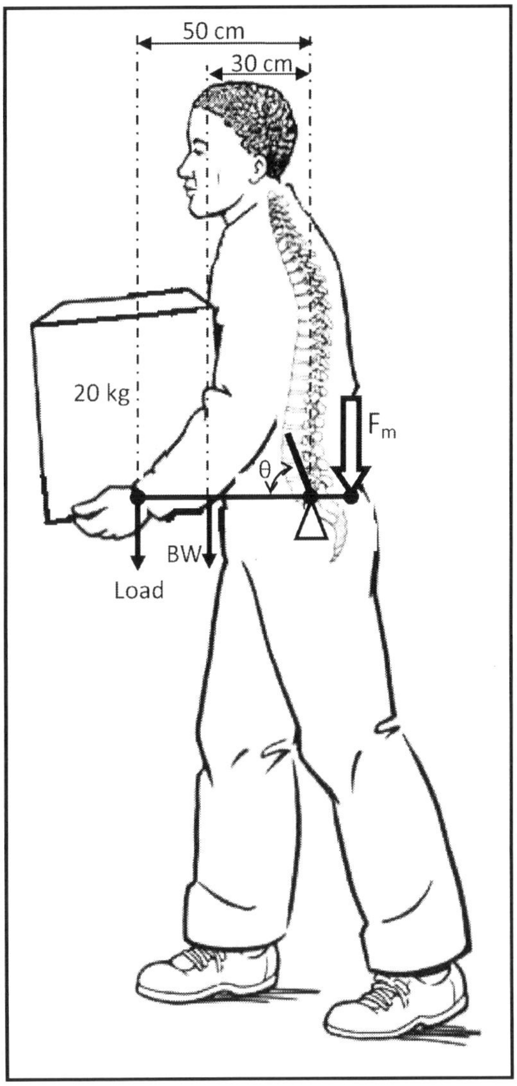

Figure 31.4 — Lever system at L5/S1 in the spine during lifting.[10]

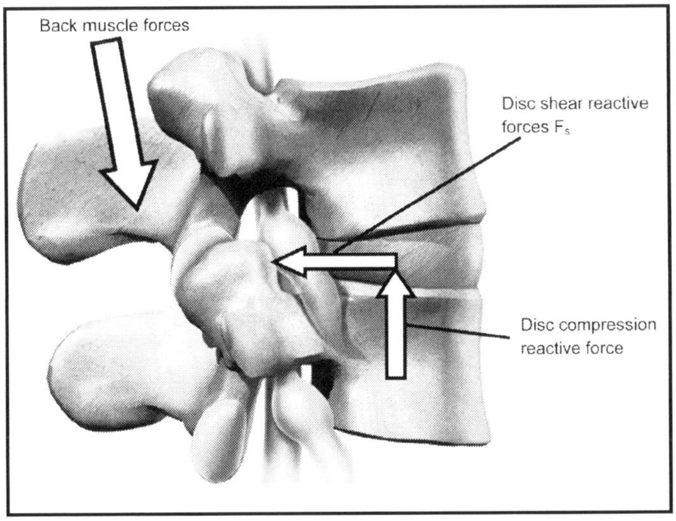

Figure 31.5 — The resultant forces developed in the spine due to compressive forces acting on the spine.[11]

3. Antagonistic muscle forces (forces that act against the main muscle force) are sometimes generated, particularly when the torso is flexed or torsionally rotated. These antagonistic forces further increase the compression and shear on the spine.
4. Often the resultant forces during dynamic movement are higher than static forces.

The forces generated in the spine can be compared with tissue tolerance (capacity) to determine if a task is safe for the worker.

Compression Force Tolerance Limits

The tolerance of the lumbar spine to withstand compressive forces had been determined through extensive cadaveric testing. Compressive strength is defined as the maximum axial load that can be sustained during the test without a permanent loss in disc height, and the results vary widely due to biological variability and differences in the test procedure. Measured compressive failure strength from cadaver testing ranged from approximately 2 kN to 11 kN[12,13] (Figure 31.6). The mean lumbar spine compressive strength was found to be 4.9 ± 2.2 kN.[12] The large variance in measured compressive failure strength makes it difficult to determine a definitive failure criterion.

In 1981, the National Institute for Occupational Safety and Health (NIOSH) established a biomechanical criterion of 3.4 kN for compression on the low back.[15] Later, a 1991 committee revised the NIOSH equation but decided to keep 3.4 kN as the recommended compression limit (RCL), which most young, healthy workers can tolerate.[12,16]

Repetitive Loading of Spine

Injuries to the spine can occur through acute trauma or as the result of the accumulation of damage over time. "It is when this loading accumulates by repeated exposures, or exposures of sufficiently long duration, that the internal tolerances of tissues are eventually exceeded."[6]

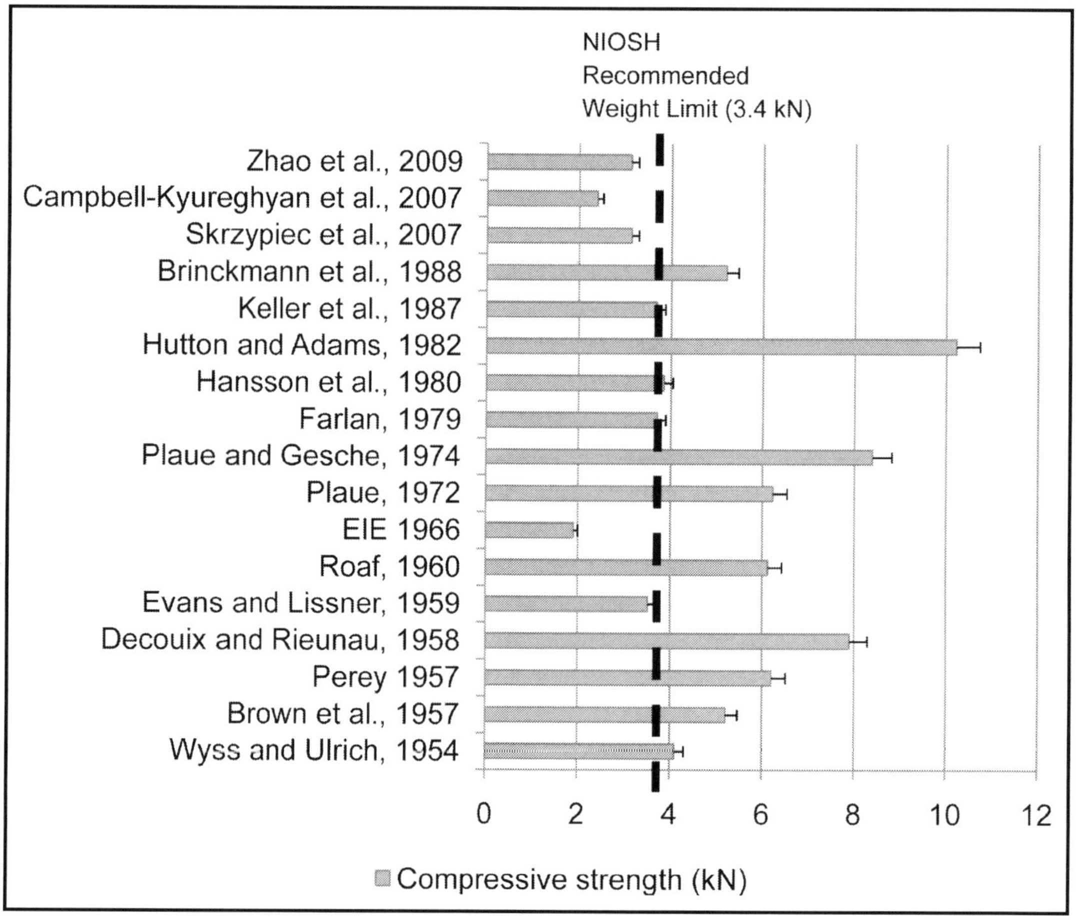

Figure 31.6 — Lumbar compressive failure strength values from cadaveric studies (1954–2009).[12–14]

In addition to failure due to a single large load, motion segments can fail due to repeated loading at lower force levels, called a fatigue failure.[17–19] As the load is applied and removed repeatedly, the motion segment height decreases as a result of viscoelastic deformation and creep. Brinckmann et al.[18] showed that fatigue failure probability varies based on the load magnitude and the number of cycles. Most studies have attempted to determine a fatigue failure limit based on number of cycles to failure. However, this approach has several drawbacks, the most serious being that (1) it does not account for the variability in the applied load in real-world applications, and (2) frequency of force applications representing manual materials handling is often observed in industry.[20–22] Recent research[23,24] suggests that energy dissipation may be a fatigue failure measure that eliminates some of the problems associated with the number of cycles.

Relationship Between Back Pain and Compressive Force

Chaffin and Park[25] reported an association between the incidence of LBP and compressive force. In addition, compression forces greater than 6.5 kN resulted in an incidence rate of LBP that was nine times higher than the LBP incidence rate when the compressive force was less than 2.5 kN. In a study of 6912 workers in industrial jobs, Herrin et al.[26] found that peak compressive force on the spine is a good predictor of not only back pain but also of overall overexertion injuries. Herrin and colleagues showed that the incidence rate of LBP was highest when the compressive force was greater than 1500 lbs (680 kg) and the lowest when the compressive force was less than 1000 lbs (453 kg). Anderson et al.[27] reported a 40% increase in LBP incidence rates if the compressive force was greater than 3.4 kN.

In a study of 109 cases of overexertion injuries, 10 back injuries were reported including eight muscle strains and two disc injuries.[28] The average compressive force for the muscle strain injuries was 5.34 kN, while compressive force associated with disc injuries averaged 7.97 kN.

Creep

When subjected to compressive loads, the pressure generated in the intervertebral disc forces out fluid resulting in a change in volume and, hence, height of the disc. This process is termed creep. During a normal day, the body will shrink in stature by approximately 1.1% due to body weight and other loads. Heavier loads will cause additional loss in stature, but recovery will occur in approximately 10 minutes after the load is removed.[29,30] The overall diurnal shrinkage recovers overnight.

Creep also occurs as a result of repetitive loading and has been used as a measure of the damage resulting from the load.[31,32] Although creep is subject to saturation (a limit on its value no matter how much load is applied or how long the load is maintained) and is not a particularly good damage predictor, creep itself has significant impacts on the behavior of a motion segment.[33] The narrowing of the space between the vertebrae changes the areas of contact between the facets joints.

Shear Force

In addition to compression, the spine is also subject to shear forces. The annulus fibrosis in the disc and the posterior elements of the vertebrae are the primary mechanisms by which the shear force is resisted. The shear capacity of the spine is not well defined. An ultimate shear force of 2000 to 3000 N was reported by several researchers.[34–37] McGill et al.[38] and Norman et al.[39] determined anterior shear force limits from porcine tissue and industrial injury reporting data, termed University of Waterloo Action Limits (UW AL), for shear forces generated in the lumbar spine. More than 500 N of shear force was considered to be risky and 1000 N to be hazardous for men, while more than 330 N was considered risky and 660 N was set to be hazardous for women.

The shear forces in the spine, particularly in the posterior elements when the disc is compressed, can be quite high.[40] It has been proposed that the facet joints, with their concentration of nerves and rich blood supply, can be a significant source of pain.

Physiological Criteria

There is no universal definition of muscle fatigue.[41] There are, however, two types of fatigue: (1) a general feeling of exhaustion or tiredness known as whole body fatigue or central fatigue, and (2) a more location-specific muscle fatigue limited to specific muscle groups (for example, back, neck and shoulder) known as localized muscle fatigue (LMF).

The two most commonly used physiological measurements in manual material handling include energy expenditure and heart rate to quantify whole body physical fatigue.

Energy Expenditure

The ability to perform physical work mostly depends on the ability to transform chemical energy from food into mechanical energy. Primarily, the energy stored in the form of glucose is metabolized to provide the muscles with contractile tension and body heat. Oxygen must be supplied to the working muscles at sufficient rates to allow complete metabolism. In addition, the muscle's enzymes and ability to utilize oxygen must be sufficient. If these requirements are not met, muscles lose their ability to produce tension. This is sensed by the neural system, which then results in sensations of discomfort and loss of strength (physical fatigue). In addition, if the supply of oxygen is not sufficient it can lead to accumulation of lactic acid in the working muscles, leading to symptoms of fatigue. The mechanics of energy expenditure are shown in Figure 31.7. If there is sufficient supply to the working muscles it is called aerobic metabolism and CO_2 is the end product. If O_2 supply is not sufficient, lactic acid is produced as a byproduct, and it is called anaerobic metabolism.

Energy expenditure increases linearly with an increase in work intensity (Figure 31.8). However, this relationship holds true for a given type of work under given environmental conditions and for a given individual. A change in the nature of work will affect this relationship. Similarly, different individuals will exhibit different relationships based primarily on their body weight and physical fitness. Less physically fit individuals and/or heavier individuals will expend greater energy for performing the same work.

Maximum Oxygen Uptake

Maximum aerobic power is defined as the highest attainable rate of aerobic metabolism during performance of rhythmic dynamic muscular exertions. Maximum aerobic power is often expressed either in liters/min or Kcal/min (for all practical purposes, 1 L/min = 5 Kcal/min). Maximum aerobic power or maximum aerobic capacity of U.S. males and females is estimated to be 15 Kcal/min and 10.5 Kcal/min, respectively.[43–47] These values were measured on a treadmill or bicycle ergometer. Petrofsky and Lind[48] showed that each type of task has its own maximum aerobic capacity level, and it was significantly lower for lifting (free style method) than that measured using a bicycle ergometer. Maximum aerobic capacity for lifting of loads ranged from 54% to 80% of that for bicycle ergometer. Therefore, it may be more appropriate to use maximum oxygen uptake (VO_2 max) than aerobic power or aerobic capacity, as it is task independent.

Lifting as Percentage of Aerobic Capacity

Several studies performed in the 1960s and 1970s recommended 33% of maximum

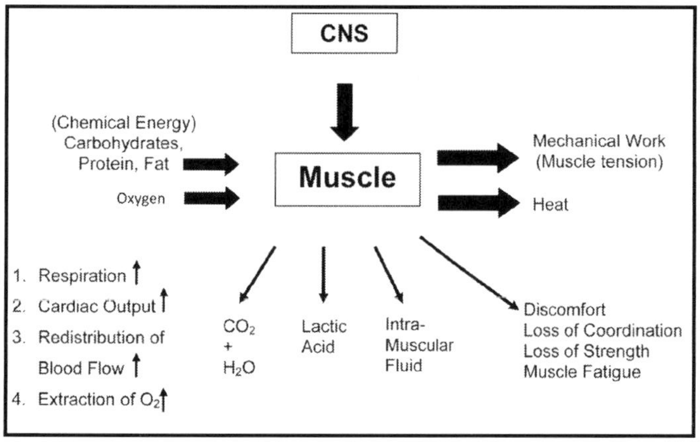

Figure 31.7 — Schematic diagram of mechanics of energy expenditure.[42]

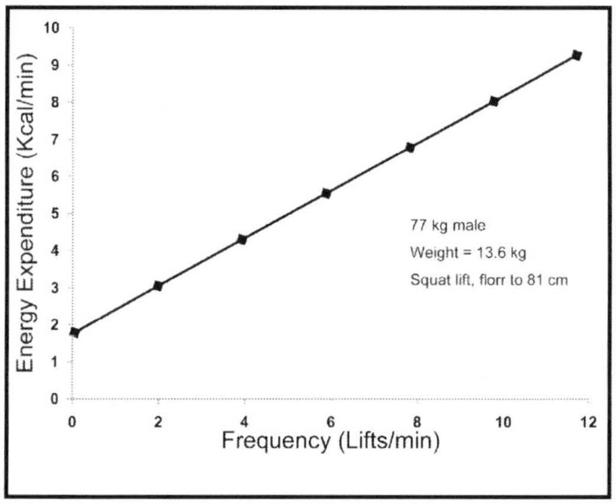

Figure 31.8 — Relationship between work intensity and energy expenditure.[42]

aerobic capacity (measured on treadmill or bicycle ergometer) of a normal healthy person as the maximum energy expenditure rate for an 8-hour workday.[45,48–52] Still others recommended 5 Kcal/min as the maximum energy expenditure rate for an 8-hour workday.[49, 53–56] Others have recommended a lower limit.[57–61]

From the literature review,[62,63] it is apparent that there are three major factors for determining acceptable levels of energy expenditure: (1) design limits (DL) vs. maximum permissible limits (MPL), (2) lifting location (below or above 30 inch or 76 cm height, and (3) duration of continuous lifting. At the design limit, most of the men and at least half the women should find the task acceptable; at the maximum permissible limit, about 25% of the men and even fewer women will find the task acceptable.[63] The recommended energy expenditures for the design and maximum acceptable limits, as recommended by Garg[62], are summarized in Table 31.1.

Determining Energy Expenditure Requirements of a Job

There are three different options available to determine the energy expenditure requirements of a job. These include (1) direct measurement of energy expenditure by measuring the amount of oxygen consumed and carbon dioxide produced, (2) estimating energy expenditure from heart rate, and (3) using models to estimate energy expenditure. Direct measurement of energy expenditure in the field requires sophisticated and portable equipment and training. The relationship between energy expenditure and heart rate depends on the nature of job, temperature and humidity, mental stress, gender and physical fitness. Thus, estimating energy expenditure from a worker's heart rate may include significant errors. Regarding models, the most comprehensive model for estimating energy expenditure requirements of manual material handling jobs is the model developed by Garg et al.[64] The authors reported a correlation coefficient of 0.95 and a standard error of 0.61 between the predicted and the measured values.

Heart Rate

Heart rate is a measure of circulatory load. The following factors affect working heart rate:

Table 31.1 — Design and maximum permissible limits for energy expenditure for frequent lifting[63]

Lift Location Height in Inches (cm)	*Duration of Lifting* 1 Hour DL	1 Hour MPL	1–2 Hours DL	1–2 Hours MPL	2–8 Hours DL	2–8 Hours MPL
V ≤ 30" (75 cm)	4.72	6.75	3.78	5.40	3.12	4.45
V > 30" (75 cm)	3.30	5.40	2.65	4.05	2.18	3.12

Source: A. Garg, *Applied Ergonomics* (Milwaukee, WI: University of Wisconsin–Milwaukee, Department of Industrial & Manufacturing Engineering, in cooperation with University of Utah Department of Family and Preventive Medicine, 2006).[42]

1. Work intensity
2. Mental stresses
3. Environmental stresses (temperature and humidity)
4. Nature of work (static versus dynamic)
5. Physical fitness

It is worth mentioning that while mental stress has a pronounced effect on heart rate, it has little effect on energy expenditure. Similarly, environmental stresses have a much greater effect on heart rate than on energy expenditure, which is also true for physical fitness at submaximal loads. For example, physically fit workers would have a lower heart rate than physically unfit workers while working at the intensity of physical exertion. In general, females and older workers performing the same work at the same intensity will exhibit a higher heart rate than their young male counterparts.

Heart rate response to exercise is shown in Figure 31.9. With exercise or physical work heart rate increases from a resting value and will reach a steady-state

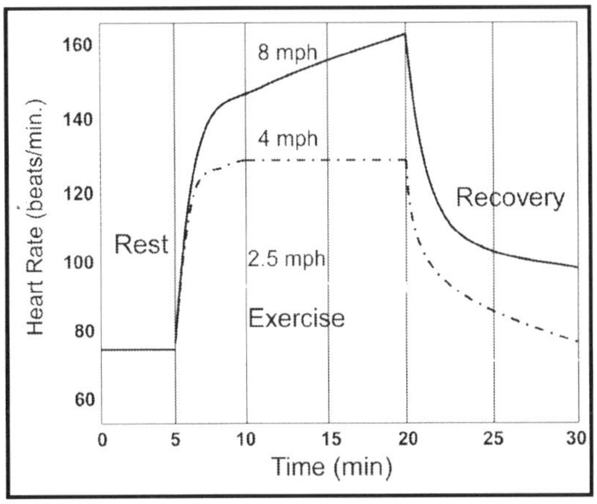

Figure 31.9 — Heart rate response to physical work.[42]

value as shown in the figure. However, if one keeps increasing the level of exercise the heart rate may keep rising with time and may not reach a steady-state depending on the individual, environmental conditions, nature of work, and intensity of work (Figure 31.9). An increase in heart rate with time (upward slope) is considered an indication of excessive physical fatigue, indicating full recovery does not occur between work cycles.[65]

Maximum Heart Rate

Maximum attainable heart rate depends on age and type of work. For highly dynamic work such as running, swimming, bicycling, etc., maximum heart rate can be calculated from the following equation:

$$\text{Maximum Heart Rate} = 206\text{–}0.62 \times \text{Age} \qquad (31\text{-}4)$$

This equation implies that for each year increase in age, maximum heart deceases by 0.6 beat/min. Petrofsky and Lind[48] showed that maximum attainable heart rate also depends on the nature of work. For example, the average maximum heart rate for bicycling was 187 beats/min, and maximum heart rates for lifting 2-, 15-, 50-, and 80-lb weights were 144, 160, 164, and 182 beats/min, respectively.

Recommended Heart Rate

Earlier studies recommended an average heart rate of 110 beats/min for an 8-hour workday. This was based on 33% of VO_2 max measured on a treadmill or bicycle ergometer. However, several studies have suggested that 110 beats/min may be too high and the expectation might result in undue fatigue.[48,58,66,67] In light of these studies, it appears that more reasonable heart rates that can be maintained for an 8-hour workday are 100–105 beats/min for leg work and 90–95 beats/min for arm work.

Rodgers[68] and Rodahl and Issekutz[44] and recommend a percentage of heart rate reserve (%HR Reserve) to determine circulatory strain. For work involving large muscle groups (whole body work), Rodgers suggested a maximum value of 33% of percentage of heart rate reserve. Otherwise, the work is likely to cause physical fatigue. Percentage of heart rate reserve can be computed from the following equation:

$$\%HR \text{ Reserve} = \frac{(\text{Avg. HR on the job} - \text{Resting HR})}{(\text{Predicted max. HR} - \text{Resting HR})} \qquad (31\text{-}5)$$

Localized Muscle Fatigue

Localized muscle fatigue is generally defined as the inability of a muscle to maintain a required or desired force even with an increased effort due to previous muscle exertions.[69–71]

An understanding of localized muscle fatigue is important because LMF shows the physiological manifestation of strain in the affected muscle-tendon units caused by the task's or job's biological stressors. Some of the current job analysis methods, such as the Strain Index, use localized muscle fatigue physiology as the end point of interest.[72] At present, the injury pathways from localized muscle fatigue to musculoskeletal disorders are not fully understood. Further, time period for development of work-related musculoskeletal disorders is not clear, ranging from hours to months.[73] However, these authors suggested that under certain exertion conditions, persistent fatigue and discomfort may result in a disease state. Some believe that hypoxia, anaerobic metabolism, and accumulation of metabolites from localized muscle fatigue may cause muscle disorders.[74–79] Moore and Garg[80] suggest that localized muscle fatigue may lead to persistent localized pain; persistent pain may lead to tendonitis/tenosynovitis, and further complications may lead to more severe diseases, such as carpal tunnel syndrome. Several other researchers have suggested that under certain conditions, static muscular work as well as repetitive work with low applied force may cause muscle injury.[73,78,81,82] In addition, there are many biomechanical theories for work-related musculoskeletal disorders based on the cumulative trauma load-tolerance model for tendons. Detailed discussions can be found in Moore and Garg [80], Moore[83], Gordon et al. [American Academy of Orthopaedic Surgeons][84], Amiel et al.[85], Woo and Xerogeanes,[86] Krausher and Nirschl[87], and the National Research Council and the Institute of Medicine.[6]

During static work as well as repetitive exertions, intramuscular tissue pressure (hydrostatic pressure) increases in proportion to muscle force (%MVC). This results in reduced blood flow through the muscle (Figure 31.10), blood flow is completely blocked at 60% MVC, and normal blood supply is maintained if the applied force <10% MVC. Reduced blood flow results in hypoxia and changes from aerobic to anaerobic metabolism. This leads to accumulation of metabolites (lactic acid), lowering of ph value (acid metabolism), and an increase in calcium and potassium ions concentration in the extra-cellular fluid. Accumulation of metabolites and increase in Ca+ concentration are believed to cause muscle fatigue. Incidentally, Sjögaard et al.[88] reported that the muscle was fatigued after 1 hour of isometric knee-extension at 5% MVC even though the normal blood supply to the exercising muscle was maintained.

Symptoms of localized muscle fatigue include discomfort (including soreness, aching, tingling, pain, and stiffness); increased perceived exertion; decreased strength; increased muscle tremor; increase in eye-hand coordination time; and/or loss of neuromuscular control.[72,89,90] An increase in systolic, diastolic, and mean arterial pressures, as well as an increase heart rate, has also been reported with localized muscle fatigue. It has been suggested that fatigue may be a "safety factor" to protect muscles from damage due to overexertion.[69]

Job physical variables that are relevant to localized muscle fatigue include concentric or static work, weight of the object or applied force, duration of force, duration of recovery time, frequency of exertions, speed of work, and posture (Figure 31.11). Examples of static work include holding objects in hands; pushing and pulling heavy loads; working in trunk bent-over posture forward, sideways, or twisted; working with arms raised; working with arms held out horizontally in front or sideways; working with neck bent over or bent back; sitting without back support; prolonged standing in one place; putting weight on one leg while the other foot operates a foot pedal; and/or working in constrained postures.

The following are recommendations for reducing localized muscle fatigue:

1. Minimize static muscular effort.
2. Reduce %MVC (weight, force).
3. Provide adequate rest periods for sustained exertions and frequent exertions.

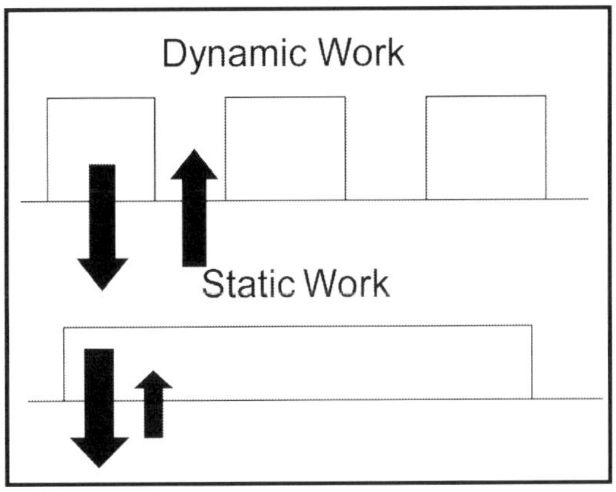

Figure 31.10 — Blood supply to muscles during dynamic and static work.[42]

4. Provide frequent, short rest breaks as these are more effective than few, long rest breaks.
5. Use jigs, fixtures, clamps, etc., to support objects.
6. Raise, tilt, and/or rotate work surface height to reduce trunk and neck flexion.
7. Minimize forward and backward reaches. If possible keep forward reach <15 inches.
8. Keep shoulder flexion <25° and shoulder abduction <15°–20°.
9. Avoid carrying material especially when weight >15 lb and time >1 minute.
10. Avoid operating foot pedals with one foot.

Two of the most commonly used methods to study localized muscle fatigue are (1) electromyography (EMG), and (2) subjective measures of fatigue using fatigue scales and the Borg RPE and CR-10 scales.[91] EMG analysis requires monitoring changes in the frequency spectrum characteristics and RMS amplitude.[70,89,92–94]

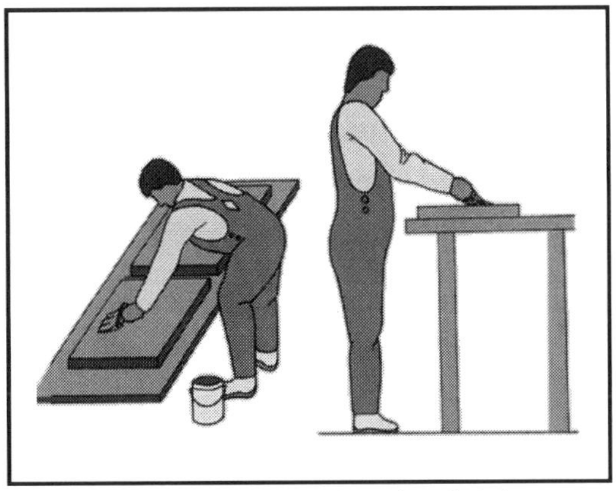

Figure 31.11 — Raising work surface height to minimize postural stresses.[42]

The frequency spectrum of the EMG is generally analyzed by determining changes in median (50% of the frequencies below it and 50% above it) or mean power frequency (average of all frequencies within the spectrum). Some researchers have used the ratio of high to low frequencies and zero crossings. When muscles are fatigued, median and mean power frequencies shift toward the lower end of the spectrum (i.e., they are lower) because the amplitude of the high frequency components of the EMG power spectrum starts to decrease and the low frequency components increase.[41,70,71,93–100] The slope of the graph shift is usually linear[100], more intense exertions have a steeper slope than less intensive exertions.

Epidemiological Criteria

Epidemiology is the study of identifying risk factors affecting the health of population(s) of interest. Traditionally, epidemiologic criteria are used in ergonomics to support or validate biomechanical, physiological, and/or psychophysical criteria. This is the case with low back disorders (LBD), where it is difficult to assign a direct cause for low back pain in most cases.[6,101,102] Epidemiology examines the conditions under which a disorder exists and does not exist and identifies risk factors based on statistical relationships.

Three types of studies are generally used in epidemiologic research. Cross-sectional studies look for correlation between potential risk factors and outcomes. Case-control studies start with two groups: one group that has the disorder of interest (cases) and the other group that is free of that disorder (controls). The investigators then dig backward in time to determine which potential risk factors the subjects have been exposed to. Cohort studies can be either retrospective (looking backward) or prospective (forward looking, following the cohort over a period of time). Prospective cohort studies also begin with two groups: one group that has been exposed to specific risk factor(s) (exposed group), and the other group that does not have exposure to that risk factor (or those risk factors). Cohort studies then follow subjects over a period of time and determine which subjects develop the disorder during the follow-up period. Prospective cohort studies investigate the association between proposed risk factors and disorders of interest.

Strength of association is used to measure the magnitude of the association between the risk factor and disorder. Strength of association provides more confidence that the relationship is causal. Temporal association measures whether or not the risk factor preceded the disorder and is, therefore, causal rather than a result of the disorder. Consistency of association refers to finding the same association across studies or between subgroups within the same study. High consistency of association also provides greater confidence that the association is causal.

If an association is found between a risk factor and the disorder, two additional issues should be considered. The first is the dose-response relationship. Dose-response provides a measure of the association between the level of the exposure and the development and/or severity of the disorder. Of particular interest is whether a reduction in exposure (lower dose) reduces the rate of development of the disorder. Biological plausibility is the other issue to be considered. Regardless of the statistical relationship between a factor and the disorder, there must be some plausible explanation as to why the factor might cause the disorder. For example, hair color cannot be plausibly explained as a risk factor for LBD and, therefore, should be rejected even if a statistical analysis shows a correlation.

Two methods are often used to explain the strength of the relationship between a risk factor and disorder. These are odds ratio (OR) and relative risk (RR). The odds ratio is the ratio of the odds of an event occurring in one group to the odds of it occurring in another group. It is a measure of association commonly used in case-control studies. *Relative risk* is a ratio of the probability of the event occurring in the exposed group vs. a nonexposed group. It is a measure of association used in cohort studies and clinical trials. An odds ratio or relative risk greater than one indicates that exposure increases the risk of developing the disorder, and higher numbers indicate a greater risk. Similarly, odds ratios or relative risk less than one suggest that the risk factor actually provides a protective effect. Neither term should be confused with the actual risk of developing a disorder.

Epidemiologic risk factors identified for low back disorders include force, posture, repetition, and duration. Force, an instantaneous measure, and posture directly affect the biomechanical forces on the spine. Repetition and duration do not have an effect on the total force experienced by the spine, but they do affect spine's tolerance to force. Since the effect of load is often cumulative rather than acute, how often and for how long a load is imposed on the spine will affect the risk of LBD.

Risk Factors for LBD

There are many single contributors, otherwise known risk factors, that are associated with the development of work-related low back pain. Generally, risk factors are divided into job physical, psychosocial, and personal risk factors. Personal risk factors may include age, gender, body mass index, anthropometry, and physical fitness, etc. (Table 31.2).

Heavy physical work, lifting, pushing/pulling, bending, twisting, and reaching while lifting are believed to be some of the job physical risk factors for LBP (Table 31.3). There is a complex interaction between these factors, and therefore, many job analysis methods quantify the combined effect of some of these factors rather than using a single quantifier for each individual factor. In addition, hobbies and leisure activities at home may cause or contribute to low back disorders. Therefore, workers may experience significant impairment in their work activities due to the LBD that was not the direct result of those work activities. The solution may include modifying their work activities so as to reduce or eliminate low back pain, which has an effect on productivity and may induce injuries to other body parts.

It is believed that the risk of LBP increases when the strain, as shown below, is greater than 1. It should be noted that worker capacity is not a fixed number and depends on type of stress and how the body is loaded.

$$\text{STRAIN} = \frac{\text{JOB PHYSICAL DEMANDS}}{\text{WORKER CAPACITY}}$$

Table 31.2 — Potential individual risk factors for LBP.[103,104]

Individual Risk Factors	*Risk Level*
Age	High
Gender	High
Anthropometry	Low (extreme cases)
Strength and physical fitness	High (job specific)
Spine mobility and range of motion	Low
Medical history	High
Smoking	Low
Years of employment	Low
Marital status	Low
Psychosocial factors	Low (treatment, return to work)

Table 31.3 — Job risk factors for LBP reported in the literature.[105]

Job Risk Factors	*Possible LBP Outcome*
Heavy physical work	Higher incidence of LBP Higher risk of compensable back injury Severity of LBP significantly greater Back symptoms interfere with work much more Greater need to report LBP
Sudden or unexpected maximal effort	Higher incidence of low back injury
Haste, speed and inattention	18% of all high cost LB injuries Greater than $10,000/case
Bending, stretching and reaching	Higher incidence of LBP Higher risk of compensable back injury Increase in severity of LBP
Lifting, lowering, holding and carrying	Higher incidence of LBP
Pushing and pulling	9%–18% of LB strains and sprains
Static posture	Higher incidence of LBP
Prolonged exposure to whole body vibration	Higher incidence of LBP Long term back problems Prolonged sickness due to back disorders
Cold Temperature	Makes muscles less efficient Extra clothing may impede efforts Higher energy expenditure
Confined Work Space	Higher possibility for LBP

Ergonomic Job Analysis

Biomechanical Models

The primary purpose of biomechanical models is to quantify forces and moments on body joints. Biomechanical models are often used to estimate compressive and shear forces on lumbar spine. Some biomechanical models can determine static strength requirements of jobs in occupational settings. Chaffin[106] has provided an excellent discussion on historical perspective and how occupational biomechanics principles and models have evolved over the last 40 years.

Biomechanical models range from simple 2- and 3-dimensional, static biomechanical models[25,107–109] to quasi-static and dynamic 3-dimensional, anatomically complex and/or EMG driven models to predict individual lumbar tissue loads.[110–121] Simple biomechanical models often do not account for antagonistic muscle activity.[122,123] Co-contraction provides joint stiffening, stability, and controlled movement. However, co-contraction often substantially increases mechanical load, such as compressive and shear forces on the lumbar spine.

Complex biomechanical models have been used primarily to simulate industrial manual material handling tasks in a controlled laboratory environment. At present, it is still very challenging to apply these complex biomechanical models in industrial settings as they require data such as EMG measurements, postural data in three dimensions as a function of time in an industrial setting, and other individual variables.

The most commonly used biomechanical model in occupational settings is the 3-D Static Strength Prediction Model from the University of Michigan developed by Chaffin and Baker.[107] The model is used to estimate compressive force on the lumbar spine and to determine the static strength requirements of a job. This software-based biomechanical model requires (1) gender specification, (2) subject's height and weight, (3) body posture data provided as body joint angles for various body joints, (4) magnitude of hand force, and (5) direction of hand force. The model provides options for simulating different percentile male and female populations, such as the 50th percentile male population. The output from the model includes an estimate of compressive and shear forces on the lumbar spine and the percentage of the population capable of performing the task based on the static strength requirements of the simulated job for different joint locations and affected muscle groups. In addition, the model provides many other calculations, such as body joint locations, resultant forces, and moments at various body joints and forces in trunk flexor and extensor muscles, etc.

Two different epidemiologic studies have shown the effectiveness of these biomechanical models in industry by demonstrating a relationship between job physical stresses estimated from these models and incidence of back and other musculoskeletal injuries in the workplace. Chaffin and Park[25] showed that the low back pain incidence rate increased by more than 900% when compressive force on the spine increased from under 113 kg to greater than 635 kg. Herrin et al.[26] found that the incidence and severity rates of back injuries increased with an increase in compressive force on the low back from less than 450 kg to more than 680 kg. The same study also reported that describing extreme job requirements such as the most stressful task seemed more predictive of back and other musculoskeletal injuries than using those indices that represent aggregations (averaging or pooling of stressful and non-stressful aspects of a job). However, others have suggested that cumulative spine load in the workplace may be more predictive of work-related low back pain.[39,124]

Some of the limitations of the 3-D Static Strength Prediction Model include that it does not account for stresses associated with repetitive work, i.e., it does not differentiate whether the task is performed once or several hundred times per day. And, while the model accounts for stresses on body joints due to varying anthropometry, the volitional strength of body joints for a given gender does not adjust with a change in anthropometry in the model.

Example of 2-D Static Biomechanical Analysis

As a simple example, consider a worker who is lifting a 40-lb (18.14-kg) box using a semi-squat posture. Body postures are measured for this worker according to the diagram in Figure 31.12(a) (Table 31.4). Posture measurements as well as the weight held in each hand (20 lb per hand = 40 lb total) are then entered into the biomechanical model, and the model software will provide a simulated figure for visual comparison (Figure 31.12(b).

The 3-D SSPP model offers a variety of results in the form of report. Most commonly, analysts will review compressive and shear forces on the L_5/S_1 disc and static strength capabilities by body part. These results, based on the input from Table 31.4, are shown in Figure 31.13.[127] These results show that 91% of the male working population have sufficient strength to perform this lift. The 3-dimensional low back compression on the L_5/S_1 joint for the 50th percentile male is 813 lb (368.7 kg). NIOSH[15,126] recommends a maximum compressive force of 770 lb (349.2 kg or 3.4 kN).

The above example is for a simple 2-dimensional (sagittal plane) lift. Two-dimensional analyses are appropriate when the task being analyzed requires symmetrical posture from the worker. Unfortunately, most tasks in industry are not performed with symmetrical postures. For these asymmetrical posture tasks, a 3-dimensional analysis is preferred.

Example of 3-D Static Biomechanical Analysis

Consider a worker loading parts into a machine center. Rough castings weigh 40 lb (18.14 kg) and, on average, two castings are loaded into the machine center every 10 minutes. Because of general machine size and cutting fluid shields, the worker must lean into the machine to place the rough casting on the platen. Finished parts have a smooth top and can be unloaded using a vacuum hoist. The company would like to

Table 31.4 — Summary of 2-D posture and force measurements entered into 3-D SSPP software[125]

Body Part	*Posture (angle) and Weight Lifted*
Upper arm angle	–80°
Lower arm angle	–50°
Upper leg angle	155°
Lower leg angle	60°
Trunk flexion angle	50°
Left hand lifting weight	20 lbs
Right hand lifting weight	20 lbs

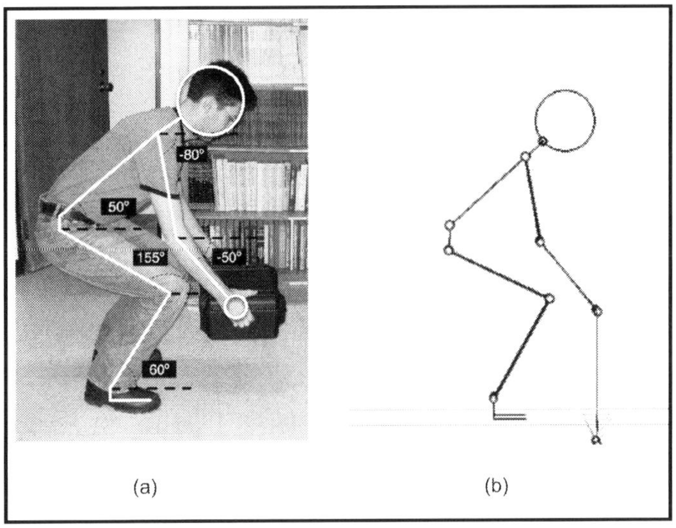

Figure 31.12 (a,b) — body posture angles entered into 3-D SSPP for 2-D analysis (a) Body joint angles from the picture; (b) 2-D software-generated model.[125]

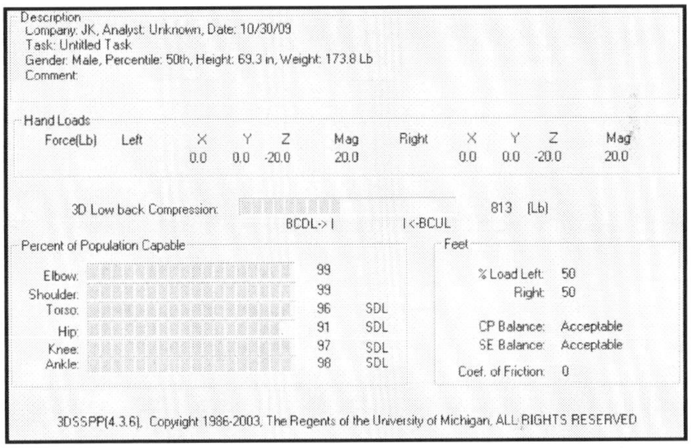

Figure 31.13 — Summary results from 3-D SSPP software for 2-D analysis based on input from Table 31.4.[127]

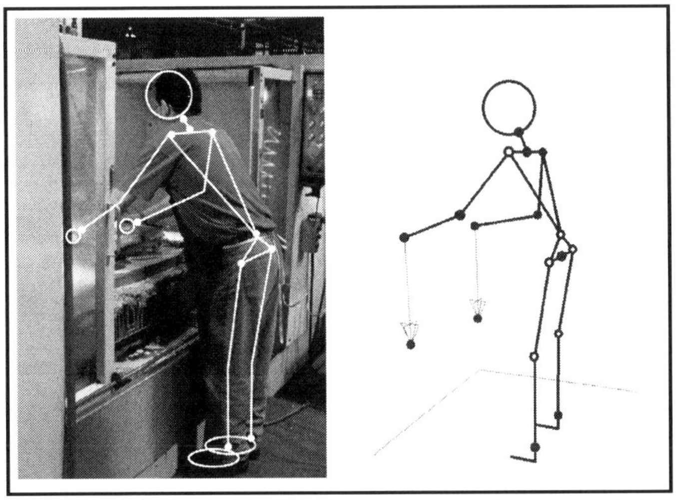

Figure 31.14 — Worker loading casting into machine center (left) and 3-D model generated body posture (right) for example in Table 31.5.[128]

Table 31.5 — Body segment angles used for 3-D analysis example using static strength prediction model.[129]

	Left		Right			
	Horz	*Vert*	*Horz*	*Vert*	*Trunk*	*Angles*
Forearm	100°	–20°	100°	–10°	Flexion	70°
Upper arm	65°	–50°	35°	–70°	Axial rotation	0°
Upper leg		100°		100°	Lateral bending	0°
Lower leg		90°		90°		

determine the biomechanical stresses due to loading these parts.

Figure 31.14 shows a worker loading a casting into the machine. Body segment angles for the 3D model are complex and difficult to measure in the workplace. Common practice is to take photographs of a worker performing the task and then use the 3DSSPP software to mimic the posture seen in the photos. Table 31.5 shows the body segment angles used to generate the comparison figure shown in Figure 31.14.

Results of the biomechanical analysis of the task shown in Figure 31.14 are shown in Figure 31.15. These results are based on the 50th percentile male anthropometric measurements, the body joint angles in Table 31.5, and hand force levels of 20 lb (9.1 kg) lifting with each hand.

These results show that the low back compression for lifting in this posture for a 50th percentile male is 594 lb (269.4 kg), below the limit of 770 lb (349 kg or 3.4 kN) recommended by NIOSH.[15,126] For this task, 84% of the male working population have sufficient shoulder strength to perform the lift. Regarding the strength requirements for the task, it is generally recommended that jobs be designed to accommodate at least 75% of the female working population.

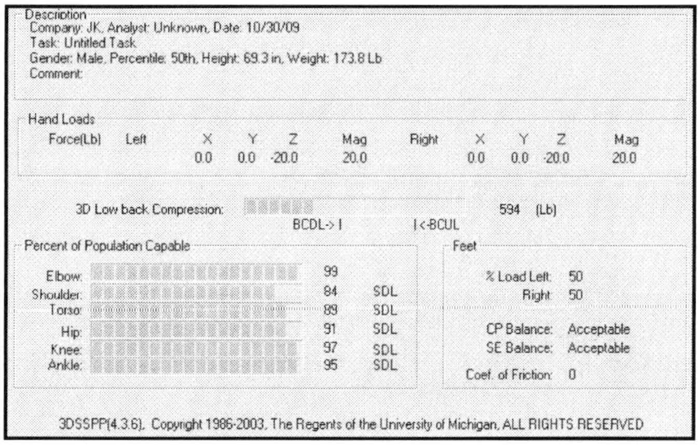

Figure 31.15 — Summary results from 3-D SSPP software based on input from Table 31.5.[130]

Lumbar Motion Monitor

The Lumbar Motion Monitor (LMM) is a triaxial electrogoniometer. The LMM measures the position of the thoracolumbar spine in three-dimensional space with time and calculates its position, velocity, and acceleration. Marras et al.[131] used the LMM to conduct a cross-sectional study of 403 repetitive industrial jobs from 48 manufacturing companies. The jobs were divided into two groups for low back pain based on OSHA 200 logs: (1) high risk, and (2) low risk. Low-risk group jobs had no injuries and no turnover for at least 3 years. High-risk group jobs had at least 12 back injuries per 200,000 hours of exposure. Among different job physical exposure variables tested, maximum load moment was the most powerful single variable that correlated with high-risk jobs (OR = 5.17). Marras et al.[132] developed a multiple logistic regression model for predicting the probability of a job falling in the high-risk group. The LMM driven model output includes maximum load moment, maximum sagittal trunk flexion angle, lifting frequency, average twisting velocity, and maximum lateral velocity. This model was able to distinguish between high- and low-risk jobs (OR =10.7). It should be clarified that the model does not predict the risk of developing low back pain, but it predicts the probability of belonging to the high-risk group for low back pain.

Maximum Acceptable Weights and Forces

Psychophysical measures, such as maximum acceptable weights (MAWs), and forces are often used to analyze manual materials handling tasks to determine what percentages of male and female populations are capable of performing a given task. These weights and forces are determined experimentally in laboratories by simulating the manual materials handling task of interest. During the experiments, all job physical exposure variables are fixed except one. Often the subject has control over either the weight of the object (or force for pushing/ pulling) or frequency of exertion. For example, during a lifting experiment, the size of box, couplings on the box (type of grasp), lifting origin, lifting destination, lifting technique, and frequency of lifting are fixed. The subject has control over the weight in the box. The subject is then given specific instructions such as "work as hard as you can without straining yourself, or without becoming unusually tired, weakened, overheated, or out of breath."[133] The subject is asked to adjust the weight in the box being lifted as often as he/she desires. If the subject finds the weight is too heavy, they should reduce the weight, or increase the weight if the subject feels the work is too light. Experiments are typically conducted for 25 to 45 minutes, but subjects are asked to select a weight they feel they could lift, under the specified conditions, for an entire 8-hour work shift. Push/pull forces are determined using a similar protocol.

Snook and Ciriello[133] have conducted extensive experiments for lifting, lowering, pushing/pulling, and carrying tasks. The results of these experiments are published in tables that provide the percentage of male and female populations capable of performing tasks under given conditions. Several other researchers have also used psychophysical methodology to determine maximum acceptable weights and forces.

Maximum acceptable weights have been used to assess jobs in industry for risk of back injuries. Snook[1] reported that workers were three times more likely to suffer a back injury if they performed a job that was acceptable to less than 75% of the working population. Herrin et al.[26] found that risk of back injury increased when workers performed a job that was acceptable to less than 90% of the working population.

One advantage of psychophysical methodology is that the maximum acceptable weights and forces provide a realistic simulation of industrial work. The results represent an integrated response of the body accounting for strength requirements, fatigue, and discomfort/pain. Disadvantages include that psychophysically determined maximum acceptable weights may exceed recommended compressive force limits, particularly when lifting near the floor or when reaching and lifting. Similarly, MAWs may exceed energy expenditure recommendations, particularly when lifting frequencies exceed six lifts/min.[133] And, maximum acceptable weights based on 25–45 minutes of experiments may overestimate the maximum weights that would be actually acceptable to workers for an 8-hour shift.[135,136]

Maximum Acceptable Weight Example

Workers load large aluminum castings into machine centers. The castings are 8 centimeters thick, 25 centimeters wide, 45 centimeters long and weigh 17 kilograms. The castings are delivered to the workstations in crates where the castings are stored vertically. Workers must lift the castings out of the crate and set them flat on top of the crate. From there the workers use a vacuum hoist to lift the castings and set them in the machine center. Machine time is 20 minutes per part, and there are four machines; thus, workers lift parts at an average of one lift every 5 minutes. Measurements show the following lifting parameters:

- Object weight = 17 kg
- Object width = 25 cm
- Initial hand height = 50 cm
- Final hand height = 102 cm
- Task frequency = One lift every 5 minutes

For this example, use the maximum acceptable weight lifting table for lifting task performed once every 5 minutes and lift ending between knuckle and shoulder height (there are separate tables for males and females) was used. The first step is to locate the column of data associated with lifting, where the end of the lift is occurring between knuckle height and shoulder height (this corresponds to an end of lift height of 102 cm). Next, the row of data associated with a box width of 25 cm (Figure 31.16) must be determined.

The tables provide data only for boxes 34 cm and larger, therefore, a 34-cm box width is assumed. (Note: Box width is defined as the dimension of the box *extending away from the body.*) For convenience, the data from Figure 30.16 are reproduced in Table 30.6a. Next, the maximum acceptable weight in the column for "one lift every 5 minutes" that is closest to the actual object weight of 17 kg is identified. For men, this will be 18 kg (highlighted in Table 31.6a).

Looking to the left across this row, the data shows that 90% of male workers can lift a 34 cm wide box weighing 18 kg a distance of 51 cm, between knuckle height and shoulder height, once every 5 minutes. Similarly, the sample data provided in Table 30.6b[134], shows that 25% of female workers are capable of performing such a task. Thus, since our target is ≥ 75% of workers being capable of performing the task, this task is believed to pose an increased risk for injury to female workers.

Width‡	Distance§	Percent¶	Floor level to knuckle height One lift every								Knuckle height to shoulder height One lift every								Shoulder height to arm reach One lift every							
			5 s	9 s	14 s	1 min	2 min	5 min	30 min	8 h	5 s	9 s	14 s	1 min	2 min	5 min	30 min	8 h	5 s	9 s	14 s	1 min	2 min	5 min	30 min	8 h
75	76	90	*6*	7	9	11	13	14	14	17	8	10	12	13	14	14	16	17	6	8	9	10	10	11	12	13
		75	*9*	11	13	16	19	20	21	24	10	14	16	18	18	19	21	23	8	10	12	14	14	14	16	17
		50	*12*	*15*	17	22	25	27	28	32	13	17	20	22	23	24	26	29	10	13	15	17	17	18	20	22
		25	*15*	*18*	*21*	28	31	34	35	41	16	*21*	*24*	27	27	28	32	35	11	16	18	21	21	22	24	27
		10	*18*	*22*	*25*	33	37	40	41	48	*19*	*24*	*28*	31	32	33	37	40	*14*	18	21	24	24	25	28	31
	51	90	6	8	9	12	13	15	15	17	8	11	13	15	15	16	18	19	6	8	9	12	12	12	14	15
		75	*9*	11	13	17	19	21	22	25	11	15	17	20	20	21	23	25	8	11	12	15	15	16	18	20
		50	*13*	15	18	23	26	28	29	34	14	19	21	25	25	26	29	32	10	14	16	19	20	20	23	25
		25	*16*	*19*	22	29	33	35	36	42	*17*	*23*	26	30	31	32	36	39	13	17	19	23	24	25	27	30
		10	*19*	*22*	*26*	34	38	42	43	50	*20*	*26*	*30*	35	36	37	41	45	*15*	19	22	27	27	29	32	35
	25	90	8	9	11	13	15	16	17	20	10	13	15	18	18	19	21	23	7	10	11	14	14	14	16	18
		75	*11*	13	15	19	22	24	24	28	13	17	20	23	24	25	27	30	10	13	15	18	18	19	21	23
		50	*15*	18	21	26	29	32	33	38	17	22	25	30	30	31	35	38	12	16	19	23	23	24	27	29
		25	*18*	*22*	26	33	37	40	41	48	*20*	27	*30*	36	36	38	42	46	15	20	22	28	28	29	32	35
		10	*22*	*26*	*31*	38	44	47	49	57	*23*	*31*	*35*	42	42	44	49	53	*17*	*23*	26	32	32	34	38	41
49	76	90	7	8	10	13	15	16	17	20	8	10	12	13	14	14	16	17	7	9	10	12	12	13	14	16
		75	*10*	12	14	19	22	24	24	28	10	14	16	18	18	19	21	23	9	11	13	16	16	17	19	21
		50	*14*	*16*	19	26	29	32	33	38	13	17	20	22	23	24	26	29	11	15	17	20	21	21	24	26
		25	*17*	*20*	*24*	33	37	40	41	48	16	21	24	27	27	28	32	35	13	18	20	25	25	26	29	31
		10	*20*	*24*	*28*	38	43	47	48	57	*19*	*24*	*28*	31	32	33	37	40	*15*	*21*	23	28	29	30	33	36
	51	90	7	9	10	14	16	17	18	20	8	11	13	15	15	16	18	19	7	9	11	14	14	14	16	18
		75	10	13	15	20	23	25	25	30	11	15	17	20	20	21	23	25	9	12	14	18	18	19	21	23
		50	*14*	17	20	27	30	33	34	40	14	19	21	25	25	26	29	32	12	15	18	23	23	24	27	29
		25	*18*	*21*	25	34	38	42	43	50	17	23	26	30	31	32	36	39	14	19	21	28	28	29	32	35
		10	*21*	*25*	*29*	40	45	49	50	59	*20*	*26*	*30*	35	36	37	41	45	*16*	*22*	25	32	32	34	37	41
	25	90	8	10	12	16	18	19	20	23	10	13	15	18	18	19	21	23	9	11	12	16	16	17	19	21
		75	12	15	17	23	26	28	29	33	13	17	20	23	24	25	27	30	11	14	16	21	21	22	25	27
		50	*16*	20	23	30	34	37	38	45	17	22	25	30	30	31	35	38	14	18	21	27	27	28	32	35
		25	*21*	*25*	29	38	43	47	48	56	*20*	*27*	30	36	36	38	42	46	16	22	25	33	33	34	38	42
		10	*24*	*29*	*34*	45	51	56	57	67	*23*	*31*	*35*	42	42	44	49	53	*19*	*25*	*29*	38	38	40	44	48
34	76	90	8	10	11	15	17	19	19	23	8	11	13	15	15	16	18	19	8	10	12	14	14	15	16	18
		75	*12*	14	17	22	25	28	28	33	11	15	17	20	20	21	23	25	10	14	16	18	19	19	22	24
		50	*16*	*19*	22	30	34	37	38	44	14	19	21	25	25	26	29	32	13	17	20	23	24	25	27	30
		25	*20*	*24*	*28*	37	42	47	47	55	17	*23*	26	30	31	32	36	39	*16*	*21*	24	28	29	30	33	36
		10	*24*	29	*33*	44	50	54	56	65	*20*	*26*	*30*	35	36	37	41	45	*18*	*24*	*28*	33	33	34	38	42
	51	90	9	10	12	16	18	20	20	24	9	12	14	17	17	18	20	22	8	11	13	16	16	17	18	20
		75	*12*	15	18	23	26	28	29	34	12	16	18	22	23	23	26	29	11	14	17	21	21	22	24	26
		50	*17*	20	24	31	35	38	39	46	15	20	23	28	29	30	33	36	14	18	21	26	27	28	31	34
		25	*21*	*25*	*30*	39	44	48	49	57	18	24	27	34	35	36	40	44	*17*	22	25	32	32	33	37	41
		10	*25*	*30*	*35*	46	52	57	58	68	*21*	*28*	*32*	40	40	42	46	51	*19*	*26*	*29*	37	37	39	43	47
	25	90	10	12	14	18	20	22	23	27	11	14	16	20	20	21	23	26	10	13	15	19	19	19	22	24
		75	*15*	18	21	26	30	32	33	38	14	18	21	26	27	28	31	34	13	17	20	24	25	26	29	31
		50	*20*	24	28	35	40	43	44	52	18	23	27	33	34	35	39	43	16	22	25	31	31	33	36	40
		25	*26*	*30*	*35*	44	50	54	55	65	*21*	*28*	32	40	41	42	47	52	*20*	*26*	*30*	37	38	39	44	46
		10	*29*	*35*	*41*	52	59	64	66	76	*25*	*33*	*37*	47	47	49	55	60	*23*	*30*	*35*	43	44	45	51	55

‡ Box width (the dimension away from the body) (cm).
§ Vertical distance of lift (cm).
¶ Percentage of industrial population.
Italicized values exceed 8 h physiological criteria (see text).

Figure 31.16 — Example table for males from Liberty Mutual Insurance Manual Materials Handling Guidelines.[137]

Table 31.6 a,b — Maximum acceptable weight tables for (a) male workers (kg) (b) female workers (kg).[133]

Width	Distance	Percent Capable	Knuckle Height to Shoulder Height One Lift Every: 5 sec	9 sec	14 sec	1 min	2 min	5 min	30 min	8 hr
		90	9	12	14	17	17	***18***	20	22
		75	12	16	18	22	23	23	26	29
34	51	50	15	20	23	28	29	30	33	36
		25	18	24	27	34	35	36	40	44
		10	21	28	33	40	40	42	46	51

(b)

Width	Distance	Percent Capable	Knuckle Height to Shoulder Height One Lift Every: 5 sec	9 sec	14 sec	1 min	2 min	5 min	30 min	8 hr
		90	8	8	9	10	11	11	12	14
		75	9	10	11	12	13	13	14	17
34	51	50	10	11	13	14	15	15	17	19
		25	12	13	14	16	17	***17***	19	22
		10	13	14	16	18	19	19	21	24

Revised NIOSH Lifting Equation

In 1981, NIOSH developed the *Work Practices Guide for Manual Lifting*. The objective was to provide a simple and quantitative job design and analysis tool for manual lifting and lowering tasks. The NIOSH *Work Practices Guide* became one of the most widely used job analysis tools in industry worldwide. Studies by Liles and Mahajan[138], Huang et al.[139], and Marras et al.[131] demonstrated that the *Guide* was able to differentiate between safe and hazardous jobs .

In 1991, NIOSH revised the lifting equation[16,140] and added twisting of the trunk (asymmetry) and type of hand grasp (coupling). It also expanded the frequency table to allow for different job durations over a working shift. And, the 1991 equation provided a new methodology to study complex lifting jobs, i.e., jobs where one or more job physical variables changed during the job cycle.

The Revised Lifting Equation (RLE) is applicable to two-handed lifting and lowering tasks. It is not applicable if:

- The task requires one-handed lifting;
- There is significant energy expenditure;
- There are unexpected heavy loads or slips and falls;
- Lifting is performed in a seated, kneeling, or restricted work space;
- There is high speed lifting;
- The center of mass changes significantly during lifting;
- The surface is slippery;
- There are added environmental stresses due temperature and/or humidity, or
- The individual is lifting/lowering for over 8 hours.

The Recommended Weight Limit (RWL) represents a load weight that nearly all healthy male workers and at least 75% of female workers could perform without increased risk of an overexertion injury or low back pain. It is based on the four criteria listed in Table 31.7.

RWL is computed from the following equation:

$$RWL = LC \times HM \times VM \times DM \times AM \times FM \times CM$$

where

LC = load constant (51 lb)
HM = horizontal multiplier = (10/H)

Table 31.7 — Criteria used for recommended weight limit in NIOSH-revised lifting equations.[15,41]

Criteria	*Limit*
Compressive force	770lbs (350 kg)
Strength	≥ 75% Females 99% Males
Energy expenditure	
Near floor level	3.12 Kcal/min
Bench height	2.18 Kcal/min
Epidemiologic	Nominal risk

VM = vertical multiplier = (1–0.0075 × I V-30 I)
DM = distance multiplier = (0.82 + 1.8/D)
AM = asymmetric multiplier = (1–0.0032 × A)
FM = frequency multiplier = From Table 31.10
CM = coupling multiplier = From Table 31.11

Each multiplier is computed from the appropriate formula or the value is obtained from a table look-up. Multipliers are penalties and their values can never exceed 1.0. Under ideal lifting conditions, each multiplier is equal to 1.0 and the RWL is 51 lbs. As one deviates from ideal conditions such as when lifting near the floor, reaching and lifting, and/or twisting and lifting, etc., the multipliers will be less than 1.0 and the RWL will be less than 51 lbs.

Lifting Index (LI) is a term that provides an estimate of the level of physical stress associated with a manual lifting/lowering task. It is computed from the following equation:

$$LI = \frac{\text{Load Weight (kg)}}{\text{RWL (kg)}} \qquad (31\text{-}6)$$

A LI ≤ 1.0 implies that the job is safe. If LI > 1.0 the job is believed to be unsafe to some workers, and the higher LI, the more unsafe the job. Thus, LI can be used as a criterion for prioritizing jobs for ergonomic improvements.

Definitions and Measurements

Lifting Task is the act of grasping an object of definable size and weight with two hands and vertically moving the object without mechanical assistance.

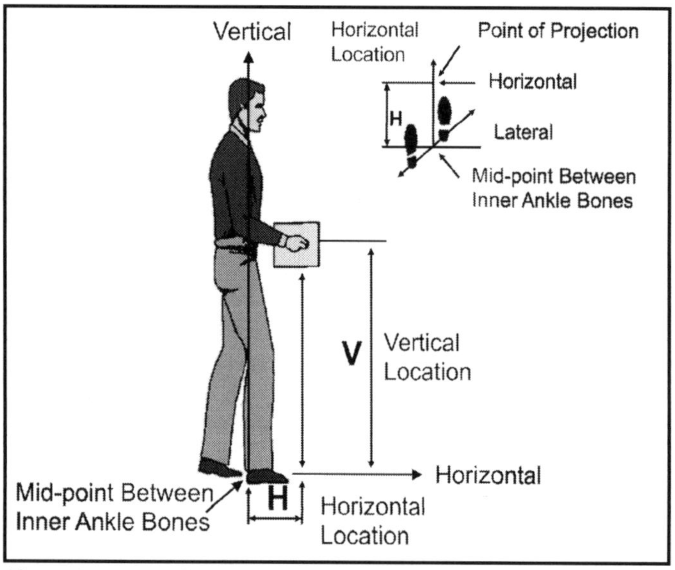

Figure 31.17 — Schematic representation of lifting task and measurements of variables of interest for revised NIOSH lifting equation (modified).[140]

Load Weight (W) is the weight of the object in kg.

Horizontal Distance (H) is the distance in inches of the hands away from the midpoint between the ankles. It can be measured as shown in Figure 30.17. Alternatively, one could measure the horizontal distance of the right hand from the right ankle and left hand from the left ankle and take the average of the two distances. NIOSH has set a minimum value of 10 inches (25 cm) for H and a maximum value of 25 inches (63 cm).

Table 31.8 — NIOSH lifting equation data collection worksheet.[16]

To determine the Recommended Weight Limit (RWL), multiply 51 pounds by each multiplier for a lifting/lowering task's origin and destination.

	ORIGIN		DESTINATION	
	Observed	Multiplier	Observed	Multiplier
HM = Horizontal Distance from the Ankles	in		in	
VM = Vertical Distance from the Floor	in		in	
DM = Vertcal Distance the Load is Moved	in		in	
AM = Assymetry (deg)	°		°	
FM = Frequency (lifts/min)				
CM = Load Coupling: Good, Fair, Poor	G F P		G F P	
Recommended Weight Limit (RWL) = 51 lbs x HM x VM x DM x AM x FM x CM				

To calcualte the Lifting Index divide the load lifted by the Recommended Weight Limit (RWL)

	ORIGIN	DESTINATION
Recommended Weight Limit (RWL)	lbs	lbs
Load (W) Lifted	lbs	lbs
Lifting Index (LI) = W/RWL		

Vertical Location (V) is defined as the vertical height of the hands (midpoint of knuckles) above the floor in inches (cm). Alternatively, V can be measured for the right and left hands separately and the average of the two heights can be used. The value for V is between 0 and 70 inches (175 cm) (Figure 31.17).

Travel Distance (D) is defined as the vertical travel distance of the hands between the origin of the lift and the highest point during the lift. The highest point often is the end point or the destination. D is assumed to be between 10 and 70 inches (25 to 175 cm) (Figure 31.17).

Asymmetric Angle (A) is defined as the angle between the asymmetry line and the mid sagittal line. It accounts for twisting of the trunk, legs, and/or shoulders. The range for A is between 0° and 135°.

Couplings (C) refers to the grasp at hand-object interface. It is subjectively classified as good, fair, or poor. NIOSH provides guidelines for good, fair, and poor classifications.

Frequency (F) is defined as the number of lifts per minute. In those cases where F changes with time, NIOSH recommends that F should be averaged over a 15-minute period. The range for F is between 0.2 (one lift every 5 minutes) and 15 lifts/min (maximum allowable frequency).

Duration of Lifting is defined as the amount of time spent lifting loads during a shift.

Duration of Continuous Lifting is defined as the amount of time spent lifting loads without a significant break.

Depending on duration of continuous lifting, the Revised NIOSH Lifting Equation recommends rest allowances that can range from 0 to 120% of work time. Rest time does not imply that a worker has to be idle during this time. Light work can be performed during rest time.

Origin and Destination Analysis

All measurements for task variables are made at the origin (beginning) of the lifting/lowering task. However, in those situations where it is more difficult to set a load down than to pick it up, the RLE recommends that (1) RWLs be computed both at the origin and destination of lifts/lowers, and (2) the lower of the two values should be used to compute the Lifting Index (LI).

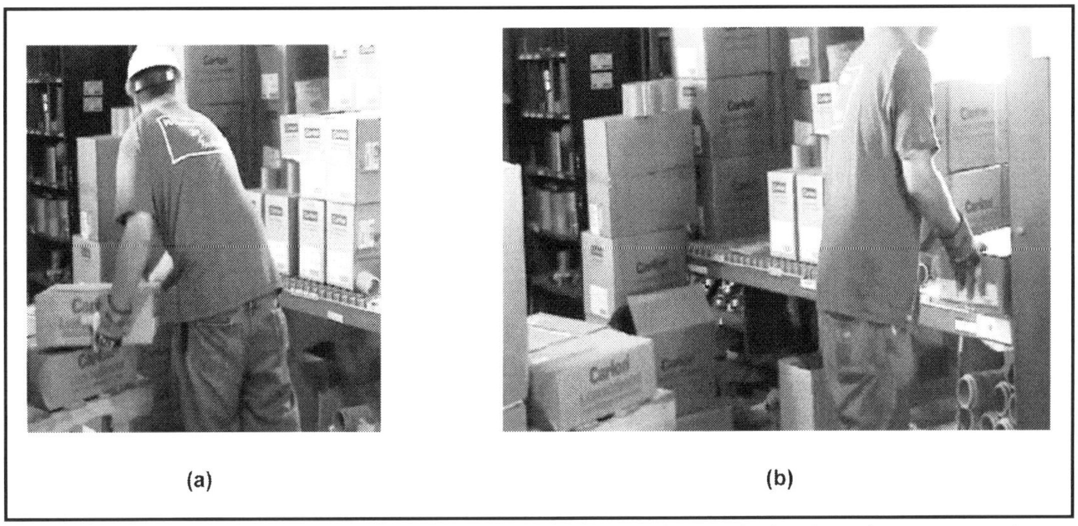

Figure 31.18 — (a) Worker lifting the box off a pallet; (b) worker placing the box into the storage rack.

Multiple Task Analysis

A job may comprise multiple tasks. A multitask is defined when one or more of the six task variables are different in different lifts performed by the worker. For example, weight, horizontal location, and/or vertical location of the hands may be different for lifts performed by the worker. In these situations a complex procedure must be used to analyze these jobs.[140]

A few studies have been performed to determine the validity of the RLE.[132,141,142] These studies support the conclusion that the RLE has the ability to differentiate between safe and hazardous jobs. For example, Marras et al.[132] evaluated the effectiveness of the RLE in its ability to predict risk of low-back injuries. The study involved 353 industrial jobs representing more than 21 million person-hours of exposure. The results indicated that the NIOSH Lifting Equation was predictive of low back injuries (OR = 3.1).

Table 31.9 — Interpretation of lifting index.[16]

Lifting Index	*Task is probably...*
LI < 1	Safe
1< LI < 3	Increased Risk
LI > 3	Not Safe

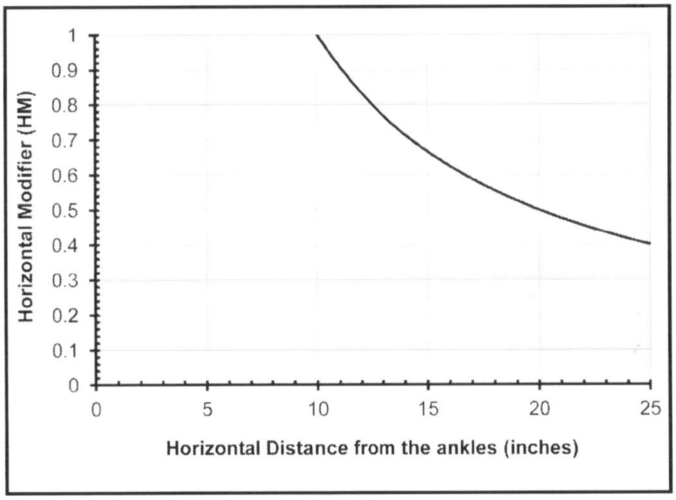

Figure 31.19 — Horizontal multiplier (HM).

Revised NIOSH Lifting Equation Example A

An example data collection sheet for the NIOSH lifting equation is shown in Table 31.8.

The resulting LI falls into one of the ranges as shown in Table 31.9.

The worker lifts a box weighing 10 lb. from a pallet and onto a storage rack (Figure 31.18). The worker's vertical position of the hands is 28 in. from the floor and 12 in. away from the body (horizontal distance). The hands vertical location at the destination is 38 in. and 12 in. away from the body. The worker twists 45° while picking up the box but has little to no twisting while placing the box on the shelf. This task is performed between 3 to 4 hours per day, lifting one box every 10 seconds. The coupling of this box is fair, since the box does not have any handles.

Multiplier Figures and Tables

To determine the HM, find the observed (measured) horizontal distance from the person's ankles to the center of the hands for the origin and destination. *The example's origin and destination, HM = 0.83 (Figure 31.19).*

To determine the VM, find the observed (measured) vertical distance from the person's center of the hands to the floor for the origin and destination. *The example's VM at the origin, VM = 0.99 and at the destination, VM = 0.94 (Figure 31.20).*

To determine the DM, find the observed (measured) distance multiplier, take the travel distance of the load, from the origin and destination. *The example's DM = 1.0 (Figure 31.21).*

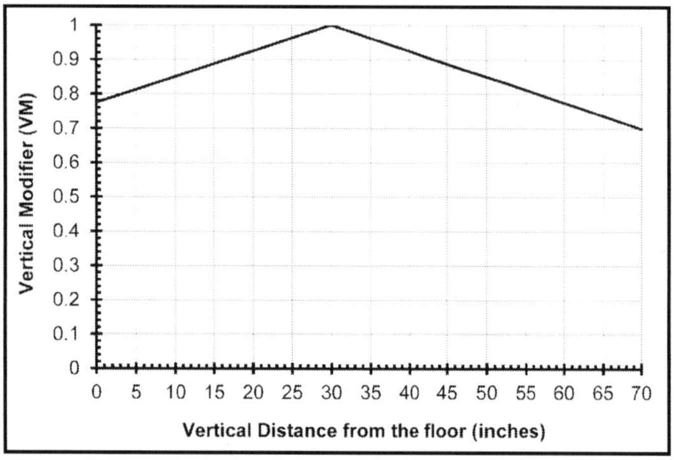

Figure 31.20 — Vertical multiplier (VM).

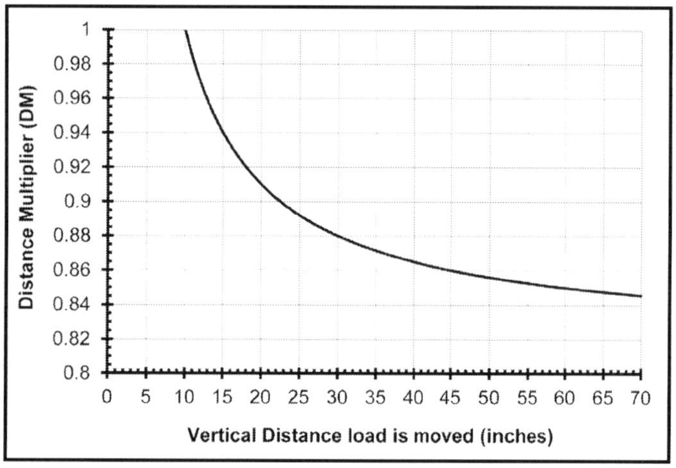

Figure 31.21 — Distance multiplier (DM).

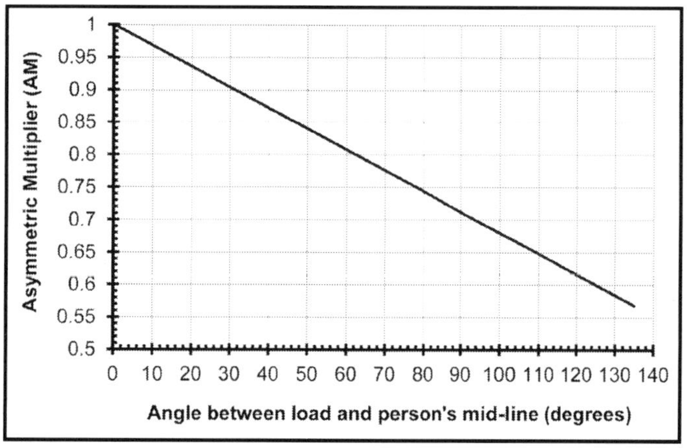

Figure 31.22 — Asymmetric multiplier (AM).

To determine the AM, find the angle between the location of the load and person's midline where A is measured in degrees. The AM is measured at the destination only if the destination's placement requires control. *At the origin, A = 45°, AM = 0.86 (Figure 31.22).*

To determine the FM, look up the frequency of lifts per minute, by the duration of task and at the vertical distance (V) at the origin and destination.

The lifting frequency is set at two lifts per minute and the task time is between 3–4 hours (Table 31.10).

> *At the origin, the VM origin value <30 in., FM = 0.27*
> *At the destination, the VM destination value >30 in., FM = 0.27*

To determine the CM, look up the type of hand coupling and the Vertical distance (V) in Table 31.11. *In the example, both origin and destination have fair coupling. At the origin, the value is <30 in., resulting in a CM = 0.95; and at the destination, the value is >30 in., with a CM = 1.00 (Table 31.11).*

The data collection worksheet for the NIOSH lifting equation is filled from the above calculations (Table 31.12).

To determine the LI, use the equation, LI = W/RWL

> *At the origin, LI = 10 / 9.3 =* ***1.07***
> *At the destination, LI = 10 / 10.7 =* ***0.93***

Theoretically, the LI at origin is more than 1.0, exceeding NIOSH recommendations for RWL. One would interpret that this job might be too unsafe to some workers. However, for practical purposes the job appears to be safe for most workers. If efforts are needed to improve the task, one first must identify the problem using the resulting multiplier values (Table 31.13).

To identify the problem(s), the multipliers (Table 31.13) are listed in ascending order to get:

FM = 0.27
HM = 0.83
AM = 0.86
CM = 0.95
DM = 1.0
VM = 0.99

Table 31.10 — Frequency multiplier (FM).

	Work Duration					
	<= 1 Hour >		*1 but <= 2 Hours*		*>2 but <=8 Hours*	
Frequency Lifts/min (F)	*V<30+ (cm)*	*V>=30 (cm)*	*V<30 (cm)*	*V>=30 (cm)*	*V<30 (cm)*	*V>=30 (cm)*
<=0.2	1	1	0.95	0.95	0.85	0.85
0.5	0.97	0.97	0.92	0.92	0.81	0.81
1	0.94	0.94	0.88	0.88	0.75	0.75
2	0.91	0.91	0.84	0.84	0.65	0.65
3	0.88	0.88	0.79	0.79	0.55	0.55
4	0.84	0.84	0.72	0.72	0.45	0.45
5	0.8	0.8	0.6	0.6	0.35	0.35
6	0.75	0.75	0.5	0.5	0.27	0.27
7	0.7	0.7	0.42	0.42	0.22	0.22
8	0.6	0.6	0.35	0.35	0.18	0.18
9	0.52	0.52	0.3	0.3	0	0.15
10	0.45	0.45	0.26	0.26	0	0.13
11	0.41	0.41	0	0.23	0	0
12	0.37	0.37	0	0.21	0	0
13	0	0.34	0	0	0	0
14	0	0.31	0	0	0	0
15	0	0.28	0	0	0	0
>15	0	0	0	0	0	0

Clearly, the first thing to do is alter the lifting frequency multiplier. However, in some cases this may not be possible, so the next several smallest multipliers — in this sample HM and AM — would need to be considered for modification. Both of them may require some minor layout changes that in the end should result in reduced risk of injury.

Revised NIOSH Lifting Equation Example B

Workers load parts onto an automated powder coat paint line for 8 hours per day. Parts weight 28 lb (12.7 kg) and arrive on pallets containing 24 total parts across six layers. The pallets are delivered by fork truck and placed onto a height adjustable pallet lift. As each pallet layer is unloaded, the lift raises the pallet; thus, workers are always lifting from the same height. Workers lift the parts with two hands and place them on a hook. The hooks are hanging from a chain driven track that continuously moves at 18 feet per minute. Hooks are spaced every 3 feet along the line, thus six parts are loaded per minute onto the line (18 ft per minute ÷ 3 ft per hook = 6 hooks per minute). Two workers load parts simultaneously (one from each side of the pallet); thus, each worker loads parts at a rate of three lifts per minute. The hook line is located 90° adjacent to the pallet. Workers typically stand slightly askew to both the line of hooks and the pallet such that workers are twisting approximately 45° to their right and 45° to their left while lifting and hanging parts.

Since this job requires placing parts carefully and precisely onto the paint line, both origin and destination analyses are required. The lifting parameters for this job are provided in Table 31.14 below.

Table 31.11 — Coupling multiplier.

	VM Value at Origin or Destination	
Coupling	*< 30 in. or 75 cm*	*> 30 in. or 75 cm*
Good	1.00	1.00
Fair	0.95	1.00
Poor	0.90	0.90

Table 31.12 — NIOSH lifting equation data collection worksheet for Example A.

To determine the Recommended Weight Limit (RWL), multiply 51 pounds by each multiplier for a lifting/lowering task's origin and destination.

	ORIGIN		DESTINATION	
	Observed	Multiplier	Observed	Multiplier
HM = Horizontal Distance from the Ankles (in)	12	0.83	12	0.83
VM = Vertical Distance from the Floor (in)	28	0.99	38	0.94
DM = Vertcal Distance the Load is Moved (in)	10	1.0	10	1.0
AM = Assymetry (deg)	45	0.86	0	1.0
FM = Frequency (lifts/min)	6	0.27	6	0.27
CM = Load Coupling: Good, Fair, Poor	Fair	0.95	Fair	1.0
Recommended Weight Limit (RWL) = 51 lbs x HM x VM x DM x AM x FM x CM	9.3		10.7	

To calcualte the Lifting Index divide the load lifted by the Recommended Weight Limit (RWL)

	ORIGIN	DESTINATION
Recommended Weight Limit (RWL) (lb)	9.3	10.7
Load (W) Lifted (lb)	10	10
Lifting Index (LI) – W/RWL	1.07	0.93

Table 31.13 — Resulting multiplier values.

HM = Horizontal distance from the ankles (cm)	30	0.83
VM = Vertical distance from the floor (cm)	71	1.0
DM = Vertical distance load is moved (cm)	25	1.0
AM = Asymmetry (deg)	45°	0.86
FM = Frequency (lifts/min)	6	0.27
CM = Load coupling: good, fair, poor	Fair	0.95

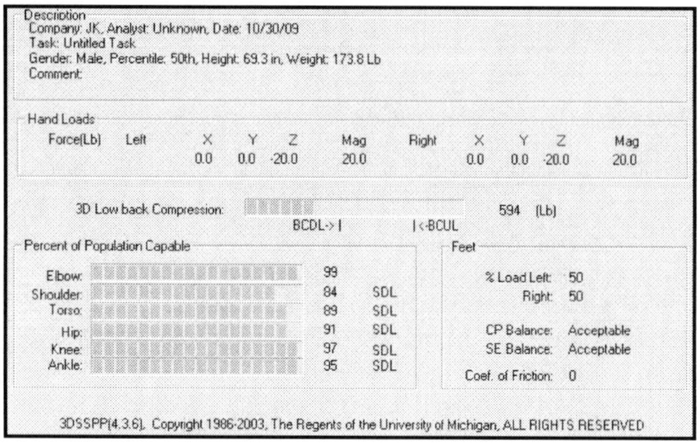

Figure 31.15 — Origin and destination multipliers associated with loading single part onto paint line conveyor.

Using Table 31.14, the lift parameters are converted to the multipliers found in Table 31.15.

Using the multipliers in the RLE yields the following Recommended Weight Limits (RWLs) for origin and destination of lift:

RWL = LC * HM * VM * DM * AM * CM * FM

RWL_{ORIGIN} = 51 * 0.61 * 0.93 * 0.95 * 0.86 * 1.00 * 0.55

RWL_{ORIGIN} = 13 lb.

$RWL_{DESTINATION}$ = 51 * 0.67 * 0.82 * 0.95 * 0.86 * 1.00 * 0.55

$RWL_{DESTINATION}$ = 12.6 lb.

Because the destination of the lift results in a lower RWL (12.6 < 13 lbs.), the RWL from the destination is taken as the RWL for the job. Recall that the actual weight lifted is 28 lbs.. The actual weight and the RWL for the job may now be used to calculate the LI for the job as follows:

LI = Actual Weight / RWL

LI = 28 / 13 lbs.

LI = 2.15

Since the lifting index is greater than 1.0, the job is classified as hazardous to some workers.

An examination of the multipliers shows the frequency multiplier (0.55) to be the lowest (i.e. contributes to the greatest single reduction in RWL). Therefore, one alternative would be to reduce the frequency of lifts to reduce the risk for injury.

Lifting Guidelines

Transferring heavy parts, working in highly repetitive tasks, etc., can be physically demanding

- Tasks should be designed to minimize trunk flexion
- Keep objects close to the body
- Minimize twisting and bending
- Pre-plan the placement of the parts/product to reduce corrections needed
- Use jib cranes to move heavy objects

Lifting Technique

Loads of either moderate or heavy weight can be lifted in several different ways. The most common lifting recommendations generally observed in industrial tasks are to

- Bend the knees
- Keep the back straight
- Lift with the legs

It was assumed that squatting would lower the compressive forces on the spine and, hence, would be a suggested technique for lifting. Studies on squatting during lifting found higher muscle activity[143]

Table 31.14 — Origin and destination parameters of loading single part onto paint line conveyor.

	Weight (W)	Horizontal Location (H)	Vertical Location (V)	Travel Distance (D)	Asymmetry (A)	Coupling (C)	Frequency (F)
Origin	28 lbs	16.5"	40"	14"	45°	Fair	3 /min
Destination	28 lbs	15"	54"	14"	45°	Fair	3 /min

of the back muscles when compared to stooping. Moreover, squatting when compared to stooping during lifting might increase quadriceps fatigue[144,145] and generate greater compressive loads on the spine.[64,146,147] It was also found that workers rarely use the recommended lifting techniques.[148]

Keeping the back straight might result in a much larger horizontal distance if the load is bulky and cannot be brought in-between the knees. Ortengren et al.[149] compared lifting using the back muscle activity with lifting using leg muscles and found no considerable difference in muscle activity between the two types of lifting.

Bending the knees and keeping the back straight (squatting) is more fatiguing during repetitive lifting than bending the trunk (stooping). Productivity might decrease when workers are forced to squat while lifting. But, excessive stooping is not desirable either, since it might produce greater stresses in ligaments and higher shear forces on the spine.[147] Therefore, during lifting, the following recommendations might be more useful and practical (Figure 31.23):

- Stand close to the load with legs comfortably apart (a)
- Do not overexert and get a feel of the load (b), if it's too heavy, get help
- Keep the load as close to body as possible (b)
- Preferably bend from hips and minimize bending your back. Otherwise, bend your knees and back up to an comfortable level (c)
- Lift the load slowly and steadily, keeping it close to the body (c)
- Avoid twisting while lifting (d)

Job Strength Requirements

Several studies have measured job physical requirements and compared those with workers' job-specific strengths to determine the risk of low back and other musculoskeletal injuries. The hypothesis is that back and other musculoskeletal injuries occur because the job physical requirements exceed the job-specific strengths of the workers performing those jobs. In other words, there is a mismatch between the strength requirements of the jobs and workers' strength capabilities. To test the hypothesis requires (1) identifying the most stressful tasks performed by the workers, (2) quantifying the physical strength requirements of those tasks and (3) measuring the physical strength capabilities of the workers performing those tasks. Some studies have used static strength prediction biomechanical models to analyze the strength requirements of the jobs to identify and quantify the most stressful tasks.[25,26,150–152] Workers' job-specific, static strengths were also measured. By comparing the job strength requirements with the workers' strengths, the studies were able to identify those workers whose job physical strength requirements exceeded the workers' strength capabilities.[25,150,152,153]

Two different studies have demonstrated that both future low back pain incidence rates and severity rates increased when the maximum weight lifted by the workers on

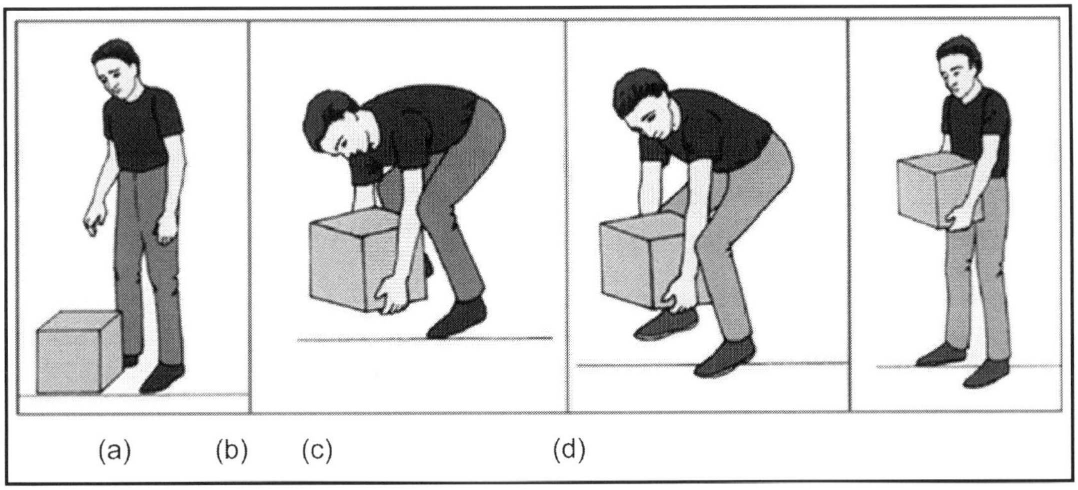

Figure 31.23 — Gradual lifting recommendations.

the job exceeded the workers' job specific isometric strength.[153,154] These studies suggested that (i) weaker workers are at a higher risk of experiencing a low back-related injury than stronger workers, and (ii) weaker workers are more likely to have lost workdays.

Snook and Ciriello[133] and Herrin et al.[26] analyzed jobs using maximum acceptable weights and forces to determine percent of workers that were capable of performing jobs based on these data. Snook and Ciriello reported that those jobs that were acceptable to less than 75% of workers have higher incidence of low back pain than jobs that were acceptable to at least 75% of workers. Similarly, Herrin et al. found that jobs that were acceptable to less than 90% of workers had higher incidence and severity of low back injuries than jobs that were acceptable to at least 90% of workers.

Pushing/Pulling

Pushing/pulling tasks are common in industries and services such as shipping and receiving, moving, warehousing, garbage collection, agriculture, fire fighting, construction, gardening, and nursing.[155–157]

Pushing is defined as an application of force directed away from the body and pulling is defined as force directed toward the body. Often, the direction of exerted force is not strictly horizontal. Pushing and pulling of objects involve an initial force to start the movement of an object, a lower force to sustain the movement and a stopping force to stop the movement of an object.

Pushing and pulling of objects exposes workers to two types of hazards: (1) stresses to the musculoskeletal system from the applied hand force, and (2) accidents due to slipping or tripping.[158,159] Pushing and pulling activities are associated with shoulder injuries and LBP. It is estimated that 9–18% of low back injuries are associated with pushing and pulling.[1,15,160–166] Similarly, several studies have reported increased shoulder pain from workers pushing/pulling wheeled equipment.[155,167,168]

The following factors should be considered when designing and analyzing pushing/pulling tasks:

1. **Friction:** Friction between the floor and shoes (as well as wheels) affects an individual's ability to push/pull an object and the subsequent risk of MSDs. A person needs the right flooring and shoe combination to apply sufficient pushing/pulling force without the risk of slipping. However, the lower the coefficient of friction, the easier the object will slide on a surface.
2. **Wheels:** In general, less pushing/pulling force is required with harder wheels of a cart pushed/pulled over a harder surface. Similarly, wheels with a large diameter require lower pushing/pulling forces. In addition, it is less likely that larger wheels will get stuck or hung up on humps, holes, cracks, and other floor obstruction. Swiveling of wheels is another consideration. A cart with all four swiveling casters requires more force to turn.[169,170]
3. **Maintenance:** Maintenance of the wheels and wheel bearings affect the amount of pushing/pulling force required to move a cart.
4. **Floor:** Large ridges between uneven floors and between two floors (for example, floor and elevator) can require substantially higher forces when pushing and pulling carts. Similarly, it is much harder to push/pull a cart on an inclined surface than on a horizontal surface. It is also more difficult to control a loaded cart on an inclined surface.
5. **Weight of the cart:** For a given cart and floor surface, as the weight of the cart increases, the force required to push/pull the cart also increases. However, what is important is the force required to push/pull a cart rather than the total weight of the cart. A heavier, well-designed cart might require a lower pushing/pulling force than a lighter poorly designed cart.
5. **Handle height:** In general, pushing and pulling strengths decrease with an increase in handle height from the floor. However, compressive forces on the low back could be high with handles placed at lower heights. Karawowski and Marras[156] recommended hip-to-elbow handle height for pushing tasks and is knee-to-hip height for pulling tasks. Hoozemans et al.[171] suggested that the hands should be at shoulder height for two-handed pushing. Lee et al.[160]

recommended hands should be at 109 cm from floor for pushing and 152 cm for pulling. Lett and McGill[172] recommended that the optimum height for pushing is shoulder height, and the optimum height for pulling is waist height.

7. It does not appear that there are major differences between pushing and pulling strengths. However, several studies have shown that pulling results in higher compressive force than pushing of carts. Conversely, Lett and McGill[172] reported that pushing tasks produced greater peak compression and peak posterior shearing forces than pulling trials under the same conditions.

Acceptable Pushing/Pulling Forces

Snook and Ciriello[133] have provided extensive data for pushing and pulling acceptable forces to different percent capable male and female populations. These data include acceptable levels of both initial and sustained forces for males and females. Acceptable levels of pushing and pulling forces are provided for three different hand heights, seven different pushing/pulling frequencies, and six different pushing/pulling horizontal distances.

Workstation Design Recommendations

Design of a workstation for a job should be within the acceptable limits (Table 31.16) and should

- Fit the job to the worker
  - Snook et al.[134] showed that the risk of low back injury is three times greater if less than 75% of workers cannot perform the job without overexertion.
- Design jobs so that they are within the physical capability of at least 75% to 90% of the working population.

Benefits of Ergonomic Job Design

Some of the benefits of ergonomic job design may include:

- Improved quality
- Increase in productivity
- Decrease in injuries
- Reduction in incidence of LBP
- Reduction in severity of LBP (lost and restricted workdays)
- Decrease in cost

Whole Body Vibration

Vibration is the motion resulting from oscillating force acting on an object. If the force is present after the onset of motion, the resulting vibration is considered forced, and if the force is removed the remaining motion is called free vibration. The amount of motion depends on the magnitude and frequency of the applied force and the mass and stiffness properties of the body. The motion is greatly increased if the frequency of the load and the body are matched. This condition is called resonance and can lead to very large motions. Energy can be removed from the system through damping, a property of the specific materials, and higher amounts of damping lead to reduced motions. Damping can be due to a combination of factors, including viscoelastic behavior and friction.

The human body reacts in a complex way to vibration through sensory mechanoreceptors controlling motor performance. Vibration affects the body in many ways, such as sensorimotor, physiological, mechanical, and psychological functions. Vibratory motions are transmitted to the tissue and organs and are absorbed (damped) internally. The motion is often resisted by muscle activity, leading to fatigue due to continuous muscle contractions.

One of the most important parameters for determining the effects of vibration is frequency. There are three major ranges of frequency when dealing with human whole body vibrations: low (up to 2 Hz), medium

Table 30.16 — Recommended acceptable limits for the different criteria of job design.

Criteria	*Acceptable Limit*
Compressive force	770 lbs
Strength	75% capable
Energy expenditure	3.1 Kcal/min (whole body exertion) 2.2 Kcal/min (arm work)
Heart Rate	100–105 beats/min 90–95 beats/min (arm work)
Postural stress	%MVC, exertion time and recovery time
Perceived Stress	Somewhat hard

Table 31.17 — Human response to different vibration frequencies.(173)

Frequency (Hz)	*Symptoms*
4–10	Discomfort Abdominal pain Influence on breathing Muscle contraction
5–7	Chest pain
10–18	Urge to urinate
13–20	Head symptoms
13–20	Influence on the speech
20–23	Increased muscle tone

(2 to 20 Hz), and high (above 20 Hz). Each frequency range has different affects on the body. Table 31.17 shows typical human responses to vibration at different frequencies. The severity of the response depends upon the magnitude of the vibration (amplitude) as well as the frequency. In addition, the biomechanical properties of human body segments and tissue vary with the direction of the motion.

The International Standards Organization (ISO) has defined limits for human exposure to whole body vibration (ISO 2631).(174) The limits are defined in terms of the allowable time exposure to equivalent vibration acceleration (Table 31.8). The standard defines three levels of exposure: (1) a reduced comfort boundary, (2) a fatigue-decreased proficiency boundary, and (3) an exposure health limit. Table 31.18 shows the fatigue-decreased proficiency boundary. The acceleration values are multiplied by 2 to get exposure limits, while dividing by 3.15 results in the reduced comfort boundary condition. Although the typical industrial work environment has a work period of 8 hours or less, exposure to vibration for more than 8 hours can be found in occupations like commercial flight operators, crew onboard ships, submarines, etc. The standard is applied by measuring acceleration of vibration in different frequencies and determining the acceleration in one-third octave bands from 1–80 Hz. The one-third octave band accelerations are combined into a single equivalent acceleration from.

$$a_w = \sqrt{\left[\sum_i (w_i\, a_i)^2\right]} \qquad (31\text{-}7)$$

Table 31.18 — ISO 2631 Whole-body vibration fatigue decreased proficiency boundary duration values for Z Axis RMS acceleration for frequency or center frequency of the third octave ranging from 4 to 8 Hz.(174)

Acceleration RMS (m/sec²)	*Duration*
0.14	24 h
0.19	16 h
0.32	8 h
0.53	4 h
0.72	2.5 h
1.19	1 h
1.80	25 min
2.13	16 min
2.83	1 min

Table 31.19 — Approximate comfort level in public transportation to frequency-weighted vibrations.(175)

Frequency Weighted Vibration Magnitude RMS (m/sec²)	*Comfort level*
< 0.315	High
0.315 to 1	Moderate
> 1	Low

Where a_w is the weighted acceleration, and w_i and a_i are the weighting factor and the RMS acceleration for the i-th 3rd octave band.

ISO 2631(174) provides approximate reactions due to exposure of vibration levels during transport as shown in Table 31.19. RMS acceleration values greater than 2 m/sec^2 could be extremely uncomfortable when generated by a vehicle such as a truck.

Measurement and Limits

Vibrations accelerations are measured along three orthogonal axes as shown in Figure 31.24. The most common measurement tools are piezo-resistive for low frequencies and piezoelectric for high frequencies. The measured accelerations are divided into one-third octave bands for further processing. One key to obtaining accurate measurements is to limit the mass of the accelerometer to a maximum of one-tenth of the mass of the object being evaluated.

The European Union has adopted guidelines (ISO 2631) for determining worker exposure to vibration and has set limits on the exposure. The maximum of 1.4 times the x-direction or y-direction horizontal weighted acceleration, or the vertical weighted acceleration, is used as the exposure acceleration. The exposure acceleration is then combined with the exposure time to determine whether the level of vibration is acceptable.

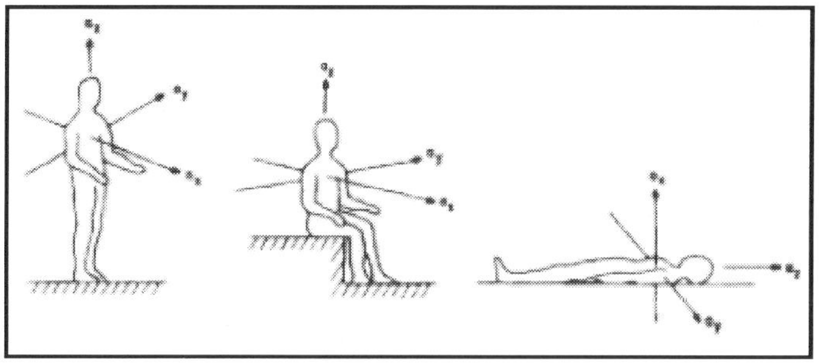

Figure 31.24 — Orthoganol coordinate system for whole body.(174)

Control and Prevention

Controlling and preventing injuries due to whole body vibration is a multistage and ongoing process. To provide the most protection to workers, and make the most efficient use of resources, the following steps should be taken:

1. Identify the main sources of vibration
2. Rank the sources according to their contribution to the overall exposure
3. Determine the acceptable exposure level
4. Identify potential solutions and rank them according to effectiveness and cost
5. Implement the chosen solutions
6. Evaluate the impact of the solutions and modify/extend the program as needed

Vibration control can be achieved at one of two locations: the source, or the target (worker). Reducing vibrations at the source reduces the problem for all workers and is desirable but may not always be feasible or cost-effective. The other option is to reduce vibration exposure to the worker by reducing exposure time (job rotation) or providing appropriate personal protective devices (seat cushions, floor mats, etc.).

Approaches for reducing vibration at the source include choosing equipment that inherently produces less vibration or using vibration isolators. Vibration isolators are springs or pads that are placed between the equipment and its supports to reduce the transmission of vibration and can be retrofit on many types of equipment.

Reducing vibration exposure at the worker can also take one of several options. Job rotation can be one of the most effective means of reducing vibration exposure, provided the other tasks do not also involve excessive vibration. Special mats or pad on which the worker stands or sits can reduce vibration for ground or seat borne vibration. Similarly, gloves are available that reduce vibrations from hand-held tools. When choosing a vibration reduction product it is extremely important to consider the frequency of the vibrations. Incorrectly chosen products can actually amplify the vibration exposure due to resonance.

References

1. **Snook, S.H., R.A. Campanelli, and J.W. Hart:** A study of three preventive approaches to low back injury. *J. Occup. Med. 20*:478–481 (1978).
2. **Bigos, S.J., D. Spengler, N.A. Martin, et al.:** Back injuries in industry: A retrospective study: II. Injury factors. *Spine 11*:246 (1986).
3. **Liles, D.H., S. Deivanayagam, M.M. Ayoub, and P. Mahajan:** A job severity index for the evaluation and control of lifting injury. *Hum. Factors. 26*:683–693 (1984).
4. **Webster, B.S., and S.H. Snook:** The cost of 1989 workers' compensation low back pain claims. *Spine 19*:1111 (1994).
5. **National Research Council/Institute of Medicine (NRC/IOM):** "Musculoskeletal Disorders and the Workplace: Low Back and Upper Extremities." Panel on Musculoskeletal Disorders and the Workplace. Washington, D.C.: Commission on Behavioral Social, Sciences Education, NRC/IOM, 2001.
6. **National Research Council/Institute of Medicine (NRC/IOM):** "BLS Occupational Injury and Illness Data." Presentation to the NRC/IOM Panel on Musculoskeletal Disorders and the Workplace, Washington D.C.: National Academy Press, 1999.
7. **Cedars-Sinai Health Systems** The Human Spine: Vertebrae and Curvatures, 2000. www.csmc.edu/images/468459_Lumbar_vertebrae.jpg.
8. **Bogduk, N., and L.T. Twomey:** Schematic representation of the human vertebrae. In *Clinical Anatomy of the Lumbar Spine*. New York: Churchill Livingstone, 1987.
9. **Co, A.C.:** Cross sectional view of the inter*vertebral disc along with the vertebrae. In The Anatomical Chart Series,* Classic Library Edition, A.C. Co (ed.). Skokie, Ill. 1993.

10. **National Institute for Occupational Safety and Health (NIOSH):** Lever system at L5/S1 in the spine during lifting. In *Simple Solutions: Ergonomics for Construction Workers.* (DHHS/NIOSH Publication no. 2007-122). Cincinnati, Ohio: NIOSH, 2007. www.cdc.gov/niosh/docs/2007-122/materials.html. [Accessed on July 18, 2011.]
11. **Medical Multimedia Group, LLC:** *The Resultant Forces Developed in the Spine Due to Compressive Forces Acting on the Spine.* Missoula, Mont.: Medical Multimedia Group, LLC, 2002.
12. **Jäger, M., and A. Luttmann:** The load on the lumbar spine during asymmetrical bi-manual materials handling. *Ergonomics 35*:783–805 (1992).
13. **Campbell-Kyureghyan, N.H., S.V. Yalla, M.J. Voor, and D.R. Burnett:** "Effect of Orientation on Failure Criteria for Lumbar Spine Segments." *Proceedings of Annual Meeting of the American Society of Biomechanics,* Stanford, Calif. 2007.
14. **Chaffin, D.B., G. Andersson, and B.J. Martin:** *Occupational Biomechanics,* 3rd ed. New York: Wiley-Interscience, 1999.
15. **National Institute for Occupational Safety and Health (NIOSH):** *Work Practices Guide for Manual Lifting,* Technical Report 81-122. Cincinnati, Ohio: DHHS/NIOSH, 1981.
16. **Waters, T.R., V. Putz-Anderson, A. Garg, and L.J. Fine:** 1993. Revised NIOSH equation for the design and evaluation of manual lifting tasks. *Ergonomics 36*:749–776 (1993).
17. **Hansson, T.H., T.S. Keller, and D.M. Spengler:** Mechanical behavior of the human lumar spine. II: Fatigue strength during dynamic compressive loading. *J. Orthop. Res. 5*:479–487 (1987).
18. **Brinckmann, P., M. Biggemann, and D. Hilweg:** *Fatigue Fracture of Human Lumbar Vertebrae.* Oxford, UK: Butterworth-Heinmann, 1988.
19. **Gallagher, S., W.S. Marras, A.S. Litsky, and D. Burr:** Torso flexion loads and the fatigue failure of human lumbosacral motion segments. *Spine 30*:2265 (2005).
20. **Campbell-Kyureghyan, N.H., and W.S. Marras:** Cumulative effects of load frequency and velocity on the lumbar spine response during a repetitive lifting task. In *Human Factors and Ergonomics Society's 49th Annual Meeting, Orlando, Fla.* 2005.
21. **Yalla, S.V., N.H. Campbell-Kyureghyan, and M.J. Voor:** Frequency dependence of strain and energy dissipation during thoracolumbar spine cyclic loading. In *Proceedings of SE American Society of Biomechanics Annual Conference, April 27–29, Birmingham, Ala., 2008.*
22. **Campbell-Kyureghyan, N.H., and W.S. Marras:** Combined experimental and analytical model of the lumbar spine subjected to large displacement cyclic loads. Part II. Model validation. *Int. J. Computat. Vision Biomech. 2*:95–104 (2009).
23. **Campbell-Kyureghyan, N.H.:** "Computational Analysis of the Time-Dependent Biomechanical Behavior of the Lumbar Spine." PhD diss., The Ohio State University, Columbus, Ohio, 2004.
24. **Campbell-Kyureghyan, N., S.V. Yalla, P. Cerrito, and M. Voor:** Stiffness and energy density variation with respect to frequency in a thoracolumbar spine during cyclic loading. *Proceedings of XXII Congress of the International Society of Biomechanics, July 5–9,* Cape Town, South Africa, 2009.
25. **Chaffin, D.B., and K.S. Park:** A longitudinal study of low-back pain as associated with occupational weight lifting factors. *Am. Ind. Hyg. Assoc. J. 34*:513-525 (1973).
26. **Herrin, G.D., M. Jaraiedi, and C.K. Anderson:** Prediction of overexertion injuries using biomechanical and psychophysical models. *Am. Ind. Hyg. Assoc. J. 47*:322 (1986).
27. **Anderson, C.K., D.B. Chaffin, G.D. Herrin, and L.S. Matthews:** A biomechanical model of the lumbosacral joint during lifting activities. *J. Biomech. 18*:571–584 (1985).
28. **Bringham, C.J., and A. Garg:** The role of biomechanical job evaluation in the reduction of overexertion injuries: A case study. In *Proceedings of the 23rd Annual American Industrial Hygiene Association Conference,* May 22–27, pp. 138–144. Philadelphia, Pa., 1983.
29. **Adams, M.A., P. Dolan, W.C. Hutton, and R.W. Porter:** Diurnal changes in spinal mechanics and their clinical significance. *J. Bone Joint Surg. Br. 72*:266–270 (1990).
30. **Dolan, P., E. Benjamin, and M. Adams:** Diurnal changes in bending and compressive stresses acting on the lumbar spine. *J. Bone Joint Surg. Br. 75-B(Suppl 1)*:22 (1993).
31. **Kazarian, L.E.:** Creep characteristics of the human spinal column. *Orthop. Clin. N. Am. 6*: 3–18 (1975).
32. **Gallagher, S., W.S. Marras, A.S. Litsky, D. Burr, J. Landoll, and V. Matkovic:** A comparison of fatigue failure responses of old versus middle-aged lumbar motion segments in simulated flexed lifting. *Spine 32*:1832 (2007).
33. **Campbell-Kyureghyan, N.H., and W.S. Marras:** Combined experimental and analytical model of the lumbar spine subjected to large displacement cyclic loads. Part I. Model development. *Int. J. Computat. Vision Biomech. 2*:87–93 (2009).
34. **Cyron, B.M., and W.C. Hutton:** Articular tropism and stability of the lumbar spine. *Spine 5*:168 (1980).

35. **Farfan, H.F.:** The pathological anatomy of degenerative spondylolisthesis: A cadaver study. *Spine 5*:412 (1980).
36. **van Dieen, J.H., A. van der Veen, B.J. van Royen, and I. Kingma:** I. Fatigue failure in shear loading of porcine lumbar spine segments. *Spine 31*:E494 (2006).
37. **Marras, W.S., and K.P. Granata:** Changes in trunk dynamics and spine loading during repeated trunk exertions. *Spine 22*:2564 (1997).
38. **McGill, S.M., R.W. Norman, V.R. Yingling, R.P. Wells, and P. Neumann:** Shear happens! Suggested guidelines for ergonomists to reduce the risk of low back injury from shear loading. In *Proceedings of 30th Annual Conference of the Human Factors Association of Canada, Mississauga, Ontario, Canada, 1998.*
39. **Norman, R., R. Wells, P. Neumann, J. Frank, H. Shannon, and M. Kerr:** A comparison of peak vs cumulative physical work exposure risk factors for the reporting of low back pain in the automotive industry. *Clin. Biomech. 13*:561–573 (1998).
40. **Frei, H., T.R. Oxland, and L.P. Nolte:** Thoracolumbar spine mechanics contrasted under compression and shear loading. *J. Orthop. Res. 20*:1333–1338 (2002).
41. **National Institute for Occupational Safety and Health (NIOSH):** *Selected Topics in Surface Electromyography for use in the Occupational Setting: Expert Perspectives.* DHHS (NIOSH) Publication No. 91-100. Cincinnati, Ohio: U.S. Department of Health and Human Services, 1992.
42. **Garg, A.:** *Applied Ergonomics.* Milwaukee, Wisc.: University of Wisconsin - Milwaukee, Department of Industrial & Manufacturing Engineering in coperation with University of Utah Department of Family and Preventive Medicine, 2006.
43. **Kamon, E., and N.L. Ramanathan:** Estimation of maximal aerobic power using stairclimbing- A simple method suitable for industry. *Am. Ind. Hyg. Assoc J. 35*:181–188 (1974).
44. **Rodahl, K., and B. Issekutz:** Physical performance capacity of the older individual. In *Muscle as a Tissue.* New York: McGraw-Hill, 1962.
45. **Chaffin, D.B.:** "Some Effects of Physical Exertion." Ann Arbor, Mich.: Dept. of Industrial Engineering, The University of Michigan, 1972.
46. **Garg, A.:** Physiological responses to one-handed lift in the horizontal plane by female workers. *Am. Ind. Hyg. Assoc. J. 44*:190 (1983).
47. **Cummings, E.G.:** Breath holding at beginning of exercise. *J. Appl. Physiol. 17*:221 (1962).
48. **Petrofsky, J.S., and A.R. Lind:** Comparison of metabolic and ventilatory responses of men to various lifting tasks and bicycle ergometry. *J. Appl. Physiol. 45*:60 (1978).
49. **Bink, B.:** Additional studies on physical working capacity in relation to working time and age. *Ergonomics 7*:83 (1964).
50. **Andrews, R.B.:** The relationship between measures of heart rate and rate of energy expenditure. *AIIE 1(1)*:2–10 (1969).
51. **Michael, E.D.:** Cardiorespiratory responses during prolonged exercise. *J. Appl. Physiol. 16*:997 (1961).
52. **National Institute for Occupational Safety and Health (NIOSH):** "Metabolic Indices in Material Handling Tasks." Rodgers, S.H. In *Safety in Manual Material Handling.* Drury, C.G. (ed.) DHEW (NIOSH), Publication No. 78-185, 1986.
53. **Bink, B.:** The physical working capacity in relation to working time and age. *Ergonomics 5*:25–28 (1962).
54. **Barnes, R.M.:** *Motion and Time Study: Design and Measurement of Work.* New York: Wiley, 1980.
55. **Lehmann, G.:** Physiological measurements as a basis of work organization in industry. *Ergonomics 1*:328–344 (1958).
56. **Muller, E.A.:** The physiological basis of rest pauses in heavy work. *Exp. Physiol. 38*:205 (1953).
57. **Karger, D.W., and W.M. Hancock:** *Advanced Work Measurement.* New York: Industrial Press, 1982.
58. **Garg, A., G. Hagglund, and K. Mericle:** A physiological evaluation of time standards for warehouse operations as set by traditional work measurement techniques. *IIE Trans. 18*:235–245 (1986).
59. **Ekblom, B., P.O. Astrand, B. Saltin, J. Stenberg, and B. Wallstrom:** Effect of training on circulatory response to exercise. *J. Appl. Physiol. 24*:518 (1968).
60. **Williams, C.A., J.S. Petrofsky, and A.R. Lind:** Physiological responses of women during lifting exercise. *Eur. J. Appl. Physiol. Occup. Physiol. 50*:133–144 (1982).
61. **Legg, S.J., and C.M. Pateman:** A physiological study of the repetitive lifting capabilities of healthy young males. *Ergonomics 27*:259 (1984).
62. **Garg, A.:** Occupational biomechanics and low-back pain. *Occup. Med. 7*:609–628 (1992).
63. **Garg, A., S.H. Rodgers, and J.W Yates:** The physiological basis for manual lifting. In S. Kumar (ed.), *Advances in Industrial Ergonomics and Safety IV.* Boca Raton, Fla.: CRC Press, 1992.
64. **Garg, A., D.B. Chaffin, and G.D. Herrin:** Prediction of metabolic rates for manual materials handling jobs. *Am. Ind. Hyg. Assoc. J. 39*:661–674 (1978).

65. **Brouha, L.:** Physiology in industry. New York: Pergamon Press, 1960.
66. **Astrand, I.:** Aerobic work capacity in men and women with special reference to age. *Acta Physiol. Scand. Suppl. 49(169)*:192 (1960).
67. **Ciriello, V.M., and S.H. Snook:** A study of size, distance, height, and frequency effects on manual handling tasks. *Hum. Factors 25*:473-483 (1983).
68. **Rodgers, S.H.:** *Kodak's Ergonomic Design for People at Work*, Volume 2. New York: Van Nostrand Reinhold, 1986.
69. **Dugan, S.A., and W.R. Frontera:** Muscle fatigue and muscle injury. In *Phys. Med. Rehab. Clin. N. Am. 11(2)*:385 2000.
70. **Blackwell, J.R., K.W. Kornatz, and E.M. Heath:** Effect of grip span on maximal grip force and fatigue of flexor digitorum superficialis. *Appl. Ergon. 30*:401–405 (1999).
71. **Jurell, K.C.:** Surface EMG and fatigue. *Phys. Med. Rehab. Clin. N. Am. 9(4)*:933 (1998).
72. **Moore, J.S., and A. Garg:** The strain index: a proposed method to analyze jobs for risk of distal upper extremity disorders. *Am. Ind. Hyg. Assoc. J. 56*:443–458 (1995).
73. **Kuorinka, I., and L. Forcier:** *Work Related Musculoskeletal Disorders (WMSDs): A Reference Book for Prevention.* Boca Raton, Fla.: CRC Press, 1995.
74. **Maeda, K.:** Occupational cervicobrachial disorder and its causative factors. *J. Hum. Ergol. 6*:193–202 (1977).
75. **Bjelle, A., M. Hagberg, and G. Michaelson:** Occupational and individual factors in acute shoulder-neck disorders among industrial workers. *Br. Med. J. 38*:356 (1981).
76. **Henriksson, K.G.:** Muscle pain in neuromuscular disorders and primary fibromyalgia. *Eur. J. Appl. Physiol. Occup. Physiol. 57*:348–352 (1988).
77. **Kilbom, A., F. Gamberale, J. Persson, and G. Annwall:** Physiological and psychological indices of fatigue during static contractions. *Eur. J. Appl. Physiol. Occup. Physiol. 50*:179–193 (1983).
78. **Hagg, G.M.:** Static workloads and occupational myalgia-a new explanation model. In P.A. Anderson, D.J. Hobart, and J.V. Danhoff, editors, *Electromyographical Kinesiology*, pp. 141-144. Amsterdam: Elsevier Science Publishers, P.V., 1991.
79. **Hagberg, M., and D.H.:** Prevalence rates and odds ratios of shoulder-neck diseases in different occupational groups. *Br. Med. J. 44*:602 (1987).
80. **Moore, J.S., and A. Garg:** *Occupational Medicine: State of the Art Reviews.* Philadelphia, Pa.: Hanley & Belfus, Inc., 1992.
81. **Lieber, R.L., and J. Friden:** Skeletal muscle metabolism, fatigue and injury. In S.L. Gordon, S.J. Blair, and L.J. Fine, editors, *Repetitive Motion Disorders of the Upper Extremity.* Rosemont, Ill.: American Academy of Orthopedic Surgeons, 1995.
82. **Hikida, R.S., R.S. Staron, F.C. Hagerman, W.M. Sherman, and D.L. Costill:** Muscle fiber necrosis associated with human marathon runners. *J. Neurol. Sci. 59*:185 (1983).
83. **Moore, J.S.:** Carpal tunnel syndrome. In J.S. Moore and A. Garg, editors, *Occup. Med. 7(4)*:741–764. 1992.
84. **Gordon, S.L., S.J. Blair, and L.J. Fine (eds.):** *Repetitive Motion Disorders of the Upper Extremity.* Rosemont, Ill.: American Academy of Orthopaedic Surgeons. 1995.
85. **Amiel, D., C.R. Chu, and J. Lee:** Effect of loading on metabolism and repair of tendons and ligaments. In S.L. Gordon, S.J. Blair, and L.J. Fine, editors, *Repetitive Motion Disorders of the Upper Extremity*, pp. 217–230. Rosemont, Ill.: American Academy of Otrhopaedic Surgeons, 1995.
86. **Woo, S.L.Y., and J.W. Xerogeans:** The biomechanics of soft tissue: Normal, injured and healed states. In S.L. Gordon, S.J. Blair and L.J. Fine, editors, *Repetitive Motion Disorders of the Upper Limb.* Rosemont, IL: American Academy of Orthopedic Surgeons. 1995.
87. **Kraushaar, B.S., and R.P. Nirsciil:** Tendinosis of the elbow(tennis elbow): Clinical features and findings of histological, immunohistochemical, and electron microscopy studies. *J. Bone Joint Surg. Am. 81*:259–278.
88. **Sjogaard, G., B. Kiens, K. Jorgensen, and B. Saltin:** Intramuscular pressure, EMG and blood flow during low-level prolonged static contraction in man. *Acta Physiol. Scand. 128*:475–484 (1986).
89. **Radwin, R.G., and B.A. Ruffalo:** Computer key switch force-displacement characteristics and short-term effects on localized fatigue. *Ergonomics 42*:160–170 (1999).
90. **Kuorinka, I.:** Subjective discomfort in a simulated repetitive task. *Ergonomics 26*:1089 (1983).
91. **Borg, G.:** Psychophysical scaling with applications in physical work and the perception of exertion. *Scand. J. Work, Environ. Health 16*:55 (1990).
92. **Krivickas, L.S., A. Taylor, R.M. Maniar, E. Mascha, S.S. Reisman:** Is spectral analysis of the surface electromyographic signal a clinically useful tool for evaluation of skeletal muscle fatigue? *J. Clin. Neurophysiol. 15*:138 (1998).
93. **Lowery, M., P. Nolan, and M. O'Malley:** Electromyogram median frequency, spectral compression and muscle fibre conduction velocity during sustained sub-maximal contraction of the brachioradialis muscle. *J. Electromyogr. Kinesiol. 12*:111–118 (2002).

94. **Chaffin, D.B.:** Localized muscle fatigue-definition and measurement. *J. Occup. Environ. Med. 15*:346 (1973).
95. **Elfving, B., G. Nemeth, I. Arvidsson, and M. Lamontagne:** Reliability of EMG spectral parameters in repeated measurements of back muscle fatigue. *J. Electromyogr. Kinesiol. 9*:235–243 (1999).
96. **Petrofsky, J.S.:** Quantification through the surface EMG of muscle fatigue and recovery during successive isometric contractions. *Aviat. Space, Environ. Med. 52*:545 (1981).
97. **Moritani, T., M. Muro, A. Nagata:** Intramuscular and surface electromyogram changes during muscle fatigue. *J. Appl. Physiol. 60*:1179 (1986).
98. **Esposito, F., C. Orizio, and A. Veicsteinas:** Electromyogram and mechanomyogram changes in fresh and fatigued muscle during sustained contraction in men. *Eur. J. Appl. Physiol. 78*:494–501 (1998).
99. **Dimitrova, N.A., and G.V. Dimitrov:** Interpretation of EMG changes with fatigue: Facts, pitfalls, and fallacies. *J. Electromyogr. Kinesiol. 13*:13–36. 2003.
100. **Pease, W.S., and M.A. Elinski:** Surface and wire electromyographic. Recording during fatiguing exercise. *Electromyogr. Clin. Neurophysiol. 43*:267 (2003).
101. **Deyo, R.A., M. Battie, A. Beurskens, et al.:** Outcome measures for low back pain research: A proposal for standardized use. *Spine 23*:2003 (1998).
102. **Deyo, R.A., S.K. Mirza, and B.I. Martin:** Back pain prevalence and visit rates: Estimates from US national surveys, 2002. *Spine 31*:2724 (2006).
103. **Garg, A., and J.S. Moore:** Epidemiology of low-back pain in industry. *Occup. Med. 7(4)*:593 (1992).
104. **Frymoyer, J.W., M.H. Pope, J.H. Clements, D.G. Wilder, B. MacPherson, and T. Ashikaga:** Risk factors in low-back pain. An epidemiological survey. *J. Bone Joint Surg. 65*:213 (1983).
105. **National Research Council (NRC):** *Musculoskeletal Disorders and the Workplace: Low Back and Upper Extremities.* Washington, D.C.: National Academy Press, 2001.
106. **Chaffin, D.B.:** Digital human modeling for workspace design. *Rev. Hum. Factors Ergon. 4*:41–74 (2008).
107. **Chaffin, D.B., and W.H. Baker:** A biomechanical model for analysis of symmetric sagittal plane lifting. *IIE Trans. 2*:16–27 (1970).
108. **Martin, J.B., and D.B. Chaffin:** Biomechanical computerized simulation of human strength in sagittal-plane activities. *IIE Trans. 4*:19–28 (1972).
109. **Garg, A., and D.B. Chaffin:** A biomechanical computerized simulation of human strength. *IIE Trans. 7*:1–15 (1975).
110. **Marras, W.S., and K.P.:** The development of an EMG-assisted model to assess spine loading during whole-body free-dynamic lifting. *J. Electromyogr. Kinesiol. 7*:259–268 (1997).
111. **Granata, K.P., and W.S. Marras:** An EMG-assisted model of loads on the lumbar spine during asymmetric trunk extensions. *J. Biomech. 26*:1429–1438 (1993).
112. **Granata, K.P., and W.S. Marras:** The influence of trunk muscle coactivity on dynamic spinal loads. *Spine 20*:913 (1995).
113. **McGill, S.M.:** A myoelectrically based dynamic three-dimensional model to predict loads on lumbar spine tissues during lateral bending. *J. Biomech. 25*:395 (1992).
114. **Marras, W.S., and C.M. Sommerich:** A three-dimensional motion model of loads on the lumbar spine: II. Model validation. *Hum. Factors 33*:139–149 (1991).
115. **McGill, S.M., and R.W. Norman:** Dynamically and statically determined low back moments during lifting. *J. Biomech. 18*:877 (1985).
116. **Marras, W.S., and C.M. Sommerich:** A three-dimensional motion model of loads on the lumbar spine: I. Model structure. *Hum. Factors 33*:123–137 (1991).
117. **McGill, S.M.:** Electromyographic activity of the abdominal and low back musculature during the generation of isometric and dynamic axial trunk torque: Implications for lumbar mechanics. *J. Orthop. Res. 9*:91–103 (1991).
118. **Cholewicki, J., and S.M. McGill:** Lumbar posterior ligament involvement during extremely heavy lifts estimated from fluoroscopic measurements. *J. Biomech. 25*:17 (1992).
119. **Granata, K.P., and W.S. Marras:** An EMG-assisted model of trunk loading during free-dynamic lifting. *J. Biomech. 28*:1309–1317 (1995).
120. **Marras, W.S., and K.P. Granata:** A biomechanical assessment and model of axial twisting in the thoracolumbar spine. *Spine 20*:1440 (1995).
121. **van Dieën, J.H., and I. Kingma:** Total trunk muscle force and spinal compression are lower in asymmetric moments as compared to pure extension moments. *J. Biomech. 32*:681–687 (1999).
122. **Marras, W.S., and G.A. Mirka:** A comprehensive evaluation of trunk response to asymmetric trunk motion. *Spine 17*:318 (1992).
123. **Cholewicki, J., S.M. McGill, and R.W. Norman:** Comparison of muscle forces and joint load from an optimization and EMG assisted lumbar spine model: towards development of a hybrid approach. *J. Biomech. 28*:321–331 (1995).

124. **Kumar, S.:** Cumulative load as a risk factor for back pain. *Spine 15*:1311 (1990).
125. **3D Static Strength Prediction Program (3D SSPP):** "Body Posture Angles Similar to 2D Posture as Entered into 3D SSPP (a) 2D Model Superimposed on the Real-Time Scenario (b) 2D Software-generated Model." Ann Arbor, Mich.: Center for Ergonomics, University of Michigan, 2008.
126. **3D Static Strength Prediction Program (3D SSPP):** Revisions in *NIOSH Guide to Manual Lifting*. 1991.
127. **3D Static Strength Prediction Program (3D SSPP):** Summary results from 3D SSPP software based on input from Table 4. 2008.
128. **3D Static Strength Prediction Program (3D SSPP):** Worker loading castings into machine center (left) and analysis image from 3D SSPP for comparison (right). 2008.
129. **3D Static Strength Prediction Program (3D SSPP):** Body segment angles used for 3-dimensional analysis example. 2008.
130. **3D Static Strength Prediction Program (3D SSPP):** Summary results from 3D SSPP software based on input from Table 5. 2008.
131. **Marras, W.S., S.A. Lavender, S.E. Leurgans, et al.:** The role of dynamic three-dimensional trunk motion in occupationally-related low back disorders. *Spine 18*:617–628 (1993).
132. **Marras, W.S., K.G. Davis, B.C. Kirking, K.P. Granata:** Spine loading and trunk kinematics during team lifting. *Ergonomics 42*:1258–1273 (1999).
133. **Snook, S.H., and V.M. Ciriello:** The design of manual handling tasks: revised tables of maximum acceptable weights and forces. *Ergonomics 34*:1197 (1991).
134. **Snook, S.H.:** The design of manual handling tasks. *Ergonomics 21*:963 (1978).
135. **Mital, A.:** Comprehensive maximum acceptable weight of lift database for regular 8-hour shifts. *Ergonomics 27*:1127–1138 (1984).
136. **Fernandez, J.E., M.M. Ayoub, J.L. Smith:** Psychophysical lifting capacity over extended periods. *Ergonomics 34*:23 (1991).
137. **Snook, S.H.:** Snook tables. In *Liberty Mutual Manual Materials Handling Guidelines*. Hopkinton, Mass.: Liberty Mutual Research Institute for Safety, 1978.
138. **Liles, D.H., and P. Mahajan:** Using NIOSH lifting guide decreases risks of back injuries. *Occup. Health Saf. 54*:57 (1985).
139. **Huang, J., Y. Ono, E. Shibata, Y. Takeuchi, and N. Hisanaga:** Occupational musculoskeletal disorders in lunch centre workers. *Ergonomics 31*:65–75 (1988).
140. **U.S. Department of Health and Human Services (DHHS), National Institute for Occupational Safety and Health (NIOSH):** *Applications Manual for the Revised NIOSH Lifting Equation,* DHHS (NIOSH) Publication no. 94-110, by T.R. Waters, V. Putz-Anderson, and A. Garg. Cinncinati, Ohio: DHHS, NIOSH, Division of Biomedical and Behavioral Science, 1994.
141. **Wang, M.J.J., A. Garg, Y.C. Chang, Y.C. Shih, W.Y. Yeh, and C.L. Lee:** The relationship between low back discomfort ratings and the NIOSH lifting index. *Hum. Factors 40*:509–516 (1998).
142. **Waters, T.R., S.L. Baron, L.A. Piacitelli, et al.:** Evaluation of the revised NIOSH lifting equation: a cross-sectional epidemiologic study. *Spine 24*:386 (1999).
143. **Vakos, J.P., A.J. Nitz, A.J. Threlkeld, R. Shapiro, and T. Horn:** Electromyographic activity of selected trunk and hip muscles during a squat lift: Effect of varying the lumbar posture. *Spine 19(6)*:687 (1994).
144. **Trafimow, J.H., O.D. Schipplein, G.J. Novak, and G.B. Andersson:** The effects of quadriceps fatigue on the technique of lifting. *Spine 18*:364 (1993).
145. **Burgess-Limerick, R., B. Abernethy, R.J. Neal, V. Kippers:** Self-selected manual lifting technique: Functional consequences of the interjoint coordination. *Hum. Factors 37(2)*:395–411 1995.
146. **Lindbeck, L., and U.P. Arborelius:** Inertial effects from single body segments in dynamic analysis of lifting. *Ergonomics 34*:421 (1991).
147. **Garg, A., and G.D. Herrin:** Stoop or squat: A biomechanical and metabolic evaluation. *IIE Trans. 11*:293–302 (1979).
148. **Kuorinka, I., M. Lortie, and M. Gautreau:** Manual handling in warehouses: The illusion of correct working postures. *Ergonomics 37*:655–661 (1994).
149. **Ortengren, R., G.B.J. Andersson, and A. Nachemson:** Studies of relationships between lumbar disc pressure, myoelectric back muscle activity, and intra-abdominal (intragastric) pressure. *Spine 6*:98 (1981).
150. **Chaffin, D.B.:** Human strength capability and low-back pain. *J. Occup. Environ. Med. 16*:248 (1974).
151. **Chaffin, D.B., G.D. Herrin, W.M. Keyserling, and A. Garg:** A method for evaluating the biomechanical stresses resulting from manual materials handling jobs. *Am. Ind. Hyg. Assoc. J. 38*:662 (1977).
152. **McMahan, P.B.:** Strength testing may be an effective placement tool for the railroad industry. *Trends in Ergonomics/Human Factors V*, pp. 787–794. Amsterdam: Elsevier Science Publishers B.V., 1988.
153. **Chaffin, D.B., G.D. Herrin, and W.M. Keyserling:** An updated position. *J. Occup. Environ. Med. 20*:403 (1978).
154. **Keyserling, M.W., G.D. Herrin, and D.B. Chaffin:** Isometric strength testing as a means of controlling medical incidents on strenuous jobs. *J. Occup. Environ. Med. 22*:332–336 (1980).

155. **Hoozemans, M.J.M., A.J. van der Beek, M.H.W. Frings-Dresen, L.H.V. van der Woude, and F.J.H. van Dijk:** Low-back and shoulder complaints among workers with pushing and pulling tasks. *Scand. J. Work Environ. Health 28*:293–303 (2002).
156. **Karwowski, W., and W.S. Marras:** *The Occupational Ergonomics Handbook*. Boca Raton, Fla.: CRC Press, 1999.
157. **Baril-Gingras, G., and M. Lortie:** The handling of objects other than boxes: univariate analysis of handling techniques in a large transport company. *Ergonomics 38*:905–925 (1995).
158. **Chaffin, D.B.:** Biomechanical strength models in industry. *Ergonomic Interventions to Prevent Musculoskeletal Injuries in Industry*, pp. 27–45. Cincinnati, Ohio: ACGIH, 1987.
159. **Grieve, G.P.:** Treating backache — A topical comment. *Physiotherapy 69*:316 (1983).
160. **Lee, K.S., D.B. Chaffin, G.D. Herrin, and A.M. Waikar:** Effect of handle height on lower-back loading in cart pushing and pulling. *Appl. Ergon. 22*:117–123 (1991).
161. **Frymoyer, J.W., M.H. Pope, M.C. Costanza, J.C. Rosen, J.E. Goggin, and D.G. Wilder:** Epidemiologic studies of low-back pain. *Spine 5*:419 (1980).
162. **Pope, M.H.:** Risk indicators in low back pain. *Ann. Med. 21*:387–392 (1989).
163. **Garg, A., and J.S. Moore:** Prevention strategies and the low back in industry. *Occup. Med. 7*:629–640 (1992).
164. **Metzler, F.:** Epidemiology and statistics in Luxembourg. *Ergonomics 28*:21–24 (1985).
165. **Klein, B.P., R.C. Jensen, and L.M. Sanderson:** Assessment of workers' compensation claims for back strains/sprains. *J. Occup. Environ. Med. 26*:443 (1984).
166. **Delleman, N.J., M.P. Vander Griten, and V.H. Hilderandt:** *Handmatig Duwen/Trekken en Gezondheidseffecten*. The Hague: Ministerie van Sociale zaken en Werkgelegenheid. 1995.
167. **Van der Beek, A.J., M.H.W. Frings-Dresen, F.J.H. Van Dijk, H.C.G. Kemper, and T.F. Meijman:** Loading and unloading by lorry drivers and musculoskeletal complaints. *Int. J. Ind. Ergon. 12(1-2)*:13–23 (1993).
168. **Harkness, E.F., G.J. Macfarlane, E.S. Nahit, A.J. Silman, and J. McBeth:** Mechanical and psychosocial factors predict new onset shoulder pain: a prospective cohort study of newly employed workers. *Occup. Environ. Med. 60*:850 (2003).
169. **Al-Eisawi, K.W., C.J. Congleton, J.J. Kerk, A.A. Amendola, O.C. Jenkins, and W. Gaines:** Factors affecting minimum push and pull forces of manual carts. *Appl. Ergon. 30*:235–245 (1999).
170. **Das, B., and J. Wimpee:** Ergonomics evaluation and redesign of a hospital meal cart. *Appl. Ergon. 33*:309–318 (2002).
171. **Hoozemans, M., P.P. Kuijer, I. Kingma, et al.:** Mechanical loading of the low back and shoulders during pushing and pulling activities. *Ergonomics 47*:1–18 (2004).
172. **Lett, K., and S. McGill:** Pushing and pulling: personal mechanics influence spine loads. *Ergonomics 49*:895–908 (2006).
173. **Rasmussen, G.:** "Human Body Vibration Exposure and Its Measurement," Bruel & Kjaer *Technical Review No. 1*. Norcross, Ga.: Bruel & Kjaer, 1982.
174. **International Organization for Standardization (ISO):** *Mechanical Vibration and Shock — Evaluation of Human Exposure to Whole Body Vibration — Part 1: General Requirements* (ISO Standard 2631-1:1997). Geneva: 1997.
175. **Mansfield, N.J.:** *Human Response to Vibration*. Boca Raton, Fla.: CRC Press LLC, 2004.

Outcome Competencies

After completing this chapter, the reader should be able to:

1. Define the underlined terms used in this chapter.
2. Describe and define the various types of upper extremity disorders.
3. Identify the risk factors associated with the development of an upper extremity disorder.
4. Use appropriate job analysis methods and tools to evaluate tasks.
5. Discuss recommended hand tool design characteristics.
6. Consider proper design characteristics when evaluating of or designing tasks and work stations.
7. Understand basic anatomy and physiology of the shoulder.
8. Describe risk factors and risk reduction strategies for an office environment.

Prerequisite Knowledge

Basic anatomy and physiology

Prior to beginning this chapter, the reader should review the following chapters:

Chapter Number	Chapter Topic
30	Ergonomics
31	Musculoskeletal Disorders, Job Evaluation and Design Principles

Key Terms

carpal tunnel syndrome • cubital tunnel syndrome • De Quervain's tenosynovitis • Guyon's Canal Syndrome • nerve compression • pronator syndrome • radial tunel syndrome • strain index • tendonitis • upper extremity • zone of convenient reach

Key Topics

I. Introduction
II. Definition and Diagnosis of Distal Upper Extremity Disorders
  A. Nerve-Related Disorders
  B. Tendon Disorders (Tendonitis/Tenosynovitis)
  C. Delayed-Onset Muscular Soreness
III. Risk Factors for Distal Upper Extremity Disorders
IV. Distal Upper Extremity Job Analysis Methods
  A. WISHA Checklist
  B. ACGIH® Threshold Limit Value (TLV®) for Hand Activity Level (HAL)
  C. The Strain Index
V. Hand Tool Design
  A. Tool Weight
  B. Tool Shape
VI. Workstation Design
  A. Workstation Design Factors
  B. Design Principles
  C. Zone of Convenient Reach
  D. Workstation Design Process
  E. Seated Workstation Design
  F. Standing Workstation Design
VII. Shoulder
  A. Epidemiologic Findings
  B. Risk Factors
  C. Job Analysis and Design
VIII. Officer Ergonomics
  A. VDT Workstation Design
IX. References

32

Upper Extremities

By Arun Garg, PhD, Naira Campbell-Kyureghyan, PhD, Na Jin Seo, PhD, Sai Vikas Yalla, PhD, and Jay Kapellusch, PhD

Introduction

The upper extremities include the shoulder, upper arm, elbow, lower arm, wrist and hand. Commonly, the upper extremity is divided into shoulder and distal upper extremities (DUE), from elbow to fingers. Musculoskeletal disorders and risk factors for the shoulder and distal upper extremity are covered in separate sections. First, distal upper extremity disorders are introduced, followed by DUE risk factors and commonly used job analysis methods to determine risk of developing DUE disorders. It should be noted that some of the topics presented, such as localized muscle fatigue and workstation design, are applicable to both upper extremities and low back, which is covered in Chapter 31. Recommendations for hand tool design are presented. This is followed by workstation design principles and recommendations. Then, epidemiological findings on shoulder pain, shoulder disorders and overhead work are presented followed by risk factors and job analysis for overhead work. Relevant data on shoulder girdle strength, endurance time and overhead repetitive work are provided. Lastly, recommendations for office ergonomics are provided.

Definition and Diagnosis of Distal Upper Extremity Disorders

Nerve-Related Disorders

Entrapment or "pinching" of a nerve by either direct pressure or mechanical compression can cause interference in nerve conduction signals. Repetitive stress applied to the nerve over a period of time can cause nerve compression. Occupations such as assemblers and chicken cutters report higher incidence of compression neuropathy.[1] Nerve compression can also occur from other extrinsic events such as fractures and trauma that result in bony compression or dislocations as well as from rheumatoid arthritis that results in synovial thickening of the bursa at the tendon and bone junction.[1]

Specific symptoms vary depending on the site of nerve entrapment. In general, nerve compression in the distal upper extremity is accompanied by distal sensory and then motor deficits. Symptoms include numbness and tingling of the area of the limb innervated by the affected nerve as well as weakness of the muscles that are innervated by the affected nerve.[1]

The nerve disorders based on sites of nerve compression from the proximal to the distal upper extremity include[1]:

Cubital Tunnel Syndrome

Ulnar nerve entrapment at the medial side of the elbow (also referred to as cubital tunnel syndrome) (Figure 32.1a) causes numbness and tingling in the little finger and ulnar half of the ring finger, usually accompanied by atrophy of the intrinsic muscles of the hand and weakness of grip.[2] Resting upon the elbow or repetitive flexing of the elbow may cause the symptoms.[3,4]

Radial Tunnel Syndrome

Radial tunnel syndrome is defined as the entrapment of the posterior interosseous nerve, a continuation of the deep branch of the radial nerve after the

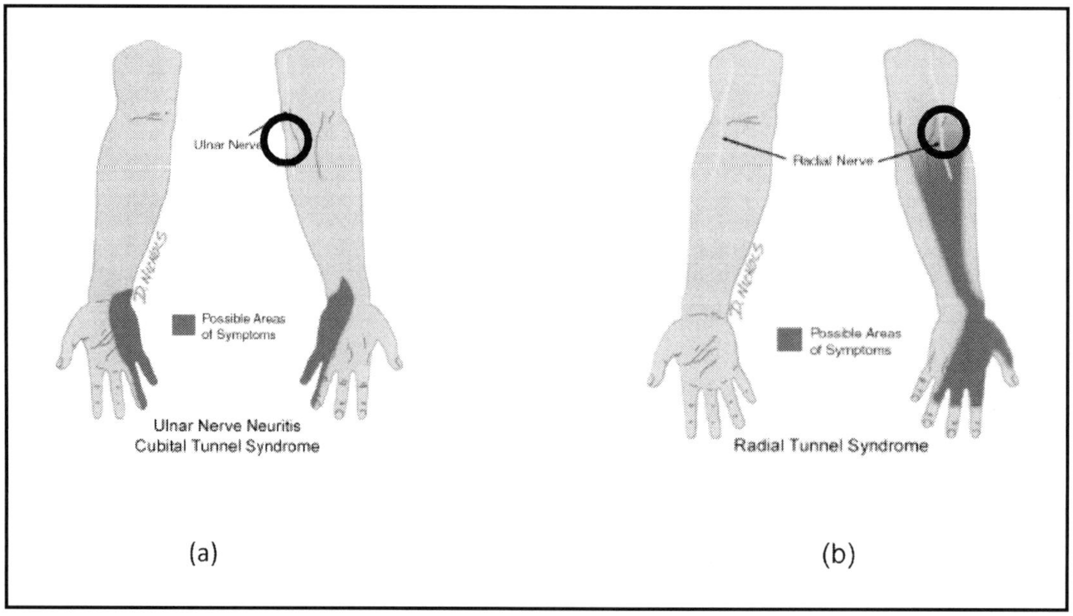

Figure 32.1 a,b — (a) Entrapment of the ulnar nerve and affected body part; (b) Entrapment of the posterior interosseous nerve and affected body part.[5]

supinator muscle, in the lateral aspect of the proximal forearm. This is also referred to as radial tunnel syndrome and posterior interosseous syndrome, see Figure 32.1b. It could be caused by repetitive movements of the wrist and forearm.[6] Symptoms include pain at the dorsal aspect of the upper forearm, about 1.5 cm distal to the lateral epicondylitis and weakness and early fatigue of the extensor digitorum communis muscle group.[7]

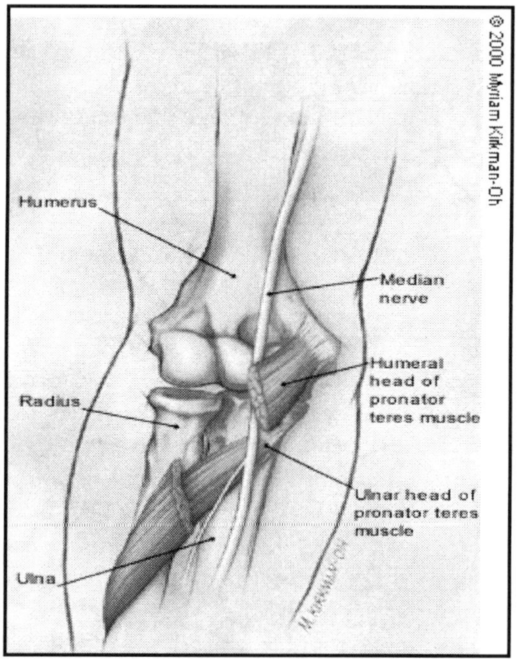

Figure 32.2 — Schematic representation of the median nerve in the proximal forearm.[12]

Pronator Syndrome

Pronator syndrome is defined as entrapment of the median nerve in the proximal forearm (Figure 32.2).[8] Pronator syndrome is often reported as repetitive strain injury among athletes, carpenters, mechanics, and writers, possibly due to overuse of the pronator muscle.[4,9,10] Symptoms include abnormal sensitivity in volar thumb, index, and middle fingers, weakness of finger flexor muscles, and pain in the proximal forearm.[11]

Guyon's Canal Syndrome

Guyon's canal syndrome refers to ulnar nerve entrapment in the canal of Guyon at the wrist (Figure 32.3), also known as ulnar tunnel syndrome, or handlebar palsy. Compressive injuries may be related to both single and repeated trauma.[11] Tasks requiring use of the hand as a hammer, heavy gripping, and recurrent pressure such as from pizza cutters or cycling may compress the ulnar nerve.[13–15]

Carpal Tunnel Syndrome (CTS)

Carpal tunnel syndrome (CTS) is defined as the compression neuropathy of the median nerve at the wrist (Figure 32.4).[17] It is the most common peripheral mono-neuropathy in the distal upper extremity.[18] The incidence is three times more common in women than in men and it usually occurs among individuals older than 30 years of age.[19]

The carpal tunnel is a packed fibro-osseous tunnel at the wrist, bounded by the carpal bones and the flexor retinaculum (transverse carpal ligament). The median nerve and nine long extrinsic digital flexor tendons to the fingers and thumb pass through the carpal tunnel.[21] Elevation of carpal tunnel pressures greater than 20 to 30 mm Hg may cause ischemia to the nerve segment and decreased nerve conduction, resulting in demyelination and eventually in axonal death.[1]

The median nerve inside the carpal tunnel, shown in Figure 32.4, may be compressed either due to elevated pressure inside of the tunnel or by the contents within carpal tunnel such as the transverse carpal ligament or non-specific thickening of tendon sheaths. Some of the tasks and occupations that have been reported to be associated with CTS include gardening, house painting, meat cutting and packaging, manufacturing, logging, construction work, and poultry work.[22] The most common generic job-related physical risk factors associated with CTS include forceful exertion, high repetition and awkward hand/wrist posture. Other factors reported in the literature include exposure to hand/arm vibration, pinch grasp, static work, cold temperature, poorly fitting gloves and possibly unaccustomed work.[22] Other factors may include use of the palm as a hammer, acute trauma and fractures. In addition, obesity, pregnancy, hypothyroidism, diabetes, and arthritis can either cause or aggravate the symptoms.[23,24]

The early symptoms may include numbness, tingling and paresthesias, and may be accompanied with pain (Figure 32.4). Numbness and/or tingling are often more pronounced at night.[1] Patients may find relief of symptoms by shaking their hands to relieve ischemia.[25] Progressively, further nerve impairment may result in subsequent sensory and motor deficit causing muscle weakness of the thumb, index, middle, and part of the fourth fingers, clumsiness, and a tendency to drop objects.[1,26]

According to the National Institute of Occupational Safety and Health (NIOSH), carpal tunnel syndrome may be diagnosed when the following criteria are met[27]:

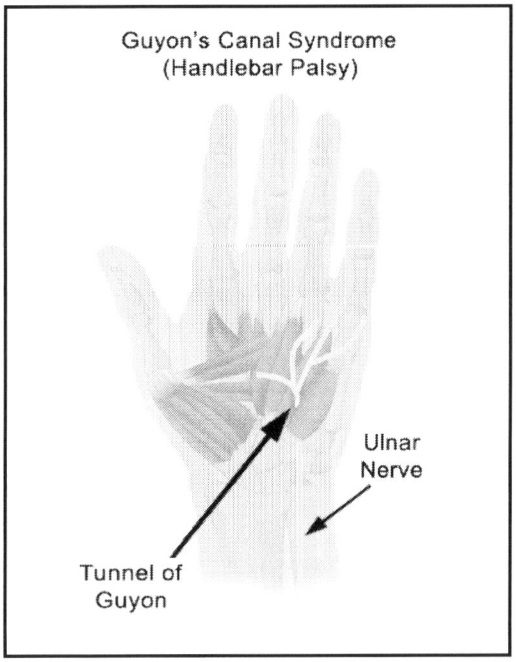

Figure 32.3 — Schematic representation Guyon's canal syndrome.[16]

1. Paresthesia, hyperesthesia, pain, or numbness affecting at least part of the median nerve distribution of the hand, and
2. Positive evidence of median nerve compression across the carpal tunnel based on either clinical evaluation (e.g., positive Tinel's sign, positive Phalen test result) or nerve conduction testing (electro-diagnosis).[28]

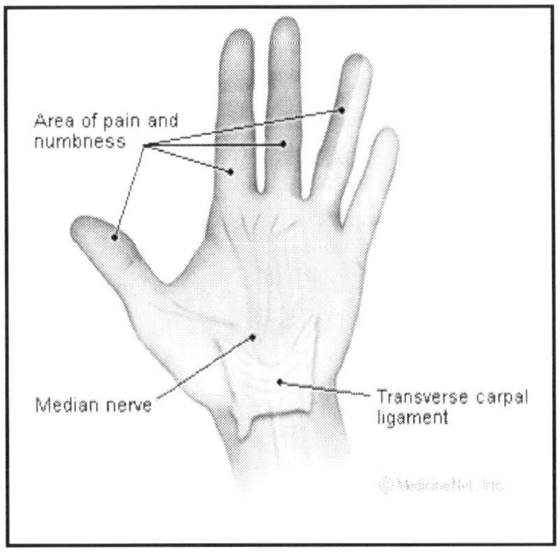

Figure 32.4 — Schematic representation of carpal tunnel syndrome and possible areas of pain.[20]

It is commonly accepted that for a diagnosis of CTS a person must have both numbness/ tingling in the fingers affected by the median nerve, and an abnormal nerve conduction study consistent with median mononeuropathy at the wrist.

Tendon Disorders (Tendonitis/Tenosynovitis)

Tendonitis refers to inflammation in tendons. Clinically, the term tendinitis is rather widely and vaguely used to refer to localized tenderness to palpation and localized soreness in response to passive stretching, or active contraction in a muscle-tendon unit. Similarly, tenosynovitis refers to any tendon sheath disorder regardless of etiology or the state of inflammation.[29]

Common sites of tendinitis in the distal upper extremity include the elbow and wrist. Two common tendinitis near the elbow are lateral epicondylitis (tennis elbow) on the lateral side of the arm near the elbow, and medial epicondylitis (golfer's elbow) on the medial side of the arm.[30] Wrist tendinitis includes wrist extensor tendinitis (dorsal wrist pain with positive resisted wrist extension) and digital flexor tendinitis (volar wrist pain and digital flexor tenderness). Digital flexor tendinitis include flexor carpi radialis tendinitis with its symptoms on the volar radial aspect of the wrist, and flexor carpi ulnaris tendinitis with its symptoms on ulnar side.[31]

The common tenosynovitis includes de Quervain and trigger finger and/or trigger thumb. De Quervain's tenosynovitis is also called as stenosing tenosynovitis of the radial styloid process, stenosing tenosynovitis of the first dorsal compartment, De Quervain's disease, de Quervain's tendonitis, and de Quervain's stenosing tenosynovitis. It refers to an inflammatory process on the radial aspect of the wrist involving the first dorsal retinacular compartment containing the tendons of the abductor pollicis longus and extensor pollicis brevis.[32] Trigger finger or trigger thumb (also called as digital stenosing tenosynovitis) refers to an inflammatory process of the digital flexor tendon sheaths affecting the fingers. It results in painful locking of the involved digit.

The reported causes for tendinitis and tenosynovitis include both acute trauma and chronic trauma related to overexertion or extensive use.[33–36] Tendinitis is most common among middle-aged to older adults.[37] Some of the common DUE disorders and their diagnoses are summarized in Table 32.1.[27,28,30–32]

Delayed-Onset Muscular Soreness

Delayed-onset muscular soreness is defined as muscle soreness due to microscopic tearing

Table 32.1 — Common DUE disorders and their diagnoses

Disorder	*Symptoms and Physical examinations*
Carpal tunnel syndrome	• Numbness/Tingling in digits (1–4) • Abnormal nerve conduction study consistent with median mononeuropathy at the wrist.
Lateral Epicondylitis	• Lateral elbow pain • Pain upon palpation of 1 or more lateral tender points • Resisted wrist extension test (optional)
Medial Epicondylitis	• Medial elbow pain • Pain upon palpation of 1 or more of 2 medial tender points • Resisted wrist flexion (optional)
DeQuervain's	• Radial wrist pain • Tenderness over 1st extensor compartment • Positive Finkelstein test
Wrist Extensor Tendinitis	• Dorsal wrist pain • Tenderness over 2–6 extensor compartment • Positive resisted wrist extension
Digital Flexor Tendinitis	• Volar wrist pain • Digital flexor tendon tenderness
Trigger Finger / Trigger Thumb	• Triggering of finger(s) and/or thumb • Tenderness over A-1 pulley • Pain in the finger

of the muscle fibers from 24 to 48 hours after high-force application, especially eccentric muscle contractions.[38–44] The cause for delayed-onset muscular soreness is believed to be unaccustomed, vigorous physical activity with eccentric muscle contractions.[41–45] Symptoms include muscle pain, swelling, decreased muscle endurance, muscle soreness and/or stiffness hours or days after exercise.[38–40] The symptoms subside after 5 to 7 days.[38,40]

Muscle strain is defined an injury to a muscle such as overstretching of a muscle or tears in muscle fibers. It can be caused by an accident or excessive physical activity or effort. Symptoms include pain, difficulty in moving the injured muscle, discoloration, bruised skin, and/ swelling. When damage or injury such as tearing occurs to a ligament it is called ligament sprain. Non specific pain is defined as reported pain in a body part with no diagnosed specific disorder.

Risk Factors for Distal Upper Extremity Disorders

There is substantial evidence that physical work is associated with DUE disorders. The most commonly studied DUE disorder is carpal tunnel syndrome (CTS).[26–29,46,47] Generic risk factors for DUE disorders include forceful exertion, high repetition and awkward hand/wrist posture.[22,48] In a review of epidemiological literature, NIOSH[49] found that there was insufficient evidence for posture alone to be a risk factor, though other studies have indicated posture as a risk factor. Many people believe that lack of job rotation is a risk factor but there is little data on job rotation and risk of DUE disorders. Keyboard activities have been found to have either no association or at most a weak association with DUE disorders. Other generic risk factors for DUE disorders mentioned in the literature include unaccustomed work, stress concentration, hand/wrist/forearm contact with sharp surfaces, duration of task per day, insufficient recovery time, static work, pinch grasp, exposure to hand/arm vibration, exposure to cold temperature and poorly fitting gloves. There are insufficient epidemiological studies on many of these potential risk factors except hand/arm vibration. Several studies have shown that hand/arm vibration is associated with DUE disorders.

Epidemiological literature suggests that certain individual factors are associated with DUE disorders. These include age (with peak incidence around the sixth decade), BMI, history of arthritis, pregnancy, diabetes and thyroid disease. Consistent associations between DUE disorders and smoking status, birth control pill use or hormone replacement therapy and gout are less well established.

There are relatively few studies on psychosocial factors and DUE disorders and no consistent associations have been reported.

Distal Upper Extremity Job Analysis Methods

WISHA Checklist

Checklists are generally used as a surveillance tool. They tend to have high sensitivity and low specificity. One of the most comprehensive checklists is from the Washington State Department of Labor & Industries.[50] The purpose of this checklist is to identify employee exposure to specific workplace hazards that can cause or aggravate work-related musculoskeletal disorders (WMSDs). A "caution zone job" is a job where an employee's typical work activities include any of the specific physical risk factors shown in Table 32.2 a,b,c. Typical work activities are those that are a regular and foreseeable part of the job and occur on more than one day per week, and more frequently than one week per year. To use this checklist the evaluator first determines whether any physical risk factors that apply are present that would cause categorization as a "caution zone job". If all the conditions for a caution job are satisfied, a WMSC hazard exists.

ACGIH® Threshold Limit Value (TLV®) for Hand Activity Level (HAL)

In 2001, the ACGIH® Worldwide, a private, non-profit professional organization, published a Threshold Limit Value for Hand Activity Level (TLV® for HAL).[51] The TLV® for HAL is based on two job physical exposure factors: (1) hand activity level (HAL) and (2) normalized peak hand force (Figure 32.5). The guideline includes both a TLV® and a lower limit called the 'Action Limit.' Physical exposure above the TLV® is believed to be

Table 32.2 — WISHA checklist (a) specific risk factor for each body posture (b) high hand force (c) highly repetitive motion (d) repeated impact.(50)

(a)

Body Part	*Risk Factor*	*Duration*	*Visual*	
Shoulders	Working with the hand(s) above the head or the elbow(s) above the shoulders	> 4 hours total per day	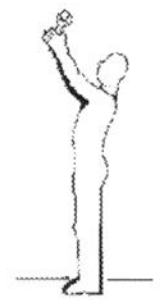	☐
Shoulders	Repetitively raising the hand(s) above the head or the elbow(s) above the shoulder(s) more than once per minute	> 4 hours total per day	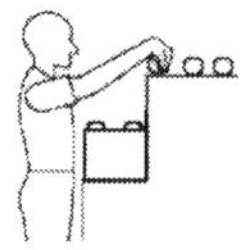	☐
Neck	Working with the neck bent more than 45° (without support or the ability to vary posture)	> 4 hours total per day	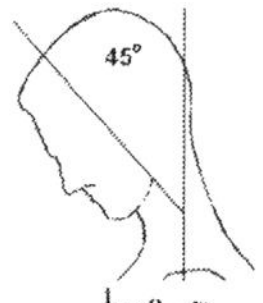	☐
Back	Working with the back bent forward more than 30° (without support or the ability to vary posture)	> 4 hours total per day	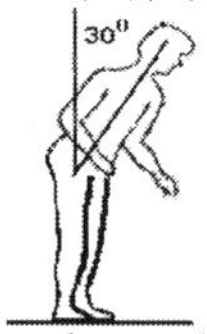	☐
Back	Working with the back bent forward more than 45° (without support or the ability to vary posture)	> 2 hours total per day	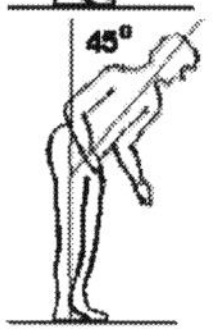	☐
Knees	Squatting	> 4 hours total per day	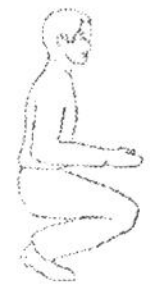	☐
Knees	Kneeling	> 2 hours total per day	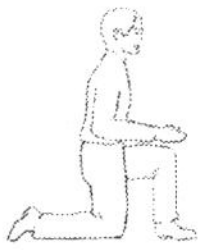	☐

(b)

Risk Factor	*Combined with*	*Duration*	*Visual*
Gripping an un-supported object(s) weighing 10 or more pounds per hand, or gripping with a force of 10 or more pounds per hand (comparable to clamping light duty automotive jumper cables onto a battery)	Highly repetitive motion	> 3 hours total per day	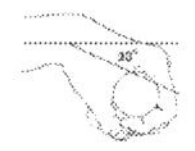
	Wrist flexion ≥ 30° or extension ≥ 45° or ulnar deviation ≥ 30 °	> 3 hours total per day	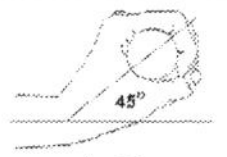 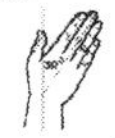 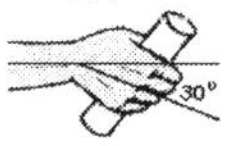
	No other risk factors	> 4 hours total per day	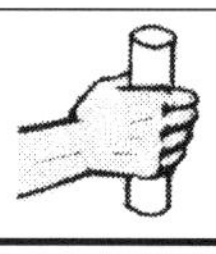

Table 32.2 — WISHA checklist (a) specific risk factor for each body posture (b) high hand force (c) highly repetitive motion (d) repeated impact (continued).[50]

(c)

Risk Factor	*Combined with*	*Duration*	
Using the same motion with little or no variation every few seconds (excluding keying activities)	No other risk factors	> 6 hours total per day	☐
Using the same motion with little or no variation every few seconds (excluding keying activities)	Wrist flexion ≥ 30° or extension ≥ 45° or ulnar deviation ≥ 30 ° AND High, forceful exertions with the hands	> 2 hours total per day	☐
Intensive keying	Wrist flexion ≥ 30° or extension ≥ 45° or ulnar deviation ≥ 30°	> 4 hours total per day	☐
Intensive keying	No other risk factors	> 7 hours total per day	☐

(d)

Risk Factor	*Duration*	*Visual*	
Using the hand (heel/base of palm) as a hammer > 1 per minute	> 2 hours total per day	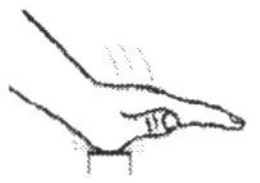	☐
Using the knee as a hammer > 1 per minute	> 2 hours total per day	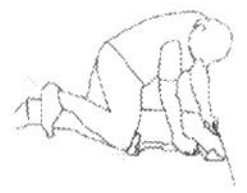	☐

unsafe. The Action Limit represents a set for conditions to which it is believed that nearly all workers may be repeatedly exposed without adverse health effects. Physical exposure above the Action Limit and below the TLV® is treated as concern zone.

There are two options for determining Hand Activity Level (HAL). The first method is to use at least three trained observers. Observers rate the Hand Activity Level using the scale shown in Figure 32.6.

Consensus among three or more trained observers is used to assign the HAL rating. The second option is to use the HAL Table (Table 32.3) that utilizes frequency (number of exertions per second) and duty cycle (% duration of exertion).

There are many different methods for determining normalized peak force. The simplest method is to use the following equation:

$$RPE_{50th\ \%\ M/F} = (RPE_{subject}) \times \left(\frac{\text{Max Strength}_{subject}}{\text{Max Strength}_{50th\ \%\ M/F}} \right) \quad (32\text{-}1)$$

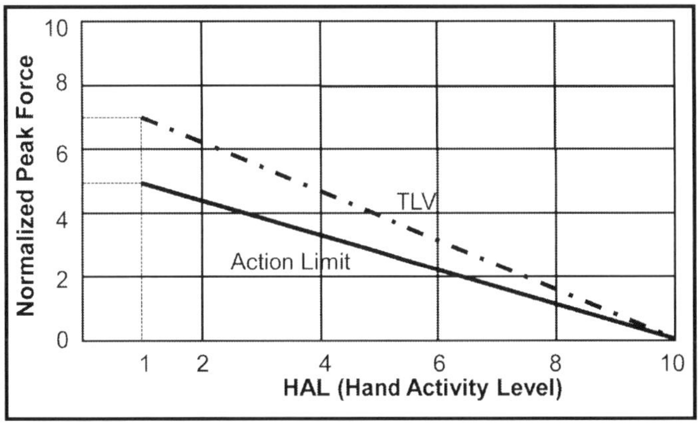

Figure 32.5 — TLVs® and action Limit for hand activity level (HAL) and normalized peak hand force.[51]

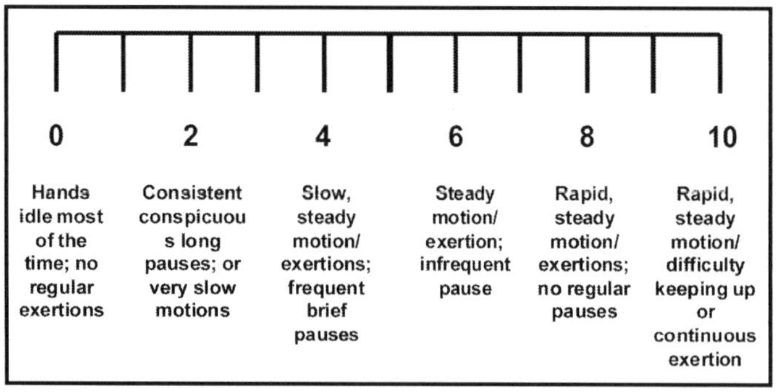

Figure 32.6 — Hand activity level scale.[51]

where RPE represents the subject's rating of perceived exertion for peak force using the Borg CR-10 scale.[52] Some studies have used observer rating to determine normalized peak force.

The TLV® is only intended to apply to "mono-task jobs" performed four or more hours per day. A "mono-task job" is defined as one that "involves performing a similar set of motions or exertions repeatedly, such as working on an assembly line or using a keyboard and mouse."

Epidemiological studies performed with the TLV® for Hand Activity have shown conflicting results. Studies by Gell at al.[53] and Werner et al.[54] found that TLV® for HAL did not predict the risk of CTS.[53,55] Similarly, a study of cashiers was negative.[46] However, a cohort study demonstrated that the TLV® for Hand Activity predicted a 3-fold risk of CTS among a cohort of 2,092 workers followed for 1 year.[47]

TLV® for HAL example

Workers were observed assembling wiring harnesses. The job included stripping and cutting wire, twisting exposed wire ends, applying wire nuts, and applying plastic cable ties. Automated equipment was provided to cut and strip wire, a pneumatic hand-tool was provided to apply wire nuts, and a power-grip actuated hand-tool was provided to apply cable ties. The work pace was brisk and there were few opportunities for more than a second or so of "rest."

Three analysts observed the job and provided their ratings of hand activity level (HAL) and normalized peak force (NPV, using the Borg CR-10 scale). Based on consensus, they agreed to use the hand activity level verbal anchor scale, the hand activity level for the job was rated as "rapid steady motion/exertions; no regular pauses;" this corresponds to a HAL rating of 8. After each analyst tried the job for several cycles, they agreed that the effort required to perform the job was "light" on the Borg CR-10 scale (corresponding to a normalized peak force of 2). The combination of peak force with a rating of 2 (vertical axis) and HAL rating of 8 (horizontal axis) falls above TLV® in Figure 32.5) Therefore, this job would be classified as hazardous.

Table 32.3 — The HAL Table with frequency (number of exertions per second) and duty cycle (% duration of exertion)

Frequency (exertions per second)	*Period (seconds per exertion)*	*Duty Cycle (% of duration of exertion)*				
		0–20	*20–40*	*40–60*	*60–80*	*80–100*
0.125	8.0	1	1	—	—	—
0.25	4.0	2	2	3	—	—
0.5	2.0	3	4	5	5	6
1.0	1.0	4	5	5	6	7
2.0	0.5	—	5	6	7	8

The Strain Index

The Strain Index is a job analysis tool to identify jobs that do and do not expose workers to an increased risk of developing a distal upper extremity (DUE) disorder.[48] The Strain Index is a semi quantitative job analysis method that provides a numerical score (SI score) that is believed to be related to the risk of developing DUE musculoskeletal disorders (MSDs). The Strain Index was derived from principles related to the physiology, biomechanics, and the epidemiology of DUE disorders.[48] The SI score is the product of six multipliers that correspond to six job physical variables. The six job variables are: Intensity of Exertion, Duration of Exertion per Cycle, Efforts per Minute, Hand/Wrist Posture, Speed of Work, and Duration of Task per Day to describe the exertional demands of a job.[48] All six job variables are rated on a scale of 1 to 5 (Tables 32.4 and 32.5).

The Intensity of Exertion is the most critical variable in the Strain Index. It describes the force requirements of a job and reflects the magnitude of muscular effort required to perform the task once. It does not reflect stresses related to fatigue from repetitive work. The Intensity of Exertion rating can be determined either by using the verbal descriptors listed in Table 32.4, or expressing the force requirements of the task as a percentage of the worker's maximum voluntary contraction (%MVC).

The Duration of Exertion task variable is defined as the percentage of the cycle time that exertions are applied. To determine Duration of Exertion (Eq. 32-2), the cycle time and the total time of all exertions must be measured. Percent duration of exertion, the percentage of the job cycle spent applying force, is calculated by dividing the average duration of exertion per cycle by the average cycle time and multiplying by 100.

$$\%\text{ Duration of Exertion} = \frac{(\text{Average Duration of Exertion per Cycle})}{(\text{Average Exertional Cycle Time})} \times 100 \quad (32\text{-}2)$$

The task variable Efforts per Minute is the number of force exertions per minute and represents the repetitiveness of the job being analyzed. To measure effort/min., the number of exertions that occur during an average, exertional cycle time is counted and then this count is divided by the cycle time.

Hand/Wrist Posture refers to the anatomical position of the hand or wrist relative to the anatomical neutral position. It reflects the stresses to the distal upper extremity when working in a non-neutral hand/wrist posture. Often, hand/wrist posture is rated qualitatively rather than measuring it directly. A rating for hand/wrist posture is assigned using the verbal anchors in Table 32.5.

Speed of Work refers to the pace of a task or job. It is subjectively estimated using the verbal anchors provided in Table 32.5. A "fast" speed of work means that a worker is working at a rapid pace higher than "normal" but is not overtly rushed. The rating "very fast" implies that the worker is either unable or barely able to keep up with the required pace of job and appears overly rushed.

Table 32.4 — Percent MVC or the verbal descriptors used to determine the rating for Intensity of Exertion task variable in the Strain Index.

Rating Category	*Verbal Descriptor*	*% MVC*
1	Light	< 10
2	Somewhat Hard	10 to 29
3	Hard	20 to 49
4	Very Hard	50 to 79
5	Near Maximal	> 80

Duration of Task per Day refers to the total time that a job is performed per day. The objective is to account for beneficial effects of task diversity such as job rotation, assuming the other job(s) do not load the same muscle tendon units to the same extent. It also accounts for the adverse effects of performing the same job for a prolonged period of time. Duration of Task per Day is measured and expressed in hours/day. A rating for Duration of Task per Day is assigned according to Table 32.5.

Strain Index Multipliers and Strain Index Score

Corresponding to each task variable and its rating in the Strain Index there is a multiplier value, given in Table 32.6. The Strain Index Score is the product of all six multipliers. After each of the six task variables are assigned ratings, the Strain Index Score is calculated by multiplying the six multipliers for each of the six task variables as shown in Equation 32-3.

Strain Index (SI) = (32-3)
(Intensity of Exertion Multiplier) ×
(Duration of Exertion Multiplier) ×
(Exertions per Minute Multiplier) ×
(Posture Multiplier) × (Speed of Work Multiplier) ×
(Duration per Day Multiplier)

The Strain Index Score is used to assign the hazard classification. Moore and Garg[48]

Table 32.5 — Rating scales for the six Strain Index task variables (ordinal ratings varying from one to five for the six Strain Index task variables).[48]

Rating	*Intensity of Exertion*	*%Duration of Exertion*	*Efforts per Minute*	*Hand/Wrist Posture*	*Speed of Work*	*Duration per Day (hrs)*
1	Light	< 10%	< 4	Very Good	Very Slow	< 1
2	Somewhat Hard	10% – 30%	4 – 8	Good	Slow	1 – 2
3	Hard	30% – 50%	9 – 14	Fair	Fair	2 – 4
4	Very Hard	50% – 80%	15 – 19	Bad	Fast	4 – 8
5	Near Maximal	> 80%	20	Very Bad	Very Fast	> 8

Table 32.6 — The Strain Index multipliers for the six task variables.[48]

Rating	*Intensity of Exertion*	*Duration of Exertion*	*Efforts per Minute*	*Hand/Wrist Posture*	*Speed of Work*	*Duration per Day*
1	❑	0.5	0.5	1	❑	0.25
2	3	1	1	1	1	0.5
3	6	1.5	1.5	1.5	1	0.75
4	9	2	2	2	1.5	1
5	13	3	3	3	3	1.5

recommended a threshold value of five. A Strain Index score of five or greater suggests that a job is hazardous.[48] Knox and Moore[56] supported a SI Score criterion of 5.0 for hazard classification, but the study suggested that the 5.0 criterion value might be too high. Moore et al.[57] found a cut off value of 5.0 to be predictive. Rucker and Moore[58] substantiated the use of 5.0 as the criterion Strain Index Score for classifying jobs as "hazardous" versus "safe", but the study suggested that a more appropriate criterion might be about 9 for manufacturing jobs. Moore et al.[59] concluded that a SI Score of 6.1 worked the best when the analysis was performed on combined jobs from all three previous studies.

Example of Strain Index Analysis

A worker was assembling small electronics parts. With her left hand, she held an assembly using a loose oblique grip with her wrist extended approximately 45° from anatomical neutral. The assembly weighed only a few ounces (< 1 lb). With her right hand she picked up small plastic lenses and placed them in the assembly. She held each lens using a multipoint pinch; her right wrist was typically extended approximately 30° from anatomical neutral. Each lens weighed less than one ounce. On average she placed one lens in the assembly every 4 seconds, thus she performed an average of 15 efforts per minute with her right hand. Each assembly held 20 lenses. On average it took 80 seconds to insert all the lenses into an assembly. Of those 80 seconds approximately 50 seconds were spent with her right hand holding a lens and 30 seconds were spent with her hand empty (preparing to pick up a new lens). The total cycle time was typically 85 seconds per assembly, including the time it took to place a finished assembly and pick up a new finished assembly. Since approximately 50 seconds of that cycle were spent with the right hand holding a lens, duration of exertion for the right hand is 50s ÷ 85s = 59%. Similarly, since her left hand held each assembly until it was complete and then picked up a new, empty assembly, her left hand performed approximately 0.7 efforts per minute (1 effort every 85 seconds) and has a duration of exertion of 82s ÷ 85s = 96%. The work was self-paced and while she did not "hurry," she did work quickly to be productive. She typically performed her job for 4 hours of an 8 hour shift.

Table 32.7 summarizes job parameters as well as the corresponding Strain Index ratings and multipliers for the right and left hand of the worker.

Using the multipliers from this table find the Strain Index score for the left hand is determined:

Table 32.7 — Strain Index ratings and multipliers for the right and left hand of the worker for the Strain Index example.

	Intensity of Exertion	*Duration of Exertion*	*Efforts per Minute*	*Hand/Wrist Posture*	*Speed of Work*	*Duration per Day*
Left Hand						
Parameter	<10% MVC	96%	0.7	30° Ext.	Fair	4hrs
SI Category	Light	> 80%	< 4	Fair	Fair	2-4
Rating	1	5	1	3	3	2
Multiplier	1	3	0.5	1.5	1	0.5
Right Hand						
Parameter	<10% MVC	59%	15	45° Ext.	Fair	4hrs
SI Category	Light	50 - 80%	15 - 19	Bad	Fair	2-4
Rating	1	4	4	4	3	2
Multiplier	1	2	2	2	1	0.5

$SI = 1 \times 3 \times 0.5 \times 1.5 \times 1 \times 0.5 = 1.13$

Since this score is less than 6.1, the job is determined to be low risk for DUE injuries. Similarly, the Strain Index score for the right hand is

$SI = 1 \times 2 \times 2 \times 2 \times 1 \times 0.5 = 4.0$

Once again the score is less than 6.1 and the job is determined to be low risk for DUE injuries.

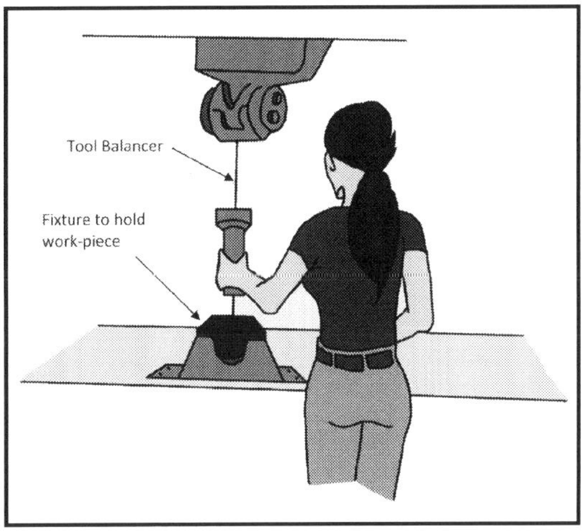

Figure 32.7 — Tool balancer for heavy tools.[60]

Hand Tool Design

The following are the recommendations for hand tool design:

Tool Weight

- Whenever possible, use lightweight hand tools (0.5–1.5 kg). Avoid tools heavier than 1.7 kg.
- For heavy tools, and or tools used with high repetition, use a tool balancer to support the tool weight, together with a fixture to hold the work piece (Figure 32.7).
- When selecting hand tools remember that heavier tools and/or higher applied forces require longer rest breaks than lighter hand tools and/or lower applied forces (see DUE Job Analysis Methods for further information).

Tool Shape

- Keep the center of gravity of a tool as close to the center of grip as possible to reduce the bending moment on the wrist and to avoid rotation and slipping of the tool from the hand (Figure 32.8a).
- Minimize torque on the wrist by keeping the applied force and tool thrust force in the same line (Figure 32.8b).
- Use long handles (> 11.4 cm) on wrenches (Figure 32.9a), shears, or pliers to utilize mechanical advantage and to reduce the applied force (AF).
- Avoid stress concentration in the palm (Figure 32.9b) :
    - Use a T-shaped handle to pull toward the body.
    - Use a cylindrical handle with flange at the base to apply downward force.

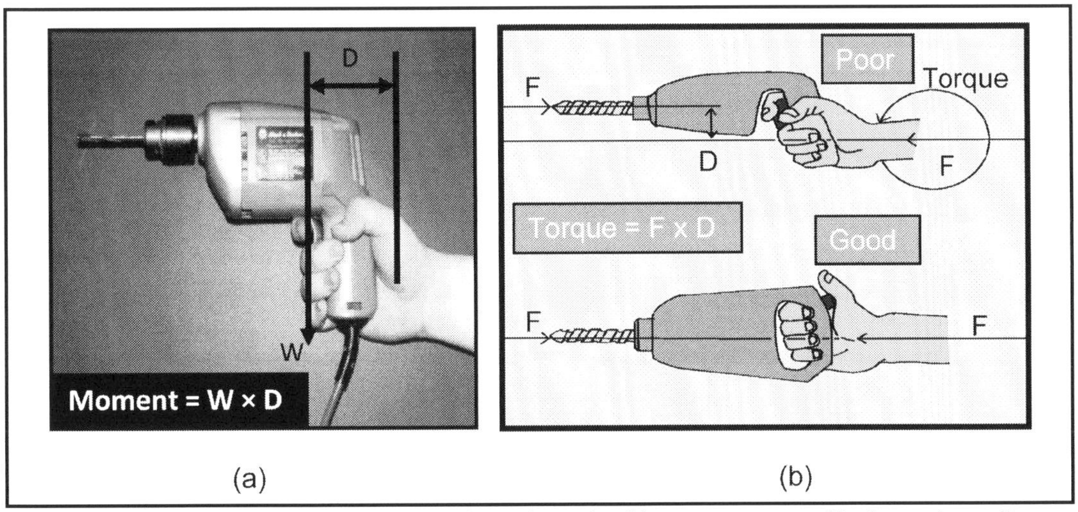

Figure 32.8 — (a) The moment generated by the tool weight; (b) Torque generated by force, depending on the alignment of the forearm with the force application point.[60]

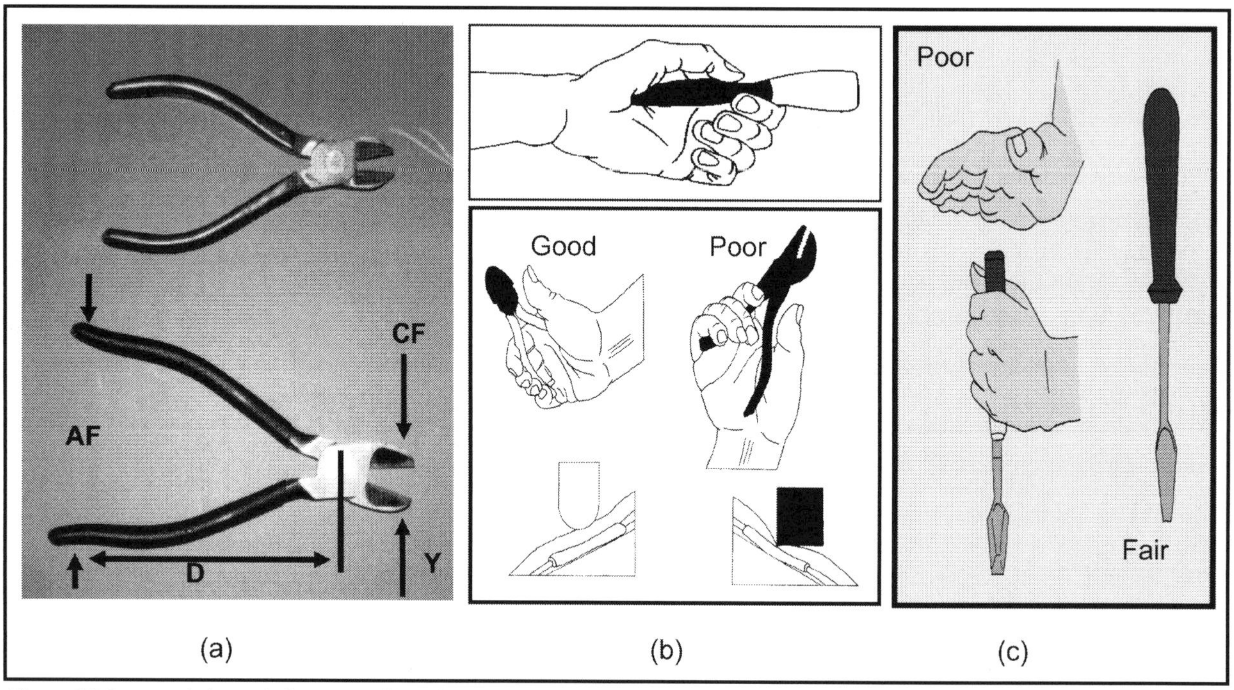

Figure 32.9 — Tool shape is better with (a) long handles; (b) avoid stress concentration on the palm; and (c) rounded and cushioned handle top is less harmful when using hand as a hammer.[60]

- Use pneumatic, electric or battery powered hand tools rather than manually powered tools.
- Avoid using square handles.

- Avoid use of the palm as a hammer. If palm of the hand must be used to apply force, provide a rounded and cushioned handle top (Figure 32.9c).
- Recommended handle design dimensions:
  - Refer to Figure 32.10a for handle grip dimensions.
  - Use sleeves on the handle (Figure 32.10b) to provide soft surfaces to reduce contact pressure on the hand and to provide high friction with the hand to increase manipulability.
  - Bend the tool to reduce deviation of the wrist (Figure 32.10c).
  - Choose a tool or orient the work surface to reduce awkward posture of the shoulder and upper extremity (Figure 32.11).
  - Use a tool extension to reduce reaching (see Figure 32.12a).

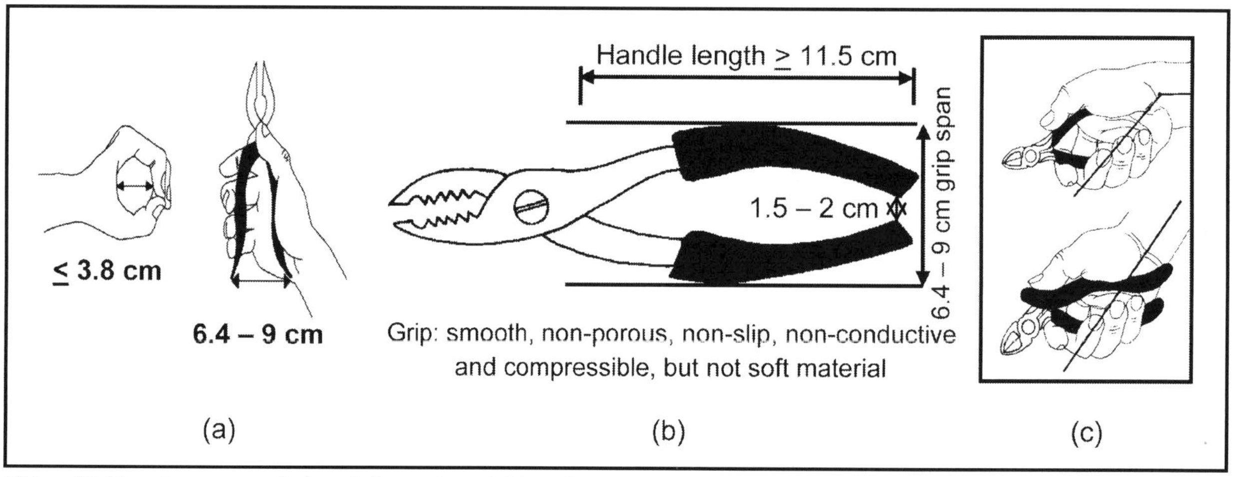

Figure 32.10 — Recommended tool dimensions: (a) handle grip dimensions; (b) handle length dimensions; and (c) reduced wrist ulnar deviation by tool handle design.[60,61]

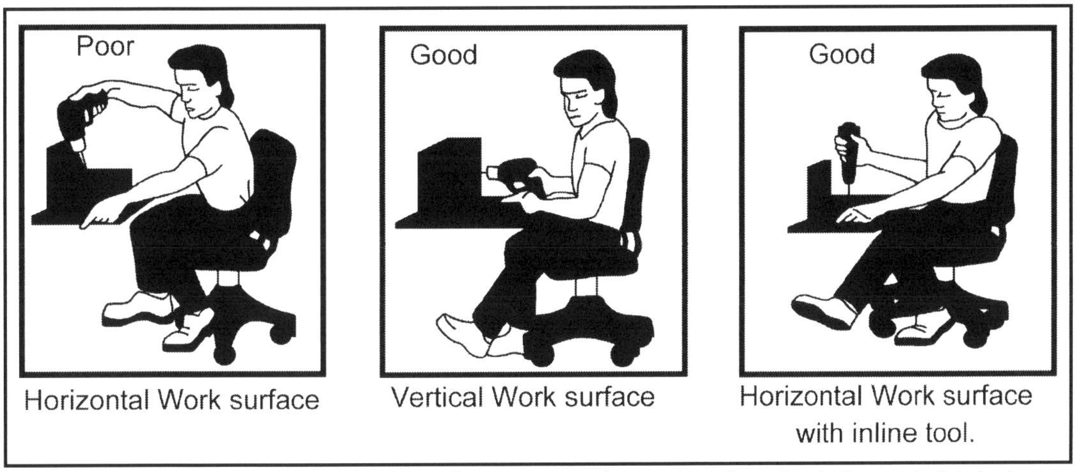

Figure 32.11 — Reducing awkward wrist and upper extremity postures by using inline and pistol grip tools appropriately.[60]

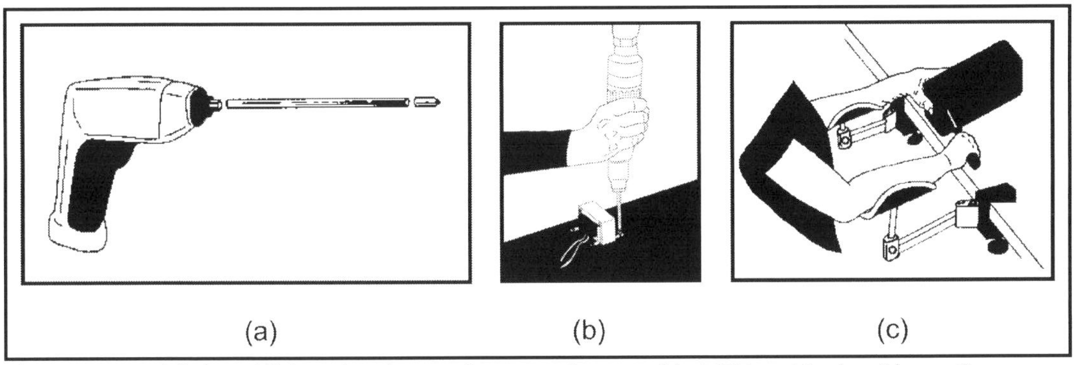

Figure 32.12 — (a) The addition of tool extensions to reduce reaching; (b) hand tools with reaction torque; and (c) the addition of arm supports to workstations for tasks that require non-varying repetitive tasks or assembly work.[60]

- Avoid tool reaction torque (Figure 32.12b) (force required to prevent the tool from rotating in the hand at the end of final tightening) from nut runners by using shut-off tools with:
  - Preset torque shut off
  - Automatic mechanical clutch
  - Hydraulic pulse system
  - Air-flow shut-off
- Tool maintenance
  - Replace worn-out tools with new tools (blades, bits, brushes, blunt edges, etc.). Worn-out tools require more force.
- Workstation design
  - Provide arm supports for assembly work (Figure 32.12c)
  - For overhead work, use a hand tool that is attached to a fixture and can be operated with controls located at elbow height to reduce shoulder flexion and abduction.
  - Reduce elbow extension and shoulder flexion.
  - Keep shoulder abduction angle at 20° or less (Figure 32.15a).

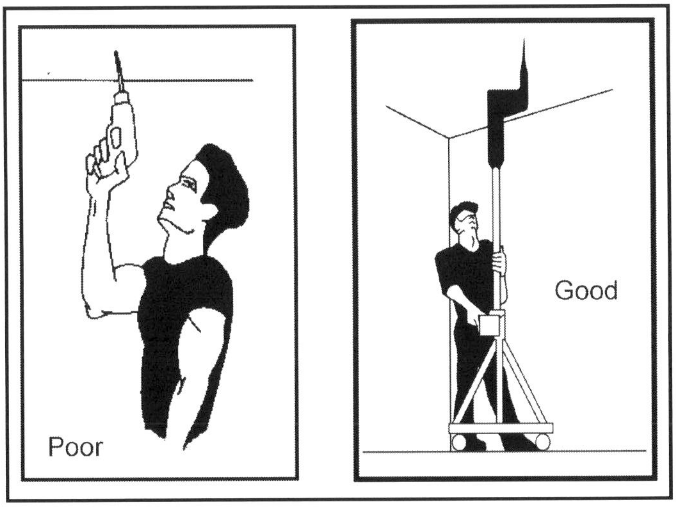

Figure 32.13 — Tool adaption with controls at the elbow height to reduce shoulder flexion.[60]

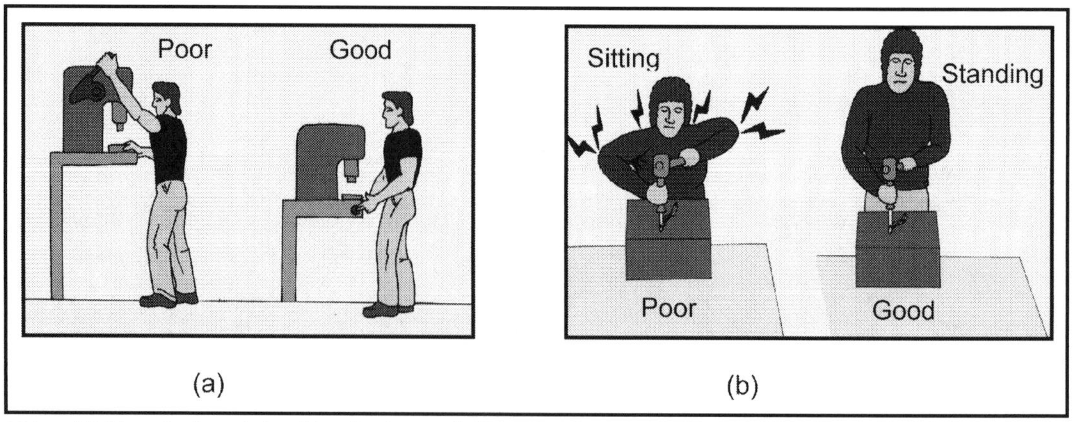

Figure 32.14 — Reduced shoulder flexion and abduction by (a) relocating controls and (b) changing sitting workstation to standing workstation position.[60]

- Avoid sustained trunk flexion greater than 20° (Figure 32.15b).
- Avoid contact with sharp or hard surfaces (Figure 32.16) (base of the wrist, forearm, and elbow).
- Provide frequent rest breaks of short duration.
- Minimize unaccustomed work.
- Reduce highly repetitive movements and encourage task and workstation rotations (Figure 32.17).

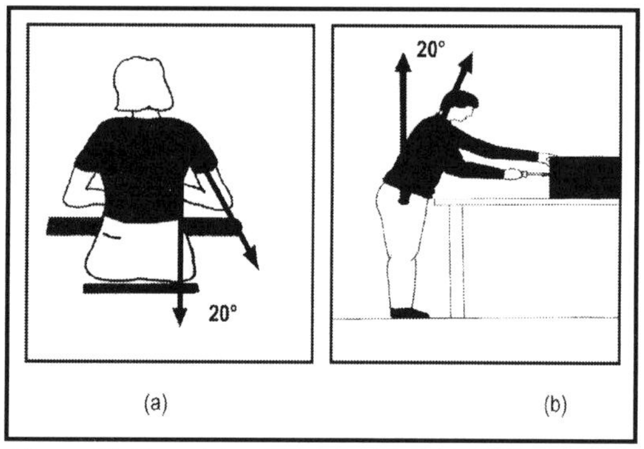

Figure 32.15 — (a) Minimize shoulder abduction angle to 20° or less. (b) Avoid sustained trunk flexion of greater than 20°.[60]

- Limit overtime.
- Frequent breaks of shorter duration are preferred over fewer breaks of longer duration.

Workstation Design

The proper design of a workstation should consider many factors, individually as well as jointly: work space, work surfaces, seats, and design and layout of the equipment.

The workspace should be large enough to enable dynamic movement and provide room for worker's manipulation with tools. Implementing appropriate workplace design principles can help to improve work habits and thereby reduce the risk of developing musculoskeletal disorders (MSDs) such as back, neck, shoulder and/or hand/wrist pain and associated disorders.

What factors need to be considered and how do they affect the design? When is a seated or standing workstation more appropriate? What are the effects of poor workstation design? These issues are discussed below.

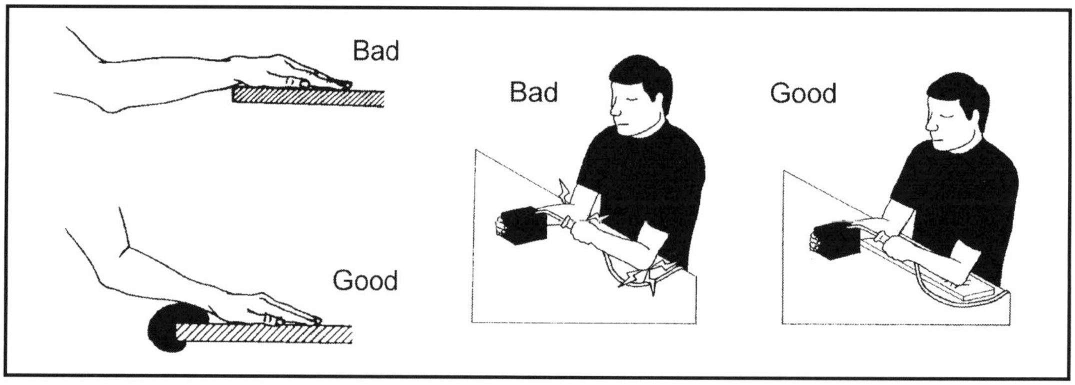

Figure 32.16 — Providing cushioned surface to rest forearm to avoid sharp or hard contact surfaces.[60]

Workstation Design Factors

Many factors contribute to proper workstation design and, conversely, many of these factors, if improperly handled, can lead to a workstation contributing to the development of MSDs. The factors affecting workstation design fall into two broad categories, namely task requirements and user characteristics.

Task Requirements: A workstation should be designed to accomplish the intended tasks. Since tasks can vary greatly in their requirements, the workstation design must consider all of the tasks for which it is to be used, and weigh the requirements of the various tasks to arrive at the best possible design. Typical task requirements to be evaluated include: visual, positional, force, time constraints, repetitive motion, and work pace.

User Characteristics: It is obvious that the characteristics of a workstation user will affect the ideal design. However, it is often true that the user is ignored in the design process. Failure to account for the range of typical user characteristics will probably result in a workstation that is suited to the task, but not to the person performing the task. A partial list of the user characteristics affecting workstation design includes: age, gender, height, body weight, strength, range of motion, eyesight, handedness, and existing MSDs. The designer must determine which characteristics are most important in performing the task and which are most likely to result in injury or lead to the development of an MSD if not correctly accounted for.

Design Principles

Three basic principles are normally employed in workstation design: design for the extreme, design for the average, and design for adjustability. Designing for the extreme or an average person results in a fixed workstation with, at most, limited adjustability. Each method has advantages and disadvantages, and none is the best solution for all situations.

Design for the Extreme: As the name implies, designing for the extreme involves determining the anthropometric characteristic that is most important for the specific workstation and then designing to accommodate either the person with the smallest percentile (such as 5th percentile reach) or the person with the largest percentile (such as 95th percentile height). Designing for the extreme requires compromise between the requirement to fit the entire population and needs of some people with either small dimensions or large dimensions. For example, a workstation height designed to fit the 5th percentile person by height will be extremely low for the 95th percentile height user. This paradox is sometimes overcome by using two (or more) designs where appropriate. A bathroom may be fitted with two sinks, one designed for the 5th percentile height and another at a higher level for taller individuals.

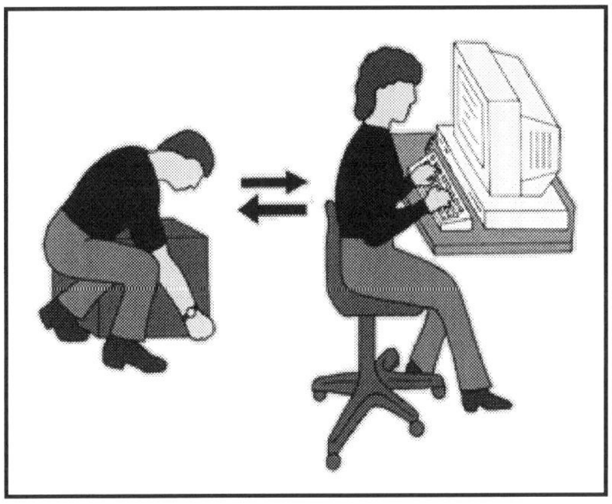

Figure 32.17 — Reducing physical fatigue by encouraging job rotation.

Design for the Average: A workstation may be designed to fit the "average" person, with the assumption that the design will also work, although it will not be ideal, for people on the extreme range of the anthropometric measure. The major difficulty in designing for the average is to determine what is meant by average in terms of anthropometry. A person with average arm length may not have the average shoulder height, and designing for the average for both dimensions may not produce a design that is particularly suited to anyone.

Design for Adjustability: Adjustable workstations can be designed to accommodate most individuals such as 5th percentile to 95th percentile. The parameters that must be adjustable, for example table height and tilt, are determined. For each parameter, the required range of adjustability is determined and that range is built into the workstation design. The use of commercially available equipment may somewhat limit the available range, but most items will accommodate most individuals. The biggest limitation on adjustability is cost. While it may be desirable to allow all features to be adjustable, it is often not practical. The designer must carefully choose which parts of a workstation really need to be adjustable.

Zone of Convenient Reach

A useful concept in workstation design is the zone of convenient reach (ZCR). ZCR was described by Pheasant[62] as the working area or horizontal or vertical space within which a worker can reach objects without bending forward. If the tasks to be performed and the required equipment and supplies all fall within the ZCR, the user will be able to maintain correct posture. The risk of MSDs may be reduced if the user does not have to bend excessively. In addition, Lim and Hoffman[63] reported a 10% increase in the worker efficiency resulting from a reduction in performance time when the arrangement of the workspace was within the ZCR.

The ZCR is easily calculated from the user anthropometry and the workstation dimension. ZCR depends upon two variables, the user's horizontal reach (*r*) and the vertical distance from the shoulder to the workstation (*d*) as illustrated in Figure 32.19 for 5th and 95th percentile female and male workers, respectively. If the arm is considered to be the hypotenuse of a triangle then:

$$ZCR^2 = r^2 - d^2 \qquad (32\text{-}4)$$

ZCR also does not determine whether a task can be performed at that reach, just that the worker will not need to bend forward. There are many postures within the ZCR that will have other restrictions such as the force required to perform the task, etc. It is also important to consider the visual constrains of the task. Visual requirements can be defined as an optimal visual distance or zone (OVZ) as illustrated in Figure 32.20 for the 5th percentile female and 95th percentile male.

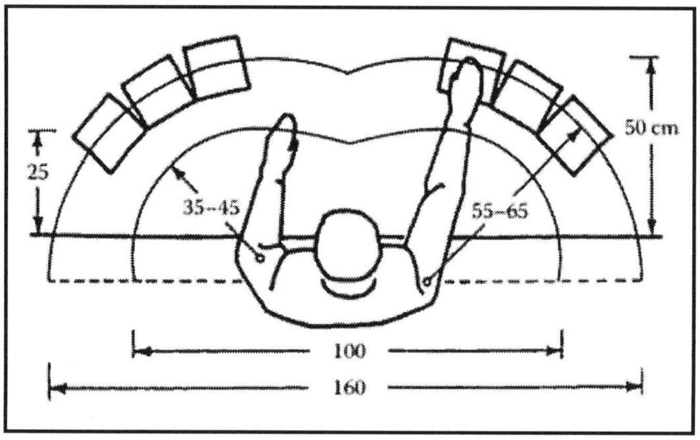

Figure 32.18 — Horizontal working area dimensions at the tabletop height.[64]

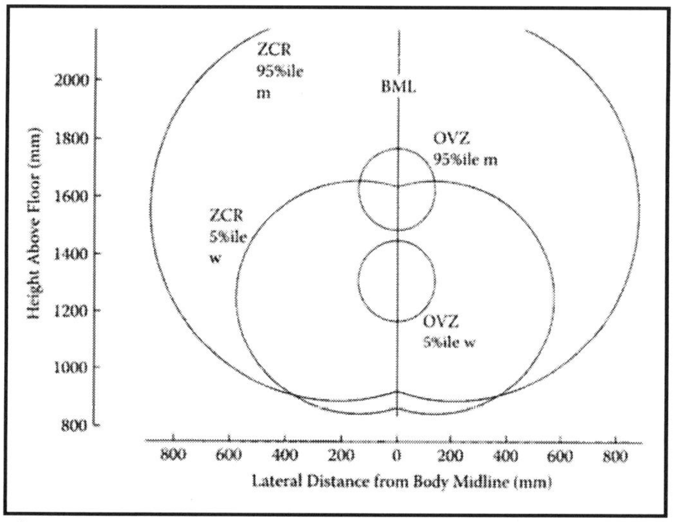

Figure 32.19 — Zone of convenient reach (ZCR) and optimal visual zone (OVZ) calculated from the body midline(BML) at the vertical distance of 500mm in front of the shoulders.[65]

Workstation Design Process

The workstation design process begins with an evaluation of the task requirements and user characteristics. Three issues that need to be considered are: what work is to be done, how it will be done, and who will be doing it. These questions provide the starting point for the design. For example, if a task requires the worker to lift a heavy item, and the worker is drawn from the general population, this will impose specific constraints on the workstation design. Task requirements can be further divided into visual requirements, postural requirements, and time constraints.

Visual Requirements: Tasks and objects that require frequent viewing should be kept at or below eye level with the head erect. For frequent viewing the user should not be required to extend their neck to look at objects above eye level. Similarly, if the objects need to be viewed frequently, the user should not have to look downward more than 30 degrees. Frequent neck flexion and maintaining the neck in a flexed posture may lead to neck pain. The visual requirements of a task also include the amount of lighting necessary to perform the task. Inadequate lighting (low level of lighting as well as too much lighting) may lead to poor posture and eye strain as the user struggles to see the work properly. The lighting requirements of a task depend upon the nature of the task. In general, tasks requiring fine manipulation require much more lighting than material handling tasks.

Postural Requirements: The position of the hands, arms, and feet, and the force requirements of the task have an impact on the risk of developing MSDs. The workstation must be designed to keep the extremities within their ZCR during task performance. If the workstation cannot be designed to accomplish this for all users, adjustability should be considered.

Time Constraints: Time constraints include both the time available to complete a specific task (i.e., how quickly the work must be performed) and the total amount of time spent on a task. Work that must be done quickly or that requires intense concentration may require frequent short breaks. Efforts should be made to place this type of work in the ZCR to minimize object retrieval time as well to reduce stresses to different body parts due to time constraint.

Based on an evaluation of the specific requirements for the workstation, either a seated or standing configuration should be chosen. Seated workstations are recommended when a task requires large force application with foot controls, use of both feet to control an action, precise foot control action, a high degree of stability and equilibrium, precise manual work, and/or long work periods. Conversely, standing workstations are indicated when legroom is not available, the task requires mobility.

Seated Workstation Design

If a seated workstation is indicated, the first step is to determine the correct height for the work surface. The correct seated working height depends on the nature of the task being performed and the user characteristics. In general, tasks requiring precision require a higher work surface height and tasks requiring exertion of forces require a lower work surface height. It is important to provide, at minimum, a height adjustable seat so that a single workstation can accommodate a wide range of users. Other adjustments may include back support, arm rests and foot support for increasing comfort and productivity.

Several guidelines regarding the desired position or work methodology help with designing other aspects of a seated workstation:

- Keep shoulder flexion and abduction angles to 20° or less. (Figure 32.15)
- Avoid hyperextension of the shoulder. Repeated reaching behind the body may cause shoulder tendonitis.
- Use arm supports for fine assembly work. (Figure 32.12c)
- Avoid contact with sharp or hard surfaces (wrist, forearm, and elbow). (Figure 32.16)
- Provide frequent rest breaks of short duration. Light work can be performed during rest time.

Standing Workstation Design

As with seated workstation design, standing workstation design begins with an evaluation of the tasks and users. It is usually recommended to keep the standing work surface height somewhere between knuckle and elbow height. However, for precision work, the surface height should be higher than elbow height. Workers vary in height, therefore it is preferable, when possible, to have an adjustable (manually or electrically) work surface height. Lighting is also very important, since it may affect the whole body posture. Several other factors to consider during standing workstation design include:

- Standing workstation design should reduce shoulder flexion (Figure 32.14)
- Properly adjust work surface height so the arms can be lowered, especially for tasks requiring application of forces (Figure 32.14)
- Avoid contact with sharp surfaces (Figure 32.16)
- Avoid sustained trunk flexion greater than 20° (Figure 32.15b)
- Avoid twisting of the trunk, especially when under heavy load.

Shoulder

There is a high prevalence of shoulder musculoskeletal disorders (MSDs) in the general population. Increased risk for shoulder pain and disorders is reported in those with jobs requiring overhead work.[48,66–71] Shoulder MSDs are also associated with a large proportion of lost or restricted days (median = 12).[70,72] Shoulder MSDs are costly, having an average total direct cost of $11,565 per shoulder claim and over $24,626 per case of rotator cuff tendinitis in Washington State.[73]

There are two primary theoretical biomechanical concerns for overhead work: (1) mechanical compression and (2) impaired blood supply. The compression of the supraspinatus tendon occurs between the humeral head and acromion process (mechanical impingement). Reduced blood flow, especially to the supraspinatus and infraspinatus muscles, is believed to occur due to an increase in intramuscular pressure, particularly when the upper arm is elevated. Since the pathophysiology of shoulder disorders is unclear, the actual mechanism for these disorders is also unclear.[74,75]

It is believed that the suprapsinatus and/or infraspinatus are the most vulnerable muscles when working with the arms elevated.[76–84] High activity in the shoulder muscles (EMG), especially in the supraspinatus and infraspinatus muscles, has been reported in elevated arm positions.[79–82,85–95] However, most studies have used trapezius EMG to study total shoulder muscle load.[89–93,95–99]

Prolonged work with elevated arms will impede muscle blood flow in the rotator cuff muscles and this might lead to localized muscle fatigue.[100] However, it is unclear what combination of arm position, duration of maintaining that posture and applied force is harmful.[49,101] At present, generally acceptable methods to quantify shoulder muscle load in relation to shoulder pain and shoulder impairment and disability are lacking.[77,99,101,102] It is difficult to recommend guidelines to prevent work-related shoulder pain and shoulder disorders due to lack of sufficient knowledge.

Epidemiologic Findings

Most studies have investigated shoulder disorders in aggregate. Further, many studies have not made a distinction between shoulder and neck pain or disorders. Despite the relatively large number of studies, NIOSH[49] did not find strong evidence for association of job-related risk factors and shoulder disorders. Further, most generic job physical risk factors were categorized as having "Insufficient evidence."[49] There is some evidence that rotator cuff (supraspinatus) tendinitis is related to job physical factors.[49] It is reported psychosocial risk factors play a major role for muscle tension syndrome.[103,104]

Punnett et al.[105] reported that shoulder flexion or abduction > 90° for 10% or more of the work cycle was predictive of chronic or recurrent shoulder disorders. Use of hand held tools increased the risk. However, mild shoulder flexion or abduction (46° to 90°) and peak shoulder torque were not associated with an increased risk of shoulder disorders. Similarly, Svendsen et al.[101] also found that arm elevations > 90° were related to shoulder disorders. Harkness et al.[106] reported that the following job physical requirements were predictive of shoulder pain defined as lasting at least 24 hours in the past month: lifting weights with one or two hands, pushing or pulling heavy weights, working with hands above shoulder level, monotonous work, and other pain.

A significant increase in shoulder injuries occurs with an increased load-shoulder strength ratio. Further, 50% of shoulder injuries occurred to those workers whose load-shoulder strength ratio exceeded 0.7. Bloswick and Villnave[107] proposed using the ratio of the shoulder moment required by the task and the gender-specific maximum strength in that posture. They proposed that a ratio less than 0.5 would not be a hazard for most workers unless high frequency was present and that a ratio greater than 1.0 would present a hazard for most workers. Thus, it appears that shoulder strength is related to shoulder injuries and the jobs should be designed to keep the weight or force well below the shoulder strength of the workers.

From the above brief review of epidemiological studies, it appears that (1) there is a lack of consistency in results from different epidemiological studies on shoulder pain and shoulder disorders and (2) the epidemiological results are not always consistent with biomechanical findings.

Risk Factors

Various researchers have reported "risk" factors for shoulder musculoskeletal disorders. These risk factors include: (1) highly repetitive work, (2) shoulder posture, especially shoulder flexion and/or abduction > 60 degrees, (3) force and (4) cumulative load.[25,71,108–113]

Sigholm et al.[81] studied the effects of hand tool weight (0, 1 and 2 kg) and arm position (shoulder flexion/abduction of 0, 45 and 90° with elbow flexed at 90 or 120°) on six shoulder muscles using intramuscular EMG. The study concluded that the most important variable in determining shoulder muscle load was the degree of upper arm elevation. Based upon the current literature it appears that following are potential risk factors for shoulder pain and shoulder disorders:

- Posture (shoulder flexion and abduction)
  - Maximum stresses appear to be at shoulder flexion of ≈ 90˚ or shoulder abduction of ≈ 90°
- Elbow extension
- Force
- Frequency (number of exertions/min)
- Amount of time spent in flexion and/or abduction
- Acromion shape (burrs in acromion process)
- Age
- Smoking

Job Analysis and Design

There are limited experimental data available for shoulder strength, endurance time and repetitive work affecting the shoulder girdle. Snook and Ciriello[114] published a series of tables containing maximum acceptable weights and pushing/pulling forces for males and females. The tables contain weights and pushing/pulling forces that are acceptable to different percentiles of the population for two handed lifting, lowering, pushing, pulling, etc. Though the tables were not developed to specifically assess risk of upper extremity disorders, the information provides insight into the interaction between task, load, and posture. The maximum acceptable weight limits may have been limited by the shoulder strength for certain lifting, lowering, pushing and pulling tasks.

Strength

The Three-Dimensional Static Strength Prediction Program (3DSSPP), developed by Chaffin and associates at the University of Michigan[115], predicts the proportion of a population that would be capable of performing a specific task based on segmental static strength. Garg et al.[116] have provided measured one-handed shoulder strength for overhead work as a function of shoulder posture for females (Figure 32.20). The study concluded that (1) shoulder posture has significant effect on one-handed lifting shoulder strength, (2) the strongest posture is upper arm at the side (0/90) and the weakest posture is with 90 degree of shoulder flexion (90/120) and (3) females have fairly low shoulder strength for jobs requiring overhead work.

Endurance Time

Rohmert[117,118] published data and graphs depicting the effects of weights , expressed as percent maximum voluntary contraction, on endurance time. The 'Rohmert's curve' has subsequently been widely cited as a guideline to determine endurance time. A common interpretation of Rohmert's curve for endurance time has been an exertion requiring less than or equal to 15–20% of maximum voluntary contraction can be maintained indefinitely, i.e., this does cause undue fatigue. However, several studies have shown that Rohmert's curve overestimates endurance time at low %MVCs.[119–122] These authors and others have reported that light workloads (corresponding to small %MVCs) may cause either muscle fatigue or musculoskeletal complaints, especially in the shoulder, neck and lower back regions.[68,93,97,119,120,123] Garg et al[122] measured endurance time for overhead work as a function of %MVC and shoulder posture (Figure 32.21). They concluded that:

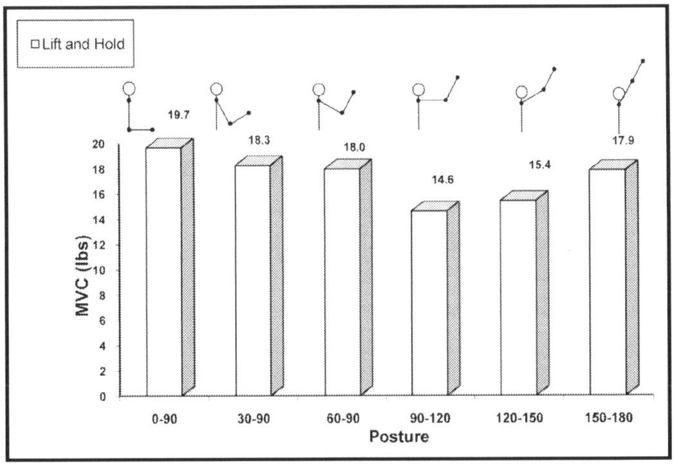

Figure 32.20 — Mazimum one-handed shoulder strength for overhead work as a function of shoulder posture in females.[116]

1. Shoulder posture (shoulder flexion angle) has a significant effect on endurance time,
2. Endurance time decreases with an increase in shoulder flexion angle up to 120° and then it increases,
3. There is a continuous non-linear decrease in endurance time with an increase in %MVC,
4. The endurance time decreases rapidly with an increase in %MVC up to about 30% MVC and then it decreases at a slower rate all the way up to 90% of MVC, and
5. The curve does not become asymptotic even at 5% of MVC (Figure 32.21).

Repetitive Work

As stated earlier Snook and Ciriello[114] have provided maximum acceptable weights for two-handed overhead lifting as a function of box size, lifting frequency and distance of lift (travel distance) for males and females. Garg et al.[124] studied the maximum acceptable frequency for one-handed lifting as a function of object weight and shoulder posture. Their findings are summarized in Figure 32.22. They concluded that the maximum frequency acceptable to the female subjects decreased both with an increase in weight of the load and an increase in the shoulder flexion angle. The weight effect was more pronounced than the posture effect. Increasing the weight from 0.91 to 2.72 kg decreased the maximum acceptable frequency from an average of 7.2 to 5 lifts/min (a 30% decrease). Increasing the shoulder flexion angle from 60° to 120° decreased the maximum acceptable frequency from an average of 6.5 to 5.6 lifts/min (a 14% decrease).

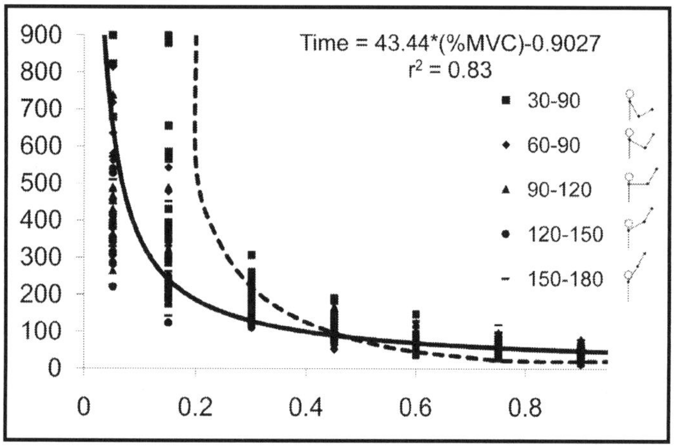

Figure 32.21 — Endurance time for females for holding weights with one hand as a function of % MVC.[122]

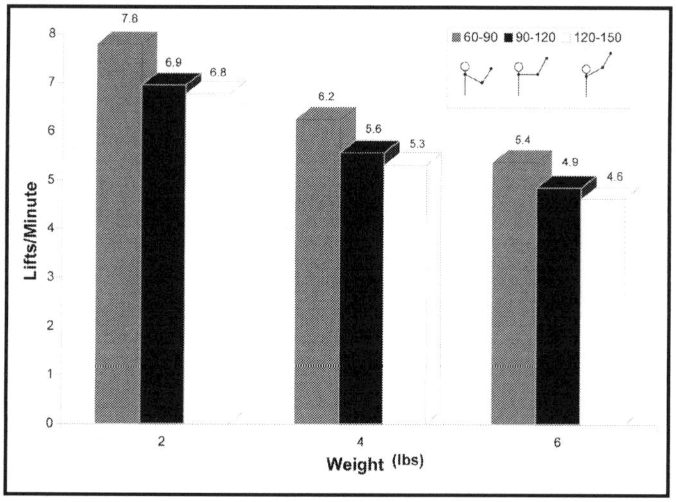

Figure 32.22 — Maximum acceptable lifting frequency for one-handed overhead work — posture and weight effects.[124]

Design Recommendations

1. Avoid all shoulder abduction/flexion ≥ 90°
2. Minimize exposures with shoulder abduction/flexion from 45°–90°
3. Avoid static loading of the shoulder muscles in the above postures.
4. Minimize forearm rotation with elbow extension and shoulder flexion.
5. Minimize shoulder torque.
6. For females, weight should be ≤ 2 lbs for repetitive lifting
7. Lift with the center of gravity of the object horizontally close to the body.

Office Ergonomics

VDT Workstation Design

Designing a visual display terminal (VDT) requires more than just providing a comfortable chair and putting a computer on the desk. Office workers spend a large amount of time working at the computer. Although in some ways similar to seated workstation design, VDTs have their own set of special requirements. In addition to the chair, work surface, and possible footrest, a VDT station requires a keyboard, keyboard shelf, document holder, and leg space. Each of these has special requirements in order to maximize efficiency and minimize the risk of MSDs. The adjustment of VDTs has received a significant amount of attention, and much information is available for use in design.

Figure 32.23 below describes a step-by-step procedure for adjusting a VDT station.

Several concerns have been identified in VDT station design including

- Whole body posture
- Wrist extension and ulnar deviation
- Finger extension
- Hours spent using keyboard & mouse
- Rest breaks
- Typing speed
- Overtime
- Unaccustomed work

In order to alleviate the identified concerns the following recommendations should be implemented (Table 32.8).

Apart from the above recommendations, it is preferred to maintain

- Frequent, short rest breaks
- Worker involvement in selecting equipment and setting up the work station and assistive devices

A recent study[132] identified several specific VDT station adjustments that might lead to lower risk of developing MSDs. The study concluded that having the keyboard low and some distance away from the operator is associated with reduced risk of injury compared to one at elbow height and close to the operator. Specifically the study recommended that:

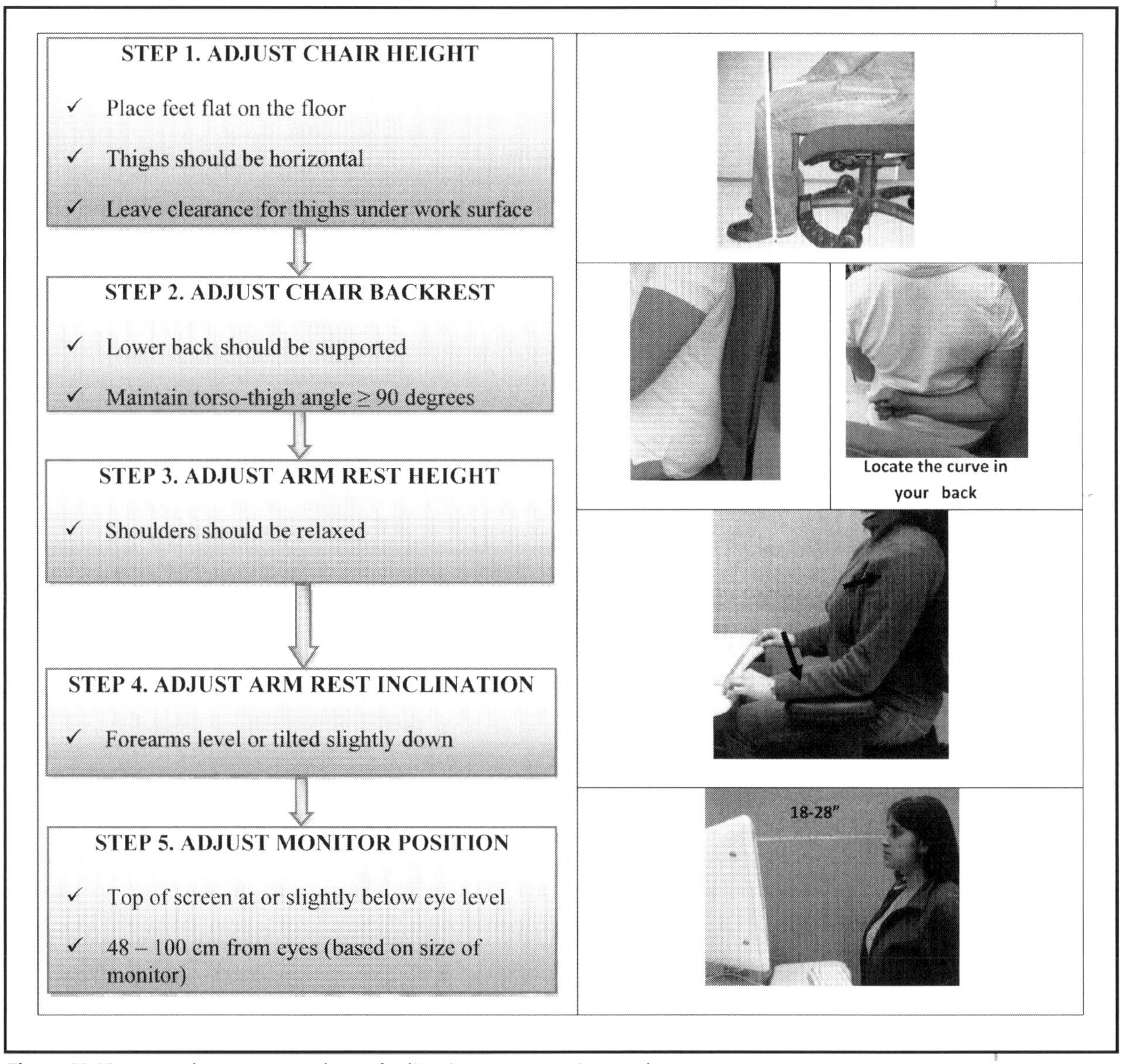
STEP 1. ADJUST CHAIR HEIGHT
✓ Place feet flat on the floor
✓ Thighs should be horizontal
✓ Leave clearance for thighs under work surface
STEP 2. ADJUST CHAIR BACKREST
✓ Lower back should be supported
✓ Maintain torso-thigh angle ≥ 90 degrees
STEP 3. ADJUST ARM REST HEIGHT
✓ Shoulders should be relaxed
STEP 4. ADJUST ARM REST INCLINATION
✓ Forearms level or tilted slightly down
STEP 5. ADJUST MONITOR POSITION
✓ Top of screen at or slightly below eye level
✓ 48 – 100 cm from eyes (based on size of monitor)
Locate the curve in your back
18-28"

Figure 32.23 — Step by step procedure of adjusting a VDT station to the user.

Table 32.8 — Recommendations in order to alleviate identified concerns of VDT station.(125–131)

	Should	*Should Not*
Adjustable Chair	• have lumbar support • backrest that reclines and has tension adjustment • have height and tilt adjustments for seat pan	• force torso-thigh angle to be less than 90 degrees (Chaffin and Anderson, 1984)
Foot rest	• be provided when feet cannot be supported by floor	• be used when clearance for thighs is limited
Work surface	• prevent inadvertent movement through fail safe mechanism • prevent inadvertent operation through control locking mechanism	• be less than 27.6 inches wide (ANSI/HFES, 2007)
Ergonomic keyboard	• be placed within forearm reach • be level with or lower than elbow height • should aid neutral posture of the wrists • preferably use a split keyboard	• be greater than 30mm height (ISO, 1998)
Wrist support and/ or Arm support	• have height and tilt adjustments • aid in maintaining neutral posture (Albin, 1997)	• be less than 1.5 in deep (Paul and Menon, 1994)
Document holder	• be at the same height and distance as the monitor • be stable while loading intended materials	• allow users to read materials at awkward postures (Bauer and Wittig, 1998)
Augmented lighting	• range between 200 and 500 lux (Illuminating Engineering Society, 1989,1993)	• degrade image quality on the display (ANSI/HFES, 2007)

- Elbow height should be ≥ the "J" key height
- Keep inner elbow angle > 120°.
- Keep shoulder flexion angle = 38°
- Keep the "J" key at least 12 cm from the table edge. The "J" key height should not be more 3.5 cm above the work surface
- Support the arms either on the desk surface or chair arm rests
- Avoid downward tilting of the head
- Avoid telephone handset shoulder rests
- Keep wrist radial deviation less than 5° when using a mouse
- Keep hours of keying ≤ 20 hours/week
- Avoid key activation force > 48g

References

1. **Netscher, D. and Fiore, N.:** Hand Surgery (Chapter 74). In *Sabiston Textbook of Surgery*, 18th ed. Townsend, C.M., et al. (eds.). Philadelphia, PA: Saunders Elsevier, 2008.
2. **Blair, W.F.:** Cubital Tunnel Syndrome in the Work Environment (Chapter 31). In *Repetitive Motion Disorders of the Upper Extremity.* Gordon, S.L., Blair, S.J. and Fine, L.J. (eds.). Rosemont, IL: American Academy of Orthopaedic Surgeons, 1995.
3. **Malabar, F.L.:** Ulnar nerve. In *Peripheral Entrapment Neuropathies*, 2nd ed. Kopell, H.P. and Thompson, W.A.L. (eds.). Huntington, NY: Robert E. Krieger Publishing Co., 1976.
4. **Feldman, R.G., Goldman, R. and Keyserling, W.M.:** Classical syndromes in occupational medicine: Peripheral nerve entrapment syndromes and ergonomic factors. *Am. J. Ind. Med.* 4:661-681 (1983).
5. **Nichols, D.:** (a) Entrapment of the ulnar nerve and possible areas of symptoms (b) Entrapment of the posterior interosseous nerve and possible areas of symptoms. [Online] Available at http://denver-sportsmed.com. [Accessed Nov. 2009]
6. **Harter Jr., B.T.:** Indications for surgery in work-related compression neuropathies of the upper extremity. *Occup. Med.* 4:485-495 (1989).

7. **Kim, R.Y., Wolfe, V.M. and Rosenwasser, M.P.:** Entrapment Neuropathies around the Elbow (Section I). In *Delee & Drez's Orthopaedic Sports Medicine*, 3rd ed. Delee, J.C., Drez Jr., D. and Miller, M.D. (eds.). Philadelphia, PA, Elsevier, 2009.
8. **Kopell, H.P. and Thompson, W.A.L.:** Pronator Syndrome: A confirmed case and its diagnosis. *N. Engl. J. Med. 259*, 713-715 (1958).
9. **Thompson, J.S. and Phelps, T.H.:** Repetitive strain injuries: How to deal with "the epidemic of the 1990's." *Postgrad. Med. 88*:143-149 (1990).
10. **Spinner, M.:** The anterior interosseous-nerve syndrome, with special attention to its variations. *J. Bone Joint Surg. Am. 52A*:84-94 (1970).
11. **Terzis, J.K. and Noah, E.M.:** Anatomy and Morphology of Upper Extremity Nerve and Frequent Sites of Compression. In *Repetitive Motion Disorders of the Upper Extremity*. Gordon, S.L., Blair, S.J. and Fine, L.J. (eds.). Rosemont, IL, American Academy of Orthopaedic Surgeons, 1995.
12. **Kirkman, M.:** Schematic representation of the median nerve in the proximal forearm. *American Family Physician*. February 1, 2000.
13. **Russell, W.R. and Whitty, C.W.M.:** Traumatic neuritis of the deep palmar branch of the ulnar nerve. *Lancet 1*:828-829 (1947).
14. **Smail, D.F.:** Handlebar palsy. *N. Engl. J. Med. 292*:322 (1975).
15. **Jones Jr., H.R. Letter:** Pizza cutter's palsy. *N. Engl. J. Med. 319*, 450 (1988).
16. Therapy, P.P.: Schematic representation Guyon's canal syndrome. [Online] Available at http://www.progressivept.net/library_wrist_38. [Accessed July 2011].
17. **Phalen, G.S. and Kendrick, J.I.:** Compression neuropathy of the median nerve in the carpal tunnel. *J. Am. Med. Assoc. 164*:524-30 (1957).
18. **Trumble, T.E.:** Compressive neuropathies. In *Principles of Hand Surgery and Therapy*. Trumble, T.E. (ed.). Philadelphia, PA: WB Saunders, 2000.
19. **Stevens, J.C., Sun, S., Beard, C.M., O'Fallon, W.M. and Kurland, L.T.:** Carpal tunnel syndrome in Rochester, Minnesota, 1961 to 1980. *Neurology 38*:134-8 (1988).
20. **Medicine Net:** Schematic representation of carpal tunnel syndrome and possible areas of pain. [Online] Available at http://images.medicinenet.com/images/illustrations/carpal_tunnel.jpg. Accessed July 2011].
21. **Wright, P.E.:** Carpal Tunnel, Ulnar Tunnel, and Stenosing Tenosynovitis (Chapter 73). In *Campbell's Operative Orthopaedics*, 11th ed. Canale, S.T. & Beaty, J.H. (eds.). Philadelphia, PA: Mosby Elsevier, 2007.
22. **Bernard, B.:** *Musculoskeletal disorders and workplace factors: a critical review of epidemiologic evidence for work-related musculoskeletal disorders of the neck, upper extremity, and low back.* DHHS (NIOSH) Publication No. 97-141, 1997.
23. **Solomon, D., et al.:** Nonoccupational risk factors for carpal tunnel syndrome. *J. Gen. Intern. Med. 14*:310-314 (1999).
24. **Stevens, J., et al.:** Conditions associated with carpal tunnel syndrome. *Mayo Clin. Proc. 67*:541-548 (1992).
25. **Pryse-Phillips, W.:** Validation of a diagnostic sign in carpal tunnel syndrome. *J. Neurol. Neurosurg. Psychiatry 47*:870-872 (1984).
26. **Katz, J. and Simmons, B.:** Carpal tunnel syndrome. *N. Engl. J. Med. 346*:1807-1812 (2002).
27. **Desai, G.J., Dalton, A.J. and LaFavor, K.M.:** Carpal Tunnel Syndrome (Chapter 66). In *Integrative Medicine*, 2nd ed. Rakel, D. (ed.). Philadelphia: Saunders Elsevier, 2007.
28. **Cummings, K., Maizlish, N., Rudolph, L., Dervin, K. and Ervin, A.:** Occupational disease surveillance: carpal tunnel syndrome. *Morb. Mortal Wkly. Rep. 38*:485-489 (1989).
29. **Moore, J.S. and Garg, A.:** *Occupational Medicine: State of the Art Reviews.* Philadelphia, PA: Hanley & Belfus, Inc., 1992.
30. **Geiderman, J.M. and Katz, D.:** General Principles of Orthopedic Injuries (Chapter 46). In *Rosen's Emergency Medicine*, 7th ed. Marx, J.A., et al. (eds.), Mosby, Inc., 2009.
31. **Ingari, J.V.:** Wrist and Hand (Chapter 20). In *Delee & Drez's Orthopaedic Sports Medicine*, 3rd edition. Delee, J.C., D. Drez, Jr., and M.D. Miller (eds.). Philadelphia, PA: Elsevier, 2009.
32. **Brady, M.:** Diseases and Disorders (Section I). In *Ferri's Clinical Advisor 2010*, 1st ed. Ferri, F. F. (ed.). Philadelphia, PA, Mosby, Inc., 2009.
33. **Rettig, A.C.:** Wrist and hand overuse syndromes. *Clin. Sports Med. 20*:591-611, 2001..
34. **Guidotti, T.L.:** Occupational repetitive strain injury. *Am. Fam. Physician 45*:585-92 (1992).
35. **Nirschl, R.P.:** Elbow tendinosis/tennis elbow. *Clin. Sports Med. 11*:851-70 (1992).
36. **Regan, W.D., Grondin, P.P. & Morrey, B.F.:** Elbow and Forearm, Section B Tendinopathies around the Elbow (Chapter 19). In *Delee & Drez's Orthopaedic Sports Medicine*, 3rd ed. Delee, J.C., Drez Jr., D. and Miller, M.D. (eds.). Philadelphia, PA: Elsevier, 2009.
37. **Alfredson, H. and Lorentzon, R.:** Chronic Achilles tendinosis: recommendations for treatment and prevention. *Sports Med. 29*:135-46 (2000).
38. **Cleak, M.J. and Eston, R.G.:** 1992. Delayed onset muscle soreness: Mechanisms and management. *J Sport Sci, 10*, 325-341.

39. **Gulick, B.T., et al.:** Various treatment techniques on signs and symptoms of delayed onset muscle soreness. *J. Athl. Train. 31*:145-152 (1996).
40. **Gulick, B.T. and Kimura, I.F.:** Delayed onset muscle soreness: What is it and how do we treat it? *J. Sport Rehabil. 5*:234-243 (1996).
41. **Smith, L.L.:** Acute inflammation: The underlying mechanism in delayed onset muscle soreness? *Med. Sci. Sport Exerc. 23*:542-549 (1991).
42. **Smith, L.L.:** Causes of delayed onset muscle soreness and the impact on athletic performance: A review. *J. App. Sport Sci. Res. 6*:135-141 (1992).
43. **Cheung, K., Hume, P. and Maxwell, L.:** Delayed onset muscle soreness: Treatment strategies and performance factors. *Sports Med. 33*:145-164 (2003).
44. **Nosaka, K., Newton, M. and Sacco, P.:** Muscle damage and soreness after endurance exercise of the elbow flexors. *Med. Sci. Sport Exerc. 34*:920-927 (2002).
45. **Brinker, M.R., et al.:** Basic Science and Injury of Muscle, Tendon, and Ligament (Chapter 1). In *Delee and Drez's Orthopaedic Sports Medicine*, 3rd ed. Delee, J.C., Drez Jr., D. and Miller, M.D. (eds.). Philadelphia, PA: Saunders Elsevier, 2009.
46. **Bonfiglioli, R., et al.:** Relationship between repetitive work and the prevalence of carpal tunnel syndrome in part-time and full-time female supermarket cashiers: a quasi-experimental study. *Intl. Arch. Occup.Environ. Health 80*:248-253 (2007).
47. **Violante, F. S., et al.:** Carpal tunnel syndrome and manual work: a longitudinal study. *J. Occup. Environ. Med. 49*:1189 (2007).
48. **Moore, J. S. and Garg, A.:** The strain index: a proposed method to analyze jobs for risk of distal upper extremity disorders. *Am. Ind. Hyg. Assoc. J. 56*:443-458 (1995).
49. **Bernard, B.P.:** Musculoskeletal Disorders and Workplace Factors. *DHHS (NIOSH)* Publication No. 97-141. U.S. Department of Health and Human Services. Cincinnati, OH: NIOSH, 1997.
50. **Washington State Department of Labor and Industries:** 296-62-05174, W. Washington State Department of Labor and Industries WISHA Checklist. 2001. Available at http://www.lni.wa.gov/wisha. [Accessed July 15, 2011].
51. **American Conference of Governmental Industrial Hygienists (ACGIH®):** *Threshold Limit Values® for Chemical Substances and Physical Agents and BEIs.* Cincinnati, OH: ACGIH®, 2001.
52. **Borg, G.:** Psychophysical scaling with applications in physical work and the perception of exertion. *Scandinavian J. Work Environ. Health 16*:55 (1990).
53. **Gell, N., Werner, R.A., Franzblau, A., Ulin, S.S. and Armstrong, T.J.:** A longitudinal study of industrial and clerical workers: incidence of carpal tunnel syndrome and assessment of risk factors. *J. Occup. Rehab. 15*:47-55 (2005).
54. **Werner, R.A., Franzblau, A., Gell, N., Ulin, S.S. and Armstrong, T.J.:** Predictors of upper extremity discomfort: a longitudinal study of industrial and clerical workers. *J. Occup. Rehab. 15*:27-35 (2005).
55. **Franzblau, A., Armstrong, T.J., Werner, R.A. and Ulin, S.S.:** A cross-sectional assessment of the ACGIH TLV for hand activity level. *J. Occup. Rehab. 15*:57-67 (2005).
56. **Knox, K. and Moore, J.S.:** Predictive validity of the strain Index in turkey processing. *J. Occup. Environ. Med. 43*:451 (2001).
57. **Moore, J.S., Rucker, N.P. and Knox, K.:** Validity of generic risk factors and the strain index for predicting nontraumatic distal upper extremity morbidity. *Am. Ind. Hyg. Assoc. J. 62*:229-235 (2001).
58. **Rucker, N. and Moore, J.S.:** Predictive validity of the strain index in manufacturing facilities. *Appl. Occup. Environ. Hyg. 17*:63-73 (2002).
59. **Moore, J.S., Vos, G.A., Stephens, E. and Garg, A.:** The validity and reliability of the Strain Index. *Proceedings of IEA 2006: 16th World Congress on Ergonomics. Masstricht, Netherlands, 2006.*
60. **Garg, A.:** *Applied Ergonomics*, University of Wisconsin - Milwaukee, Department of Industrial and Manufacturing Engineering in cooperation with University of Utah Department of Family and Preventive Medicine, 2006.
61. **Tichauster, E.R.:** Biomechanical basis of ergonomics. Anatomy applied to the design of work situation, 1978.
62. **Pheasant, S.:** *Bodyspace: Anthropometry Ergonomics and Design.* London, England: Taylor & Francis, 1986.
63. **Lim, J. and Hoffmann, E.:** Appreciation of the zone of convenient reach by naive operators performing an assembly task. *Intl. J. Ind. Ergon. 19*:187-199 (1997).
64. **Grandjean, E.:** *Fitting the Man to the Task: Occupational Ergonomics.* London, England: Taylor & Francis, 1988.
65. **Pheasant, S. and Haslegrave, C.M.:** *Bodyspace: anthropometry, ergonomics, and the design of work*, 3rd ed. Boca Raton, FL: CRC Press, 2006.
66. **Hagberg, M. and Wegman, D.H.:** Prevalence rates and odds ratios of shoulder-neck diseases in different occupational groups. *Brit. Med. J. 44*:602 (1987).
67. **Winkel, J. and Westgaard, R.:** Occupational and individual risk factors for shoulder-neck complaints: Part II-The scientific basis (literature review) for the guide. *Intl. J. Ind. Ergon. 10*:85-104 (1992).

68. **Sommerich, C.M., McGlothlin, J.D. and Marras, W.S.:** Occupational risk factors associated with soft tissue disorders of the shoulder: a review of recent investigations in the literature. *Ergon. 36*:697-717 (1993).
69. **Kuorinka, I. and Forcier, L.:** *Work related musculoskeletal disorders (WMSDs): a reference book for prevention.* CRC Press, 1995.
70. **U.S. Bureau of Labor Statistics:** Workplace injuries and illness in 2003. USDL – 95-508. Washington, D.C.: U.S. Department of Labor, Bureau of Labor Statistics, 2004.
71. **Miranda, H., et al.:** A population study on differences in the determinants of a specific shoulder disorder versus nonspecific shoulder pain without clinical findings. *American J. Epid. 161*:847 (2005).
72. **Kelsey, J.L., Praemer, A., Nelson, L., Felberg, A. and Rice, L.M.:** *Upper extremity disorders. Frequency, impact, and cost.* New York: Churchill Livingstone Inc., 1997.
73. **Silverstein, B., Viikari-Juntura, E. and Kalat, J.:** Use of a prevention index to identify industries at high risk for work-related musculoskeletal disorders of the neck, back, and upper extremity in Washington State, 1990-1998. *Am. J. Ind. Med. 41*:149-169 (2002).
74. **Hagberg, M.:** Occupational musculoskeletal stress and disorders of the neck and shoulder: a review of possible pathophysiology. *Intl. Arch. Occup. Environ. Health. 53*:269-278 (1984).
75. **Hegmann, K.T. and Moore, J.S.:** Common neuromusculoskeletal disorders (Chapter 2). In *Sourcebook of occupational rehabilitation.* King P.M. (ed.). New York: Plenum Press, 1998.
76. **Sporrong, H. and Styf, J.:** Effects of isokinetic muscle activity on pressure in the supraspinatus muscle and shoulder torque. *J. Ortho. Res. 17*:546-553 (1999).
77. **Järvholm, U., Palmerud, G., Kadefors, R. and Herberts, P.:** The effect of arm support on supraspinatus muscle load during simulated assembly work and welding. *Ergon. 34*:57 (1991).
78. **Hagberg, M.:** Electromyographic signs of shoulder muscular fatigue in two elevated arm positions. *Am. J. Phys. Med. 60*:111 (1981).
79. **Herberts, P., Kadefors, R. and Broman, H.:** Arm positioning in manual tasks: an electromyographic study of localized muscle fatigue. *Ergon. 23*:655-666 (1980).
80. **Bjelle, A., Hagberg, M. and Michaelson, G.:** Occupational and individual factors in acute shoulder-neck disorders among industrial workers. *Brit. Med. J. 38*:356 (1981).
81. **Sigholm, G., Herberts, P., Almström, C. and Kadefors, R.:** Electromyographic analysis of shoulder muscle load. *J. Ortho. Res. 1*:379-386 (1983).
82. **Järvholm, U., Palmerud, G., Styf, J., Herberts, P. and Kadefors, R.:** Intramuscular pressure in the supraspinatus muscle. *J. Ortho. Res. 6*:230-238 (1988).
83. **Järvholm, U.L.F., Palmerud, G., Herberts, P., Högfors, C. and Kadefors, R.:** Intramuscular pressure and electromyography in the supraspinatus muscle at shoulder abduction. *Clinical Ortho. Related Res. 245*:102 (1989).
84. **Sporrong, H., Palmerud, G. and Herberts, P.:** Hand grip increases shoulder muscle activity: An EMG analysis with static handcontractions in 9 subjects. *Acta Orthopaedica 67*:485-490 (1996).
85. **Takala, E.P. and Viikari-Juntura, E.:** Muscular activity in simulated light work among subjects with frequent neck-shoulder pain. *Intl. J. Ind. Ergon. 8*:157-164 (1991).
86. **Christensen, H.:** Muscle activity and fatigue in the shoulder muscles of assembly-plant employees. *Scand. J. Work Environ. Health 12*:582 (1986).
87. **Chaffin, D.B. and Park, K.S.:** A Longitudinal Study of Low-Back Pain as Associated with Occupational Weight Lifting Factors. *Am. Ind. Hyg. Assoc. J. 34*:513-525 (1973).
88. **Herberts, P. and Kadefors, R.:** A study of painful shoulder in welders. *Acta Orthopaedica 47*:381-387 (1976).
89. **Hagberg, M.:** Work load and fatigue in repetitive arm elevations. *Ergonomics, 24*, 543-555 (1981).
90. **Hagberg, M. and Sundelin, G.:** Discomfort and load on the upper trapezius muscle when operating a wordprocessor. *Ergonomics, 29*, 1637 (1986).
91. **Jensen, C., Nilsen, K., Hansen, K. and Westgaard, R.H.:** Trapezius muscle load as a risk indicator for occupational shoulder-neck complaints. *Intl. Arch. Occup. Environ. Health 64*:415-423 (1993).
92. **Jensen, C., Finsen, L., Hansen, K. and Christensen, H.:** Upper trapezius muscle activity patterns during repetitive manual material handling and work with a computer mouse. *Journal of Electromyography and Kinesiology, 9*, 317-325 (1999).
93. **Veiersted, K.B., Westgaard, R.H. and Andersen, P.:** Electromyographic evaluation of muscular work pattern as a predictor of trapezius myalgia. *Scand. J. Work Environ. Health. 19*:284-290 (1993).
94. **Palmerud, G., et al.** Voluntary redistribution of muscle activity in human shoulder muscles. *Ergon. 38*:806 (1995).
95. **Vasseljen, O. and Westgaard, R.H.:** A case-control study of trapezius muscle activity in office and manual workers with shoulder and neck pain and symptom-free controls. *Intl. Arch. Occup. Environ. Health 67*:11-18 (1995).

96. **Jonsson, B.:** Measurement and evaluation of local muscular strain in the shoulder during constrained work. *J Human Ergology 11*:73 (1982).
97. **Aarås, A., Westgaard, R.H. and Stranden, E.:** Postural angles as an indicator of postural load and muscular injury in occupational work situations. *Ergon. 31*:915-933 (1988).
98. **Westgaard, R.H. and Aarås, A.:** Postural muscle strain as a causal factor in the development of musculo-skeletal illnesses. *Appl. Ergon. 15*:162 (1984).
99. **Westgaard, R.H.:** Measurement and evaluation of postural load in occupational work situations. *Euro. J. Appl. Physio. 57*:291-304 (1988).
100. **Järvholm, U., Palmerud, G., Karlsson, D., Herberts, P. and Kadefors, R.:** Intramuscular pressure and electromyography in four shoulder muscles. *J. Ortho. Res. 9*:609-619 (1991).
101. **Svendsen, S.W., Bonde, J.P., Mathiassen, S.E., Stengaard-Pedersen, K. and Frich, L.H.:** Work related shoulder disorders: quantitative exposure-response relations with reference to arm posture. *Brit. Med. J. 61*:844 (2004).
102. **Sejersted, O.M. and Westgaard, R.H.:** Occupational muscle pain and injury; scientific challenge. *Eur. J. Appl. Physiol. 57*:271-274 (1988).
103. **Krantz, G., Forsman, M. and Lundberg, U.:** Consistency in physiological stress responses and electromyographic activity during induced stress exposure in women and men. *Integ. Psychol. Behav. Sci. 39*:105-118 (2004).
104. **Dainoff, M.J., Cohen, B.G. and Dainoff, M.H.:** The effect of an ergonomic intervention on musculoskeletal, psychosocial, and visual strain of VDT data entry work: the United States part of the international study. *Intl. J. Occup. Saf.Ergon. 11*:49 (2005).
105. **Punnett, L., Fine, L.J., Keyserling, W.M., Herrin, G.D. and Chaffin, D.B.:** Shoulder disorders and postural stress in automobile assembly work. *Scand. J. Work Environ. Health 26*:283 (2000).
106. **Harkness, E.F., Macfarlane, G.J., Nahit, E.S., Silman, A.J. and McBeth, J.:** Mechanical and psychosocial factors predict new onset shoulder pain: a prospective cohort study of newly employed workers. *Brit. Med. J. 60*:850 (2003).
107. **Bloswick, D.S. and Villnave, T.:** Ergonomics (Chapter 54). *Patty's Industrial Hygiene*, 5th ed., Vol. 4. New York: John Wiley & Sons, 2000.
108. **Stenlund, B., Goldie, I., Hagberg, M., Hogstedt, C. and Marions, O.:** Radiographic osteoarthrosis in the acromioclavicular joint resulting from manual work or exposure to vibration. *Brit. Med. J. 49*:588, 1992.
109. **Herberts, P., Kadefors, R., Andersson, G. and Petersén, I.** Shoulder pain in industry: an epidemiological study on welders. *Acta Orthopaedica 52*:299-306 (1981).
110. **Herberts, P., Kadefors, R., Hogfors, C. and Sigholm, G.:** Shoulder pain and heavy manual labor. *Clinic. Ortho. Related Res. 191*:166 (1984).
111. **Andersen, J.H. and Gaardboe, O.:** Musculoskeletal disorders of the neck and upper limb among sewing machine operators: a clinical investigation. *Am. J. Ind. Med. 24*:689-700 (1993).
112. **Chiang, H.C., et al.:** Prevalence of shoulder and upper-limb disorders among workers in the fish-processing industry. *Scand. J. Work Environ. Health 19*:126-131 (1993).
113. **Wells, J.A., Zipp, J.F., Schuette, P.T. and McEleney, J.:** Musculoskeletal disorders among letter carriers: a comparison of weight carrying, walking and sedentary occupations. *J. Occup. Environ. Med. 25*:814 (1983).
114. **Snook, S.H. and Ciriello, V.M.:** The design of manual handling tasks: revised tables of maximum acceptable weights and forces. *Ergonomics 34*:1197 (1991).
115. **University of Michigan, Center for Ergonomics:** T. R. o. t. U. o. 3D SSPP software. Ann Arbor, MI: University of Michigan, 2009.
116. **Garg, A., Hegmann., K.T., Kapellusch, J.:** Maximum one-handed shoulder strength for overhead work as a function of shoulder posture in females. *Occup. Ergon. 5*:131-140 (2005).
117. **Rohmert, W.:** Fixing Rest Allowances for Static Muscular Work. *Ergonomics 5*:489 (1962).
118. **Rohmert, W., Wangenheim, M., Mainzer, J., Zipp, P. and Lesser, W.:** A study stressing the need for a static postural force model for work analysis. *Ergonomics 29*:1235 (1986).
119. **Sjøgaard, G., Kiens, B., Jørgensen, K. and Saltin, B.:** Intramuscular pressure, EMG and blood flow during low-level prolonged static contraction in man. *Acta. Physiol. Scand. 128*:475-484 (1986).
120. **Rose, L., Ericson, M., Glimskär, B., Nordgren, B. and Ortengren, R.:** Ergo-Index: Development of a model to determine pause needs after fatigue and pain reactions during work, in *Computer Appliations in Ergonomics Occupational Safety and Health*, Mattila, M. and Karwowski, W. (eds.). London, England: Elsevier Science Publications, 1992.
121. **Nag, P.K.:** Endurance limits in different modes of load holding. *Appl. Ergon. 22*:185 (1991).
122. **Garg, A., Hegmann, K.T., Schwoerer, B.J. and Kapellusch, J.M.:** The effect of maximum voluntary contraction on endurance times for the shoulder girdle. *Intl. J. Ind. Ergon. 30*:103-113 (2002).

123. **Jørgensen, K., Fallentin, N., Krogh-Lund, C. and Jensen, B. :** Electromyography and fatigue during prolonged, low-level static contractions. *Euro. J. Appl. Physiol. 57*:316-321 (1988).
124. **Garg, A., et al.:** Physiological and psychophysical measurements of muscle fatigue and CTDs for short-cycle overhead work. Technical Report. Contract No. 9739-730 C4. Detroit, MI: American Automobile Manufacturers Association, 1999.
125. **Chaffin, D.B., Andersson, G.B.J. and Martin, B.J.:** *Occupational biomechanics.* New York: Wiley, 1984.
126. **Human Factors and Ergonomics Society (HFES):** *ANSI/HFES 2007 – Human Factors Engineering of Computer Workstations.* Santa Monica, CA: HFES, 2007.
127. **Paul, R. and Menon, K.K.:** Ergonomic evaluation of keyboard wrist pads. *12th Triennial Congress of the International Ergonomics Association.* Toronto, International Ergonomics Association, 1994.
128. **Bauer, W. and Wittig, T.:** Influence of screen and copy holder positions on head posture, muscle activity and user judgment. *Appl. Ergon. 29*:185-192 (1998).
129. **Illuminating Engineering Society (IES):** *I.E.S. Recommended practice for lighting offices containing VDTs.* (IESRP-24-1989). New York: IES, 1998.
130. **Illuminating Engineering Society (IES):** *I.E.S. American National Standard Practice for Office Lighting.* (ANSI/IES RP-1-1993). New York: IES, 1993.
131. **Albin, T.J.:** Effect of wrist rest use and keyboard tilt on wrist angle while keying. *Proceedings at the 13th Annual Congress of the IEA.* 4:16-18 (1997).
132. **Marcus, M., et al.:** A prospective study of computer users: II. Postural risk factors for musculoskeletal symptoms and disorders. *Am. J. Ind. Med. 41*:236-249 (2002).

Outcome Competencies

After completing this chapter, the reader should be able to:

1. Define the underlined terms used in this chapter.
2. Understand the relationship between Occupational Health Psychology and Industrial Hygiene.
3. Explain how the organization of work influences job and task level stressors.
4. Discuss the impact of chemical and physical exposures on employees' psychological health.
5. Identify contextual factors that may increase or reduce workers' exposure to psychosocial hazards or lessen or strengthen the effects of job and task level stressors on health.
6. Describe practical instruments and techniques to measure work stressors.
7. Describe occupational heath interventions organizations can implement to lessen the occurrence of and/or consequences of psychosocial hazards in the workplace.

Key Terms

Occupational Health Psychology (OHP) • psychosocial hazards • task level stressors • work stressors • interventions • primary prevention • secondary prevention • tertiary prevention • participatory action research

Prerequisite Knowledge

None

Key Topics

I. Occupational Health Psychology
II. The Organization of Work
III. Health Impacts of Job/Task Level Stressors
    A. Cardiovascular Disease (CVD)
    B. Psychological Disorders
    C. Musculoskeletal Disorders
    D. Injuries
IV. Psychological Health Impacts of Chemical and Physical Hazards
V. Economic Costs of Work Stressors
VI. Contextual Influences on Work Organization, Stress, and Health
    A. Changing Nature of Work
    B. What Does the Data Show?
    C. Changing Nature of Work and Trends in Health
VII. Work-Family Interface
VIII. Safety Climate
IX. How to Measure Work Stressors
    A. Self-Report Questionnaires
    B. Job Exposure Matrices
    C. Observer Measures of Job Stressors
X. Interventions to Reduce Work Stressors and Risk of Work Stress-Related Illness and Injury
    A. Worker Participation
    B. Improve Job/Task Characteristics
    C. Organizational Level Interventions
    D. Participatory Ergonomics
XI. Evaluations of Job/Task Redesign and Organizational Interventions
    A. Integrating Occupational Health with Health Promotion/Stress Management
    B. Collective Bargaining
    C. Legislation and Regulation
XII. Conclusions
XIII. References

Occupational Health Psychology

33

By Paul A. Landsbergis, PhD, MPH, Robert R. Sinclair, PhD, Marnie Dobson, PhD, Leslie B. Hammer, PhD, Maritza Jauregui, PhD, Anthony D. LaMontagne, ScD, MA, MEd, Ryan Olson, PhD, Peter L. Schnall, MD, MPH, Jeanne Stellman, PhD and Nicholas Warren, ScD, MAT

Occupational Health Psychology

During the 20th century, under pressure from labor organizations and social and public health reformers, workers in developed countries gained gradual improvements in working conditions, including substantial decreases in occupational fatality rates[1] and reductions in retirement age.[2] However, in recent years, global economic forces have produced significant changes in the nature of work — through new manufacturing systems and technologies (e.g., lean production and flexible manufacturing), new occupations (e.g., information processing and call center work) and new organizational practices (e.g., downsizing). Retirement age is increasing, and families are increasingly relying on two incomes, simply to make ends meet. The social and economic power of the workforce is in decline as reflected by the smaller proportion of workers who belong to labor unions. Sweatshop work has reappeared.[3] Organizational restructuring, flexible staffing and temporary or contingent work have become more common. More people work on non-standard work-schedules (not voluntarily), job insecurity is a fact-of-life for too many employees, and many, if not most workers, no longer join an employer expecting the job to be their final job, or even their final career.[4]

Some of these changes have led to increased flexibility, responsibility, and learning opportunities, which may offer some workers greater potential for self-direction, skill development, and career growth.[4] Despite these potential benefits, many workers must contend with increased exposure to workplace "psychosocial hazards" — also called "work stressors", "job stressors", "work organization stressors" or "sources of stress at work." These are threats to working people that influence health through psychological pathways, such as uncertainty, anxiety, and loss of control[5] or physiological pathways, such as sympathetic nervous system arousal or immune system responses, or influence safety through fatigue and production pressure. Management of psychosocial hazards requires awareness of both physiological pathways to health, and sociocultural influences, such as team dynamics and organizational climate that may either intensify the effects of psychosocial hazards or, when positive, may help protect workers from adverse health consequences at work.

Occupational health psychology (OHP) shares with industrial hygiene (IH) a focus on measuring workplace health and safety hazards, developing interventions to reduce exposure to hazards, and using the "hierarchy of controls" to guide interventions. However, while IH focuses on physical, chemical, and biological hazards; OHP focuses on psychosocial hazards. Psychosocial hazards represent a significant direct threat to workers' safety and health. In fact, higher levels of work stressors contribute to many of the illnesses and injuries IH seeks to prevent. In addition, the effects of physical hazards on health may depend on the nature of the psychosocial context of work and a given hazard may be more dangerous in the presence of work stressors. For example, accidents are more likely when workers experience high work demands, job insecurity, or long working hours.[6–10] Finally, psychosocial stressors may hinder the effectiveness of workplace interventions, as in the case of safety training programs that are less likely to be effective when workers feel forced to choose between working safely and maintaining excessively high productivity standards. OHP can provide IH and other disciplines concerned with work and health with theories to explain the causes and consequences of psychosocial hazards, tools to assess workers' exposure to psychosocial hazards, and a large body of scientific evidence highlighting interventions that reduce exposure to or help lessen the harmful effects of these hazards.

The National Institute of Occupational Safety and Health (NIOSH) defines OHP as the application of psychological principles to improving the quality of work-life and promoting the safety, health, and well being of people at work. OHP is multidisciplinary and draws upon public health, preventive medicine, nursing, industrial engineering, law, epidemiology, sociology, gerontology, and psychology to promote worker safety, health, and well being. According to the Society for Occupational Health Psychology:

> "OHP is concerned with the broad range of exposures and mechanisms that affect the quality of working life and the responses of workers. These include individual psychological attributes, job content and work organization, organizational policies and practices, and the economic and political environments in which organizations function. OHP research and practice explores interventions targeting the work environment as well as the individual, to create healthier workplaces and organizations and to improve the capacity of workers to protect their safety and health and to maximize their overall effectiveness (www.sohp-online.org)."

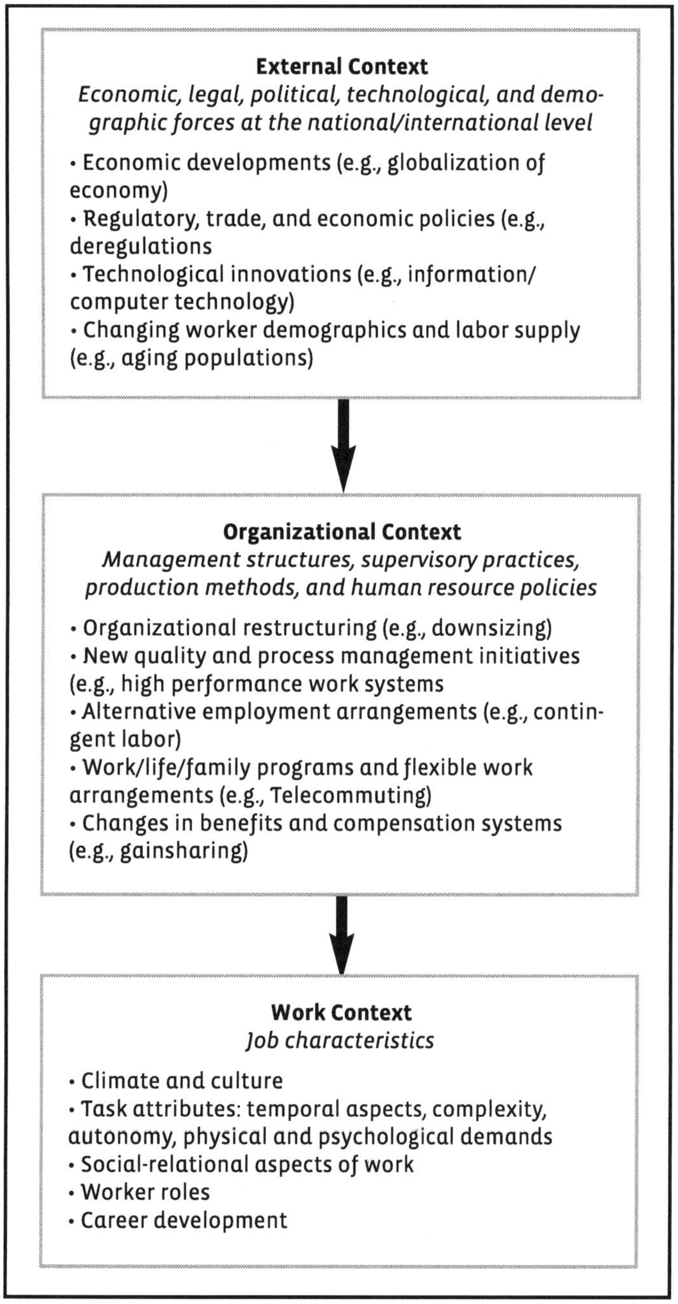
External Context
Economic, legal, political, technological, and demographic forces at the national/international level
• Economic developments (e.g., globalization of economy)
• Regulatory, trade, and economic policies (e.g., deregulations
• Technological innovations (e.g., information/computer technology)
• Changing worker demographics and labor supply (e.g., aging populations)
Organizational Context
Management structures, supervisory practices, production methods, and human resource policies
• Organizational restructuring (e.g., downsizing)
• New quality and process management initiatives (e.g., high performance work systems
• Alternative employment arrangements (e.g., contingent labor)
• Work/life/family programs and flexible work arrangements (e.g., Telecommuting)
• Changes in benefits and compensation systems (e.g., gainsharing)
Work Context
Job characteristics
• Climate and culture
• Task attributes: temporal aspects, complexity, autonomy, physical and psychological demands
• Social-relational aspects of work
• Worker roles
• Career development

Figure 33.1 — Organization of Work.

The Organization of Work

NIOSH defines the organization of work as "the work process (the way jobs are designed and performed)" and "the organizational practices (management and production methods and accompanying human resource policies) that influence job design. The organization of work also includes external factors, such as the legal and economic environment and technological factors that encourage or enable new organizational practices" (Figure 33.1).[4]

Work organization factors may affect worker health by influencing levels of psychosocial, biomechanical, chemical, biological or physical risk factors at the job level (A), through direct effects on health (C), or by modifying the relationship between risk factors and health (D) (as shown in Figure 33.2).[11]

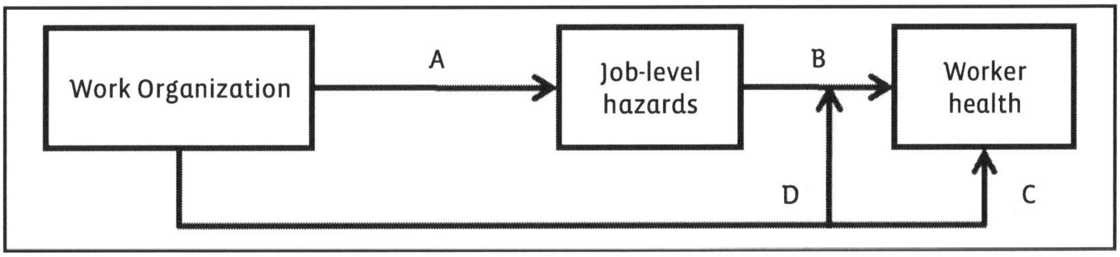

Figure 33.2 — Conceptual pathways that link organizational characteristics with workplace health and safety hazards and worker health outcomes.[11]

Table 33.1 lists some of the main work organization and job level factors which have been studied in relation to work stress and worker health and safety. Jobs with low socioeconomic status may involve increased exposure to many of these stressors, or interact with work stressors to produce illness and injury.[12]

Health Impacts of Job/Task Level Stressors

A substantial body of research has linked sources of stress at work to a variety of illnesses and injuries. The most widely studied physical health outcome is cardiovascular

Table 33.1 — Types of Work Organization and Job-level Stressors Related to Health and Safety

Organizational/Employment Level[11]

Organizational Practices/Characteristics
- "Precarious" or "contingent" work: temporary, part-time or contract work[13,14]
- Downsizing, restructuring[15]
- Lack of union protections or poor labor-management relations[16,17]
- Poor safety culture, climate[18,19]
- Poor work-family balance[260,261]

Production Characteristics
- Systems of work organization: "lean production" (Toyota Production System), continuous improvement, total quality management, process control[20]
- Incentive or "piece rate" pay systems[21]
- Electronic surveillance or performance monitoring[22,23]
- Technology[24]
- Inadequate staffing levels (numerical flexibility)[4]

Job/Task Level

Job strain: High psychological job demands combined with low job "decision latitude" or job control[25,26]
Effort-reward imbalance: "high efforts" combined with "low rewards."[27] "Rewards" include respect, support, fair treatment, promotion opportunities, income, and job security.
Organizational injustice has been defined in three ways: 1) unfair distributions of rewards and benefits at work (distributive injustice); 2) unfair decision making procedures (procedural injustice); 3) and unfair treatment by supervisors, (relational or interactional injustice).[28,29]
Lack of coworker support, social isolation.[30,31]
Bullying/mobbing: verbal abuse, threatening conduct, intimidation, humiliation, or sabotage by others that prevented work from getting done.[32]
"Threat-avoidant" vigilant work involves continuously maintaining a high level of vigilance in order to avoid disaster, such as loss of human life.[33,34]
NIOSH[35] also identifies the following six categories of job-level stressors:
The Design of Tasks. Heavy workload, infrequent rest breaks, long work hours and shiftwork; hectic and routine tasks that have little inherent meaning, do not utilize workers' skills, and provide little sense of control.
Management Style. Lack of participation by workers in decision-making, poor communication in the organization, lack of family-friendly policies.
Interpersonal Relationships. Poor social environment and lack of support or help from coworkers and supervisors.
Work Roles. Conflicting or uncertain job expectations, too much responsibility, too many "hats to wear."
Career Concerns. Job insecurity and lack of opportunity for growth, advancement, or promotion; rapid changes for which workers are unprepared.
Environmental Conditions. Unpleasant or dangerous physical conditions such as crowding, noise, air pollution, or ergonomic problems (biomechanical risk factors).

disease (CVD), along with its risk factors, such as hypertension, cigarette smoking, and diabetes.[26,28,36] CVD is the number one cause of disease and death in the industrialized world, and is projected to become the most common cause of death worldwide early in the 21st century.[37,38] Work stressors have also been associated with psychological disorders, such as depression and anxiety[39,40], musculoskeletal disorders, such as carpal tunnel syndrome and tendinitis[41–43] and acute injuries.[44,45] Some suggestive evidence links job stress with effects on the immune system[46] and gastrointestinal disorders.[47] However, further research is needed to examine those associations. Reviews on the impact of long work hours on a variety of health outcomes are also available.[48–51] (For further information on the physiology of the stress response, see references 36, 52, and 53).

Cardiovascular Disease (CVD)

Work stressors. Strong, consistent evidence of an association between job strain (high demand-low control work) and CVD has been observed in men. The data for women are more sparse and less consistent, but, as for the men, most of the studies probably underestimate existing effects.[26] CVD has also been associated with effort-reward imbalance[54–56], long work hours (60 or more hours per week)[57–60], shiftwork[61], lack of "relational justice" (primarily lack of supervisor support)[62], downsizing[15] and threat avoidant vigilance. The strongest evidence for this last risk factor comes from studies of single occupations, where professional drivers, particularly urban bus drivers, emerge as the occupation with the most consistent evidence of elevated CVD risk.[63,64]

Socioeconomic status. The association of job strain[65–67] and effort-reward imbalance[68] with CVD is stronger among workers in lower (vs higher) status jobs. Higher levels of exposure among workers in lower status jobs to physical and chemical hazards, as well as other work and life stressors, may contribute to this interaction.

Population attributable risk (PAR%) of work stressors. The proportion of CVD due to job strain may be substantial, with estimates as high as 20–30% for U.S. men[69] or 6% for men and 14% for women in Denmark (for "monotonous high paced work," a conservative proxy measure for job strain).[70] However, few studies have examined the combined or synergistic effect of multiple workplace stressors, which would increase estimates of the proportion of CVD due to work. For example, one Swedish study[71] found that the effects of combined exposure to job strain and to effort-reward imbalance upon CVD were stronger than the sum of their separate effects.

Blood Pressure

Work stressors appear to contribute to CVD risk by increasing blood pressure (BP). Work systolic ambulatory BP in workers facing job strain is typically 4–8 millimeters of mercury (mm Hg) higher than those without job strain[33,72,73], and 12 mm Hg higher when facing chronic job strain.[73] Ambulatory BP has also been associated with effort-reward imbalance[74], and work hours more than 55 hours per week[75] The impact of job strain on blood pressure appears to be greater for workers in lower status jobs.[12,76]

The importance of measuring blood pressure while working. Few studies of job strain[33,77] or long work hours[78–80] and "casual" clinic BP have shown significant associations. However, strong associations are found in studies where BP is measured by an ambulatory (portable) monitor during normal daily activities and exposure to daily stressors, including work — in other words, ambulatory BP is a more valid measure of average BP.[33] Compared to casual BP measurements, ambulatory BP monitoring provides a more reliable measure of BP, since the extended monitoring time enables many more BP readings to be gathered.[81] Ambulatory BP also is a better predictor than casual clinic BP of target organ damage, such as increases in the size of the heart's left ventricle[82] and CVD.[83]

Masked Hypertension (MH). Ambulatory BP monitoring allows for the identification of "masked" hypertension (MH), i.e., elevated ambulatory BP while working or for 24 hours, but normal in an office setting — a condition of major clinical and public health significance. About 10–30% of adults with normal clinic BP have MH.[84] People with MH often have target organ damage, such as increases in the size of the heart's left ventricle[85,86] increased carotid plaque burden[85,87], and increased CVD risk[88,89] similar to patients with a diagnosis of hypertension — and at significantly greater levels than people with normal clinic and ambulatory BP. People with MH, and no previous diagnosis of hypertension, require counseling, work stressor assessment, and possibly treatment, and but rarely receive these because their clinic-measured BP appears normal. Few studies have examined workplace predictors of MH. In recent unpublished data from a New York City hospital, MH was associated with job strain, effort-reward imbalance and shiftwork.[84]

Other Cardiovascular Risk Factors

While evidence is not always consistent, a number of studies have linked work stressors to a variety of CVD risk factors, suggesting additional pathways by which work stressors contribute to the development of CVD. Work stressors have been associated with cigarette smoking intensity and cessation[90–92], overweight[51,90,92], type II diabetes[93,94], sedentary behavior[92,95], alcohol use[51,90,92], coronary atherosclerosis[96–99], inadequate sleep[100–103] (which can lead to increased blood pressure, heart rate[50,104] and CVD risk[105], and lowered heart rate variability[74,106–109]), also a CVD risk factor.[110]

Psychological Disorders

Stressful features of work organization have been shown to substantially affect mental health. Increased overtime was associated with depression, fatigue, confusion, and impaired cognitive function in autoworkers.[111] Job strain has been associated with psychological distress[40,112–117], depression[118–120], anxiety[113–115], and burnout[40,121] — including in prospective cohort studies.[116,117,122]

Effort-reward imbalance also increases the risk for psychological distress, anxiety and depression[123–125], even after adjusting for demands and control.[126] In a population-based study in Germany, the impact of effort-reward imbalance on risk of depression was significantly greater for workers in low status (vs high status) jobs.[127]

Justice and fairness at work have also been linked to mental health, conceptualized as either *relational* justice, whether supervisors treat their employees with respect and fairness, or *procedural* justice, the fairness of organizational decision making processes.[128,129] Two prospective studies have shown higher risk for depressive symptoms or disorders due to lack of justice at work up to four or five years later[130,131], even in addition to the effect of effort-reward imbalance.[131] Four longitudinal studies showed evidence that social support at work decreased the risk of future depression.[122]

Bullying or "mobbing" is a relatively recent area of workplace research.[132] Bullying is characterized by persistent negative actions which create a perceived power imbalance and a hostile working environment. It takes on many forms, including excessive workplace monitoring, unreasonable workloads, verbal abuse or overt criticism and even isolating individuals through gossip or practical jokes.[133] Bullying has been estimated in the United States to affect 37% of the workforce or 54 million individuals[134] however other studies have found variation by occupational sector, and measurement.[135] The reported effects of bullying include decreased self-esteem in the target, lower physical and emotional health[136], depression[137], a higher incidence of post-traumatic stress disorder[138] and intent to leave an organization.[139]

One consequence of layoffs and downsizing is the redistribution of work among remaining employees resulting in increased workload and longer working hours and more days worked a year.[49,51,140,141] In a Finnish study, downsizing "survivors" (those who did not lose their jobs) had a very high risk of being prescribed psychotropic medications (including anti-depressants) compared to those who did not experience downsizing.[142]

Workers may also be subject to another psychological syndrome, post-traumatic stress disorder (PTSD) as a result of traumatic situations they may encounter or witness while at work.[143] Even among workers who have been trained and even 'hardened' for trauma, such as emergency medical technicians, or career soldiers, PTSD can be a serious and enduring problem.[144,145] However, it appears that workers who have such training are at less risk for PTSD than workers completely unprepared for traumatic experiences. The differential effect of training was seen in workers who responded to the 9/11 attacks, where the risk among civilian workers was significantly greater than among law enforcement personnel.[146] There is significant risk for traumatic exposures among untrained workers who may be subjected to violence on the job, or even witness the murder of co-workers. Workplace violence is a significant occupational hazard[147], especially in health care.[148] PTSD can be an occupational hazard for workers recovering from serious injuries on the job.[149] The extent to which this effect, or PTSD in general, occurs is not known.

Population attributable risk (PAR%) of work stressors. There are few studies estimating the fraction of psychological disorders related to work stressors.[150,151] A recent Australian study estimated that 13% of prevalent cases of depression in working men and 17% in working women were attributable to job strain.[151]

Musculoskeletal Disorders

Musculoskeletal Disorders (MSDs), Cumulative Trauma Disorders, Repetitive Strain Injuries and other, similar terms all refer to the same phenomena—disorders of the joints, muscles, and associated soft tissues: tendons, ligaments, cartilage, nerves and blood vessels (see Table 33.2). Although MSDs can occur by several mechanisms, they are hardly ever caused by a single incident. They usually reflect the accumulation (hence 'cumulative') of repeated, small injuries ("micro-trauma") to a tissue, often through occupational exposure to physically and mentally stressful work. Hence, work-related MSDs are classified as occupational diseases, to distinguish them from injuries, which are the result of a single, traumatic incident.

Biomechanical stressors. At the job level, risk factors for MSDs include repetition, force requirements, postural and motion characteristics, tissue compression, and vibration.[152,153]

Table 33.2 — Types and Examples of Musculoskeletal Disorders (MSDs)

- Muscle Disorders: spasms, ruptured fibers
- Tendon Disorders: tendonitis and tenosynovitis (inflammation of the tendon alone or with its synovial sheath); epicondylitis (inflammation of tendon insertions on bone)
- Nerve Disorders: compression of major nerve trunks: Carpal Tunnel Syndrome, sciatica
- Circulatory or Combined Circulatory/Nerve: thoracic outlet syndrome, HAVS (hand/arm vibration syndrome: damage to hand nerves and vessels from vibration)
- Skeletal/Joint/ Spine Disorders: osteo-arthritis, damage to intervertebral discs

Psychosocial stressors. Recent research has identified psychosocial stressors as contributing factors to the development of upper extremity and low back MSDs. These include: job strain[41]; effort-reward imbalance and several other stressors listed in Table 33.1. As with biomechanical stressors, risk posed by psychosocial factors depends upon magnitude and duration of exposure to the stressor. The effects of both biomechanical and psychosocial job stressors are mediated by individual anatomical, physiological, and psychological capacity. Some components of individual capacity are genetically determined (e.g., gender, basic anatomical characteristics, physiology), and some are modifiable (e.g., health behaviors, skill learning).

Mechanisms. While the mechanisms by which biomechanical exposures cause MSDs are well understood, there is still an evolving understanding of how job stress can contribute to MSD etiology. Several mechanisms have been proposed; these are not mutually exclusive and include:

- Reduction in immune function and the body's ability to heal microtrauma
- Disturbances in muscle fiber recruitment, leading to chronic overexertion of and damage to particular fibers
- Behavior changes, such as altered work technique and increased muscle tension
- Psychological changes in pain perception and reporting behavior
- Hyperventilation, resulting in increased body fluid pH, which affects nerve and muscle firing.

When physical and mental stresses are kept within the abilities of the human organism to repair the micro-trauma, work can be healthy; the body and mind may, in fact, be strengthened. This is, of course, the principle behind physical exercise. But any of the above stressors, especially in combination, can become injurious without sufficient rest and recovery time—i.e., if the rate of micro-trauma development exceeds the rate of repair.

Evidence base. MSD researchers have not always agreed on what types of work stressors to measure and include in their studies. But, a solid and growing body of evidence has demonstrated that a wide variety of biomechanical and psychosocial stressors have independent associations with MSDs. Most studies have been cross-sectional[42,154,155] but a smaller set of prospective studies indicates that the associations are causal.[156–159] Intervention studies support this conclusion; Maes et al.[160] demonstrated a reduction in sickness absence related to an intervention that reduced levels of biomechanical risk factors and job demands, while increasing job control.

Work organization and biomechanical and psychosocial stressors. As with all job/task-level stressors, levels of biomechanical and psychosocial risk factors for MSDs are strongly influenced by work organization (Arrow A in Figure 33.2). For example, MSD risk factors such as lack of rest breaks or task variety[161] and job interference with family[162] are shaped by the work organization. Downsizing has been linked to MSD symptoms partly through the mechanism of increased work demands.[163] Seemingly simple changes instituted through lean production, such as prohibiting alternating standing and seated postures, may also be associated with increased MSD symptomatology.[164] Direct links to organizational production-related decisions (Arrow C in Figure 33.2) include MSD associations with just-in-time production[165], understaffing and compressed work scheduling.

Interaction. Biomechanical and psychosocial risk factors may interact to cause MSDs—that is, their combined effect could be greater than the additive individual effects (as in the multiplicative effect of smoking and asbestos exposure in the etiology of lung cancer). Most of the studies listed above did not find statistically significant interactions between biomechanical and psychosocial stressors, however, a small number have found interactive effects. Hollmann et al.[166] found that job control buffered the effect of physical load, but only in jobs with low physical demands. A longitudinal study of retail store material handling employees[155] found low back pain to be associated with two types of interactions: high scheduling demands x job dissatisfaction and high job intensity x low supervisor support. In a laboratory study, Faucett and Rempel[167] found that the contributions of keyboard and seat back heights to symptom development were modified by psychological demands, decision latitude, and supervisor support. One difficulty in evaluating independent or interactive effects is the degree to which biomechanical and psychosocial factors are highly correlated with each other[168], and thus may be both assessed by the same measure.

Injuries

An injury is defined as the physical health consequence of a single traumatic event. A growing body of research suggests that unhealthy work organization increases an employee's risk of injury. For example, long work hours (>8 hours/day or >40 hours/week) have been associated with increased risk of work accidents in Germany[44], and work related injuries and illnesses in U.S. workers aged 23–43.[10] Very long work hours/extended shifts (≥ 24 hours) among medical interns and residents have been associated with reduced sleep, attentional failures[169], medical errors[170] and motor vehicle crashes.[171]

Injuries have been associated, among nurses, with restructuring that increases stressful working conditions[172], downsizing, and work intensification[173], understaffing, inadequate resources, and low nurse manager leadership[45], and, among hospital workers, with low job control and supervisor support.[174] A study of unionized U.S. blue-collar workers found that "safety control" (e.g., influence over organizational safety practices and procedures, safe behaviors) protected against the risk of (self-reported) injuries associated with "situational constraints" (e.g., faulty equipment, poor information, interruptions in work).[8] A study of U.S. construction laborers found that 10 of the 12 job stressors examined (e.g., job demands, low job control, job insecurity, exposure hours) were associated with either (self-reported) injuries or "near misses."[6] Work accidents have also been associated with smoking[175], obesity and sleep-disordered breathing[176], thus the promotion of unhealthy behaviors by work stressors may be one pathway by which work stressors lead to injuries.

Lower injury rates have been associated with worker empowerment, good relations between management and workers[177,178], autonomy, delegation of control, low stress, low grievance rates[177] and encouragement of long-term commitment of the workforce.[178] Several studies suggest that injury rates tend to be highest in workplaces "where there is a unilateral determination of health and safety by management and lowest where mechanisms of union-based representation are present."[17] For example, a British national study found, in workplaces with at least one injury, lower injury rates in unionized workplaces.[179] However, other studies have shown higher injury rates in unionized workplaces in the same industry.[180] Since unions tend to be organized in higher hazard industries[181], the presence of a union may be less important than the particular union's influence or the strategies it adopts. For example, another British study found that "joint consultative committees, with all employee representatives appointed by unions, significantly reduce workplace injuries relative to those establishments where the management alone determines health and safety arrangements."[182,183] In two unionized Chrysler auto assembly plants in France and England, accident rates were much lower in the plant where workers were better organized and more militant on the shop floor.[184] Unionized U.S. construction sites are more likely than non-union sites to have OSHA inspections, enforcement and compliance with OSHA standards.[185]

A barrier to research on work organization and injuries is underreporting of work injuries. A recent report from the House Committee on Education and Labor documents "chronic" and "gross" underreporting; "as much as 69 percent of injuries and illnesses may never make it into" the Bureau of Labor Statistics Survey of Occupational Injuries and Illnesses.[186] Various reasons for underreporting exist, however, a major reason cited in the report is OSHA's reliance on self-reporting by employers, who "have strong incentives to underreport" workplace injuries and illnesses. These include reduced likelihood of an OSHA inspection, lower workers compensation insurance premiums, and better chances of winning government contracts and bonuses. Strategies that result in underreporting include intimidation and harassment of workers who report injuries and illnesses, forcing workers back to work too soon after serious injuries (to reduce "lost-time" rates), absentee policies, discouraging physicians from reporting injuries or diagnosing illnesses, and safety incentive programs which provide awards for a period of time without a recordable injury.[186] A review commissioned by OSHA did not find evidence to substantiate injury reductions as the result of safety incentive programs, rather they concluded that such programs can reduce worker injury reporting.[187]

Psychological Health Impacts of Chemical and Physical Hazards

Workers can be exposed to a wide variety of chemical and physical conditions that can exert neurobehavioral effects similar to those of drugs and alcohol. Brown[188] cites diagnoses that are now recognized by the American Psychiatric Association as attributable to specific chemical exposures, which include carbon monoxide, nerve gas and organophosphate pesticides, two metals: mercury and lead; as well as several neurotoxic solvents. Typical diagnoses include substance-induced delirium, mental retardation, symptoms of dementia and intoxication, psychotic episodes, anxiety and mood alteration.[189] Cognitive impairment is another general effect that is less severe but an important factor that can be detected with early testing. Adolescent workers may be particularly vulnerable to cognitive/behavioral impacts.[190] Table 33.3 provides a list of chemical and physical agents associated with neurobehavioral toxicity.

In addition to the direct effects of chemical and physical hazards on neurobehavior, these hazards often interact with other chemical exposures and may be exacerbated by individual characteristics and susceptibilities. Schulte and co-workers recently developed conceptual models for understanding and studying the relationship between work and obesity.[191] They cite neurotoxins as one class of occupational hazards which could interact with excessive worker body mass index (BMI). They state that while no epidemiological studies have investigated the risk of neurotoxicity in workers as a function of BMI, "over the past decade, anecdotal and experimental data obtained with animals often suggest that rats and mice with increased body mass show exaggerated neurotoxic responses to diverse classes of known neurotoxic chemicals (e.g., organometals, substituted pyridines, substituted amphetamines).[192] Thus, given the linkage between obesity and

Table 33.3 — Examples of Neurotoxic Agents Found in Occupational Settings (adapted from Mergler, 1998[193] and Brown, 2007[188])

Metals: Associated with a wide range of behavioral abnormalities, including agitation and mood lability. Peripheral neuropathy is frequently observed.			
	Aluminum	Manganese	
	Arsenic	Mercury	Tin
	Lead	Thallium	
Solvents: In acute doses can lead to inebriation-like symptoms. Personality widely affected. (Other toxic effects also seen.)			
	Carbon disulfide	Perchloroethylene	
	n-Hexane, Methyl butyl ketone	Toluene	
	Methyl chloride	Trichloroethylene	
Pesticides: Interferes with normal neuronal functioning through their anticholinesterase activity. Can be fatal after acute exposure.			
	Organophosphates	Carbamates	
Physical hazards: High doses of ionizing radiation have been associated with dementia and mood alteration. Low-level behavioral effects not known. Noise elicits a typical physiological stress response at levels well below those associated with hearing loss.			

factors known or suspected to damage the nervous system, it could be hypothesized that obesity may enhance the susceptibility of the nervous system to toxic chemicals found in the work environment."[191] It is likely that neurotoxins interact with worker vulnerability and other exposures as well.

While the *acute* effects of exposure are often easily observable — as in the Mad Hatter in *Alice in Wonderland*, who exhibited symptoms of mercury poisoning found in millinery workers who used metallic mercury for treating the felt fabrics — at low exposure levels, the effects can be subtle and only detectable through sophisticated neurobehavioral testing.[194] (The diagnoses recognized by the American Psychiatric Association primarily reflect acute responses). Sophisticated neurotoxicological testing has never been carried out in a systematic way in the occupational setting nor have any major epidemiological studies been designed and carried out, despite the fact that such testing was proposed decades ago.[195] Thus, knowledge of occupational neurobehavioral toxicity is limited to observations of acute exposures or to very small sample studies — often in experimental settings. Further, given the systematic paucity of data on where chemicals are used, it is difficult to even estimate the potential extent of worker exposure, long-term health effects or increased accident rates attributable to neurological or cognitive impairment. It is also not known whether exposure to stressful working conditions exacerbates the neurochemical effects of chemical and physical exposures. To sum up, while society generally exercises wide-ranging judicial and regulatory vigilance over the use of illicit drugs and alcohol, it has not demonstrated a similar vigilance to the regulation and oversight of chemical and physical neurobehavioral toxicants or study of neurobehavioral toxicology at work.

Economic Costs of Work Stressors

One of the most common motivations for job redesign and changing the way that work is organized is to reduce costs and thereby increase profitability. However, there is a point at which the enhanced productivity, if any, that results from organizational changes will be offset by the increased costs that result from injury and illness among the workforce. For example, a study by the American Management Association found that 70% of companies that had experienced downsizings and layoffs reported a substantial increase in disability claims, even with fewer employees.[196] Those injury and illness costs not paid by employers get directly transferred to employees, their families and other taxpayers. Table 33.4 lists direct and indirect costs associated with unhealthy working conditions.

Table 33.4 — Organizational Costs of Work Stress-related Injury and Illness

Direct Costs	*Indirect Costs*
Medical, hospital and pharmaceutical	Workplace absenteeism/ sick leave
Health insurance premiums	Presenteeism
Disability	Disability management
Compensation benefits	Turnover and training
	Lawsuits related to stress

Table 33.6 — Indirect disability costs to employers

Case management
Return-to-work programs
Wellness programs
Employee assistance programs
Safety programs

Direct costs. Table 33.5 lists the top illnesses and injuries financially affecting large U.S. employers through direct costs.(197) Many of the illnesses, especially cardiovascular, musculoskeletal, anxiety disorders, depression and alcoholism have been associated with workplace stressors.

Although companies pay substantial direct health costs, so do their employees. Whereas premiums have increased between 8% and 14% every year since 2000, inflation and increases in employees' earnings were in the 3–4% range for the same period.(198) This means that workers have to spend more of their income every year on their portion of healthcare coverage and expenses. A 2007 survey of 170 of the largest Fortune 1000 companies in the U.S. found that these companies subsidized only 78% of premium costs yet reported spending over $15 billion dollars annually in health insurance(199), leaving their employees to cover $4.2 billion in premiums as well as deductibles, co-payments and co-insurance. Public and private sector employees in Connecticut with work-related musculoskeletal disorders and with health insurance still paid $15–71 million in out-of-pocket expenses.(200)

Table 33.5 — Major illness and injuries financially affecting U.S. employers

Physical
Angina Pectoris
Essential Hypertension
Diabetes Mellitus
Low back pain
Myocardial Infarction
COPD
Spinal Trauma
Sinusitis
Ear, nose, throat or mastoid disesases
Psychological
Alcoholism
Bipolar disorders
Depression
Anxiety disorders
Acute phase schizophrenia
Psychoses
Neurotic, personality and non-psychotic disorders

Psychosocial factors contribute to workers' compensation and disability claims when they play a role in producing illnesses which are recognized as compensable. In the U.S., 7% of the workforce received disability benefits in 2001. Of these, 27% were due to mental strain, depression or mood disorders, 22% from musculoskeletal disorders and 11% from cardiovascular disease.(201) These three stress-related illnesses are also the top causes of disability in other developed countries, such as the Netherlands, Denmark and Sweden, and in these countries and the U.S., the proportion of disabled adults is increasing.(202) It is unknown how many cases are not identified or reported to workers' compensation or disability systems, and these, along with denied claims, are paid for by workers and their families. A rough estimate is available from the Australian state of Victoria, where 21,437 cases of depression could be attributed to job strain, but only 696 "mental stress" workers compensation claims attributed to chronic stressors were filed that year — a 30-fold difference.(151)

Indirect costs (both disability and productivity costs) account for over half of the expenses to employers associated with employee ill health(203), and the three stress-related illnesses listed above cause the highest indirect costs to the employer.(197) Table 33.6 lists the most common indirect disability costs to employers.(204)

Productivity costs include turnover, absenteeism and "presenteeism." Up to 40% of turnover can be attributed to stressors at work.(205) Work stressors associated with turnover include lack of work-life balance(206), effort-reward imbalance(207), and job strain.(208)

Absenteeism. A meta-analysis reviewing 153 studies that examined the relationship between stress at work and absenteeism concluded that stressors cause illnesses which then results in increased absenteeism.[209] Absenteeism was an adaptive coping response by reducing exposure to work stressors at times when the individual was most vulnerable to ill health.

Presenteeism occurs when employees feel pressure to work even when not feeling well. It is characterized by decreased quality and quantity of work and time at work not working on task, and can be a response to job stressors, overwork and company policies. An analysis of several health and insurance databases found that presenteeism was most likely to be associated with the following conditions in order of economic impact to employers: arthritis, hypertension, depression/sadness/mental illness, allergies, migraine/headaches, cancer, asthma, heart disease, and respiratory infections.[197]

Total costs. The estimated annual costs to U.S. employers of employee illnesses discussed in this section are more than $1 trillion.[210] Costs to employees and to society for these conditions may well be greater, since employers pay only a proportion of the cost of work-related illnesses. Employees and society also pay costs associated with illness such as family instability, bankruptcy, divorce or substance abuse. Simply because "job stressors" is not a standard accounting line item on a financial spreadsheet does not mean that it is insignificant in its financial toll on organizations, their employees and society as a whole.

Contextual Influences on Work Organization, Stress and Health

Changing Nature of Work

Developed Countries

Sweeping changes in the organization of work in developed countries, resulting in part from economic globalization, appear to be increasing work stressors.[14] The Tokyo Declaration, a 1998 consensus document produced by occupational health experts from the European Union, Japan and the US, summarized these changes:

> "Organization restructuring, mergers, acquisitions and downsizing, the frantic pace of work and life, the erosion of leisure time, and/or the blending of work and home time. Most of these developments are driven by economic and technological changes aiming at short-term productivity and profit gain... Production practices are increasingly "leaner". New employment practices such as use of contingent workers are increasingly adopted. Concurrently, job stability and tenure is decreasing... New management models are introduced with more teamwork, just-in-time, and TQM (Total Quality Management)... This rapid change, combined with both over- and under-employment, is likely to be highly stress provoking. Occupational stress-related mental and psychosomatic complaints are very common in all 15 EU member states.[211]

Work intensification can result from teamwork structures and high performance/lean staffing work systems, overwork motivated by pay for performance job structures, vulnerability to low pay and risk of job loss among temporary workers, fear of displacement because of organizational restructuring and downsizing and work overload for workers who remain after staff reductions from downsizing.[4] According to NIOSH, "Concern exists that various worker participatory or involvement strategies may often be more ceremonial than substantive, having little meaningful influence on worker empowerment — or perhaps even eroding workers' means to influence job conditions through more traditional labor-management mechanisms such as collective bargaining."[4] Restructuring, use of contract and temporary employees, work intensification, computer technology and electronic monitoring all tend to reduce time available and opportunities for informal social networking at work, which helps build social support and collective efforts to reduce stressors.[31]

NIOSH is also concerned that people who work extended hours on a given shift may be at risk of exceeding permissible exposure limits to hazardous substances; that increased public contact and nonstandard work schedules (such as night work), common in the growing service sector, may expose workers to an increased risk of violence on the job; and that worker health and safety may be indirectly affected by cuts in occupational health services or the loss of accumulated health and safety knowledge (due to downsizing), or lack of safety training (among temporary workers).[4]

Use of **electronic performance monitoring** is increasing, with 45% of US employers reporting use in 1999.[212] Monitoring is conducted through: software to monitor computer use; by listening to calls and providing time quotas for directory assistance/customer service (call center) operators; camera surveillance; tracking of mobile workers (e.g., drivers or utility workers) by Global Positioning System (GPS)-enabled vehicles or cell phones. Employees have typically no input into the design or planning of monitoring systems.[22,212] The result is often less worker control over schedules and how work is done, and an increased emphasis on quantity and speed over quality. Such changes can create a climate of fear, threat of reprimand, constant deadline pressure and a "more coercive, stricter number-counting supervisory style" with constant negative feedback, not a "more helpful...supervisory approach."[22,23] Electronic monitoring is common in the fast growing and stressful call center industry, which currently employs about 3% of U.S. workers.[213,214]

Developing Countries

Many developing countries, over the past 30–50 years, have undergone urbanization and industrialization and enacted policies of deregulation, privatization, and reduced social protections. A recent World Health Organization (WHO) report describes the "race to the bottom" in working conditions in developing countries as they attempt to attract overseas capital to low regulation export zones, and the rural dislocation, and social and environmental health impacts that result. In developing countries, there is increasing downsizing and job insecurity in the formal economy, growth in the (unregulated) informal economy, and continuing problems of child labor and forced or bonded labor.[215]

What Does the Data Show?

European surveys show continuing increases in work intensity and job demands between 1990–2005, but no change or slight declines in job control or autonomy since 1995[216], suggesting an increase in the prevalence of job strain. Average annual **work hours** for a US worker in the paid labor force have not changed substantially in the past 25 years.[217] However, since the proportion of women in the paid labor force has increased dramatically, the combined number of hours worked by middle-income husbands and wives with children, age 25–54, has increased from about 3,000 to 3,600 per year between 1982–2002.[218] Due to dramatic declines in work hours in other developed countries, annual U.S. work hours are now among the longest in the developed world, about 5–10 more weeks per year than workers in Western Europe.[141,217] In the US, there is no legal requirement for minimum vacation time (as in EU countries), and no paid vacation or holidays are provided for 31% of low wage (vs. 12% of high wage) workers and 64% of part-time (vs. 10% of full-time) workers.[219] **Precarious work** is increasing[216] and is associated with working at higher speeds, making more repetitive movements, having less control over work pace, and receiving less training.[220]

Socioeconomic status. The increase in stressful working and employment conditions may be even greater for workers in lower status jobs. Since income for the bottom half of the income distribution has been largely stagnant for 30–35 years, income inequality (the gap between richer and poorer) has increased dramatically in the U.S. since 1970, and is the highest in the developed world.[217] Labor unions, which provide protection especially for lower status workers, now represent a smaller proportion of the workforce in the U.S. and some other developed nations.[221] Precarious or contingent (temporary and part-time) employment is more common among workers in lower status jobs.[222,223] Policies associated with economic globalization, including de-regulation, privatization of government services, weakened social protections and reduced social welfare transfer payments, such as social security or health insurance, have a greater impact on workers with less income, job skills, or fewer employment options. New organizational practices, such as lean production, downsizing and electronic monitoring, affect working conditions for most workers, although arguably a greater impact may be seen among workers in lower status jobs.

Changing Nature of Work and Trends in Health

Adverse health effects, primarily musculoskeletal disorders, psychological disorders and CVD, have been associated with privatization of public services[224], downsizing[15], labor market flexibility[225], precarious/contingent work[226,227], lean production[20], income inequality[228], and electronic monitoring.[229]

Despite large declines in CVD mortality over the past 40 years in the U.S.[230], there has been little or no decline in new cases of CVD (incidence) in the past 20 years.[231–234] While smoking prevalence and cholesterol levels have declined, there have been increases in diabetes[235], overweight[236] and hypertension[237], and increasing recognition that psychosocial stressors may contribute to these trends.[238] Increases in sleeping problems have been reported in the U.S.[239], Finland[240], and Sweden.[241] Thus, while public health efforts and advances in medical technology enable us to live longer with disease, we are not doing an adequate job of preventing stress-related diseases such as CVD and hypertension.

In **developing countries**, there has been a rapid increase in the prevalence of hypertension, smoking, obesity[242] and CVD. Anecdotal reports describe night work at call centers in India (answering calls from the U.S. and Europe) where workers face sleep disorders, heart disease, depression and family discord[243], and work at Chinese factories that supply Western companies, with high rates of injuries and illnesses, child labor and 16-hour days on fast-moving assembly lines.[244]

Socioeconomic health disparities. Stressful working conditions appear to be increasing to a greater extent among lower (vs higher) status workers, implying increases in health disparities by socioeconomic position — and the data show increasing disparities in CVD mortality (higher mortality among blue-collar than white-collar workers) since the 1960s.[245–247] Socioeconomic disparities in CVD incidence[248,249] and in the prevalence of hypertension, diabetes and smoking are also increasing.[250]

International health disparities. The longer work hours, greater income inequality, weaker unions, and weaker social protections faced by U.S. workers compared to Western European workers, may be translating into higher rates of illness. The US has the highest prevalence of any and serious psychological disorders, including anxiety disorders, mood disorders, impulse-control disorders and substance abuse, in a study comparing 14 countries[251] and higher coronary heart disease death rates than most other developed countries.[252]

Historical trends. Natural selection shaped the human physical and psychological apparatus to fit a hunter-gatherer existence. For both men and women, this involved brief periods of intense physical exertion, punctuated by long periods of rest and recuperation. Hunter-gatherer life allowed for close bonding in a small band, ample social support, varied and challenging "work", and a lot of control over one's "work process." With an evolutionary history of several million years based on this way of living, even the roughly 10,000 years of our settled agricultural past have probably not substantially changed the design features of human anatomy and psychology.[253–256]

This helps to explain why CVD and hypertension are epidemics primarily of industrial societies, with a very low prevalence in non-market agricultural or hunter-gatherer communities.[257,258] The rising prevalence of hypertension and CVD in developed countries parallels the transformation of working life during the past two centuries, away from agricultural work and relatively autonomous craft-based work towards machine-based (including computer-based) labor, characteristic of the assembly line and mass production.[259] Key characteristics of the assembly-line approach to job design are high workload demands combined with low employee control ("job strain"), and, during periods of economic growth, long work hours.

Work-Family Interface

Demographic and Social Changes. Demographic, social, technological, and economic changes in the U.S. over the past 50 years have dramatically affected the way that workers integrate their family and work lives, leading to a greater need for organizational supports and public policy oriented towards working families (for reviews see references 260 and 261). Demographic and social changes include the aging of the population, an increased proportion of women in the labor force, and an increase in multigenerational households. Technological change and economic globalization have led to changes in work hours, location of work, and control over work hours. The U.S. now has a 24/7 economy with many workers occupying low wage, high demand service jobs that frequently require them to have second jobs to make ends meet. All of these changes have led to increases in the demands of work and family and the resulting effects of such multiple role demands on the safety and health of workers and their families.(260)

These social and demographic changes require improvements in both the way that organizations are structured to provide support for working families, and improvements in government policies related to dependent care, family leave programs, and health care systems — all policies that impact working families. At present, these public policy supports for working families in the U.S. are far below those of all other industrialized nations.(260) For example, while the Family and Medical Leave Act (FMLA) of 1993 requires U.S. employers with 50 or more employees to allow workers to take family leave of up to 12 weeks per year, with a guarantee of being able to return to the same or similar job at the same pay and benefits, there is no requirement at the federal level for any of this leave to be paid. Thus, it is virtually impossible for most working families to actually afford to use the FMLA. This is in stark contrast to family leave programs in other industrialized nations in Europe and Japan that provide universal child care and paid family leave through their governments.(262) In addition, the U.S. is the only industrialized nation without some form of national health insurance for working adults.

Work-Family Integrated into OHP with a focus on Primary Prevention. Quick and Terick argue that OHP "...should develop, maintain, and promote employees' health and the health of their families."(263) Thus, the work family interface has been a central focus of OHP research. Extending the application of psychology and the public health model of prevention not only to workers' occupational safety and health, but also to their families, introduces the field of OHP as another lens through which to view work-family stressors and work-family benefits.

Furthermore, work-family interventions provide a useful set of strategies to ameliorate, or even prevent, the stress from dealing with excessive combined demands from work and family. The field of work and family has a strong focus on prevention with the development of interventions, including work-family supports, benefits, and policies, such as dependent care supports and organizational leave policies, which can be expected to improve the health and well being of workers and their families, e.g.(264,265), and the health of organizations.(266)

Increasing control over when and where work is done helps to alleviate work-family stress, e.g.(267), just as providing supervisor support for work and family can reduce work-family conflict.(268) Work schedule and location flexibility and alternative work schedules can be seen as positive or negative depending on who has control over the schedule and the location and who is making use of such policies. Flexibility in time and place of work is beneficial to workers who can take advantage of these practices, such as higher level salaried workers, and there is much literature that supports such beneficial effects of flexible scheduling on health and well being of workers.(260) It may not be an advantage, however, to lower wage hourly workers and in fact, may be used by their managers as a way of manipulating the work schedule to meet other organizational needs. For example, one management practice that is used to avoid paying overtime to current employees or paying benefits to new employees is to make frequent use of part-time workers to fill in shifts during high demand hours. In addition, industries such as retail and restaurant work often use inconsistent schedules and give employees limited advanced notice of schedules. This is a particular detriment to working parents who are in dire need of consistent schedules in order to make adequate arrangements for child care. Thus, labor unions are skeptical of words like "flexibility" and "alternative work schedules," while work-family scholars tend to focus on the benefits of flexibility and alternative work schedules to individual workers.

Work-Family Conflict and Health. The strain associated with excessive combined work and family responsibilities has been shown to lead to depression(264,269), decrements in healthy behaviors(270), and coronary heart disease.[271] Research examining the relationship between work-family conflict and physical ill health as measured by self reports shows a positive relation between the two, e.g.[269,272–275] Furthermore, Thomas and Ganster[276] found that extensive work-family conflict was positively related to diastolic blood pressure and cholesterol levels. Brisson et al.[277] found that, among white-collar women holding university degrees, the combined exposure of large family responsibilities and high job strain had a greater effect on blood pressure than exposure to either one of these factors alone.

Work-family benefits as measured by positive "spillover" have been related to better self-reported mental health. Positive spillover occurs when the benefits of one role (e.g., mood, values or skills related to work) transfer to benefit the other role (e.g., family). For example, Grzywacz and Bass[278] found that work-family spillover was associated with lower risk of mental illness, depression, and problem drinking. In addition, Hanson, Hammer and Colton[279] reported that the more positive the spillover, the higher their reports of mental health.

Work-Family Conflict and Safety. Little research exists on the relationship between work-family conflict and safety. One study among poultry food workers demonstrated that higher levels of perceived safety climate were related to lower levels of work-to-family conflict[280], suggesting that when supervisors value safety, this helps to reduce stress and the impact of work-family conflict on workers.

Workers who are experiencing high levels of work-family conflict can be more stressed, and thus, are not able to concentrate on doing their jobs as effectively because of limited cognitive resources, e.g.[281] A recent study of nurses by Cullen and Hammer[282] demonstrated that higher levels of organizational work performance norms were related to work-family conflict, which in turn, was related to lower levels of safety compliance. Pressures for production (i.e., work performance norms) were directly related to work overload which in turn impacted work-family conflict. Furthermore, Daniels, Hammer, and Truxillo[283] found that high levels of work-family conflict increased workers' cognitive load, leading to decreased safety performance among a group of construction workers. This is the first study to demonstrate that the stress and strain associated with work-family conflict can reduce one's cognitive recourses, making individuals less able to focus on safety. One solution to such potential safety hazards is changing the organization of work in ways that would alleviate work-family conflict through mechanisms of increased control, reduced demands, and increased support at work.

Safety Climate

According to the hierarchy of controls for occupational hazards, the first priority for employers, and the most effective injury prevention method, is to eliminate relevant hazards from the work environment. However, not every hazard can be completely eliminated through engineering or job design. Thus, it is crucial that hazard control efforts identify aspects of work organization that may be modified to further reduce or eliminate worker exposures. To facilitate this approach, organizational leaders, including management and labor, should also create a strong social context for safety that encourages technical competence, hazard recognition and control, and prevention behaviors.

Personnel selection and training are both essential to maintaining a workforce with the necessary knowledge, skills, and abilities to perform tasks competently and safely. However, a technically competent workforce is necessary, but not sufficient, for creating a strong social environment for safety. In the absence of adequate government regulation, workers' compensation, or labor-management agreements, pressure to compete in the marketplace can encourage employers to favor production over safety and neglect safety priorities.[284,285] Many social processes may be relevant to the success of a safety program, including warning design and hazard communication[286,287], observational learning processes[288–294], and safety communication and feedback.[7,295–302] Although it is beyond the scope of this chapter, we note that safety feedback processes can be misused and applied with inappropriate incentive systems, and are therefore a subject of debate within OHP and other disciplines.[303–309] Within OHP, the concept of organizational safety climate has received the most attention from researchers interested in the social context for safety, and is therefore the main focus of this section.

As with other organizational phenomena, the social environment for safety is best understood through a multi-level perspective that includes inputs from line workers, union representatives, supervisors, and upper level management. Inputs from crucial supporting departments are also relevant, such as maintenance, human resources, and environmental health and safety. Although all employees' actions impact organizational safety priorities and outcomes, decisions and actions at higher levels of the organization have broad and powerful effects on working conditions and pressures experienced by line workers. From this perspective, hazards and behaviors observed on the ground can be viewed as "the final common pathway" to injuries rather than the fundamental causes of injuries.(310) For example, an upper level salesperson at a construction company may win jobs for his or her firm by bidding unrealistic cost-estimates and timelines to clients, which could then create pressures on supervisors to emphasize speed and implement extended work hours, which might lead to elevated fatigue, decision errors, or "cutting corners" by line workers (as well as increased biomechanical and psychosocial risk factors for MSDs and other occupational illnesses). Production pressure may be intense "... when pay systems are tied to production, so that lost time is lost pay, or where there are quotas, with penalties for not achieving the quota."(307) To illustrate, the U.S. Chemical Safety Board found that causes of the 2005 explosion at a Texas refinery that killed 15 workers included cost-cutting at the top of the corporation that affected safety conditions, worker fatigue, poor training, and ignoring numerous warnings and "near misses."(311)

The terms organizational safety "culture" and "climate" are often used interchangeably in the workplace, but researchers discourage this practice and distinguish between the concepts.(312) Organizational safety *culture* is the broader of the two concepts.(313) Most definitions of culture include the shared basic assumptions, values, and observable practices of a group (rites, rituals, symbols, stories, work methods), as well as the socialization methods used to sustain those values and practices over time in order to succeed and survive as a group.(314–316) To illustrate the broad and complex meaning of culture, consider two organizations that share the same basic value that "safety priorities supercede production priorities." Workers surveyed about the priority of safety would produce similar average scores in each organization. However, the two organizations could use very different cultural practices to promote and sustain those values, including stories, slogans, signs, training, and safety policies and practices. Therefore, assessing culture needs to involve both sampling the self-reported values of workers *and* sampling/observing the rites, rituals, practices, stories (etc.) used by the organization to sustain and promote those values. In contrast, safety *climate* is focused exclusively on perceptions of the relative priority of safety within the organization at a given point in time, and is measured by assessing workers' shared perceptions about safety policies, procedures, and practices.(18,299,312) Many organizational factors impact employees' perceptions of safety priorities, including cultural practices, the intensity of management commitment to safety at all levels of the organization, the adequacy of safety control systems, the quality of safety communication, the freedom to voice concerns about hazards and exercise health and safety rights without penalty, and the work practices of line supervisors and peer groups.

The formal concept of safety climate was developed by Zohar.(317,318) Based on a review of research literature on characteristics of organizations with the best safety records, Zohar developed a 40-item safety climate survey that asked workers for their perceptions about seven dimensions of safety, including perceived management attitudes towards safety and the status of the safety officer. The survey was tested with stratified random samples from 20 industrial organizations in Israel. Results showed that variance in climate scores between factories was greater than variance within factories, which demonstrated that workplaces can in fact possess a shared psychological climate for safety. Moreover, the total climate score for these organizations correlated with independent expert rankings of factory safety resulting from site inspections.

Since Zohar's seminal paper, over 200 journal articles listed in the PsychInfo database have been published on safety climate, and over 20 climate surveys have been developed and validated, with management safety values being the most commonly assessed dimension.[319] A meta-analysis of 32 studies showed that the construct of safety climate is moderately correlated with self-reported safe behaviors (r = .43 for safety compliance, r = .50 for safety participation) and modestly inversely correlated with injuries (r = -.22 for retrospective studies, r = -.35 for prospective studies).[18] There is also evidence that organizations with poor safety climates experience significant underreporting of injuries[320], which suggests that the climate-injury relationship could currently be underestimated. The sum of current evidence suggests that safety climate is a valid predictor of safe behaviors and injury rates, and encourages the use of safety climate surveys as diagnostic tools.

Several models have been proposed to explain the relationship between safety climate and injury rates.[6,8,321–325] Zohar[312] proposed a multi-level model of safety climate, where both organization level and subgroup level safety climates affect workers' behavior-outcome expectancies, which then in turn affect actual safety behaviors and injury outcomes. In the model, enforced safety policies are proposed to have a direct positive effect on climate at the organizational level and on supervisory safety practices. In turn, supervisory safety practices are shown to have a direct effect on climate at the sub-group level (see Figure 33.3). Workers have limited control over the organization of their work tasks and implementation of organizational priorities, so the multi-level model of climate also shows direct pathways from leadership levels in the organization to injury outcomes.

Current trends in safety climate research include multi-level investigations of climate at both the organizational and subgroup levels, and interactions between moderators/mediators of the relationship between climate and safety outcomes, such as leadership style[326,327], employee safety control[328] and psychological strain.[329,330] An example of a potential moderator of safety climate is union status, which was found to have a positive correlation with climate level in a study of injured construction workers in California (r = .23). The authors suggested that this relationship might be explained by factors such as involvement of union members in enforcement of safety

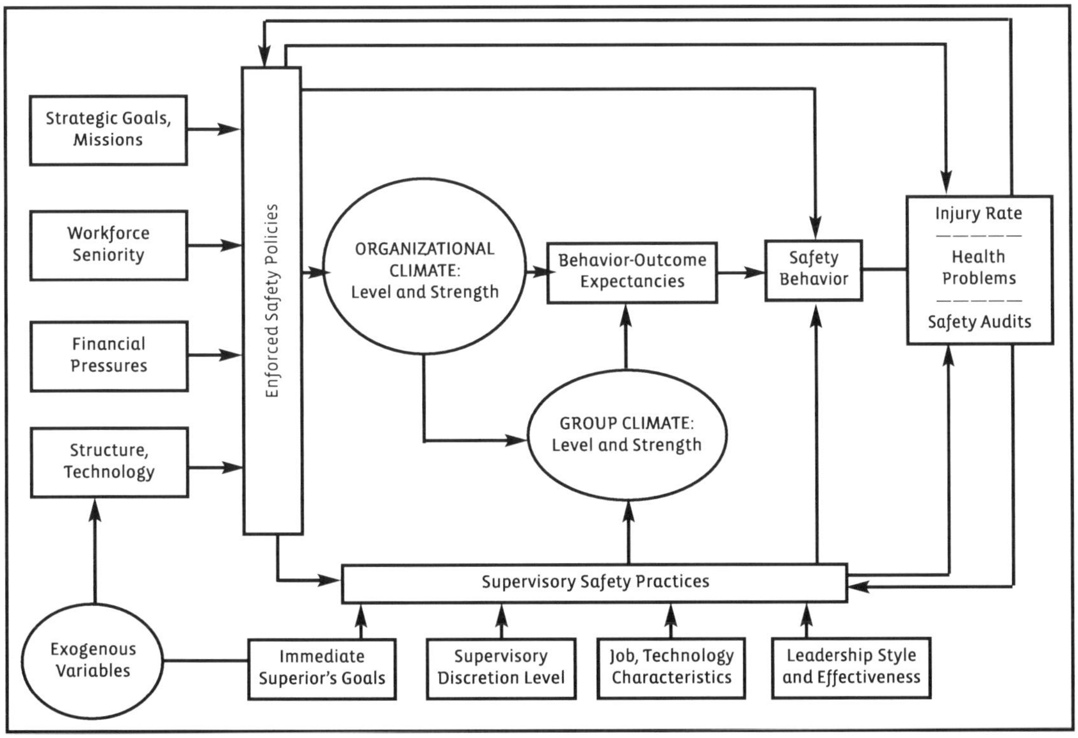

Figure 33.3 — Model of safety climate.[312]

policies, increased formal training through the union, introduction of safety language into negotiated contracts, and more vigorous monitoring of large unionized construction sites by OSHA.[7]

Lone Workers: A Special Safety Climate Challenge. Creating a strong social context for safety with lone workers in dangerous and demanding occupations, such as commercial trucking and home care nursing, is a socially significant challenge. For example, truck drivers account for 15% of all occupational fatalities[331], 8% of all musculoskeletal injuries[332], and have elevated levels of serious health conditions that cause early mortality, such as heart disease.[333] Relative to more traditional work environments, lone workers are exposed to highly variable work environments, and have less exposure to important safety support and social influence, such as physical and technical assistance from peers and supervision, and social modeling. Social isolation at work is also considered stressful, increasing risk of cardiovascular disease[334], and interferes with opportunities to build social networks and support and collective efforts to reduce stressors.[31]

Little is currently known about the development of safety climates under isolated work arrangements. However, research with professional drivers highlights potential leverage points for establishing safety as a high priority, including the involvement of key administrative personnel in the safety program, such as dispatchers or fleet managers who are known to impact drivers' perceptions of safety priorities[335] and turnover rates.[336] As in standard, location-based workplaces, decisions about work organization have an impact on injury rates as well as safety climate. For instance, since long work hours are associated with injury rates in other industries[51], as well as driving[337], reducing pressure to work long hours would be a key component to improving safety and health among drivers. Other promising strategies to reduce injury risk include providing professional drivers with opportunities to track and report hazards[338], participate in the development of safety processes and goals[339], receive safety-related feedback about driving behaviors from on-board computers[340,341], bargain over work hours and schedules, and provide greater opportunities for co-worker social interaction.[31]

How to Measure Work Stressors

As part of worksite screening/surveillance programs, industrial hygienists can contribute to the assessment of exposures to work stressors and help identify jobs, departments or facilities at high-risk of work stressor-related illness or injury. Ideally, this would be conducted in collaboration with clinicians, ergonomists, psychologists, epidemiologists or other health professionals. However, basic work stressor assessment surveys (and scoring instructions) are available on-line (Table 33.7). National averages for comparison purposes are available, for example, for NIOSH's Quality of Work Life module.[341] In addition, for further assistance, industrial hygienists can obtain professional advice on work stressor assessment through organizations such as NIOSH, the Society for Occupational Health Psychology, or the Center for Social Epidemiology.

Self-Report Questionnaires

Work stressors are typically measured using self-report questionnaires.[343] Most of the questionnaires focus on workers' perceptions of their exposure to stressors — the conditions that can lead to harmful consequences at work. Stressors may be distinguished from "strain" — the adverse cognitive, emotional, or physical harms that workers experience as a result of stressors. Due to adaptation, people working in a stressful job may not report feelings of stress. For example, blood pressure elevation at work due to stressors may not be associated with perceived anxiety or distress.[344]

Some questionnaires ask about stressors specific to a particular occupation, for example, nurses[345], teachers[346] or bus drivers.[347] Such measures provide detailed information, and along with focus groups and interviews, are especially useful for designing interventions.

However, to help identify high-risk job titles or workplaces, the standard approach is the use of generic measures of job characteristics such as demands, control, and support, using language general enough to be used across a variety of occupations and industries.

Table 33.7 — Widely used work stressor questionnaires

Questionnaire	*Number of Scales*	*Number of Questions*	*Comments*
Job Content Questionnaire (JCQ) http://www.jcqcenter.org/	8	49	v. 2.0 includes new questions on emotional work demands, change and flexibility at work, organizational level employee influ ence, and collective control
Effort-Reward Imbalance (ERI) http://www.uni-duesseldorf.de/ medicalsociology/ Questionnaire_ psychometric_in.117.html http://www.uni-duesseldorf.de/ medicalsociology/Effort-reward_ imbalance_at_wor.112.0.html	4	17	"Reward includes respect, support, fair treatment, promotion opportunities, income, and job security
Quality of Work Life Questionnaire (NIOSH) http://www.cdc.gov/niosh/topics/stress/ qwlquest.html	36	67	Used in national U.S. surveys in 2002, 2006; national averages in[341]
Generic Job Stress Questionnaire (NIOSH) http://www/cdc.gov/niosh/topics/workorg/ tools/niosh-job-stress-questionnaire.html	21	116	
Copenhagen Psychosocial Questionnaire (COPSOQ) http://www/arbejdsmiljofoskning.dk/ Sp%C3%B8rgeskemaer/Psykisk%20 arbejdsmilj%C3%B8.aspx	8;26;30	44(short); 95(med); 141(long)	
Occupational Stress Index (OSI) http://www2a.cdc.gov/niosh-working/ detail.asp?id=85 http://www.workhealth.org/OSI%20Index/ OSI%20Home%20Page.html	7	58	Includes occupational Specific questions based on generic questions; version for professional drivers

Job Exposure Matrices

In some studies in the U.S. and Sweden, a job-exposure matrix (based on national surveys) has been used to assign exposure to work stressors to individuals on the basis of their job titles — a more objective method of work stressor assessment than self-report. Despite the likelihood of individual differences between workers who hold the same job title in terms of their exposure to and reactions to stressors, such studies have shown associations between job stressors and cardiovascular disease.[66,69,348,349] The U.S. Dept. of Labor's O*NET job characteristics system (http://online.onetcenter.org/) has shown promise as a job exposure matrix in health studies.[350–352]

Observer Measures of Job Stressors

A system of work assessment, using worksite observational interviews conducted by trained observers, was developed by researchers in Germany.[353] Observers record obstacles/barriers that hinder work performance, time pressure (work pace), worker control over time handling, and monotonous working conditions. In a study of San Francisco transit operators, after adjustment for age, gender and other confounders, objective stressors (job barriers and time pressure) were significantly associated with hypertension[34] and with musculoskeletal disorders.[354]

Interventions to Reduce Work Stressors and Risk of Work Stress-related Illness and Injury

Programs to improve the organization of work and reduce work stressors and their health effects can be conducted in a wide variety of ways. Changes can be made at the level of the job, at the level of the organization, at a more individual level, or from outside the organization through laws and regulations. NIOSH developed a framework of levels of intervention and stages of prevention[355], which we have expanded upon (see Table 33.8).

Within each level, interventions can be considered primary, secondary, or tertiary prevention[356]: primary prevention means preventing disease before it develops, for example, through changing stressful job characteristics, organizational changes, or changes in the economic or political context in which people work; secondary prevention involves early detection and prompt efforts to correct the beginning stages of illness, for example, reversing high blood pressure, buildup of plaque in the arteries, or chronic insomnia, before a heart attack occurs through health promotion, stress management or Employee Assistance Programs; tertiary prevention consists of measures to reduce or eliminate long-term impairments and disabilities and minimize suffering after illness has occurred, for example, rehabilitation and return-to-work after a heart attack.[355,357,358] Included in Table 33.8 are features of the IH's "hierarchy of controls" which correspond to the three levels of prevention.

NIOSH has urged OHP to "give special attention to the primary prevention of organizational risk factors for stress, illness, and injury at work. OHP concerns the application of psychology to improving the quality of work life, and to protecting and promoting the safety, health and well-being of workers. The notion of health "protection" in this definition refers to intervention in the work environment to reduce worker exposures to workplace hazards, while health "promotion" refers to individual-level interventions to equip workers with knowledge and resources to improve their health and thereby resist hazards in the work environment" (http://www.cdc.gov/niosh/topics/stress/ohp/ohp.html). Although both of these types of interventions can be the focus of primary prevention efforts, the NIOSH definition of OHP emphasizes health protection.

Worker Participation

"Participatory action research", used in some job stress intervention studies, involves a partnership between employees, unions, management and outside experts to: 1) meet both research and intervention objectives, and 2) work together to define problems, develop strategies, introduce changes that benefit employees, measure outcomes, evaluate changes[359,360], and develop their own capacities to solve problems. This approach was developed in the 1950s–60s in Scandinavia, and contributed to the development of work

Table 33.8 — Levels of work organization interventions and stages of prevention

<table>
<tr><th>Levels of Intervention</th><th>Primary (preventive)</th><th>Secondary (protective)</th><th>Tertiary (reactive)</th><th>Typical intervention methods</th></tr>
<tr><td>GOAL</td><td>Reduce or eliminate job stressors</td><td>Reduce or eliminate job stressors; Alter ways that people respond to job stressors</td><td>Treat compensate, rehabilitate workers with stress-related illnesses</td><td></td></tr>
<tr><td rowspan="2">Legislative/Policy</td><td rowspan="2">Work hour limits, ban mandatory overtime, staffing requirements</td><td colspan="2">Workers compensation</td><td rowspan="2">Legislation, regulation</td></tr>
<tr><td></td><td>Social Security Disability</td></tr>
<tr><td>Employer/Organization</td><td>Work-family programs; Workplace health & safety programs; New systems of work organization; Work site surveillance</td><td>Health promotion programs; Work-site surveillance; Health screenings surveillance</td><td>Company provided long-term disability; Return to work programs</td><td>Collective bargaining; Employer-initiated programs/policies, including contingent work, downsizing, new systems of work organization</td></tr>
</table>

environment laws in Scandinavia in the 1970s. Those laws emphasized not only reducing chemical and physical hazards at work but also reducing job stressors, increasing worker influence and a joint labor-management approach to new technology and the work environment to improve both worker health and organizations.[361,362] This success of this approach also spurred the development of labor-management-researcher and labor-researcher programs on occupational health and safety in the U.S.[363]

NIOSH points out that worker participation should be judged based on how well workers understand how to safely perform their jobs, are fully cognizant of the potential hazards associated with those jobs and are trained on each of the engineering, administrative, and personal protective equipment controls that are in place to protect them from those hazards. This knowledge also includes ensuring that workers understand and are able to verify the proper functioning of each control measure.[364]

Discussed below are examples of interventions at the various levels of Table 33.8.

Improve Job/Task Characteristics

The effectiveness of interventions at the *job/task* level to improve job design, reduce job stressors, and create a more healthy work organization have been documented.[365–367] One program was initiated by the Stockholm municipal transit agency to reduce traffic congestion and improve passenger service. During planning, there was interest by the municipal workers union and researchers to also study job stress and the health of bus drivers.[368] Bus routes were changed; the number and length of bus lanes were increased; automatic green lights were provided for buses; bus stops were moved and rebuilt; and a computerized passenger information system was provided on the bus and at bus stops. As a result, on "intervention" bus routes, drivers reported fewer job "hassles" and less distress after work compared to workers on other routes that had not been changed. There was objective evidence for reduced hassles such as: fewer illegally parked cars, fewer delays due to passenger obstruction or information requests, and less risky behavior by pedestrians/cyclists. Finally, there was a large decline in the systolic blood pressure of drivers in the intervention group (-10.7 mm Hg), larger than the decline among bus drivers on control routes (-4.3 mm Hg).[368]

Between 1999–2004, more than 200 interventions to improve the health, well-being and work environment of 3,500 Copenhagen bus drivers were conducted using a process of labor-management-researcher cooperation.[369] The interventions focused on: *life style* (smoking cessation, healthy diet courses, and fresh fruit available in garages); *job characteristics/work organization* (more flexible schedules, meeting drivers wishes on rotation and schedules, and better communication between management and drivers); *education and training* (personnel management and communication for managers, handling threats and violence, and "knowing your bus"); and the *physical work environment* (more resources for bus preventive maintenance and joint labor-management meetings). Surveys at baseline and 4 years later show benefits of these efforts: decreases in job stress and fatigue, decreases in drivers reporting that they "can't take their full break", the "rush hour schedule is too tight", and "managers do not treat drivers well"; and, more exercise and better diet among the drivers.[369]

An intervention among Swedish office workers involved individual stress management (relaxation training), and worker committees which developed and helped carry out "action plans" to reduce sources of stress at work. Compared to a control group, the intervention group reported increases in work challenge and autonomy over eight months, increases in supervisor support, and, interestingly, improvements in their lipid profile (cholesterol), a change not explained by changes in diet, exercise, smoking, or weight.[370]

A team of employees, union representatives, management, and researchers helped to guide an intervention study among hospital workers in Quebec, Canada.[371–373] Interviews provided specific and practical recommendations, for example, consultation with nurses on staffing, schedules and a plan for training; ergonomic improvements; improvements in team communication and support; some task rotation between nurses and nurses' aides; job enrichment and training for nurses' aides; reducing delays in filling open staff positions (for example, nurses and clerks); and better guidance and training of new staff.[371] Some improvements in psychological distress and job characteristics (by survey) were seen at one-year follow-up.[372]

In the U.S., studies conducted by the hotel workers union (UNITE-HERE) in cooperation with academic researchers have indicated a high prevalence of working in pain among hotel room cleaners, and a combination of high workload and biomechanical stresses on the job.[374] In a 1998 study in San Francisco, many hotel room cleaners reported constant time pressure, skipping breaks, lack of supervisor respect, and an increase in workload in the past five years.[375] Study results were presented to a union-management contract negotiating committee, and, as a result, in the 1999 contract, the quota for rooms to be cleaned in a day was reduced from 15 to 14 and, in special cases, to 13.[375]

Other U.S. studies include efforts to reduce "burnout" symptoms among state child protection agency employees through a labor-management committee and new technology[376], increase participation in decision-making through labor-management committees at an auto manufacturer[372], and reduce work-related musculoskeletal disorders through job redesign at a meat-packing plant.[377]

The New York City Worksite Blood Pressure Study was not an intervention study, however, blood pressure, job characteristics and health behaviors were measured at baseline and three-year follow-up in eight workplaces. Men who reported job strain at baseline but no job strain three years later had significant decreases in their blood pressure at work (-5.3 mm Hg systolic, -3.2 mm Hg diastolic).[378] In addition, men who quit smoking during these three years had a much larger increase in levels of job control than men who did not quit smoking, non-smokers or those who started smoking.[91] These findings suggest that interventions to reduce job strain or increase job control could achieve similar benefits.

Organizational Level Interventions

Work-family programs. We know anecdotally that formal work-family interventions such as the implementation of alternative work schedules and the provision of dependent care supports appear to be beneficial to workers. However, there is a lack of systematic, well-designed intervention studies to draw firm conclusions.[266,379] Formal work-family interventions in U.S. organizations are needed due to the lack of support for working families at the national level.[380–382] However, the majority of employers are small business owners who may find it difficult to afford such formal work-family supports. Some research suggests that the informal support that an organization provides may be more important than the formal supports.[383] Informal support includes improving the culture and climate for work and family through training supervisors on being more family–supportive and positioning support for working families as part of the mission of the organization. Recently, systematic intervention research by Hammer and colleagues[384,385] has demonstrated that training grocery store supervisors on family-supportive supervisor behaviors led to improved health, work and well-being outcomes for workers.

Worksite surveillance/screening programs. NIOSH has called for increasing surveillance research to: document exposures to known hazardous work stressors, detect emerging trends that may pose a risk, and describe the distribution of these exposures and trends by industry, occupation or demographic group.[4] In the US, occupational and environmental medicine clinics can play a key role in such surveillance efforts. In addition to clinical care, such clinics conduct research, and provide patient education, industrial hygiene and ergonomics services, and social work and support groups.[386] Thus, a team approach is recommended in which industrial hygienists work together with clinicians, health educators, ergonomists, psychologists, epidemiologists and other health professionals to identify high-risk workplaces and jobs, facilitate the provision of clinical care, and design and implement workplace interventions.

Workplace screenings should be conducted for job stressors using the survey instruments described in Table 33.7, and for biomedical risk factors, such as high blood pressure, masked hypertension, and lowered heart rate variability, using ambulatory (portable) monitors.[387] This can help to identify clusters of work-related disease and help target jobs and work sites for primary and secondary prevention programs. Such surveillance is a key component of the newly developing field of occupational cardiology, which links cardiologists, health promotion experts and occupational health specialists, and involves developing return-to-work guidelines for cardiac patients, including workplace modifications.[388]

New systems of work organization. Employers have implemented more controversial "interventions" (new systems of work organization) in order to improve productivity, product quality, and profitability. These include "lean production" (the Toyota Production System), which can have negative effects on employee health.[20,389,390] The traditional assembly line system of work organization, known as Taylorism or "scientific management", was based on the idea that management planned work while workers carried out those plans. Taylorism contributes to workers' stress-related illnesses, "burnout"[20,361], and high rates of absenteeism in tight labor markets.[391]

In the past 50–60 years, various prescriptions for "reforming" Taylorism, reducing worker stress and improving product quality have been proposed, including "high involvement human resource management", "high-performance work organizations", "team concept", and "modular manufacturing." However, worker teams in lean production, the most well known new system, have limited authority and an intensified work pace. Increases in stress are often reported by workers when lean production is introduced. In physically demanding jobs, the intensification of labor appears to increase musculoskeletal disorders.[20,392] Lean production and related systems, such as continuous improvement, total quality management, kaizen, Six Sigma, and 5S, originally developed for manufacturing, are becoming more commonplace in many sectors, including health care, construction and government.[31]

An alternative system, called "socio-technical systems" (STS) design, developed in England and Scandinavia in the 1950s and 60s, has similar roots to "action research" methods. Developed in the context of a unionized workforce, STS promotes the idea of worker teams that have a great deal of control over the pace and content of work. Jobs have a longer "cycle time" and require greater skill. It produces a more flexible work organization.[20,361,393] Evaluations of thousands of work life programs in Sweden and Norway provide evidence of increased job control, increased employee health and satisfaction, and increased productivity.[394] For example, in a Swedish study, auto assembly workers in an STS-style flexible work organization reported more autonomy, more learning of new skills and more variety than workers on a traditional Taylorist assembly-line.[395] Their adrenalin and fatigue levels did not increase over the work day, while adrenalin and fatigue increased on the traditional assembly-line. After work, adrenalin levels of workers on the traditional assembly-line continued to rise (especially for women workers), however, adrenalin levels declined for workers in the flexible work organization.[395] This ability to "unwind" after work for workers in STS designed jobs suggests improved cardiovascular health for workers in such jobs.

Participatory Ergonomics

Given the evidence implicating combined biomechanical and psychosocial exposures in the etiology of MSDs and identifying work organization as a root cause of these exposures and their health effects, practitioners are developing participatory ergonomics (PE) interventions (Sidebar 33.1, Figure 33.4). PE is simultaneously a "microergonomic" (fitting job characteristics to the worker) and a "macroergonomic" approach, involving a multilevel identification and remediation of job-level and work organization risk factors, and requiring input from all levels of the organization.[396] The approach is based on participatory employee "design teams", trained to identify job-level and work organization risk factors, with wide program responsibilities that include surveillance, solution design and piloting, evaluation of intervention effectiveness, training, and program diffusion. Many programs have a higher level steering or oversight committee, with management representation, to provide guidance and resources to front-line teams. (It should be remembered that the National Labor Relations Act (NLRA) that prohibits "employer domination" of teams, groups or committees that "deal" with health and safety issues. For example, NLRA Section 8(a)(2) restricts management from selecting which bargaining unit workers are on these design teams, or controlling the agenda, time and place and length of meetings.)

Sidebar 33.1 — Addressing work stressors through Participatory Ergonomics

Effective PE programs extend employee influence from the traditional testing of ideas and prototypes supplied by management or consultants to broader involvement in all aspects of the control process. This promotes a dynamic, flexible and sustainable program of ergonomic improvement:

- Identification of problems, using employer administrative data and active surveillance of MSD symptoms and disease, and proactive identification of risk factors.
- Development of solution strategies, testing prototypes and alternative approaches, and adjusting solutions to address unanticipated problems resulting in more practical solutions and better acceptance by employees. In contrast, a common barrier in "top-down" approaches is "non-compliance", which is then generally blamed on employee behavioral problems, rather than inappropriate solutions.
- Involvement of employees in training other employees and participating in diffusion of new equipment, techniques, and work organization throughout the company.
- Participation in evaluation and improvement of intervention activities as well as long- term cost-benefit analysis of program effectiveness.

Ideally, PE does not separate job level biomechanical and psychosocial and work organization risk factors; they are treated as parts of an integrated, organizational whole. In developing a participatory approach to design or re-design of the sociotechnical system (the fit of human physical and psychological capabilities with the engineering design of the production system), PE simultaneously addresses the multilevel influences on employee health while improving job-level physical characteristics and psychosocial characteristics: increasing decision latitude and social support, and moderating psychological workload demands. The PE approach has shown promising results.[392–394]

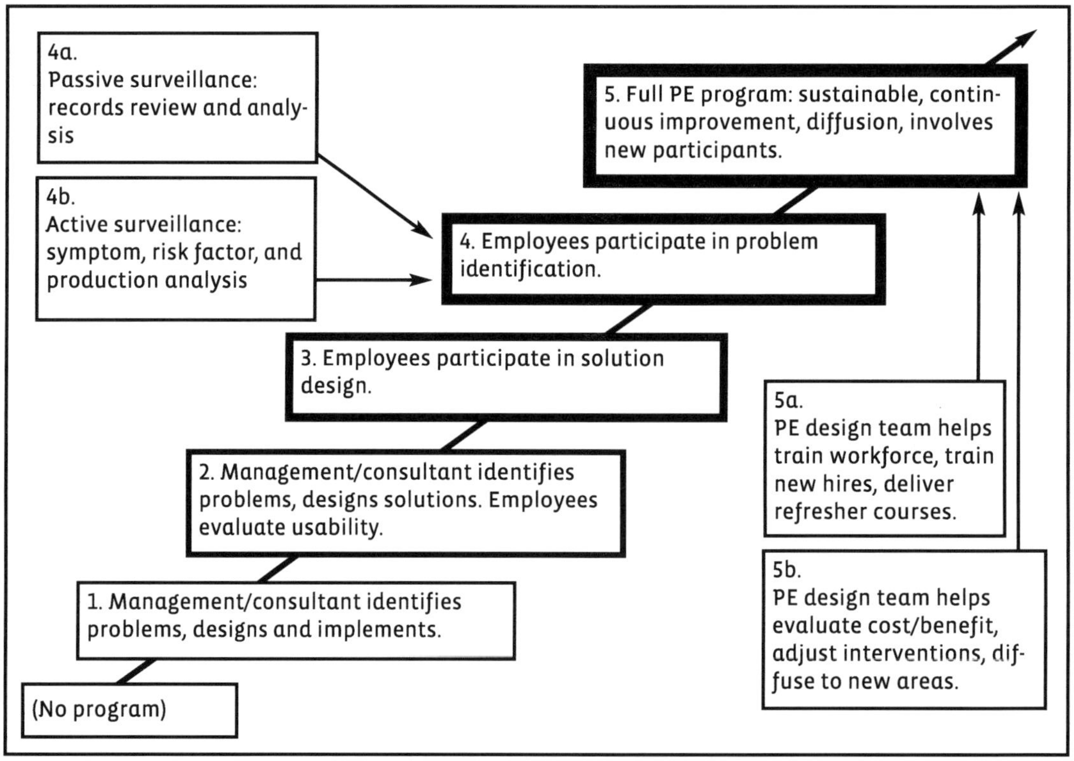

Figure 33.4 — Participatory ergonomics process: hierarchical framework, showing progressive implementation of PE elements to create fully participatory program (Diagram used with permission from Public Health Reports).

Evaluations of Job/Task Redesign and Organizational Interventions

The most comprehensive review, published in 2007, evaluated 90 job stress intervention studies.[357] About half of the studies focused on stress management — helping the individual cope with job stress (a "low systems" approach). Some attempted to make changes only at the organizational level. But about 1/3 used a "high systems" approach, that is, they focused on both organizational change and strengthening individual capacity to withstand stressors — for example, the Swedish office worker[370] or the Copenhagen bus driver[369] studies described above. Those studies represent a growing proportion of published intervention studies. The time needed in these studies for the intervention and for evaluation (follow-up) is long, usually months or years (versus hours to months for "low systems" approaches). "High systems" approach studies were more likely than individual change studies to have worker participation in the development or implementation of the intervention.

Overall, of the 31"low systems" approach studies with control or comparison groups included (highest quality), 25 of 30 found favorable changes at the individual level (as expected), but only 10 measured organizational level changes and only 3 of those found favorable changes at that level. In contrast, of the 19 highest quality "high systems" approach studies, 17 measured individual level health with 13 of those finding favorable changes; 18 measured organizational level factors, with 17 of those finding favorable changes.[357]

The most common organizational outcome in these studies, sickness absence, declined as a result of the intervention in 8 of the 9 highest quality "high systems" approach studies.[357]) For example, in a study of 217 Finnish work sites, there was less sickness absence when there was more participatory and customer service-oriented interventions.[400] In a study of 52 Danish worksites, sickness absence increased a much smaller amount in intervention workplaces (that did most to improve the psychosocial work environment) than "control" workplaces.[401]

Two other relevant systematic reviews were published by the Cochrane Collaboration in 2007[402,203], which included "natural experiments", or unintended changes in stressors, such as from downsizing and restructuring. The previous systematic review[357] excluded natural experiments, focusing only on those interventions in which an organization purposefully intervened on job stress. The review of organizational-level interventions to increase job control[403] found some evidence of health benefits (e.g., reductions in anxiety and depression) when employee control increased or (less consistently) when demands decreased or support increased. They also found that two participatory interventions that occurred alongside downsizing reported worsening employee health.[403] The review of task restructuring interventions[402] found that interventions that increased demand and decreased control tended to have an adverse effect on health, while those that decreased demand and increased control resulted in improved health.

Integrating Occupational Health with Health Promotion/Stress Management

Blue-collar workers tend to have more cardiovascular risk factors such as smoking, unhealthy diet or lack of exercise. They are also exposed to more physical, chemical and psychosocial occupational hazards. This makes a compelling case for integrating occupational health and workplace health promotion interventions.[404] However, blue-collar workers tend to participate less in health promotion programs, in part because they have less control over their work schedules. As the 2002 Barcelona Declaration on Developing Good Workplace Health in Europe pointed out, smoking and alcohol use are also work-related and "can only be tackled through health promoting workplaces."[357]

One U.S. study attempted to address this problem by giving blue-collar workers time-off of work for participation in such programs.[405] The study found that when workers were aware of changes being made by their employer to reduce workplace hazards, workers were more likely to participate in smoking cessation and nutrition programs and occupational health programs.[406]

Eight of the studies in the 2007 job stress intervention review involved integrating occupational health with health promotion efforts.[357] In one example, a program provided to Dutch manufacturing employees included individual-level exercise, health education and social skills training programs as well as organizational-level support for lifestyle improvement (for example, an exercise facility, smoking policy, and healthier cafeteria food); in terms of addressing psychosocial hazards, the intervention also aimed to provide workers with greater influence over production decisions, greater task variety, job rotation, and training.[160] The results were reduced cardiovascular disease risk, greater job control and reduced job demands, improved ergonomics and reduced absenteeism.[160]

While such an integrated approach is not yet common in the U.S., some positive developments exist. A new type of "health risk appraisal" has been developed and is being used by the New York State Department of Health. It goes beyond asking workers about their health behaviors and reviews companies' support for exercise programs, smoking cessations programs or healthy food in their cafeterias, and policies on organizational level "interventions", such as flexible work schedules and collective bargaining (see Sidebar 33.2).[407]

Collective Bargaining

Organizational and job/task level change can also occur as a result of collective bargaining. Many negotiated contracts not only address chemical and physical hazards and shiftwork, but also workload demands[16,408], for example, bans on mandatory overtime or minimum staffing levels for hospital nurses, or reductions in the number of hotel rooms cleaned per day by workers in San Francisco. Job control is addressed through flexible work schedules, voluntary overtime, less repetitive work, participation in decision-making, skills training and promotion opportunities. Social support at work can be improved by supervisor training programs or by schedules which provide opportunities for social interaction among workers.[31] Contracts can provide for job security, protect workers against harassment and discrimination, and provide for programs to help workers balance work and family, such as childcare, elder care, family leave and flexible work schedules.[409–411] The San Francisco-based Labor Project for Working Families provides unions with resources to assist with contract negotiations specific to the development of family-friendly workplaces (http://www.working-families.org/index.html). Finally, contracts provide processes to resolve conflicts, such as a grievance procedure and labor-management safety and health committees.[16,408]

Collective bargaining has modified lean production to some extent — through more moderate work demands (e.g., adding staff, increasing worker control over line speed and production standards), by increasing job control (by electing team leaders, ability to transfer, joint committees), ergonomics programs and less arbitrary access to training.[20] The stresses of electronic performance monitoring have also been addressed through collective bargaining. For example, at an Arizona

Sidebar 33.2 — Questions on "organizational foundations" of worksite supports for cardiovascular health from "Heart Check", used by the New York State Department of Health[407]

- Did the worksite use some form of negotiated management by objective format between the employee and supervisor for determining workload (either through collective bargaining or individual negotiation)?
- Did the worksite use a formal employee appraisal process for the supervisor to assess employee performance?
- Does the worksite have a formal employee grievance procedure?
- Does the worksite provide flexible work scheduling policies (flextime schedule/work at home)?
- Does the worksite provide leave/vacation time allowances?
- Does the worksite provide extended disability coverage or sick time allowances?
- Does the worksite have a strategy to address dependent (child/elder) care?
- Does the worksite subsidize the employee's health insurance by at least 50%?

call center, the Communications Workers of America and AT&T eliminated individual measurement and secret monitoring. Average time per call was measured only for the group. Supervision was conducted in the traditional way by peers sitting beside the operator, listening to calls, and discussing results with the employee. This method produced fewer customer complaints, and a lower grievance rate and absenteeism.[22] Similarly, at Federal Express, after customer complaints of poor service, less importance was placed on the number of calls a person handled and more on service quality. In Chicago, city employees won the right to turn off GPS-enabled cell phones during breaks and after work. The Teamsters Union agreed to United Parcel Service (UPS) demands to use GPS only if its use was limited to tracking packages and not for discipline of workers.[212]

Legislation and Regulation

Historically, legislative/policy interventions have been more common in Europe[403] and Japan[412] than the U.S.[413], with exceptions, such as U.S. state laws banning mandatory overtime or providing minimum staffing levels for nurses, or the California paid family leave law.[414] In the U.S., ergonomic regulations have also addressed work organization.[413] The only existing state regulation, in California, requires that "the employer shall consider engineering controls..., and administrative controls, such as job rotation, work pacing or work breaks." The OSHA Ergonomics Program Standard, rescinded in 2001, described administrative controls for MSD risk including "employee rotation, rest breaks, alternative tasks, job task enlargement, redesign of work methods and adjustment of work pace."[413]

Work environment laws enacted in Scandinavia in the 1970s went much further.[394] For example, the Swedish law stated that "The employee shall be given the opportunity of participating in the design of his own working situation. Technology, work organization and job content shall be designed in such a way that the employee is not subjected to physical or mental strains which can lead to illness or accidents"; and that work should provide "opportunities for variety, social contact and co-operation, and personal and professional development."[415]

Other developed countries (including Europe, Canada and Japan) also have national health insurance, and universal child care and paid family leave through their governments.[262] For example, in Finland, government-provided day care is available to all children under the age of seven, regardless of the family's financial or employment status.

In addition to national laws, European-wide initiatives have included: a 1989 European Union directive to "alleviate monotonous work at predetermined pace to reduce health effects"; the 1993 European Union Working Time Directive limiting the maximum length of a working week to 48 hours in 7 days, and a minimum rest period of 11 hours in each 24 hours; a European Commission Guidance document on work-related stress in 2000[416]; and an agreement on work-related stress by major employer and union federations in Europe on October 8, 2004, which states that "all employers have a legal obligation to protect the occupational safety and health of workers. This duty also applies to problems of work-related stress in so far as they entail a risk to health and safety."[417]

Work organization and job stressors are shaped by the competition employers face in the global economy. Thus, solutions will likely need to be international in scope. The European-wide regulations and labor-management agreements that deal with job stress are one example of international solutions — by encompassing all countries in the European Union. In addition, international trade agreements have consequences that affect the psychosocial work environment, and thus are additional targets for research and negotiation.

Conclusions

In summary, industrial hygienists, as part of their workplace observations, should include descriptions of all hazardous conditions. Thorough job hazard evaluations should identify chemical, biological, physical and psychosocial hazards. Industrial hygienists should collect information about worker injuries or symptoms that have not been reported and identify barriers to collecting accurate hazard and injury data. They can inform health care providers to screen for cardiovascular problems related to job stressors. Production changes (for example, just-in-time delivery), downsizing or use of temporary workers should be assessed regarding employee stress and strain, and job schedules should be evaluated for the opportunity to reduce family and work stress. Attention to preserving psychological health, and designing sustainable jobs, will allow the industrial hygienist to help prevent workplace injuries and illnesses.

The theories, tools and evidence base of OHP, described in the chapter, will hopefully allow industrial hygienists to expand their repertoire in this manner. The field of OHP has also benefitted from research on the behavioral/psychological effects of workplace chemical exposures, as well as the IH model of the "hierarchy of controls", which OHP has applied to psychosocial hazards at work. We hope this chapter helps to stimulate collaboration between these fields and we strongly encourage IH and OHP professionals (and other occupational health professionals) to continue to seek ways to share our knowledge and expertise toward our shared goal of a safer and healthier workplace. Table 33.9 provides a summary of recommended resources for IH professionals to learn more about OHP.

Table 33.9 — Recommended resources for Occupational Health Psychology

Articles

Adkins, J.A.: Promoting organizational health: The evolving practice of occupational health psychology. *Prof. Psych.: Res. and Practice, 30*:129–37 (1999).
Grosch, J.W. and S.L. Sauter: (2005). Psychological stressors and work organization. In *Textbook of Clinical Occupational and Environmental Medicine*, 2nd edition. Rosenstock, L., M.R. Cullen, C.A. Brodkin, and C.A. Redlich (eds.). Philadelphia, PA: Elsevier Saunders, 2005. pp. 931–942.
Quick, J.C.: Occupational Health Psychology: Historical roots and future directions. *Health Psych. 18*:82–88 (1999).
Quick, J.C.: Occupational Health Psychology: The convergence of health and clinical psychology with public health and preventative medicine in an organizational context. *Prof. Psych.: Res. and Practice 30*:123–28 (1999).
LaMontagne, A.D., T. Keegel, A.M. Louie, A. Ostry, and P.A. Landsbergis: A systematic review of the job stress intervention evaluation literature: 1990–2005. *Int. J. Occup. Env. Health 13(3)*:268–280 (2007). Full details of reviewed studies available from first author upon request (alamonta@unimelb.edu.au).
LaMontagne, A.D., T. Keegel, A.M. Louie, and A. Ostry: Job stress as a preventable upstream determinant of common mental disorders: A review for practitioners and policy-makers. *Advances in Mental Health 9*:17–35 (2010).
Sauter, S.L. and J.J. Hurrell, Jr.: Occupational health psychology: Origins, content, and direction. *Prof. Psych.: Res. and Practice 30*:117–22 (1999).
Sauter, S.L., J.J. Hurrell, Jr., H.R. Fox, L.E. Tetrick, and J. Barling: Occupational health psychology: An emerging discipline. *Ind. Health 37*:199–211 (1999).
Semmer N.: Job stress interventions and the organization of work. *Scand. J. Work, Env. and Health 32(6)*:515–27 (2006).

Books

Barling, J., and M.R. Frone: *The Psychology of Workplace Safety.* Washington, D.C.: APA Books, 2004.
Barling, J., E.K. Kelloway, and M.R. Frone (eds.): *Handbook of Work Stress.* Thousand Oaks, CA: Sage, 2005.
Hofmann, D.A. and L.E. Tetrick (eds.): *Health and Safety in Organizations: A Multilevel Perspective.* San Francisco, CA: Jossey Bass, 2003.
Keith, M., J. Brophy, P. Kirby, and E. Rosskam: Barefoot research: A Workers' Manual for Organizing on Work Security. Geneva, Switzerland: International Labour Office, 2002.
National Institute for Occupational Safety and Health (NIOSH): *The Changing Organization of Work and the Safety and Health of Working People.* (Publication Number 2002-116). Cincinnati, OH: NIOSH, 2002.
National Institute for Occupational Safety and Health (NIOSH): *Guide to Evaluating the Effectiveness of Strategies for Preventing Work Injuries: How to Show Whether a Safety Intervention Really Works.* (Publication Number 2001-119). Cincinnati, OH: NIOSH, 2001.
Thomas, J. and M. Hersen (eds.): *Handbook of Mental Health in the Workplace.* Thousand Oaks, CA: Sage, 2002.
Quick, J.C. and L.E. Tetrick: *Handbook of Occupational Health Psychology, 2nd edition.* Washington, D.C.: APA Books, 2010.
Quick, J.C., J.D. Quick, D.L. Nelson, and J.J. Hurrell: *Preventative Stress Management in Organizations.* Washington, D.C.: APA Books, 1997.
Schnall, P., M. Dobson, E. Rosskam, D. Gordon, P. Landsbergis, and D. Baker (eds.): *Unhealthy Work: Causes, Consequences, Cures.* Amityville, NY: Baywood, 2009.
Schnall, P, K. Belkic, P.A. Landsbergis, and D. Baker (eds.): The workplace and cardiovascular disease. *Occup. Med.: State of the Art Reviews* 15(1):(2000).

(continued on next page)

Table 33.9 — Recommended resources for Occupational Health Psychology (continued)

Professional Organizations

The Society for Occupational Health Psychology (www.sohp-online.org)
European Academy-OHP (www.ea-ohp.org)

Journals

Work & Stress
Journal of Occupational Health Psychology

Work Stressor Measurement

http://www.cdc.gov/niosh/topics/workorg/tools/
http://www2a.cdc.gov/niosh-workorg/results.asp
http://www.workhealth.org/OMSTAR/OMSTAR%20chapter%206.pdf
Landsbergis, P.A. and T. Theorell: Measurement of psychosocial workplace exposure variables. *Occup. Med.: State of the Art Reviews 15(1)*:163–88 (2000).

Web Sites

National Institute for Occupational Safety and Health (NIOSH) resources:
OHP: http://www.cdc.gov/niosh/topics/stress/ohp/ohp.html
Work stress: http://www.cdc.gov/niosh/topics/stress/
Organization of work: http://www.cdc.gov/niosh/programs/workorg/
Work stress surveys: http://www.cdc.gov/niosh/topics/workorg/tools/
Wikipedia OHP Page (http://en.wikipedia.org/wiki/Occupational_health_psychology)
Job Stress Network, Center for Social Epidemiology: www.workhealth.org
Workplace Bullying Institute: http://bullyinginstitute.org/
Unhealthy Work (book): http://www.baywood.com/books/previewbook.asp?id=978-0-89503-335-2
American Psychological Association, Psychologically Healthy Workplace Program: http://www.phwa.org/
Sloan Work and Family Research Network: http://www.bc.edu/wfnetwork
Work, Family, and Health Network: https://www.kpchr.org/workplacenetwork
Labor Project for Working Families: www.working-families.org
Hazards magazine: http://www.hazards.org/

References

1. **Stout, N. and H. Linn:** Occupational injury prevention research: progress and priorities. *Injury Prevention 8(Suppl IV)*:iv9–iv14 (2002).
2. **Wegman, D. and J. McGee (eds.):** *Health and Safety Needs of Older Workers.* Washington, D.C.: The National Academies Press, National Research Council, 2004.
3. **Bonacich, E. and R. Appelbaum:** The Return of the Sweatshop. In *Cities and Society.* Kleniewski, N. (ed.). New York: Blackwell Publishing, 2005. pp. 127–143.
4. **National Institute for Occupational Safety and Health (NIOSH):** *The Changing Organization of Work and the Safety and Health of Working People.* Cincinnati, OH: NIOSH, 2002. Report No.: 2002–116.
5. **Yassi ,A., T. Kjellström, T. de Kok, and T. Guidotti:** *Basic Environmental Health.* London, England: Oxford University Press, 2001.
6. **Goldenhar, L.M., L.J.Williams, and N.G. Swanson:** Modelling relationships between job stressors and injury and near-miss outcomes for construction labourers. *Work & Stress 17(3)*:218–240 (2003).
7. **Gillen, M., D. Baltz, M. Gassel, L. Kirsch, and D. Vaccaro:** Perceived safety climate, job demands, and coworker support among union and nonunion injured construction workers. *J. Safety Res. 33*:33–51 (2002).
8. **Snyder, L.A., A.D. Krauss, P.Y. Chen, S. Finlinson, and Y. Huang:** Occupational safety: Application of the job demand-control-support model. *Accident Anal. and Prev. 40(5)*:1713–1723 (2008).
9. **Probst T.:** Job insecurity: Exploring a new threat to employee safety. In *The Psychology of Workplace Safety.* Barling, J. and M. Frone (eds.).Washington, D.C.: American Psychological Association, 2004. pp. 63–80.
10. **Dembe, A.E., J.B. Erickson, R.G. Delbos, S.M. Banks:** The impact of overtime and long work hours on occupational injuries and illnesses: new evidence from the U.S. *Occup. Environ. Med. 62(9)*:588–97 (2005).
11. **MacDonald, L., A. Harenstam, N. Warren, L. Punnett:** Incorporating work organisation into occupational health research: an invitation for dialogue. *Occup. Env. Med. 65*:1–3 (2008).

12. **Landsbergis, P., P. Schnall, T. Pickering, K. Warren, and J. Schwartz:** Lower socioeconomic status among men in relation to the association between job strain and blood pressure. *Scan. J.Work Env. and Health 29(3)*:206–215 (2003).
13. **Benach, J., C. Muntaner, F.Benavides, M. Amable, and P. Jodar:** A new occupational health agenda for a new work environment. *Scan. J. Work Env. and Health 28*:191–96 (2002).
14. **Kompier, M.:** New systems of work organization and workers' health. *Scand. J. Work Env. and Health 32(6)*:421–30 (2006).
15. **Vahtera, J., M. Kivimaki, J. Pentti, A. Linna, M. Virtanen, P. Virtanen, and J. Ferrie:** Organisational downsizing, sickness absence, and mortality: 10-town prospective cohort study. *BMJ 328(7439)*:555 (2004).
16. **Landsbergis, P.A., and J. Cahill:** Labor union programs to reduce or prevent occupational stress in the United States. *Internatl. J. of Health Serv. 24*:105–129 (1994).
17. **James, P. and D. Walters:** Worker representation in health and safety: options for regulatory reform. *Ind. Relations J. 33(2)*: 141–156 (2002).
18. **Clarke S.:** The relationship between safety climate and safety performance: A meta-analytic review. *J. Occup. Health Psych. 11(4)*:315–327 (2006).
19. **Reason. J.:** *Human Error: Causes and Consequences*. New York: Cambridge University Press, 1990.
20. **Landsbergis, P.A., J. Cahill, and P. Schnall:** The impact of lean production and related new systems of work organization on worker health. *J. Occup. Health Psych. 4(2)*:108–130 (1999).
21. **Brisson, C., A. Vinet, M. Vezina,and S. Gingras:** Effect of duration of employment in piecework on severe disability among female garment workers. *Scan. J. Work Env. and Health 15*:329–34 (1989).
22. **Office of Technology Assessment:** The Electronic Supervisor: New Technology, New Tensions, OTA-CIT-333. Washington, D.C.: U.S. Government Printing Office, 1987.
23. **Smith, M. and B. Amick:** Electronic monitoring at the workplace: Implications for employee control and job stress. In *Job Control and Worker Health*. Sauter, S., J. Hurrell, Jr. and C. Cooper (eds.). New York: Wiley, 1989. pp. 275–289.
24. **European Foundation:** *Use of Technology and Working Conditions in the European Union*. Dublin: European Foundation for the Improvement of Living and Working Conditions; 2008.
25. **Karasek, R. and T. Theorell:** *Healthy Work: Stress, Productivity, and the Reconstruction of Working Life*. New York: Basic Books, 1990.
26. **Belkic, K., P. Landsbergis, P. Schnall, and D. Baker:** Is job strain a major source of cardiovascular disease risk? *Scan. J. Work Env. and Health 30(2)*:85–128 (2004).
27. **Siegrist, J., D. Starke, T. Chandola, I. Godin, M. Marmot, I. Niedhammer, and R. Peter:** The measurement of Effort-Reward Imbalance at work: European comparisons. *Soc. Sci. & Med. 58(8)*:1483–99 (2004).
28. **Kivimaki, M., M. Virtanen, M. Elovainio, A. Kouvonen, A. Vaananen, and J. Vahtera:** Work stress in the etiology of coronary heart disease—a meta-analysis. *Scan. J. Work Env. and Health 32(6)*:431–42 (2006).
29. **Cropanzano, R., B. Goldman, and L. Benson:** Organizational justice. In *Handbook of Work Stress*. Barling, J., E. Kelloway, and M. Frone (eds.). Thousand Oaks, CA: Sage, 2005. pp. 63–87.
30. **Johnson, J.V.:** Collective control: Strategies for survival in the workplace. *Internatl. J. Health Serv. 19(3)*:469–480 (1989).
31. **Richardson, C.:** Working alone: The erosion of solidarity in today's workplace. *New Labor Forum 17(3)*:69–78 (2008).
32. **Workplace Bullying Institute and Zogby International:** *U.S. Workplace Bullying Survey*. Bellingham, WA: Workplace Bullying Institute and Zogby International, 2007.
33. **Belkic, K., P.A. Landsbergis, P. Schnall, D. Baker, T. Theorell, J. Siegrist, R. Peter, and R. Karasek:** Psychosocial factors: review of the empirical data among men. In *The Workplace and Cardiovascular Disease*. Occupational Medicine: State of the Art Reviews. Schnall, P., K. Belkic, P.A. Landsbergis, and D. Baker (eds.). Philadelphia, PA: Hanley and Belfus, 2000. p. 24–46.
34. **Greiner, B., N. Krause, D. Ragland, and J. Fisher:** Occupational stressors and hypertension: a multi-method study using observer-based job analysis and self-reports in urban transit operators. *Soc. Sci. Med. 59*:1081–94 (2004).
35. **National Institute for Occupational Safety and Health (NIOSH):** *Stress... at Work*. Report No.: 99-101. Cincinnati, OH: NIOSH, 1999.
36. **Schnall, P., K. Belkic, P.A. Landsbergis, and D. Baker:** The workplace and cardiovascular disease. In *Occupational Medicine: State-of-the-Art Reviews*. Philadelphia, PA: Hanley and Belfus, 2000.
37. **World Health Organization (WHO):** *The Atlas of Heart Disease and Stroke*. Geneva, Switzerland: WHO, 2004.
38. **Graziano, J.:** Global burden of cardiovascular disease. In *Heart Disease*. Zipes, D.,P. Libby, R. Bonow, E. Braunwald (eds.). London: Elsevier, 2004. pp. 1–19.

39. **Stansfeld, S. and B. Candy:** Psychosocial work environment and mental health — a meta-analytic review. *Scan. J. Work Env. and Health 32(6)*:443–462 (2006).
40. **Van Der Doef, M. and S. Maes:** The job demand-control(-support) model and psychological well-being: a review of 20 years of empirical research. *Work & Stress 13(2)*:87–114 (1999).
41. **Rugulies, R. and N. Krause:** Job strain, iso-strain, and the incidence of low back and neck injuries. A 7.5-year prospective study of San Francisco transit operators. *Soc. Sci. and Med. 61*:27–39 (2005).
42. **Bongers, P., A. Kremer, and J. ter Laak:** Are psychosocial factors, risk factors for symptoms and signs of the shoulder, elbow, or hand/wrist?: A review of the epidemiological literature. *Am. J. Ind. Med. 41*:315–42 (2002).
43. **Sauter, S. and N. Swanson:** An ecological model of musculoskeletal disorders in office work. In Beyond Biomechanics: Psychosocial Aspects of Musculoskeletal Disorders in Office Work. Moon, S. and S. Sauter (eds.). London: Taylor & Francis, 1996. pp. 3–21.
44. **Hanecke, K., S. Tiedemann, F. Nachreiner, and H. Grzech Sukalo:** Accident risk as a function of hour at work and time of day as determined from accident data and exposure models for the German working population. *Scand. J. Work Environ. Health 24(Suppl 3)*:43–48 (1998).
45. **Clarke, S., D. Sloane, and L. Aiken:** Effects of hospital staffing and organizational climate on needlestick injuries to nurses. *Am. J. Public Health 92(7)*:1115–19 (2002).
46. **Nakata, A., et al.:** Decrease of suppressor-inducer (CD4+ CD45RA) T lymphocytes and increase of serum immunoglobulin G due to perceived job stress in Japanese nuclear electric power plant workers. *J. Occup. Env. Med. 42(2)*:143–50 (2000).
47. **Suls, J.:** Gastrointestinal problems. In *Encyclopedia of Occupational Health and Safety*. Stellman, J. (ed.). Geneva, Switzerland: International Labor Office, 1998. pp. 34.59–34.60.
48. **Spurgeon, A., J.M. Harrington, and C.L. Cooper:** Health and safety problems associated with long working hours: a review of the current position. *Occup. Env. Med. 54(6)*:367–75 (1997).
49. **Sparks, K., C. Cooper, Y. Fried, and A. Shirom:** The effects of hours of work on health: A meta-analytic review. *J. Occup. Org. Psych. 70*:391–408 (1997).
50. **van der Hulst, M.:** Long workhours and health. *Scan. J. Work Env. and Health 29(3)*:171–188 (2003).
51. **Caruso, C., E. Hitchcock, R. Dick, J. Russo, and J. Schmit:** Overtime and extended work shifts: Recent findings on illnesses, injuries, and health behaviors. Report No.: 2004-143. Cincinnati, OH: NIOSH, 2004.
52. **Frankenhaeuser, M. and G. Johansson:** Stress at work: psychobiological and psychosocial aspects. *Internatl. Rev. Appl. Psych. 35*:287–99 (1986).
53. **Theorell, T.:** Anabolism and catabolism—antagonistic partners in stress and strain. *Scan. J. Work Env. Health 6*:136–143 (2008).
54. **Siegrist, J.:** Adverse health effects of high-effort/low-reward conditions. *J. Occup. Health Psych. 1*:27–43 (1996).
55. **Bosma, H., R. Peter, J. Siegrist, and M. Marmot:** Two alternative job stress models and the risk of coronary heart disease. *Am. J. Public Health 88*:68–74 (1998).
56. **Kivimaki, M., P. Leino-Arjas, R. Luukkonen, H. Riihimaki, J. Vahtera, and J. Kirjonen:** Work stress and risk of cardiovascular mortality: prospective cohort study of industrial employees. *BMJ 325*:857 (2002).
57. **Russek, H.I. and B.L. Zohman:** Relative significance of heredity, diet, and occupational stress in coronary heart disease of young adults. *Am. J. Med. Sci. 235*:266–75 (1958).
58. **Falger, P.R.J. and E.G.W. Schouten:** Exhaustion, psychologic stress in the work environment and acute myocardial infarction in adult men. *J. Psychosomatic Res. 36*:777–86 (1992).
59. **Liu, Y. and H. Tanaka:** Overtime work, insufficient sleep, and risk of nonfatal acute myocardial infarction in Japanese men (The Fukuoka Heart Study Group). *Occup. Env. Med. 59*:447–451 (2002).
60. **Sokejima, S. and S. Kagamimori:** Working hours as a risk factor for acute myocardial infarction in Japan: case-control study. *Br. Med. J. 317*:775–80 (1998).
61. **Steenland, K.:** Shift work, long hours, and CVD: A Review. *Occupational Medicine: State-of-the-Art Reviews. 15(1)*:7–17 (2000).
62. **Kivimaki, M., et al.:** Justice at work and reduced risk of coronary heart disease among employees: the Whitehall II Study. *Arch. Internal Med. 165*:2245–51 (2005).
63. **Belkic, K., R. Emdad, and T. Theorell:** Occupational profile and cardiac risk: possible mechanisms and implications for professional drivers. *Internatl. J. Occup. Med. Env. Health 11*:37–57 (1998).
64. **Tuchsen, F.:** High-risk occupations for cardiovascular disease. In *The Workplace and Cardiovascular Disease*. Schnall, P., K. Belkic, P.A. Landsbergis, and D. Baker (eds.). Philadelphia: Hanley & Belfus, 2000. pp. 57–60.

65. **Johnson, J.V. and E.M. Hall:** Job strain, workplace social support, and cardiovascular disease: a cross-sectional study of a random sample of the Swedish working population. *Am. J. Public Health 78(10)*:1336–42 (1988).
66. **Theorell, T., et al.:** SHEEP Study Group. Decision latitude, job strain and myocardical infarction: a study of working men in Stockholm. *Am. J. Public Health 88*:382–88 (1998).
67. **Hallqvist, J., F. Diderichsen, T. Theorell, C. Reuterwall, and A. Ahlbom:** The SHEEP Study Group. Is the effect of job strain on myocardial infarction due to interaction between high psychological demands and low decision latitude? Results from Stockholm Heart Epidemiology Program (SHEEP). *Social Sci. and Med. 46(11)*: 1405–1415 (1998).
68. **Kuper, H., A. Singh-Manouz, J. Siegrist, and M. Marmot:** When reciprocity fails: effort-reward imbalance in relation to coronary heart disease and health functioning in the Whitehall II study. *Occup. Env. Med. 59*:777–784 (2002).
69. **Karasek, R.A., T. Theorell, J.E. Schwartz, P.L. Schnall, C.F. Pieper, and J.L. Michela:** Job characteristics in relation to the prevalence of myocardial infarction in the U.S. Health Examination Survey (HES) and the Health and Nutrition Examination Survey (HANES). *Am. J. Public Health 78(8)*:910–918 (1988).
70. **Kristensen, T.S., M. Kronitzer, and L. Alfedsson:** *Social Factors, Work, Stress and Cardiovascular Disease Prevention.* Brussels, Belgium: The European Heart Network; 1998.
71. **Peter, R., J. Siegrist, J. Hallqvist, C. Reuterwall, and T. Theorell:** The SHEEP Study Group. Psychosocial work environment and myocardial infarction: improving risk estimation by combining two complementary job stress models in the SHEEP Study. *J. Epi. Community Health 56(4)*:294–300 (2002).
72. **Brisson, C.:** Women, work and cardiovascular disease. In *The Workplace and Cardiovascular Disease. Occupational Medicine: State of the Art Reviews.* Schnall, P., K. Belkic, P.A. Landsbergis, and D. Baker (eds.). Philadelphia, PA: Hanley and Belfus, 2000. pp. 49–57.
73. **Schnall, P.L., P.A. Landsbergis, J. Schwartz, K. Warren, and T.G. Pickering:** A longitudinal study of job strain and ambulatory blood pressure: results from a three-year follow-up. *Psychosomatic Med. 60*:697–706 (1998).
74. **Vrijkotte, T.G., L.J. van Doornen, and E.J. de Geus:** Effects of work stress on ambulatory blood pressure, heart rate, and heart rate variability. *Hypertension 35(4)*:880–86 (2000).
75. **Hayashi, T., Y. Kobayashi, K. Yamaoka, and E. Yano:** Effect of overtime work on 24-hour ambulatory blood pressure. *J. Occup. Environ. Med. 38(10)*:1007–11 (1996).
76. **Landsbergis, P., P. Schnall, R. Chace, L. Sullivan, and R. D'Agostino:** Psychosocial job stressors and cardiovascular disease in the Framingham Offspring Study: A prospective analysis (poster). In 4th ICOH Conference on Work Environment and Cardiovascular Disease. Newport Beach, CA, 2005.
77. **Schnall, P.L., P.A. Landsbergis, and D. Baker:** Job strain and cardiovascular disease. *Annual Rev. Public Health 15*:381–411 (1994).
78. **Iwasaki, K., T. Sasaki, T. Oka, and N. Hisanaga:** Effect of working hours on biological functions related to cardiovascular system among salesmen in a machinery manufacturing company. *Ind. Health 36*:361–367 (!998).
79. **Park. J., et al.:** Regular overtime and cardiovascular functions. *Ind. Health 39(3)*:244–49 (2001).
80. **Nakanishi, N., H. Yoshida, K. Nagano, H. Kawashimo, K. Nakamura, and K. Tatara:** Long working hours and risk for hypertension in Japanese male white collar workers. *J. Epi. Comm. Health 55(5)*:316–322 (2001).
81. **Pickering, T., D. Shimbo, and D. Haas:** Ambulatory blood pressure monitoring. *N.E. J. Med. 354*:2368–74 (2006).
82. **Verdecchia, P., D. Clement, R. Fagard, P. Palatini, and G. Parati:** Task force III: Target-organ damage, morbidity and mortality. *Blood Pressure Mon. 4*:303–317 (1999).
83. **Pierdomenico, S., et al.:** Cardiovascular Outcome in Treated Hypertensive Patients with Responder, Masked, False Resistant, and True Resistant Hypertension. *Am. J. Hypertension 18*:1422–28 (2005).
84. **Landsbergis, P., P. Schnall, K. Belkic, J. Schwartz, D. Baker, T. Pickering:** Work conditions and masked (hidden) hypertension—insights into the global epidemic of hypertension. *Scand. J. Work Env. and Health 6(6)*:41–51 (2008).
85. **Liu, J.E., M.J. Roman, R. Pini, J.E. Schwartz, T.G. Pickering, and R.B. Devereux:** Cardiac and arterial target organ damage in adults with elevated ambulatory and normal office blood pressure [see comments]. *Ann. Intern. Med. 131(8)*:564–72 (1999).
86. **Sega, R., et al.:** Alterations of cardiac structure in patients with isolated office, ambulatory, or home hypertension: data from the general population. Pressione Arteriose Monitorate E Loro Associazioni (PAMELA) Study. *Circulation 104(12)*:1385–92 (2001).
87. **Hara, A., et al.:** Detection of carotid atherosclerosis in subjects with masked hypertension and whitecoat hypertension by self-measured blood pressure at home: The Ohasama Study. *J. Hypertens. 25*:321–327 (2007).

88. **Fagard, R. and V. Cornelissen:** Incidence of cardiovascular events in white-coat, masked and sustained hypertension versus true normotension: a meta-analysis. *J. Hypertens. 25(11)*:2193–98 (2007).
89. **Pierdomenico, S., et al.:** Prognostic Relevance of Masked Hypertension in Subjects With Prehypertension. *Am. J. Hypertens. 21(8)*:879–83 (2008).
90. **Siegrist, J. and A. Rodel:** Work stress and health risk behavior. *Scand. J. Work Env. and Health 32(6)*:473–481 (2006).
91. **Landsbergis, P.A., P.L. Schnall, D.K. Deitz, K. Warren, T.G. Pickering, and J.E. Schwartz:** Job strain and health behaviors: results of a prospective study. *Am. J. Health Promotion 12(4)*:237–245 (1998).
92. **Kouvonen, A., et al.:** Effort-reward imbalance at work and the co-occurrence of lifestyle risk factors: cross-sectional survey in a sample of 36,127 public sector employees. *BMC Public Health 6*:24 (2006). doi:10.1186/1471-2458-6-24.
93. **Kawakami, N., S. Araki, N. Takatsuka, H. Shimizu, and H. Ishibashi:** Overtime, psychosocial working conditions, and occurrence of non-insulin dependent diabetes mellitus in Japanese men. *J. Epi. Comm. Health 53(6)*:359–63 (1999).
94. **Kumari, M., J. Head, and M. Marmot:** Prospective study of social and other risk factors for incidence of Type 2 diabetes in the Whitehall II Study. *Arch. Intern. Med. 164*:1873–80 (2004).
95. **Johansson, G., J.V. Johnson, and E.M. Hall:** Smoking and sedentary behavior as related to work organization. *Social Sci. and Med. 32*:837–46 (1991).
96. **Muntaner, C., F.J. Nieto, L. Cooper, J. Meyer, M. Szklo, and H.A. Tyroler:** Work organization and artherosclerosis: findings from the ARIC study. Atherosclerosis Risk in Communities. *Am. J. Prev. Med. 14*:9–18 (1998).
97. **Lynch, J., N. Krause, G.A. Kaplan, R. Salonen, and J.T. Salonen:** Workplace demands, economic reward and progression of carotid atherosclerosis. *Circulation 96(1)*:302–07 (1997).
98. **Hintsanen, M., et al.:** Job strain and early atherosclerosis: the Cardiovascular Risk in Young Finns study. *Psychosom. Med. 67(5)*:740–47 (2005).
99. **Rosvall, M., P.-O. Ostergren, B. Hedblad, S.-O. Isacsson, L. Janzon, and G. Berglund:** Work-related psychosocial factors and carotid atherosclerosis. *Internatl. J. Epi. 31(6)*:1169–78 (2002).
100. **Knudsen, H.K., L.J. Ducharme, and P.M. Roman:** Job stress and poor sleep quality: data from an American sample of full-time workers. *Soc. Sci. Med. 64(10)*:1997–2007 (2007).
101. **Jansson, M. and S.J. Linton:** Psychosocial work stressors in the development and maintenance of insomnia: a prospective study. *J. Occup. Health Psychol. 11(3)*:241–48 (2006).
102. **Dahlgren, A., G. Kecklund, and T. Akerstedt:** Overtime work and its effects on sleep, sleepiness, cortisol and blood pressure in an experimental field study. *Scand. J. Work Env. Health 32(4)*:318–27 (2006).
103. **Nomura, K., M. Nakao, T. Takeuchi, and E. Yano:** Associations of insomnia with job strain, control, and support among male Japanese workers. *Sleep Med. 10(6)*:626–29 (2009).
104. **Harma M.:** Are long workhours a health risk? *Scand. J. Work Env. Health 29(3)*:167–69 (2003).
105. **Ferrie, J.E., et al.:** A prospective study of change in sleep duration: associations with mortality in the Whitehall II cohort. *Sleep 30(12)*:1659–66 (2007).
106. **Collins, S.M., R.A. Karasek, and K. Costas:** Job strain and autonomic indices of cardiovascular disease risk. *Am. J. Ind. Med. 48*:182–93 (2005).
107. **van Amelsvoort, L.G.P.M., E.G. Schouten, A.C. Maan, C.A. Swene, and F.J. Kok:** Occupational determinants of heart rate variability. *Int. Arch. Occup. Env. Health 73*:255–62 (2000).
108. **Kageyama, T., N. Nishikido, T. Kobayashi, Y. Kurokawa, T. Kaneko, and M. Kabuto:** Long commuting time, extensive overtime and sympathodominant state assessed in terms of short-term heart rate variability among male white-collar workers in the Tokyo megapolis. *Ind. Health 36(3)*:309–17 (1998).
109. **Kobayashi, F., H. Furui, Y. Akamatsu, T. Watanabe, and H. Horibe:** Changes in psychophysiological functions during night shift in nurses: influences of changing from a full-day to a half-day work shift before night duty. *Int. Arch. Occup. Env. Health 69*:83–90 (1997).
110. **Task Force of the European Society of Cardiology and the North American Society of Pacing and Electrophysiology:** Heart rate variability standards of measurement, physiological interpretation and clinical use. *Eur. Heart J. 17*:354–81 (1996).
111. **Proctor, S.P., R.F. White, T.G. Robins, D. Echeverria, and A.Z. Rocskay:** Effect of overtime work on cognitive function in automotive workers. *Scand. J. Work Env. Health 22*:124–32 (1996).
112. **Ahola, K., et al.:** Contribution of Burnout to the Association Between Job Strain and Depression: the Health 2000 Study. *J. Occup. Env. Med. 48(10)*:1023–30 (2006).
113. **Bourbonnais, R., C. Brisson, J. Moisan, and M. Vezina:** Job strain and psychological distress in white-collar workers. *Scand. J. Work Env. Health 22*:139–45 (1996).

114. **Cropley, M., A. Steptoe, and K. Joekes:** *Job Strain and Psychiatric Morbidity.* Cambridge, U.K.: Cambridge University Press, 1999.
115. **D'Souza, R.M., L. Strazdins, L.L.Y. Lim, D.H. Broom, and B. Rodgers:** Work and Health in a Contemporary Society: demands, control, and insecurity. *J. Epi. Commun. Health 57*:849–54 (2003).
116. **Stansfeld, S., R. Fuhrer, M. Shipley, and M. Marmot:** Work characteristics predict psychiatric disorders: prospective results from the Whitehall II study. *Occ. Env. Med. 56*:302–07 (1999).
117. **Clays, E., D. De Bacquer, F. Leynen, M. Kornitzer, F. Kittel, and G. De Backer:** Job Stress and depression symptoms in middle-aged workers—prospective results from the Belstress Study. *Scand. J. Work Env. Health 33(4)*:252–59 (2007).
118. **Wang, J.:** Work stress as a risk factor for major depressive episode(s). *Psychol. Med. 35*:865–71 (2005).
119. **Rugulies, R., U. Bultmann, B. Aust, and H. Burr:** Psychosocial Work Environment and Incidence of Severe Depressive Symptoms: Prospective Findings from a 5-Year Follow-up of the Danish Work Environment Cohort Study. *Am. J. Epi. 163(10)*:877–887 (2006).
120. **Paterniti, S., I. Niedhammer, T. Lang, and S.M. Consoli:** Psychosocial factors at work, personality traits and depressive symptoms: Longitudinal results from GAZEL study. *Br. J. Psych. 181*:111–17 (2002).
121. **Schaufeli, W.B. and D. Enzmann:** *The Burnout Companion to Study and Practice: A Critical Analysis.* London, England: Taylor & Francis, 1998.
122. **Netterstrom, B., et al.:** The relation between work-related psychosocial factors and the development of depression. *Epi. Rev. 30(1)*:118–132 (2008).
123. **Calnan, M., D. Wainwright, and S. Almond:** Effort-Reward Imbalance and Mental Distress: a study of occupations in general medical practice. *Work and Stress 14(4)*:297–311 (2000).
124. **Siegrist, J.:** Social Reciprocity and Health: New Scientific evidence and policy implications *Psychoneuroendocrinol. 30(10)*:1033–38 (2005).
125. **van Vegchel, N., J. de Jonge, H. Bosma, and W. Schaufeli:** Reviewing the effort-reward imbalance model: drawing up the balance of 45 empirical studies. *Soc. Sci. Med. 60*:1117–31 (2005).
126. **Tsutsumi, A., et al.:** The Effort Reward Imbalance and Mental Distress: Experience in Japanese Working Population. *J. Occup. Health 44*:398–407 (2002).
127. **Wege, N., N. Dragano, R. Erbel, K.H. Jockel, S. Moebus, A. Stang, and J. Siegrist:** When does work stress hurt? Testing the interaction with socioeconomic position in the Heinz Nixdorf Recall Study. *J. Epidemiol. Comm. Health 62(4)*:338–41 (2008).
128. **Elovainio, M., M. Kivimaki, and J. Vahtera:** Organizational justice: Evidence of a new psychosocial predictor of health. *Am. J. Public Health 92(1)*:105–08 (2002).
129. **Bourbonnais, R.:** Are job stress models capturing important dimensions of the psychosocial work environment? *Occup. Env. Med. 64*:640–41 (2007).
130. **Ferrie, J., J. Head, M. Shipley, J. Vahtera, M. Marmot, and M. Kivimaki:** Injustice at work and incidence of psychiatric morbidity: the Whitehall II study. *Occup. Env. Med. 63*:443–50 (2006).
131. **Kivimäki, M., J. Vahtera, M. Elovainio, M. Virtanen, and J. Siegrist:** Effort-reward imbalance, procedural injustice and relational injustice as psychosocial predictors of health: complementary or redundant models? *Occ. Env. Med. 64*:659–65 (2007).
132. **Lutgen-Sandvik, P., S. Tracy, and J. Alberts:** Burned by Bullying in the American Workplace: Prevalence, Perception, Degree and Impact. *J. Mgmt. Studies 44*:6 (2007).
133. **Salin, D.:** Ways of explaining workplace bullying: A review of enabling, motivating and precipitating structures and processes in the work environment. *Human Rel. 2003;56*:1213–32 (2003).
134. **Namie, G.:** U.S. Workplace Bullying Survey, September 2007. Workplace Bullying Institute and Zogby International, 2007.
135. **Ortega, A., A. Hogh, J. Hyld-Pejtersen, and O. Olsen:** Prevalence of workplace bullying and risk groups: a representative population study. *Internatl. Arch. Occ. Env. Health 82(3)*:417–26 (2008).
136. **Einarsen, S. and A. Skogstad:** Bullying at work: epidemiological findings in public and private organizations. *Eur. J. Work and Org. Psych. 5*:185–202 (1996).
137. **Niedhammer, I., S. David, and S. Degioanni:** Association between workplace bullying and depressive symptoms in the French working population. *J. Psychosom. Res. 61*:251–259 (2006).
138. **Leymann, H. and A. Gustafsson:** Mobbing at work and the development of post-traumatic stress disorders. *Eur. J. Work and Org. Psych. 5(2)*:251–275 (1996).
139. **Simons, S.:** Workplace Bullying Experienced by Massachusetts Registered Nurses and the Relationship to Intention to Leave the Organization. *Adv. in Nursing Sci. 31(2)*:E48–E59 (2008).

140. **Lee, S., D. McCann, and J.C. Messenger:** *Working Time Around the World: Trends in Working Hours, Laws, and Policies in a Global Comparative Perspective.* London and Geneva: Routledge and ILO, 2007.
141. **International Labour Organization (ILO):** *Key Indicators of the Labour Market.* Geneva, Switzerland: ILO, 2007.
142. **Kivimaki, M., et al.:** Organizational Downsizing and increased use of psychotropic drugs in employees who remain in employment. *J. Epi. Comm. Health (61):*154–58 (2007).
143. **Penk, W.:** Post-traumatic Stress Disorder (PTSD). In *Handbook of Mental Health in the Workplace.* Beverly Hills, CA: Sage, 2002. pp. 215–247.
144. **Hoge, C.W., C.A. Castro, S.C. Messer, D. McGurk, D.I. Cotting, and R.L. Koffman:** Combat duty in Iraq and Afghanistan, mental health problems, and barriers to care. *N. Eng. J. Med. 351(1):*13–22 (2004).
145. **Koenen, K.C., S.D. Stellman, J.F. Sommer, Jr., and J.M. Stellman:** Persisting posttraumatic stress disorder symptoms and their relationship to functioning in Vietnam veterans: a 14-year follow-up. *J. Trauma Stress 21(1):*49–57 (2008).
146. **Perrin, M.A., L. DiGrande, K. Wheeler, L. Thorpe, M. Farfel, and R. Brackbill:** Differences in PTSD prevalence and associated risk factors among World Trade Center disaster rescue and recovery workers. *Am. J. Psychiatry 164(9):*1385–94 (2007).
147. **National Institute for Occupational Safety and Health (NIOSH):** NIOSH Current Intelligence Bulletin #57: Violence in the Workplace: Risk Factors and Prevention Strategies. Cincinnati, OH: NIOSH, 1996.
148. **National Institute for Occupational Safety and Health (NIOSH):** Violence: Occupational Hazards in Hospitals (Publication No. 2002-101). Cincinnati, OH: NIOSH, 2002.
149. **Schottenfeld, R.S., and M.R. Cullen:** Recognition of occupation-induced post-traumatic stress disorders. *J. Occ. Med. 28(5):*365–69 (1986).
150. **Nurminen, M. and A. Karjalainen:** Epidemiologic estimate of the proportion of fatalities related to occupational factors in Finland. *Scand. J. Work Env. Health 27(3):*161–213 (2001).
151. **LaMontagne, A., T. Keegel, D. Vallance, A. Ostry, and R. Wolfe:** Job strain-attributable depression in a sample of working Australians: Assessing the contribution to health inequalities. *BMC Pub. Health 8:*181–89 (2008).
152. **Kuorinka, I. and L. Forcier (eds.):** *Work-Related Musculoskeletal Disorders (WMSDs): A Reference Book for Prevention.* London, England: Taylor & Francis, 1995.
153. **Bernard, B. (ed.):** *Musculoskeletal Disorders and Workplace Factors.* U.S. Department of Health and Human Services, Public Health Service, Centers for Disease Control, National Institute for Occupational Safety and Health. DHHS (NIOSH) Publication #97–141; 1997.
154. **Huang, G.D., M. Feuerstein, W.J. Kop, K. Schor, and F. Arroyo:** Individual and combined impacts of biomechanical and work organization factors in work-related musculoskeletal symptoms. *Am. J. Ind. Med. 43(5):*495–506 (2003).
155. **Johnston, J.M., D.P. Landsittel, N.A. Nelson, L.I. Gardner, and J.T. Wassell:** Stressful psychosocial work environment increases risk for back pain among retail material handlers. *Am. J. Ind. Med. 43(2):*179–87 (2003).
156. **Feveile, H., C. Jensen, H. Burr:** Risk factors for neck-shoulder and wrist-hand symptoms in a 5-year follow-up study of 3,990 employees in Denmark. *Internatl. Arch. Occ. Env. Health 75(4):*243–51 (2002).
157. **Fredriksson, K., et al.:** Risk factors for neck and shoulder disorders: a nested case-control study covering a 24-year period. *Am. J. Ind. Med. 38(5):*516–28 (2000).
158. **Viikari-Juntura, E., R. Martikainen, R. Luukkonen, P. Mutanen, E.P. Takala, and H. Riihimaki:** Longitudinal study on work related and individual risk factors affecting radiating neck pain. *Occ. Env. Med. 58(5):*345–52 (2001).
159. **Canivet, C., et al.:** Sleeping problems as a risk factor for subsequent musculoskeletal pain and the role of job strain: results from a one-year follow-up of the malmo shoulder neck study cohort. *Int. J. Behav. Med. 15(4):*254–62 (2008).
160. **Maes, S., C. Verhoeven, F. Kittel, and H. Scholten:** Effects of a Dutch work-site wellness-health program: the Brabantia Project. *Am. J. Pub. Health 88(7):*1037–41 (1998).
161. **Roquelaure, Y., S. Mechali, C. Dano, S. Fanello, F. Benetti, and D. Bureau:** Occupational and personal risk factors for carpal tunnel syndrome in industrial workers. *Scand. J. Work Env. Health 23:*364–69 (1997).
162. **Shannon, H., et al.:** Changes in general health and musculoskeletal outcomes in the workforce of a hospital undergoing rapid change: A longitudinal study. *J. Occ. Health Psych. 6(1):*3–14 (2001).
163. **Kivimaki, M., J. Vahtera, J. Ferrie, H. Hemingway, and J. Pentii:** Organizational downsizing and musculoskeletal problems in employees: a prospective study. *J. Occup. Env. Med. 58(12):*811–17 (2001).
164. **Messing, K., F. Tissot, and S. Stock:** Distal Lower-Extremity Pain and Work Postures in the Quebec Population. *Am. J. Pub. Health 98(4):*705–13 (2008).

165. **Leclerc, A., P. Franchi, M. Cristofari, B. Delemotte, P. Mereau, and C. Teyssier-Cotte:** Carpal tunnel syndrome and work organization in repetitive work: a cross sectional study in France. *Occ. Env. Med. 55*:180–87 (1998).
166. **Hollmann, S., H. Heuer, and K.-H. Schmidt:** Control at work: a generalized resource factor for the prevention of musculoskeletal symptoms? *Work & Stress 15(1)*:29–39 (2001).
167. **Faucett, J. and D. Rempel:** VDT-related musculoskeletal symptoms: interactions between work posture and psychosocial work factors. *Am. J. Ind. Med. 26*:597–612 (1994).
168. **MacDonald, L.A., R.A. Karasek, L. Punnett, and T. Scharf:** Covariation between workplace physical and psychosocial stressors: evidence and implications for occupational health research and prevention. *Ergo. 44(7)*:696–718 (2001).
169. **Lockley, S.W., et al.:** Effect of reducing interns' weekly work hours on sleep and attentional failures. *N. Eng. J. Med. 351(18)*:1829–37 (2004).
170. **Landrigan, C.P., et al.:** Effect of reducing interns' work hours on serious medical errors in intensive care units. *N. Eng. J. Med. 351(18)*:1838–48 (2004).
171. **Barger, L.K., et al.:** Extended work shifts and the risk of motor vehicle crashes among interns. *N. Eng. J. Med. 352(2)*:125–34 (2005).
172. **Aiken, L.H. and C.M. Fagin:** Evaluating the consequences of hospital restructuring. *Med. Care 35:10 Suppl*:OS1–OS4 (1997).
173. **Shogren, E. and A. Calkins:** *Findings of Minnesota Nurses Association Research Project on Occupational Injury/Illness in Minnesota between 1990–1994.* St. Paul, MN: Minnesota Nurses Association, 1997.
174. **d'Errico, A., et al.:** Hospital injury rates in relation to socioeconomic status and working conditions. *Occ. Env. Med. 64(5)*:325–33 (2007).
175. **Stoohs, R., C. Guilleminault, A. Itoi, and W. Dement:** Traffic accidents in commercial long-haul truck drivers: The influence of sleep-disordered breathing and obesity. *Sleep 17(7)*:619–23 (1994).
176. **Sacks, J. and D. Nelson:** Smoking and injuries: an overview. *Prev. Med. 23*:515–20 (1994).
177. **Hale, A. and J. Hovden:** Management and culture: the third age of safety. A review of approaches to organizational aspects of safety, health and environment. In *Occupational Injury: Risk, Prevention and Intervention.* Feyer, A.-M. and A. Williamson (eds.). London: Taylor & Francis, 1998.
178. **Shannon, H., J. Mayr, and T. Haines:** Overview of the relationship between organizational and workplace factors and injury rates. *Safety Sci. 26(3)*:291–317 (1997).
179. **Litwin, A.:** *Trade Unions and Industrial Injury in Great Britain.* London: London School of Economics and Political Science, 2000.
180. **Shannon, H.S., et al.:** Workplace organizational correlates of lost-time accident rates in manufacturing. *Am. J. Ind. Med. 29(3)*:258–68 (1996).
181. **Leigh, J.:** Are Unionized Blue Collar Jobs More Hazardous Than Non-unionized Blue Collar Jobs? *J. Labor Res. 3(3)*:349–57 (1982).
182. **Reilly, B., P. Paci, and P. Holl:** Unions, Safety Committees and Workplace Injuries. *Br. J. Ind. Rel. 33 (2)*:275–88 (1995).
183. **Nichols, T., D. Walters, and A. Tasiran:** Trade Unions, Institutional Mediation and Industrial Safety Evidence from the UK. *J. Ind. Rel. 49(2)*:211–25 (2007).
184. **Grunberg, L.:** The Effects of the Social Relations of Production on Productivity and Workers' Safety: An Ignored Set of Relationships. *Internatl. J.Health Svcs. 13(4)*:621–34 (1983).
185. **Weil, D.:** Assessing OSHA performance: New evidence from the construction industry. *J. Policy Anal. and Mgmt. 20(4)*:651–74 (2001).
186. **Committee on Education and Labor:** Hidden Tragedy: Underreporting of Workplace Injuries and Illnesses. Washington, D.C.: U.S. House of Representatives, 2008.
187. Dennison Associates, in association with Ruth Ruttenberg and Associates: Review of the literature on safety incentives prepared for the Office of Evaluation, Directorate of Policy, Occupational Safety and Health Administration. Washington, D.C.: Occupational Safety and Health Administration; 1998.
188. **Brown, J.S., Jr.:** Psychiatric issues in toxic exposures. *Psych. Clin. North Am. 30(4)*:837–54 (2007).
189. **Association AP:** *Diagnostic and Statistical Manual of Mental Disorders,* 4th edition. Washington, D.C.: American Psychiatric Association, 2000.
190. **Rohlman, D.S., M. Lasarev, W.K. Anger, J. Scherer, J. Stupfel, and L. McCauley:** Neurobehavioral performance of adult and adolescent agricultural workers. *Neurotox. 28(2)*:374–80 (2007).
191. **Schulte, P.A., et al.:** Work, obesity, and occupational safety and health. *Am. J. Public Health 97(3)*:428–36 (2007).
192. **Mayeux, R.C.R., et al.:** Reduced risk of Alzheimer's disease among individuals with low caloric intake. *Neurol. 52*:A296 (1999).
193. **Mergler, D.:** Nervous System. In *Encyclopaedia of Occupational Health and Safety,* 4th edition. Stellman, J. (ed.). Geneva, Switzerland: International Labor Office, 1998.

194. **Mergler, D., et al.:** Surveillance of early neurotoxic dysfunction. *Neurotoxicol. 17(3-4)*:803–12 (1996).
195. **Melius, J.M. and P.A. Schulte:** Epidemiologic design for field studies: occupational neurotoxicity. *Scand. J. Work Env. Health (Suppl 4)*:34–39 (1981).
196. **Auman, J. and B. Draheim:** The Downside to Downsizing. In *Benefits Canada*; May 1997. p. 31–33.
197. **Goetzel, R.Z., S.R. Long, R.J. Ozminkowski, K. Hawkins, S. Wang, and W. Lynch:** Health, absence, disability, and presenteeism cost estimates of certain physical and mental health conditions affecting U.S. employers. *J. Occup. Env. Med. 46(4)*:398–412 (2004).
198. **Kaiser Family Foundation (KFF) and Health Research and Educational Trust (HRET):** Employer Health Benefits 2006 Annual Survey. Washington, D.C.: KFF and HRET, 2006.
199. **Towers Perrin:** 2007 Healthcare Cost Survey. In http://www.towersperrin.com/tp/getwebcachedoc?webc=HRS/USA/2007/200703/07HCSSfinal.pdf; March 2007.
200. **Morse, T.F., C. Dillon, N. Warren, C. Levenstein, and A. Warren:** The economic and social consequences of work-related musculoskeletal disorders: the Connecticut Upper-Extremity Surveillance Project (CUSP). *Int. J. Occup. Env. Health 4(4)*:209–16 (1998).
201. **Social Security Administration:** Annual Statistical Report of the Social Security Disability Insurance Program. Washington, D.C.: SSA, 2001.
202. **Karasek, R.:** *The Stress-Disequilibrium Theory of Chronic Disease Development: Low Social Control and Physiological Deregulation.* Lowell, MA: University of Massachusetts, 2005.
203. **Goetzel, R.Z., A.M. Guindon, J.J. Turshen, R.J. Ozminkowski:** Health and productivity management: establishing key performance measures, benchmarks, and best practices. *J. Occup. Env. Med. 43(1)*:10–17 (2001).
204. **Chelius, J., D. Galvin, and P. Owens:** Disability: it's more expensive than you think. *Business and Health 11(4)*:78–84 (1992).
205. **Hoel, H., K. Sparks, and C. Cooper:** *The Cost of Violence/Stress at Work and the Benefits of a Violence/Stress-free Working Environment.* Geneva, Switzerland: International Labour Organisation (ILO), 2001.
206. **Hobson, C.J., L. Delunas, and D. Kesic:** Compelling Evidence of the need for Corporate Work/Life Balance Initiatives: Results from a National Survey of Stressful Life Events. *J. Employ. Couns. 38*:38–44 (2001).
207. **Hasselhorn, H., P. Tackenberg, and R. Peter:** Effort-reward imbalance among nurses in stable countries and in countries in transition. *Internatl. J. Occup. Env. Health 10(4)*:401–08 (2004).
208. **de Croon, E., et al.:** Stressful Work, Psychological Job Strain, and Turnover: a 2-year Prospective Study of Truck Drivers. *J. Appl. Psych. 89(3)*:442–54 (2004).
209. **Darr, W. and G. Johns:** Work strain, health, and absenteeism: A meta-analysis. *J. Occup. Health Psych. 13(4)*:293–318 (2008).
210. **Jauregui, M. and P. Schnall:** Work, Psychosocial Stressors and the Bottom Line. In *Unhealthy Work: Causes, Consequences and Cures*. Schnall, P., M. Dobson, and E. Rosskam (eds.). Amityville, NY: Baywood Publishing, 2009.
211. The Tokyo Declaration. *J. Tokyo Med. Univ. 56(6)*:760–67 (1998).
212. **Gruber, J.:** GPS monitoring and the global workforce. Labor and Employment Law Summer 2005.
213. **Batt, R., V. Doellgast, and H. Kwon:** The U.S. Call Center Industry 2004: National Benchmarking Report. Ithaca, NY: Cornell University; 2004.
214. **Luce, S. and T. Juravich:** *Stress in the Call Center: A Report on the Worklife of Call Center Representatives in the Utility Industry.* Amherst, MA: University of Massachusetts, 2002.
215. **Benach, J., C. Muntaner, and V. Santana:** Employment Conditions and Health Inequalities. Final Report to the WHO Commission on Social Determinants of Health. Barcelona, 2007.
216. **European Foundation:** Fifteen years of working conditions in the EU: Charting the trends. Dublin: European Foundation for the Improvement of Living and Working Conditions, 2006.
217. **Mishel, L. and J. Bernstein:** *The State of Working America.* Washington, D.C.: Economic Policy Institute, 2006.
218. **Economic Policy Institute:** *The State of Working America 2004/2005.* Washington, D.C.: Economic Policy Institute, 2005.
219. **Ray, R. and J. Schmitt:** *No-Vacation Nation.* Washington, D.C.: Center for Economic and Policy Research, 2007.
220. **Paoli, P. and D. Merllié:** Third European Survey on Working Conditions. Dublin: European Foundation for the Improvement of Living and Working Conditions; 2001.
221. **Kwon, H. and J. Pontusson:** Globalization, union decline and the politics of social spending growth in OECD countries, 1962–2000: Yale University; 2006.

222. **Robertson, R., et al.:** Employment Arrangements: Improved Outreach Could Help Ensure Proper Worker Classification [GAO-06-656]. Washington, D.C.: U.S. Government Accountability Office, 2006.
223. **Hipple, S.:** Contingent work in the late 1990s. *Monthly Labor Rev. 124(3)*:3–27 (2001).
224. **Ferrie, J.E., M.J. Shipley, M. Marmot, S. Stansfeld, and G.D. Smith:** The health effects of major organizational change and job insecurity. *Soc. Sci. Med. 46*:243–54 (1998).
225. **Ferrie, J., H. Westerlund, M. Virtanen, J. Vahtera, and M. Kivimäki:** Flexible labor markets and employee health. *Scand. J. Work Env. Health Suppl. (6)*:98–110 (2008).
226. **Quinlan, M., C. Mayhew, and P. Bohle:** The global expansion of precarious employment, work disorganization, and consequences for occupational health: a review of recent research. *Internatl. J. Health Svcs. 31(2)*:335–414 (2001).
227. **Cummings, K.J. and K. Kreiss:** Contingent workers and contingent health: risks of a modern economy. *JAMA 299(4)*:448–50 (2008).
228. **Kaplan, G. and J. Lynch:** Socioeconomic considerations in the primordial prevention of cardiovascular disease. *Prev. Med. 29*: S30–S35 (1999).
229. **Smith, M.J., P. Carayon, K.J. Sanders, S.-Y. Lim, and D. LeGrande:** Employee stress and health complaints in jobs with and without electronic performance monitoring. *Applied Ergo. 23*:17–27 (1992).
230. **Liao, Y. and R.S. Cooper:** Continued adverse trends in coronary heart disease mortality among blacks, 1980-91. *Pub. Health Reports 110*:572–79 (1995).
231. **Rosamond, W.D., et al.:** Trends in the incidence of myocardial infarction and in mortality due to coronary heart disease, 1987 to 1994 [abstract]. *N. Eng. J. Med. 339*:863 (1998).
232. **Goldberg, R.J, J. Yarzebski, D. Lessard, and J.M. Gore:** A two-decades (1975 to 1995) long experience in the incidence, in-hospital and long-term case-fatality rates of acute myocardial infarction: A community-wide perspective. *J. Am. College Cardiol. 33(6)*:1533–39 (1999).
233. **McGovern, P.G., et al.:** Trends in acute coronary heart disease mortality, morbidity, and medical care from 1985 through 1997: The Minnesota Heart Survey. *Circ. 104*:19–24 (2001).
234. **Rosamond, W.D., A.R. Folsom, L.E. Chambless, and C.-H. Wang:** Coronary heart disease trends in four United States communities. The Atherosclerosis Risk in Communities (ARIC) Study 1987–1996. *Internatl. J. Epi. 30*:S17–S22 (2001).
235. **Harris, M.I., et al.:** Prevalence of diabetes, impaired fasting glucose, and impaired glucose tolerance in US adults — The third National Health and Nutrition Examination Survey, 1988–1994. *Diabetes Care 21(N4)*:518–24 (1998).
236. **Kuczmarski, R.J., K.M. Flegal, S.M. Campbell, and C.L. Johnson:** Increasing prevalence of overweight among U.S. adults. *JAMA 272*:205–11 (1994).
237. **Hajjar, I., and T. Kotchen:** Trends in Prevalence, Awareness, Treatment, and Control of Hypertension in the United States, 1988–2000. *JAMA 290(2)*:199–206 (2003).
238. **Gornel, D.L.:** Rates of death from coronary heart disease: Letter to the Editor. *N. Eng. J. Med. 340(9)*:730–32 (1999).
239. **National Sleep Foundation:** Sleep in America Poll. Washington, D.C.: National Sleep Foundation, 2005.
240. **European Foundation for the Improvement of Living and Working Conditions:** Finnish quality of work life surveys. Dublin, Ireland: European Foundation for the Improvement of Living and Working Conditions, 2005.
241. **Gustafsson, R. and I. Lundberg:** Working Life and Health. Stockholm, Sweden: National Institute of Work Environment, 2004. [In Swedish].
242. **Hajjar, I., J. Kotchen, and T. Kotchen:** Hypertension: Trends in Prevalence, Incidence, and Control. *Annual Rev. Public Health 27*:465–90 (2006).
243. **Mahapatra, R.:** A cry for help at India's call centers. The Associated Press January 1, 2008.
244. **Barboza, D.:** In Chinese factories, lost fingers and low pay. *New York Times.* January 5, 2008.
245. **Marmot, M. and T. Theorell:** Social class and cardiovascular disease: the contribution of work. In *The Psychosocial Work Environment: Work Organization, Democratization and Health.* Johnson, J.V. and G. Johansson (eds.). Amityville, NY: Baywood Publishing Company, 1991. pp. 33–48.
246. **Gonzalez, M.A., F.R. Artalejo, and J.R. Calero:** Relationship between socioeconomic status and ischaemic heart disease in cohort and case-control studies: 1960–1993. *Internatl. J. Epi. 27(3)*:350–58 (1998).
247. **Singh-Manoux, G.K. and M. Siahpush:** Increasing inequalities in all-cause and cardiovascular mortality among US adults aged 25–64 years by area socioeconomic status, 1969–1998. *Internatl. J. Epi. 31*:600–13 (2002).
248. **Hallqvist, J., M. Lundberg, F. Diderichsen, and A. Ahlbom:** Socioeconomic differences in risk of myocardial infarction 1971–1994 in Sweden: time trends, relative risks and population attributable risks. *Internatl. J. Epi. 27*:410–15 (1998).

249. **Tuchsen, F. and L.A. Endahl:** Increasing inequality in ischaemic heart disease morbidity among employed men in Denmark 1981-1993: the need for a new preventive policy. *Internatl. J. Epi. 28*:640–644 (1999).
250. **Kanjilal, S., et al.:** Socioeconomic status and trends in disparities in 4 major risk factors for cardiovascular disease among U.S. adults, 1971–2002. *Arch. Intern. Med. 166(21)*:2348–55 (2006).
251. **Demyttenaere, K., et al.:** Prevalence, severity, and unmet need for treatment of mental disorders in the World Health Organization World Mental Health Surveys. *JAMA 291(21)*:2581–90 (2004).
252. **Nolte, E. and C.M. McKee:** Measuring the health of nations: updating an earlier analysis. *Health Aff. (Millwood) 27(1)*:58–71 (2008).
253. **Braithwaite J.:** Hunter-gatherer human nature and health system safety: an evolutionary cleft stick? *Internatl. J. Qual. in Health Care 17(6)*:541–45 (2005).
254. **Diamond, D.:** *The Third Chimpanzee*. New York: HarperCollins; 2006.
255. **Margulis, L. and D. Sagan:** *Acquiring Genomes*. New York: Basic Books, 2002.
256. **Pinker, S.:** *How the Mind Works*. New York: W.W. Norton & Company, Inc., 1997.
257. **Schnall, P.L. and R. Kern:** Hypertension in American Society: An Introduction to Historical Materialist Epidemiology. In *The Sociology of Health and Illness: Critical Perspectives*. Conrad, P. and R. Kern (eds.) New York: St. Martin's Press, 1981. pp. 97–122.
258. **Waldron, I., M. Nowatarski, M. Freimer, J.P. Henry, N. Post, and C. Witten:** Cross-cultural variation in blood pressure: A qualitative analysis of the relationship of blood pressure to cultural characteristics, salt consumption and body weight. *Soc. Sci. and Med. 16*:419–30 (1982).
259. **Schnall, P., K. Belkic, P.A. Landsbergis, and D. Baker:** Why the workplace and cardiovascular disease? *Occup. Med.-State Art. 15(1)*:1–5 (2000).
260. **Hammer, L.B. and K.L Zimmerman:** Quality of work life. In *APA Handbook of Industrial and Organizational Psychology,* Volume 3. Zedeck, S. (ed.). Washington, D.C.: American Psychological Association, 2011, pp. 399-431.
261. **Neal, M.B. and L.B. Hammer:** *Working couples caring for children and aging parents: Effects on work and well-being*. Mahwah, NJ: Lawrence Erlbaum Associates, Inc., 2007.
262. **Davis, M.F. and R. Powell:** The International Convention of the Rights of the Child: A catalyst for innovative childcare policies. *Hum. Rights Quart. 25*:689–719 (2003).
263. **Quick, J.C. and L.E. Tetrick:** *Handbook of Occupational Health Psychology*. Washington, D.C.: American Psychological Association, 2003.
264. **Hammer, L.B., J.C. Cullen, M.B. Neal, R.R. Sinclair, and M. Shafiro:** The longitudinal effects of work-family conflict and positive spillover on depressive symptoms among dual-earner couples. *J. Occup. Health Psychol. 10*:138–54 (2005).
265. **Hammer, L.B., M.B. Neal, J.T. Newsom, K.J. Brockwood, and C. Colton:** A longitudinal study of the effects of dual-earner couples' utilization of family-friendly workplace supports on work and family outcomes. *J. Appl. Psychol. 90*:799–810 (2005).
266. **Kelly E., et al.:** Getting there from here: Research on the effects of work-family initiatives on work-family conflict and business outcomes. *The Academy of Management Annals. 2(1)*:305–49 (2008).
267. **Kelly, E.L. and P. Moen:** Rethinking the clockwork of work: Why schedule control may pay off at work and at home. *Adv. Dev. Hum. Res. 9(4)*:487–506 (2007).
268. **Hammer, L.B., E.E. Kossek, and N.L. Yragui:** Effects of family supportive supervision on work-family conflict over time. In: *Work, Stress & Health Conferenc*e, Washington, D.C., 2008.
269. **Frone, M.R., M. Russell, and M.L. Cooper:** Antecedents and outcomes of work-family conflict: Testing a model of the work-family interface. *J. Appl. Psychol. 77*:65–78 (1992).
270. **Allen, T.D. and J. Armstrong:** Further examination of the link between work-family conflict and physical health: The role of health-related behaviors. *Am. Behav. Sci. 49(9)*:1204–21 (2006).
271. **Eaker, E.D., S.G. Haynes, and M. Feinleib:** Spouse behavior and coronary heart disease: Prospective results from the Framingham Heart Study. *Activitas Nervosa Superior 25(2)*:81–90 (1983).
272. **Burke, R.J. and E.R Greenglass:** Work-family conflict, spouse support, and nursing staff well-being during organizational restructuring. *J. Occup. Health Psychol. 4*:327–36 (1999).
273. **Frone, M.R., M. Russell, and G.M. Barnes:** Work-family conflict, gender, and health-related outcomes: A study of employed parents in two community samples. *J. Occup. Health Psychol. 1(1)*:57–69 (1996).
274. **Gryzwacz, J.G.:** Work-family spillover and health during midlife: Is managing conflict everything? *Am. J. Health Promot. 14*:236–43 (2000).
275. **Netemeyer, R.G., J.S. Boles, and R. McMurrian:** Development and validation of work-family conflict and family-work conflict scales. *J. Appl. Psychol. 81(4)*:400–10 (1996).
276. **Thomas, L.T. and D.C. Ganster:** Impact of family-supportive work variables on work-family conflict and strain: A control perspective. *J. Appl. Psychol. 80(1)*:6–15 (1995).

277. **Brisson, C., et al.:** Effect of family responsibilities and job strain on ambulatory blood pressure among white-collar women. *Psychosom Med. 61(2)*:205–13 (1999).
278. **Grzywacz, J.G. and B.L. Bass:** Work, family, and mental health: Testing different models of work-family fit. *J Marriage Fam. 65*:248–62 (2003).
279. **Hanson, G.C., L.B. Hammer, and C.L. Colton:** Development and validation of a multidimensional scale of perceived work-family positive spillover. *J. Occup. Health Psychol. 11(3)*:249–65 (2006).
280. **Grzywacz, J.G., et al.:** Work-family conflict: Experiences and health implications among immigrant Latinos. *J. Appl. Psychol. 92*:1119–30 (2007).
281. **Hobfoll, S.E.:** Conservation of resources: A new attempt at conceptualizing stress. *Am Psychol. 44(3)*:513–24 (1989).
282. **Cullen, J.C., and L.B. Hammer:** Developing and testing a theoretical model linking work-family conflict to employee safety. *J. Occup. Health Psychol. 12*:266–78 (2007).
283. **Daniels, R.J., L.B. Hammer, and D.M. Truxillo:** The relationship between work-family conflict and safety among construction workers. Unpublished Manuscript, 2008.
284. **Platt, J.:** Social traps. *Am. Psychol. 28*:641–51 (1973).
285. **Herrnstein, R.J., G.F. Loewnstein, D. Prelec, and W. Vaughan:** Utility maximization and melioration: Internalities in individual choice. *J. Behav. Dec. Making. 6*:149–85 (1993).
286. **Tan-Wilhelm, D., et al.:** Impact of a worker notification program: Assessment of attitudinal and behavioral outcomes. *Am. J. Ind. Med. 37*:205–13 (2000).
287. **Wogalter, M.S., V.C. Conzola, and T.L. Smith-Jackson:** Research-based guidelines for warning design and evaluation. *Appl. Ergo. 33*:219–30 (2002).
288. **Alvero, A.M. and J. Austin:** The effects of conducting behavioral observations on the behavior of the observer. *J. Appl. Behav. Anal. 37*:457–68 (2004).
289. **deTurck, M.A., I. Chih, and Y. Hsu:** Three studies testing the effects of role models on product users' safety behavior. *Hum. Factors 41(3)*:397–412 (1999).
290. **deTurck, M.A., R.A. Rachlin, and M.J. Young:** Effects of a role model and fear in warning label on perceptions of safety and safety behavior. *Adv. Consum. Res. 21*:208–12 (1994).
291. **Olson, R., A. Grossheusch, and S. Schmidt:** The effects of social modeling on the use of personal protective equipment. In: *Association for Behavior Analysis International Conference; 2008*. Chicago, IL, 2008.
292. **Racicot, B.M. and M.S. Wogalter:** Effects of a video warning sign and social modeling on behavioral compliance. *Accident Anal. Prevent. 27*:57–64 (1995).
293. **Sasson, J.R., J. Austin, and A.M Alvero:** Behavioral observations: Effects on safe performance. *Prof. Safe. 52*:26–32 (2007).
294. **Wogalter, M.S., N.A. McKenna, and S.T. Allison:** Warning and compliance: Behavioral effects of cost and consensus. In: *Human Factors Society 32nd Annual Meeting*, 1988.
295. **Alavosius, M. and B. Sulzer-Azaroff:** Acquisition and maintenance of health-care routines as a function of feedback density. *J. Appl. Behav. Anal. 23(2)*:151–62 (1990).
296. **Cooper, M.:** Reducing accidents using goal setting and feedback: A field study. *J. Occup. Org. Psychol. 67*:219–40 (1994).
297. **Hofmann, D.A. and A. Stetzer:** The role of safety climate and communication in accident interpretation: Implication from negative events. *Acad. Mgmt. J. 41*:644–57 (1998).
298. **Hofmann, D.A. and F.P Morgeson:** Safety-related behavior as a social exchange: The role of percieved organizational support and leader-member exchange. *J. Appl. Psychol. 84(2)*:286–96 (1999).
299. **Griffin, M.A. and A. Neal:** Perceptions of safety at work: A framework for linking safety climate to safety performance, knowledge, and motivation. *J. Occup. Health Psychol. 5(3)*:347–58 (2000).
300. **Glasgow, R.E., G. Sorensen, C. Giffen, R.H. Shipley, K. Corbett, and W. Lynn:** Promoting worksite smoking control policies and actions: the community intervention trial for smoking cessation (COMMIT) experience. *Prevent Med. 25*:186–94 (1996).
301. **Komaki, J., K.D. Barwick, and L.R. Scott:** A behavioral approach to occupational safety: Pinpointing and reinforcing safe performance in a food manufacturing plant. *J. Appl. Psychol. 63(4)*:434–45 (1978).
302. **Zohar, D. and G. Luria:** The use of supervisory practices as leverage to improve safety behavior: A cross-level intervention model. *J. Safety Res. 34*:567–77 (2003).
303. **Brown, G. and J. Barab:** Cooking the Books—Behavior-Based Safety at the San Francisco Bay Bridge. *New Solutions. 17(4)*:311–24 (2007).
304. **DeJoy, D.:** Behavior change versus culture change: Divergent approaches to managing workplace safety. *Safety Sci. 43*:105–29 (2005).
305. **Frederick, J. and N. Lessin:** Blame the Worker; The Rise of Behavioral-based Safety Programs. *Multinat. Mon. 21(11)* (2000).

306. **Krause, T., K. Seymour, and K. Sloat:** Long-term evaluation of a behavior-based method for improving safety performance: a meta-analysis of 73 interrupted time-series replications. *Safety Sci. 32*:1–18 (1999).
307. **Hopkins, A.:** What are we to make of safe behaviour programs? *Safety Sci. 44*:583–597 (2006).
308. **Sulzer-Azaroff, B. and J.Austin:** Behavior-based safety and injury reduction: A survey of evidence. *Prof. Saf. July*:19–24 (2000).
309. **Tuncel, S., L. Harshad, S. Salem, and N. Daraiseh:** Effectiveness of behaviour based safety interventions to reduce accidents and injuries in workplaces: Critical appraisal and meta-analysis. *Theor. Iss. Ergo. Sci. 7(3)*:191–209 (2006).
310. **Krause, T.R.:** *The behavior-based safety process: Managing involvement for an injury-free culture.* New York: Van Nostrand Reinhold, 1997.
311. **U.S. Chemical Safety and Hazard Investigation Board:** Investigation Report: Refinery Explosion and Fire, Report No. 2005-04-I-Tx. Washington, D.C.: U.S. Chemical Safety Board, 2007.
312. **Zohar, D.:** Safety climate: Conceptual and measurement issues. In *Handbook of Occupational Health Psychology.* Tetrick, L.E. and J.C. Quick (eds.). Washington, D.C.: American Psychological Association, 2003.
313. **Guldenmund, F.W.:** The nature of safety culture: A review of theory and research. *Safety Sci. 34(1–3)*:215–57 (2000).
314. **Schein, E.H.:** Organizational culture. *Am. Psych. 45(2)*:109–19 (1990).
315. **Harris, M.:** *Cultural materialism: The struggle for a science of culture.* New York: Random House, 1979.
316. **Skinner, B.F.:** Selection by consequences. *Sci. 213(4507)*:501–04 (1981).
317. **Zohar, D.:** Safety climate in industrial organizations: Theoretical and applied implications. *J. Appl. Psychol. 65(1)*:96–102 (1980).
318. **Zohar, D.:** Thirty years of safety climate research: Reflections and future directions. *Accident Anal. Prev. 42(5)*:1517–522 (2010).
319. **Flin, R., P. Mearns, R. O'Connor, and R. Bryden:** Measuring safety climate: Identifying the common features. *Safety Sci. 34*:177–92 (2000).
320. **Probst, T.M., T.L. Brubaker, and A. Barsotti:** Organizational injury rate underreporting: the moderating effect of organizational safety climate. *J. Appl. Psych. 93(5)*:1147–54 (2008).
321. **Zohar, D. and G. Luria:** A multi-level model of safety climate: Cross-level relationships between organization and group-level climates. *J. Appl. Psych. 90(4)*:616–28 (2005).
322. **Seo, D.:** An explicative model of unsafe work behavior. *Safety Sci. 43(3)*:187–211 (2005).
323. **Neal, A. and M.A. Griffin:** Safety climate and safety at work. In *The Psychology of Workplace Safety.* Barling, J. and M.R. Frone (eds.). Washington, D.C.: American Psychological Association, 2004.
324. **Zohar, D.:** A group-level model of safety climate: Testing the effect of group climate on microaccidents in manufacturing jobs. *J. Appl. Psych. 85(4)*:587–96 (2000).
325. **Cheyne, A., S. Cox, A. Oliver, and J.M. Tomas:** Modelling safety climate in the prediction of levels of safety activity. *Work Stress 12(3)*:255–71 (1998).
326. **Zohar, D. and O. Tenne-Gazit:** Transformational leadership and group interaction as climate antecedents: A social network analysis. *J. Appl. Psych. 93(4)*:744–57 (2008).
327. **Barling, J., C. Loughlin, and E.K. Kelloway:** Development and test of a model linking safety-specific transformational leadership and occupational safety. *J. Appl. Psych. 87(3)*:488–96 (2002).
328. **Huang, Y., M. Ho, G. Smith, and P. Chen:** Safety climate and self-reported injury: Assessing the mediating role of employee safety control. *Accident Anal. Prevent. 38(3)*:425–33 (2006).
329. **Fogarty, G.J.:** Psychological strain mediates the impact of safety climate on maintenance errors. *Int. J. Appl. Avia. Stud. (5)*:1 (2005).
330. **Siu, O., D.R. Phillips, and T. Leung:** Safety climate and safety performance among construction workers in Hong Kong: The role of psychological strains as mediators. *Accident Anal Prevent. 36(3)*:359–66 (2004).
331. **Bureau of Labor Statistics:** *Fatal occupational injuries by occupation and event or exposure.* Washington, D.C.: U.S. Department of Labor, 2006.
332. **Bureau of Labor Statistics:** *Nonfatal occupational injuries and illnesses requiring days away from work.* Washington, D.C.: U.S. Department of Labor, 2007.
333. **Leigh, J.P. and T.R. Miller:** Occupational illnesses within two national data sets. *Int. J. Occup. Env. Health 4(2)*:99–13 (1998).
334. **Johnson, J.V., E.M. Hall, and T. Theorell:** Combined effects of job strain and social isolation on cardiovascular disease morbidity and mortality in a random sample of the Swedish male working population. *Scand. J. Work Env. Health 15(4)*:271–79 (1989).
335. **Newnam, S., M.A. Griffin, and C. Mason:** Safety in work vehicles: A multilevel study linking safety values and individual predictors to work-related driving crashes. *J. Appl. Psych. 93(3)*:632–44 (2008).
336. **Keller, S.B. and J. Ozment:** Managing driver retention: Effects of the dispatcher. *J. Bus. Log. 20(2)*:97–118 (1999).

337. **Braver, E., et al.:** Long hours and fatigue: a survey of tractor trailer drivers. *J. Pub. Health Policy 13*:341–366 (2002).
338. **Olson, R., D.I. Hahn, and A. Buckert:** Predictors of severe trunk postures among short-haul truck drivers during non-driving tasks: an exploratory investigation involving video-assessment and driver behavioural self-monitoring. *Ergo. 52(6)*:707–22 (2009).
339. **Ludwig, T.D. and E.S. Geller:** Managing injury control among professional pizza deliverers: Effects of foal setting and response generalization. *J. Appl. Psych. 82*:253–61 (1997).
340. **Hickman, J.S. and E.S. Geller:** Self-management to increase safe driving among short-haul truck drivers. *J. Org. Behav. Mgmt. 23(4)*:1–20 (2003).
341. **Roetting, M., Y. Huang, J. McDevitt, and D. Melton:** When technology tells you how to drive-truck drivers' attitudes towards feedback by technology. *Trans. Res. Part F, 6*:275–87 (2003).
342. **Waters, T., R. Dick, J. Davis-Barkley, and E. Krieg:** A Cross-Sectional Study of Risk Factors for Musculoskeletal Symptoms in the Workplace Using Data From the General Social Survey (GSS). *J. Occ. Env. Med. 49(2)*:172–84 (2007).
343. **Landsbergis, P.A. and T. Theorell:** Measurement of psychosocial workplace exposure variables. *Occup. Med.-State Art 15(1)*:163–88 (2000).
344. **Friedman, R., et al.:** Psychological variables in hypertension: relationship to casual or ambulatory blood pressure in men. *Psychosom. Med. 63*:19–31 (2001).
345. **Lake, E.T.:** Development of the Practice Environment Scale of the Nursing Work Index. *Res. Nursing Health 25(3)*:176–88 (2002).
346. **Schonfeld, I.:** Psychological distress in a sample of teachers. *J. Psych. 123*:321–38 (1990).
347. **Krause, N., D.R. Ragland, B.A. Greiner, S.L. Syme, and J.M. Fisher:** Psychosocial job factors associated with back and neck pain in public transit operators. *Scand. J. Work Env. Health. 23(3)*:179–86 (1997).
348. **Johnson, J.V., W. Stewart, E.M. Hall, P. Fredlund, and T. Theorell:** Long-term psychosocial work environment and cardiovascular mortality among Swedish men. *Am. J. Pub.Health 86(3)*:324–31 (1996).
349. **Hammar, N., L. Alfredsson, and J.V. Johnson:** Job strain, social support at work, and incidence of myocardial infarction. *Occup. Env. Med. 55*:548–53 (1998).
350. **Alterman, T., et al.:** Examining associations between job characteristics and health: Linking data from the occupational information network (O*NET) to two U.S. National Health Surveys. *J. Occup. Env. Med. 50(12)*:1401–13 (2008).
351. **Cifuentes, M., J. Boyer, D.A. Lombardi, and L. Punnett:** Use of O*NET as a job exposure matrix: A literature review. *Am. J. Ind. Med. 53*:898–914 (2010).
352. **Meyer, J.D., M. Cifuentes, and N. Warren:** Association of self-rated physical health and incident hypertension with O*NET factors: Validation using a representative national survey. *J. Occup. Env. Med. 53(3)*:139–45 (2011).
353. **Greiner, B.A. and N. Krause:** Expert-observer assessment of job characteristics. *Occup. Med.-State Art 15(1)*:175–83 (2000).
354. **Greiner, B.A. and N. Krause:** Observational stress factors and musculoskeletal disorders in urban transit operators. *J. Occup. Health Psych. 11(1)*:38–51 (2006).
355. **Murphy, L. and S. Sauter:** Work Organization Interventions: State of Knowledge and Future Directions. *Soz.-Praventivmed. 49*:79–86 (2004).
356. **Last, J.:** *A Dictionary of Epidemiology,* 4th edition. Oxford: University Press, 2001.
357. **LaMontagne, A., T. Keegel, A. Louie, A. Ostry, and P. Landsbergis:** A Systematic Review of the Job Stress Intervention Evaluation Literature: 1990–2005. *Int. J. Occup. Env. Health 13*:268–80 (2007).
358. **Landsbergis, P.:** Interventions to reduce job stress and improve work organization and worker health. In *Unhealthy Work: Causes, Consequences and Cures.* Schnall, P.L. et al. (eds.). Amityville, NY: Baywood Publishing, 2009.
359. **Susman, G. and R. Evered:** An assessment of the scientific merits of action research. *Admin. Sci. Quart. 23*:582–603 (1978).
360. **Israel, B., S. Schurman, and J. House:** Action research on occupational stress: Involving workers as researchers. *Int. J. Health Serv. 19(1)*:135–55 (1989).
361. **Gardell, B., and B. Gustavsen:** Work environment research and social change: current developments in Scandinavia. *J. Occup. Behav. 1*:3–17 (1980).
362. **Deutsch, S.:** The contributions and challenge of participatory action research. *New Solutions 15(1)*:29–35 (2005).
363. **McQuiston, T.:** Empowerment evaluation of worker safety and health education programs. *Am. J. Ind. Med. 38*:584–97 (2000).
364. **Robson, L., H. Shannon, L. Goldenhar, and A. Hale:** *Guide to Evaluating the Effectiveness of Strategies for Preventing Work Injuries: How to Show Whether a Safety Intervention Really Works.* Cincinnati, OH: National Institute for Occupational Safety and Health, 2001.
365. **Murphy, L., J. Hurrell, S. Sauter, and G.E. Keita:** *Job Stress Interventions.* Washington, D.C.: American Psychological Association, 1995.

366. **International Labor Office. Conditions of Work Digest:** *Preventing Stress at Work.* Geneva, Switzerland: International Labor Office, 1992.
367. **Landsbergis, P.A., et al.:** Job stress and heart disease: Evidence and strategies for prevention. *New Solutions. Summer*:42–58 (1993).
368. **Rydstedt, L.W., G. Johansson, and G.W. Evans:** The human side of the road: Improving the working conditions of urban bus drivers. *J. Occ. Health Psych. 3*:161–71 (1998).
369. **Poulsen, K., S. Jensen, E. Bach, and J. Schostak:** Using action research to improve health and the work environment for 3500 municipal bus drivers. *Educ. Act. Res. 15(1)*:75–106 (2007).
370. **Orth-Gomer, K.:** International epidemiological evidence for a relationship between social support and cardiovascular disease. In *Social support and cardiovascular disease.* Shumaker, S. and S. Czajowski (eds.). New York: Plenum Press, 1994.
371. **Bourbonnais, R., C. Brisson, A. Vinet, M. Vezina, and A. Lower:** Development and Implementation of a Participative Intervention to Improve the Psychosocial Work Environment and Mental Health in an Acute Care Hospital. *Occ. and Env. Med. 63*:326–34 (2006).
372. **Bourbonnais, R., C. Brisson, A. Vinet, M. Vezina, and A. Lower:** Effectiveness of a participatory intervention on psychosocial work factors to prevent mental health problems in a hospital setting. *Occ. and Env. Med. 63*:335–42 (2006).
373. **Bourbonnais, R. C. Brisson, and M. Vezina:** Long-term effects of an intervention on psychosocial work factors among healthcare professionals in a hospital setting. *Occup. Env. Med. 68*:479-86 (2011).
374. **Frumin, E. et al.:** *Workload-related musculoskeletal disorders among hotel housekeepers.* New York: UNITE-HERE, 2006.
375. **Lee, P. and N. Krause:** The impact of a worker health study on working conditions. *J. Pub. Health Pol. 23*:268–85 (2002).
376. **Cahill, J., L.H. Feldman:** Computers in child welfare: planning for a more serviceable work environment. *Child Welfare. 72*:3–12 (1993).
377. **Israel, B.A., S.J. Schurman, and J.S. House:** Action research on occupational stress: involving workers as researchers. *Int. J. Health Serv. 19*:135–55 (1989).
378. **Smith, M. and D. Zehel:** A stress reduction intervention programme for meat processors emphasizing job design and work organization. *Condit. Work Digest. 11(2)*:204–13 (1992).
379. **Casper, W.J., L.T. Eby, C. Bordeaux, A. Lockwood, and D. Lambert:** A review of research methods in IO/OB work-family research. *J. Appl. Psych. 92*:28–43 (2007).
380. **Hammer, L.B., J.C. Cullen, and M. Shafiro:** Work-family best practices. In *Work-life Balance: A Psychological Perspective.* Jones, F., R. Burke and M. Westman (eds.). East Sussex, UK: Psychology Press, 2006.
381. **Kelly, E.L.:** Work-family policies: The United States in International Perspective. In *The Work and Family Handbook: Multi-disciplinary perspectives and approaches.* Pitt-Catsouphes, M., E.E. Kossek, and S. Sweet (eds.). Mahwah, NJ: Lawrence Erlbaum Associates, 2006.
382. **Kossek, E.E.:** Work and family in America: Growing tensions between employment policy and a changing workforce. In *America at Work: Choices and Challenges.* Lawler, E. and J. O'Toole (eds.). New York: Palgrave MacMillan; 2006.
383. **Allen, T.D.:** Family-supportive work environments: The role of organizational perceptions. *J. Vocat. Behav. 58*:414–35 (2001).
384. **Hammer, L., E. Kossek, N. Yragui, T. Bodner, and G. Hanson:** Development and validation of a multi-dimensional scale of family supportive supervisor behaviors (FSSB). *J. Mgmt. 35*:837–56 (2009).
385. **Hammer, L.B., E.E. Kossek, W.K. Anger, T. Bodner, and K. Zimmerman:** Clarifying work-family intervention processes: The roles of work-family conflict and family supportive supervisor behaviors. *J. Appl. Psych. 96*: 34–150. (2011)..
386. **Herbert, R., et al.:** The union health center: A working model of clinical care linked to preventive occupational health services. *Am. J. Ind. Med. 31*:263–73 (1997).
387. **Schnall, P. and K. Belkic:** Point estimates of blood pressure at the worksite. *Occ. Med.-State Art. 15(1)*:203–08 (2000).
388. **Belkic, K., P. Schnall, P. Landsbergis, and D. Baker:** The workplace and CV health: Conclusions and thoughts for a future agenda. *Occup. Med.-State Art. 15(1)*:307–22 (2000).
389. **Babson, S.:** Lean or mean: The MIT model and lean production at Mazada. *Labor Studies J. 18*:3–24 (1993).
390. **Mehri, D.:** The Darker Side of Lean: An Insider's Perspective on the Realities of the Toyota Production System. *Acad. Mgmt. Perspect. 20(2)*:21–42 (2006).
391. **Ramsay, H.:** From Kalmar to Koromo. In *International Workshop on Worker Participation: What Can We Learn from the Swedish Experience?* Cressey, P. (ed.). Dublin: European Foundation for the Improvement of Living and Working Conditions, 1992.
392. **Lewchuk, W., and D. Robertson:** Working conditions under lean production: A worker-based benchmarking study. *Asia Pacific Business Review. 2*:60–81 (1996).

393. **Gardell, B.:** Worker participation and autonomy: a multilevel approach to democracy at the workplace. *Int. J. Health Serv. 12*:527–58 (1982).
394. **Levi, L.:** Legislation to protect worker CV health in Europe. *Occ. Med.-State Art 15(1)*:269–73 (2000).
395. **Melin, B., U. Lundberg, J. Soderlund, and M. Granqvist:** Psychophysiological stress reactions of male and female assembly workers: a comparison between two different forms of work organization. *J. Org. Behav. 20*:47–61 (1999).
396. **Kuorinka, I.:** Tools and means of implementing participatory ergonomics. *Int. J. Ind. Ergo. 19*:267–70 (1997).
397. **Eklof, M., A. Ingelgard, and M. Hagberg:** Is participative ergonomics associated with better working environment and health? A study among Swedish white-collar VDU users. *Int. J. Ind. Ergo. 34*:355–66 (2004).
398. **Laing, A.C., et al.:** Effectiveness of a participatory ergonomics intervention in improving communication and psychosocial exposures. *Ergo. 50(7)*:1092–109 (2007).
399. **Cole, D., et al.:** *Effectiveness of participatory ergonomics interventions: A systematic review.* Toronto, Ontario: Institute for Work & Health, 2005.
400. **Lindstrom, K., K. Schrey, G. Ahonen, and S. Kaleva:** The effects of promoting organisational health on worker well-being and organisational effectiveness in small and medium-sized enterprises. In *Healthy and Productive Work: An International Perspective.* Murphy, L.R. and C. Cooper (eds.). London: Taylor & Francis, 2000.
401. **Nielsen, M.L., T.S. Kristensen, and L. Smith-Hansen:** The Intervention Project on Absence and Well-being (IPAW): Design and results from the baseline of a 5-year study. *Work Stress 16(3)*:191–206 (2002).
402. **Bambra, C., M. Egan, S. Thomas, M. Petticrew, and M. Whitehead:** The psychosocial and health effects of workplace reorganisation. 2. A systematic review of task restructuring interventions. *J. Epidemiol. Comm. H. 61(12)*:1028–37 (2007).
403. **Egan, M, et al.:** The psychosocial and health effects of workplace reorganization. 1. A systematic review of organisational-level interventions that aim to increase employee control. *J. Epi. Commun. H. 61(11)*:945–54 (2007).
404. **Sorensen, G., et al.:** Preventing chronic disease at the workplace: A workshop report and recommendations. *Am. J. Pub. Health* 2011. [In press].
405. **Sorensen, G., et al.:** A model for worksite cancer prevention: integration of health protection and health promotion in the WellWorks Project. *Am. J. Health Promot. 10(1)*:55–62 (1995).
406. **Sorensen, G., A. Stoddard, J.K. Ockene, M.K Hunt, and R. Youngstrom:** Worker participation in an integrated health promotion/health protection program: Results from the WellWorks Project. *Health Educ. Quart. 23*:191–203 (1996).
407. **Golaszewski, T., and B. Fisher:** Heart check: The development and evolution of an organizational heart health assessment. *Am. J. Health Promot. 17(2)*:132–53 (2002).
408. **Landsbergis, P.:** Collective bargaining to reduce CVD risk factors in the work environment. *Occup. Med.-State Art. 15(1)*:287–92 (2000).
409. **AFL-CIO Working Women's Department:** Bargaining Fact Sheet: Control Over Work Hours and Alternative Work Schedules. Washington, D.C.: AFL-CIO Working Women's Department, 2001.
410. **Grundy, L., L. Bell, N. Firestein:** Labor's Role In *Addressing The Child Care Crisis.* New York: Foundation for Child Development, 1999.
411. **Dones, N. and N. Firestein:** Labor's Participation in Work Family Issues: Successes and Obstacles. In *Learning from the Past - Looking to the Future.* Beem, C. and J. Heymann (eds.). Racine, WI: The Work, Family and Democracy Project, 2002.
412. **Shimomitsu, T., and Y. Odagiri:** Working life in Japan. *Occup. Med.-State Art. 15(1)*:280–81 (2000).
413. **Warren, N.:** U.S. regulations for work organization. *Occup. Med.-State Art. 15(1)*:275–80 (2000).
414. **Milkman, R., and E. Appelbaum:** Paid family leave in California: new research findings. In: *The State of California Labor 2004.* Berkeley, CA: University of California Press, 2004.
415. **Levi, L.:** Work stress and health: Research approaches and health promotion strategies. In *Behavioral Medicine: An Integrated Biobehavioral Approach to Health and Illness.* Araki, S. (ed.). New York: Elsevier, 1992.
416. **Levi, L.:** The European Commission's Guidance on Work-Related Stress and Related Initiatives: From words to action. In *Stress and Quality of Working Life: Current Perspectives in Occupational Health.* Rossi, A.M., P.L. Perrewe, and S.L. Sauter (eds.). Greenwich, CT: Baywood, 2005.
417. **European Trade Union Confederation, Union of Industrial and Employers Confederations of Europe, European Association of Craft Small and Medium-Sized Enterprises, European Centre of Enterprises with Public Participation and of Enterprises of General Economic Interest:** *Framework Agreement on Work-Related Stress.* Brussels, Belgium: European Trade Union Confederation, 2004.

Outcome Competencies

After completing this chapter, the reader should be able to:

1. Define underlined terms used in this chapter.
2. Explain risk reduction methods.
3. Explain the framework needed to prevent accidental releases.
4. Recall regulations related to chemical releases.
6. Describe the difference between hazard evaluation and hazard identification.
7. List the important models to evaluate chemical releases.
8. Summarize disasters of historical importance.

Prerequisite Knowledge

Prior to beginning this chapter, the reader should review the following chapters:

Chapter Number	Chapter Topic
3	Legal Aspects of Industrial Hygiene
4	Occupational Exposure Limits
7	Principles of Evaluating Worker Exposure
44	Emergency Planning and Crisis Management in the Workplace
48	Hazardous Waste Management
49	Laboratory Health and Safety

Key Terms

disasters • emergency response • exposure assessment • extrinsic safety • hazard and operability (HAZOP) surveys • hazard analysis (HAZAN) • hazard evaluation • hazard identification • human factors • intrinsic safety • risk analysis • risk management • toxic chemical releases

Key Topics

I. Historical Background
   A. Characteristics of Disasters
   B. Evolution of Planning, Prevention, and Response
II. Purpose
   A. Framework
   B. Sources of Information
   C. Roles
III. Principles of Prevention
   A. Hazard Management
   B. Community Interaction
IV. Legislation
   A. Hazardous Materials Transportation Act
   B. Superfund
   C. Emergency Planning and Community Right to Know Act of 1986
   D. OSHA
   E. EPA
   F. CSB
   G. FEMA
   H. Other U.S. Legislation
   I. Seveso Directive
   J. Control of Industrial Major Accident Hazards (CIMAH)
V. Hazard Identification
   A. Data Collection
   B. Hazard Indices
   C. Dow and MOND Indexes
   D. HAZOP
   E. HAZAN
   F. Fault Tree Analysis
   G. Event Tree Analysis
   H. Cause-Consequence Analysis
   I. Root Cause Analysis
   J. Human Error Analysis
VI. Environmental Hazards
VII. Hazard Evaluation
   A. Release Characteristics
   B. Dispersion Models
   C. Biological Effect Prediction
   D. Integrated Systems
VIII. Risk Reduction
   A. Intrinsic Safety
   B. Extrinsic Safety
   C. Human Factors
IX. Planning and Response
   A. Scope
   B. Planning Process
   C. Health Planning Considerations
   D. Casualty Handling
   E. Exposure Assessment
   F. Organizational Communication
   G. Drills

Prevention and Mitigation of Accidental Chemical Releases

34

Jeremiah R. Lynch, CIH, CSP, PE

Historical Background

Characteristics of Disasters

Natural disasters such as earthquakes and floods have been occurring since before recorded history, but the advent of man-made disasters, other than war, required the development of cities, factories, and transportation systems. Some significant natural and man-made disasters are listed in Table 31.1.[1] In each case the disaster and the subsequent public reaction resulted in improved means of detection and prevention. This also is likely to happen in the aftermath of examples such as the Exxon Valdez oil spill on March 24, 1989, and the explosion and fire at the Phillips Petroleum Co. plant in Pasadena, Tex., on October 23,

Table 34.1 — Disasters and Results

Type	*Location and Date*	*Total Deaths*	*Results*
Earthquake	Chicago, IL; 10/9/1871	250	building codes prohibiting wooden structures; water reserve
Flood	Johnstown, PA; 5/31/1889	2209	inspections of dams
Tidal wave	Galveston, TX; 9/8/1900	6000	sea wall built
Fire	Iroquois Theater, Chicago, IL 12/30/03	575	stricter safety standards
Marine fire	*General Slocum*, East River, NY 6/15/04	1021	stricter ship inspections; revision of statutes (life preservers, experienced crew, fire extinguishers)
Earthquake	San Francisco, CA; 4/18/06	452	widened streets; limited heights of buildings; steel frame and fire-resistant buildings
Mine	Monongah, WV; 12/6/07	361	creation of Federal Bureau of Mines; stricter mine inspections
Fire	N. Collinwood School; Cleveland, OH; 3/8/08	176	need realized for fire drills and planning of school structures
Fire	Triangle Shirt Waist Co. New York, NY; 3/25/11	145	strengthening of laws concerning alarm signals, sprinklers, fire escapes, fire drills
Marine	*Titanic* struck iceberg, Atlantic Ocean; 4/15/12	1517	regulation regarding number of lifeboats; all passenger ships equipped for around-the-clock radio watch; International Ice Patrol
Explosion	New London School, TX; 3/18/37	294	odorants put in natural gas
Fire	"Coconut Grove," Boston, MA; 11/28/42	492	ordinances regulating aisle space, electrical wiring, flameproofing of decorations
Explosion	Caprolactam factory; Flixborough, England, 6/1/74	28	increased emphasis on hazard analysis
Toxic release	Union Carbide plant, Bhopal, India, (methyl isocyanate); 12/3/84	2500	tighter laws and regulations to prevent toxic chemical releases
Nuclear	Chernobyl, Russia (nuclear plant burns, releases radiation over Russia and Europe); 4/86	31+	re-evaluation of nuclear power safety

Source: Reference 1.

1989. Although it is natural to tighten precautions following a disaster, it would be better to recognize and evaluate the potential for a disaster before it happens and thus prevent it and others like it. The development of modern disaster prevention technology has as its focus (1) methods of hazard analysis that allow the prediction of the potential for a disaster in the absence of the event; and (2) the application of preventive measures not learned by experience.

Evolution of Planning, Prevention, and Response

The space shuttle *Challenger* disaster made it apparent that even sophisticated agencies such as the National Aeronautics and Space Administration were not uniformly applying the most advanced risk analysis technology. Although the many acknowledged uncertainties in the input data limit the precision of all risk analysis techniques, it is possible to calculate the bounds on the probability of an event with useful levels of certainty. These techniques include fault tree analyses, failure mode and effect analysis, vulnerability analysis, what-if studies, and the Bayesian statistics of decision analysis, which will be briefly discussed later in this chapter. Other more advanced methods are described in the books and journals listed in the references. In the future, man-made disasters may not be considered unavoidable accidents unless the probability of their occurrence has been shown to be vanishingly small by a preevent risk analysis.

Advances in control technology are not so much scientific breakthroughs as the application of many small measures, the value of which has long been recognized. These measures are discussed under the headings Intrinsic Safety, Extrinsic Safety, and Human Factors. The important advances in prevention are the use of such techniques as hazard and operability (HAZOP) surveys, coupled with risk analysis, to determine and prioritize what needs to be done to control risk in each situation.

Prevention is obviously preferable to response, but prudence requires that workable response plans exist wherever a disaster could occur. Spurred by experience and legislation, plans are evolving to become multisite/community-based designs that are rationalized by exacting studies of response experience and tested and refined by realistic drills.

Purpose

Framework

The prevention and mitigation of the nonroutine chemical releases that may result in a disaster are exercises in risk management. In occupational hygiene the risk management process has traditionally been divided into the categories of recognition, evaluation, and control. This same framework is applicable to the present topic except that the real recognition and evaluation phases are often combined, and control activities are divided into those measures taken to prevent the event and those taken to mitigate or minimize the consequences of the event. In this chapter the categories of hazard identification, hazard evaluation, risk reduction, mitigation, and response are used.

Identification begins with a data collection activity that asks the question, "What chemicals are present in sufficient quantities to create a disaster if the entire amount was released?" HAZOP, hazard analysis (HAZAN), and various failure mode analyses are done next to develop release scenarios for credible releases. There are techniques to quantitatively estimate probabilities, but these are used less often. In the evaluation phase the possible consequence is estimated from the scenario assumptions, dispersion models, and biological effect criteria. Interaction between the identification and evaluation phases is necessary to be sure that the most serious consequence scenarios are identified.

A value judgment regarding risks applied to the results of the hazard evaluations may lead to the conclusion that risk reduction is necessary. The best way to reduce risk is to build plants so that disastrous events cannot happen. Where such events are still possible, equipment (scrubbers, alarms) and procedures are added to reduce risk. In some high hazard industries such as explosives manufacturing, isolation and distance are used to reduce the consequences of events.

If an event does occur, the consequence depends on what actions are taken to respond to the emergency. Emergency forces must be available and properly used. People at risk must be evacuated or protected. Casualties must be properly moved and attended. All of this requires intelligent planning tested by frequent realistic drills.

Sources of Information

The body of knowledge on disaster prevention and response is enormous. The literature is filled with lessons learned from emergencies; detailed analyses of disasters and their causes; results of experimental chemical releases; mathematical dispersion models; risk analysis techniques; engineering means of prevention; and guides to emergency planning. Consequently, this chapter is not an exhaustive coverage of the subject but an overview and source guide. Some of the major elements of technology in disaster prevention, mitigation, and response are described. Organizational sources of assistance are listed in the conclusion, and the references provide additional help. Many of these are secondary sources that can in turn provide long lists of primary resources. Taken as a whole, this body of information can provide access to essentially everything published on the subject as of the time of writing and to the main organizations and research groups working in this field. Although such a broad view is useful, it is likely that there also will be certain customary traditional approaches taken by specific industries (chemical manufacturing, transportation, nuclear power).

All of the assembled and codified experience of others is not enough. Each manager of a facility or operation that has the potential to cause a disaster has to create a unique understanding of that potential and how to control it. Much of the disaster prevention and mitigation literature deals with process tools by which the probabilities of unlikely events are examined and how to reduce those probabilities. However, no two sets of circumstances that might lead to disaster are alike, and thus, each manager must become expert in his or her own problem. This is a continuing effort, because circumstances change due to new laws, plant aging, engineering or process changes, new knowledge of chemical toxicity, and the evolving expectations of the public. The manager must be sensitive to these changes and to improvements in the understanding of how accidents happen and to the near-miss events that provide performance experience without major loss. The literature is helpful, but only learning by evaluation will lead to safety.

Roles

The manager of any process or operation has the actual and legal responsibility for what happens. Management delegates, depending on the size of the organization, the responsibility for planning and coordinating disaster prevention, mitigation, and response activities. These coordinators rely on internal and external experts to advise them and to perform certain tasks. Engineers need to describe in detail how the equipment operates, so that HAZOP analysts can ask "what if." The network of firefighters, first responders, and hospitals need to consider what they would do in a disaster. In this multidisciplinary effort the health professional (physician/occupational hygienist) is not usually in the lead role but performs a key specialist role, particularly in toxic disasters. Some of these contributions are as follows.

- Expert advice on the potency and acute and chronic health effects of chemicals that might be released
- Response strategies (evacuation versus "button-up," or sealing off those who may be exposed) for various release scenarios
- Planning and drilling for casualty handling involving all available resources
- Technical health and environmental hazard information to help inform authorities and the public
- Exposure assessment before, during, and after a release event by modeling and/or measurement
- Planning, auditing, and drilling the health and environmental components of the overall response plan

These may be new roles for some health professionals, but they derive from their basic skills and from increasing concern for toxic chemical releases. This chapter addresses the full range of roles in disaster prevention, mitigation, and response but does so from the point of view of the health professional with the background needed to ease integration into the overall disaster planning team.

Principles of Prevention

Hazard Management

A systematic approach to chemical process hazard management requires that the means for preventing catastrophic release, fire, and explosion are understood, and that the necessary preventive measures and lines of defense are installed and maintained.[2,3] A schematic representation of this management system is shown in Figure 34.1.[4] Although the process is logical and technically correct, the successful management of chemical process hazards will not occur without management commitment. This commitment takes the form of a requirement to know the magnitude of the hazards, a determination to follow through on necessary changes to reduce risk, and a reasonable and prudent criterion for what is acceptable. This last is the most difficult principle on which to achieve agreement. Historically, the threshold of acceptability was defined and reduced by public reaction to catastrophes. These criteria were not explicitly stated but could be implied from the laws, regulations, standards, codes, and practices accepted and applied. As the criteria of acceptability changes, old codes, standards, and practices need to be reexamined to see whether they achieve the currently required level of risk reduction. This is a continuing process and one that requires new risk management and analysis skills not widely used in the past.

Community Interaction

Decision-making in risk management has been broadened beyond the facility manager and owners to include the community at risk.[5–7] As a practical matter, the community

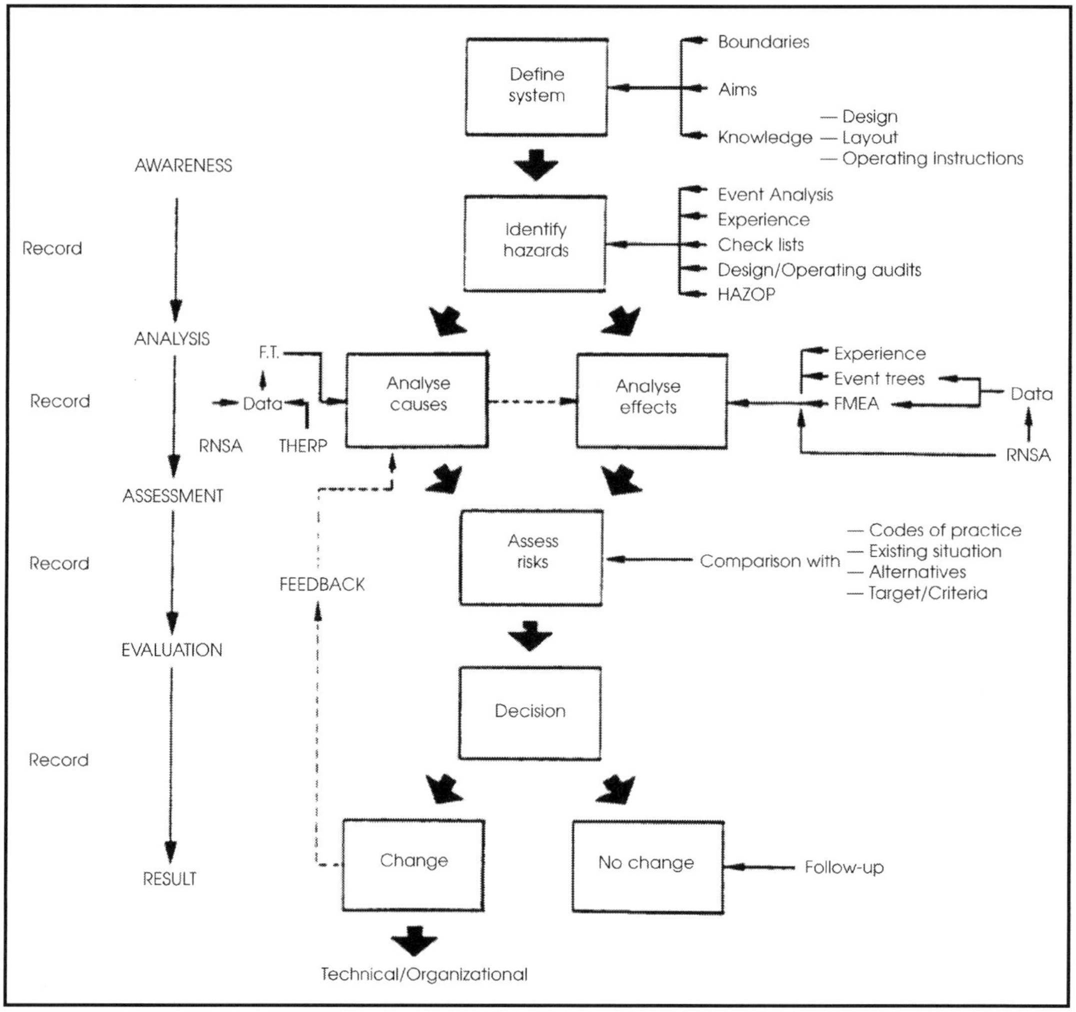

Figure 34.1 — Process hazards management. (Source: Reference 4.)

will be involved in decisions on new facilities and even on existing facilities either because the law requires it, or because intense public pressure would substantially hinder any action that did not have public acceptance. To gain this acceptance, the community needs to be involved from the earliest phase of the planning process, and the facility management needs to be completely open and accurate as the project development evolves. The local facility management needs to work closely with community leaders to understand and resolve their concerns. The principles of risk communication teach that it is not only the magnitude of the risk that determines acceptability but also how decisions about the imposition of risks and benefits are made. Failure to observe these principles can result in the failure of a project that would otherwise have met pure objective risk acceptability criteria.

Even within the enterprise there can be problems of risk communication. For example, the design of a new or modified facility will be in the hands of engineers who are in the habit of dealing with concepts that can be quantified with some accuracy. The risks to be considered can rarely be well quantified, and the health risks in particular have an added level of uncertainty. Beyond this, there is the uncertain question of public reaction. There is no fixed formula for managing the engineer-health professional-public interaction. The universal principle of openness, respect, and sensitivity are the best guides.

Legislation

Hazardous Materials Transportation Act

The U.S. Department of Transportation (DOT) is responsible for administering the Hazardous Materials Transportation Act[8] as well as the Natural Gas Pipeline Safety Act[9] and the Hazard Liquid Pipeline Safety Act.[10,11] All of these acts are intended to adequately protect the public against the risk to life and property that are inherent in the transportation of hazardous materials in commerce. They give the secretary of transportation the authority to regulate any safety aspect of the transportation of hazardous materials including packing, handling, labeling, marking, placarding, and routing. Regulations on packing cover the manufacture, marking, maintenance, repairing, and testing of packages. Regulations on handling cover number of personnel, level of training, frequency of inspection, and safety assurance procedures for handling of hazardous materials. The requirements are promulgated in a series of regulations in *Code of Federal Regulations* (CFR) Title 49, Parts 171-199. They incorporate by reference a long series of guides and standards developed by some of the organizations listed in Table 34.2.

In 49 CFR 172 are listed hazardous materials subject to labeling and other requirements of law. This list gives the hazard class, the United Nations or North American identification numbers, labeling and packaging requirements, and quantity restrictions. It is supplemented by the Reportable Quantities list for hazardous substances designated under the Comprehensive Environmental Response, Compensation and Liability Act of 1980 (CERCLA) as published by the U.S. Environmental Protection Agency (EPA). To aid those who must comply with these complex laws and regulations, DOT publishes a series of information bulletins for shippers, carriers, freight handlers, and container manufacturers. These bulletins cover duties of employees, shipping documents, labels, container specifications, quality control, violation reporting, and incident investigations. For example, the 2000 *Emergency Response Guidebook*[12] provides initial response recommendations for first responders to hazardous materials emergencies. However, the main thrust of DOT's activity is accident prevention rather than emergency response.

Table 34.2 — Organizations Involved in Hazardous Materials Transportation Safety

American Society of Mechanical Engineers (ASME)
American National Standards Institute (ANSI)
American Society for Testing and Materials (ASTM)
Compressed Gas Association (CGA)
The Chlorine Institute (CI)
American Iron and Steel Institute (AISI)
Chemical Manufacturers Association (CMA)
National Fire Protection Association (NFPA)
Institute of Makers of Explosives (IME)
The Fertilizer Institute (TFI)
International Maritime Organization (IMO)
Society of the Plastics Industry (SPI)
International Organization for Standardization (ISO)

In addition to DOT, the Nuclear Regulatory Commission regulates radioactive materials transport (10 CFR 71), the Federal Aviation Administration regulates aircraft carriage enforcement procedures (14 CFR 13), and the Coast Guard regulates hazardous cargo on board ships and in ports (33 and 46 CFR).

Superfund

CERCLA,[13] more commonly known as Superfund, was enacted "to provide for liability, compensation, cleanup and emergency response for hazardous substances released into the environment and the cleanup of inactive hazardous waste disposal sites." Although Superfund is best known for its efforts to deal with hazardous waste sites, there are several provisions relevant to nonroutine chemical releases.[14,15]

Response. Superfund regulations[16] establish the list of extremely hazardous substances, threshold planning quantities, and facility notification responsibilities necessary for the development and implementation of state and local emergency response plans. Section 104 provides the authority for the removal of any hazardous substance that may be released into the environment and the authority to respond to a release as necessary to "protect the public health or welfare of the environment."

Planning. Section 105 calls for the revision of the National Contingency Plan[17] to include the requirements of CERCLA.

Liability. Section 107 establishes a standard of strict liability for incidents involving the release of hazardous substances and provides for fines of up to $50,000,000 plus response costs plus triple punitive damages. Of interest to first responders to hazardous materials incidents is a provision stating that "no person shall be held liable . . . for damages as a result of actions taken or omitted in the course of rendering care, assistance, or advice in accordance with the National Contingency Plan or at the direction of an on-scene coordinator appointed under such plan with respect to an incident creating a danger to public health or welfare or the environment as a result of any release of a hazardous substance or the threat thereof unless there was gross negligence."

CERCLA was amended by the Superfund Amendments and Reauthorization Act (SARA), which is discussed in the following paragraphs.

Emergency Planning and Community Right to Know Act of 1986

This broad piece of legislation, known as Title III of SARA,[18] establishes a number of emergency planning, notification, reporting, and training requirements. The law requires that states establish emergency response commissions, emergency planning districts, and local emergency planning committees (LEPCs) consisting of representatives of government, police and fire departments, hospitals, the media, community groups, and industry. Each LEPC writes an emergency plan covering hazardous substance facilities; emergency response and coordination; notification; release warning and dispersion; emergency equipment and facilities; evacuation; training; and drills. The LEPC is guided by publications from the national response team established by the National Contingency Plan (Section 105 of CERCLA). Local personnel are to be trained in hazard mitigation, emergency preparedness, fire prevention and control, disaster response, and other emergency training topics.

The act also requires facilities to notify the community emergency coordinator and the LEPC in the event of a release of certain hazardous chemicals in excess of specified amounts. The notification must identify the substance; the amount released; time and duration of the release; media (air, water); anticipated health risks; medical advice; precautions; and a telephone contact. To avoid releases of extremely hazardous substances, EPA will review systems for monitoring, detecting, and preventing such releases, including perimeter alert systems. Facilities are also required to provide material safety data sheets (MSDSs) or lists of MSDSs to LEPCs.

Other major sections of this act provide for the reporting of routine nonemergency releases of certain toxic chemicals (Section 313). SARA provisions also require (Section 126) that the Occupational Safety and Health Administration (OSHA) issue standards for the heath and safety of employees in hazardous waste operations (HAZWOPER).

OSHA

In 1985 OSHA initiated a special emphasis program for the chemical industry (ChemSEP). As part of this program OSHA inspected facilities to study current practices for the prevention of catastrophic incidents and the mitigation of releases. At the same time, EPA conducted a review of emergency systems for monitoring, detecting, and preventing releases of extremely hazardous substances as required by Section 305 of SARA. These two efforts led OSHA and EPA to cooperate on the development of standards for the prevention of chemical release disasters. Because workers at a facility are usually the population most immediately and seriously impacted by a release, and because OSHA has more experience in inspecting safety hazards at industrial facilities, the coordinated regulations will be issued and enforced by OSHA.

On June 1, 1992, OSHA issued a final rule, "Process Safety Management of Highly Hazardous Chemicals."[2] This rule has its antecedents in OSHA's ChemSEP effort, EPA's SARA review, and the Chemical Manufacturers Association's (CMA's) Chemical Awareness and Emergency Response (CAER) program.[19] Input from Organization Resources Counselors,[20] the American Petroleum Institute, the Oil Chemical and Atomic Workers, and the United Steelworkers of America was also considered. The rule is performance oriented and requires that process safety management (PSM) systems be put in place in covered workplaces.

In its Appendix A the rule includes a list of highly hazardous chemicals with threshold quantity amounts that trigger the provisions of the rule. In addition, the rule applies to flammable liquids or gases (except certain fuels) in excess of 10,000 lb. Appendix C of the rule is a compliance guideline for PSM, and Appendix E provides further sources of information.

EPA

On January 6, 1999, EPA issued an amended final rule, "Accidental Release Prevention Requirements; Risk Management Programs Under the Clean Air Act, Section 112(r)(7)."[3] The purpose of the regulation is to prevent accidental releases of regulated substances and reduce the severity of those releases that do occur. The rule requires a risk management plan and one of three levels of management system programs depending on the degree of risk as determined by a hazard assessment. This rule covers stationary sources, which includes those establishments covered by OSHA's PSM rule. The highest (most stringent) level of risk management program required by the EPA rule is fundamentally identical to OSHA PSM requirements; so any establishment that meets PSM will meet all three EPA levels.

The chemicals regulated under this rule are appear in the "List of Regulated Substances and Threshold Quantities for Accidental Release Prevention."[21] The list gives the name of the chemical, the Chemical Abstract Service number, the threshold quantity, and the basis for the listing.

CSB

The U.S. Chemical Safety and Hazard Investigation Board (CSB) is an independent, scientific investigatory agency, not a regulatory or enforcement body. The Clean Air Act Amendments of 1990 created CSB. However, the board was not funded and did not begin operations until January 2000. The principal role of the new chemical safety board is to investigate accidents to determine the conditions and circumstances that led up to the event and to identify the cause or causes so that similar events might be prevented. It has a unique statutory mission, and the law explicitly states that no other agency or executive branch official may direct the activities of the board. In addition to its reports of investigations[22] CSB also issues guidelines. A safety bulletin from CSB[23] concerning "Management of Change" discusses two incidents (one in Maryland and the other in Washington State) that occurred in the United States in 1998. The first incident involved a fire at an oil refinery in Anacortes, Wash. The fire in the delayed coking unit caused six fatalities. The second incident involved a reactor vessel explosion and fire at a detergent alkylate plant in Baltimore, Md., that injured four people and caused extensive damage. Each case history offers valuable insights into the importance of having a systematic method for management of change (i.e., managing changes in chemical processes using a formal management of change [MOC] program). An MOC methodology should be applied to operational deviations and variances, as well as to planned changes, such as those involving technology, processes, and equipment.

FEMA

The Federal Emergency Management Agency (FEMA) is an independent agency of the federal government, reporting to the president. Since its founding in 1979, FEMA's mission has been to reduce loss of life and property and protect our nation's critical infrastructure from all types of hazards through a comprehensive, risk-based, emergency management program of mitigation, preparedness, response, and recovery.[24] Although disasters such as floods and earthquakes are FEMAs main concerns, the agency would get involved in a chemical event such as Bhopal where there was major community involvement, and has published planning guidance.

Other U.S. Legislation

Several other U.S. laws have provisions that relate to nonroutine chemical releases.

Resource Conservation and Recovery Act. This law lists certain hazardous wastes and requirements for their treatment, disposal, and storage.

Clean Water Act. The Clean Water Act sets limits on the release of hazardous substances into water.

Toxic Substance Control Act. Under certain circumstances, EPA may require health and environmental properties testing of new and existing chemicals. In addition, if releases may present substantial risk to health or the environment, in some instances such releases are reportable to the EPA administrator.

Seveso Directive

The Council of the European Communities adopted the Seveso Directive, named after an accidental release of dioxin in Italy in 1976, on June 30, 1982.[25,26] On December 9, 1996, Council Directive 96/82/EC on the control of major-accident hazards called the Seveso II Directive was adopted.[27] These directives set up an approach to the prevention of major chemical release disasters in Europe and cover many of the same requirements as the U.S. regulations.[28]

Control of Industrial Major Accident Hazards (CIMAH)

Following the Seveso disaster the European Community issued in 1983 a directive on major accident hazards of certain industrial activities. Each member country was required to implement this directive by means of national laws. The United Kingdom issued the CIMAH regulations in 1984[29] to control fire, explosion, and toxic hazards. The regulations require safety study, notification, emergency plans, and public information when listed chemicals are held in excess of stated quantities.

Hazard Identification

Hazard identification is the first step in the risk assessment and management process. It starts with data collection to define the system and proceeds through the identification of hazards and the analysis of causes and effects. The output of the hazard identification step leads to hazard evaluation and risk reduction, as needed. Many formal techniques have been developed for the systematic analysis of complex systems. Some of the most commonly used methods (HAZOP and HAZAN) and some specialized methods such as human error analysis are discussed later in this chapter. Some others are listed in the references.[30–42] They all attempt to consider all reasonable possibilities and all suffer from the drawback that the probability of future events can only be guessed.

Data Collection

A necessary first step in all hazard identification and analysis procedures is the collection of accurate data about the substances present; the process and equipment; and the layout, topography, meteorology, and demographics of the plant and surrounding community. A complete inventory of substances present would include raw materials, additives, catalysts, intermediates, products, and wastes. The inventory should specify quantities, locations, use, and marking and type of storage. Chemicals used in utilities (hydrazine, chlorine) should also be listed. For each substance on the inventory the substance-specific information listed in Table 34.3 should be obtained. No single source (e.g., MSDS) will have all of this information, and measurements may need to be made to collect some of the data.

Plant and process equipment data collection starts with an up-to-date set of process and instrumentation drawings (P&ID). As plants age and are modified, the engineering details of plant changes are not always carried over to the P&ID, so it becomes out of date. This can be a serious problem when conducting hazard analyses if the plant is not, in fact, what the analysts think it is. In addition to accurate P&IDs, additional detail should be collected on the age and condition of equipment, the state of maintenance, and the actual process operating procedures and practices used. What is known about the degree of corrosion of pipes and vessels? Are battery limit block valves operable? Have safety valves been tested, and are rupture disks properly installed? Have prescribed operating procedures been modified by short cuts? Will remote sensors work?

To predict the consequences of a release, it is necessary to know how the land lies, which way the wind blows, and where the people are. Simple dispersion models make worst case assumptions and need little data, whereas complex models require a lot of data, as discussed later. Demographic data, transportation routes, and the location of fire stations and hospitals are also needed for casualty care planning.

The collection and continuous updating of this assembly of information is a difficult task and a burdensome effort. Companies need to assure by means of their audit or review process that the job is being done wherever it is needed.

Table 34.3 — Substance Specific Information

Health effects
Exposure limits—TLV, IDLH, ERPG, Community Exposure Guides
Effects—irritancy, systems organ, cancer reproduction effect, neurotoxicity
Toxicity—oral, dermal LD50
Odor—threshold, persistence
Physical/chemical properties
Physical—solubility, vapor pressure, melting/boiling point, density
Chemical—formula, structure, molecular weight, corrosivity
Fire and explosion properties
Flammability—flash point, autoignition temperature
Explosivity—upper and lower explosive limits, detonation, explosive decomposition, pyrophoric
Reactivity—auto reaction, incompatibilities, effect of impurities
Environmental
Fate—biodegradation, bioconcentration, hydrolysis, photolysis, volatility
Effects—terrestrial, aquatic

Hazard Indices

A complete inventory lists a few substances that have the potential to cause a catastrophic incident and many that do not. A necessary step in going from the inventory to the development of event scenarios is a ranking of the list by hazard potential. Several hazard indices have been developed for this purpose.[43,44] The vapor hazard index[45] is a ratio of the concentration of saturated vapor divided by the threshold limit value (TLV®)[46] times 1000. However, the TLVs® are based on a variety of end points rather than the acute toxicity of primary concern in chemical release incidents. The substance hazard index[20] is the ratio of the vapor pressure of a substance to its acute toxicity concentration, which is calculated from either the American Industrial Hygiene Association (AIHA®) Emergency Response Planning Guideline Level™ Three (ERPG-3; see below), the EPA Levels of Concern, or the Acute Toxic Concentrations developed by the State of New Jersey. Substances with substance hazard indexes over 5000 are considered dangerous. Both of these indexes consider only intrinsic human toxicity. Other ranking systems have been developed[47] that consider both human and environmental endpoints.

EPA has proposed a screening index in its rulemaking under SARA. The index is equal to a "level of concern" value (usually the National Institute for Occupational Safety and Health [NIOSH] immediately dangerous to life or health [IDLH] value in milligrams per liter) divided by V, the vapor fraction (1 for gases). EPA uses this index to determine threshold quantities for the planning and notification provisions of their rules. An obvious weakness of this index is that it depends on IDLH values that may not be consistent and accurate measures of intrinsic hazard.

Dow and MOND Indexes

The Dow Chemical Co. Fire and Explosion Index[48] was originally intended as an aid to fire protection by calculating a fire and explosion index. It also calculates the maximum probable property damage and the maximum probable days outage. It also considers general and special process hazards such as toxicity hazards and arrives at a toxicity index. A simplified flow diagram is shown in Figure 34.2.

The American Institute of Chemical Engineers Center for Chemical Plant Safety[49] has summarized this relative ranking procedure as follows.

(1) Identify on the plot plan those process units that would have the greatest effect or contribute the most to a fire, explosion, or release of toxic material.
(2) Determine the material factor for each unit.
(3) Evaluate the appropriate contributing hazard factors, considering fire, explosion, and toxicity.
(4) Calculate the unit hazard factor and damage factor for each unit.
(5) Determine the fire and explosion index and area of exposure for each unit.
(6) Calculate maximum probable property damage.
(7) Evaluate maximum probable days outage and business interruption costs.

Based on the nature and severity of the hazard, various preventive and protective features are selected and the process repeated to calculate new indexes.

The MOND fire, explosion, and toxicity index, which is a variation of the Dow Index and was developed by the MOND division of Imperial Chemical Industries (ICI) in the United Kingdom, has been extended to consider more operations and equipment and to evaluate the hazards from materials and reactions more extensively.

Both methods can be used during the design stage of a project or on an existing unit. A team of specialists in engineering, fire, safety, and health will best be able to conduct them.

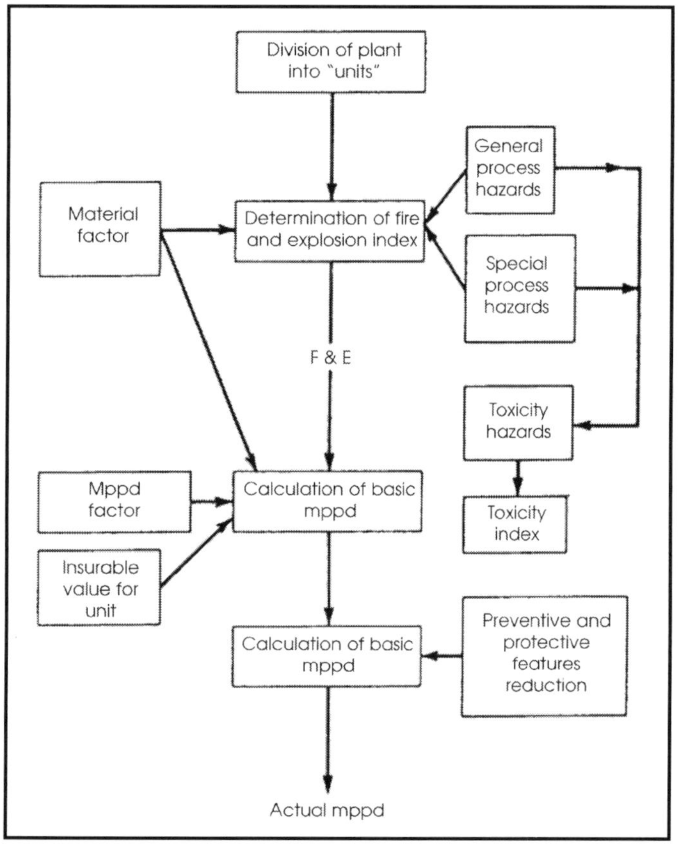

Figure 34.2 — Dow index procedure. (Source: Reference 4.)

HAZOP

A HAZOP survey is one of the most common and widely accepted methods of systematic qualitative hazard analysis. It is used for both new and existing facilities and can be applied to a whole plant, a production unit, or a piece of equipment. It uses as its database the usual sort of plant and process information and relies on the judgment of engineering and safety experts in the areas with which they are most familiar. The end result is reliable, therefore, in terms of engineering and operational expectations, but it is not quantitative and may not consider the consequences of complex sequences of human errors.

The objectives of a HAZOP study can be summarized as follows:[50]

- Identify areas of the design that may possess a significant hazard potential.
- Identify and study features of the design that influence the probability of a hazardous incident occurring.
- Familiarize the study team with the design information available.
- Ensure that a systematic study is made of the areas of significant hazard potential.
- Identify pertinent design information not currently available to the team.

- Provide a mechanism for feedback to the client of the study team's detailed comments.

A HAZOP study is conducted in the following steps.

Specify the Purpose, Objective, and Scope of the Study. The purpose may be the analysis of a plant yet to be built or a review of the risk of an existing unit. Given the purpose and the circumstances of the study, the above objectives can be made more specific. The scope of the study includes the boundaries of the physical unit and also the range of events and variables considered. For example, at one time HAZOPs were mainly focused on fire and explosion end points, but now the scope usually includes toxic release, offensive odor, and environmental end points. The initial establishment of purpose, objectives, and scope is very important and should be precisely set down so that it will be clear, now and in the future, what was and was not included in the study. These decisions need to be made by an appropriate level of responsible management.

Select the HAZOP Study Team. The team leader should be skilled in HAZOP and in the interpersonal techniques to facilitate successful group interaction. As many other experts as needed should be included in the team to cover all aspects of design, operation, process chemistry, and safety. The team leader should instruct the team in the HAZOP procedure and should emphasize that the end objective of a HAZOP survey is hazard identification; solutions to problems are a separate effort.

Collect Data. Theodore[50] listed the following materials that are usually needed: (1) process description; (2) process flow sheets; (3) data on the chemical, physical, and toxicological properties of all raw materials, intermediates, and products; (4) P&IDs; (5) equipment, piping, and instrument specifications; (6) process control logic diagrams; (7) layout drawings; (8) operating procedures; (9) maintenance procedures; (10) emergency response procedures; and (11) safety and training manuals.

Conduct the Study. Using the information collected, the unit is divided into study nodes, and the sequence diagramed in Figure 34.3 is followed for each node. Nodes are points in the process at which process parameters (i.e., pressure, temperature, and composition) have known and intended values. These values change between nodes as a result of the operation of various pieces of equipment such as distillation columns, heat exchangers, or pumps. Various forms and worksheets have been developed to help organize the node process parameters and control logic information.

When the nodes and parameters are identified, each node is studied by applying the specialized guide words to each parameter. These guide words and their meanings are key elements of the HAZOP procedure. They are listed in Table 34.4.[48]

Repeated cycling through this process, which considers how and why each parameter might vary from the intended and what the consequence would be, is the substance of the HAZOP study.

Write the Report. As much detail about events and their consequences as is uncovered by the study should be recorded. Obviously, if the HAZOP identifies a credible sequence of events that would result in a disaster, appropriate follow-up action is

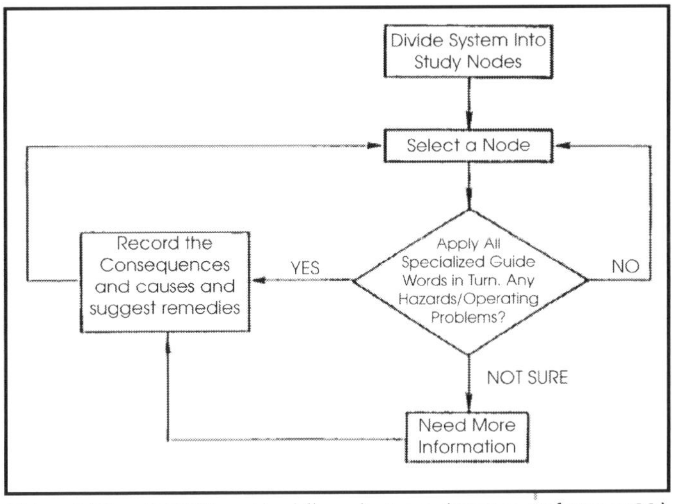

Figure 34.3 — HAZOP method flow diagram. (Source: Reference 38.)

Table 34.4 — HAZOP Guide Words and Meanings

Guide Word	*Meaning*
No	negation of design intent
Less	quantitative decrease
More	quantitative increase
Part of	qualitative decrease
As well as	qualitative increase
Reverse	logical opposite of the intent
Other than	complete substitution

needed. Thus, although risk reduction action is not a part of the HAZOP per se, the HAZOP may trigger the need for such action.

HAZOP studies are time-consuming and expensive. Just getting the P&IDs up to date on an older plant may be a major engineering effort. Still, for processes with significant risk, they are cost-effective when balanced against the potential loss of life, property, business, and even the future of the enterprise that may result from a major release.

HAZAN

The acronym "HAZAN" is a generic term for a variety of quantitative hazard and risk analysis methods. A logical sequence for the systematic examination of a facility is to use hazard identification and ranking techniques first. If there are possible scenarios that could lead to unacceptable consequences, then qualitative techniques (HAZOP) can be applied next. Where a qualitative hazard exists, HAZAN methods can be used to estimate the quantitative probability of adverse events. How much analysis is worthwhile is a function of the consequence of the adverse event and the difficulty in preventing it.

Fault Tree Analysis

Fault tree analysis is a logical method of analyzing how and why a disaster could occur. It is a graphical technique that starts with the end event—the accident or disaster, such as a nuclear fuel meltdown—and works backward to find the initiating event or combination of events that could lead to the final event. If the probabilities of each potential initiating event are known or can be estimated, then the probability of the end or top event can be calculated.

The following example of fault tree analysis is taken from Accident and Emergency Management.[50] A water pumping system consists of two pumps, A and B, where A is the pump ordinarily operating, and B is a standby pump that automatically takes over if A fails. Flow of water through the pump is regulated by a control valve in either case. Suppose that the top event is no water flow, resulting from the following initiating events: failure of Pump A and failure of Pump B, or failure of the control valve. The fault tree diagram for this system is shown in Figure 34.4. This diagram shows

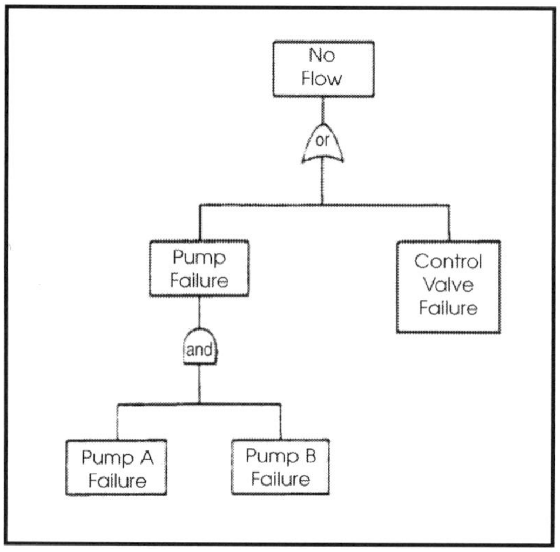

Figure 34.4 — Fault tree diagram. (Source: Reference 39.)

the logical relationship of the events and allows the calculation of the probability of the top event if the probabilities of the initiating events are known. Let A, B, and C represent the failure of Pump A, the failure of Pump B, and the failure of the control valve, respectively. Then it can be seen from the diagram that the top event, T (no water flow), occurs if both A and B occur or if C occurs. A, B, and C can be assumed to be independent events unless they have a common cause or are otherwise related. From the basic theories of probability:

P(T) = P(AB) + P® - P(ABC)

and $P(AB) = P(A)P(B)$

and $P(ABC) = P(A)P(B)P(C)$

Therefore: $P(T) = P(A)P(B) + P(C) - P(A)P(B)P(C)$.

If the individual initiating event probabilities P(A), P(B), and P(C) are known, then the probability of P(T), the top or end event, can be calculated.

The output of fault tree analysis (and of several other methods of reliability analysis described below) is a list of the minimum combinations of events sufficient to cause the outcome. This list of events is called the minimal cut set and can be ranked in terms of likelihood and consequence as a means of prioritizing safety improvement programs.

Event Tree Analysis

Another technique for applying the basic concepts of probability to the evaluation of reliability of actual systems that have the potential to cause disasters is event tree analysis.[38] This technique is similar to fault tree analysis in that it examines, in a probabilistic manner, the consequences of a series of logically connected events. Event tree analysis, however, differs from fault tree analysis in that it starts with the initiating event rather than working backward from the end event. As in fault tree analysis, a diagram is constructed showing the logical relationship between events and outcomes. Event tree analysis may be qualitative or, if reasonably accurate probabilities can be assigned to events, a quantitative estimate of reliability can be obtained. In practice, the analyst reads off the diagram the sequences of events that result in disaster and then describes and examines the events in these sequences to describe how an accident may occur. As with fault tree analysis, the result is useful both in the design of safe new plants and to improve the safety of existing facilities.

Cause-Consequence Analysis

Fault tree analysis and event tree analysis have been combined into cause-consequence analysis so that sequences can be worked out either from the event to the outcome or from the outcome back to the initiating events. The result can be either qualitative or quantitative depending on the nature of the input data. Because the analysis, although in some ways more complex, is more intuitively obvious, the display and description of sequences better serves the purposes of communication and of training those who can influence or control events. The output is usually a ranking of accident sequences based on their consequences and a ranking of minimal cut sets to evaluate important initiating events.

Root Cause Analysis

Several of the attributes of the analytical methods described above have been combined in a variety of methods under the rubric "root cause analysis."[51] In general these are methods to aid in identifying, understanding, and preventing chronic problems and improving the reliability of the plant and equipment. These methods can be automated using various computer programs such as PROACT.

Human Error Analysis

The preceding methods of analysis are easiest to do if the initiating events can be accurately assumed to be independent. Indeed, this assumption is often implicit in analyses, as they are usually performed even if the independence of initiating events is not stated. Yet it is obvious that equipment failure events often have common causes (a storm, a power failure) and thus are not independent. Another potential common cause is when operating personnel have an erroneous assessment of the situation or a mindset about what is happening, sometimes persisting in the face of evidence to the contrary. This human error then becomes the common cause of a series of initiating events that, if looked at as independent events, would seem to have a very low probability of occurring simultaneously. At Three Mile Island, the operator's misunderstanding of the cooling water status led to several actions or inactions that formed a part of a sufficient minimal cut set to result in the accident. In the case of the Ocean Ranger oil rig disaster,[52] the operators did not appreciate the damage that sea water had done to the ballast control panel. Because of confusing and conflicting information presented by the system, their attempts to operate the ballast controls became a common cause in a series of unlikely events that resulted in the capsizing of the rig and the loss of 84 lives.

The techniques previously described can be used to analyze the reliability of complex systems even when common causes and man-machine interactions are involved.[53–55] Human error analysis is a specialized subdiscipline of hazard evaluation that adds considerations of human performance to the hazard evaluation process. It is specialized and complex because of the difficulty in understanding the multitude of factors that influence human error rates and their variability, the high degree of interaction between human and system failure (lack of independence), and the nature of the options for altering human error rates.[56] Yet, human behavior must be factored into reliability analysis for it to be accurate in the increasing number of systems where errors in man-machine interaction can be an initiating event in a disaster.

The most commonly used quantitative method for the measurement and assessment of personnel-induced errors is the technique for human error prediction (THERP).[4] This procedure involves (1) identification of human activities that create a hazard, (2) estimation of failure rates; and (3) effect of human failures on the system.

The output of THERP is an input to fault tree or other methods of hazard analysis. Although THERP can estimate failure rates for the routine performance of tasks, it cannot cope with error in human decisions and has difficulty with task error rates altered by stress, as in an emergency.

Environmental Hazards

In addition to fire, explosion, or the sudden release of a toxic gas, an emergency may be precipitated by the sudden release of an environmentally hazardous material.[57] A large oil spill can threaten aquatic organisms, birds, and those who depend on them for food. Chemicals released into rivers can threaten fish and drinking water supplies. Spills on land can reach and contaminate streams and aquifers and be transported to human or animal receptors or be taken up by plants and enter the food chain.

The identification of the potential for environmental disasters is similar in some respects to that of other kinds of disasters. Critical facilities that could potentially release environmentally toxic substances should be identified. Release scenarios and the pathways by which the substance would reach environmentally sensitive locations can be described and the consequences of each release-pathway combination analyzed. The engineering risk analysis methods described above for releases of substances toxic to humans can be applied to these environmental release scenarios.

The variety of transport media and the chemical and biological changes that may occur, as illustrated in Figure 34.5, complicate prediction of human or environmental receptor exposure and consequent harm. These complex processes can result in a delay of years before the consequences of a release are manifest. Also, because of the many uncertainties associated with each leg of a pathway, it is very difficult to predict consequence with any accuracy.

Human health consequences are predicted based on exposure of the human receptor compared with certain accepted exposure limits for food or drinking water. For risk management purposes, these human health consequences are valued in the same way as human health consequences resulting from air contaminants. For environmental damage, the situation is more complex. There is a substantial lack of data on the effects of a wide variety of chemicals on an even wider variety of organisms. Further, there is no accepted system for making environmental value judgments across different species.

Hazard Evaluation

Hazard evaluation, in this context, means estimation of the harm that might be done by a toxic release.[58] The preceding section discussed how to identify hazards and analyze the likelihood of release events. Based on this analysis, various release scenarios can be developed. This section discusses the methods used to estimate the consequences of a release. Basically, there are five steps: (1) scenario definition (part of hazard identification); (2) release rate amount and physical state estimation, (3) transport and dispersion modeling, (4) biological effects prediction, and (5) consequence estimation. Each of these steps is based on a combination of scientific theory, empirical data, and judgment. As a result, there is considerable uncertainty associated with the final conclusion(s).

Release Characteristics

In the preceding section a number of methods for identifying scenarios that could result in a disaster were discussed. These events would result in a release of a hazardous material. The release would have certain physical, chemical, and biological characteristics that need to be known or modified to predict the consequence of the events and thus develop appropriate mitigation in response plans. Specifically, some event will result in a loss of containment of a substance that will then be released at some rate for some time. The release may be a gas, a liquid, or a two-phase mixture. All of the characteristics of the release are taken into account in source models to predict the source terms that are inputs to various dispersion models.

Loss of containment is any event that allows substances normally contained in the tanks and piping of a facility to be released into the environment. In emergencies the concern is not so much about losses of containment that result in a slow release, such as the leaks that produce fugitive emissions (although these are important in the prevention of air pollution). The loss of containment events that produce disastrous releases are those capable of releasing large amounts of material or energy in a short time.

In general, properly designed, intact, undisturbed pipes and vessels do not spontaneously fail. Failure and release occur as a result of improper design, as in the case of the flexible coupling between reactors used at Flixborough[59], or because of some unintended event. Pipes may fail as a consequence of unintended stress brought on by weather or physical forces compounded by corrosion, fatigue, or embrittlement. Vessels fail in fires or because there is either too much or too little pressure. In the transportation of chemicals by road or rail, vehicle accidents can cause loss of containment. Storms, groundings, or collisions of tankers can cause the release of their cargoes.

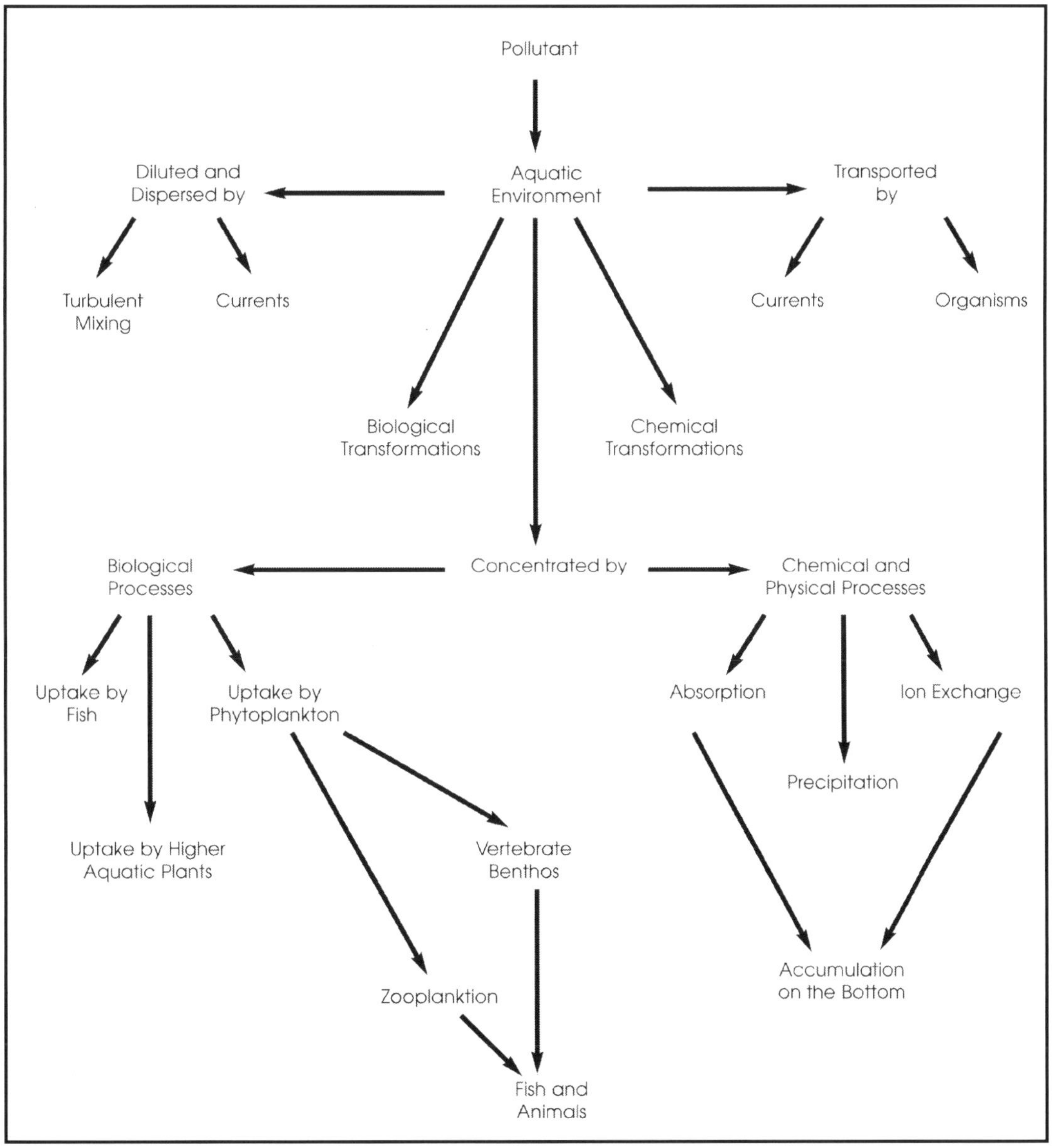

Figure 34.5 — Environmental distribution processes affecting pollution. (Source: Reference 46.)

The manner in which containment is lost will determine the release mechanism. Figure 34.6 illustrates several ways in which containment could be lost. The type and location of rupture and the phase, pressure, and temperature of the material determine the rate, period, and velocity of the release. The release could be a pressurized jet resulting in a momentum plume of gas or a rapidly expanding vapor cloud of a positively or negatively buoyant gas. Two-phase releases can be a mix of a gas and a bulk liquid that may subsequently evaporate or a liquid aerosol in a gas stream that is dispersed with or without complete evaporation.[60]

Loss of containment can also result in a spill of a substance in water, such as an oil spill, or on the ground where soil or groundwater contamination may be a problem unless appropriate remedial action is taken.

Depending on all of these factors, releases may be divided into four general time/area classes.[61]

(1) Continuous point release: a prolonged, small area release; a hole or broken pipe on a large vessel.
(2) Term point release: a brief period release from sudden and complete loss of a container of a gas. When the release duration is less than one-tenth of a minute, it is considered to be spontaneous or a "puff."
(3) Continuous area release: a prolonged release over some area, as from a spill of a volatile liquid on the ground or water.
(4) Term area release: a rapid release over some area, as from the evaporation of a pool of spilled refrigerated liquid.

Modeling of the source terms for a release requires knowledge of the class of release, the geometry of the release aperture and surroundings (contaminant wall, pond), the physical chemical properties of the material at the time of the release, and the

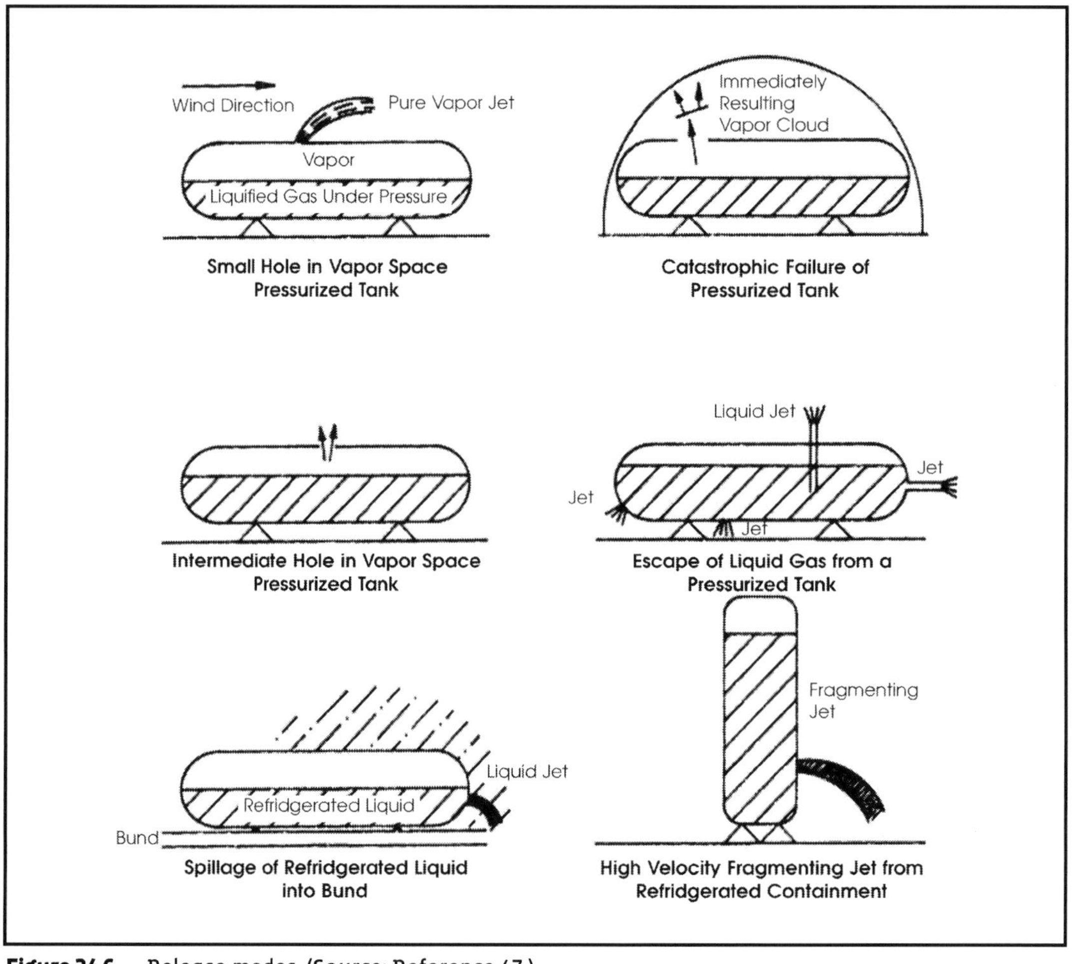

Figure 34.6 — Release modes. (Source: Reference 47.)

environmental conditions. All of these data are brought together as input to a source emission model, as shown in Figure 34.7.

A large number of models have been developed to estimate release rates and source terms as inputs to subsequent dispersion models. Release of a gas, liquid, or two-phase mixture from a hole in a pressurized container can be modeled from first principles and from fluid dynamics, assuming the size and shape of the hole.[62] For buoyant gases these models yield dispersion model input source terms directly. For heavy gases and liquids the situation is more complicated, and empirical models based on test data developed at Edgewood Arsenal and Thorney Island are used.[63] A number of evaporation models have been developed by the states, the U.S. government, and by other governments and private concerns. These models deal adequately with the most frequently expected accident conditions.

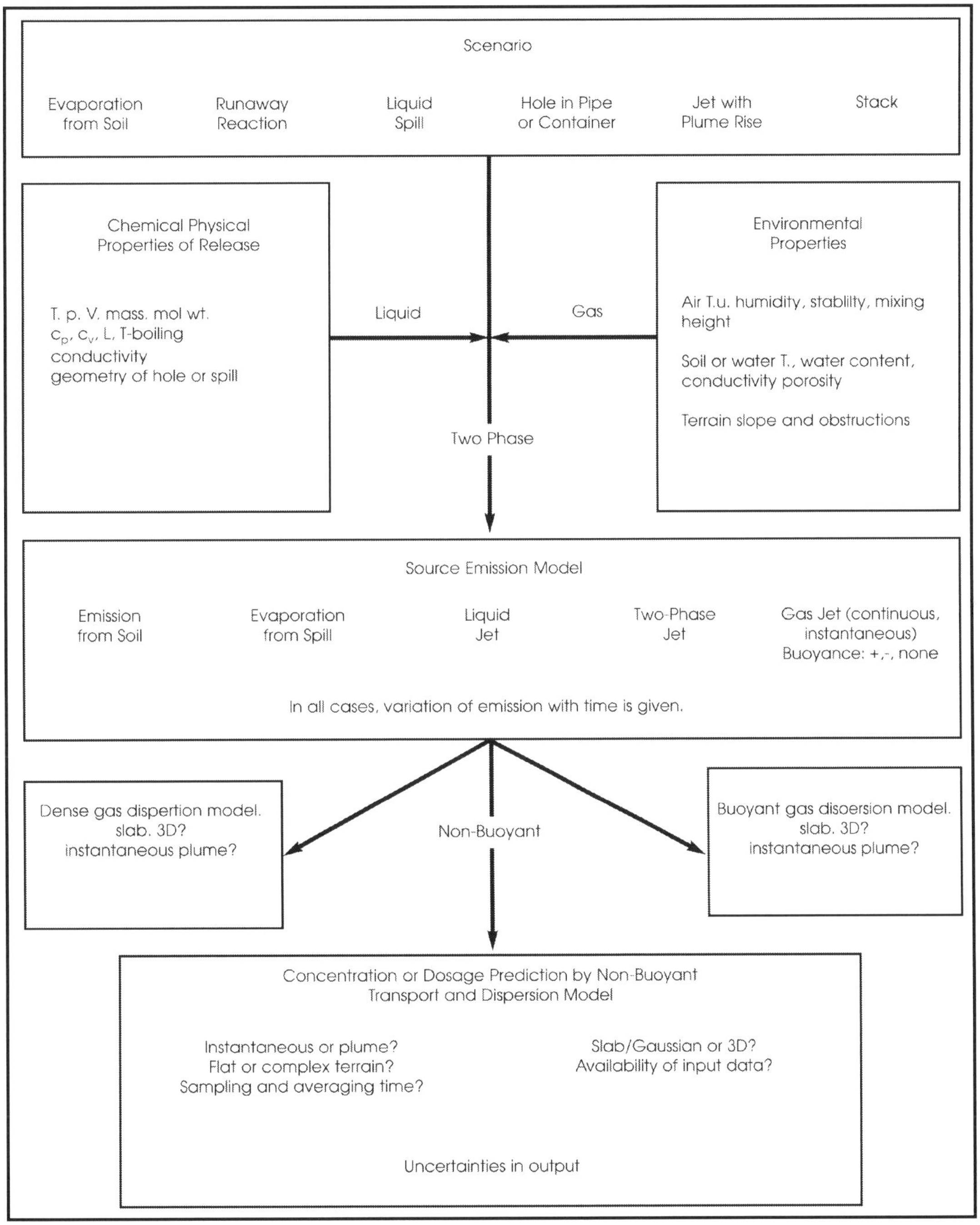

Figure 34.7 — Generalized vapor cloud model logic sequence. (Source: Reference 56.)

However, additional work is needed for such unique conditions as chemical reaction after release, evaporation of mixtures, vadose layer release, and terrain effects. Toxic releases resulting from fires are a special case of loss of containment. The release and subsequent ignition of a flammable liquid or gas can result in the formation of a toxic gas or aerosol that can then be dispersed. Release can be modeled as in the noncombustible gases, but the products of combustion are difficult to predict quantitatively, particularly when they vary with temperature and the availability of oxygen. Fires can also cause the destruction of toxic materials and can in those cases reduce the hazard to the general population. Another concern for fires in plants where radioactive materials are used for gauges, radiography, or other purposes is that the fire will destroy the radioactive material shielding and possibly disperse the material. This needs to be considered in facility design[64] and in disaster planning.

Dispersion Models

When a toxic substance is released into the atmosphere, it moves or spreads as carried by its own momentum, by gravity, and by the wind. This dispersion of the gas cloud will both dilute it and cause it to cover or involve a wider area. It is necessary to predict the concentration of the toxic substance that may occur at any location and time to predict the consequences to people and the protective measures necessary to avoid those consequences.[65–67] Although long-range transport of clouds may be best described by box or compartment models, the intermediate range (100–1000 m) movement of a toxic substance is usually dealt with by dispersion modeling.

Methods of modeling the dispersion of a release of gas in the atmosphere are based on the following premises.[19,59]

- The gas is not lost or losses are taken into account (conservation of matter).
- Through the action of turbulence in the atmosphere, the gas is distributed horizontally and vertically according to a Gaussian (normal) distribution, the parameters of which are a function of distance from the source.
- The parameters of the distribution are derived from experiments and are described by empirical equations.

These premises lead to the idealized Gaussian plume model for a continuous source shown in Figure 34.8. Because this is an idealized model, it has a number of limitations. The model is valid only for a continuous source over flat open ground. It assumes that meteorological conditions are constant in time and space, that there is some wind, and that the gas is the same density as air.

Hanna[68] noted that there were over 100 hazardous materials transport and dispersion models, that the number was growing at the rate of about 10 per year, and that only a few have been adequately evaluated with field data. He listed the characteristics of 40 of these (Table 34.5) and characterized the models in terms of the phenomena they treat. Four models are discussed here to illustrate the basic principles important for the transport and dispersion of hazardous gases.

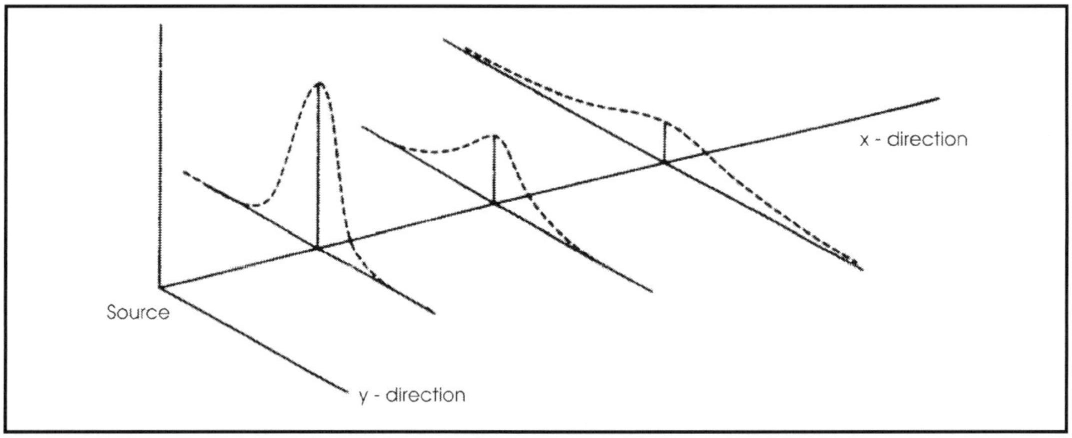

Figure 34.8 — Gaussian distribution. (Source: Reference 50.)

AIRTOX

The AIRTOX model for the release and dispersion of toxic air contaminants can account for single-phase denser-than-air releases. It is a hybrid model that incorporates various theoretical models, and it uses a slab model approach to calculate air dispersion. It assumes a pseudo-instantaneous dense gas cloud to calculate instantaneous sources. Continuous sources are also modeled, and the passive plume is assumed to disperse according to standard Gaussian formulas with a wind shear component. The model has been shown to compare fairly well with field data.

Table 34.5 — Models for Hazardous Gas Transport and Dispersion

Model	*Reference*[A]	*Instantaneous Puff*	*Continuous Plume*	*Dense Gas*	*Slab Similarity*	*Numerical (Grid)*	*Winds Vary*
AIRTOX	Paine et al. (1986)	X	X	X	X		
AVACTA II	Zannetti et al. (1986)	X	X		X		X
Britter	Britter (1979, 1980)		X	X	X		
CARE	Verholek (1986)	X	X	X	X		X
CHARM	Radian (1986); Balentine & Eltgroth (1985)	X	X	X	X	X	X
Chatwin	Chatwin (1983s)	X		X	X		X
CIGALE 2	Crabol et al. (1986)	X		X	X		
COBRA III	Oliverio et se. (1986)	X	X	X	X		
CRUNCH	Fryer (1980); Jagger (1983)		X	X	X		
3D-MERCURE	Riou & Saab (1985)	X	X	X		X	X
D2PC	Whitacre et al.	X	X		X		
DEGADIS	Havens & Spicer (1985)	X	X	X	X		
DENS20	Meroney (1984)	X	X	X	X		
DENZ	Fryer & Kaiser (1979)	X		X	X		
Fay & Zemba	Fay & Zemba (1985, 1986)	X	X	X	X		
FEM3	Chan (1983)	X	X	X		X	X
HAZARD	Drivas et al. (1983)	X	X	X	X	X	X
HEAVY GAS	Deaves (1985)	X	X	X		X	X
HEAVYPUFF	Jensen (1983)	X		X	X		
HEGADAS	Colenbrander & Puttock (1983)	X	X	X	X		
HEGDAS	Morrow		X	X	X		
Hoot et al.	Hoot et al. (1973)		X	X	X		
INPUFF 2.0	Peterson & Lavdas (1986)	X			X		X
MADICT	Ludwig (1985)	X			X	X	X
MESOPUFF 11	Scire and Lurmann (1983)	X			X		X
MIDAS	Woodward (1987)	X	X	X	X		X
NILU	Eidsvik (1980)	X		X	X		
Ooms et al.	Ooms et al. (1974)		X	X	X		
Port Comp. System	MOE (1983, 1986)	X	X	X	X		
RIMPUFF	Mikkelsen et al. (1984)	X	X		X		X
SAFEMODS	Raj (1981, 1986)	X	X	X	X		
SAFER	Personal correspondence	X	X	X	X	X	X
SIGMET	England et al. (1978)	X	X	X		X	X
SLAB	Morgan et al. (1983)	X	X	X	X		
SPILLS	Fleischer (1980)	X	X		X		
TOXGAS	McCready et al. (1986)	X			X		
Van Ulden	Van Ulden (1974)	X		X	X		
VAPID	Jensen (1983)	X	X	X	X		
Webber	Webber & Brighton (1986)	X		X	X		
Wilson	Wilson (1981)	X	X		X		
Zeman	Zeman (1982)	X	X	X	X		

Source: Reference 46.
[A]References refer to the source article (Hanna 1987).

DEGADIS

The dense gas dispersion (DEGADIS) model assumes that the crosswind distribution is uniform in the middle of the cloud and Gaussian at the edges, and that the vertical distribution follows a modified power law. The model deals with the dilution of a dense gas cloud by entrainment as the cloud moves under the influence of wind and gravity. It can calculate the initial cloud behavior near its source (the source blanket) and can simulate both steady-state and transient spills. Transient spills are modeled as a series of pseudo steady-state releases with a coordinate system that moves with the wind over the transient gas source. This moving observer concept and the source blanket concept are unique to DEGADIS, but there are several aspects of the model that need further evaluation.

FEM3

The FEM3 model is representative of three-dimensional models. Although simpler two-dimensional models provide great insight into the physical processes important for the transport and dispersion of hazardous gases and agree fairly well with the limited databases, the physical event is three-dimensional; therefore, two-dimensional models cannot model much of what is happening. FEM3, like most three-dimensional models, is extremely complex, and its computer code requires a long time to execute even on a supercomputer. Yet, as complex as it is, it is necessary to neglect certain processes, such as interphase heat exchange, to keep the run time within reason. Obviously, FEM3 is not suitable for real-time simulations. Its best application is as a means of understanding what is happening.

INPUFF 2.0

The INPUFF model is typical of a group of puff trajectory models for nondense emissions. The model cannot deal with the negative buoyancy of a dense gas cloud close to the source. It can model plume rise from positively buoyant plumes using standard formulas found in EPA UNAMAP models. INPUFF uses a Gaussian puff to calculate the distribution of concentrations in each puff. Dispersion coefficients are based on extensive experimental evidence, and the rate of dispersion can change with time. Multiple sources can be handled by summing the contribution from individual puffs at the receptor.

Model Uncertainty

Uncertainty in model predictions is an important consideration when models are used to predict the consequences of toxic chemical releases. The causes of uncertainty can be divided into three components.

Model Assumptions. As noted above in the discussion of FEM3, all models that attempt to approximate reality can take a very long time to run on a supercomputer; consequently, useful models contain some simplifying assumptions and therefore are only approximations of reality. How much error these assumptions introduce depends on how far they are from true and how robust the model is. One reason there are so many models is that each model is a better or worse fit of an event to be modeled. Therefore, it is incumbent on the risk assessor to select the best model for the release scenario.

Input Errors. All models require the input of values for certain parameters that describe the physical, chemical, and meteorological conditions. These input parameters may not be single fixed values but may be variables that are functions of time and space. Often, they are not well known and must be approximated or assumed, which introduces error. There is a trade-off between model accuracy and input error. The more realistic the model, the greater the number of less accurately known input parameters it will require. At some point short of maximum possible reality, an optimum combination of model detail and input error results in minimum overall error. When models are used for planning purposes to predict the consequences of a hypothetical future event, it is of course necessary to assume all of the input parameters. Often, worst-case assumptions are made so that the predicted consequence will be conservative. Unfortunately, the selection of a series of worst-case values for the input parameters can result in an excessive but unknown degree of conservatism.

Random Error. Turbulence of a fluid is an inherently chaotic process and thus cannot be usefully predicted. This stochastic uncertainty is dealt with as a random variable with a variance roughly equal to the square of the mean of the predicted concentration. It is usually the smallest of the three components of error.

Validation

Comparing predicted results with actual data from field tests validates models.[69,70] The number of models has increased much more rapidly than the quantity of field-test data, so most models are not validated. When a complex model is validated using a carefully assembled mass of accurate input data, the agreement between predicted and actual can be quite good (less than a factor of two difference). When assumptions are substituted for data, the agreement is not as good, and the best that can be said is that the predicted concentration is not inconsistent with the actual concentration given the anticipated level of error. In general, models that predict long-term averages are more accurate than dynamic models of instantaneous concentrations, because errors in parameters tend to be averaged out.

Biological Effect Prediction

The modeling technology and techniques described in previous paragraphs can predict with some error the concentration time pattern of the released chemical as it moves out from a point or area of release. People at locations where this cloud passes may be exposed and as a result may suffer adverse effects. The exposure may be by inhalation or by skin contact with or without absorption through the skin. The degree of adverse effect depends on the dose, which in turn depends on the concentration and duration of the exposure and on whether the person is out of doors, in a car, or inside a house.

The prediction of the effects of exposure is a classic question of toxicology. When little information is available on the toxicity of the chemical or only gross estimates of exposure concentrations are available, it may be adequate to classify chemicals according to relative toxicity using some estimate such as the median lethal dose (LD_{50}). A number of such schemes are shown in Table 34.6. The LD_{50} is the dose at which half of the animals in an experiment would be expected to die as a result of a short-term exposure. It is a common reference point for acute toxicity and may be the only data point available for some less common chemicals. In some cases the best adverse effects prediction that can be done will be based on a judgment of concentration from the amount released and some simple box model applied to a lethality class for the chemical to arrive at a consequence prediction suitable for emergency response.

Table 34.6 — Classification Systems for Acute Toxicity

Textbook (Hodge & Sterner)	*Industrial Chemicals (EEC)*	*Poison Law (Japan)*	*Pesticide Act (US)*	*Transport of Goods (United Nations)*	*Pesticide (WHO)*
Extremely toxic (< 1)	very toxic (< 25)	designated poison (< 15)	category I (< 50)	group I (< 5)	extremely hazardous < 5
Highly toxic (> 1–50)	toxic (< 25–200)	poisonous (< 30)	category II (< 5-500)	group II (< 5-50)	highly hazardous (> 5–50)
Moderately toxic (> 50–500)	harmful (< 200–2000)	deleterious substance (< 300)	category III (> 500–5000)	group III solids (> 50–500)	moderately hazardous (> 50–500)
Slightly toxic (> 500–5000)			category IV (> 5000)	liquids (> 50–2000)	slightly hazardous (> 500)
Practically nontoxic (> 5000–15,000)					
Relatively harmless (> 15,000)					

Note: Based on LD_{50} (mg/kg body weight)
Source: Institution of Chemical Engineers (ICE). Risk Analysis in the Process Industries. (Pub. series 45). London: ICE, 1985.

The time-concentration relationship to adverse effect may be divided into three domains. At the most distant fringe of the area touched by the cloud the concentration may be below an actual or practical biological threshold such that no effect occurs regardless of the duration of the exposure. In this region, effect is predicted by whether the concentration alone is over or under some threshold. Closer in, where the concentration is somewhat higher, the effect may depend on the product of the time and the concentration. Still closer to the source, where the concentration is highest, and the adverse effects of some substances such as chlorine or ammonia[71] may include death, the adverse effect is best predicted by the square of the concentration times the time. This more complex biological behavior, which occurs in the zone of exposure of greatest concern in disasters, requires that both the modeling and the effects prediction guidelines include a time component.

A simple way of relating exposure concentration-time-effect is shown in Table 34.7. This table divides the exposure concentration ranges into hazard bands and gives some indication of the proportion of people affected (e.g., lethal for 50%). This type of data presentation based on direct human experience is only possible for a few chemicals such as chlorine. For most chemicals only animal data are available; therefore, some process of extrapolation must be used, and only the most serious end points are estimated.

Various organizations have set emergency exposure limits or guidelines for use in hazard evaluation, remediation, and emergency response planning. To be useful, such guidelines should be developed both for substances for which human experience is known and for those for which only animal data are available. They should have uniform effect criteria (e.g., threshold of lethality) and should specify the exposure duration. It is also helpful if a process of consensus among experienced scientists sets the guidelines so they have broad credibility.

The Committee on Toxicology of the National Research Council set out to develop emergency exposure limits in the early 1960s. These levels, later called Emergency Exposure Guidance Levels (EEGLs) were defined as

> *a ceiling limit for an unpredicted single exposure, usually lasting 60 minutes or less and never more than 24 hours, whose occurrence is expected to be rare in the lifetime of any person. It reflects an acceptance of the statistical likelihood of the occurrence of a non-incapacitating, reversible effect in an exposed population. It is designed to avoid substantial decrements in performance during emergencies and might contain no uncertainty factor.*[72]

The National Research Council's (NRC's) EEGL effort was sponsored by the military, and the exposed population was healthy

Table 34.7 — Hazardous Bands for Chlorine Gas

Hazard Band	*Exposure (ppm)*	*Effect*
Distress (3–15 ppm)	3–6	Causes stinging or burning sensation but tolerated without undue ill effect for up to 1 hour
	10	Exposure for less than 1 min causes coughing
Danger (15–150 ppm)	10–20	Dangerous for 1/2–1 hour exposure Immediate irritation to eyes, nose, and throat, with cough and lachrymation
	100–150	5–10 min exposure fatal for some vulnerable victims
Fatal (> 150 ppm)	300–400	A predicted average lethal concentration for 50% of active healthy people for 30 min exposure
	1000	Fatal after brief exposure (few breaths)

Source: Reference 53.

adults. Recognizing that the EEGLs were not applicable to the general population, the NRC introduced the concept of Short-Term Public Emergency Guidance Levels. These guidelines are intended for public emergencies, but the NRC has recommended few of them.

During the 1970s NIOSH developed a set of IDLH exposure levels as part of an effort known as the Standards Completion Program. The concept and the term "IDLH" came from respiratory protection regulations that made a distinction between respiratory protection devices that are suitable for life-threatening environments and those that are not. The IDLHs were occupational exposure levels based on a 30-min exposure time. Because they were never intended as general public exposure limits, and because some of them were set by simply taking 100 times the TLV in effect at the time, they are not suitable as community emergency guidelines.

Increased concern over accidental chemical releases following the Bhopal disaster prompted AIHA® to establish the Emergency Response Planning Committee. This committee was charged with the development of a set of levels that could be used as boundaries between different degrees of an emergency. They are not recommended exposure levels in any sense, because the existence of exposure over any of them is an unwanted event. As indicated by the name, they are intended for response planning purposes but are also useful in prioritizing disaster prevention measures. They are developed according to a protocol initially developed by the Organizational Resource Counselors and are defined as follows.(73)

Emergency Response Planning Guideline 3 (ERPG-3) is the maximum airborne concentration below which it is believed that nearly all individuals could be exposed for up to 1 hour without experiencing or developing life-threatening health effects. The ERPG-3 level is a worst-case planning level above which there is the possibility that some members of the community may develop life-threatening health effects. This guidance level could be used to determine whether a potentially releasable quantity of a chemical could reach this level in the community, thus demonstrating the need for steps to mitigate the potential for such a release.

ERPG-2 is defined as the "maximum airborne concentration below which it is believed that nearly all individuals could be exposed for up to one hour without experiencing or developing irreversible or other serious health effects or symptoms which could impair an individual's ability to take protective action."(73) Above ERPG-2, for some members of the community, there may be significant adverse health effects or symptoms that could impair an individual's ability to take protective action. These symptoms might include severe eye or respiratory irritation or muscular weakness.

ERPG-1 is defined as the "maximum airborne concentration below which it is believed that nearly all individuals could be exposed for up to one hour without experiencing other than mild, transient adverse health effects or without perceiving a clearly defined objectionable odor."(73) ERPG-1 identifies a level that does not pose a health risk to the community but that may be noticeable due to slight odor or mild irritation. In the event that a small, nonthreatening release has occurred, the community could be notified that they might notice an odor or slight irritation, but that concentrations are below those that could cause health effects. For some materials, because of their properties, there may not be an ERPG-1. Such cases would include substances for which sensory perception levels are higher than the ERPG-2 level. In such cases no ERPG-1 level would be recommended.

Human experience takes precedence in developing ERPGs™, but they can also be developed from animal data. The documentation recognizes that human response is not precise, and that there are uncertainties in the data on which the limits are based. Although limits could be set for a range of exposure times, the committee chose the single time of 1 hour based on the available toxicology information and typical exposure scenarios.

Guidance on acutely hazardous chemicals has also been provided by other organizations. The World Bank and the European Economic Community have used Lethal Concentration for 50% (LC_{50}) to arrive at acutely hazardous quantities rather than concentrations.(74) The National Fire Protection Association (NFPA) has developed a health hazard rating scale for use by emergency service personnel. The U.K. Health and Safety Executive sets specified level of toxicity exposure concentrations as an aid in calculating individual risk from major hazards.(75)

Finally, the Clean Air Act Amendments of 1990 required EPA to promulgate an initial list of 100 substances that, in the case of an accidental release, are known to cause death, injury, or serious adverse effects to the environment, and to set threshold quantities for these substances. This list includes chlorine; ammonia; methyl chloride; ethylene oxide; vinyl chloride; methyl isocyanate; hydrogen cyanide; hydrogen sulfide; toluene diisocyanate; phosgene; bromine; hydrogen chloride; hydrogen fluoride; sulfur dioxide; and sulfur trioxide. The threshold quantities are based on the toxicity, reactivity, volatility, dispersibility, combustibility, or flammability of the substance.

Integrated Systems

The risk manager needs to have the whole risk assessment process summarized so that prevention and response options will be clear. The crisis center director needs a system that takes all the available data on the conditions and circumstances at the time of a release and predicts the consequences fast enough and clearly enough for proper response decisions to be made. A number of integrated risk assessment systems have been developed for these purposes.

Manual Systems. The few most likely scenarios can be modeled for several weather conditions or a worst-case set of conditions. The predicted concentration time patterns can be plotted as isopleths at the ERPG or other effect boundary concentrations. These plots can be on separate pages for different wind directions or as movable transparent overlays that can be oriented on a map for the site of release and the current wind direction. These consequence prediction systems have the advantage of being easy to understand and use and do not depend on the availability of a computer and a source of electricity. They have the disadvantage of being very approximate and of covering only a limited number of possibilities. For these reasons a number of rather sophisticated computer systems have been developed; but even when a computer-based integrated risk assessment system is used, it is prudent to have a manual backup available.

Computer Systems. Several integrated risk assessment commercial computer programs have been developed (Table 34.8). Although the capabilities of the various systems are different, and newer versions generally add capabilities, the following attributes are found in at least one system.

- Accepts substance, circumstance, and meteorology input
- Provides substance hazard data
- Includes source term/initial dispersion modeling
- Does air dispersion modeling
- Provides models for site-specific terrain
- Analyzes sensor data
- Provides a real-time graphical display
- Assesses risk

Computer systems have been used for risk assessment, planning, training, drills, accident critiques, and response to emergencies. Although the systems are capable of real-time operation, they are most commonly used to provide simulations for planning and training purposes.

Risk Reduction

The material presented in preceding paragraphs describes systems that allow the prediction of the likelihood and consequence of various chemical releases of various event scenarios. These predictions can be made for either an existing plant or a projected new plant during the design phase. Given the uncertainties of the modeling and estimation methods used, qualitative descriptions of probability and consequence are usually appropriate. Thus, the probability varies from frequent (meaning likely to occur repeatedly) to very unlikely (meaning not likely to occur in hundreds or thousands of years). The consequences range from minor odor or discomfort events to very serious events that may cause multiple deaths. These probability consequence combinations for each release scenario can be displayed on a graph or matrix that can serve as a graphical aid to mitigation priority setting. Obviously, an event that is predicted to

Table 34.8 — Integrated Risk Assessment Computer Systems

System	*Source*
CARE	Environmental Systems Corp.
CAMEO	National Safety Council
EPI Code	Homann Associates, Inc.
HASTE	Environmental Research and Technology Inc.
SAFER	SAFER Emergency Systems, Inc.

occur frequently with very serious consequences is an unacceptable situation, and a design or operation that results in such a prediction must be modified to reduce the risk before proceeding. For existing facilities, probabilities are more likely to be infrequent and consequences moderate. Mitigation effort priorities in this zone may be set based on a judgmental estimate of the degree of unacceptability of each probability consequence combination. At some low probability/low consequence point, it will be decided based on criteria derived either from policy or law that nothing further needs to be done. This scheme for deciding whether something needs to be done leads logically to consideration of the mitigation options available.[76,77]

Intrinsic Safety

Case histories of incidents have shown that some plants tend to be intrinsically safe. Kletz[59] analyzed plant safety in terms of attributes that make the plant "friendly," or forgiving of error. These plants are designed so that departures from normal tend to be self-correcting or at most lead to minor events rather than major disasters. Plants designed to be forgiving and self-correcting are inherently safer than plants where equipment has been added to control hazards or where operators are expected to control them. Some characteristics of friendly plants are as follows.

- Low inventory: smaller equipment and vessels and less intermediate product in storage means less hazardous material on site.
- Substitution: hazardous materials can sometimes be replaced with less hazardous materials.
- Attenuation: if hazardous materials must be handled, they can be used in their least hazardous forms.
- Simplification: operators are less likely to make mistakes if the plant and its instrumentation are easy to understand.
- Domino effects: an event should self-terminate rather than initiating other events.
- Incorrect assembly impossible: equipment design can make assembly mistakes impossible.
- Obvious status: an operator should be able to look at a piece of equipment and know if it is correctly installed or if a valve is open or shut.
- Tolerance: small mistakes need not create big problems.
- Low leak rates: leaks should be small and easy to control.

The application of these principles is summarized in Table 34.9.

Extrinsic Safety

Friendly plants as described by Kletz are designed to avoid major problems, and this approach to plant safety should be taken whenever possible. When it is not, external features of the plant should be arranged to minimize the undesirable consequences of a release. The most obvious means of reducing the exposure of community populations is to locate high-hazard facilities remote from communities. In general, siting is a major design consideration both within a facility and in the relation of the facility to population centers. LeVine[78] provides some guidelines for the layout of plants storing highly toxic hazardous materials (HTHM).

High-integrity storage tank design is essential for HTHM. Consideration should be given to overdesign or the use of double integrity storage tanks, for example, with a concrete outer tank or berm.

If the liquid storage tank for HTHM is diked, it is good practice that the same dike does not contain inventories of other materials that are flammable, reactive, or incompatible with the HTHM. If located next to a diked area containing flammable and/or reactive chemicals, the toxic storage may have to be provided with fixed fire protection for cooling. Factors to be considered include drainage in the diked areas, response time, adequacy of the site fire brigade or public fire department that would respond, and the flammability and reactivity of the nearby materials. The impounding area should be designed to minimize the vaporization rate of volatile HTHM. Installed means of evaporation suppression should be considered (e.g., foam).

HTHM should not be stored in proximity to explosive/flammable/reactive materials that might affect the storage tank. Diking for materials that are flammable or reactive should be sloped or drained to carry spilled material to a separate impoundment tank or area and away from any nearby HTHM tank.

Table 34.9 — Characteristics of Friendly Plants

Characteristic	*Examples* *Friendliness*	*Hostility*
Low inventory		
Heat transfer	miniaturized	large
Intermediate storage	small or nil	large
Reaction	vapor phase	liquid phase
	tubular reactor	pot reactor
Substitution		
Heat transfer	media nonflammable	flammable
Solvents	nonflammable	flammable
Carbaryl production	Israeli process	Bhopal process
Attenuation		
Liquefied gases	refrigerated	under pressure
Explosive powders	slurried	dry
Runaway reactants	diluted	neat
Any material	vapor	liquid
Simplification		
	hazards avoided	hazards controlled by added equipment
	single stream	multistream with many crossovers
	dedicated plant	multipurpose plant
	one big plant	many small plants
Domino Effects		
	open construction	closed buildings
	fire breaks	no fire breaks
Tank roof	weak seam	strong seam
Horizontal cylinder	pointing away from other equipment	pointing at other equipment
Incorrect assembly impossible		
Compressor valves	noninterchangeable	interchangeable
Device for adding water to oil	cannot point upstream	can point upstream
Obvious status	rising spindle valve or ball valve with fixed handle	nonrising spindle valve
	figure-8 plate	spade
Tolerant of maloperation or poor maintenance	continuous plant	batch plant
	spiral-wound gasket	fiber gasket
	expansion loop	bellows
	fixed pipe	hose
	articulated arm	hose
	bolted arm	quick-release coupling
	metal	glass, plastic
Low leak rate		
	spiral-wound gasket	fiber gasket
	tubular reactor	pot reactor
	vapor phase reactor	liquid phase reactor

Source: Adapted from Reference 47.

For HTHM the impoundment system should be designed to minimize the surface area and move material away from other hazard areas.

The concept and design of a designated dump tank should be investigated at the earliest stages of site layout. Depending on the potential hazard and the time required to empty the HTHM storage tank, it may be desirable to keep some storage vessels empty or at low levels for such emergency transfers. The possible need to empty a leaking tank is one important reason for providing a submerged pump or other transfer method.

The momentum of the tank contents might overflow a traditionally designed dike wall if the tank were to burst. A dike wall of about one-half tank height is required for containment of this scenario. Full-height, close-in dikes or berms have been provided for some cryogenic ammonia (and liquefied natural gas) storage tanks. The dike must be sized to contain at least the volume of the largest tank within the dike.

In case all means of containment fail, releases should be controlled through safety valves or other pressure relief systems and directed by vent headers to a safe release point or to an emergency relief treatment system. These end-of-pipe systems act as release countermeasures by means of secondary containment or by destroying the released materials. They include scrubbers, flares, incinerators, absorbers, condensers, and any other device placed in the vent stream to prevent release to the atmosphere. Even when release to the atmosphere has occurred, some mitigation is possible by means of such vapor release countermeasures as water sprays or curtains, steam or air curtains, or deliberate ignition.

The operation of secondary containment and vapor release countermeasures are triggered by some release warning system. This warning may come from observation of process parameters as displayed in the control room; from the detection of odor or the sighting of a cloud of smoke, fume, or colored gas; or from a signal from an installed vapor detection sensor. The early warning that can be provided by an installed detection system can trigger a quick response that may prevent most or all of a release. The detectors sense and measure gases and vapors by combustion, catalytic, electrochemical, and solid-state devices. They may alarm locally or remotely in the control room or be part of a network connected to a computer that analyzes the information from a number of locations and presents the results in a way that highlights response options. For early warning vapor detection systems to be useful tools they must be reliable and well maintained. Also, they must be specific enough for the chemical of concern and sufficiently sensitive to differentiate between routine releases (fugitives) and emergencies.

Human Factors

The best-designed plant can fail if improperly operated. Case histories of plant disasters[79,80] have shown that human error was often involved in the chain of events that led to the outcome. At Three Mile Island it was a persistent misunderstanding by the operators of the status of the cooling system that led them to overriding of automatic safety systems.

The possibility of human error cannot be eliminated, so plants should be designed to be forgiving of operator mistakes. Operator training and motivation can substantially reduce human error. OSHA has listed operating procedures necessary to control plants that handle highly hazardous chemicals.[2] These operating procedures should be detailed in readily available operating manuals that are kept evergreen as plant equipment or procedures change. Operators should be thoroughly trained in the operating procedures before they assume responsibility for plant operations, and supplemental and refresher training should be provided as needed-typically annually. Some form of testing or qualification should be set up to ensure that each operator has learned the procedures. Periodically, management should compare prescribed and actual operating procedures. When there are differences, they should be analyzed to determine whether it is because of an employee lapse or because the written procedures are impractical or could be improved.

Contractors present a special concern in the control of human factors related to chemical releases. Teams of contractor employees often work on site under the supervision of their own company with only indirect control by the site owner. The training of contractor employees is the responsibility of the contractor and is complicated by relatively high turnover in some jobs. When contractors hire skilled trades from a hiring hall, the contractor may not know who will be working on a job until the day of the assignment. Even when all of a contractor's regular employees are trained and aware of safe operating procedures, the contractor may subcontract specific tasks and thus bring on site people who are not trained and aware. Frequently, there are multiple contractors on a site doing jobs that may affect each other's safety. Some major disasters appear to be related to a lack of a clear division of responsibilities and close coordination between the owner and the several contractors.[59,81] Although the legal consequences of owner-contractor interaction complicate the matter, at least one jurisdiction has stated that "where . . . a special risk is likely to arise due to the nature of the work performed (and the owner of the premises has special knowledge of it), the owner must retain sufficient control of the operator to ensure that contractors' employees are properly protected against the risk."[75] In the United States an owner has the responsibility under OSHA to ensure that the contractor is informed of hazards and that the contractors' employees are trained.

A typical program addressing the contractor issue might include the following.

- The contract must include the site safety and health manual and the operating procedures to be followed.
- The contractor must attend a work review before the job starts, at which specifications, safety, process hazards, and employee training is detailed.
- The contractor must be provided with MSDSs for all hazardous materials to be encountered.
- The contractor must train his or her employees and provide the owner with a list of trained employees. The contractor must understand that only trained employees will be admitted to the site.
- The contractor must obtain any necessary work permits (hot work, confined space entry) before starting such work.
- The contractor must keep accident records and inform the owner of any accidents.
- The contractor is subject to safety reviews and inspections.
- Any violation of safety rules can be cause for termination of the contract.

The above list is not intended to cover all requirements and may not fully apply to certain contractors who have little involvement with hazardous processes, but it gives an example of the level of interaction some owners have found necessary to ensure adequate control of contractors.

Planning and Response

Even when all reasonable measures to prevent a chemical release have been taken, the risk or probability of a release occurring is not zero. A prudent management practice, therefore, is to anticipate that an emergency may occur eventually and to plan for it. A well-developed and implemented emergency plan can minimize loss and help protect people, property, and the environment. To accomplish this requires planned procedures, clearly understood responsibilities, designated and accepted authority and accountability, and trained and drilled people. When an emergency occurs, it will be too late to plan, so it must be done ahead of time based on the kinds of emergencies that might occur.[49,82–84]

Scope

An emergency response plan must be tailored to fit the facility, community, and the types of emergencies that can occur.[85] Michael[86] divided emergency response functions to consider in planning into the following five categories: (1) accident assessment, which includes detecting abnormal conditions, assessing the potential consequences, and immediately taking appropriate measures to mitigate the situation; (2) notification and communication, which includes the physical and administrative means whereby plant operators can rapidly notify plant management, off-site emergency response agencies, and the public; (3) the command and coordination function, which clearly establishes who is in charge of the emergency response in the plant and in off-site communities; (4) protective actions, which are those taken to protect the health and safety of plant personnel and the public, such as release mitigation, sheltering, and evacuation; and (5) support actions, include fire fighting, emergency medical care, social services, and law enforcement.

Plan evaluators should expect to find the attributes listed in Table 34.10 considered in the plan.[87] Not all of these attributes will be required in every plan, but it is useful to consider all of them to ensure that the plan is complete.

Planning Process

Successful planning requires the cooperation and support of all involved. For this reason, planning should be under the direction and overview of a committee that includes those groups with a significant interest or stake in the successful implementation of the plan in the event of an emergency. The CAER program developed by CMA recognizes the importance of community involvement and seeks to achieve two goals:[83] (1) development of a community outreach program and means to provide the public with information on chemicals manufactured or used at local chemical plants; and (2) improvement of local emergency response planning by combining chemical plant emergency plans with other local planning to achieve an integrated community emergency response plan.

In the United States, SARA established LEPCs for each planning district. These committees facilitate the preparation and implementation of emergency plans and must include representatives from key public and private groups or organizations.

Regardless of the composition of the planning committee, it must have a commitment to work together on a common goal to be successful. The group must have the ability, authority, and resources to do the job. It must have access to all the industrial, community, transportation, and planning skills needed. Most important, the group must agree on its purpose and be able to work together cooperatively.

Health Planning Considerations

The planning process proceeds through various situations and contingency and resource assessment steps to arrive at a set of options that is incorporated into a plan that can be tested and refined. Each of the members of the planning committee has special considerations to input to the planning process. Facility medical and occupational hygiene members of the planning committee have specialized considerations involving casualty handling, exposure assessment, and external communications.

Table 34.10 — Plan Evaluation Attributes

Scope and provenance
Emergency response organization
Emergency alarm
Operational communications
Control centers
Evacuation sheltering
Accounting for people
First aid
Transportation
Security
Fire fighting
Chemical release detection and mitigation
Community notification and information
Shutdown of operations
Continuity of utilities and services
Mutual (industry) aid organizations
Outside agency notification and coordination
Public affairs
Governmental relationships
Restoration to normal operations
Clean up and rehabilitation
Legal issues
Training
Drills
Detailed action plans and standard operating procedures
Critique and plan revision

Casualty Handling

Adequate provision must be made in the plan to ensure that optimum treatment is provided or made available for all individuals who experience either injury, illness, or psychological distress as a consequence of an emergency.[88,89] A well-developed plan for handling medical emergencies should be integrated into the facility emergency plan and, where appropriate, the local community plan.

Provisions for handling casualties vary significantly depending on such factors as the nature of the operation, associated hazards, size of the work force, and proximity to major hospital facilities. Staffing, training, equipment, facilities, and transportation needs must be considered in a comprehensive plan to minimize the effects of illness and injury resulting from an emergency.

It is unlikely that a plant will equip itself with staffing and facilities capable of definitively treating all illness or injury arising from a major incident. Appropriate use of outside specialized medical units is, in general, most likely to result in optimum clinical care for ill or injured employees. The proximity of these specialized facilities, which will determine the levels of initial treatment or stabilization required on site, can be described as follows.

(1) Patient can be delivered to a hospital within 10 min. Only triage, resuscitation, first aid treatment of serious injuries or illnesses, basic stabilization, and definitive treatment of minor casualties are needed on site.
(2) Patient can be delivered to a hospital within 60 min. Formal stabilization may be required and, in some cases, treatment may need to be initiated on site.
(3) Patient cannot be delivered to a hospital within 60 min. On-site facility must be equipped to provide more definitive treatment before patient is transferred.

Treatment Locations

Treatment for injuries may need to be provided at various locations. The casualty handling provisions of the medical plan need to identify these locations and the level of care available at each.

- Incident site: Because the casualty should be moved to a safe place of treatment at the earliest possible opportunity, only lifesaving procedures are normally conducted at the incident site.
- Site facility: This is the first medical unit where equipment and conditions are conducive to assessment, stabilization, and/or initial treatment of casualties.
- Safe facility: It may be necessary to designate a location outside the site for use if the incident or gas release requires evacuation of the site medical facility.
- Minor injury facility: In the event of multiple casualties with minor injuries, transfer to a local satellite center may be appropriate.
- General hospital: The usual location of surgical teams and facilities for continuing patient care.
- Specialized medical units: Definitive care centers for burns, plastic surgery, and neurosurgery are often available.

Transportation

It is unlikely that the site will be able to provide all the vehicles necessary to remove casualties to the hospital or even transport multiple casualties within the site. Arrangements should be made with external agencies to provide multiple ambulances and to move casualties in such a way that therapy can continue during transit. For rapid transport from remote sites consideration should be given to helicopter evacuation of casualties. Transport of equipment may be necessary in the event the site medical facility must be evacuated. Minor casualties can be discharged to home or to other treatment facilities by car or taxi. In all transport cases a fellow worker or supervisor should give consideration to providing escort.

Close liaison with the ambulance services must be maintained, and it is advisable that there should be a shared communications network. Accurate records of all patients in transit must be kept and the need for escorts taken into account when determining emergency response staffing. Signs to direct ambulances to the treatment center/triage area, escorts for ambulances on site, and police escorts for ambulances in the community may also be required.

Staffing

Staffing requirements for emergencies depend on the potential number of casualties from each credible event scenario and the probable nature and severity of the illnesses or injuries. The goal is to ensure that the sum of in-house and external staff is enough to deal with credible emergencies at each stage of the incident. Plans that maximize the likelihood of stabilizing and maintaining the patient until transfer can be affected must be developed. The proximity of specialized medical units and ease of transportation will influence these plans. Identification of appropriate external specialized medical units should be made on the basis of anticipated types of illness and injury. Staff must have an understanding of these facilities and their medical capabilities, and in turn the external medical units need to be made familiar with the operations and hazards at the facility. Both staff and the medical facilities also need to be equipped with adequate toxicity and treatment data on relevant materials.

In addition to trauma and burn specialists, consideration should be given to the provision of neurosurgeons for head and spinal injuries, plastic surgeons, and other physicians to handle patients affected by the inhalation of chemicals or combustion products. In the absence of ready availability of such medical specialists, consideration should be given to the training needs of site and community medical staff.

Equipment

Decisions on the appropriate level of emergency medical equipment also depend on the evaluation of the scenarios that may follow a major incident. The nature of the materials handled, anticipated injury or illness outcome, number of potential casualties, on-site staffing levels, and proximity to local hospitals and specialized medical units are factors to be considered.

Record Keeping

Adequate record keeping is essential in any clinical situation, and it is no less important when there may be a significant number of casualties arriving in a short space of time and being rapidly transferred for further treatment. Patients must, where possible, be adequately identified and records kept of their arrival and departure times at the treatment center, together with details of their clinical condition. This information is necessary to monitor the developing staffing requirements; control the flow of patients through the center; provide adequate information to hospitals of anticipated number and extent of injuries; provide transport groups with anticipated requirements; answer requests from distraught relatives; and provide management with an overview for internal and media information.

Exposure Assessment

A significant contribution to disaster response planning and execution can be made by the assessment of the magnitude and impact of exposures resulting from the release of chemicals into the environment or from the toxic products of fires. Exposure assessment may be defined as the estimation or measurement of the exposure of a population in terms of concentration and duration, evaluation of that exposure by comparison with health effects criteria, and estimation of the health consequences. This assessment should be made for both toxic chemical releases and for toxic decomposition products generated by fires. It may be needed for both on-site and off-site populations including rescue and emergency personnel. Effective emergency response requires that exposure for all involved populations be quickly and accurately assessed, interpreted, and communicated so that it can form a basis for management decision making.

The focus of emergency planning for toxic chemical release is on those releases that could cause serious acute effects or death. Other less serious releases can, however, have a major impact. Experience has shown that major odor incidents, although not harmful to health, can cause serious aggravation and hostility in local communities. Releases of chemicals that are chronic health hazards or carcinogens can also have serious consequences even when the release is barely detected by local communities and is of such short duration that no health effect is anticipated.

There are several distinct situations and purposes that may need either a predicted, contemporary, or retrospective assessment of exposure by either dispersion modeling or air contaminant concentration measurement.

Prevention. As discussed earlier, exposure patterns for various scenarios are predicted by dispersion modeling for the purpose of prioritizing risk reduction measures.

Emergency Action. In the event of a toxic release into a community, people may need to be advised to evacuate or button-up (seal themselves indoors) as appropriate.[90,91] Because this decision must be made quickly (usually in minutes), exposure assessment for all plausible scenarios is usually estimated in advance by modeling. Affected areas, predicted by map overlays or similar means, are typically communicated to local authorities that advise the public.

Declaring the Emergency Over. Exposure assessment is needed to decide when people can return to an affected area or "unbutton." Because the time constraints on the emergency decision no longer apply, and because modeling is not much use in predicting where pockets of gas may remain, actual measurement is often the best way to make the decision that it is safe to return.

Event Record. Documentation of the time course of exposure for various population segments can serve several purposes.

In the event of claims for injury, this record can be used to show where injurious concentrations did and did not occur. It is also useful as an aid to understanding any symptoms seen and as part of the critique of emergency prevention and response actions. This record is based on model predictions supplemented by measurements.

Public Reassurance. Releases of odorous or small quantities of toxic materials not requiring emergency action may still need exposure assessment for public reassurance. A public perception of harm can sometimes be as much of a problem as actual harm.

Emergency and rescue crews operating near a release automatically use self-contained breathing apparatus, so no measurement is needed at that time. At some distance away, contamination will be low enough so that other respirators could be used or that no respirators are needed. These areas could be better defined by measurements if necessary. For reentry and other post emergency purposes, the objective is to be sure that no pockets remain. A wide net of measurements that takes into account weather conditions is needed. Familiarity with the modeling results and the map overlay predictions will help decide where to measure. Measurement teams need to be provided with and trained in the use of personal protective equipment.[92]

The direct-reading instruments and detector tubes necessary for near-term measurements should be on hand before an emergency arises, and these instruments must be kept in a state of readiness. Batteries go dead and detector tubes expire. Long-term measurements may be made with sorbent tubes or filters sent to an outside laboratory for analysis. In some circumstances even gas bags may be useful. Supplies should be kept in reserve and a fast, accurate laboratory identified.

Because the measurement data collected may be needed later, careful records should be kept. A form that is easily completed by measurement crews working under the severe time constraints of the field would be useful.

Organizational Communication

Fast, reliable, accurate operational communication is the hallmark of a good emergency plan. It is also very difficult to achieve if left until an emergency actually occurs. Things happen so fast, and there are so many people who have or need information, that careful preparation, training, and discipline is needed for the communication system to work effectively.

Initial Notification. It is essential that there be early communication with the medical group concerning the occurrence of an emergency situation, even when there are no immediate casualties. This notice allows decisions to be made about appropriate short-term staffing requirements and the alerting of other agencies of the potential need for support.

Lines of Communication. The lines of flow for information and instruction are derived from the organization and command structure of the emergency response organization. Open communication channels are needed with the incident manager, transport organization, hospitals, and public relations manager. Reliable, redundant links are needed for information to flow out. Because the disaster organization is usually different from the routine organization, many of these communications links are not routinely staffed. It is necessary for response team members to get to their posts, report in, and test primary and backup communication systems as quickly as possible.

Communication Roles. Because members of the emergency response team may not be on site at the time of an emergency, it is necessary to assign responsibility for calling in medical/health personnel needed at the appropriate times. Names and telephone numbers should be kept up to date. Once the plan is in operation, it may be necessary to designate individuals whose only role is to ensure that all messages are immediately handled without tying up the communications network or distracting other people from their duties. Everyone who needs to communicate during an emergency needs to be trained and drilled in the operation of the equipment and in the strict communication discipline necessary to avoid system overload.

Critical operational communications often are to and from external resources (hospitals, ambulance services, fire departments, government offices, etc.); therefore, the external resources should be contacted in advance to determine their communication capabilities and expectations. Frequently, these organizations have backup systems of communication available that are not widely known. In the case of a natural disaster involving both the community and the plant, the external resources are also operating in an emergency mode and may not have the same resources and communications ability as in normal times.

Public Information. Serious incidents involving employee or public exposure to toxic chemicals are likely to receive intensive mass media coverage in many countries. Public concern over safety has increased, so it is important that the facts of an emergency are properly communicated to the media. For purposes of communication, an emergency can be divided into three time phases.

(1) Initial response: Because an emergency may occur at night or on a weekend, there could be an initial period (30 min to 1 hour) when no senior managers will be present. Decisions and communications during this phase must be planned.
(2) Management control: When senior managers and the designated spokesperson arrive (usually within an hour), decisions and communications can be matched more exactly to the situation and fixed planned procedures modified.
(3) Expert input: Within 8 to 24 hours of the emergency it should be possible to enlist outside experts to help with complex technical or scientific issues that may arise.

It is important that spokespersons be aware of the toxic hazards present on site and have access to information concerning their health effects. They should have at least MSDS-type information available. Some facilities have developed briefer, more focused fact sheets for emergency use. Health professionals should become involved in developing this communication reference material and in helping the designated spokesperson understand the data and be able to anticipate media questions. Particular attention needs to be given to technical terminology that may be unfamiliar to the spokesperson and to the media.

Drills

Realistic tests of plan execution are necessary to evaluate the plan, for preparations to implement the plan, and as a means of training.[93,94] Experience has shown that only the simplest of plans are likely to work the first time they are tested. Consequently, a facility should not assume that it is prepared to deal with an emergency unless the emergency response plan has been realistically exercised. Drills can be broad or specialized and can vary in depth of involvement of the facility and community. Some specific types of drills include the following.

- Tabletop: a step-by-step read-through of the emergency response plans by key controllers
- Notification test: an exercise for communication facilities, notification procedures, call-lists, and backups
- Organization test: covers assembly, team makeup, understanding responsibilities, and response time
- Rolling equipment test: involves emergency equipment call-up and movement, security and access, off-site responders, mobile communications
- Full-scale test: involves casualty simulation, off-site response, community involvement, and media

One test drill or another should test command and control, communications, casualty handling, mediation, and all other significant aspects of the plan. The drills should be carefully planned so that they are realistic within their scope. Drill evaluators should make observations and contribute later to the comprehensive critique. Drills often detect some common emergency response plan failures such as the following.

- Designated individuals who do not have the training, time, or resources to carry out their duties
- Delayed notification because of inadequate on-site authority at the time of the event
- Communications overloads that block access to local authorities
- Security breakdowns that inhibit access by responders and/or allow unauthorized access
- Difficult decisions (e.g., sacrifice property to avoid a toxic release) not being made quickly enough
- Incorrect casualty handling decisions being made because of confusion and inadequate communication among emergency crews, first responders, and hospitals

- Control rooms becoming isolated and providing inadequate protection
- Media/external communication needs interfering with operational communications
- Chemical exposure effects and treatment information not being communicated to the hospital that receives the chemical casualties
- Support function (transportation, utilities, etc.) responsibilities listed in site plan that are not reflected and detailed by function plans

The objective of drilling is to find these potential defects by realistic exercises so that the plan can be revised and training improved to maximize the likelihood that an actual emergency can be responded to without any critical errors.

Transportation Emergencies

Planning for successful response to chemical release emergencies that occur while a chemical is in transit involves some special considerations.[95–97] The first responders will not necessarily know what chemical is involved, and it may take some time at the critical early stage of the emergency to obtain that information. When the required information is on hand, it may be that special skills or equipment are needed to deal with the situation, so arrangements must be made to bring these to the scene. For these reasons, planning for transportation emergencies is more complex, and response often takes longer than for site emergencies.

The first item of information that may be available to firefighters, police, rescue workers, or other emergency services is the DOT placard on the side of the vehicle. A four-digit number on the placard or on an orange panel is the identification number for a material in the DOT guidebook.[98] This guidebook also provides a series of generic guides for each material that describe potential hazards and initial emergency actions.

The DOT identification number and the name of the material also is shown on the shipping papers that should be on the truck, train, ship, or aircraft. In the case of a tank truck the driver should also have a copy of the MSDS that gives more specific hazard, precaution, and emergency information for the material.

Additional information and assistance is available from the Chemical Transportation Emergency Center (CHEMTREC), a public service of CMA. CHEMTREC provides immediate advice by telephone and also contacts the shipper of the hazardous material for detailed assistance and appropriate response. CHEMTREC needs to know either the identification number or name of the material and the nature of the accident. CHEMTREC operates continuously and should be called as soon as immediate needs have been met and the facts ascertained.

Backing up CHEMTREC is another CMA service, the Chemical Emergency Network or CHEMNET. This network consists of about 240 response teams representing about 100 chemical companies. These CHEMNET teams can provide on-site experts to assist local emergency services with advice on the best way to handle a specific chemical accident. A similar network in Canada is called the Transportation Emergency Assistance Plan and is operated out of 11 regional response centers.

Summary

Sources of Information

The body of information and technology relating to the subject of this chapter is very large, far larger than could be covered in the space available. Consequently, this chapter does not attempt to instruct the reader on how to do the many tasks involved in disaster prevention and response planning. Instead, this chapter should be regarded as an overview of the subject that identifies the sources the reader may consult to expand on each detailed topic. Many of these sources are referenced in the text. In addition, there are some institutions that have a continuing involvement in this field and can be looked to for the latest information and technology.

DOT. The DOT Office of Hazardous Materials Transportation has developed an *Emergency Response Guidebook* (ERG) (DOT P 5800.4), which is a manual primarily for initial response to hazardous materials incidents that occur in the transport of hazardous materials. The ERG, which is updated periodically, gives the name of the material corresponding to the identification number displayed on the placard on the vehicle and listed on the shipping paper. Each identification/substance listing refers the user to a numbered guide that briefly describes potential hazards (fire, explosion, health hazards) and emergency action (fire fighting, dealing with spills or leaks, first aid). The ERG is a means of quickly providing critical information to first responders. The guide advises the responder to immediately contact CHEMTREC for additional assistance beyond the initial phase of the incident. In addition to the ERG, DOT is the lead agency in transportation safety research, guidance, and regulation.

NFPA. The NFPA is primarily concerned with fire protection and suppression systems but is also an authority on certain aspects of hazardous materials. Their *Fire Protection Guide on Hazardous Materials*(64) contains the complete texts of the four NFPA documents that classify most common hazardous materials: NFPA 325M: "Fire Hazard Properties of Flammable Liquids, Gases and Volatile Solids"; NFPA 49: "Hazardous Chemicals Data"; NFPA 491M: "Manual of Hazardous Chemical Reactions;" and NFPA 704: "Identification of the Fire Hazards of Materials." In addition to the full texts of *NFPA 49, NFPA 325, NFPA 491, and NFPA 704,* the guide also includes the following information.

- NFPA 497: parameters to determine the degree and extent of hazardous locations for liquids, gases, and vapors including NEC® groups
- NFPA 432: storage requirements, including organic peroxide classification and "diamond" ratings for 160 chemicals
- Data from NFPA 77: combustibility parameter and static electric characteristics
- NFPA 499: parameters to determine degree and extent of hazardous locations for dusts, including NEC groups
- NFPA 430: oxidizer classification for 90 chemicals

This consolidated guide includes information on fire and explosion hazards, life hazards, personal protection, fire fighting, and other facts needed to make informed decisions in an emergency.

American Institute of Chemical Engineers Center for Chemical Process Safety (CCPS). A number of manuals developed by CCPS(49,78,99,100) were used as a basis for this chapter. The CCPS and its committees maintain an awareness of the technology, and their handbooks reflect the state of the art.

CMA. The CMA CHEMTREC and CAER programs have been described above. These programs and other activities are the responsibility of CMA staff and committees who stay current on developments related to chemical emergencies. They are available to assist member chemical companies and the general public as appropriate.(19,87,101)

University of Delaware Disaster Research Center (DRC). This center provides a unique resource that "engages in a variety of sociological and social science research on group and organizational preparations for, responses to, and recovery from community-wide emergencies, particularly natural and technological disasters."(102,103) The DRC conducts studies, sends teams to disaster sites, and maintains a publication collection of over 20,000 items related to the social and behavioral aspects of disasters.

References. The list of publications at the end of this chapter contains a number of general and specialized references to the modern literature on this subject.

Future Trends

Presently proposed governmental regulations will require process hazard risk assessment for many facilities that have not done it in the past. Because of these regulations and as a consequence of expansion of the risk assessment field, the process will become more formal and detailed. New practitioners will enter the field, and it will be increasingly important for the facility manager to be sure of the qualifications of those who would provide this service. Some 5 or more years ahead, as the results of a number of risk assessments become known, it is probable that new regulations, at least in the United States, will establish expectations for the results of the risk assessment process and will try to define more precisely what risk is acceptable.

The technology of process hazard risk assessment, in addition to being more formal and detailed as mentioned above, is likely also to become more probabilistic. The analogy to health risk assessment that claims to calculate the likelihood of an adverse consequence will be persuasive.

The lack of credible input data (e.g., mean time to failure) will be partly relieved by expanded databases developed in the course of increased regulatory activity. A need will be seen for a measure of the actual or limiting probability on chemical releases of various magnitudes, so that there will be a number to compare with acceptable risk criteria or bright-lines. A challenge to all involved in process hazard analysis will be to try to ensure that the databases support the outcome both in quantity and quality. Further, it must be assured that the assumptions of independence of causes typically made are carefully considered, and that the consequences of multiple human errors be included in any analyses.

Community involvement in disaster prevention and response planning is already a fact in the United States and is likely to spread. In the future the public will expect to be even more involved and to participate in decision-making. As a consequence, some situations that were considered to constitute an acceptable level of risk will need to be revisited and new consensus criteria of acceptability applied. Risk assessors and the public will need to educate each other to achieve common understandings and expectations.

References

1. **Thygerson, A.L.:** *Accidents and Disasters: Causes and Countermeasures.* Englewood Cliffs, N.J.: Prentice-Hall, 1977.
2. "Process Safety Management of Highly Hazardous Chemicals." *Code of Federal Regulations* Title 29, Part 1910.119. 1992.
3. "Accidental Release Prevention Requirements." *Code of Federal Regulations* Title 40, Part 68. 1996.
4. **Concawe:** *Concawe Methodologies for Hazard Analysis and Risk Assessment in the Petroleum Refining and Storage Industry.* The Hague: Concawe, 1982.
5. **O'Reilly, J.T.:** *Emergency Response to Chemical Accidents. Planning and Coordinating Solutions.* New York: McGraw-Hill, 1987.
6. **Wilson, E.A.:** Selected annotated bibliography and guide to sources of information on planning for and response to chemical emergencies. *J. Haz. Mater. 4* (1981).
7. **Elkins, C.L., and J.L. Makris:** Emergency planning and community right-to-know. *J. Air. Pollut. Control Assoc. 38* (1988).
8. *Hazardous Materials Transportation Act. U.S. Code 49,* sec. 1801–1819 (1975).
9. *Natural Gas Pipeline Safety Act of 1968 as amended. U.S. Code 49,* sec. 1671–1686 (1968).
10. *Hazardous Liquid Pipeline Safety Act of 1979 as amended. U.S. Code 49,* sec. 2001–2014 (1979).
11. **Solomon, C.H.:** The Exxon chemicals method of identifying potential process hazards. *Inst. Chem. Eng. Loss Preven. Bull. 52* (1983).
12. **Department of Transportation (DOT):** *2000 Emergency Response Guidebook.* Washington, D.C.: DOT, 2000.
13. *Comprehensive Environmental Responses, Compensation and Liability Act of 1980. U.S. Code 42,* sec. 9601 et seq. (1980).
14. **DePol, D.R., and P.N. Cheremisinoff:** *Emergency Response to Hazardous Materials Incidents.* Lancaster, Pa.: Technomic Publishing, 1984.
15. **U.S. Environmental Protection Agency (EPA):** *Chemical Emergency Preparedness Program: Interim Guideline.* Washington, D.C.: EPA, 1985.
16. "Emergency Planning and Notification." *Code of Federal Regulations* Title 40, Part 355. 2002. pp. 440–445.
17. **Federal Emergency Management Agency (FEMA):** *Planning Guide and Checklist for Hazardous Materials Contingency Plan* (FEMA-10). Washington, D.C.: U.S. Government Printing Office, 1981.
18. *Superfund Amendments and Reauthorization Act of 1986. U.S. Code 42,* sec. 11001 et seq. (1986).
19. **Chemical Manufacturers Association (CMA):** *Community Awareness and Emergency Response Program Handbook.* Washington, D.C.: CMA, 1985.
20. **Organization Resources Counselors (ORC):** *Recommendations for Process Hazards Management of Substance with Catastrophic Potential.* Washington, D.C.: ORC, 1988.
21. "List of Regulated Substances and Thresholds for Accidental Release Prevention." *Code of Federal Regulations* Title 40, Part 68.130. 1999.
22. **U.S. Chemical Safety and Hazard Investigation Board (CSB):** *Chemical Accident Investigation Report, Tosco Avon Refinery, Martinez, California.* Washington, D.C.: CSB, 1998.
23. **U.S. Chemical Safety and Hazard Investigation Board (CSB):** *Management of Change* (No. 2001-04-SB). Washington, D.C.: CSB, 2001.
24. **Federal Emergency Management Agency (FEMA):** *National Environmental Policy Act: FEMA Desk Reference.* Washington, D.C.: FEMA, 1996.

25. **European Economic Communities (EEC):** *Council Directive of 24 June 1982 on the Major Hazards of Certain Industrial Activities* (Seveso Directive; 85/501/EEC). Brussels: EEC, 1982.
26. **European Communities (EC):** *Council Common Position on the Control of Major Accident Hazards Involving Dangerous Substances* (96/C120/03/EC). Brussels: EC, 1996.
27. **European Communities (EC):** *Council Directive 96/82/EC on the Control of Major-Accident Hazards* (OJ No L 10; Seveso II Directive). Brussels: EC, 1997.
28. **Lykke, E.:** *Avoiding and Managing Environmental Damage from Hazardous Industrial Accidents.* Pittsburgh, Pa.: Air and Waste Management Association, 1986.
29. **Health and Safety Executive (HSE):** *A Guide to the Control of Industrial Major Accident Hazards Regulations of 1984* [HS(R)21] London: HSE, 1985.
30. **Air Pollution Control Association:** *Avoiding and Managing Environmental Damage from Major Industrial Accidents.* Pittsburgh, Pa.: AWMA (1986).
31. **Apostolakis, G.:** The concept of probability in safety assessments of technological systems. *Science 250* (1990).
32. **Clifton, J.J.:** Risk analysis and predictive techniques. *Major Haz.* (UK) July 1987.
33. **Frankel, E.G.:** *Systems Reliability and Risk Analysis.* Amsterdam, The Netherlands: Martinus Nijhoff, 1984.
34. **Freeman, R.A.:** Use of risk assessment in the chemical industry. *Plant Oper. Prog. 4* (1985).
35. **Gressel, M.G., and J.A. Gideon:** An overview of process hazard evaluation techniques. *Am. Ind. Hyg. Assoc. J. 52*:158–163 (1991).
36. **Institution of Chemical Engineers (ICE):** *Risk Analysis in the Process Industries* (Pub. series no. 45). London: ICE, 1985.
37. **Institution of Chemical Engineers (ICE):** *The Assessment and Control of Major Hazards* (EFCE Pub. series no. 42). London: ICE, 1985.
38. **Lees, F.A.:** *Loss Prevention in the Process Industries*, vol. 2. London: Butterworth, 1980.
39. **Lees, F.A.:** Some aspects of hazard survey and assessment. *Chem. Engin.* (UK) 1980.
40. **American Institute of Chemical Engineers (AIChE):** *Evaluating Process Safety in the Chemical Industry: A Users Guide to Quantitative Risk Analysis.* New York: AIChE, 2000.
41. **American Institute of Chemical Engineers (AIChE):** *Guidelines for Chemical Process Quantitative Risk Analysis,* 2nd ed. New York: AIChE, 2000.
42. **American Institute of Chemical Engineers (AIChE):** *Layer of Protection Analysis: Simplified Process Risk Assessment.* New York: AIChE, 2001.
43. **Coppock, R.:** *Regulating Chemical Hazards in Japan, West Germany, France, the United Kingdom and the European Community: A Comparative Examination.* Washington, D.C.: National Academy Press, 1986.
44. **Harris, N.C., and A.M. Moses:** *The Use of Acute Toxicity Data in the Risk Assessment of Accidental Releases of Toxic Gases* (Symp. Series 80, 136). London: Institute of Chemical Engineers, 1983.
45. **Pitt, M.J.A.:** Vapour hazard index for volatile chemicals. *Chem. Ind.* (1982).
46. **American Conference of Governmental Industrial Hygienists (ACGIH®):** *Threshold Limit Values for Chemical Substances and Physical Agents.* Cincinnati, Ohio: ACGIH®, 2001.
47. **Institution of Chemical Engineers:** Bhopal: The company report. Loss Prevent. *Bull. 63(1)* (1985).
48. **Dow Chemical Co.:** *Fire and Explosion Index Hazard Classification Guide*, 5th ed. Midland, Mich.: Dow Chemical Co., 1981.
49. **American Institute of Chemical Engineers (AIChE):** *Guidelines for Hazard Evaluation Procedures.* New York: AIChE, 1992.
50. **Theodore, L., J.P. Reynolds, and F.B. Taylor:** *Accident and Emergency Management.* New York: John Wiley & Sons, 1989.
51. **Latino, K., and R. Latino:** *Root Cause Analysis: Improving Performance for Bottom Line Results,* 2nd ed. Boca Raton, Fla.: CRC Press, 2002.
52. **Royal Commission on the Ocean Ranger Marine Disaster:** *Report One: The Loss of the Semi Submersible Drill Rig Ocean Ranger and its Crew* (Pub. Z1-1982/1-IE). Toronto: Canadian Government Publishing Center, 1984.
53. **Heising, C.D., and W.S. Grengebach:** The Ocean Ranger oil rig disaster: A risk analysis. *Risk Anal. 9* (1989).
54. **Bell, B.J., and A.D. Swain:** *A Procedure for Conducting Human Reliability Analyses* (NUREG/CR-2254). Washington, D.C.: U.S. Nuclear Regulatory Commission, 1983.
55. **McCormick, N.J.:** *Reliability and Risk Analysis.* New York: Academic Press, 1981.
56. **Rasmussen, J.:** *Approaches to the Control of the Effects of Human Error in Chemical Plant Safety* (Riso-M2638). Roskilde, Denmark: Riso National Laboratory, 1987.
57. **Hart, G.S.:** Avoiding and managing environmental damage from major industrial accidents. Executive summary of the international conference. *J. Air Pollut. Control Assoc. 36* (1986).
58. **American Institute of Chemical Engineers (AIChE):** *Guidelines for Consequence Analysis of Chemical Releases.* New York: AIChE, 1999.

59. **Kletz, T.A.:** Friendly plants. *Chem. Eng. Prog.* (1989).
60. **Ramskill, P.M.:** *Discharge Rate Calculation Methods for Use in Plant Safety Assessment* (SRD R 352). Culcheth, UK: Safety and Reliability Directorate, 1986.
61. **Beddows, N.A.:** Emergency prediction information. *Prof. Safety* (1990).
62. **van den Bosch, C.J.H.:** *Methods for the Calculation of the Physical Effects Due to Releases of Hazardous Materials (Liquids and Gases)* (Yellow Book; CPR-14E), 3rd ed. The Hague, The Netherlands: TNO, 1997.
63. **McNaughton, D.J., C.G. Wirly, and P.M. Bodner:** Evaluating emergency response models for the chemical industry. *Chem. Eng. Prog.* (1987).
64. **National Fire Protection Association (NFPA):** *Fire Protection Guide on Hazardous Materials*, 13th ed. Quincy, MA: NFPA, 2001.
65. **Baxter, P.J., P.C. Davies, and V. Murray:** Medical planning for toxic release into the community: The example of chlorine gas. *Brit. J. Ind. Med. 46* (1989).
66. **Coleman, R.J.:** Evacuation planning: crisis or control. *Fire Chief Mag.* (1983, Feb.).
67. **Cooney, W.D.C.:** The role of public services-off-site arrangements. *Major Haz.* (UK) (1987).
68. **Hanna, S.R., and P.J. Drivas:** *Guidelines for the Use of Vapor Cloud Dispersion Models.* New York: American Institute of Chemical Engineers, 1987.
69. **McQuaid, J.D. (ed.):** Heavy gas dispersion trials at Thorney Island-2. *J. Haz. Mater. 16* (1987).
70. **Nielson, M., and N.O. Jensen:** Research on continuous and instantaneous gas clouds. *J. Haz. Mater. 21* (1989).
71. **Pedersen, F., and R.S. Seleg:** Predicting the consequences of short-term exposure to high concentrations of gaseous ammonia. *J. Haz. Mater. 21* (1989).
72. **National Research Council:** *Emergency and Continuous Exposure Guidance Levels for Selected Airborne Contaminants.* Washington, D.C.: National Academy Press, 1985.
73. **American Industrial Hygiene Association (AIHA®):** *Emergency Response Planning Guides.* Akron, Ohio: AIHA®, 1987.
74. **World Health Organization:** *Rehabilitation Following Chemical Accidents: A Guide for Public Officials.* Copenhagen, Denmark: FADL, 1989.
75. **Health and Safety Executive:** *Annual Report of the Chief Inspector of Factories for 1974.* London: Her Majesty's Stationary Office, 1975.
76. **Edmundson, J.N.:** The use of risk results in planning and design. *Major Haz.* (UK) (1987).
77. **Prugh, R.W., and R.W. Johnson:** *Guidelines for Vapor Release Mitigation.* New York: American Institute of Chemical Engineers, 1987.
78. **LeVine, R.:** *Guidelines for Safe Storage and Handling of High Toxic Hazard Materials.* New York: American Institute of Chemical Engineers, 1987.
79. **Kletz, T.A.:** *What Went Wrong?* London: Gulf, 1985.
80. **American Institute of Chemical Engineers (AIChE):** *Chemical Process Safety: Learning from Case Histories*, 2nd ed. New York: AIChE, 1999.
81. **Suro, R.:** *Plastics plant explodes; many missing.* New York Times (24 October 1989).
82. **Brown, G.N.:** Disaster planning for industry. *Occup. Health (UK)* (1977).
83. **Eberlein, J.:** Emergency plans—the industry approach. *Chem. Ind. 82* (1987).
84. **Krikorian, M.:** *Disaster and Emergency Planning.* Loganville, Ala.: International Loss Control Institute, 1982.
85. **National Response Team (NRT):** *Hazardous Materials Emergency Planning Guide* (NRT 1). Washington, D.C.: NRT, 2001.
86. **Michael, E.J., O.W. Bell, J.W. Wilson, and G.W. McBride:** Emergency planning considerations for chemical plants. *Environ. Prog.* (1988).
87. **Chemical Manufacturers Associations (CMA):** *Site Emergency Response Planning.* Washington, D.C.: CMA, 1986.
88. **Fulde, G.W.O. (ed.):** *Emergency Medicine, the Principles of Practice.* Sydney, Australia: Williams and Williams, 1988.
89. **Laing, G.S.:** *Accidental and Emergency Medicine.* New York: Springer Verlag, 1988.
90. **Duclos, P., S. Binder, and R. Riester:** Community evacuation following the Spencer Metal Processing plant fire, Nanticoke, Pennsylvania. *J. Haz. Mater. 22* (1989).
91. **Rogers, G.O., and J.H. Sorensen:** Warning and response in two hazardous materials transportation accidents in the U.S. *J. Haz. Mater. 22* (1990).
92. **American Conference of Governmental Industrial Hygienists (ACGIH®):** *Guidelines for the Selection of Chemical Protective Clothing*, 3rd ed. Cincinnati, Ohio: ACGIH®, 1987.
93. **Merriman, M.:** *Not a drill. Occup. Health Safety* (March 1990).
94. **Michael, E.J., and R.E. Vanesse:** *Planning and Implementation of Emergency Preparedness Exercises Including Scenario Preparation.* Boston: Stone and Webster, 1985.
95. **Bennett, G.F., F.S. Feates, and J. Welder:** *Hazardous Materials Spills Handbook.* New York: McGraw-Hill, 1982.

96. **Maloney, D.M., A.J. Policastro, L. Coke, and W. Dunn:** The development of initial isolation and protective action distances for U.S. DOT publication 1990 *Emergency Response Guidebook*. In *Proceedings of HAZMAT CENTRAL*. Rosemont, Ill.: Hazardous Waste Management, 1990.
97. **Student, P.J. (ed.):** *Emergency Handling of Hazardous Materials in Surface Transportation*. Washington, D.C.: Association of American Railroads, 1981.
98. **U.S. Department of Transportation (DOT):** *Emergency Response Guidebook* (DOT P 5800.4). Washington, D.C.: DOT, 1987.
99. **American Institute of Chemical Engineers (AIChE):** *Guidelines for the Technical Management of Chemical Process Safety*. New York: AIChE, 1989.
100. **American Institute of Chemical Engineers (AIChE):** *Plant Guidelines for the Technical Management of Chemical Process Safety*. New York: AIChE, 1992.
101. **Chemical Manufactures Association (CMA):** *Evaluating Process Safety in the Chemical Industry*. New York: CMA, 1992.
102. **Disaster Research Center:** *Publication List*. [Booklet] Newark: University of Delaware, 1989.
103. **Hughes, M.A.:** A selected annotated bibliography of social science research on planning for and responding to hazardous material disasters. *J. Haz. Mater. 27* (1991).

Outcome Competencies

After completing this chapter, the reader should be able to:

1. Define and understand important terms and concepts used in this chapter.
2. Identify examples of workplaces and operations that require controls.
3. List and define various kinds of emission and exposure control methods.
4. Recognize and use engineered controls
5. Identify the goals and mechanisms of ventilation including local exhaust and dilution.
6. Recognize and use administrative controls.
7. Recognize the role of respiratory controls.
8. Recognize the limitations of various control approaches.
9. Understand the importance of cost effectiveness when choosing controls.

Prerequisite Knowledge

In conjunction with this chapter, the user should read or review the following chapters.

Chapter Number	Chapter Topic
7	Principles of Evaluating Worker Exposure
8	Occupational and Environmental Health Risk Assessment/Risk Management
18	Indoor Air Quality
22	Biohazards and Associated Issues
40	Respiratory Protectiony

Key Terms

administrative controls • control • dilution ventilation • emission • exposures • engineered (or engineering) controls • local exhaust ventilation (LEV) • PPE controls • prevention • problem characterization

Key Topics

I. Introduction

II. The Industrial Hygienist's Role

III. General approaches to Control
- A. Fundamental Control Assumptions
- B. Prevention
- C. Control Begins at the Design Stage
- D. Problem Characterization
- E. Application of Controls

IV. Emission and Exposure Control in Nonindustrial Environments
- A. Types of Emissions

V. Emission and Exposure Control in Industrial Environments
- A. Aerosol Emission Source Behavior
- B. Vapor Emission Source Behavior

VI. Engineered Controls
- A. Substitution of a Less Hazardous Material
- B. Process Change
- C. Isolation and enclosure
- D. Wet Methods
- E. Ventilation
- F. Types of Ventilation
- G. Employee Rotation and Reduction of Exposure Times
- H. Housekeeping
- I. Personal Hygiene
- J. Maintenance

VII. Personal Protective Equipment (PPE): Respirators

VIII. Cost, Energy, and Sustainability Considerations

IX. Successful Controls

X. Summary

XI. References

General Methods for the Control of Airborne Hazards

35

By D. Jeff Burton, CIH, PE

Introduction

This chapter introduces the general subject of the control of airborne contaminants for the purpose of minimizing employee exposures. Control of emissions and employee exposures may be accomplished by many methods. Chapters 36 and 37 cover the important emission and exposure controls of dilution and local exhaust ventilation. Respirators, personal protective equipment and other hazard controls are discussed in the chapters dealing with those topics.

The industrial hygienist (IH) has a responsibility to choose controls that are compatible with (and acceptable to) the employee and the process or task, and that are cost-effective and energy-efficient. The type of control chosen also depends on regulatory requirements (some operations require specific controls, e.g., welding stainless steel indoors requires local exhaust ventilation), the nature of the hazard, and the affect on the employee. The selection of controls must consider the control's effect on operations and maintenance; controls should not materially interfere with normal operations and productivity, and maintenance should be possible with little effect on ease of access and safety.

The Industrial Hygienist's Role

Traditionally, the industrial hygienist's role was to anticipate, recognize, evaluate, and control occupational health hazards. In recent years the actual control of emissions and hazardous conditions often has become a joint effort by the IH and engineering departments, maintenance departments, or others. The IH must continue to be an active team player as a consultant, reviewer, information provider, conceptual designer, and final authority for employee exposure control. In most cases the engineering/maintenance staff should rely on the industrial hygienist for guidance, calculations, and even design assistance. The industrial hygienist should be involved in the review and commissioning of all emission and exposure controls during design, installation, operation, and maintenance. Otherwise, employee exposure control may be compromised.

General Approaches to Control

Administrative actions, engineered (or, engineering) controls, and PPE are the three traditional approaches used to control emissions and employee exposures. Each of these is discussed in more detail in this and other chapters of the book. In-depth coverage may be found in the references listed at the end of this chapter. Samples of these control approaches are shown in Table 35.1 and Figure 35.1.

Fundamental Control Assumptions

There are five fundamental assumptions that the industrial hygienist should recognize:

1. All hazards can be controlled to some degree and by some method.
2. There are multiple alternative approaches to control.
3. More than one control may be useful or required.

Table 35.1 — Approaches and Examples of the Major Control Methods

Type of Control	*Approaches and Examples*
Administrative controls	Management involvement, training of employees, rotation of employees, air sampling, biological sampling, medical surveillance
Engineering controls	Process change, substitution, isolation, ventilation, source modification
PPE	Gloves, aprons, rubberized clothing, hard hats
Source modification	Changing a hazard source to make it less hazardous (e.g, wetting dust particles or lowering the temperature of liquids to reduce off-gassing and vaporization)
Substitution	Substituting a less hazardous material, equipment, or process for a more hazardous one (e.g., use of soap and water in place of solvents, use of automated instead of manually operated equipment)
Process change	Changing a process to make it less hazardous (e.g., paint dipping in place of paint spraying)
Isolation	Separating employees from hazardous operations, processes, equipment, or environments (e.g., use of control rooms, physically separating employees and equipment, barriers placed between employees and hazardous operations)
Ventilation	Two fundamental approaches: general exhaust (dilution of air contaminants) and local exhaust (of air contaminants)
Process controls	Continuous processes typically are less hazardous than intermittent processes
Isolating techniques	Storage of hazardous materials (e.g., use of ventilated storage cabinets for chemicals, size of storage container)
	isolating equipment (e.g., physical isolation of valves and pump seals, barriers around equipment)
	isolating employees (e.g., use of closed control rooms, isolation booths, supplied-air islands)

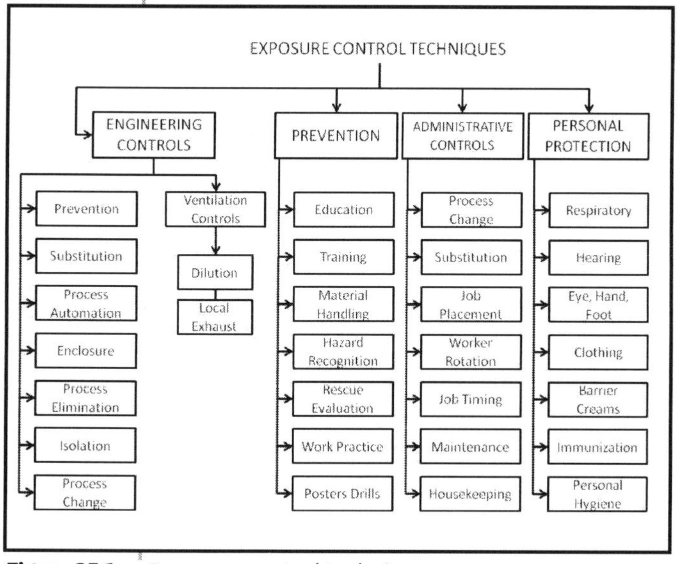

Figure 35.1 — Exposure control techniques.

4. Some control methods are more cost-effective and energy-efficient than others.
5. General dilution ventilation of some form must be provided for every area with human occupancy.

Controls based on these assumptions are more likely to be both realistic and cost-effective.

Prevention

The use of prevention is important to the overall application of controls. The industrial hygienist should cultivate an attitude of prevention in every situation where the risk of employees being exposed to air contaminants exists. Every control evaluation should begin with the question, "Is it possible to *prevent* the condition or potential exposure with a control?"

Case Study 1. Part-time welders in a plant were exposed to welding smoke while welding parts for a machine manufactured in the plant. The industrial hygienist was asked to research emission and exposure control options. Reviewing the literature, the IH found that traditional exposure control approaches included local exhaust ventilation, dilution ventilation, and respirators.

Outcome. However approaching the situation with the intent of prevention, resulted in suggestion to find an alternative method of bonding the metals. Would chemical bonding be feasible? What about riveting, bolting, or automated welding in a closed system? A report was prepared listing all options. A management team eventually selected bolting of parts as the most cost-effective control.

Control Begins at the Design Stage

It is generally more difficult and expensive to apply emission or exposure controls after an operation or process has already been installed or constructed. The industrial hygienist should be involved from the very beginning of any project in which emissions and exposures are likely to occur. Design criteria found in good occupational health programs are shown in Table 35.2.

Problem Characterization

The first five steps shown in Table 35.3 have traditionally been called problem characterization. Today all nine steps would be considered part of risk assessment and risk management, which is a broad approach to determining hazards and controls. Without the first five steps, the chances of finding and implementing cost-effective controls is minimal. Problem characterization and risk assessment are two of the most important functions, and critical competencies, of the industrial hygienist.

As controls are being considered, the IH must know everything about the behavior of the emission source, the worker, the air, and their relationships to each other. Figure 35.2 shows the relationship that must exist in any exposure problem.

In Figure 35.3, consider which employee is more likely to be exposed. Based on the proximity of the worker to the emission

Table 35.2 — Occupational Hygiene Design Criteria for Projects with Emission/Exposure Potential

(1) Meet all applicable codes, regulations, and standards
(2) Obtain occupational hygiene input
(3) Design processes to be as enclosed as possible, or to be remote from employees
(4) Design to maintain employee exposures as low as possible—below the action level if possible, and never to exceed the permissible exposure limit
(5) Use low-hazard materials and processes
(6) Design with employee safety and health as a major objective
(7) Make process equipment as maintenance-free as possible
(8) Automate systems as much as possible
(9) Obtain occupational hygiene review of proposed plans and specifications
(10) Include the occupational hygienist in the commissioning process

Table 35.3 — Approach to the Implementation and Application of Controls

(1) Identify/characterize hazard
(2) Identify emission/exposure sources
(3) Characterize sources
(4) Characterize worker involvement with sources
(5) Characterize air movement
(6) Identify all alternative controls available
(7) Choose the most effective control(s) considering compliance requirements, costs, and ethics
(8) Implement controls
(9) Follow up with testing and maintenance of control systems

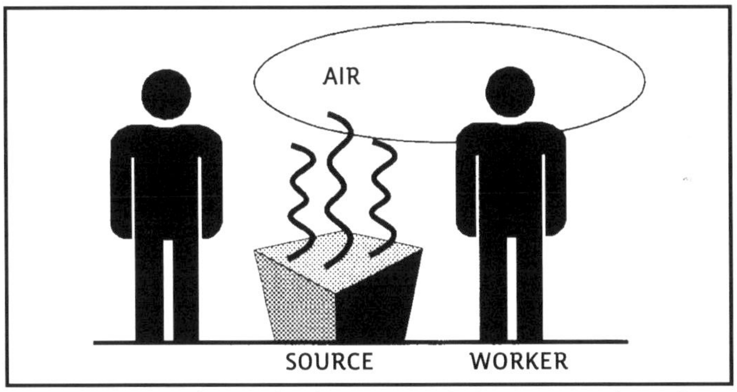

Figure 35.2 — Relationship between emission source, air, and employee.

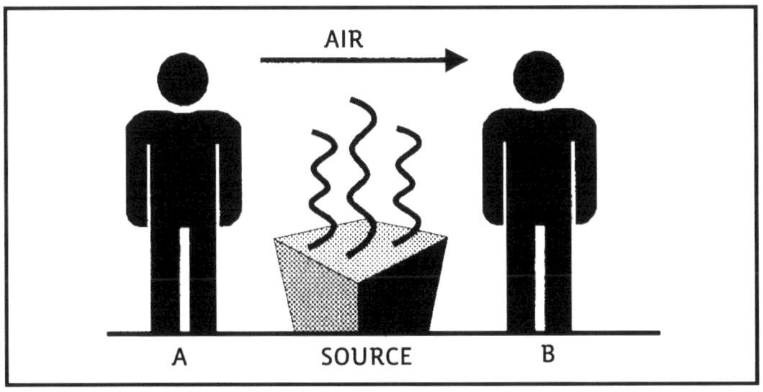

Figure 35.3 — Evaluation of source, employee, and air assists in strategy development.

Table 35.4 — Information Needs for Problem Characterization

Emission source behavior
- Where are emission sources or potential emission sources?
- Which emission sources actually contribute to exposure?
- What is the relative contribution of each source to exposure?
- Characterize each contributor (e.g., chemical composition, temperature, rate of emission, direction of emission, initial emission velocity, continuous or intermittent, time intervals of emission).

Air behavior
- How does the air move (e.g., direction, velocity)?
- Characterize the air (e.g., air temperature, mixing potential, supply and return flow conditions, air changes per hour, effects of wind speed and direction, effects of weather and season).

Worker behavior
- How do workers interact with emission sources?
- Characterize employee involvement (e.g., worker location, work practices, worker education and training, cooperation).

source and the direction of air movement, it appears that Employee B is at greater risk of over exposure. Obviously, employee exposures do not occur unless a hazard source is located somewhere in the workplace, and air must move the contaminant or hazard into the occupied space of the worker (or the worker must move into the contaminated or hazardous area.) Table 35.4 lists the questions that must be answered to evaluate employee risk. Some of these cannot be answered with certainty, but the IH should develop an estimate for each, even if the estimate only borders on the quantitative.

Exposure is directly related to the amount of airborne contaminant that reaches the breathing zone (BZ) of the worker and the time duration of exposure. Controls must attempt to reduce the transfer of contaminants into the BZ and/or reduce the time of exposure. Problem characterization is the primary technique used to identify and evaluate these parameters.

Application of Controls

Once an airborne hazard has been anticipated (or recognized) and the problem characterization data have been gathered, the application of controls usually follows the implementation steps shown in Table 35.3. A team consisting of the industrial hygienist

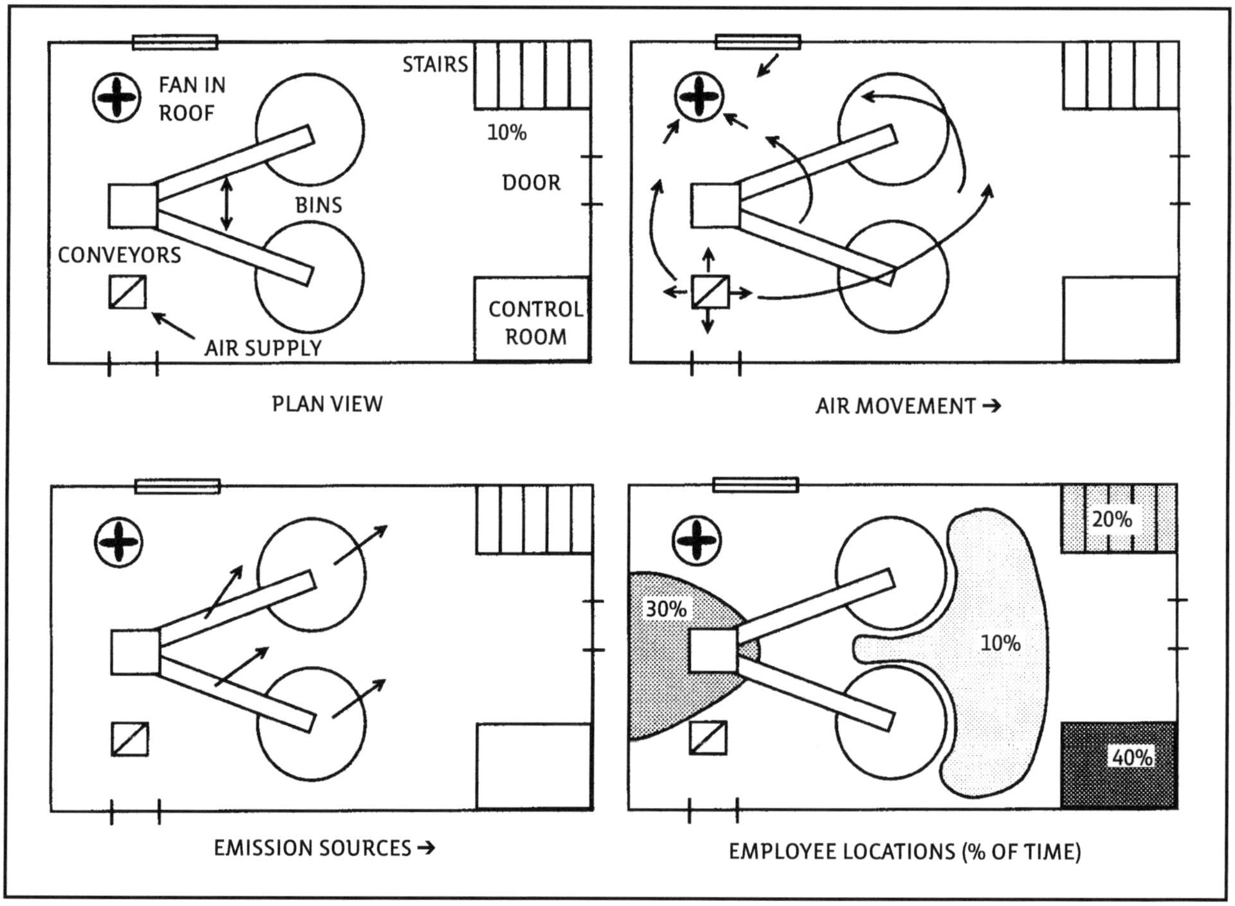

Figure 35.4 — Problem characterization of a grain-handling operation.

and others (e.g., facilities engineering, designers, maintenance supervisors, fire marshal, safety professional, operations) usually will generate an application plan consisting of control options.

Case Study 2. Figure 35.4 shows a simple problem characterization. The top figure shows a plan view (looking down on the floor plan) of a grain handling system in a food manufacturing plant. Grains are dried and then stored in two bins. Two employees work in the building. Dust exposure has created the need for emission and exposure control.

Outcome. Note that all three aspects of the emission and exposure problem are presented on three more plan views. Emission sources are identified by arrows—direction and magnitude are suggested by the arrows. Worker locations show proximity to emission sources. Airflow is indicated by arrows and volume flow rates. For example, air flows out of the building through a roof-penetrating exhaust fan, as shown in Figure 35.4. This simple data provides the input information that the IH and the control team need to evaluate and select cost-effective controls.

The remainder of this chapter is devoted to describing the application of various control approaches. The first section deals with source control in nonindustrial environments. Subsequent sections present control strategies found primarily in industrial environments, but the general principles apply to all control projects.

Emission and Exposure Control in Nonindustrial Environments

Employee groups traditionally have been divided into two categories: blue-collar workers and white collar workers. Blue collar workers work in industrial and production-type plants. These employees are often exposed to airborne chemical contaminants related to plant processes and materials. White-collar workers are those who work in commercial establishments such as stores and warehouses, office environments, hospitals and schools.

In its infancy industrial hygiene concentrated on the control of emissions and exposures to blue-collar workers (e.g., control of exposures to silica and coal dust in mines, solvents and acid mists in manufacturing facilities, and heavy metals in smelters and foundries). In recent decades it has been recognized that white-collar workers also are exposed to airborne hazards (e.g., ozone, formaldehyde, mold spores). Today, airborne contaminants control in the commercial/office environment is as important as controlling exposures in traditional industrial environments.

In the nonindustrial environment two primary controls are used: emission source control and dilution ventilation. This section introduces source control. Dilution ventilation is covered in the Chapter 36.

There are two basic approaches to emission source control in office buildings, commercial establishments and other employee environments where exposure problems exist: (1) use, specify, and/or install equipment, materials, and furnishings with low emissions; and (2) limit or minimize emissions once equipment, materials, or furnishings are in place and the building has been occupied.

Types of Emissions

Emissions can be separated into two families: the wet emitters and the dry emitters. Table 35.5 shows the various types. When selecting or specifying building materials, equipment, or furnishings, follow the useful approaches found in Table 35.6.

Emission and Exposure Control in Industrial Environments

The majority of life and health-threatening employee exposures to airborne chemicals occur in the industrial environment. However, emission sources and their controls as described in the remainder of this chapter can be applied in both the industrial and nonindustrial occupational environments.

Aerosol Emission Source Behavior

Particulate air contaminants become airborne by a number of mechanisms in industrial environments. This emission activity is called pulvation. Table 35.7 and Figure 35.5 show typical mechanisms of pulvation. Control of particle emissions must recognize

Table 35.5 — Types of Emission Sources Found in the Nonindustrial Environment

Type of Emission	*Description*
Wet materials emitting into the building air construction	These include solvents, paints, adhesives, and sealers applied during the construction or during remodeling of a building. Most of the emissions occur during the first few hours or days after application, but some may continue to emit at low rates for days, weeks, or months after. Exposure may be controlled by applyingmaterials well before the building or space is (re)occupied.
Wet materials emitting into the building air during occupancy	These include such materials as cleaners, waxes, disinfectants, and biocides. Because the building may be occupied during application, the potential for exposure and complaints is high. Another source is the use of boiler steam, which contains water treatment chemicals, for humidification.
Dry materials emitting into the building air	These include materials such as the latex backing found on many carpets, styrene monomer from plastics, or formaldehyde from pressed wood. The offending emission is usually a material that was added during the manufacturing process. When the product is unpacked at the site, a large emission may occur, decaying quickly as time passes. Others may emit for months or years (e.g., formaldehyde from wood products.)
Dry materials emitting adsorbed chemicals (sink materials)	Surfaces can absorb/adsorb and desorb chemicals from the air adjacent to the material (sinks). The rate of take-up and desorption is a function of the sink material, the surface area, the temperature, the chemical, and the chemical's concentration in the air. Materials with rough or fleecy surfaces (such as cloth or paper) adsorb more readily than smooth materials (such as glass or steel). Sinks can become loaded with chemicals during high air concentrations (i.e., during construction) and may off-load slowly during occupancy.

Table 35.6 — Approaches to the Emission Control of Building Materials and Furnishings

Emissions	Select materials with lowest emission rates and toxicity, least potential for creating irritation, and highest odor detection threshold (zero emissions is ideal). Where not available, choose materials with low long-term emission rates, or materials with high emission decay factors. Some materials may emit low quantities initially but may emit over a long term.
Environment	Choose materials not adversely affected by temperature or humidity. Materials that significantly increase emissions with increases in temperature or humidity will likely create indoor air quality (IAQ) episodes eventually.
Sink potential	Choose materials that are least likely to become sinks, and as such, secondary emission sources. Factors affecting sink adsorption, absorption, and desorption include the following. *Roughness:* Smooth materials are less likely to become sinks than fleecy or rough materials. *Temperature:* Affects rate of uptake and desorption, diffusion, and rates of evaporation. *Humidity:* Affects rates of emission of formaldehyde from pressed wood and other carriers. *Air movement:* Affects concentrations of chemicals in air; affects size of boundary layer of air (a tiny layer of quiet air on the surface that controls the rate of gas-phase mass transfer at the sink).
Maintenance	Maintenance-free materials are less likely to become emitters. Materials that can be cleaned with water are less likely to becomesources of IAQ complaints.
Supplier	Choose suppliers and manufacturers who have information and IAQ programs. Manufacturers who have conducted emission testing and can provide the above information—along with testing results—should be supported. Without good information from suppliers and manufacturers, it is difficult to provide good IAQ through source control.
Aging	Many specifiers require newly manufactured equipment and furnishings to be "aired out" or "aged" before installation or before building occupation. Aging creates an opportunity for the initial burst of emissions to occur remote from the building and its occupants. For example, carpet can be rolled out for several days or weeks in a warehouse before installation. "Baking out" has not been shown be cost-effective.

these characteristics and attempt to minimize the pulvating energy (e.g., reduce wind, vibration, and heat.)

Vapor Emission Source Behavior

Vapor contaminants can evaporate from a liquid surface or be emitted from liquid-containing pressurized vessels. The emission rate from evaporation is related to the vapor pressure (P_v) of the material. Vapor pressures vary with temperature (T). Higher temperatures create higher vapor pressures. For example, the vapor pressure of water at sea level and T = 20°C is approximately 20 mmHg. P_v increases 760 mmHg at 100°C. At the boiling point of a liquid, the vapor pressure equals the atmospheric pressure.

The maximum concentration a vapor can attain in air (saturated condition) is given by the ratio of the vapor pressure (sometimes called the partial pressure) to atmospheric pressure. For water at standard conditions the maximum concentration of water vapor in air is approximately 2.5% by volume (determined by dividing 20 mmHg by 760 mmHg). When additional water vapor is added to air, existing water vapor will condense somewhere in the space to maintain the vapor equilibrium.

$$CR = \frac{P_v}{P_B} \qquad (35\text{-}1)$$

Table 35.7 — Pulvation Mechanisms and Resulting Airborne Particles

Mechanism	*Particle*
Agitated liquids	mist
Liquids in which bubbles rise to the surface and break	mist
Heated viscous liquids	vapor, then solidified/ condensed particles
Heated solids or metals	fume
Sprayed materials	particles, condensed particles
Conveyor-transferred dry materials	dust
Tumbled, abraded, or agitated dry materials	dust
Materials through which air passes	dust
Materials over which air passes	dust
Materials that fall from one level to another	dust
Vibrated materials	dust

Source: British Occupational Hygiene Society, Controlling Airborne Contaminants in the Workplace (London: Science Reviews Ltd, 1987).

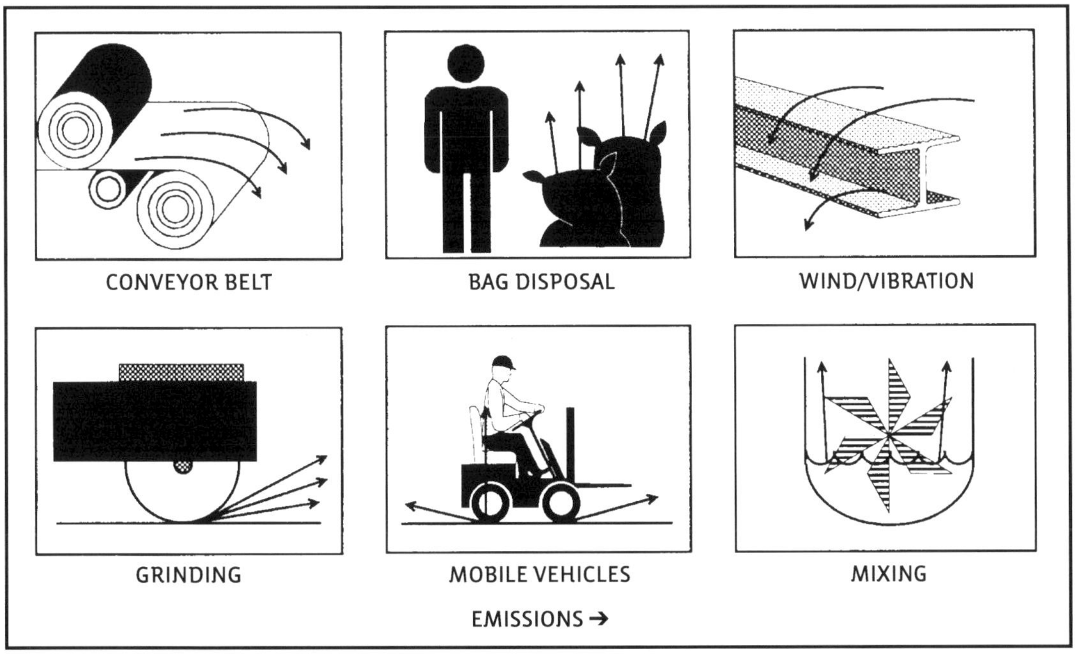

Figure 35.5 — Particle emitting process found in industrial occupancies.

where CR is concentration ratio, P_v is the vapor pressure of the contaminant, and P_B is the barometric (atmospheric) pressure. Multiplying CR by 100 will provide the concentration in percent, multiplying by 10^6 will provide the concentration in ppm.

Gases generally emit to the environment from closed systems (e.g., vessels, pipes, process equipment) or from processes that generate gases (e.g., carbon monoxide from combustion). The Vapor Hazard Index (VHI) suggested by the British Occupational Hygiene Society (Equation 35-2) is a method to estimate the relative hazard potentials of vaporous materials by comparing the concentration at saturated vapor pressure (C_{sPv}) with the appropriate occupational exposure limit (OEL), with both values imputed using consistent units (e.g., ppm).

$$VHI = \frac{C_{sPv}}{OEL} \qquad (35\text{-}2)$$

The vapor hazard index is an interesting approach, but must not be the sole criterion for decision making. Other factors may include work practices; cost of materials; difficulty of separation at the air cleaner; permit requirements; routes of entry; usage; open or closed process; specific gravity of the materials; final product performance; quality; costs; and so forth. The industrial hygienist must use all such criteria when making a final decision regarding emission and exposure control.

Case Study 3. Two chemicals were being considered for an open cleaning operation. The two chemicals' properties were: Chemical A with a P_v of 3 mmHg and an OEL of 100 ppm; and Chemical B with a P_v of 6 mmHg and an OEL of 350 ppm. The industrial hygienist was asked to recommend which chemical would be more appropriate.

Outcome. The atmospheric pressure (P_B) at the plant averages 650 mmHg. Concentration ratio at saturation for Chemical A was 4620 ppm (calculated by CR = Pv/P_B = 3/650 = 0.00462) and for Chemical B was 9230 ppm (calculated by CR = P_v/P_B = 6/650 = 0.00923). The indexes were calculated as follows. The VHI for Chemical A was calculated to be 46.2 (VHI = C_{sPv}/OEL = 4260/100), and the VHI for chemical B was 26.3 (VHI = C_{sPv}/OEL = 9230/350). Based on this outcome and other considerations related to the properties of the chemicals and the process, the industrial hygienist recommended the use of Chemical B.

Settling. Many gases and vapors are heavier than air in their pure states. A saturated air/vapor mixture (such as generated on the top of a tank of solvent) will often be heavier than air and will settle or flow downward in response to gravity. However, its rapid mixing with air and the quick dilution of such saturated air/vapor mixtures retards settling almost as soon as the air/vapor cloud leaves the source. Settling is a function of the relative density of the air/vapor mixture to air, as shown in the last column of Table 35.8. A good rule of thumb is that in percentage quantities, a heavier-than-air, air/vapor mixture will settle, but in parts-per-million quantities, the air/vapor mixture will behave like the air.

Open and Closed Industrial Processes

All industrial processes are either open or closed. Open systems are more apt to emit contaminants routinely to the air shared by employees. Closing an open system can be a primary emission control approach, for example, totally enclosing an open surface

Table 35.8 — Densities of Air/Vapor Mixtures

Chemical	VP (20 C)	MW/MW_{air}	SG (Re air)	Relative Density at 5000 ppm (Re: Air)
Acetone	185	2.0	2.7	1.005
Toluene	22	3.2	1.06	1.011
n-hexane	150	3.0	1.4	1.010
Xylene	10	3.7	1.04	1.014

Note: VP = vapor pressure in mmHg; MW = molecular weight, unitless; SG = specific gravity, unitless

Source: British Occupational Hygiene Society, *Controlling Airborne Contaminants in the Workplace.* London: Science Reviews Ltd., 1987.

tank containing sulfuric acid. However, enclosing a chemical emission source inside a building may concentrate airborne chemicals and create a higher-exposure experience for workers in the building. Additionally, a closed system may give a false sense of security because a closed system invariably leaks, or creates fugitive emissions, and these emissions must be evaluated and controlled.

Open systems include such processes or conditions as (1) stockpiles of chemicals or materials that can be pulvated (or evaporated) by vibration, wind, or other mechanical action; (2) open conveyor belts that emit because of the vibration of the equipment and the movement of material; (3) tanks and kettles that contain evaporating chemicals; (4) open containers; (5) spray painting; and (6) hand welding.

The industrial hygienist should evaluate each real or potential exposure problem and its potential control by asking the following questions.

- Is the process or equipment open or closed?
- Is there an opportunity for the material within the process or equipment to be emitted to the air shared by employees?
- Will employees be (or are they) exposed?
- Can the process, equipment, or system be closed (or opened, if the employee is required to be within the enclosure)?
- What effect on exposure will the closure (or opening) have?

Case Study 4. An employee spray paints small metal parts with an air-powered spray gun. The painter's complaints and air monitoring both suggest that the painter is exposed to solvent vapors and paint particles at about 50% of the permissible exposure limit (PEL). The industrial hygienist has been asked to evaluate the situation and make recommendations for reducing exposures to below 10% of the PEL.

Outcome. The industrial hygienist begins the investigation by answering the suggested questions: The process is open; there is an opportunity for the material to be emitted into air; employees will be exposed; and the process can be partially enclosed in a small spray booth. Because the booth will be enclosed on five sides (top, bottom, two sides, and back), there is a very good chance that emissions and exposures can be controlled if the ventilation is adequate and the painter uses good work practices. The amount of reduction can be mathematically estimated using formulas described in References 2–8. Proper work practices must be used as well, for example the painter must remain entirely outside the enclosure and in the upwind position. This will help assure that the enclosure is effective as an exposure control method. Since paint booths are designed to contain paint overspray to be effective as employee protection, other measures must be taken.

Continuous Operations. Closed systems often are used in chemical and refining industries when production processes are continuous (as opposed to batch processes). Closed production systems are almost universal in the semiconductor industry. Health hazards may arise when a closed system fails to maintain containment. In such cases secondary control measures are required. Secondary systems may include the following:

- Secondary LEV (e.g., around flanges, pumps, gas cylinders, or other closed systems)
- Dilution ventilation
- Isolation of the employee in a controlled atmosphere such as a separately ventilated control room
- Personal protective equipment (e.g., emergency respirators worn on the belt)
- Warning systems to alert employees.

No closed system can be assumed to provide perfect control. Accidents, poor design, and/or faulty equipment invariably create fugitive emissions. The industrial hygienist must anticipate such events and prepare to prevent exposures from these events.

Case Study 5. The labor union safety committee expressed concern that employees would be exposed to silane if a particular flange in a piping system failed. The industrial hygienist was asked to investigate and provide recommendations for control of any potential fugitive emissions.

Outcome. On investigation the industrial hygienist found manufacturer data that the flange had been shown to fail about 10% of the time within 10,000 hours when used with silane. The flange had never failed catastrophically; it was most likely to leak up to

0.001 lbs/hour when used at the pressure found in the piping system. Control options included using a different, more expensive flange, secondary ventilation around the valve, air monitoring systems to warn when the flange failed, automated shutoff valves operating upstream of the flange which activate in the event of a failure, and employee respirators. The industrial hygienist mathematically modeled the situation to determine how much air was required under the worst case accident to maintain air concentrations in the exhaust air to below 1 ppm and gathered information on the cost-effectiveness of each available control option (see References 2 and 5 for detailed approaches). A report was written, and management made a control choice, which in this case, was the use of secondary ventilation.

Engineered Controls

The industrial hygienist may institute engineered (or, "engineering") controls at the source, the air path, and/or at the worker. Many of these control strategies are described in more detail in Figure 35.6 and in the following paragraphs.

Substitution of a Less Hazardous Material

Eliminating a toxic emitter is generally the best approach to control, since it comes close to the ideal concept of prevention. Many toxic materials have suitable substitutes with lower toxicity ratings or lower evaporation rates. Historic examples include using walnut shells for sand in blasting, hydrochlorofluorcarbons for fluorinated or chlorinated hydrocarbons in solvent usage, toluene for benzene in paint thinners, titanium dioxide for white lead in paint, calcium silicates for asbestos, and oil for mercury in gauges.

When substituting a less toxic material, always consider the resulting hazard. Substituting acetone for toluene, for example, while providing a less toxic material, increases emissions (acetone has a lower boiling point) and increases the fire hazard (acetone has a lower flash point). In this case the hazard may actually increase. Sometimes a material's properties may be changed to reduce emissions (e.g., lowering the temperature of a solvent, wetting a dry powder, pelletizing dusty powders). The industrial hygienist should evaluate potential substitutes during the planning phase of control application and consider costs and suitability in the process.

Case Study 6. Perchloroethylene (PCE) was being used to clean metal parts in a parts cleaner. The commercial cleaner had been intended for use with Stoddard Solvent, but PCE was found to be more effective. Unfortunately, emissions had increased and employee exposures were close to the

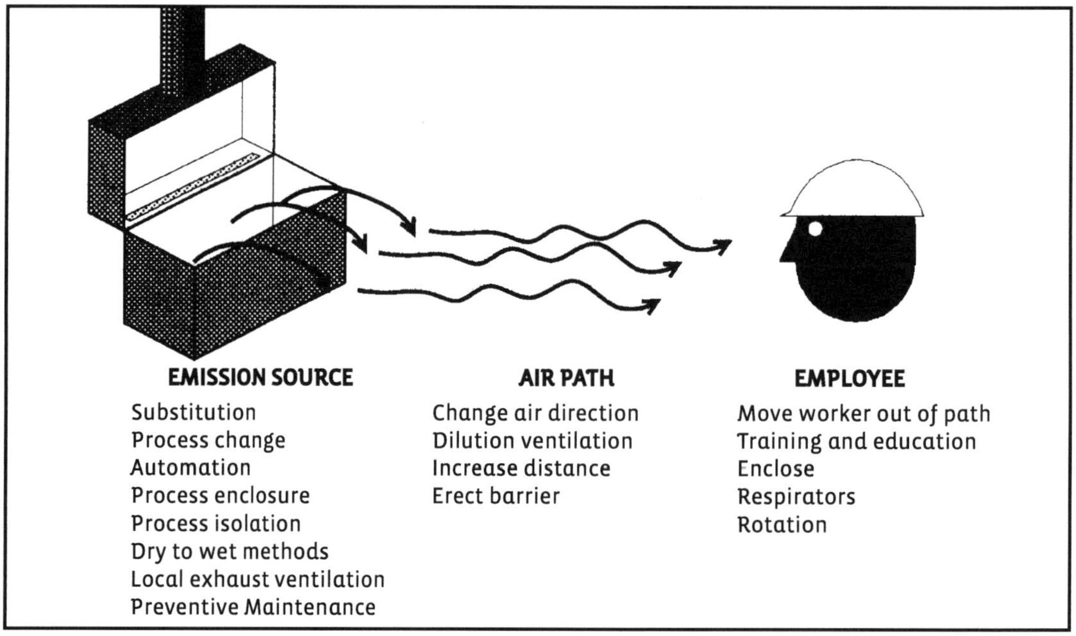

Figure 35.6 — General control strategies at the source, path, and the worker.

PEL. The industrial hygienist was called to evaluate the process.

Outcome. The industrial hygienist investigated the situation and tried several different cleaning materials and strategies. In the end plain soap and water proved to be as effective in cleaning the parts when one step in the manufacturing process was altered to eliminate coating the part with oil. In this case the successful control included both substitution and process change, which is a common occurrence.

Process Change

Process change, like substitution, attempts to replace more hazardous equipment or processes with less hazardous approaches. Historic examples include paint dipping for paint spraying, polyester resin sealants for lead solder in automobile body seams, low-speed oscillating grinders for high-speed rotary grinders, bolting for welding, cooling-coil vapor degreasing tanks for hand-washing of parts, and continuous closed processes for open batch processes.

Again, the industrial hygienist should evaluate the proposed change with regard to the final hazard being created by the change and its effects on productivity and product quality. Fortunately, process or equipment changes used for hazard control often result in increased productivity and product quality.

Case Study 7. Lead-contaminated dust was collected from a baghouse and placed in drums for shipment to an approved landfill. Exposures to employees handling the dust exceeded the PEL for lead, so the constant use of respirators was required. The industrial hygienist was asked to evaluate the process and recommend changes that could reduce the exposures and eliminate the need for respiratory protection.

Outcome. After thorough study the industrial hygienist recommended that a small sintering furnace be installed at the discharge of the baghouse. This would agglomerate the dust into chunks of material, and therefore reduce the dust levels. The exhaust for the furnace was routed into the baghouse inlet ductwork, eliminating any emissions from the furnace. Exposures to employees handling the resulting chunky materials were reduced to well below the PEL.

Isolation and Enclosure

The principle of isolation is found in almost every production plant. It may be as simple as erecting a wall between a process and an employee (e.g., separating office from production employees by a wall), or as complicated as automated processes using robotic techniques (e.g., used to spray paint automobile body frames). Enclosure, closely related to isolation, usually includes building an airtight enclosure around the process or the employee. Examples of isolation and enclosure include building around open storage of dusty materials; enclosing asbestos in airtight containers; enclosing a sandblasting operation in an airtight housing; enclosing a chemical operation in a totally enclosed system; enclosing crane operators in an air-supplied cab; consolidating chemical pipes and lines into an enclosed and exhausted area; pneumatic conveying of material; enclosing and exhausting sampling and view ports; and so forth.

The principle of isolation includes separation by time as well as space. For example, foundry shakeout can be scheduled during the evening when most employees have left the workplace, or maintenance can be performed during regular shutdown periods when production employees are not present.

Case Study 8. Two employees were overexposed to lead dust in a ball mill. Their jobs consisted of periodically inspecting each mill during the operation. The industrial hygienist was asked to recommend control strategies.

Outcome. The most cost-effective control turned out to be isolating the employees in a control room adjacent to the ball mill operation and providing closed-circuit TV cameras at the mouth of each ball mill. The control room was provided with a dedicated air handling system isolated from the air in the ball mill area. During subsequent infrequent in-person visits to the ball mill area, employees wore PPE. These controls reduced exposures by more than 500%.

Wet Methods

Wetting a dusty material reduces pulvation, but must be compatible with the process. Adding humidity to a material is also effective because it may create agglomeration among small particles and add weight.

Table 35.9 — Ventilation Types

Type	*Usage/Approach*
HVAC	Mechanically provides clean, tempered, fresh air for comfort and health. Traditionally known also as "general ventilation."
General exhaust or dilution	Controls the air environment by removing and replacing contaminated air before chemical concentrations reach unacceptable levels.
Local exhaust	Removes chemical contaminants at or near the emission source.
Local supply	Provides clean, fresh air for cooling, exclusion of contaminated air, or to replace exhausted air. Also called supplied-air island, or SAI.
Natural ventilation	Uses wind or temperature differences to induce airflow through the building, creating dilution of air contaminants.
Make-up	Replaces exhausted air.

Examples of wetting to reduce particle emissions include fogging sprays at conveyor belt transfer points, water washing of dusty surfaces, wetting of sand in sand blasting, and wetting paint overspray particles. In HVAC systems adding water moisture to dry air can reduce indoor air quality complaints by raising the relative humidity to the comfort range of 40–60%.

Ventilation

Ventilation is a widely used and time-tested approach to emission and exposure control. Think about it — ventilation is required in every human occupancy. No matter what other forms are control are used, ventilation is always required. Within the broad category of ventilation the IH will find a number of useful approaches. These are listed in Table 35.9 and covered in more depth in Chapters 33 and 34. See References for more detailed information on all ventilation topics.

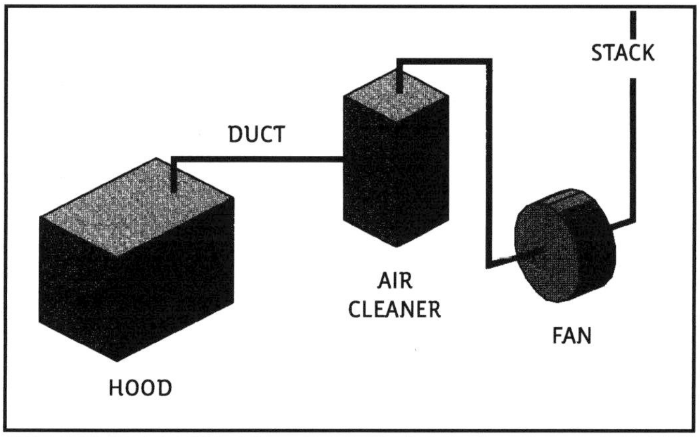

Figure 35.7 — Components of an LEV system.

Types of Ventilation

Dilution (General Exhaust) Ventilation and Local Exhaust Ventilation (LEV)

Emissions and subsequent employee exposures often are controlled with fresh dilution air in both industrial and nonindustrial environments. Dilution ventilation systems are covered in Chapter 36. LEV systems are designed to contain, control, or capture emissions at or near their sources. Typical LEV systems consist of control structures (hoods, exhausted enclosures), ductwork, air cleaners, fans, and stacks. See Figure 35.7. The LEV approach attempts to eliminate emissions to the workroom air, as opposed to dilution ventilation systems, which allow emissions to occur and dilute contaminants to some acceptable concentration before the contaminated air reaches the employee breathing zone. LEV systems are covered in more detail in Chapter 37.

Clean Outdoor Air Makeup, Replacement Air or Supply Ventilation

Makeup air systems (industrial ventilation) and supply air systems (HVAC) both provide fresh clean air, usually from outside the building, to replace air exhausted through general exhaust and LEV systems. Makeup air and supply air should be cleaned and tempered to provide healthy and comfortable conditions.

Administrative Controls

Engineered controls that eliminate or reduce the hazard are generally preferable to administrative or PPE controls. Administrative controls place at least part of the burden of responsibility for protection on the worker. However, administrative controls often are used effectively in conjunction with or in addition to engineered controls. Indeed, very few airborne hazards are controlled by one control measure alone, and some types of administrative controls are always required (e.g., training and education).

A successful control strategy for a welding operation might include implementation of LEV (which automatically provides some dilution), substitution of a less toxic material, good housekeeping of the welding area to prevent secondary pulvation of dust, preventive maintenance of welding equipment, and training and education of the welders so they can work with minimum exposure. Actually, something as simple as adjusting the welder's head position can reduce potential exposures.

Traditional administrative controls include rotation; reduction of exposure times; instituting exposure-reducing work practices; developing preventive maintenance programs; good housekeeping programs; training and education of employees; and teaching and requiring good personal hygiene.

Employee Rotation and Reduction of Exposure Times

Exposure is generally reported as a time-weighted average, or TWA (for compliance purposes). An employee's TWA exposure is a function of both the concentration of the contaminant and the length of the exposure. Although this chapter has concentrated on reducing emissions and therefore the concentration of the contaminant, TWA exposures also can be lowered by reducing the length of time the worker is exposed. The downside to this approach is that more employees are exposed. This goes against the traditional industrial hygiene philosophy of reducing exposures as much as possible for as many as possible. For example, using the evaluation in Table 35.10, eight employees must be exposed for a shorter time period to achieve an average TWA exposure of 13 ppm. The increase in worker doing this task would lead to eight people being trained to do the job safely, eight sets of PPE being supplied, eight medical exams being given, and so forth. Consideration related to the cost-effectiveness alone may disqualify the use of this type of worker rotation.

Table 35.10 — Selection Criteria for Dilution Ventilation

Conditions that lend themselves to dilution with outdoor air

- Major air contaminants are of relatively low toxicity.
- Contaminant concentrations are not hazardous.
- Smoking is not allowed in the occupied space.
- Emission sources are difficult or expensive to remove.
- Emissions occur uniformly in time.
- Emission sources are widely dispersed.
- Emissions do not occur close to the breathing zone of people.
- Moderate climatic conditions prevail.
- The outside air is less contaminated than the inside air.
- The HVAC system is capable of conditioning the dilution air.

Dilution ventilation is less effective and more expensive in the following conditions

- Air contaminants are highly toxic materials.
- Contaminant concentrations are hazardous.
- Smoking is allowed in the occupied space.
- Emission sources are easy to remove.
- Emissions vary with time.
- Emission sources consist of large point sources.
- People's breathing zones are in the immediate vicinity of emission sources (i.e., 2–3 feet).
- The building is located in severe climates.
- The outside air is more contaminated than the inside air.
- The existing HVAC system is not capable of treating the air.

Case Study 13. In spite of excellent LEV, workers hand-soldering industrial battery terminals were exposed to lead fume concentrations near the TWA PEL of 50 mg/m^3. Although workers were being adequately protected through the additional use of respirators, medical exams, good personal hygiene, and so forth, the plant desired to reduce TWA air exposures to below the action level, 30 mg/m^3. The industrial hygienist was asked to provide suggestions.

Outcome. In the end, the most cost-effective approach involved worker rotation. A similar work crew in a plastics fabricating section of the plant was trained to perform the soldering operation safely. Eventually both crews worked a half-day in each department, and resulting TWA exposures averaged 25 mg/m^3.

Housekeeping

Emitted particulate materials must go somewhere: out the stack, out the window, or onto horizontal surfaces in the plant. Settled materials become secondary emission sources, often with as much or more impact on exposures as the primary source. For example, sweeping—although a small source compared, say, with a vibratory conveyor—can be a significant source of exposure because the breathing zone of the sweeper is only a few feet away from the emission point. All buildings vibrate, and such vibration is the energy source—along with wind and traffic—to pulvate settled dust into the air.

Some Occupational Safety and Health Administration (OSHA) standards require good housekeeping (e.g., the standard for inorganic lead). All industrial hygiene guidelines for good practice mention housekeeping as an important control.

Dust may be removed and controlled by wet cleaning methods and vacuum systems. Dry sweeping and blowing simply create unwanted emissions. Spilled liquids should be cleaned up before evaporation causes a problem. Rags and absorbent materials should be disposed of following local fire and hazardous waste requirements.

Personal Hygiene

Personal hygiene is important to the overall protection of the worker but can also impact the inhalation exposure. For example, if a worker smokes without washing his or her hands, hazardous chemicals may be inhaled through contaminated cigarettes. Similarly, if dirty clothes are taken home, additional exposure may result during clothes handling and washing.

Maintenance

As noted previously, emissions may be planned or unplanned and continuous or intermittent. All are impacted by the quality of maintenance applied to the emitting process or equipment. Insufficient maintenance increases the likelihood of both catastrophic emissions (e.g., rupture failure of pipe flange) and fugitive emissions (e.g., slowly increasing rates of leaks from flanges, seals, joints, access doors). Poor maintenance practices may increase emissions when normal emission controls are detached or impaired (e.g., during filter replacement, fan seal repair, or equipment repair).

Maintenance itself may lead to elevated emissions in the vicinity of maintenance personnel. In these cases training and PPE are required to minimize exposures to maintenance personnel.

Preventive maintenance (PM) of emission controls evaluates the potential for increased emissions over time (e.g., the seal fails within 3 months of installation). PM attempts to repair, replace, or correct potential deficiencies before the problem occurs (e.g., the seal will be replaced every 2 months). Because of its great potential to impact emission sources, positively or negatively, maintenance should be a primary concern of the industrial hygienist.

Personal Protective Equipment (PPE): Respirators

Although considered to be part of the third tier of controls, respirators are often used to provide employee exposure protection. However, respirator use should not substitute for engineered and administrative controls because (1) it places the responsibility of protection on the worker and (2) the hazard is not actually reduced in the workplace.

The four generally accepted occasions for respirator use are (1) during the time other control measures are being installed or instituted; (2) during maintenance and repair work; (3) when other controls are not feasible; and (4) during emergencies. The subject of respirators is covered in depth in Chapter 40.

Cost, Energy, and Sustainability Considerations

Costs are related to (1) types of controls applied and (2) the level of control desired, e.g., the "acceptable concentration." One can control emissions, for example, such that resulting employee exposures are at the OEL, the action level (usually 50% of the OEL), 25% of the OEL, 10% of the OEL, and so forth. All of the above target levels are used by practicing industrial hygienists, although the most common target is probably 10% of the OEL. Much of the semiconductor industry has adopted standards that call for target exposures at 1% of the OEL. Other philosophical approaches to control include the following:

- *Maximum Achievable Control.* These approaches are expensive and do not include cost-effectiveness as a primary concern. Such approaches regularly

include post-installation measures such as air monitoring, reporting and record keeping procedures, medical exams, and so forth. This is the most effective for exposure control but also potentially the most expensive.
- *Maximum Financially Feasible Achievable Control.* This approach takes the attitude of achieving the lowest exposures possible within financial feasibility. This is a popular approach but makes control strategies difficult to model mathematically because no set exposure level is targeted. Establishments using this approach often attain exposure levels well below the PEL.
- *Reasonably Achievable Control.* This approach says, "We'll do the best we can, but within reason," where "reason" is defined by the user. This approach is probably less desirable than selecting a target exposure concentration.

Energy considerations are closely related to costs. Generally, if costs are low, energy consumption will also be low. If LEED certification and other "green" procedures are followed, costs, energy and environmental conditions will be optimized.

Successful Controls

Emission and exposure controls must demonstrate the following characteristics to be considered successful:

- The control must be able to achieve the target exposure concentration.
- It must be accepted by the employee and be compatible with his or her work.
- Protection must be reliable and consistent throughout its life.
- The effectiveness of control must be measurable throughout its life.
- The control must minimize the need for worker responsibility for his or her own protection.
- It must not create additional uncontrolled hazards.
- The control must protect against all routes of entry (e.g., skin and eye, gastrointestinal tract, and lung).
- It should be cost effective and financially feasible for the organization.
- Costs, energy consumption and sustainability issues will be considered and optimized.

Summary

The fundamental assumptions considered in this chapter were that (1) all hazards can be controlled to some degree; (2) there are alternative approaches to control; (3) more than one control may be useful or required; and (4) some control methods are more cost-effective and energy-efficient than others. Major families of control include engineered, administrative, and personal protective equipment.

Engineered controls include process change, substitution, isolation, ventilation, and source modification. Administrative controls include management involvement, training of employees, rotation of employees, air sampling, biological sampling, and medical surveillance. Personal protective equipment include respirators, special clothing and equipment, and other protective equipment.

Control implementation methods include:

- Identifying/characterizing of the hazard
- Identifying emission/exposure sources
- Characterizing sources
- Characterizing worker involvement with sources
- Characterizing air movement
- Identifying all alternative controls available
- Selecting the most effective control(s) considering compliance requirements, costs, and ethics
- Implementing controls
- Testing and maintaining of control systems

References

1. **American Conference of Governmental Industrial Hygienists (ACGIH®):** *Industrial Ventilation—A Manual of Recommended Practice for Design,* 26th edition. Cincinnati, Ohio: ACGIH®, 2007.
2. **American Industrial Hygiene Association™:** *ANSI/AIHA Z9.2-2006, Fundamentals Governing the Design and Operation of Local Exhaust Systems.* Fairfax, VA.: AIHA, 2006.
3. **American Society of Heating, Refrigerating and Air Conditioning Engineers (ASHRAE):** *ASHRAE 55-2004, Thermal Environmental Conditions for Human Occupancy.* [Standard] Atlanta, Ga.: ASHRAE, 1992.

4. **American Society of Heating, Refrigerating and Air Conditioning Engineers (ASHRAE):** *ASHRAE 62-2007, Ventilation for Acceptable Indoor Air Quality*, [Standard] Atlanta, Ga., 2007.
5. **Burton, D.J.:** *Industrial Ventilation Workbook*, 6th edition. Salt Lake City, UT: IVE, Inc., 2009.
6. **Cralley, L.V. and L.J. Cralley (eds.):** *In-Plant Practices for Job Related Health Hazards Control*, Vol. 2. New York: Wiley Interscience, 1989.
7. **Institut de Recherche en Santé et en Sécurité du Travail du Québec (IRSST):** *Guide for the Prevention of Microbial Growth in Ventilation Systems.* Montreal, PQ, Canada: IRSST, 1995.
8. **National Institute for Occupational Safety and Health and the Environmental Protection Agency:** *Building Air Quality—A Guide for Building Owners and Facility Managers* (EPA/400/1-91-033). Washington, D.C.: Government Printing Office, 1991.
9. **Talty, J.T. (ed.):** General Methods of Control. *In Industrial Hygiene Engineering.* Noyes Data Corporation, Park Ridge, NJ., 1988. pp 70–77.

Outcome Competencies

After completing this chapter, the reader should be able to:

1. Understand and apply important terms and concepts introduced in this chapter.
2. Identify dilution ventilation goals.
3. Identify examples of workplaces and operations compatible with dilution ventilation controls.
4. Determine appropriate dilution air volume flowrates.
5. Estimate the amount of dilution air being delivered to a space.
6. Recognize dilution ventilation limitations and alternatives.

Prerequisite Knowledge

In conjunction with this chapter, the user should read or review the following chapters.

Chapter Number	Chapter Topic
7	Principles of Evaluating Worker Exposure
9	Occupational and Environmental Health Risk Assessment
18	Indoor Air Quality
35	General Methods for the Control of Airborne Hazards

Key Terms

acceptable concentration • AHU • ASHRAE 62 • control • density correction factor • dilution ventilation • emission factors • emission rate • exposures • HVAC • general exhaust ventilation • IAQ • mixing factor • OA, SA, RA, EA • occupancy • thermal comfort • ventilation controls

Key Topics

I. All Human Occupancies Require Ventilation
II. Correcting for Non-Standard Air Density
III. Fundamental Relationships
IV. Selection Criteria: Is Dilution Ventilation the Best Primary Control Option?
V. Implementing Dilution Ventilation
VI. Special Considerations When Ventilating for Comfort and Maintaining Good IAQ in Commercial Buildings
VII. Common Problems with HVAC Systems
VIII. Estimating the Amount of Outdoor Air (OA) Required
IX. Estimating the Amount of outdoor Air (OA) Being Delivered
X. References

Dilution Ventilation

36

By D. Jeff Burton, CIH, PE

All Human Occupancies Require Ventilation

Ventilation is the use of supply and exhaust air to replenish oxygen, to dilute or remove air contaminants and odors, and to provide thermal conditioning. All occupied spaces require ventilation of some kind.

One important type of ventilation — local exhaust ventilation (LEV) — contains controls, or captures emitted air contaminants at or near their sources and is covered in Chapter 37. This chapter covers the other major type of ventilation, dilution ventilation, for both industrial and non-industrial occupancies. Dilution ventilation systems are sometimes called general exhaust ventilation or turbulent air mixing ventilation. Non-mixing types of dilution ventilation, e.g., plug flow, displacement ventilation are not included.

This chapter is written to help the practicing IH apply basic dilution ventilation principles. Theory, derivation of equations and more technical details can be found in the References. Materials presented in this chapter are thought to be compatible with current standards of good practice. However, the IH should always review current standards and consult with experts before actually applying the principles presented herein.

A good dilution ventilation system allows and encourages emissions of air contaminants to thoroughly mix with surrounding air and then provides fresh outdoor air to mix with and dilute contaminants to some safe acceptable concentration *before* the contaminated air reaches occupant or employee breathing zones.

Table 36.1 shows common properties and definitions of air used in all ventilation systems. Air has many of the same measurable properties as many other materials, e.g., weight, density, volume, viscosity, temperature, and so forth. The standard weight density of air is about 0.075 lbs per cubic foot, for example. This compares to water, as shown in Figure 36.1, which weighs about 62.4 lbs/cubic foot. The industrial ventilation definition of STP is shown in Table 36.1.

Correcting for Non-Standard Air Density

With every type of ventilation operating at non-standard conditions, an air density correction factor, d_c, can be employed to account for air density and volume changes

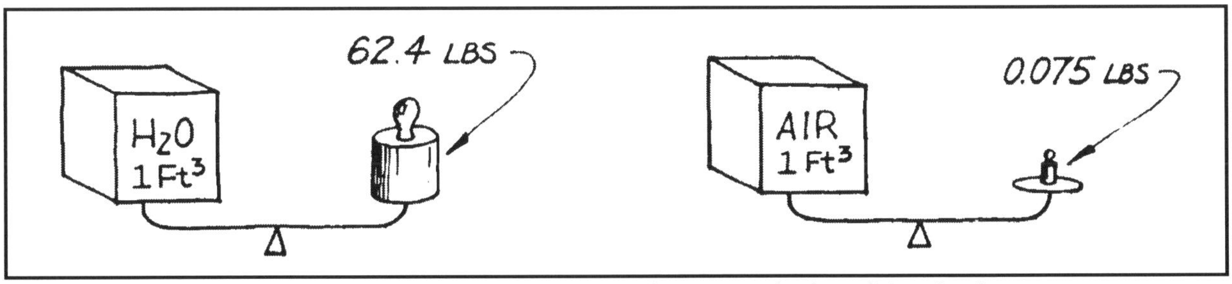

Figure 36.1 — Comparison of the Weight Densities of Water and Air at Standard Conditions (STP).

Table 36.1 — Common Properties of Air

Molecular Weight (MW) = 29 g/mole
Standard air weight density = 0.075 lb/ cu ft (1.2 kg/cubic meter) at STP
STP = Standard Temperature and Pressure
Traditional industrial ventilation definition of STP: T = 70F, BP = 29.92 inches Hg, dry air (T = 21C, BP = 760 mm Hg, dry air)
Traditional HVAC definition of STP: T = 68F, BP = 29.92 inches Hg, 50% Relative Humidity (T = 20C, BP = 760 mm Hg, 50% RH)

when the temperature or pressure is different than the standard condition. As the air moves to a higher altitude, for example, its weight density is reduced and its volume increases as shown in Figure 36.2. The magnitude of this difference can be calculated.

Air density is related to pressure and temperature through the *perfect gas equation of state*:

$$P = \rho RT \quad (36\text{-}1)$$

where:

- P = absolute pressure, lbs/sq ft (psfa)
- ρ = density, lbs/ft^3
- R = gas constant, 53.35 ft-lb/lbm-°R
- T = absolute temperature, °R

When all other conditions are equal, changes in air density and volume, V, vary linearly with changes in absolute temperature, T. Similarly, air density varies linearly with the change in air pressure, P (e.g., if the pressure increases by 5%, the density will increase by 5%). These two relationships are combined into an equation called the *Perfect or Ideal Gas Law*, derived from Equation 36-1, which is often represented as:

$$\frac{P_1V_1}{T_1} = \frac{P_2V_2}{T_2} \quad (36\text{-}2)$$

The factor d_c is derived by transposing terms in the Ideal Gas equation. A widely used definition of d_c is shown in the following equation:

$$d_c = \frac{T_{STP}}{T_{actual}} \times \frac{P_B}{P_{BSTP}} \quad (36\text{-}3)$$

where:

- P_B = absolute barometric pressure.
- T = absolute temperature in R or K
- R = degrees Rankine, R = °F + 460
- K = degrees Kelvin, K = °C + 273

The actual air density can be calculated using Equation 36-4:

$$\rho_{actual} = \rho_{STP} \times d_c \quad (36\text{-}4)$$

Example 36.1. At a plant near Salt Lake City at an altitude of 5000 feet, the summertime air temperature is 90°F and the barometric pressure is 24.89 in Hg. What is the air density correction factor, d_C? The actual air density?

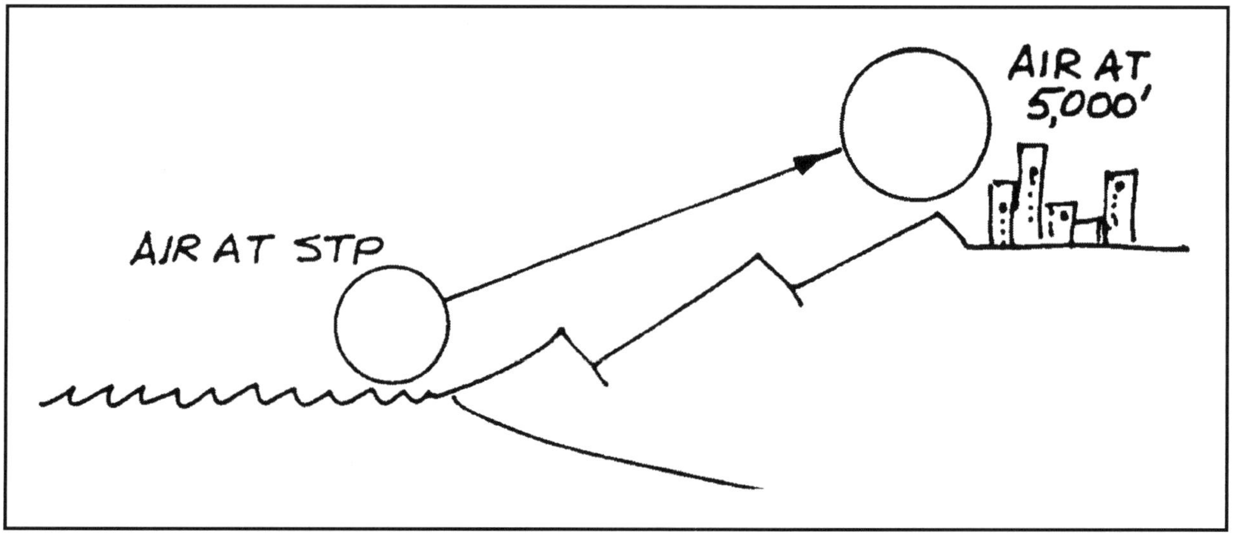

Figure 36.2 — Atmospheric Air Expands as Temperature Increases or Pressure Decreases.

Using Equation (36-3), the density correction factor can be calculated:

$$d_C = \frac{(460 + 70)}{(460 + 90)} \times \frac{P_B}{29.92} = 0.802$$

And, the actual air density can be determines with Equation 36-4:

$$\rho_{actual} = 0.075 \frac{lb}{cu\ ft} \times 0.802 = 0.060 \frac{lb}{cu\ ft}$$

Information on determining the air density correction factor and handling unusual density corrections for high static pressures in ductwork and high moisture content in hot air is presented in References 1 and 2.

Fundamental Relationships

As mentioned above, emissions and subsequent employee or occupant exposures are often controlled with fresh dilution air in both industrial and nonindustrial environments. For a constant emission source, no contaminant sinks, perfect air mixing, and a constant dilution air flowrate, the following basic ratios describe the resulting equilibrium concentration in a ventilated space (e.g., chamber, room, building, space, lab, workroom, plant, hood, etc.).

$$C = \frac{E}{Q} \qquad (36\text{-}5)$$

where:

E = emission rate
C = concentration
Q = dilution ventilation rate in the same units as E

Emission and ventilation rates are usually expressed as cubic feet per minute (cfm), actual feet per minute (acfm) when the air density correction factor has been applied or standard cubic feet per minute (scfm) when standard air conditions (STP) are assumed. In the SI system, the traditional units are cubic meters per second.

Contaminants in air must be diluted to below some acceptable concentration, C_a. C_a is usually chosen by the industrial hygienist as some fraction of a published OEL or other exposure standard.

Selection Criteria: Is Dilution Ventilation the Best Primary Control Option?

Dilution ventilation is not always the most appropriate *primary* control. Table 36.2 shows typical selection criteria for dilution ventilation as the primary approach to emission and exposure control. When conditions in the second category of the table prevail, costs and energy consumption will be high. If the outside air is more contaminated, for example, dilution cannot be achieved unless the outdoor air is scrubbed of those air contaminants. Source removal, LEV, generation control, substitution, or other forms of primary control should be considered, possibly with dilution ventilation as a secondary control.

In the vast majority of cases the outside air will be less contaminated than indoor air. Researchers report, however, that outdoor concentrations of the reactive gases sulfur dioxide and ozone often are greater than indoor concentrations in commercial buildings. Another exception occurs when there is an outdoor source near an air intake, such as a truck idling next to a building air intake, in which case the outdoor concentrations of carbon monoxide, nitrogen oxides, and smoke may be higher than those in indoor air. Also, summertime concentrations of mold spores and pollen are often greater outdoors than indoors.

Air contaminants emitted from an industrial process, plus carbon monoxide, nitrogen oxides, and respirable dust concentrations are usually greater inside the building. But this may be reversed if significant outdoor sources exist. For example, when the wind blows in a dry climate, outdoor levels of dust may exceed indoor dust concentrations. Or, if a parking garage is attached to a building, outside air concentrations of carbon monoxide may be higher. Air concentrations of total volatile organic compounds (TVOC), carbon dioxide, formaldehyde, radon, and environmental tobacco smoke concentrations are almost always greater indoors than outdoors.

Table 36.2 — Conditions Favorable and Unfavorable for Dilution Ventilation as the Primary Control

Certain conditions lend themselves to dilution with outdoor air:

Indoor air contaminants are of relatively low toxicity or cause minor irritation.
Contaminant concentrations in occupant air are not hazardous.
Smoking is not allowed in the occupied space.
Emission sources are difficult or expensive to remove or control.
Emission rates occur uniformly over time.
Emission sources are widely dispersed.
Emissions do not occur close to the breathing zone of occupants (using the IH definition of breathing zone).
Moderate climatic conditions prevail.
The outside air is less contaminated than the inside air.
The HVAC system is capable of conditioning the dilution air required.

This means dilution ventilation is less effective and more expensive when:

Air contaminants are highly toxic or irritating materials.
Contaminant concentrations are hazardous or cause great discomfort.
Smoking is allowed in the occupied space.
Emission sources are easy to remove or control.
Emission rates vary with time.
Emission sources consist of large, point sources.
People's breathing zones are in the immediate vicinity of emission sources (using the IH definition of a breathing zone).
The building is located in severe climates.
The outside air is more contaminated than the inside air.
The existing HVAC system is not capable of conditioning the outside air.

Case Study 1. Employees of a new office building were complaining about "bad air." Specific complaints included headache, watery eyes, irritation of the nose and throat, and dry, itchy skin. The industrial hygienist was asked to investigate and determine if additional dilution ventilation was appropriate.

Outcome. The industrial hygienist found that at the end of the day carbon dioxide totaled about 1200 ppm in the return air plenum. No specific chemical or biogenic sources, indoors or outdoors, were immediately obvious. However, the building was only six weeks old. The measured carbon dioxide concentration suggested insufficient outside air to dilute airborne contaminants. The fact that this was a new building suggested the problem of off-gassing. Recently built heating, ventilating, and air conditioning (HVAC) systems are usually capable of providing more air and better distribution than in the past. The industrial hygienist recommended that during the first 4–6 months of occupancy, the system be set to deliver 100% fresh air.

Case Study 2. A Los Angeles-based computer components firm operated 15 small dip tanks in a room adjacent to a set of offices. Although the dip tanks were enclosed and provided with local exhaust ventilation, both plant and office employees were concerned about potential exposure because the building's air handling unit (AHU) served both the office and the production area. An occasional "chemical" odor infiltrated the office area from the tank room. Plant employees were concerned about fugitive emissions from the tanks and office employees were asking for more dilution air. The industrial hygienist performed an problem characterization study following the procedure outlined in Chapter 35.

Outcome. Traditional IH testing determined that the fugitive emissions from the tanks were at a concentration above the odor threshold, but employee exposures were well below appropriate OELs. Improving the local exhaust ventilation with additional baffles alongside the tanks helped reduce fugitive emissions but did not entirely eliminate them. Complaints in the office were alleviated by additional dilution ventilation which reduced exposure concentrations to below odor and irritation thresholds. Other control solutions could have included isolating the office HVAC system from the tank area AHU, isolating the tank area from the rest of the building, and moving the tank operation or the offices to another building but none were considered cost-effective.

Implementing Dilution Ventilation

If preliminary indications point to dilution as a primary control measure, the industrial hygienist should develop the following information: (1) a profile of the contaminant sources; (2) an estimate of emission rates; (3) a description of the space (e.g, volume); (4) an acceptable concentration for exposure; and (5) an appropriate air dilution flowrate.

Sources. A basic understanding of emission sources should be obtained, if possible. Any information is better than none; intelligent professional judgment is better than no estimate. This information-gathering task includes descriptions of emission sources; chemical description of emissions to include chemical composition, size and shape, and temperature; current airborne concentrations; and rates of generation or evaporation over time.

Steady State Emission Rates. Estimating generation or evaporation rates for air contaminants requires ingenuity, detective work, and skill. Published emission factors are often used.

Once an estimate of the evaporation or generation rate is established, it is possible to estimate an emission rate as shown in Equation 36-6 which is based on the fundamental natural relationship that one pound-molecular weight (lb-mole) of a material will evaporate to fill 387 cubic feet of space. In SI units, one gram-mole evaporates to fill about 24.1 liters of air. These constants are true at the ventilation definition of STP. Dividing the emission volume by the time over which it evaporates provides the units of cubic feet per minute (or cubic meters per second), the same units used in ventilation for airflow.

$$E = \frac{387 \times G}{MW \times t \times d_C}\text{, in US Units} \qquad (36\text{-}6a)$$

$$E = \frac{0.0241 \times G}{MW \times t \times d_C}\text{, in SI Units} \qquad (36\text{-}6b)$$

Where:

E = volume rate of vapor emitted at STP conditions, $d_c = 1$; US units = ft^3/min, SI units = m^3/sec

G = generation or evaporation quantity; US units = lbs, SI units = grams

MW = molecular weight or molecular mass

t = approximate time of generation or evaporation, minutes (seconds)

d_c = density correction factor, unitless

Accuracy. Note that these calculations are considered to be "approximate" in most cases. Always use good judgment about the answers obtained.

The Space. Obtain all of the physical parameters of the building, its equipment and processes, and its occupants. Gather data on the occupied space, width, height, length, barriers, obstructions, and so forth. Building plans are often helpful.

Existing Ventilation and Air Movement. Identifying and understanding existing ventilation is important. This might include general heating and air conditioning ventilation, location of space heaters, open doors and windows, use of freestanding fans, LEV systems, and other dilution systems already in place. Prevailing air movement in the space, including the directions and velocities, should be identified. Ask about other times of the day, other seasons, and when the operation is running differently (for instance, what happens during very cold weather or when the local exhaust system is turned off).

Occupants. Obtain a thorough understanding of the physical locations of people; time considerations, such as how much time people spend in particular locations and how they interact with emission sources; and training, education, and cooperativeness.

Acceptable Concentration. As mentioned above, the industrial hygienist must determine an acceptable level of exposure. Usually it is some fraction of existing exposure standards (e.g., 10% of the OEL). Without an acceptable concentration, modeling is impossible, and predicting the benefits of dilution ventilation is difficult.

Dilution Ventilation Rates. Dilution air volumes should be based on the information developed above. The volume flow rate of air required to dilute a constant volume flow rate of emitted vapor can be approximated as follows:

$$Q_d = \frac{E \times K_{eff} \times 10^6}{C_a} \quad (36\text{-}7)$$

Where:

Q_d = volume flowrate of dilution air, scfm
E = emission rate of vapor, scfm
C_a = the acceptable exposure concentration, ppm
K_{eff} = a mixing factor to account for incomplete or poor delivery of dilution air to occupants

Air Mixing. The mixing of air is sometimes called the ventilation efficiency or the ventilation effectiveness factor. Mathematically, it can be stated as:

$$K_{eff} = \frac{\text{Actual } Q_d}{\text{Ideal } Q_d} \quad (36\text{-}8)$$

The value of K_{eff} ranges from 1.0 to 2 in most cases, with excursions to K =3 in some industrial applications. If it seems likely that $K_{eff} > 2$, improving mixing or identifying another form of control should be considered because dilution is likely to be too expensive, and the uncertainties are too high. Typical values for K_{eff} in commercial buildings are shown in Table 36.3.

Dilution will be more effective, and lower values of the mixing factor, K_{eff}, can be selected when (1) dilution air is routed through the occupied zone; (2) supply air is distributed where it will be most effective (e.g., a supply register serves every office); (3) returns are located as close to contaminant sources as possible; and (4) auxiliary or freestanding fans are used to enhance mixing.

Air Changes. Once the required dilution ventilation is known, the number of air changes per hour that will occur in the space being ventilated can be calculated. The concept of an air change does not imply that a complete change of all air in the space will occur. The percentage of air in the space which is exchanged depends on the airflow within the space, which will be influenced by the distribution and locations of the incoming and exiting air. In order to achieve equilibrium pressure, incoming and exiting air volumes must be balanced. Equation 36-9 shows how to calculate the number of air changes per hour (N) within a defined space.

$$N = \frac{Q_d \times 60}{V} \quad (36\text{-}9)$$

Where:

N = the number of air changes per hour
V = the volume of the space being ventilated

Example 36.2. Toluene evaporates into the workroom air from multiple locations of a coating process. An industrial hygienist is asked to evaluate and determine the requirements for adequate dilution ventilation.

Table 36.3 — Typical Mixing Factors for Commercial Buildings (for dilution of air contaminants)

K_{eff}	*Typical Conditions*
1.0	Wide open office spaces with good supply and return locations, all HVAC equipment function adequately; no point sources of emission.
1.1	Supply and return conditions not ideal but use of freestanding fans to create mixing; no point sources of emission.
1.2–1.4	Poor placement of supply and return registers; partitioned offices with generally adequate distribu tion of supply and return locations; discernable but small point sources; warm air supply and return in ceiling.
1.4 –2.0	Crowded spaces with tight partitions; poor supply and return locations; point sources of emission close to people; people located close to interior walls. Steps should be taken to improve mixing or use other emission and exposure control approaches.

Outcome. A problem characterization study produced the following estimates: Nine pounds of toluene are uniformly evaporated from the process during an 8-hour period. The workroom has excellent air mixing in its 125,000 cubic foot space. The air density correction factor for the location was determined to be 0.95. The IH suggested an acceptable concentration of 5% of the published OEL of 100 ppm.

Estimates for the volume flow rates (Q_d) required for dilution to the Ca are shown in the following equations using: G = 9 lbs; t = 480 minutes; OEL = 100 ppm; C_a = 5 ppm; K_{eff} = 1.0; d_c = 0.95; MW = 92.1; and workroom volume = 125,000 cubic feet. Using Equations 36-6 and 36-7:

$$E \approx \frac{387 \times 9}{92.1 \times 480 \times 0.95} \approx 0.08293 \text{ acfm}$$

And,

$$Q_d \approx \frac{0.08293 \times 1 \times 10^6}{5} \approx 16{,}600 \text{ acfm}$$

Then, the resulting number of air changes per hour can be determined:

$$N \approx \frac{16{,}600 \times 60}{125{,}000} \approx 8 \text{ air changes per hour}$$

Example 36.3. New particleboard wood shelving has been proposed for installation in a large office bay. The industrial hygienist was asked to estimate the volume flow rate of formaldehyde (HCHO) emitted and the dilution air volume flow rate required to keep background concentrations of HCHO at or below 0.05 ppm. Assume: STP, MW = 30, A = 250 m^2 of particleboard, C_a = 0.05 ppm, K_{eff} = 1.25.

Outcome. After searching product literature the industrial hygienist found the supplier's published emission rate for particleboard ranged from 2000 to 25,000 microgram per m^2 per day (24 h). To evaluate the worst case the IH assumed an HCHO emission rate for the first few weeks after installation of 25,000 micrograms/m^2/day.

Converting the units from micrograms/m^2/day to lbs/min:

$$\text{Emission rate} \approx \frac{(25{,}000\ \mu g/m^2/day) \times 250 m^2}{1{,}000{,}000 \frac{\mu g}{g} \times 454 \frac{g}{lb} \times \left(1440 \frac{min}{day}\right)}$$

$$\approx 9.56 \times 10^{-6} \text{ lb/min}$$

The emission rate is the weight of the generated contaminate over a period of time; this is equivalent to G/t in Equation 36-6. Therefore, the volume rate of vapor emitted can be determined by substituting this value into Equation 36-6:

$$E = \frac{387 \times G}{MW \times t \times d_c} = \frac{387}{MW \times d_c} \times \frac{G}{t}$$

$$E = \frac{387}{30 \times 1} \times 9.56 \times 10^{-6} = 1.23 \times 10^{-4} \text{ scfm}$$

The volume flow of dilution air required to maintain the background concentration below 0.05 ppm with this emission fate of contaminant can be determined using Equation 36-7.

$$Q_d = \frac{(1.23 \times 10^{-4}) \times 1.25 \times 10^6}{0.05} \approx 3{,}080 \text{ scfm}$$

Note that Example 36-3 considers the *worst case* scenario. The practical meaning of this calculation is that if the existing ventilation system is not capable of providing at least 3,080 cfm of fresh dilution air then some other solution will be required (e.g., emission-retarding coatings, alternative shelving materials, pre-installation airing, etc.).

Special Considerations when Ventilating for Comfort and Maintaining Good IAQ in Commercial Buildings

Heating, ventilating and air conditioning (HVAC) equipment is used for tempering, dehumidifying, and cleaning air for comfort, safety, and health. HVAC systems also may contribute to odor control and to maintenance of air contaminant levels at acceptable concentrations.

The widely used standard ASHRAE 55 has historically applied an 80/20/10 rule to establish satisfactory *comfort* performance. In this approach, if 80% of the occupants are satisfied with all environmental conditions (e.g., temperature, humidity, odor, drafts), or if less than 20% are dissatisfied, then comfort requirements have been met. If more than 10% are dissatisfied with any one condition, then satisfactory performance is not achieved.

HVAC engineers talk in terms of "zones." Each zone usually contains a thermostat to control temperature. The more zones there are, the better chance there is of providing satisfactory comfort conditions for more people. Typically, air in perimeter zones is harder to condition because of the required filtration, heating, cooling and humidity controls. Outdoor conditions (temperature, wind, sun, rain) can greatly impact the need for thermal conditioning. Interior zones often need only filtration and cooling and are not as impacted by outdoor conditions (see Figure 36.3).

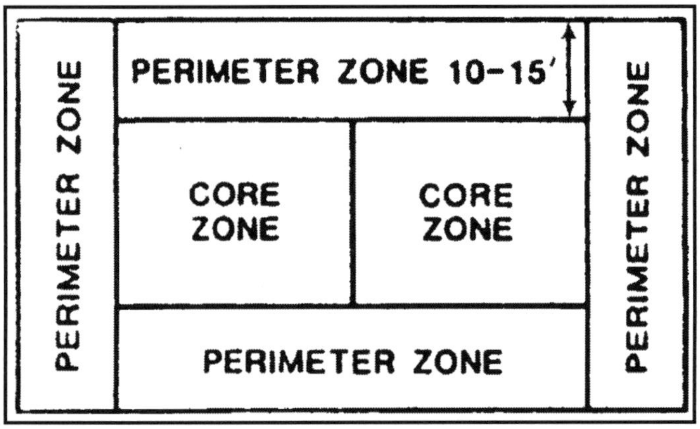

Figure 36.3 — Zones within an HVAC System.

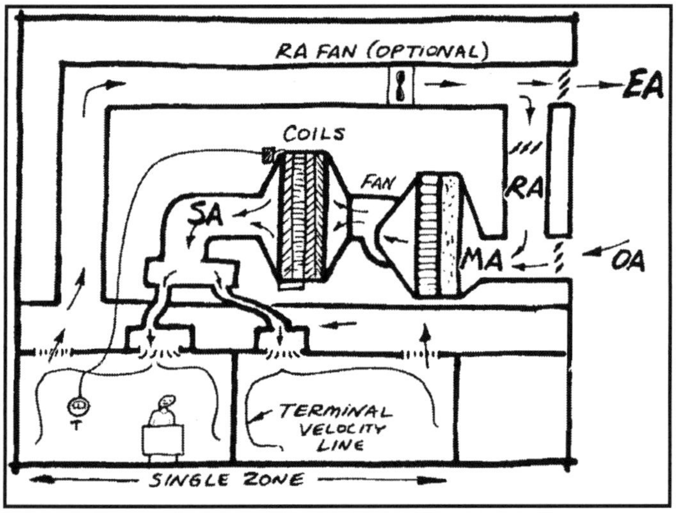

Figure 36.4 — Schematic Representatation of a Mechanical Room Containing HVAC Equipment and the Spaces It Serves.

When designing an adequate HVAC system, the combinations of air volume flowrate, temperature, humidity, and air quality which will satisfy the needs of the occupants of a space must be selected carefully. Air handling systems generally consist of:

- Outside air (OA) intakes, plenums and ducts
- Filters
- Supply air fans (SA)
- Heating and/or cooling coils
- Humidifying and/or dehumidifying equipment
- Supply air ducts (SA)
- Distribution plenums, ducts, terminal boxes or devices, supply registers
- Dampers
- Return air grilles, plenums and ducts (RA)
- Exhaust (or relief) air systems (EA)
- Controls and instrumentation

Figure 36.4 is a schematic of a simple, constant volume commercial HVAC system – a single-zone, constant air volume system (SZ-CAV) showing much of the equipment mentioned above. These systems supply a constant airflow to the space and vary the temperature and humidity.

Variable Air Volume (VAV) systems are often used because they provide energy conservation and lower operating costs. These systems supply a varying airflow to the space as a function of the need for temperature and humidity controls. Operating cost savings can be obtained, for example, when the VAV system actually reduces fan rpm. Air volume and fan rpm are linearly related; if the airflow is cut in half, then the rpm is cut in half. But horsepower and rpm are related through a third-power relationship. If the rpm is reduced by half, the horsepower (and energy costs) are reduced by about eight times. Simply reducing airflow with fan inlet dampers also results in lower motor operating costs and energy consumption, but not by the same factor as reducing fan rpm. See Reference 2 for more detail.

Common Problems with HVAC Systems

In many studies of IAQ problems, NIOSH has found that about 50% of IAQ problems and

Table 36.4 — Common Problems Found in HVAC Systems and their Typical Impacts

Inadequate design and/or poor operation - not enough dilution of air contaminants in occupied spaces
Inadequate replacement air supply - building under negative pressure, high concentrations of air contaminants
Poor distribution of supply air in the space - certain areas receive little air exchange
Insufficient air delivery, or not delivered appropriately, or not mixed in the space - stuffiness
Improper pressure differences - doors hard to open, outside air leaking into/through building envelope
Temperature extremes - too hot or too cold
Humidity extremes - too dry or too humid
Poor filtration -dirt, bugs, pollen in air delivery system
Poor maintenance - equipment not functioning correctly
Energy conservation has become No. 1 priority - reduction of outdoor air delivery rates
Settled water in system - mold
Visual evidence of slime or mold - odors, spores, complaints
Improper balance of distribution system — some areas do not receive sufficient outdoor air
Dampers at incorrect positions — some areas do not receive sufficient outdoor air
Supply terminal diffusers not at correct positions — inadequate distribution of supply air
VAV systems capable of shutting down air delivery — occupants do not receive sufficient SA and OA

complaints originated in the HVAC system itself. Common problems with HVAC systems that result IAQ complaints are shown in Table 36.4.

Estimating the Amount of Outdoor Air (OA) Required

The ASHRAE standard 62-2010 on IAQ suggests an "air per person" and "air per square foot" approach for determining the minimum amount of OA to be supplied to various occupancies for dilution purposes, see Table 36.5. The ASHRAE standard assumes excellent mixing, distribution and delivery of the outdoor air to occupants. It also assumes a certain occupant loading. Where these are not the case, additional OA may be required or better mixing and distribution provided. In cases where definitive data are not available, the designer/user can use default values.

This approach recognizes that air pollutants also arise from non-people sources: building materials, furnishings, and the HVAC equipment itself. However, the approach decreases the total amount of outdoor air historically required for some occupancies of interest to industrial hygienists. However, these are minimums and can be adjusted upward as the need arises.

In its simplest form, the amount of air to be supplied is estimated by an equation similar to that shown below.

$$Q_{OA} = Q_p + Q_b = R_pP_d + R_bA_b \qquad (36\text{-}10)$$

Where:

Q_{OA} = minimum design OA ventilation rate
Q_p = ventilation required to control "people" sources of air contaminants
Q_p = ventilation required to control "building" sources of air contaminants
R_p = minimum rate of outdoor air in cfm per person
P_d = number of people in the occupied area
R_b = minimum rate of outdoor air in cfm per square foot of occupied area
A_b = floor area in occupied portion of the building, square feet

Example 36.4. In an 2,000 sq ft office space with 14 occupants, the minimum required ventilation rate to the occupied zone can be determined using Equation 36-10.

Table 36.5 — Sample of ASHRAE 62-2010 Standard Table 6.1

Application	*Default Occupancy Persons per 1000 sf*	*Default Outdoor Air (OA) cfm/person*	*— Required Ventilation Rates — cfm OA /person + cfm/ft²*
Office Space	5	17	5 + 0.06
Conference Room	50	6	5 + 0.06
Science Lab (school)	25	17	10 + 0.18

Q_{OA} = (5)(14) + (0.06)(2000) =
190 cfm of fresh outdoor air

This results in an OA rate (OA/person) of 13.6 cfm/person, slightly less than traditional standard minimum of 15–20 cfm/person.

Example 36.5. To provide sufficient outdoor air in a conference rooms the proposed ventilation rates are 5 cfm/person and 0.06 cfm/sq ft. For a small conference room of 750 sq ft occupied by 30 occupants, the minimum required ventilation rate is:

Q_{OA} = (5)(30) + (0.06)(750) =
195 cfm of fresh outdoor air

This results in a OA rate (OA/person) of 6.5 cfm/person.

In certain circumstances, ASHRAE 62–2010 also requires the application of the ventilation effectiveness factor to account for poor mixing or distribution of the air. A typical default value for K_{eff} is 1.2. Additionally, the designer may have to take into account occupant population diversity and other factors in the space which also could increase the amount of air required. See Reference 5 for additional details.

Example 36.6. Continuing with Example 36.4, if the ventilation effectiveness factor for air distribution and mixing is estimated to be 80%, or K_{eff} =1.25, what is the required total outdoor ventilation rate?

Total $Q_{OA} = Q_{OA} \times K_{eff}$ = (190)(1.25) =
238 cfm of fresh outdoor air

This results in a total OA rate per person of 17 cfm/person.

Estimating the Amount of Outdoor Air (OA) Being Delivered

In addition to the traditional approach of for estimating the volumetric flow of air by measuring the air velocity in and the area of ductwork (see Chapter 38), it is possible to estimate the percentage of outdoor air (OA) in the supply air (SA) by measuring temperatures or carbon dioxide content of the various air streams at the HVAC equipment. The following ratios show the fractions of outdoor air (OA) in the supply air (SA). Figure 36.4 shows the locations of OA, SA, MA, and RA.

$$\%OA = \frac{Q_{OA}}{Q_{SA}} \times 100 \qquad (36\text{-}11)$$

$$\%OA = \frac{T_{RA}-T_{MA}}{T_{RA}-T_{OA}} \times 100 \qquad (36\text{-}12)$$

$$\%OA = \frac{C_{RA}-C_{SA}}{C_{RA}-C_{OA}} \times 100 \qquad (36\text{-}13)$$

Where:

Q_{OA} = volume of outdoor air (cfm)
Q_{SA} = volume of mixed return and outside air, the supply air (cfm)
T_{RA} = temperature of return air (dry-bulb)
T_{MA} = temperature of mixed return and outside air, the supply air (dry-bulb)
T_{OA} = temperature of outdoor air (dry-bulb)
C_{RA} = concentration of CO_2 in return air (ppm)
C_{SA} = concentration of CO_2 in supply air (ppm)
C_{OA} = concentration of CO_2 in outdoor air (ppm)

Example 36.8. The design air volume flow rates at an air handling unit (AHU) are as follows: Q_{SA} = 12,500 scfm, and Q_{OA} = 1600 cfm. What percentage of OA would be expected from this design? If the intended number of employees served by the AHU is 90, how much air per person will be delivered?

$$\%OA = \frac{1600}{12500} \times 100 = 12.8\%$$

The Q_{OA} per occupant (1600 cfm/90 people) from this design would be approximately 18 cfm/person.

Example 36.9. Assume the following wintertime temperatures were measured by an IH at the HVAC system in an office building: T_{RA} = 74°F, T_{MA} = 66°F, and T_{OA} = 40°F. Use these temperature measurements to estimate the percentage of outdoor air entering the system.

$$\%OA = \frac{74 - 66}{74 - 40} \times 100 \approx 24\%$$

In addition to the temperature measurements, CO_2 levels were also measured at the same locations: $C_{RA} \approx 870$ ppm, $C_{SA} \approx 750$ ppm, and $C_{OA} \approx 410$ ppm. These values also can be used to estimate the percentage of outdoor air in the system.

$$\%OA = \frac{870 - 750}{870 - 410} \times 100 \approx 26\%$$

Measured carbon dioxide concentrations can also be used to estimate the amount of OA reaching a specific area of the building. During the day, carbon dioxide tends to build up to some steady state concentration, e.g., from 450 ppm in the early morning before workers arrive to a fairly constant 950 ppm at noon. When everyone leaves the building, and the carbon dioxide sources are gone, the outside air will dilute carbon dioxide at an exponential rate depending on the volume of OA being delivered. Knowing initial and final concentrations and the time elapsed, the following formulas can be used to predict the volume flow of OA delivered. The outdoor concentration of carbon dioxide must be measured because that will affect the rate at which the inside CO_2 concentration can drop.

$$N \approx \frac{\ln C_i - \ln C_t}{T} \qquad (36\text{-}14)$$

$$Q_{OA} = \frac{N \times V_R}{60} \qquad (36\text{-}15)$$

Where:

- N = air exchange per hour of fresh outdoor air (OA), ac/hr
- C_i = Initial concentration of CO_2 at start of test (minus the outdoor air concentration, usually about 400 ppm)
- C_t = Concentration of CO_2 at end of test (minus the outdoor air concentration)
- T = time elapsed between start and end of test in hours
- V_R = volume of space in cubic feet

Example 36.10. The carbon dioxide concentration is measured at 1200 ppm at 5:30 pm, when all of the people have departed a small office building. The air handler is left to run in its normal operating mode. By 7:30 pm, the CO_2 concentration has been reduced to 500 ppm. The outside CO_2 concentration is 400 ppm. How many air changes per hour of OA does this suggest? What is the Q_{OA} for a space with a volume of 50,000 cu ft?

$$N \approx \frac{\ln(1200 - 400) - \ln(500 - 400)}{2} =$$

1.04 air changes/hr

$$Q_{OA} = \frac{1.04 \times 50000}{60} \approx 870 \text{ cfm}$$

The discussion and examples in this chapter have assumed steady state conditions for emission source and dilution ventilation rates. Additional references are available to provide information on the exponential buildup and decay of airborne concentrations during non-steady conditions. Additional information on the properties and behavior of water in air (i.e., humidity concerns; psychrometrics) is provided in Reference 2 and References 4–7.

References

1. **Burton, D.J.:** *Industrial Ventilation Workbook,* 7th edition. Bountiful, UT: IVE, Inc., 2011.
2. **Burton, D.J.:** *IAQ and HVAC Workbook,* Burton, D. Jeff, 4th edition. IVE, Inc. Bountiful, UT.
3. **American Conference of Governmental Industrial Hygienists (ACGIH®):** *Industrial Ventilation, a Manual of Recommended Practice for Design,* 27th edition. Cincinnati, OH: ACGIH®, 2010.
4. **American Society of Heating, Refrigeration, and Air-Conditioning Engineers (ASHRAE):** *ANSI/ASHRAE 55-2004, Thermal Environmental Conditions for Human Occupancy.* Atlanta, GA: ASHRAE, 1992.
5. **American Society of Heating, Refrigeration, and Air-Conditioning Engineers (ASHRAE):** *ANSI/ASHRAE 62–2010, Ventilation for Acceptable Indoor Air Quality.* Atlanta, GA: ASHRAE, 2010.

6. **National Institute for Occupational Safety and Health (NIOSH) and U.S. Environmental Protection Agency (EPA):** *Building Air Quality: A Guide for Building Owners and Facility Managers.* Washington, D.C.: NIOSH and EPA: (EPA/400/1-91-033). Government Printing Office, 1991.
7. **American Society of Heating, Refrigeration, and Air-Conditioning Engineers (ASHRAE):** *ASHRAE Fundamentals Handbook*, latest edition; American Society of Heating, Refrigerating and Air Conditioning Engineers (ASHRAE): Atlanta, GA: 2009.
8. **American Industrial Hygiene Association (AIHA):** ANSI/AIHA Z9 standards (Z9.1–2006 (Ventilation and Control of Airborne Contaminants During Open-Surface Tank Operations); Z9.2–2006 (Fundamentals Governing the Design and Operation of Local Exhaust Ventilation Systems); Z9.3–2007 (Spray Finishing Operations: Safety Code for Design, Construction, and Ventilation); Z9.5–2003 (Laboratory Ventilation); Z9.6–2008 (Exhaust Systems for Grinding, Polishing, and Buffing); Z9.7–2007 (Recirculation of Air from Industrial Process Exhaust Systems); Z9.9–2010 (Portable Ventilation Systems); Z9.10–2010 (Fundamentals Governing the Design and Operation of Dilution Ventilation Systems in Industrial Occupancies). Fairfax, VA: AIHA.

Chapter 37

Outcome Competencies

After completing this chapter, the reader should be able to:

1. Understand and use terms and concepts introduced in this chapter.
2. Describe performance characteristics of ducts, hoods, fans and stacks.
3. Apply basic approaches to local exhaust ventilation system design and operation.
4. Calculate airflow requirements for specific process hood applications.
5. Estimate pressure and air flow requirements for selecting fans.

Prerequisite Knowledge

Prior to beginning this chapter, the user should review the following chapters:

Chapter Number	Chapter Topic
7	Principles of Evaluating Worker Exposure
8	Occupational and Environmental Health Risk Assessment
35	General Methods for the Control of Airborne Hazards
36	Dilution Ventilation

Key Terms

air cleaner • baffle • capture velocity (Vc) • coefficient of entry • continuity equation • ducts • enclosing hood • exterior hood • fan • hood entry loss • hood face velocity (Vf) • local exhaust ventilation (LEV) • plenum • process hood • receiving hood • slot hood • stack • static pressure (SP) • static pressure losses • total pressure (TP) • velocity pressure (VP)

Key Topics

I. Introduction

II. Components of an LEV System
- A. Ductwork
- B. Hoods
- C. Fans
- D. Stacks
- E. Air Cleaners and Replacement and Makeup Air Systems
- F. Makeup Air Systems

Local Exhaust Ventilation

37

By D. Jeff Burton, CIH, PE

Introduction

A fundamental knowledge of common local exhaust ventilation (LEV) systems is important to every industrial hygienist. Although an IH may not have primary responsibility for designing an LEV system, most will find themselves recommending the installation of LEV systems as emission and exposure control measures, reviewing drawings and specifications for proposed LEV systems, proposing specialized LEV equipment, testing and troubleshooting existing LEV systems, and even explaining why existing LEV systems are ineffective in controlling emissions.

It is important to read or review Chapters 35 and 36 before beginning this chapter. Discussions of air density correction presented in Chapter 35, for example, are necessary to the understanding of LEV system design, operation and evaluation.

This chapter is written for the practicing IH and is intended to help the IH apply basic LEV ventilation principles. Theory and the derivation of equations are covered in more depth in the references. What is presented in this chapter is thought to be compatible with current standards of good practice as described in References 1–9. However, the IH should always review current standards and consult with experts before applying the principles presented herein.

Components of an LEV System

Traditionally, the five fundamental components of a local exhaust system have included the ductwork, hoods, an air cleaner, a fan, and a stack, as shown in Figure 37.1. Figure 37.2 shows the makeup air system as an important sixth component which is not often mentioned. This chapter introduces each of these six components. A critical seventh component, real-time performance monitoring, is covered in Chapter 38. Additional detailed information on each component is found in the References.

Ductwork

Pressure Differences Induce Airflow

Air moves under the influence of pressure differences. At sea level the standard barometric pressure is 14.73 psia (or 29.92 inches Hg or 407 inch w.g.). Within a ventilation system a fan is commonly used to create the pressure difference. See Table 36.1 and Chapter 36 for more information on standard conditions. In ventilation, the barometric pressure can be thought of as the absolute static pressure.

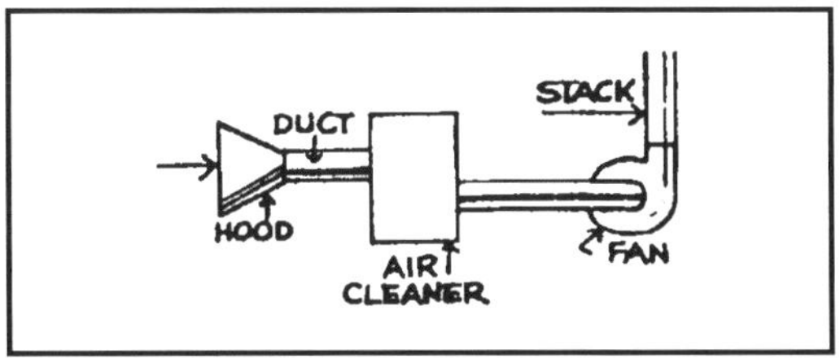

Figure 37.1 — Five basic components of an LEV system.

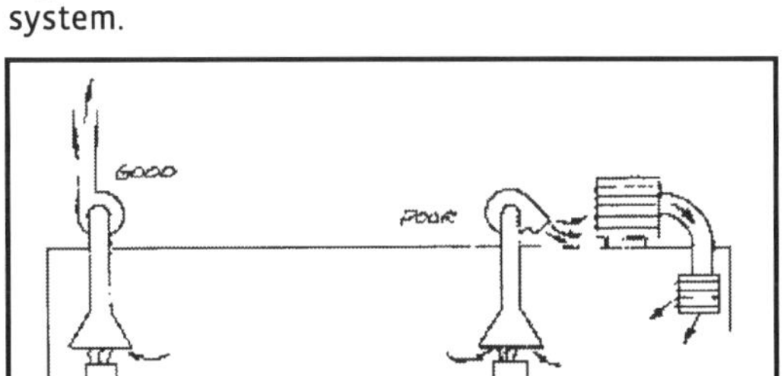

Figure 37.2 — Replacement air must be suitably provided for all air exhausted.

If a fan is capable of reducing the barometric pressure by one inch of water column (which also can be stated as creating one inch of negative static pressure, e.g., 1 inch w.g., or one inch water gauge), then the absolute static pressure in the duct will be reduced to 406 inches w.g. (or, about 29.85 inch Hg). Figures 37.3 and 37.4 show examples of the pressure changes upstream and downstream of the fan.

The absolute static pressure (SP) is created by gravity and modified by the fan. SP is felt in all directions within the duct, and is measured in a way, as shown in Figures 37.3 and 37.4, that the flow of air does not impact the measurement. It is important to note that negative static pressure tends to want to collapse the duct, while a positive static pressure wants to blow it up like a balloon.

Figure 37.5 shows some basic relationships between pressure types that can be measured with a manometer. If the manometer tube is inserted into the duct so that it faces directly into the air stream, the manometer will measure both static pressure and the pressure of the air impacting the end of the probe. This combination of pressures is known as the Total Pressure (TP). The pressure component solely attributed to the air impact is called the Velocity Pressure (VP). The velocity pressure is determined by subtracting the average static pressure from the average total pressure. The relationship between these pressures is:

$$VP = TP - SP \tag{37-1}$$

The traditional sign convention, which are relative to the absolute pressure, for each of the pressure measurements on either side of the fan are shown in Table 37.1.

An ASTM Standard Pitot Tube is the primary device used to measure TP and SP in a ventilation system. Attaching the legs of the pitot tube to a manometer in various ways allows for measurement of TP, SP, and VP. For example, attaching both legs of the pitot tube to the manometer will measure VP. The proper connections for making these pressure measurements with the pitot tube are shown in Figures 37.7 and 37.8. Arms that are

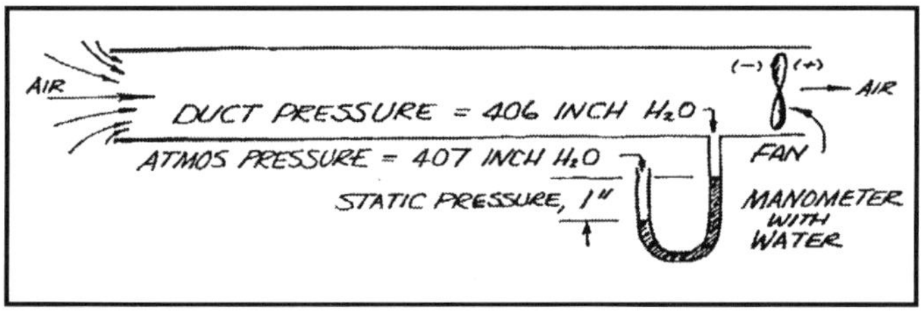

Figure 37.3 — Static pressure relationships in a duct.

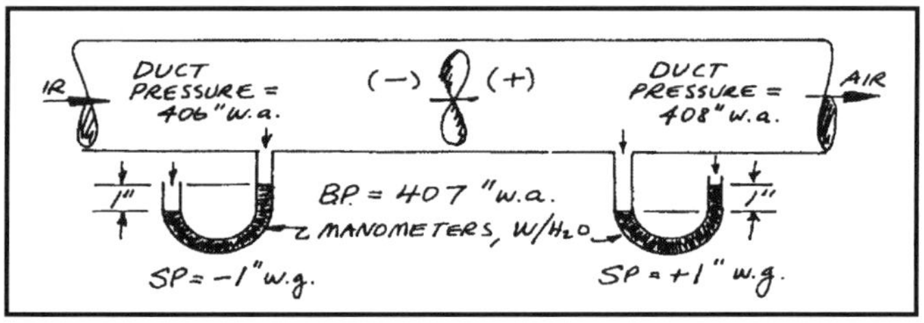

Figure 37.4 — Static pressure relationship upstream and downstream of fan.

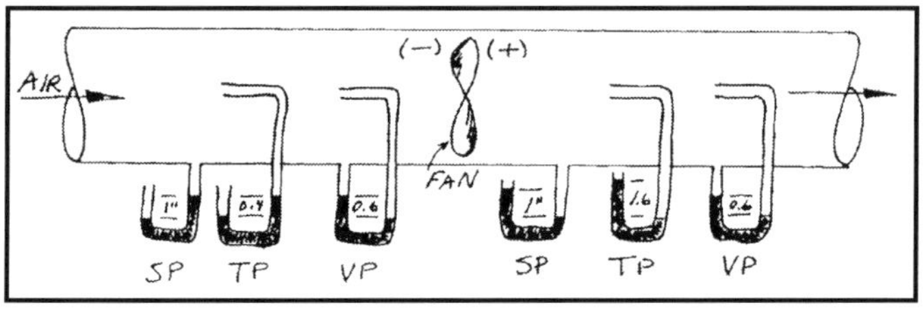

Figure 37.5 — Measuring TP, SP, and VP using manometers.

Table 37.1 — Normal Sign Convention for TP = SP + VP

	TP	*SP*	*VP*
Upstream	-	-	+
Downstream	+	+	+

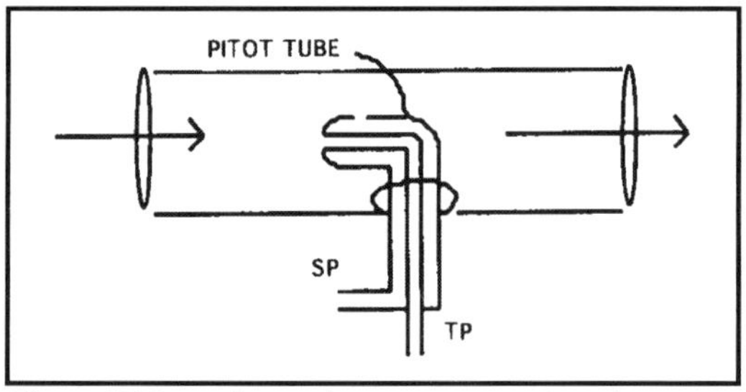

Figure 37.6 — Pitot tube measures SP and TP.

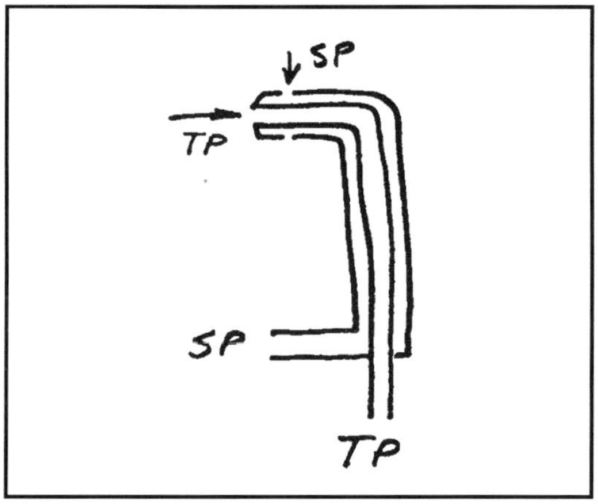

Figure 37.7 — Location of SP and TP measurements on a pitot tube.

not connected to the manometer are open to atmosphere, so the measurement is relative to the atmospheric pressure.

Additional information about testing and monitoring of ventilation systems is presented in Chapter 38.

Example 37.1. An IH measured the average values of TP and SP in a ventilation duct using a pitot tube and water manometer. How would the IH measure TP? SP? Determine the velocity pressure, VP, if the measurements for TP was –1.15" w.g., and for SP was –1.50" w.g.

Outcome. TP was measured by attaching only the top arm of the pitot tube to the manometer. Attaching only the side arm provided a measurement of SP. Equation 37.1 was used to determine the VP:

$$VP = (-1.15) - (-1.50) = 0.35\text{" w.g.}$$

In addition to providing the value for the VP, it is important to indicate that the measurements were made upstream of the fan.

Static Pressure as the Engine of the System

Static pressure can be thought of as the potential energy of the ventilation system. Similarly, it can be thought of as being converted to kinetic energy in the form of VP and other useless forms of energy, such as heat, vibration, and noise, which are known as the "losses" of the system. Losses include friction loss, turbulence losses, *vena contracta* losses, etc. Static pressure losses are discussed in more detail below.

Velocity Pressure and Velocity

Velocity pressure, VP, is directly related to the velocity of air in the duct. The relationship is a form of Bernoulli's Equation, a fundamental natural relationship discovered about 300 years ago and which relates velocity of a fluid to its velocity pressure:

$$V = 4005\sqrt{\left[\frac{VP}{d_c}\right]} \qquad (37\text{-}2)$$

Where,

- V = velocity, feet per minute (fpm)
- VP = velocity pressure (inch w.g.)
- d_c = density correction factor (unitless)

Example 37-2. The velocity pressure of an airstream in a duct is measured using a pitot tube and manometer. If the average VP was 0.22 inches w.g., then what is the average velocity in the duct? Assume a density correction factor of 0.95.

Outcome. Equation 37-2 can be used to determine the velocity from the pressure measurements.

$$V = 4005\sqrt{\left[\frac{0.22}{0.95}\right]} = 1927 \text{ fpm} \approx 1900 \text{ fpm}$$

Air Volume Flowrate

The fundamental relationship which describes air flowrate is sometimes referred to as the continuity equation or conservation of mass theorem. This relationship states that the mass rate of airflow remains constant as it moves along its path. For any two points in the air stream (e.g., in a duct), the relationship can be expressed as

$$V_1A_1\partial_1 = V_2A_2\partial_2 \qquad (37\text{-}3a)$$

where

- A = cross-sectional area through which the air moves (ft^2)
- ∂ = a measure of air density (lb/ft^3)

For almost all industrial applications, ∂ is relatively constant because the absolute (static or barometric) pressure within a ventilation system varies over a very narrow range (usually less than a few percent of ambient barometric pressure) and the air is assumed to be essentially incompressible. Therefore,

$$V_1A_1 = V_2A_2 \qquad (37\text{-}3b)$$

Note that the combination of velocity and area results in units of cubic feet per minute (cfm), a unit of flowrate designated in this chapter as Q. Therefore,

$$Q = VA \qquad (37\text{-}3c)$$

Where

- Q = volume flow rate, cubic feet per minute, cfm

The unit cfm is usually written as *scfm* for flow assumed to be at standard conditions and *acfm* for flow at actual conditions following the correction for air density.

Example 37.3. The cross-sectional area of a round 12-inch diameter duct is 0.7854 square feet. The average velocity of air flowing in the duct is 3,300 feet per minute. What is the volume flow rate (Q) through the duct? Assume a density correction factor of 1.

Outcome. The volume flow of air through the duct can be determined using Equation 37-3c.

$$Q = 3300 \text{ fpm} \times 0.7854 \text{ ft}^2 = 2591 \text{ scfm} \approx 2600 \text{ scfm}$$

Example 37.4. Using a pitot tube and manometer, an IH measures the average static and total pressures in a 14-inch diameter round duct. The IH is interested in determining the average velocity pressure, the average velocity, and the approximate air volume flow rate in the duct. The dc is assumed to be 0.95.

Outcome. The measured values for SP and TP were –1.15" w.g. and –0.85" w.g., respectively. The first step was to determine the cross sectional area of the 14 inch (1.167 ft)diameter duct in units of square feet:

$$A = \pi\left[\frac{D}{2}\right]^2 = \pi\left[\frac{1.167}{2}\right]^2 = 1.069 \text{ ft}^2$$

The velocity pressure can be determined using Equation 37.1:

$$VP = -0.85 — 1.15 = 0.30\text{" w.g.}$$

Once the VP is known, then the velocity can be determined using Equation 37-2:

$$V = 4005\sqrt{\left[\frac{0.30}{0.95}\right]} = 2250 \text{ fpm}$$

Finally, A and V can be used in Equation 37.3c to calculate the volume flow rate throught the duct:

$$Q = (2250)(1.069) = 2405 \text{ acfm} \approx 2400 \text{ acfm}$$

Ductwork and Static Pressure Losses

The duct has two functions: (1) to carry static pressure from the fan to the hood and (2) to convey or transport air contaminants through the system to the air cleaner and/or to the atmosphere through the stack. Table 37.2 provides recommended transport (or scrubbing) velocities normally thought to be necessary to carry dry particles through ventilation system without significant settling in the duct.

As the air moves through the duct and other ventilation system fittings and components, losses are created when static pressure is converted to heat, vibration, or noise. Many static pressure losses have been found to be directly related to duct velocity pressure. This means that if duct velocity pressure doubles, static pressure losses will also double for most fittings. This relationship can be expressed as:

$$SP_{loss} = F \times VP \times d_c \qquad (37\text{-}4)$$

where

SP_{loss} = loss of static pressure (inches w.g.)
F = loss factor or coefficient (unitless)

Table 37.2 — Typical Transport or Scrubbing Velocities for Particles in Ductwork

Materials	*Velocity (fpm)*
Very fine, very light dusts	2000
Fine dusts and powders	3000
Medium industrial dusts	3500
Coarse dusts	4000–4500
Heavy dusts	5000
Abrasive blasting dust	4500
Carbon black	3500
Clay	3500
Coal, fine powder	4000
Cotton dust	3000
Flour dust	2500
Foundry, general	4000
Foundry, tumbling mills	5000
Grain dust	3000
Grinding, general	4000–4500
Metal fumes	2500
Paper dust	3500
Plastics buffing dust	4000
Sandblast dust	4000
Sander dust	3000
Silica dust	4000
Soldering and tinning	2500
Tailpipe exhaust	3000

Sources: References 1-4

Major loss types include <u>hood entry loss</u>, friction loss, elbow loss, branch entry loss, system effect loss, and air cleaner loss. Published values of F (sometimes listed as K) for a wide range of fittings (elbows, branch entries, hood entries, duct friction, air cleaners, stacks) are available in the literature. Examples of these loss factors are shown in Figures 37.8 and 37.9; additional information can be found in References 1 and 2.

As mentioned in the previous section, velocity pressure is produced from the conversion of static pressure. The maximum velocity pressure possible is the available static pressure, minus any losses:

$$VP = |SP_h| - H_e \quad (37\text{-}5)$$

Where:

SP_h = hood static pressure (inch w.g.)
H_e = hood entry losses (inch w.g.)

Example 37.5. A fan, shown in Figure 37.10, is attached to connecting ductwork and a laboratory hood. It develops a negative static pressure of three inches of water at the inlet to the fan. After the losses of the duct system are deducted, one inch of negative static pressure is available in the ductwork

Type of hood	Other	Typical F	Typical Ce	Approximate Q	Notes
Duct End (round)	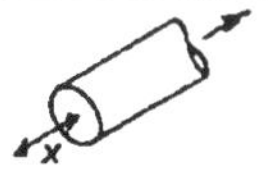	0.93	0.72	$4\pi X^2 V_c$ or $(10X^2+A_f)V_c$	Flange if possible Vc = capture velocity at distance X
Flanged Duct End (round)	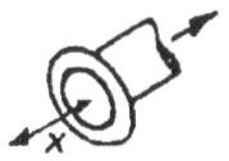	0.50	0.82	$3\pi X^2 V_c$ or $0.75(10X^2+A_f)V_c$	Flange width, W = X - 0.5D
Welding hood, portable	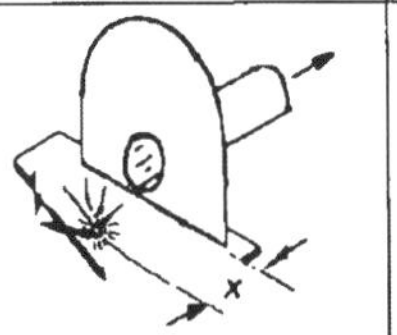	0.50	0.82	140X - 400 (cfm)	Make hood compatible with worker needs; equation is for flanged hood laying on or near welding table. empirical equation.
General dip tank hood (not in cleanroom)	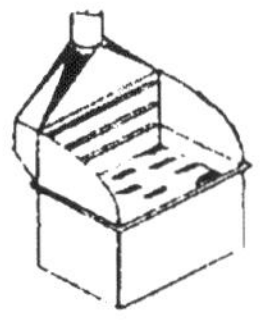 STO TTO	slot duct 1.78 0.50 1.78 0.25	--	$0.5\pi XLVc$	Vc = capture velocity at tank edge, distance X Capture velocity: 75-125 fpm Slot velocity:1500-2000 fpm TTO = tapered duct takekoff STO = straight duct takeoff Flange ends; Plenum ht ≥ 2'; Tank depth ≤ 2';
Bypass Type Lab Fume Hood	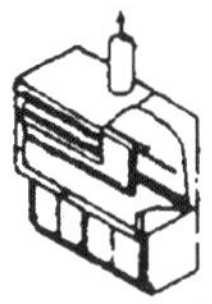	2	0.58	$80A_{face}$ to $120A_{face}$	Check w/ hood manuf. for actual F and Ce A_{face} = open area of hood face
Tapered Hood	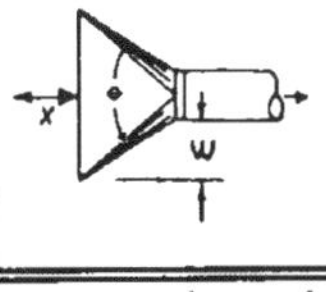 Included angle 30° 45° 60° 90° 120°	Rd Sq .08 .17 .06 .15 .08 .17 .15 .25 .26 .35	Rd Sq .96 .92 .97 .93 .96 .92 .93 .89 .89 .86	$3\pi X^2 V_c$ or $0.75(10X^2+A_f)V_c$	Flare to W where W = X - 0.5D

Figure 37.8 —Sampler of common hood parameters.

just downstream from the entry hood, this pressure is called the hood static pressure, SP_h. Based on this description and a hood entry loss of 0.40" w.g., how much velocity pressure can be produced at the hood entry to the duct?

Outcome. The velocity pressure generated from the static pressure after losses is calculated using the hood entry loss and the hood static pressure in Equation 37-5:

$$VP = |\,1\,| - 0.40 = 0.60\text{"w.g.}$$

Example 37.6. What is the static pressure loss through a mitre elbow where the average velocity pressure in the duct is 0.70 inch w.g.? Assume STP and a density correction factor of 1.

Outcome. The loss factor, F, for the mitre elbow can be found on Figure 37.8. Once F is known, then the SP_{loss} is determined using Equation 37-4.

$$SP_{loss} = 1.2 \times 0.70 \times 1 = 0.84\text{" w.g.}$$

Type:	Loss Factor, F: Smooth Transition (1)	Smooth Transition (2)	Mitre	3-piece	4-piece	5-piece
Round Duct R/D						
0.50	--	0.80	1.20	1.15	1.10	0.90
0.75	--	--	--	0.60	0.55	0.50
1.00	--	0.35	--	0.45	0.40	0.38
1.25	0.55	0.30	--	0.42	0.38	0.33
1.50	0.39	0.27	--	0.39	0.34	0.28
2.00	0.27	0.24	--	0.41	0.33	0.28
2.50	0.22	0.24	--	--	0.37	0.30

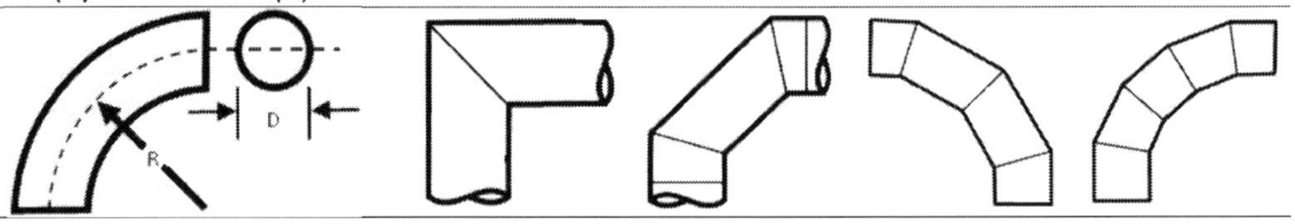

R = radius of curvature as number of duct diameters, radius to center-line of duct

(1) and (2) above represent range of sources

Loss Factor, F, includes friction loss

$SP_{loss} = F \times VP_d$

Branch Entry Losses

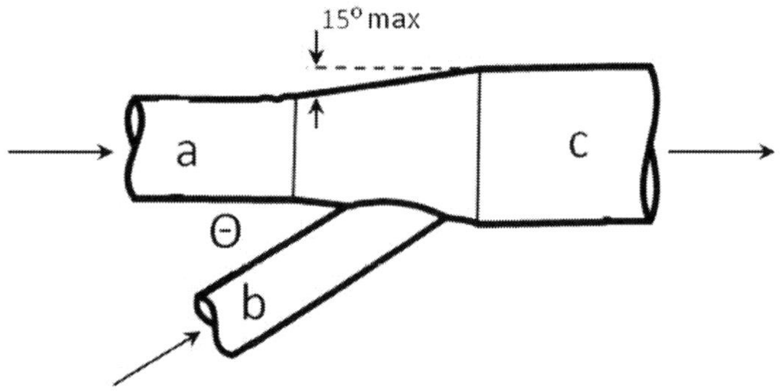

Θ	F
15	0.10
20	0.12
30	0.18
45	0.28

Loss occurs in branch B

Figure 37.9 — Sampler of loss factors for elbows and branch entries at STP.

In a similar manner, friction loss in ductwork can be approximated using the following equation.

$$SP_{loss} = F_f \times VP \times d_c \times L \times R \qquad (37\text{-}6)$$

where

SP_{Loss} = static pressure loss in ductwork due to friction (inch w.g.)
L = Length of Ductwork (feet)
R = a roughness correction factor for non-galvanized ductwork (unitless)
F_f = Loss factor per foot of length for galvanized duct (unitless)

Figure 37.11 shows a nomograph that provides flow parameters for air traveling in round ductwork at STP. The second column of each nomograph presents the friction loss factor, F, per length of duct. Typical roughness correction factors, R, are shown in Table 37.3. Reference 1 contains additional data. To use the nomograph in Figure 37.11, any two parameters must be known and plotted, then a straight line connects the two will intersect with the lines indicating the other parameter values.

Hoods

The hood must capture, contain, or receive contaminants generated at the emission source. There are three major hood types: *Enclosing, capture* (also, active, external), and *receiving* (also, passive). A lab fume hood is an enclosing hood; a welding snorkel hood is a capture hood; and a canopy hood over an hot-water open-surfaced tank is a receiving hood, for example. Additional examples of hood types are shown in Figure 37.13.

Table 37.3 — Typical Roughness Correction Factors for Ductwork.

Duct Material	*Correction Factor, R*
Galvanized duct	1.0
Smooth fiberglass, stainless steel, and ABS and PVC plastic	0.8–0.9
Spiral wound galvanized	1.1
Any flex duct (check with supplier)	2.5–8

See Reference 1, 2 and 7 for more detailed information.

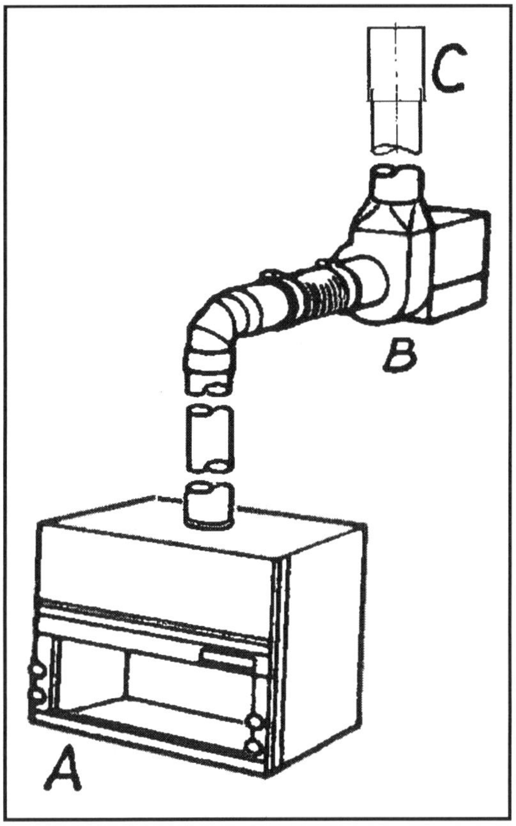

Figure 37.10 — Lab fume hood with connecting ductwork, fan, and stack.

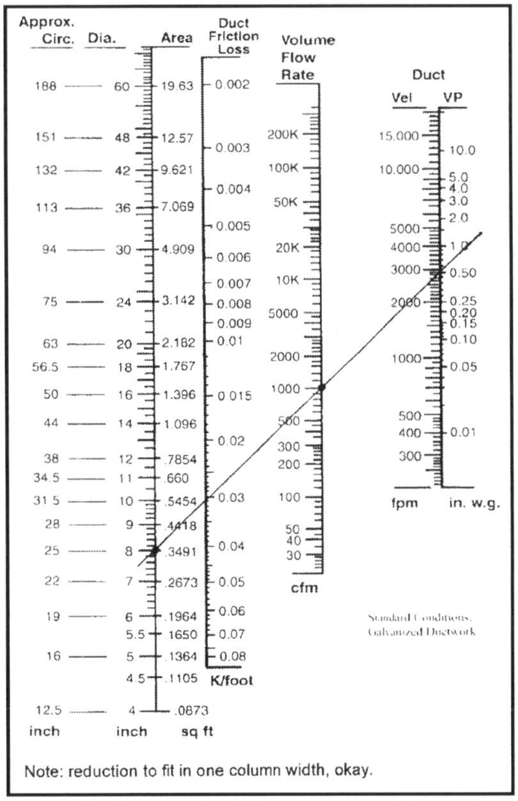

Figure 37.11 — Duct airflow nomograph including solution to Example 37.9.

Hood Entry Losses

As described above, the static pressure in the duct near the hood, usually measured a distance equal to 2-6 duct diameters downstream, is called the hood static pressure, SP_h and is shown in Figure 37.15.

The hood converts all available duct static pressure (SP_h) to duct velocity pressure (VP_{duct}) and hood entry losses, He. The entry losses may include losses associated with slots, duct entry, plenum baffles, filters and other equipment located in the air stream approaching the connecting duct. One major source of loss is the so-called *vena contracta* shown in Figure 37.14. Losses are caused by the narrowing of the airstream in a slot, duct entry or elsewhere in the entry.

Equations for estimating the hood entry loss can be expressed as a form of Equation 37-4 and Equation 37-5.

$$H_e = F \times VP \times d_c \qquad (37\text{-}7)$$

Combining Equations 37-5 and 37-7, provides another useful relationship:

$$|SP_h| = (1 + F) \times VP \times d_c \qquad (37\text{-}8)$$

The Coefficient of Entry (C_e) represents a hood's ability to convert static pressure to velocity pressure and is given by (use absolute value of SP_h):

$$C_e = \frac{Q_{actual}}{Q_{ideal}} \qquad (37\text{-}9)$$

$$C_e = \sqrt{\frac{VP}{SP_h}} \qquad (37\text{-}10)$$

$$C_e = \sqrt{\frac{1}{1 + F}} \qquad (37\text{-}11)$$

where

C_e = Coefficient of Entry (unitless)

$|SP_h|$ = absolute value of static pressure about 5 duct diameters down the duct from the hood (inch w.g.)

Q_{actual} = actual air flowrate

Q_{ideal} = ideal air flowrate if all of the SP at a hood were converted to VP

F_{hood} = loss factor F for a hood (unitless)

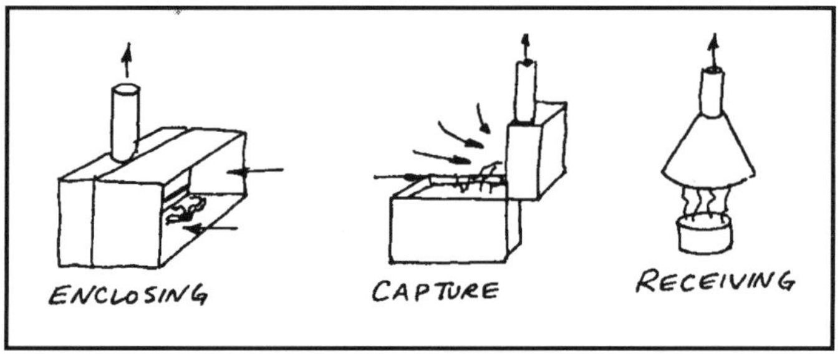

Figure 37.12 — Enclosing, capture, and receiving hoods.

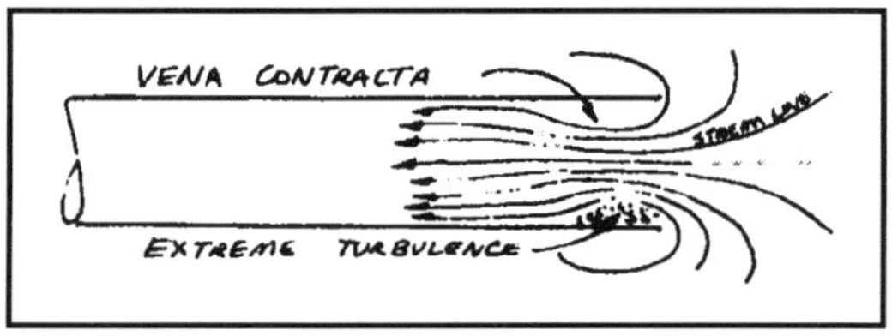

Figure 37.14 — The Vena Contracta causes static pressure losses in many fittings.

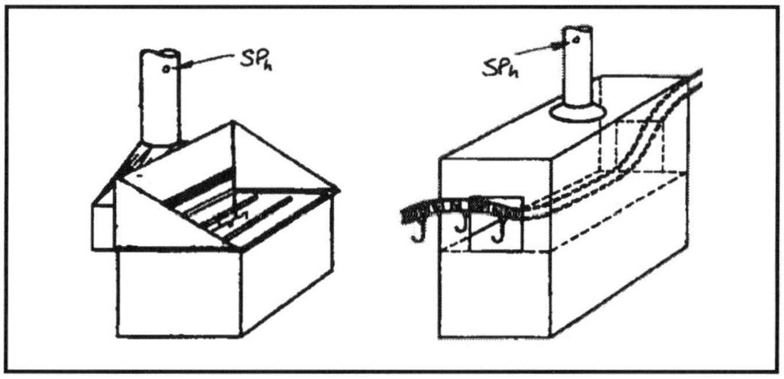

Figure 37.13 — Capture and enclosing hoods showing the location for measuring SP_h.

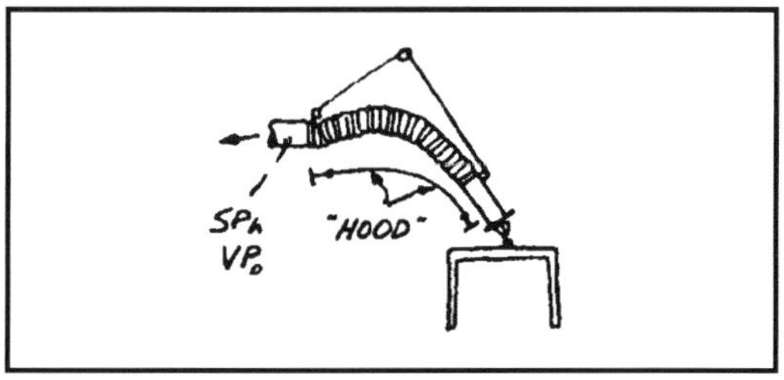

Figure 37.15 — Welding hood used in Example 37.7.

Equation 37-9 is not particularly useful in practice because an ideal flowrate cannot be measured and would not be seen in practice. Equations 37-10 and 37-11 are derived from Equation 37-9. The derivations can be found in References 1 and 2.

Example 37.7. For the welding hood shown in Figure 37.15, what is the hood static pressure, SPh, when the duct velocity pressure 0.66 inch w.g., and the hood entry loss is 0.88 inch w.g.? What is Ce for this hood?

Outcome. The coefficient of entry for this hood can be determined using Equations 37-8 and 37-11:

$$|SP_h| = VP + H_e = 0.66 + 0.84 = 1.50\text{" w.g}$$

$$C_e = \sqrt{\frac{0.66}{1.50}} = 0.66$$

Example 37.8. A new lab fume hood that is going to be installed has a published hood loss factor of 2.0. The intended velocity in the duct is 2000 fpm. Assuming a density correction factor of 0.95, what is the required hood static pressure needed to achieve the desired flowrate?

Outcome. The first step is to determine the velocity pressure associated with the intended velocity using Equation 37-2:

$$VP = \left[\frac{V}{4005}\right]^2 \times d_c = \left[\frac{2000}{4005}\right]^2 \times 0.95 = 0.24\text{" w.g.}$$

The hood static pressure then can be calculated using Equation 37-8:

$$|SP_h| = (1 + 2.0) \times 0.24 \times 0.95 = 0.68\text{" w.g.}$$

See again Figure 37.8 which provides a sampler of important design and operating parameters associated with six common hoods.

Determining Appropriate Air Volume Flowrates at a Hood

From Hood Static Pressure, SPh

The air volume flowrate is directly related to hood static pressure, SPh. This relationship allows Q to be determined when SPh is known or to determine SPh when the desired volume flowrate is known. Remember to use consistent units and the absolute value of the hood static pressure.

$$Q = 4005 \times A \times C_e \times \sqrt{\frac{|SP_h|}{d_c}} \qquad (37\text{-}12)$$

Values of C_e can be determined experimentally for existing hoods using Equation 37.10. For design, approximate values of C_e can be found on Figure 37.10 and in References 1 and 2. Hood manufacturers can also supply the value of C_e for their hoods.

Example 37.9. What is the estimated air flowrate through an existing lab fume hood, such as the one shown in Figure 37.11, if C_e is 0.58, the measured SP_h is –2.0 inch w.g., and the measured duct diameter is 12 inches? Assume a density correction factor of 0.95.

Outcome. The volume flow rate into the hood can be determined using Equation 37-13.

$$Q = 4005 \times 0.7854 \times 0.58 \times \sqrt{\frac{2.0}{0.95}} = 2650 \text{ acfm}$$

Example 37.10. A new lab fume hood, shown in Figure 37.10, is to be installed in a lab. The desired flowrate is 1,200 acfm. From Figure 37.8, C_e is determined to be 0.58. The connecting duct is a round, ten-inch diameter galvanized duct. Assuming a density correction factor 0.95, what is the approximate required hood static pressure?

Outcome. The area of the round duct can be calculated to be 0.5454 ft². Then, the static pressure at the hood can be determined using Equation 37-13.

$$SP_h = d_c \times \left[\frac{Q}{4005 \times A \times C_e}\right]^2$$

$$SP_h = 0.95 \times \left[\frac{1200}{4005 \times 0.5454 \times 0.58}\right]^2 = 0.85 \text{ inch w.g.}$$

From Published Charts

In most cases, designers choose air volume flowrates from published information. For an example, see column 5 of Figure 37.8.

References 1and 2 provide recommended flowrates for approximately 90 and 250 hoods, respectively. Table 37.4 provides a sampling of capture, control and face velocities recommended for various types of hoods.

From the Area or Hemeon Equations

Basically, air approaches a hood from all directions as it moves toward the source of negative static pressure in the connecting ductwork. Imagine a three-dimensional sphere around the end of a small, plain duct hood as shown on Figure 37.16. The velocity of air moving toward the opening is about equal at all points on the surface of the sphere centered on the opening of the hood.

Knowing the approach area and the desired capture velocity at the distance (X) from the hood opening to the surface, the volume flow rate can be estimated using Equation 37-3c. Figure 37.17 shows typical approach areas surrounding various hood types. This method of determine the volume flow rate using the velocity at a distance located on an spherical plain in front of the hood is also known as the Hemeon Method. Typical capture velocities for several common hoods are shown on Table 37.4; additional detail about capture velocities can be found in References 1 and 2.

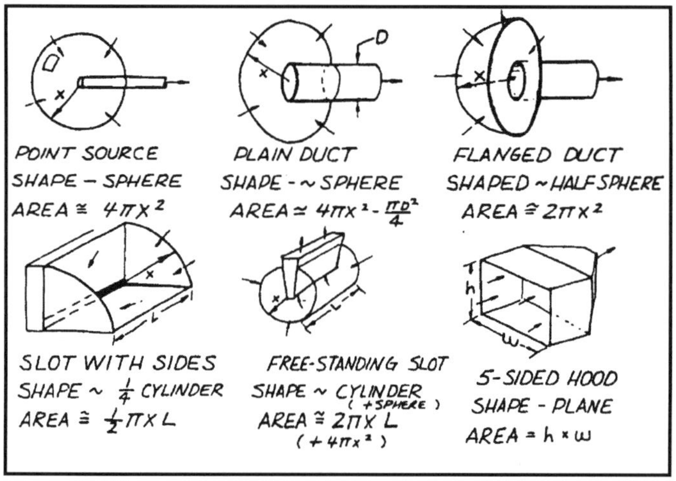

Figure 37.16 — Areas for common hoods for use with Q=VA Equation.

Example 37.11. Air enters an ideal 4" plain duct hood, similar to the one shown in Figure 37.17. What is the required volume flow rate for adequate control or capture six inches in front of the hood if the desired capture velocity is 100 fpm?

Outcome. Using the Hemeon method, the area of the sphere in front of the hood, in square feet, is calculated based on a capture distance of 6 inches or 0.5 feet.

$$A = 4\pi X^2 = 4\pi(0.5)^2 = 3.14 \text{ ft}^2$$

Using this area, the volume flow rate can be calculated from Equation 37-3c:

$$Q = 100 \times 3.14 = 314 \text{ cfm}$$

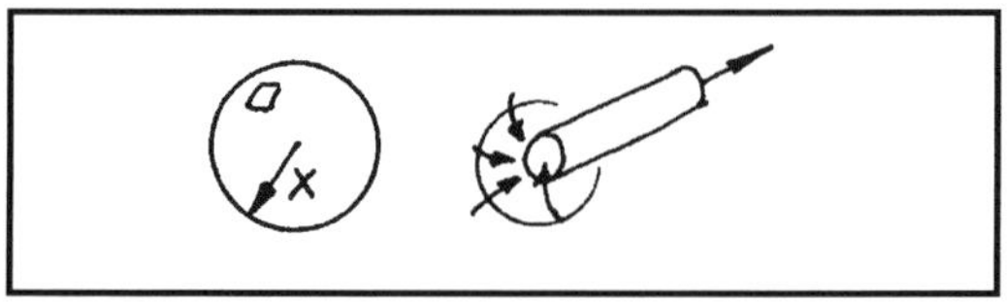

Figure 37.17 — Point source approximation of spherical approach area to plain duct entry hood.

Table 37.4 — Typical Capture and Face Velocities

Velocity Range (fpm)	*Type of Velocity*	*Operation or Typical Emission and Hoot Type*	*Environmental Conditions*
50–100	capture	degreasing	Release of emissions at no velocity into still air (e.g., no cross drafts)
75–125	face	lab fume hoods, drying ovens	Emission source is closed
	capture	soldering	Release of emissions into quiet air (e.g., less than 75 fpm cross drafts)
	capture	open surface tanks	For use with area approach to design at edge of tank.
100–200	capture	spray booths, welding, container filling, pickling, low speed conveyor transfer	Release of emission at low velocity into air with low cross drafts (e.g., both less than capture velocity)
	control	open surface tanks	For use with ANSI approach to open surface tank hood design

See References 1 and 2 for greater detail.

From the DallaValle-Silverman (DS) Equations

The DallaValle-Silverman (DS) equations suggest the following approximations for estimating air flowrates based on capture velocity. See Figure 37.18. See Reference 2 for more information.

Plain opening Hood:

$$Q = V_c(10X^2 + A) \quad (37\text{-}13)$$

Flanged opening Hood:

$$Q = 0.75V_c(10X^2 + A) \quad (37\text{-}14)$$

Slot opening :

$$Q = 3.7(LV_c X) \quad (37\text{-}15)$$

Flanged slot:

$$Q = 2.6(LV_c X) \quad (37\text{-}16)$$

Booth Hood:

$$Q = V_c \times W \times H \quad (37\text{-}17)$$

where

X = distance to source (ft)
V_c = capture velocity at distance X (fpm)
L = slot length (ft)
A = hood open face area (sq ft)
W = width of booth hood (ft)
H = height of booth hood (ft)

Example 37.12 Air enters an ideal 4 inch diameter plain duct hood. What is the required volume flow rate for if a capture velocity of 100 fpm is desires at a distance 6 inches in front?

Outcome. Using the DS method, the volume flow rate can be determined directly with the proper equation for the hood type. For a plain opening hood Equation 37-13 is used. The area of the 4 inch diameter duct is calculated to be 0.0873 ft^2.

$$Q = 100(10(0.5)^2 + 0.0873) = 259 \text{ cfm}$$

Although it is usually advisable in actual practice to the use the Hemeon equations, the DS equations are frequently used as an estimation tool and application of these equations is an expected competency for certification exams.

HOOD TYPE	DESCRIPTION	ASPECT RATIO,W/L	AIR FLOW
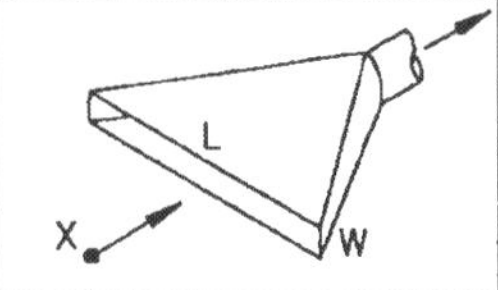	SLOT	0.2 OR LESS	Q = 3.7 LVX
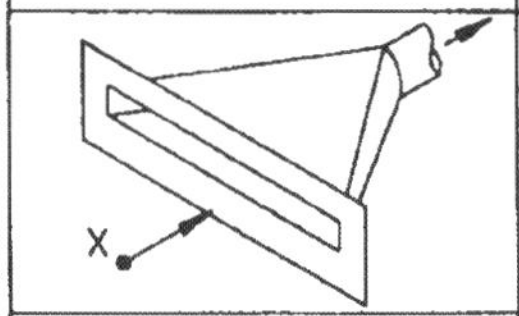	FLANGED SLOT	0.2 OR LESS	Q = 2.6 LVX
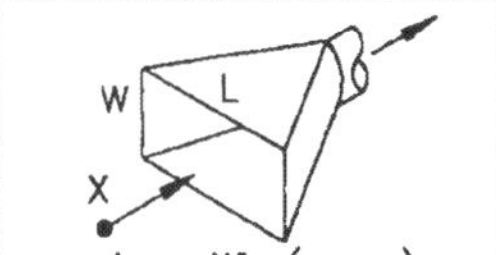 A = WL (sq.m)	PLAIN OPENING	0.2 OR GREATER AND ROUND	$Q = V(10X^2 + A)$
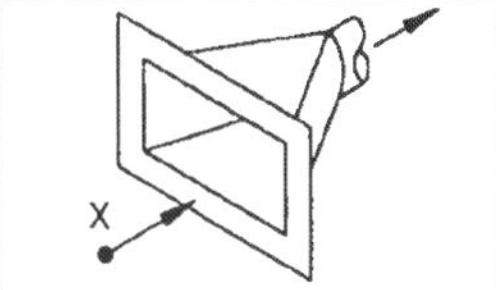	FLANGED OPENING	0.2 OR GREATER AND ROUND	$Q = 0.75V(10X^2 + A)$
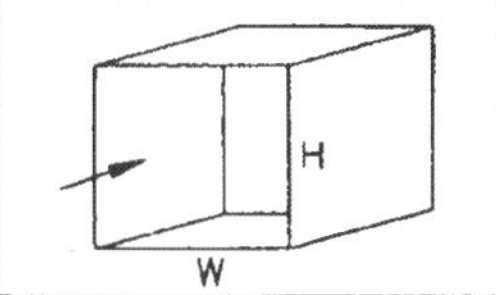	BOOTH	TO SUIT WORK	Q = VA = VWH

Figure 37.18 — DallaValle-Silverman Equations.

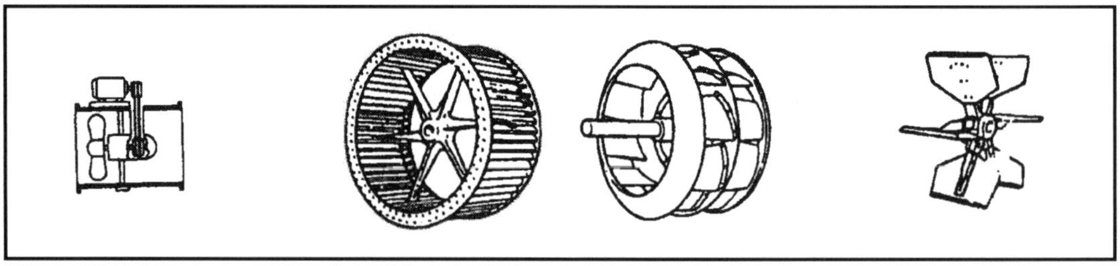

Figure 37.19 — Two major families of fans include axial and centrifugal.

Fans

The fan provides static pressure to physically move air. There are two families of fans, axial and centrifugal. These are show in Figures 37.19 and 37.20. Additionally, there are three types of centrifugal fans; forward curved, backward inclined, and radial, which are shown in Figure 37.21.

Axial fans have propeller-type blades. The wall fan, the freestanding room fan, the automobile radiator fan, the Casablanca-type fan, and the roof vent fan are all familiar types of axial fans, these are shown in Figure 37.22.

The centrifugal fan is the type found in home furnaces, swamp coolers, hair dryers, and vacuum cleaners. The radial fan (sometimes called the paddlewheel fan) is often employed in local exhaust ventilation systems because of its rugged simplicity, low initial cost, ability to generate high static pressures, and its tendency to stay clean and resist the erosive forces of dust-laden air. The backward inclined wheel is often used when the air stream is relatively clean. Its primary benefit is that it has a flat horsepower curve, i.e., it is more difficult to overload the motor. The forward curved wheel is rarely used in industrial systems. Its primary advantage is that it is quiet.

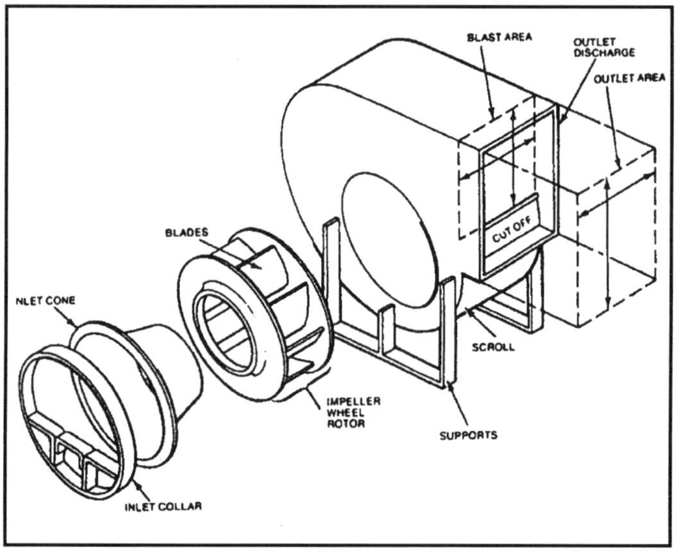

Figure 37.20 — Centrifugal fan showing important components.

Specifying Fans

Fans are usually specified by fan total pressure (FTP) and volume flow rate (Q), which help to define the "system operating point" (SOP). The fan total pressure, FTP, represents all energy requirements for moving air through the ventilation system, see Figure 37.23. According to accepted practice, FTP is calculated by adding the absolute values of the average total pressures found at the fan.

If the traditional sign convention is followed, then the formula for FTP is

$$FTP = TP_{out} - TP_{in} \quad (37\text{-}18)$$

$$FTP = SP_{out} + VP_{out} - SP_{in} - VP_{in} \quad (37\text{-}19)$$

If the velocity pressure at the outlet side of the fan equals the velocity pressure on

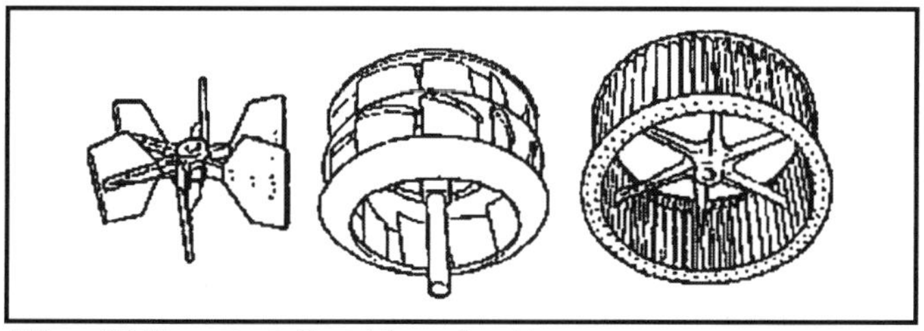

Figure 37.21 — Centrifugal fan wheel types.

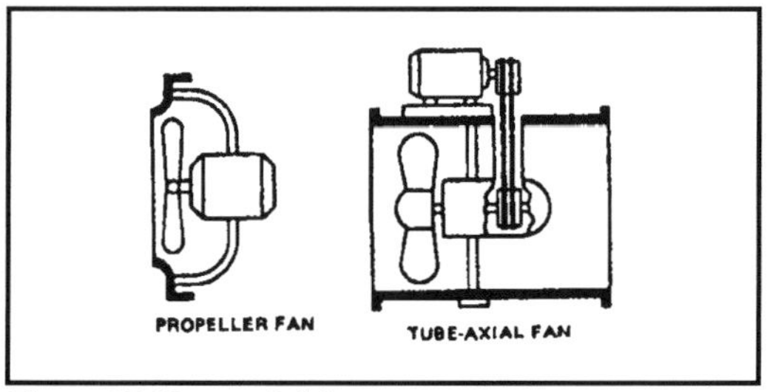

Figure 37.22 — Axial fans.

the inlet side of the fan, which will occur when the average inlet and outlet velocities are equal, then the VP terms in the above equation cancel, leaving:

$$FTP = SP_{out} - SP_{in} \qquad (37\text{-}20)$$

FTP is often referred to as the "fan total static pressure drop."

Fan Curves and Tables

Once the SOP (Q and FTP, for example) are known, the appropriate fan can be chosen from fan curves, fan tables and computer based fan selection programs. A typical curve for a fan is shown on Figure 37.24. This type of fan curve provides Q on the x-axis, FTP on the y-axis, fan rpm lines curving from upper left to lower right, and fan mechanical efficiencies (ME) along the top. The fan user plots the desired SOP on the curves to find the appropriate fan speed (rpm) and the resulting fan efficiency.

System Effect (SE) Loss and the Six and Three Rule

Like any other fitting, there are static pressure losses associated with how the ventilation system is attached to a fan. To avoid system effect losses, a straight duct length equal to six times the diameter of the duct should be provided prior to the inlet and three duct diameters at the outlet of the fan before any elbows or other fittings. If that is not possible, the appropriate loss factor can be determined using charts in References 1 and 2 and Equation 37-4 to determine the actual loss.

Example 37.20. The SE loss factor for an elbow with a radius to diameter ratio of 2.0 (R = 2.0D) placed directly on the inlet cone of a centrifugal fan is known to be 1.2. What is the static pressure loss to the system if the average velocity pressure in the connecting duct is 0.80 inch w.g.? Assume a density correction factor of 0.95.

Outcome. Using Equation 37.4:

$$SP_{loss} = 1.2 \times 0.80 \times 0.95 = 0.91\text{" w.g.}$$

Power Requirements

Once the fan is selected, the properly sized motor used to drive it must be selected. To size a motor, air horsepower (ahp), brake

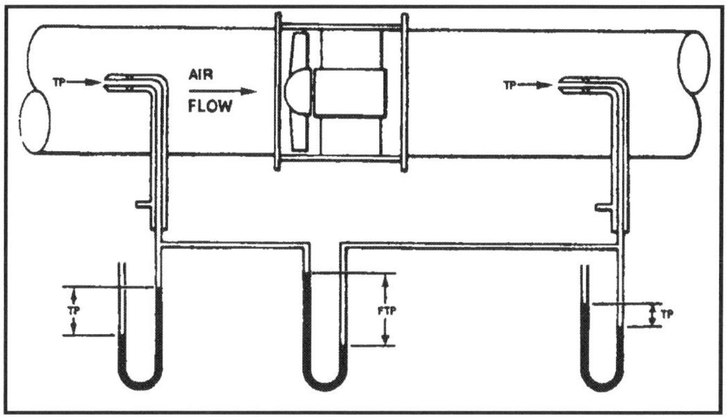

Figure 37.23 — Fan total pressure as measured using pitot tubes (Note: TP measurements are average values of TP).

horsepower (bhp), shaft horsepower (shp), and rated horsepower (rhp) need to be defined.

Air horsepower refers to the minimum amount of power to move a volume of air against the fan total pressure. It represents the power to get the air through the ventilation system. At any temperature or barometric pressure the fundamental relationship for power is given by:

$$ahp = \frac{FTP \times Q \times d_c}{6356} \qquad (37\text{-}21)$$

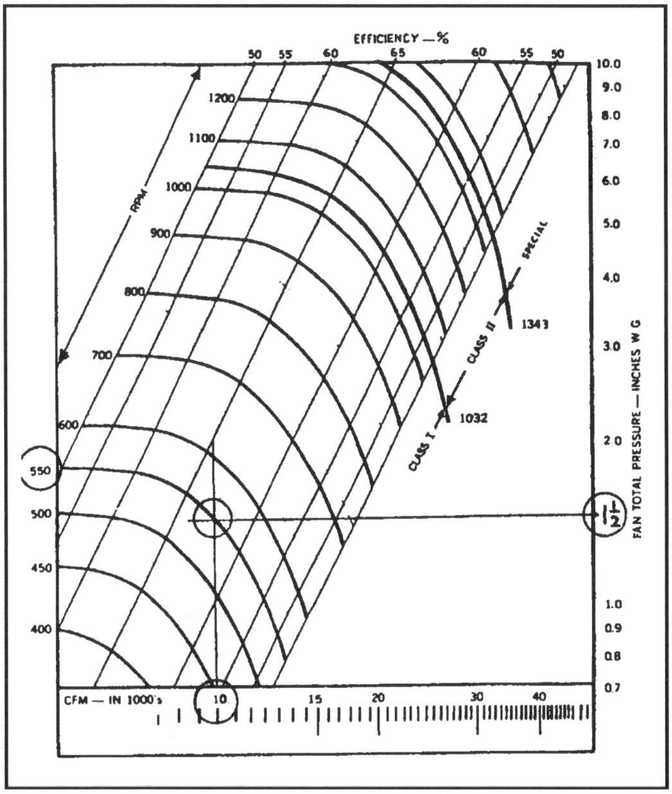

Figure 37.24 — Fan curves used for fan specification.

where

ahp = air horsepower (hp)
FTP = Fan Total Pressure (inch w.g.)

Brake horsepower refers to the actual power required to operate the fan so that it fulfills its job of moving the specified volume flow against the specified FTP. It takes into account fan inefficiencies that result from losses in the fan. The brake horsepower is air horsepower divided by a mechanical efficiency factor. The mechanical efficiency factor, ME, is determined experimentally by the fan manufacturer, and is usually provided with the fan curves.

$$bhp = \frac{ahp}{ME} \qquad (37\text{-}22)$$

where

bhp = brake horsepower (hp)
ahp = air horsepower (hp)
ME = the fan efficiency at the operating conditions (unitless)

Shaft horsepower (shp) is a combination of the brake horsepower plus any power required for drive losses, bearing losses, and pulley losses between the fan and the shaft of the motor. Generally, the fan supplier can provide the actual drive loss factor (K_{dl})for the drive system to be used. Normally, the shp can be estimated by:

$$shp = bhp \times K_{dl} \qquad (37\text{-}23)$$

Rated horsepower (rhp) is the power available from a motor. For small systems (e.g., less than 25 horsepower), rhp is usually chosen to be about one-third greater than shp. Rated horsepower motors usually come in whole sizes, e.g., 3/4 hp, 1 hp, 2 hp, 50 hp, etc.

Example 37.14. What rated horsepower motor would be appropriate to drive the fan on a ventilation system with a volume flow rate of 1200 acfm, a fan total pressure of 2.0 inch w.g., a mechanical efficiency of 0.60, a drive loss factor of 1.1, and an assumed density correction factor of 0.95.

Outcome. Equations 37-21, 37-22, and 37-23 can be combined to determine the brake horsepower:

$$bhp = \frac{FTP \times Q \times d_c \times K_{dl}}{6356 \times ME}$$

$$bhp = \frac{2.0 \times 1200 \times 0.95 \times 1.1}{6356 \times 0.60} = 0.66 \text{ hp}$$

Since this is a small system motor, the selected rated horsepower should be about 33% higher than the bhp.

$$rhp = bhp \times 1.33 = 0.66 \times 1.33 = 0.88 \text{ hp}$$

Since motor ratings are typically based on whole sizes, a one hp motor would be an appropriate selection for this system.

RPM Fan laws

The rpm fan laws are naturally occurring, fundamental mathematical relationships that describe changes in volume flow rate, pressures, and power when the fan rpm changes. They can be very helpful to the IH in troubleshooting or monitoring ventilation systems. The major fan laws are summarized below. The numbers 1 and 2 refer to conditions before and after a change in the system.

$$\frac{Q_2}{Q_1} = \frac{RPM_2}{RPM_1} \qquad (37\text{-}24)$$

$$\frac{SP_2}{SP_1} = \left[\frac{RPM_2}{RPM_1}\right]^2 \qquad (37\text{-}25)$$

$$\frac{hp_2}{hp_1} = \left[\frac{RPM_2}{RPM_1}\right]^3 \qquad (37\text{-}26)$$

Example 37.15. Assume a grinding wheel hood is exhausting 600 scfm of air and the hood static pressure is measured at –1.77 inch w.g. Three months later the hood static pressure has dropped to –1.50 inch w.g. Assuming there have been no changes in the hood and that the manometer is reading correctly, what is the approximate airflow through the hood at this new SP_h?

Outcome. Equations 37-24 and 37-25 and be combined to determine the effect of the change in the hood static pressure on the volume flow rate through the system.

$$\frac{SP_2}{SP_1} = \left[\frac{Q_2}{Q_1}\right]^2$$

$$\frac{-1.50}{-1.77} = \left[\frac{Q_2}{600}\right]^2$$

$$Q_2 = 600 \times \sqrt{\frac{-1.50}{-1.77}} = 552 \text{ scfm} \approx 550 \text{ scfm}$$

Stacks

The purpose of a stack is to disperse contaminated exhaust air into the ambient environment. This will allow contaminants to be diluted in the atmosphere to an acceptable concentration. Some re-entrainment of exhaust air almost always occurs in any building that has both intakes and stack exhausts. The amount of re-entrained air will vary depending on exhaust volumes, wind speed and direction, temperature, and the locations of intakes and stacks.

The following good practices are generally accepted among designers of stacks and air handling equipment:

- *Place the stack to avoid exhausting into the recirculation bubble,* as shown in Figure 37.25. Many designers feel that a stack height of 10 feet will provide enough height to breach the recirculation cavity on most roofs.
- *Provide ample stack height.* Check local building codes. Many use a minimum stack height of ten feet.

ASHRAE has published a diagnostic approach to stack design for shorter buildings using a "scaling length." Reference 7 provides the derivation and additional information. Figure 37.25 shows a typical example of the distribution of an exhaust plume from a stack on a roof. In the figure, H is the building height, W is the building width facing air flow, h_s is the stack height above an adjacent roof line, h_c is the height of the recirculation bubble, and L_c is the length of the recirculation bubble.

The recirculation bubble is dependent on the building shape and is generally independent of normally-encountered wind speeds. It sometimes engulfs the entire downwind side of the build. Stack heights should be sized to exhaust above the bubble. Air intakes located in the bubble have the least amount of pressure differences due to wind but are vulnerable to recirculating exhaust gases if a stack exhausts into the bubble.

To estimate L_c and h_c, a scaling length, SL, is calculated according to:

$$SL = B_S^{0.67} \times B_L^{0.33} \qquad (37\text{-}27)$$

where

B_S = smaller of H or W
B_L = larger of H or W

- *Place the stack downwind of building air intakes.* This good practice is limited because wind speed and direction vary from hour to hour, day to day, and season to season. When there is no significant prevailing wind, then the following practices take on greater importance.
- *Provide a stack velocity 1.4 time greater than the wind velocity.* This is usually sufficient to avoid downwash around the stack and to avoid reverse flow down the stack from wind pressure. It also supplies additional effective stack height. Many designers specify stacks for a 35-mph wind speed which results in a stack velocity of about 3,000 feet per minute.
- *Place the stack as far away from the intake as possible.* Fifty feet is considered adequate in most cases.

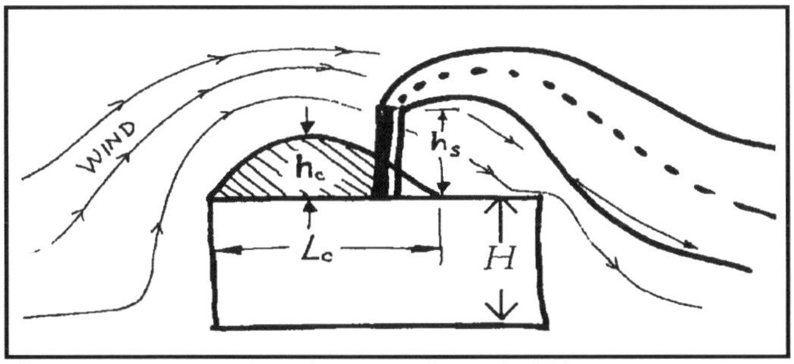

Figure 37.25 — Avoiding the recirculation bubble.

- Avoid rain caps if any building air intakes are within 50 ft. These can turn the exhaust plume back down onto the roof, minimizing effective stack height.

The 50-10-3000 Rule

A widely-used rule of thumb which incorporates many of the good practices described above is to place stacks at least fifty feet from air intakes, ten feet above adjacent roof lines and/or air intakes if within fifty feet, and to provide a stack exit velocity of 3000 fpm. This is a reasonable rule, but each stack should be designed and built to meet the needs of the situation. See Figure 37.25.

Air Cleaners and Replacement and Makeup Air Systems

Air Cleaning.

The requirements for almost all cleaning or scrubbing of industrial exhaust air is a function of the permit required by local, state, and federal air pollution control authorities. In most jurisdictions, a permit must be obtained any time a new exhaust stack is installed, or if older exhaust equipment is modified.

Typical air cleaning objectives include:

- Meeting permit requirements.
- Air pollution control; meeting air pollution standards.
- Reclaiming valuable materials.
- Enabling recirculation of exhaust air for energy conservation.
- Public relations; esthetics.

There are two families of cleaners — those for particulate and those for gases and vapors, but overlap can occur. The main types of air cleaners include:

Aerosol Collectors: Gravity separators which include balloon flues, clean out boxes, settling chambers, and impact devices like baffled ducts; filtration devices which include furnace filters, paint filters, baghouses, rolling filters; centrifugal collectors and cyclones; electrostatic precipitators; and wet scrubbers (also used with gases and vapors)

Gases and Vapors: Incinerators, absorption and adsorption collectors, catalytic scrubbers, chemical reaction scrubbers, and wet scrubbers.

Good practices to follow during the design and selection of air cleaners include choosing equipment:

- Which cleans the air stream to required levels. This also can mean not installing more equipment than necessary, for example, there's no good reason to install expensive scrubbers if a single pass water spray will suffice.
- In which the cleaning rate is not adversely effected by reasonable changes in air flow volume or contaminant loading, i.e., choose equipment with some flexibility.
- That maintains its cleaning efficiency throughout the cleaning cycle and throughout its life. The air cleaner should not need to be shut down to clean unless the process can be shut down, and the air cleaner should not have a significant loss in its cleaning efficiency as it gets older.
- That does not create heavy exposure problems for operators and maintenance people.
- And cleaning methods which will comply with other federal, state, and local requirements most easily (e.g., RCRA requirements, DOT requirements, etc.)

Makeup Air Systems

All industrial ventilation systems local exhaust or dilution require replacement air. Most makeup air systems introduce fresh, clean, outdoor air to the space occupied by people. All such air should be "conditioned" to acceptable levels of quality.

In naturally open buildings, replacement air can be supplied by atmospheric pressure through open doors, windows, cracks in walls and windows, louvers, and through roof vents. However, it is usually preferable to provide makeup air through mechanical ventilation systems.

When choosing a makeup air systems, follow these good practices:

- The correct amount of air should be supplied to the space. If the exhausted volume flowrate is 20,000 acfm, then approximately 20,000 acfm must be provided as replacement or makeup air. If slightly less is provided then the building will be under a slight negative pressure. If slightly more is provided then the building will be under a slight positive pressure.

- Proper air distribution is critical. Replacement or makeup air supply registers and grilles should be positioned so that the employee is located between the makeup air supply and the exhaust hood.
- Supply registers should be positioned to avoid disruption of emission and exposure controls
- Makeup air systems should help in the dilution of fugitive emissions.
- Makeup air unit manufacturers representatives can provide the latest information regarding local codes, availability of fuels, equipment costs, and waiting periods.
- Be wary of inadvertently recycling exhaust air. Occasionally, a makeup air unit will be placed too close to and downwind of an exhaust stack, causing inadvertent recycling of stack exhaust air.

Final Note

All aspects of industrial ventilation are a combination of engineering and art. Experience and professional judgment are still important to the success of industrial ventilation.

References and Additional Information

1. **Burton, D.J.:** *Industrial Ventilation Workbook*, 7th edition, Bountiful, UT: IVE, Inc., 2011.
2. **American Conference of Governmental Industrial Hygienists (ACGIH®):** *Industrial Ventilation, A Manual of Recommended Practice for Design*, 27th edition. Cincinnati, OH: ACGIH®, 2010.

(3) Hemeon

4. **American Society of Heating, Refrigerating and Air Conditioning Engineers (ASHRAE):** *ASHRAE 55-2004 Thermal Environmental Conditions for Human Occupancy.* [Standard]. Atlanta, GA: ASHRAE, 2004.
5. **American Society of Heating, Refrigerating and Air Conditioning Engineers (ASHRAE):** *ASHRAE 62-2010 Ventilation for Acceptable Indoor Air Quality.* [Standard]. Atlanta, GA: ASHRAE, 2010.
6. **National Institute for Occupational Safety and Health (NIOSH) and U.S. Environmental Protection Agency (EPA):** *Building Air Quality Guide for Building Owners and Facility Managers.* (EPA/400/1-91-033). Washington, D.C.: Government Printing Office, 1991. Washington, D.C.: Government Printing Office, 1991.
7. **American Society of Heating, Refrigerating and Air Conditioning Engineers (ASHRAE):** ASHRAE Fundamentals Handbook. Atlanta, GA: ASHRAE, 2009.
8. **American Industrial Hygiene Association (AIHA®):** All ANSI/AIHA® Z9 Standards 1–11. Fairfax, VA: AIHA®.

chapter 38

Outcome Competencies

After completing this chapter, the reader should be able to:

1. Understand and apply important terms and concepts introduced in this chapter.
2. Identify examples of ventilation systems that can or should be tested and monitored
3. Determine and apply appropriate testing and monitoring methods
4. Determine important system parameters through testing and monitoring
5. Establish a testing and monitoring program
6. Understand and use testing and monitoring results

Key Terms

air movement and direction • anemometer • balometer • carbon dioxide monitor • density correction factor • EA • emission rate • hood static pressure • HVAC • inspections • MA • manometer • OA • physical measurements • pitot tube • RA • SA • testing, monitoring and troubleshooting • troubleshoot • velocity pressure measurement • velometer

Prerequisite Knowledge

Prior to beginning this chapter, the user should review the following chapters:

Chapter Number	Chapter Topic
7	Principles of Evaluating Worker Exposure
8	Occupational and Environmental Health Risk Assessment
35	General Methods for the Control of Airborne Hazards
36	Dilution Ventilation
37	Local Exhaust Ventilation

Key Topics

I. Introduction
II. Ventilation System Testing and Monitoring Equipment
III. Overview of the Basic Approaches to Testing and Monitoring
   A. Physical Measurements
   B. Air Movement and Direction
   C. Capture and Hood Face Velocities
   D. Hood Static Pressure
   E. Duct Velocity Pressure Measurements
IV. Inspections as an Important Aspect of Testing and Monitoring
V. Auditing as an Important Aspect of Monitoring
VI. Monitoring of Recirculating LEV Systems
VII. Using Static Pressure Measurements to Monitor and Troubleshoot Industrial Ventilation Systems
VIII. Troubleshooting
   A. Troubleshooting LEV Systems
   B. Troubleshooting HVAC Systems
IX. Correcting, Testing, and Monitoring Results for Non-Standard Air Density
   A. Corrections to Airflow
X. Summary
XI. References and Additional Information

Testing, Monitoring and Troubleshooting of Existing Ventilation Systems

38

By D. Jeff Burton, CIH, PE

Introduction

Testing, monitoring and troubleshooting are required for all industrial ventilation and HVAC systems. The objectives of testing and monitoring for the IH usually include:

- Establishment of baseline or startup conditions.
- Periodic determination of the effectiveness of the system (e.g., emissions capture, particulate transport, employee protection, efficiency, air cleaning, comfort, compliance with standards and permit requirements)
- Monitoring of specific performance parameters in real time (e.g., filters, fans, hoods)
- Finding the sources of problems and deficiencies

It is important to read or review Chapters 36–37 before beginning this chapter. Air density correction and dilution ventilation terms and equations presented in Chapter 36, for example, are necessary for the proper interpretation of test findings. Chapter 37 defines and explains many local exhaust ventilation system terms, abbreviations and equations used in this chapter.

This chapter is written for the practicing IH and is intended to help apply basic testing and monitoring principles. Materials presented in this chapter are thought to be compatible with current standards of good practice as described in References 1–9. However, the IH should always review current standards before actually applying the principles presented herein.

Specialized knowledge of testing and balancing is required to monitor and maintain modern complex systems. Several associations train and certify people to do this work; additional information about these types of training programs are presented in Reference 1. Most IHs are not expected to conduct *in-depth* testing and monitoring of industrial ventilation and HVAC systems, however there are many basic testing, monitoring, and troubleshooting activities that are typical IH responsibilities. This chapter provides guidelines for these activities that the IH may perform, including:

- Using basic testing and monitoring instruments (e.g, smoke tubes, balometers, velometers, pitot tubes and manometers, carbon dioxide monitors, thermometers, psychrometers)
- Determining actual ventilation system operating parameters (e.g., Q, V, T, RH) using these basic instruments
- Determining primary design and operating parameters (e.g., desired Q, V, T, RH from plans and specifications)
- Locating system problem sources and deficiencies

Records should be maintained for all testing and monitoring activities. Such recordkeeping should include "as built" plans and specifications, field data forms and worksheets, methodologies used, and all reports. The use of regular field data worksheets helps assure that all of the data required to meet the project objectives are obtained and recorded and that current data collected can be compared to older data.

Ventilation System Testing and Monitoring Equipment

To conduct testing and monitoring of ventilation systems, a variety of basic and inexpensive equipment needs to be accessible. A typical IH ventilation testing kit might include:

- Tape measures and distance measuring devices to measure physical dimensions of the system and system components
- Thermometers and psychrometers for measurement of temperature, RH, and OA delivery rate
- Smoke tubes or a smoke generator to generate a method for visualizing the air movement
- Pressure sensing devices such as pitot tubes and manometers
- Velometers or anemometers for measurement of air velocity and air volume flowrate
- Balometers for measuring the air volume flowrate at registers and grilles
- Noise monitoring equipment, e.g., SPL meter
- Carbon dioxide monitors
- Other miscellaneous equipment, including rags, flashlight, drill, drill bits, mirror, tachometer, duct tape.

Basic testing devices and their primary uses are summarized below. Some devices combine functions, for example several commercially available velometers can measure a combination of temperature, pressure and air velocity.

Overview of the Basic Approaches to Testing and Monitoring

Physical Measurements

The physical measurements of the system have a significant relationship to the operating characteristics of the system. Some of the physical measurements that are significant when evaluating the operation of the system include the following. Documentation of field measurements is a significant part of the evaluation process. An example of a field data form is included as Figure 38.1. The IH should construct field data forms that meet testing and record keeping needs.

Duct diameters and duct circumferences. Duct dimensions can often be estimated from plans, drawings, and specifications. These can be used for estimating duct area. Inside duct diameter is the most important measurement, but an outside measurement is usually sufficient on large sheet metal ducts. Inside diameter can be estimated using a pitot tube. Accurate outside duct diameter measurements are often difficult to obtain. Although standard size ducts are used, ducts are often "out of round" and frequently vary from the nominal size by a small percent.

Duct lengths. Lengths can be estimated from plans, drawings, and specifications. Measurements can be made with tapes or optical devices. Often duct work is constructed from standard length pieces, so identification of the number of sections can help provide an easy estimation of total duct length. Length of the elbows, tees and other connection sections should be include determination of duct length.

PITOT TUBE TRAVERSE WORKSHEET

Date 11-8 Time 10:00 SP -2.10" w.g.
Temp 100°F B.P. 24.89" Description ROUND
df = 0.787 ρ = 0.059 lb/ft3 Name D. BURTON
Equipment PITOT Location FURNACE NO. 3
Circumference ~75" Diameter 24" Area 3.142 ft2
VP centerline 1.04" w.g. CORRECTED FOR df

	Vertical		Horizontal		NOTES
No	VP	Vel	VP	Vel	
1	0.60	3496	0.52	3255	
2	0.87	4210	0.77	3961	
3	0.90	4282	0.88	4234	
4	0.95	4399	0.94	4376	
5	1.00	4514	0.99	4491	
6	1.00	4514	1.05	4625	
7	.90	4282	0.95	4399	
8	.93	4353	0.85	4161	
9	0.80	4037	0.81	4062	
10	0.55	3347	0.61	3525	

Ave Velocity Pressure = 0.836" w.g. (RMS)
Ave Velocity = 4127 fpm
Volume Flow rate = Q = VA = 4127 x 3.142 = 13,000 acfm (ROUNDED)

Figure 38.1 — Pitot tube traverse data collection worksheet.

Sheet metal gauge. The "Mfrs Std. Gauges" for steel sheet metal is based on metal with a density of 490 pounds per cubic foot. Galvanized metal is slightly thicker than non-galvanized. Ventilation systems are often constructed of sheet metal, with typical construction in the 12–22 gauge range. A gauge size of 12 is a metal thickness of about 0.11 inches while "22 gauge" metal is about 0.034 inches thick.

Air Movement and Direction

Chemical smoke is a useful method for assisting in the evaluation of a ventilation system because it is visible. The ability to see smoke drift out of a hood or doorway, stratify in layers, or move in the wrong direction can provide a powerful tool when conducting evaluating or troubleshooting a ventilation system. As a side note, the smoke generated from many of the smoke tubes used for ventilation investigations can be irritating and annoying to building occupants.

Smoke can be used to provide a rough estimate of velocity as shown in Figure 38.2. Timing a smoke plume's travel over a known distance can provide an approximation of the velocity in feet per minute.

Capture and Hood Face Velocities

"Capture velocities" at the emission source and "face velocities" at the hood face can be estimated using velometers. Figure 38.3 shows a common method of estimating the average face velocity in a hood face, where the face is divided into an imaginary grid and measurements are made in the center of each of the grid areas and then averaged. Velometers and anemometers are appropriate instruments for collecting these types of measurements. Many velometers have velocity correction requirements for non-standard air conditions. Some correct automatically, others use the density correction factor introduced in Chapter 35. It is important to become familiar with the specific instrument to ensure that proper measurements are being collected.

Figure 38.4 shows a face velocity field data worksheet typical of those used for record keeping. The worksheet has been filled in for a hypothetical hood. Study the field worksheet carefully. Note that the measured velocity was corrected for non-standard air conditions using "VC," the velocity correction factor provided by the manufacturer.

Hood Static Pressure

Several standards recommend real-time monitoring of flowrate at exhaust hoods, including ANSI Z9.2 and ANSI Z9.5. Because hood static pressure (SP_h) and air volume flowrate are directly related and because a continuous measurement of SP_h is usually the most cost-effective approach, SP_h is often measured to comply with these standards.

When making measurements within ductwork the proper location of the measurement is typically indicated by referencing a distance from a landmark within the ventilation system. For example, the measurement may be collected "downstream from the hood" or "upstream of the fan."

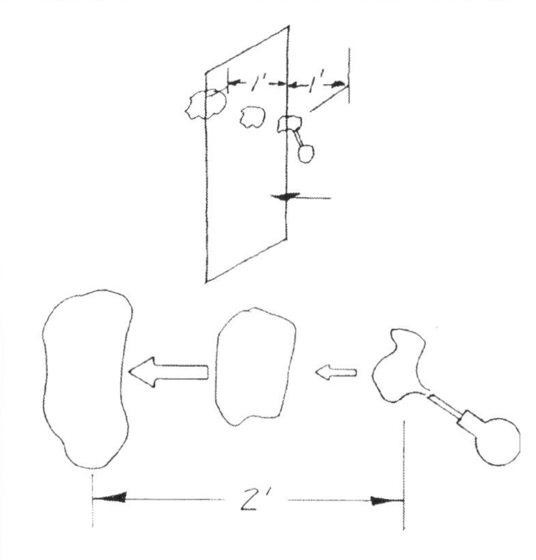

Figure 38.2 — Use of smoke to determine direction and approximate velocity of air.

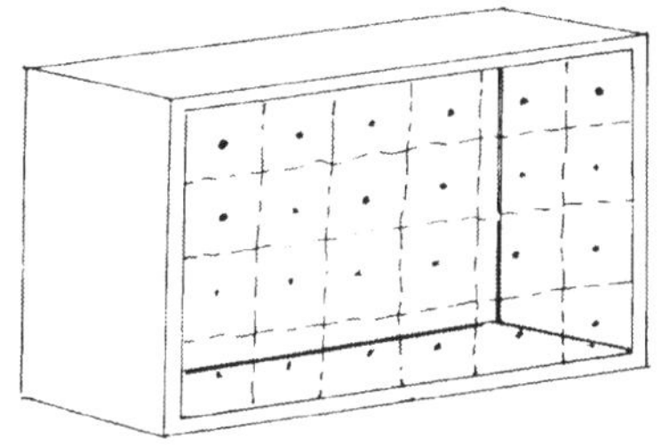

Figure 38.3 — Example of the Grid Method Used for measuring face velocity.

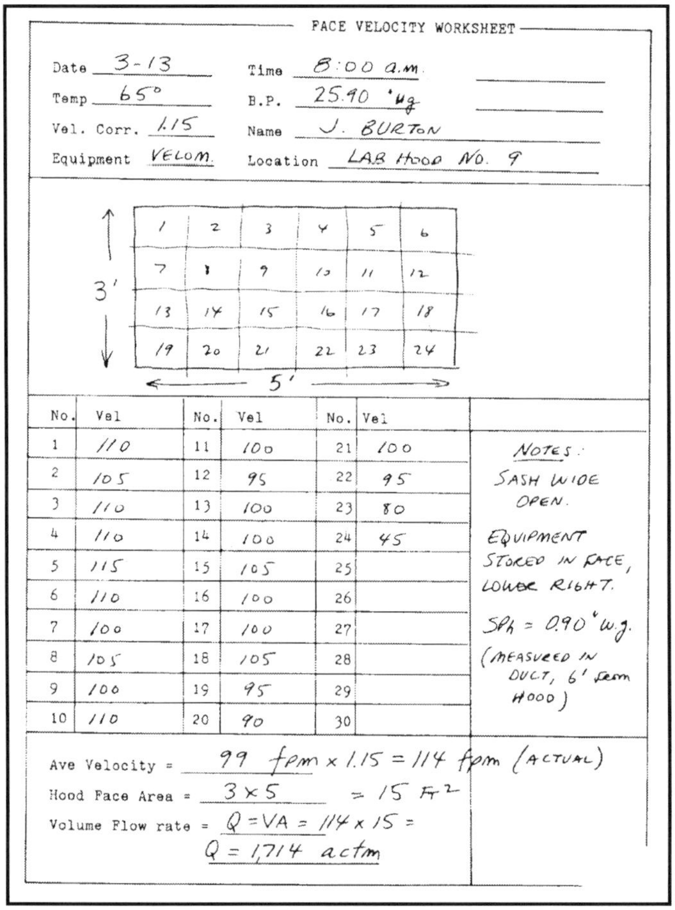

FACE VELOCITY WORKSHEET

Date 3-13 Time 8:00 a.m.

Temp 65° B.P. 25.90 "Hg

Vel. Corr. 1.15 Name J. BURTON

Equipment VELOM. Location LAB HOOD NO. 9

1	2	3	4	5	6
7	8	9	10	11	12
13	14	15	16	17	18
19	20	21	22	23	24

3' (height) × 5' (width)

No.	Vel	No.	Vel	No.	Vel
1	110	11	100	21	100
2	105	12	95	22	95
3	110	13	100	23	80
4	110	14	100	24	45
5	115	15	105	25	
6	110	16	100	26	
7	100	17	100	27	
8	105	18	105	28	
9	100	19	95	29	
10	110	20	90	30	

NOTES: SASH WIDE OPEN. EQUIPMENT STORED IN FACE, LOWER RIGHT. SPh = 0.90" w.g. (MEASURED IN DUCT, 6' from HOOD)

Ave Velocity = 99 fpm × 1.15 = 114 fpm (ACTUAL)

Hood Face Area = 3 × 5 = 15 ft²

Volume Flow rate = Q = VA = 114 × 15 =

Q = 1,714 acfm

Figure 38.4 — Face velocity data worksheet.

The actual distance between the landmark and the measurement point differs depending on the diameter of the duct; this distance is expressed as a number of "duct diameters." For example, hood static pressure should be measured about 2-6 duct diameters downstream from the hood in a straight section of the hood takeoff duct; a distance equal to two to six times the measured diameter of the duct. The measurement can be made with a pitot tube and a manometer, or with a manometer attached to a static pressure tap installed in the duct surface. An example of how these measurements can be made is shown in Figure 38.5.

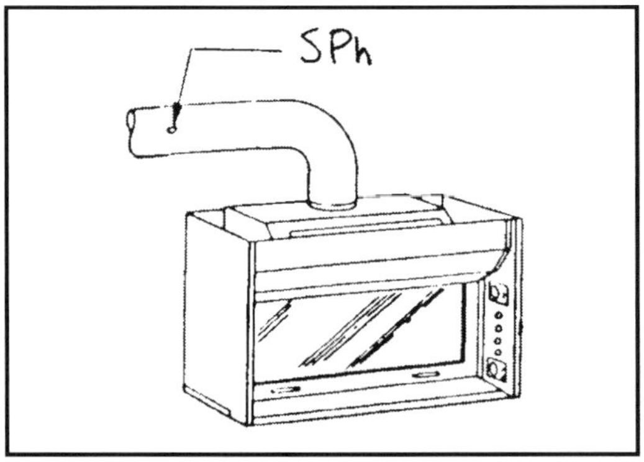

Figure 38.5 — Measurement of SPh 2-6 duct diameters downstream from the hood.

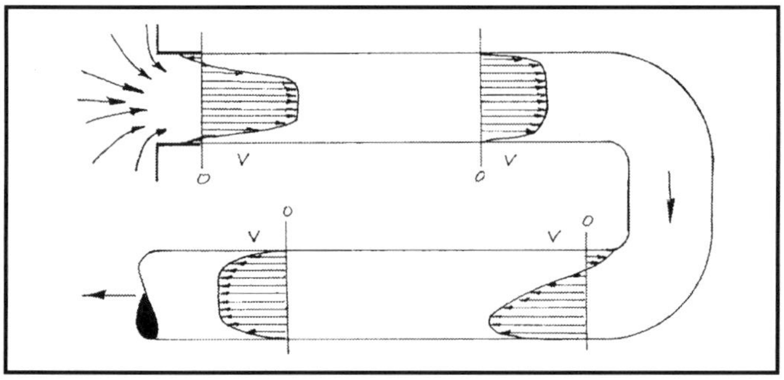

Figure 38.6 — Velocity and velocity pressure profiles at different cross sections in a duct.

Duct Velocity Pressure Measurements

Air flow in ventilation ducts is always turbulent, with a very small boundary layer of quiet air at the surface of the duct. Typical velocity pressure (VP) profiles in round ducts are shown on Figure 38.6.

The appropriate instruments for measuring VP in a ventilation system are the pitot tube and manometer.

Since velocity pressure and velocity both vary with distance from the edge of the duct, a single measurement of pressure is not usually sufficient. However, if the measurement is taken in a long straight length of duct, about six diameters downstream and three diameters upstream from obstructions or directional changes, then the average velocity pressure in the duct is approximately 81% of the measured center line velocity pressure.

Potentially, a more accurate method for determining the VP in a duct is the *pitot traverse*. In a pitot traverse, six to ten VP measurements are made on each of two traverses across the duct, 90 degrees opposed, or on each of three traverses, 60 degrees opposed. Measurements are made, for example, in the center of concentric circles of equal area as shown in Figure 38.7.

Figure 38.8 shows one simple calculation method for estimating the appropriate distance from the duct wall to the center of equal concentric circles in a round duct when conducting a pitot traverse within the

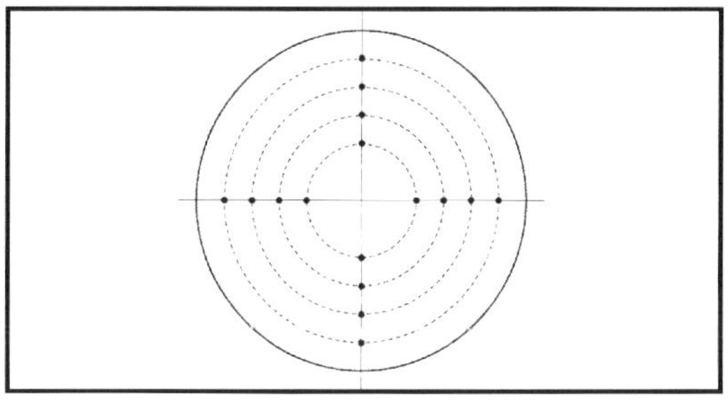

Figure 38.7— A pitot tube traverse measurement takes measurements in the center of equal concentric areas of a round duct.

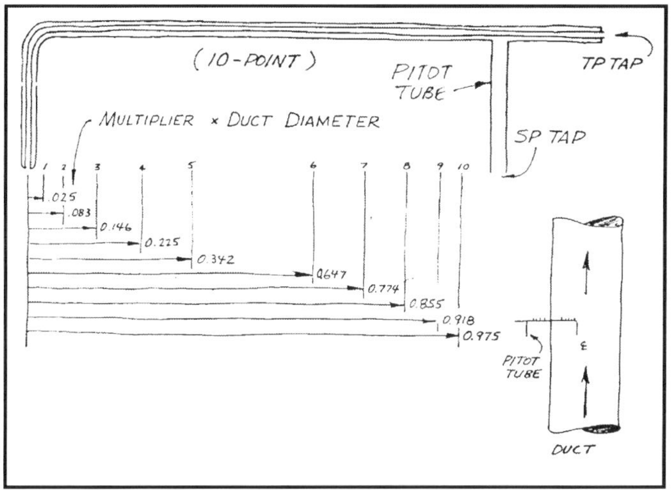

Figure 38.8 — Finding the appropriate distance from the side of the duct to take measurements.

ductwork. An example of this method is provided in Figure 38.9 which shows the appropriate measurement points for a 10-point traverse within a 12-inch diameter duct.

After calculating the measurement locations, simple markings on the pitot tube can be used to indicate the proper locations for each measurement point. To determine the average velocity through the duct, each of the VP measurements are converted to velocity, using the relationship discussed in Chapter 37, then averaged.

As mentioned above, Figure 38.4 provides an example of a VP field worksheet typical of those used for record keeping. The worksheet has been completed for a 12-inch round duct which is providing static pressure to a furnace fugitive emissions exhaust hood. Velocities shown on the sheet were estimated from velocity pressure measurements using Bernoulli's Equation corrected for non-standard conditions, as described in Chapter 35. Note that the final average velocity pressure was estimated from the final average velocity, or by using root mean square averaging of the original VP data. Additional information on calculation procedures is provided in Chapter 36 and References 1 and 2. It is normally not acceptable to average the measured velocity pressures and then calculate average velocity. The final volume flowrate was rounded to adhere to the traditional rules of significant figures.

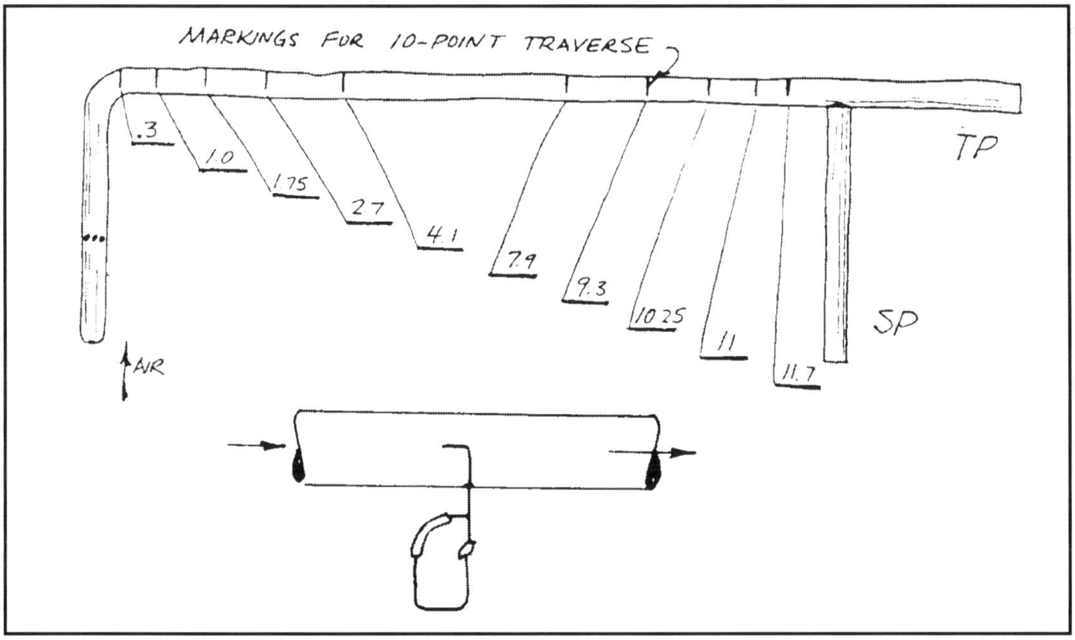

Figure 38.9 — An example showing calculated locations for pitot traverse measurements in a 12-inch diameter duct.

Inspections as an Important Aspect of Testing and Monitoring

Ventilation system testing and monitoring always includes a program of periodic inspection. The inspection frequency and items to be inspected should include a daily visual inspection of hoods, ductwork, access and cleanout doors, blast gate positions, hood static pressure, pressure drop across air cleaner, and verbal contact with users to determine their "sense" of how the system is operating. Weekly inspections should include observations of the air cleaner capacity, fan housing, pulley belts, and stack. The air cleaner components should be inspected monthly. Inspections and a full inspection of all system equipment and components should occur annually. References 2 and 5 provide additional details about inspections and inspection timing.

Table 35.1 — Sample of Audit Form for ANSI / AIHA® Z9.2-2011

Section 14. Testing, Balancing, and Operational Checklist	
( )	14.1 Performance standards and operating criteria, if not defined during design, are established by the User for every component of an LEV system.
( )	14.2 The User selects test methods and test instruments which can measure the established performance criteria of Paragraph 14.1.
( )	14.3 After construction or modification, the LEV system is tested before routine service begins to assure that the system meets the established performance criteria.
( )	14.4 The LEV system is periodically tested and monitored in accordance with a schedule determined by the User.
( )	14.5 The hood captures, receives, or contains air contaminants at some specified performance criteria established by the User.
( )	14.6 Qualitative and/or quantitative tests are adopted by the User to assure hood capture and containment performance.
( )	14.7 Each LEV system is balanced during the commissioning process and thereafter on a schedule determined by the User
( )	14.8 Persons performing testing and balancing are qualified by training, experience, or certification to perform the work.
( )	14.9 Testing and balancing instrumentation is suitable for the measurements.
( )	14.10. Testing and balancing instruments are calibrated in accordance with manufacturers= recommendations and on a schedule to be determined by the User.
( )	14.11 Records of testing and balancing are maintained by the User.
( )	14.12 Makeup or replacement air systems are also included in any LEV testing.
( )	14.13. Testing and monitoring equipment are safe for the intended use.
( )	14.14 System testing results are made available to those with a need to know.

*Copyrighted by AIHA®. Contact AIHA® for a full copy of the standard and the audit form.

Auditing as an Important Aspect of Monitoring

Ventilation system monitoring always includes a program of auditing. Table 38.1 shows part of the audit tool provided in ANSI Z9.2 for industrial ventilation systems. Reference 8 includes additional information about these important standards.

Monitoring of Recirculating LEV Systems

In recent years, energy conservation has prompted renewed interest in the recirculation of exhausted air. In some situations air removed through a ventilation system can be recirculated to the plant in order to conserve energy. Because of the high costs and potential hazards associated contaminants in LEV exhaust, the potential energy conservation savings must be balanced against other risks when considering recirculation of exhausted air. Recirculation, as a practical matter, is difficult, expensive, and challenging to maintain. Alternatives such as adding heat exchanger, selecting lower cost fuels, or implementing other energy conservation measures should be considered. Heat exchangers, for example, are often capable of recovering up to 40–60% of the heat energy of exhausted air.

If recirculation of exhausted air is included in the ventilation system design, then the system should also include monitoring equipment to help ensure continued proper operation. All hoods should be fitted with hood static pressure manometers to provide feedback to the hood user, and a control panel should monitor fan performance, bypass stack damper position, filter performance, HVAC Unit operation, and room air concentrations. Although the recirculation air volume can range up to 100% of the exhausted air, some fresh, outside air is required and should be programmed into any recirculation scheme.

Generally accepted monitoring practices on ventilation systems should provide the following:

- Real time monitoring of system performance. This could include static pressure taps, particulate counters, amperage monitors, and monitoring and testing of fail-safe systems through monitors and warning devices on critical parts and backup systems.
- Periodic inspection, testing, and preventive maintenance programs. This may include daily inspection, weekly cleaning, and preventative maintenance schedules to ensure replacement of critical parts, such as filters or sensors, on a regular basis.
- Monitoring of bypass or auxiliary exhaust systems. These are the redundant systems that would be used during system failures.
- Employees trained in the use and operation of the monitoring equipment and systems. Employees must be able to know when a system component is deficient, and the steps to take when issues occur.

Using Static Pressure Measurements to Monitor and Troubleshoot Industrial Ventilation Systems

Most ventilation systems built in recent years have sophisticated control and monitoring systems. In many systems, new or old, static pressure is used to monitor air flowrates and the performance of hoods, fans, and filters because monitoring the SP in a system is both inexpensive and reliable. By evaluating changes in SP at different points in the system, the IH can quickly identify problem location and potential causes. If the SP is known at numerous points throughout the system, changes in the VP an individual points or changes in the relative difference between the VP on opposite sides on a system component and be used to identify causes of changes that result in reduction of system performance. For example, a pressure drop, or pressure loss, across a filter based air cleaner could indicate an overloading of the filter or a tear in the filter material. Changes in the FTP could indicate changes in the fan speed, changes in the drive performance (i.e., worn belts), etc.

Troubleshooting

Invariably, something goes wrong with almost all ventilation systems. Frequently, few problems can be easily resolved unless the trouble is correctly diagnosed. Troubleshooting a ventilation system is simply a

Scenario: A computer hardware manufacturing firm exhausts a total of 24,000 acfm equally distributed through three LEV systems. The plant management wants to determine if recirculation of the LEV exhaust is an option that would lead to significant motor and heating energy savings.

One exhaust system serves light-emitting diode construction machines which emit gallium arsenide particles. Pre-baghouse air contains about 500 micrograms per cubic meter ($\mu g/m^3$) of gallium arsenide, while post-baghouse air contains about 50 mg/m^3. Another exhaust system serves a lab fume hood using nitric acid. Concentrations of nitric acid in the exhaust air are low, averaging about 0.01 mg/m^3, and the air is exhausted without scrubbing. The third exhaust system serves a simple machine shop. Iron filings and cuttings, chips, grinding dust, and other large particles are exhausted through a cyclone outside the building. No cadmium, lead or chrome-containing metals are handled in the machine shop.

The IH was included as part of a team that was asked to evaluate the systems to determine if a percentage of the exhausted air could be recirculated in to the plant.

Outcome: During the initial discussion the team agreed that each system would need to be evaluated separately. Several considerations to investigate for were identified: Would additional air cleaning be required? What types of backup systems and monitoring equipment would be required?

Further discussion and investigation showed that exhaust air from the first two systems could not be recirculated safely or economically. Gallium arsenide is highly hazardous, and arsenic is a suspected carcinogen. The lab ventilation standard, ANSI Z9.5–2003, which the plant adopted as a guidance document, effectively prohibits recirculation of lab fume hoods like the ones being used.

The team identified that because of the application of the LEV system in the machine shop there was potential for the exhaust air to be recirculated. However, to reduce the exposure risks installation of a new baghouse or HEPA filter unit attached between the cyclone and the return air plenum would be required. In addition, a static pressure monitoring device would be required across the baghouse or HEPA filter unit to assure the integrity of the air cleaning system.

type of informal investigation. It may be the first screening study in a longer-term investigation. Generally, troubleshooting is usually an individual effort over a relatively short period of time, where a formal investigation may involve many people, extensive efforts, and a longer period of time.

Troubleshooting ventilation systems usually involves three phases of study:

- Characterizing complaints and existing operating conditions plus gathering background data.
- Checking the performance of ventilation system components and their controls.
- Comparing findings to original design criteria or standards of practice

Troubleshooting LEV Systems

The following complaint scenarios describe common maladies and their potential sources.

Complaint: Excessive fugitive emissions resulting from a decreased capture velocity are present at an exhaust hood.

Possible Causes: If the process itself, and therefore, the emission rate of the contaminants, has not changed, then the cause is probably a reduced volume flowrate. Reduced flowrates can occur in the following situations: plugged or dented ducts, slipping fan belts, open access doors, holes in ducts and elbows, closed damper to branch or opened dampers to other branches, worn out fan blades, additional branches or hoods added to system , clogged air cleaners, the fan turning in the reverse direction.

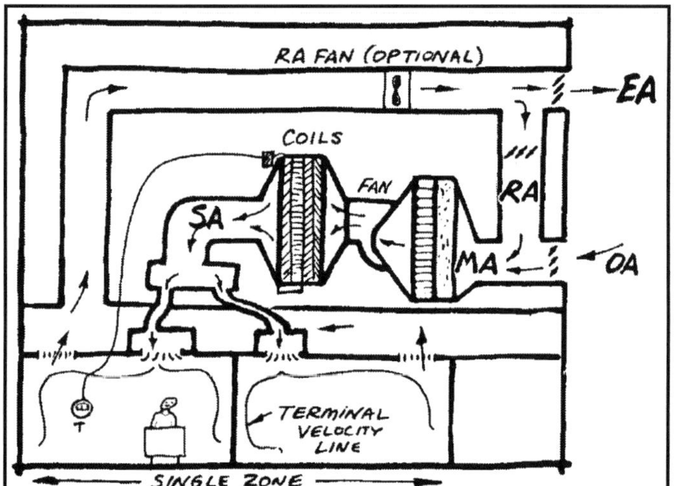

Figure 38.10 — Schematic representation of an HAVAC system serving an occupied space.

Complaint: Excessive employee exposures in an area where ventilation system is operating properly; the exhaust flow volumes and capture velocities are at design levels.

Possible Causes: In this situation, the causes could either be related to worker behaviors or to the initial system design. The work practices could be leading to the exposures. Perhaps the ventilation system interferes with the task or limits the worker's productivity to the extent that the workers avoid using the system. It is also possible that the system was based on a poor initial design that underestimated the volume air flow needed to prevent exposures.

Complaint: The ductwork within the ventilation system is consistently becoming plugged with materials.

Possible Causes: Plugging of ducts occurs when there is inadequate transport velocity, or when condensation of vapor in the duct is wetting particles, causing a build-up of material. These problem generally is the result of poor design, open access doors, fan problems.

Troubleshooting HVAC Systems

ASHRAE considers it a successful application of comfort ventilation when 80% of the occupants feel satisfied with the total comfort environment. ASHRAE 55 suggests that 90% of occupants should feel satisfied with any one parameter, such as temperature. Realistically, this means that it is possible that up to 20% of the occupants of a space will not be completely satisfied with their total environment even in "non-problem" buildings. Figure 38.10 shows a schematic representation of an HVAC system serving an occupied space. In the figure, the relationships between the supply air (SA), return air (RA), outside air (OA), the mixed (outside plus return) air (MA), and the exhaust air (EA) are depicted.

The following paragraphs list some common issues or complaints and potential causes or sources of trouble related to HVAC systems.

Complaint: Occupants complain about the work environment using descriptors like "too hot," "too cold," "too dry," or "too humid."

Potential cause: These types of complaints could be the result of simple issues like the thermostat being adjusted improperly or the adjustment of the supply diffuser leading air to blow directly on the occupants. It could also result from the supply air temperature setting too high or low, too much or too little supply air, temperature sensor malfunctioning or misplaced, or the HVAC system being defective or undersized. The humidity controls may not be operating correctly or may have been undersized in the initial system design.

Complaint: The occupants indicate that the air has a musty or "dirty sock" smell.

Potential cause: One of the primary reasons for this complaint is microbiological contamination.

Correcting Testing and Monitoring Results for Non-Standard Air Density

As introduced in Chapter 36, standard conditions for ventilation are assumed to be a barometric (atmospheric) pressure of 29.92 inches Hg, a temperature of 70°F,and dry air where air density is 0.075 lbs/cu ft. Few ventilation systems operate at standard conditions, but the adjustments can be made to account for nonstandard conditions. The equation for determining the density correction factor (d_c) was derived and explained in Chapter 36.

Corrections for water vapor in air, or relative humidity and moisture content, rarely are a concern for IH work related to ventilation systems. For room temperatures and pressures that approximate standard conditions, the effects of humidity can be ignored. However, at high air temperatures (> 100°F) the moisture content may need to be considered. Reference 1 provides additional details related to the effects of moisture content at high temperatures.

Corrections to Airflow

For a single system where the temperature remains essentially unchanged, and where static pressure changes in the system do not exceed 20 inches w.g., changes to the air density do not affect relationship between the volume air flow, the velocity of air throughout the system and the cross sectional area

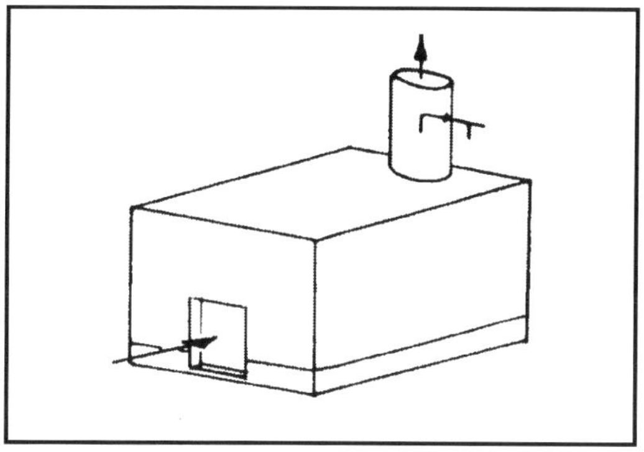

Figure 38.11 — Furnace exhaust schematic for Example 35.8.

of the ductwork (Q = VA). If the temperature in the ventilation system changes significantly (e.g., air passes through a furnace and rises 100F), then a correction to the airflow should be made.

Example 35.8. Dry air at STP conditions enters an oven at a volume flowrate of 1,000 scfm and is heated to 300°F. What is the volume flowrate exiting the oven? No water is added to the air. A basic drawing of this type of oven in shown in Figure 38.11.

Outcome. The most useful approach to this problem is to estimate the actual mass of air moving through the oven. Since the density (d) of the air at STP is 0.075 lbs/ft³, the *mass* flowrate (m) entering the oven can be calculated:

$$m = Q_{in} \times d = 1000 \times 0.075 = 75 \frac{\text{lbs}}{\text{min}}$$

The same *mass* flowrate will exit the oven but since the air density is lower, the volume flowrate will be higher. The density correction factor can be found (using Equation 36-3):

$$d_c = \frac{(460 + 70)}{(460 + 300)} \times \frac{29.92}{29.92} = 0.697 \approx 0.70$$

Using d_c the actual air density can be determined:

$$d_{actual} = d_{STP} \times d_c = 0.075 \times 0.70 = 0.0525 \text{ lb/ft}^3$$

The volume flowrate out of the oven can then be determined using the mass flowrate and the actual air density:

$$Q_{out} = \frac{m}{d_{actual}} = \frac{75}{0.0525} = 1428 \approx 1400 \text{ acfm}$$

Corrections for Velocity and Velocity Pressure Measurements

If a velometer is used to measure velocity, a density correction factor should be applied to the velocity measurement. Most commercial anemometers and velometers have an air density correction method; the individual instrument operating instructions should be consulted. If a pitot tube and manometer are used to measured velocity pressure, the density correction factor should be applied in the velocity conversion calculations (using Equation 37-2 from Chapter 37).

Summary

Proper operation of ventilation systems are necessary for conditioning of HVAC supplied air and for local exhaust system removal of contaminants from the workplace. The ability to test, monitor, and troubleshoot ventilation systems is an essential skill set for the industrial hygienist. Collaboration with engineering and maintenance professionals will help to ensure that the efforts of the IH to diagnose and recommend solutions to ventilation concerns will help to ensure that feasible, viable solutions are implemented.

References and Additional Information

1. **Burton, D.J.:** *Industrial Ventilation Workbook*, 7th edition. Bountiful, UT: IVE, Inc., 2011.
2. **American Conference of Governmental Industrial Hygienists (ACGIH®):** *Industrial Ventilation, a Manual of Recommended Practice for O&M*, 27th edition. Cincinnati, OH: ACGIH®, 2010.
3. **Burton, D.J.:** *IAQ and HVAC Workbook*, 5th edition. Bountiful, UT: IVE, Inc., 2011.
4. **American Society of Heating, Refrigerating and Air Conditioning Engineers (ASHRAE):** *ASHRAE 55-2010, Thermal Environmental Conditions for Human Occupancy*. Atlanta, GA: ASHRAE, 2010.
5. **American Society of Heating, Refrigerating and Air Conditioning Engineers (ASHRAE):** *ASHRAE 62-2007, Ventilation for Acceptable Indoor Air Quality*. Atlanta, GA: ASHRAE, 2007.
6. **National Institute for Occupational Safety and Health and the U.S. Environmental Protection Agency (NIOSH/EPA):** *Building Air Quality — A Guide for Building Owners and Facility Managers*, National Institute for Occupational Safety and Health and Environmental Protection Agency: (EPA/400/1-91-033). Washington, D.C.: Government Printing Office, 1991.
7. **American Society of Heating, Refrigerating and Air Conditioning Engineers (ASHRAE):** Fundamentals Handbook. Atlanta, GA: ASHRAE, 2009.
8. **American Industrial Hygiene Association (AIHA®):** ANSI/AIHA Z9 Standards. Fairfax, VA: AIHA®.

Outcome Competencies

After completing this chapter, the reader should be able to:

1. Define underlined terms used in this chapter.
2. Identify the significance of dermal hazards and their control in the workplace.
3. Summarize the types of protective clothing by hazard category.
4. Explain the processes of degradation, penetration, and permeation of protective clothing.
5. Summarize the test methods used to determine the effectiveness of protective clothing.
6. Explain the exposure assessment process used for selection of protective clothing.
7. Organize criteria for the selection of appropriate protective clothing.
8. Describe the process of contamination and summarize example methods of decontamination.
9. Summarize the causes, effects, and control of heat stress caused by protective clothing.
10. Identify the components of a protective clothing program.

Key Terms

breakthrough time • degradation • penetration • permeation • permeation rate

Prerequisite Knowledge

Prior to beginning this chapter, the user should review the following chapters:

Chapter Number	Chapter Topic
4	Occupational Exposure Limits
8	Occupational and Environmental Health Risk Assessment/Risk Management
19	Biological Monitoring
20	The Skin and the Work Environment
22	Biohazards and Associated Issues
26	Ionizing Radiation
27	Applied Physiology of Thermoregulation and Exposure Control
28	Thermal Standards and Measurement Techniques
34	Prevention and Mitigation of Accidental Chemical Releases
35	General Methods for the Control of Airborne Hazards
37	Local Exhaust Ventilation Systems
52	Occupational Safety

Key Topics

I. An Overview of Dermal Hazards
   A. Chemical Hazards
   B. Physical Hazards
   C. Biological Hazards

II. Types of Protective Clothing
   A. Gloves
   B. Boots
   C. Garments

III. Ergonomics of Protective Clothing

IV. Selection of Protective Clothing
   A. Determining the Hazards and Their Potential Effects
   B. Other Control Options
   C. Determining Performance Characteristics
   D. Determining the Need for Decontamination
   E. Determining the Ergonomic Constraints and Cost

V. Maintenance, Inspection, and Repair

VI. Worker Education and Training

VII. Developing and Managing a Protective Clothing Program

Personal Protective Clothing

39

By S. Zack Mansdorf, PhD, CIH, CSP, QEP and Norman W. Henry, III, MS, CIH

Introduction

Dermatological disorders are one of the National Institute for Occupational Safety and Health's (NIOSH) top 10 leading occupational health problems.[1] These disorders are primarily a result of unprotected exposures to harmful chemical, biological, and physical agents. Most of the injuries and disease risks from dermatological disorders can be prevented or reduced through the appropriate selection and use of protective clothing or other control methods.[2]

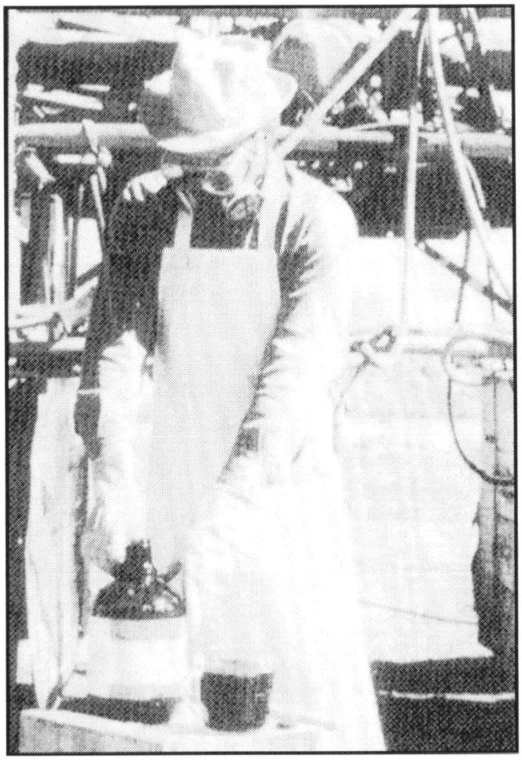

Figure 39.1 — Worker handling chemicals.

While protective clothing can be an effective control method for occupational hazards, its effectiveness depends on proper use by the wearer, and it should be used only after careful consideration of other more effective and less user-dependent control measures. Failure of the protective clothing or its improper selection and use frequently can result in injury or illness.

In this chapter the categories of dermal hazards, types of protective clothing, ergonomic considerations, selection, maintenance issues, worker education and training, and management of a protective clothing program will be reviewed.

An Overview of Dermal Hazards

There are several general categories of hazards for which specialized clothing can provide protection. These general categories include chemical, physical, and biological hazards.

Chemical Hazards

For many chemicals the dermal hazards are just one aspect of the overall potential risk factors, and some chemicals may present more than one type of dermal hazard. For example, phenol may cause both a local skin reaction and systemic damage. There are at least three key factors to be considered when assessing the dermal risk that chemical hazards pose: (1) the likely routes of exposure (e.g., inhalation, ingestion, dermal, injection); (2) potential adverse effects of unprotected exposure; and (3) the exposure potential (likely dose) associated with the

Table 39.1 — Examples of Dermal Hazard Categories

Hazard	*Examples*
Chemical	irritants allergens corrosives dermal toxins systemic toxins cancer causing agents
Physical	trauma producing thermal hazards (hot/cold) fire vibration radiation
Biological	human pathogens animal pathogens environmental pathogens

work assignment. Of the three factors, the adverse dermal effects and systemic effects through skin permeation are the most important consideration for determining the need for protective clothing.[3,4] Some exposure scenarios simply present a cleanliness issue (e.g., oil and grease) while others (e.g., skin contact with anhydrous hydrofluoric acid) could result in a situation that is immediately dangerous to life and health (see Figure 39.1).

As shown in Table 39.1, adverse effects of skin contact with chemicals can include irritation, an allergic response, corrosion (chemical burns), skin toxicity, systemic toxicity (permeation through the skin), and promotion of cancer of the skin or other body cancers. Nicotine, an example of a chemical that normally presents the greatest risk by the dermal route, has significant toxicity due to excellent skin permeability but is not generally an inhalation hazard unless vaporized and inhaled. This is only one of many instances where the dermal route offers a much more significant risk than the other routes of entry.[5] Chemicals with the potential to contribute significantly to a worker's overall dose by the dermal route are identified by a "skin" notation in the Occupational Safety and Health Administration's permissible exposure limits (PELs) and in the American Conference of Governmental Industrial Hygienists (ACGIH®) threshold limit values (TLVs®).[6] However, many other substances that do not normally present inhalation hazards can have significant adverse effects on unprotected skin.[7] For example, inorganic acids have low vapor pressures but are hazardous to the skin because of their corrosive nature. As a worst case example, a single unprotected skin exposure to anhydrous hydrofluoric acid (above 70% concentration) can be fatal. As little as a 5% acid burn can result in death from both the corrosion and the effects of the fluoride ion.[8] On the opposite end of the spectrum, inorganic lead is an example of a material that is highly toxic to humans but has little skin toxicity. In this case the concern is skin contamination that could later lead to ingestion or inhalation, since the vast majority of particulates will not permeate intact skin.

Chemical Permeation of Barriers

Research showing the diffusion of solvent through "liquid-proof" protective clothing barriers has been published for more than four decades.[9,10] Acetone, for example, has been shown to pass through neoprene rubber (of typical glove thickness) within 30 minutes of direct liquid contact on the normal outside surface of the barrier.[11] This permeation is a process by which a chemical can pass through the protective clothing without going through pinholes, pores, or other visible openings. The permeation process consists of the diffusion of chemicals on a molecular level through protective clothing. Individual chemical molecules enter the material and pass between the molecules of the protective clothing. Permeation, since it is essentially diffusion, is best described by Fick's first law.[12] The significance of Fickian diffusion within the discussion of chemical protective clothing is that the permeation rate increases with temperature and is inversely related to thickness. The permeation process occurs in three steps: (1) absorption of the chemical at the barrier surface; (2) diffusion through the barrier; and (3) desorption of the chemical on the normal inside surface of the barrier (see Figure 39.2). It should also be noted that for permeation to occur, continuous contact between the chemical and the barrier material is not required. Intermittent exposures can also result in significant permeation, as has been shown by a testing method used to model these types of exposure situations.[13]

The time elapsed from the initial contact of the chemical on the outside surface until detection on the inside surface is called the breakthrough time. The permeation rate is the rate of movement (mass flux) of the chemical through the barrier. The permeation rate is normally reported in mass per unit area per unit time (e.g., μg/cm²/min) after equilibrium is reached and may be normalized for thickness. Most current testing done for permeation resistance is for periods of up to eight hours to reflect normal work shifts.[14] However, these tests are conducted under conditions of direct liquid or gaseous contact that typically do not occur in the work environment. Therefore, it might be assumed that there would be a significant safety factor built into the test. While this point has some validity, the permeation test is static, while the work environment is dynamic (flexing of materials, pressures generated from gripping or movement, prior physical damage to the glove or garment, etc.).

Given the lack of published skin permeability and dermal toxicity data, the approach taken by most safety and health professionals is to select a barrier with no breakthrough for the duration of the job or task (usually 8 hours), which is essentially a no dose concept.[3] This is an appropriate conservative approach; however, it is important to note that there is no protective barrier currently available that provides permeation resistance to all chemicals. For situations where the breakthrough times are short, the safety and health professional should select the barrier(s) with the best performance (i.e., longest breakthrough time and/or lowest permeation rate) as well as considering other control measures (such as a clothing change).

Permeation Testing

A standard test method for determining permeation of protective clothing is F739-07, "Test Method for Resistance of Protective Clothing Materials to Permeation by Liquids or Gases Under Conditions of Continuous Contact," published by the American Society for Testing and Materials (ASTM).[15] In essence, the test consists of placing the barrier material between a reservoir of the challenge chemical (liquid or gas) and a collection cell connected to an analytical detector (see Figure 39.3). Hence, the actual reported breakthrough time is also related to the sensitivity of both the analytical method and system (i.e., collection system). Variations on this method can also be performed, such as a determination of permeation resulting from intermittent contact or a procedure for permeation of volatiles based on weight loss from evaporation through the barrier.[13,16]

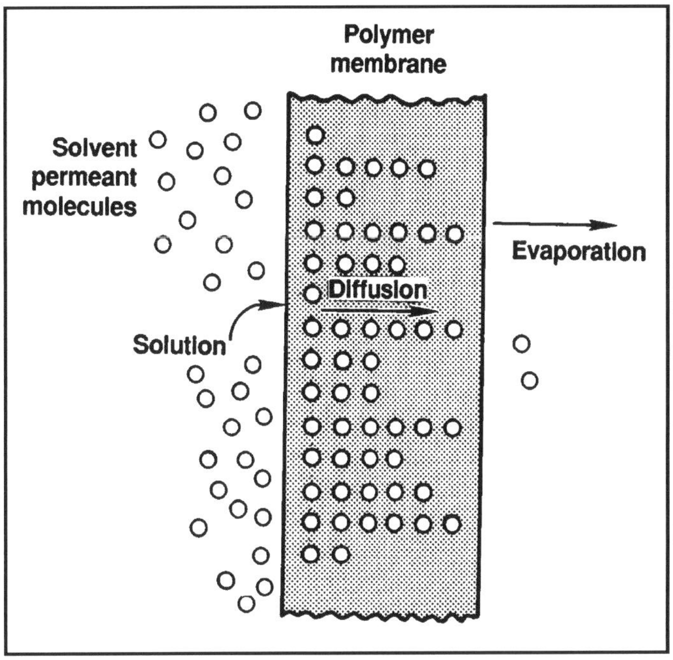

Figure 39.2 — The permeation process.

Aside from the permeation process, there are two other chemical resistance properties of concern to the health and safety professional. These are degradation and penetration. Degradation is a deleterious change in one or more physical properties of a protective material caused by contact with a chemical. For example, the polymer polyvinyl alcohol is a very good barrier to most organic solvents but swells and is degraded by water. Latex rubber, which is widely used for medical gloves, is readily soluble in toluene and hexane, as another example. Therefore, latex or natural rubber gloves would be ineffective for protection against these chemical solvents. In many cases degradation can be assumed if the barrier swells or has a change in physical appearance (wrinkles, burns, color changes, etc.). Degradation may not always be visible. Solvents can wash out the plasticizer in some polymers causing them to become brittle but not change the appearance of

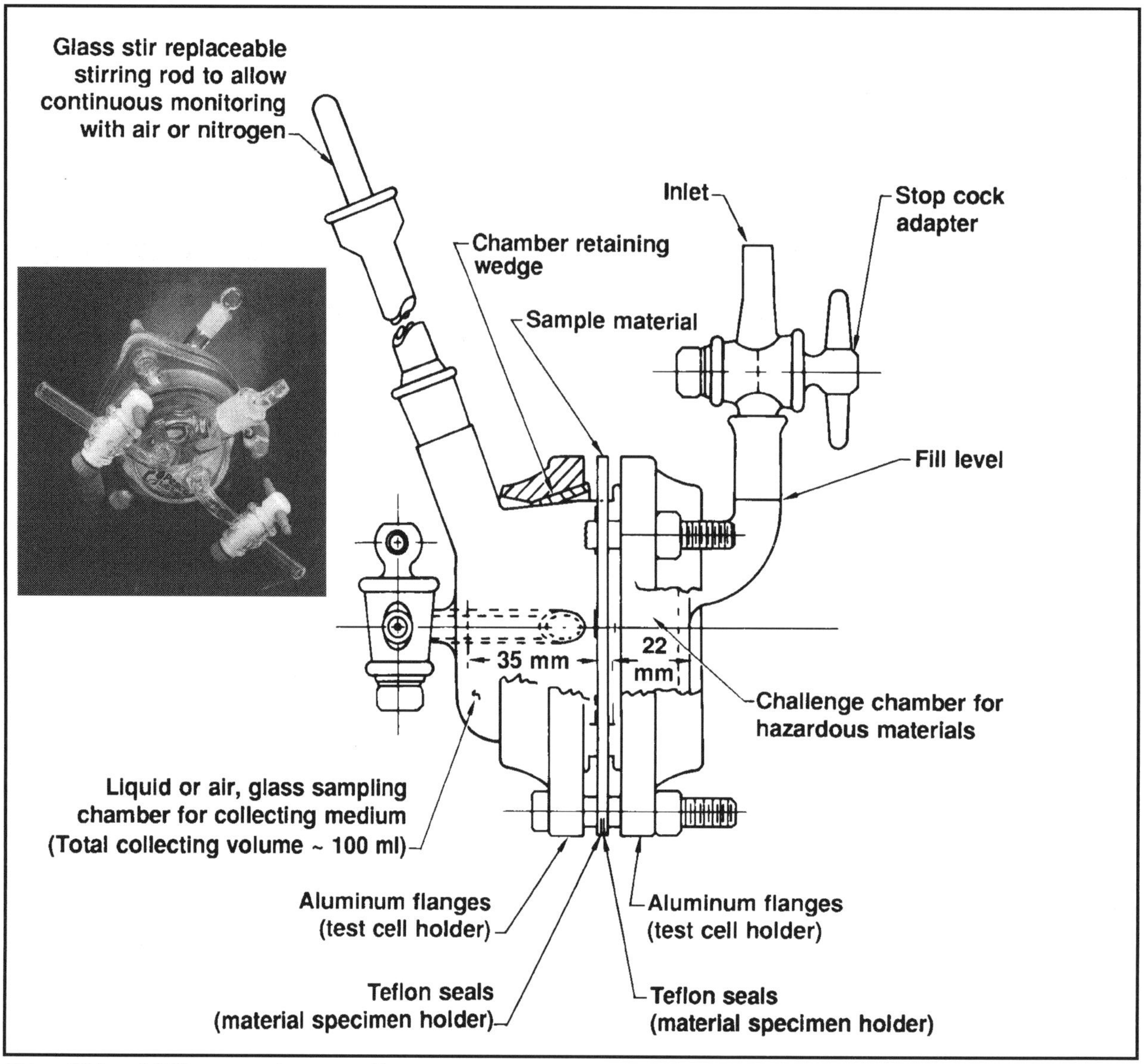

Figure 39.3 — ASTM permeation test cell.

the barrier.[17] Data showing degradation may be used to disqualify a clothing material from consideration but should not be used solely for selection, since permeation may occur without evidence of degradation.

Penetration is the flow of a chemical through zippers, weak seams, pinholes, cuts, or imperfections in the protective clothing on a non-molecular level. Even the best protective barriers will be rendered ineffective if punctured or torn. Penetration protection is important when the exposure is unlikely or infrequent and the toxicity or hazard minimal. Penetration is usually a concern in garments used for splash protection and for some applications of breathable garments that have liquid resistance.

Chemical Resistance Data and Complicating Factors

Several guides have been published listing chemical resistance data for many of the most widely used industrial chemicals; many are also available in an electronic format.[7,18,19] In addition to these guides, most manufacturers in the industrially developed countries also publish, in printed and electronic form, current chemical and physical resistance data for their products.

In general, the permeation of protective clothing can also be estimated using solubility parameters and other factors such as molecular size.[12] From this model, chemicals that are most closely related can be expected to behave most alike in terms of permeation - "like dissolves like." For example, the ketones would be expected to have similar permeation characteristics since they have similar chemical structures. Generally, this holds true, and testing supports this approximation in many instances. Hence, a barrier with good resistance to permeation by ethyl alcohol would be expected to behave in a like fashion when exposed to methyl alcohol. Nevertheless, while this is a good approximation, it is not universal. Also, most of the rubber compounds and some of the polymers contain varying mixtures of additives that can have significant effects on permeation. Neoprene rubber barriers from different manufacturers and different lots, for example, can perform quite differently.[20] The common difficulties in laboratory variability also affect permeation results. NIOSH has developed a Permeation Calculator software package which is available at the NIOSH website to persons and laboratories conducting this testing. The intent is to reduce the variables and potential errors in this testing. Finally, and to further complicate the issue, chemical mixtures can behave much differently than neat or pure compounds. For some mixtures, the breakthrough times can be much shorter than any of the individual component times.[21] This is probably because of the effects of the interactions among the components and the potential for one or more of the components to act as a vehicle. Very little published permeation data exists for mixtures. In these situations it is important to test the mixture against the barrier of choice.

Physical Hazards

As noted in Table 39.1, examples of physical hazards include those that produce trauma, those from thermal effects, and those produced by vibration or radiation. Trauma to the skin from physical hazards (cuts, abrasions, etc.) is common to many occupations, with construction and meat cutting as two examples. Thermal hazards to the skin include the adverse effects of extreme cold and heat such as those from molten metals or handling cryogenic liquids. The protective attribute of clothing for these hazards is related to the insulation provided, which generally increases with thickness. Protective clothing for flash fire and electric arc exposures requires flame resistance properties.[22] Firefighters and others with similar exposures to both heat and flame require protection that is both fire resistant and insulating.[23] They typically use a multilayered garment that also includes a vapor barrier to protect them from steam generated from the heat of a fire.

Protection from some forms of both ionizing and non-ionizing radiation can be achieved using protective clothing. In general, protective clothing intended to reduce ionizing radiation exposures is based either on the principle of shielding (e.g., lead-lined aprons and gloves) or by preventing particulate radionuclides and liquids from direct contact with the skin. Clothing for electromagnetic radiation protection, such as microwave, is based on grounding, whereas protection from light (ultraviolet, visible, and infrared) depends on the wavelength of the radiation.[24] For example, infrared protection is usually afforded by reflective clothing such as aluminumized coverings (Figure 39.4 illustrates an example of thermal hazards.)

Excessive vibration can have several adverse effects on body parts, primarily the hands. Occupations such as mining (handheld drills) and road repair (pneumatic hammers or chisels) are two examples where excessive hand vibration can lead to bone degeneration and loss of circulation in the hands (Raynaud's phenomenon).[25] Specialized protective clothing (e.g., gel, urethane or foam containing gloves) can help to damp the vibration received by the body and to keep the hands warm and dry. Selection needs to be based on knowledge of the vibration frequencies of the exposure and the effectiveness of the gloves selected at those exposure frequencies.

Biological Hazards

Biological hazards include infection from agents and diseases common to humans, those common to animals, and those common to the work environment that can have adverse effects on humans. Biological hazards common to humans have received great attention with the increasing spread of bloodborne pathogens such as AIDS (acquired immune deficiency syndrome) and hepatitis. Hence, health care work that

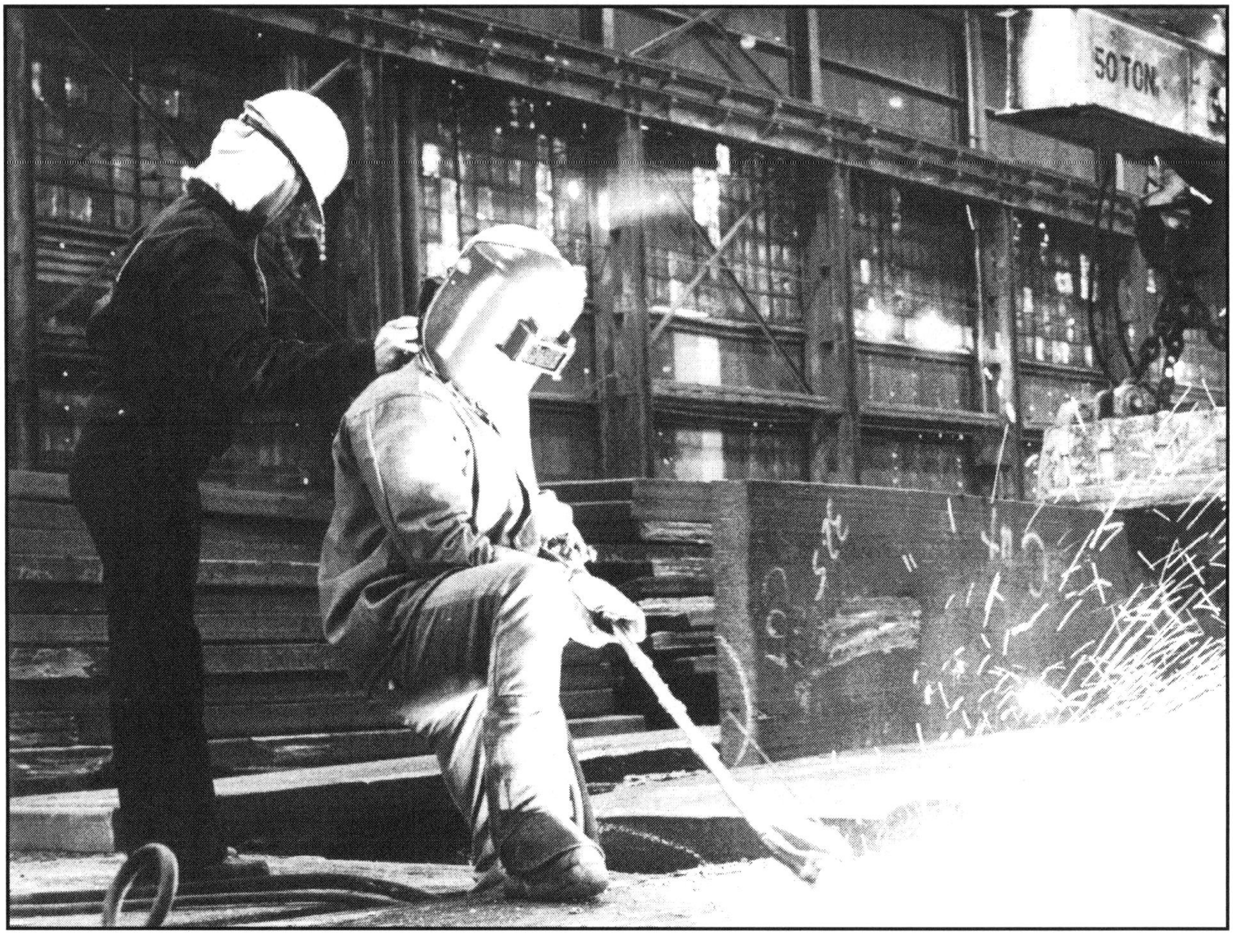

Figure 39.4 — Thermal hazards.

might involve exposure to blood or body fluids usually requires some type of liquid-resistant garment and gloves (see Figure 39.5).[26] OSHA requires that appropriate protective clothing be used for these exposure situations under its bloodborne pathogens regulation (29 CFR 1910.1030). Diseases transmitted from animals through handling (e.g., anthrax) have a long history of recognition and require protective measures similar to those used for handling bloodborne pathogens from humans.[27] Work environments that can present a hazard from biological agents include sewage treatment plants, composting facilities, and clinical and microbiological laboratories as well as other special work environments.

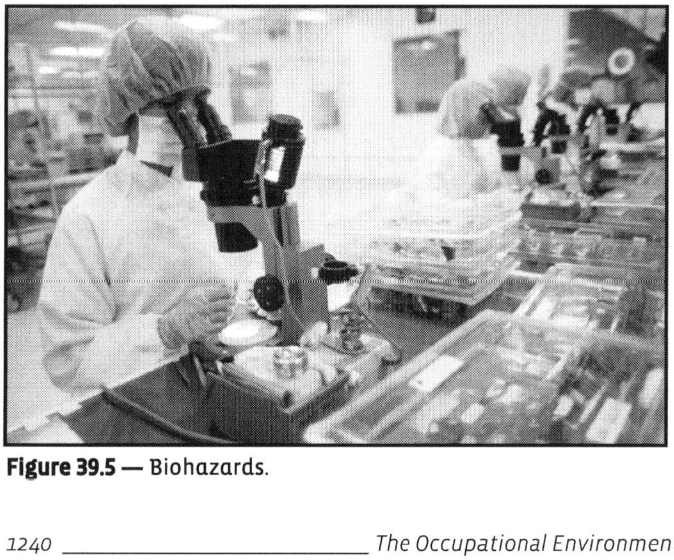

Figure 39.5 — Biohazards.

Biological Testing

Standard methods for testing the biological resistance of protective clothing have also recently been developed by ASTM Committee F-23 on Protective Clothing.[28,29] These methods were developed to determine the penetration resistance to biological liquids and blood borne-pathogens such as hepatitis and AIDS viruses. By using the same penetration test apparatus used for chemical penetration (ASTM F-903) a synthetic blood mixture with or without a serrate non-pathogenic virus particle (Phi-X 174) having the approximate size as the hepatitis virus is exposed to the outside surface of glove or garment samples to look for visual penetration of the blood. Viral particles are detected by swabbing the inside surface of the sample and platting out on a growth medium to look for viral plaques. The presence of synthetic blood and a viral plaque indicate that penetration has occurred. These pass/ fail test methods, while not quantitative in nature, help screen candidate gloves, garments and suits with physical imperfections (pin holes, etc.) that potentially would allow for dermal contact and exposure to hazardous blood-borne pathogens in biological liquids. A mechanical pressure test with synthetic blood has also been developed and added to the biological test battery for screening clothing.[30]

Types of Protective Clothing

Protective clothing in a generic sense includes all elements of a protective ensemble (e.g., garments, gloves, boots, etc.). Thus, protective clothing can include everything from a finger cot providing protection against paper cuts to a fully encapsulating suit with self-contained breathing apparatus used for an emergency response to a hazardous chemical spill.

Protective clothing can be made of natural materials (e.g., cotton, wool, leather), man-made fibers (e.g., nylon, rayon), or various polymers (plastics and rubbers such as butyl rubber, polyvinyl chloride, chlorinated polyethylene, etc.). Table 39.2 summarizes by hazard the typical physical, chemical, and biologic performance requirements and common protective materials used.

Protective clothing materials and configurations vary greatly depending on the intended use. However, for most physical hazards the normal components are analogous to personal clothing (e.g., pants, jacket, hood, boots, gloves). Special use items for applications such as flame resistance can include chaps, armlets, and aprons constructed of both treated and untreated natural (including asbestos weaves) and synthetic fibers and materials. Specially treated or inherently flame-resistant porous fabrics and materials are commonly used for flash fire and electric arc (flash over) protection (e.g., petrochemical industry and electric utility industries) but usually do not provide protection from any long-term heat or flame exposure. It should be noted that firefighting requires specialized clothing that provides flame (burning) resistance, a liquid barrier, and thermal insulation (protection from heat), while entry into fuel fires (with their strong infrared component) also requires reflective clothing (e.g., aluminumized cover). Clothing for cut protection can range from garments of aramid fibers to chain mail gloves of metal construction (including titanium) or special fiber batting for protection against chain saws. Protection from cold extremes usually includes multiple components of high insulating values that allow for the wicking and/or evaporation of perspiration. When

Table 39.2 — Common Physical, Chemical, and Biological Performance Requirements

Hazard	*Performance Characteristic Required*	*Common Protective Clothing Materials*
Thermal	insulation value	heavy cotton or other natural fabrics
Fire	insulation and flame resistance	aluminized gloves; fire retardant; aramid fiber and other special fabrics
Mechanical abrasion	abrasion resistance; tensile strength	heavy fabrics; leather with metal studding
Cuts	cut resistance	metal mesh; aromatic polyamide fiber and other special fabrics
Punctures	puncture resistance	leather; fabric coated with filled plastic; thick elastomers
Vibration	damping	natural or polymeric gloves with elastomeric linings
Chemical/toxicologic	permeation resistance	polymeric materials; elastomeric materials
Biological	"fluid-proof;" puncture resistant	latex or polymer
Radiologic	usually fluid resistant or particle	polymer gloves; lead lined resistant for radioneuclides or shield containing

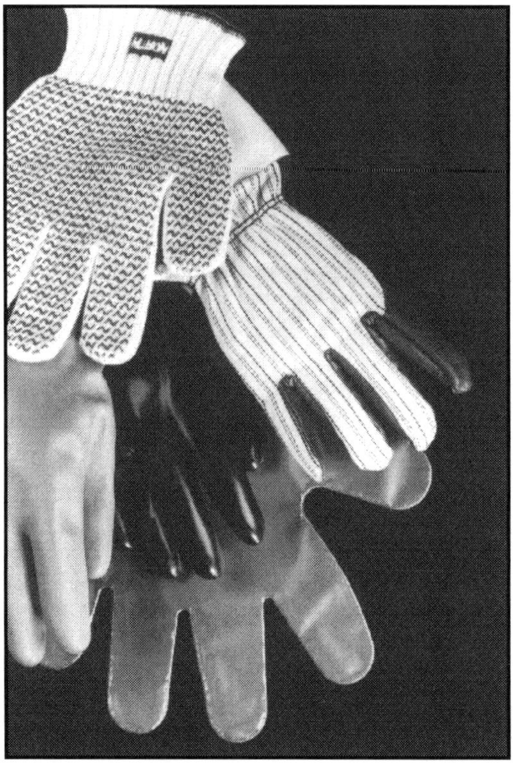

Figure 39.6 — Glove examples. (Photo courtesy of North Safety Products).

chemical protection also is needed, the clothing construction can be even more exotic.

Gloves

Protective gloves are made from a wide variety of natural and synthetic materials. Light-duty cotton gloves and heavy-duty leather gloves are used to protect against a variety of physical hazards. Synthetic gloves can be used to protect against both physical and chemical hazards. They fall into four major construction categories: knit, unsupported, supported, and laminated.

Knit synthetic gloves are typically used for cut resistance. They can be made of high strength synthetic yarns or fiber-wrapped steel yarns. Gloves of chain mail and steel-stapled leather are also available.

Chemically protective gloves (see Figure 39.6) are usually available in a wide variety of polymers and combinations such as cotton gloves coated by the polymer of interest using a dipping process during the manufacturing. Some of the foil and multi-laminate gloves are only two dimensional (flat) and therefore have some ergonomic constraints but are highly chemical resistant. These gloves typically work best when a form-fitting outer polymer glove is worn over the top of the inner flat glove (called double gloving) to conform to the shape of the hands. Polymer gloves are available in a wide variety of thicknesses ranging from very light weight (<2 mm) to heavy weight (>5 mm) with and without inner liners or substrates (called scrims). Gloves are also commonly available in a variety of lengths ranging from approximately 25 cm for hand protection to gauntlets of approximately 80 cm extending from the workers shoulder to the tip of the hand. The correct choice of length depends on the extent of protection required. However, the length should normally extend at least to the worker's wrist to prevent drainage into the glove.

Boots

Boots are available in a wide variety of heights ranging from hip height to those that only cover the bottom of the foot. Chemical protective boots are available in only a limited number of polymers since the boot heal and sole require a high degree of abrasion resistance. Common polymers and rubbers used in chemically resistant boot construction include PVC (polyvinyl chloride), butyl rubber, nitrile, and neoprene rubber. Specially constructed laminate boots using other polymers can also be obtained but are quite expensive and the polymer choices are limited at the present time. Foot coverings that are integrated into a suit and therefore use the same protective barrier are available to extend the chemical resistance properties of the barrier to the feet. They are intended as foot coverings to be used inside a boot, although some fully encapsulating suits do have integrated boots intended for contact with the ground.

Garments

Chemical protective garments can be obtained as one-piece fully encapsulating, gas-tight garments with attached gloves and boots or as multiple components (e.g., pants, jacket, hoods, etc.) (see Figure 39.7). Some protective materials used for construction of ensembles have multiple layers or laminants. Layered materials are generally required for polymers that do not have good inherent physical integrity and abrasion resistance properties (e.g., butyl rubber versus Teflon™) to permit manufacture and use as a garment or glove. Common support fabrics are nylon, polyester, aramides, and fiber glass. These substrates are coated or laminated by polymers such as PVC, Teflon, polyurethane, polyethylene, and other proprietary materials. Some suits use layering of different polymers to improve the range of chemical resistance (e.g., a layering of neoprene, nylon for support, and butyl rubber).

There has been enormous growth in the use of non-woven polyethylene- and polypropylene-based materials for disposable garment construction. These garments, sometimes incorrectly called paper suits, are made using a special process where the fibers are bonded together rather than knitted or

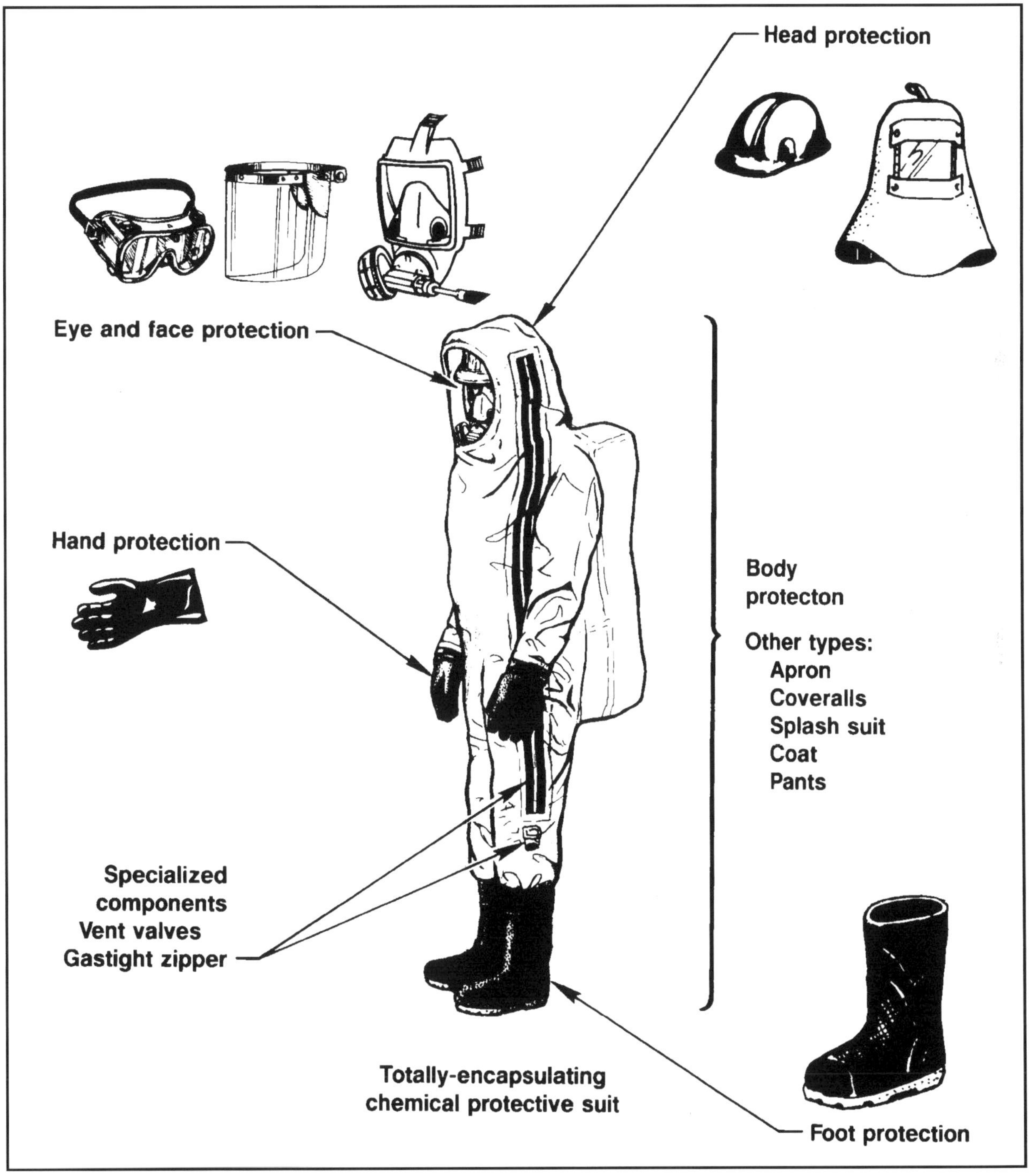

Figure 39.7 — Types of protective clothing.

woven.[31] These non-woven fabric garments are low in cost, very lightweight, and have good applications for protection against particulates, but are not normally chemical nor liquid resistant.[32] Non-woven fabric-based garments are also available with various coatings or films such as polyethylene, Saran™, and other polymers. Depending on the coating or lamination characteristics, these garments offer good chemical resistance to many common substances. Garments are also available that include construction with microporous films. These products are often considered breathable because they allow some water vapor transmission. This feature may make them less prone to producing heat stress under some conditions. However, microporous films still allow vapors to penetrate and may not always prevent liquid penetration. It should also be noted that this type of protective clothing is available for clean room applications. However, this is for protection of the product rather than the wearer. The concern here is debris from the human and lint from street clothing.

The fully encapsulating, gas-tight suit of one-piece construction provides the highest level of protection available from chemical protective clothing. In the majority of these configurations, the respiratory protection device (airline or self-contained breathing apparatus-SCBA) is worn within the suit. Protection factors for suits of this type are typically higher than those for the respiratory protection (protection factor of 10,000), provided that the suit has appropriate chemical resistance to the challenge.[33]

The U.S. Environmental Protection Agency, in cooperation with a number of other agencies such as NIOSH, has devised a scheme to describe levels of protection for protective ensembles used on hazardous waste sites.[34] Their scheme consists of four levels designated by the letters A through D.

Level A: SCBA or a positive pressure airline system with escape SCBA and a totally encapsulating chemical protective suit, gloves (double layer), chemically resistant boots, plus other safety equipment.

Level B: Same respirator as Level A with a hooded chemical-resistant suit, gloves (double layer), chemically resistant boots, plus other safety equipment.

Level C: Full-face or half-mask air-purifying respirator and the same protective clothing as in Level B, plus other safety equipment.

Level D: No respiratory protection; coveralls with an option for gloves, boot coverings, and other related safety equipment.

It should be recognized that Levels B and C require the same splash suit. Most industrial situations require a much more specific protective clothing ensemble selection beyond the generic requirement of a splash suit and gloves. The selection of the appropriate barriers for the industrial situation is usually easier to complete since the challenge chemicals and work requirements will usually be known.

Ergonomics of Protective Clothing

In all but a few cases the addition of protective clothing and equipment will decrease productivity and increase worker discomfort.[35] Some exceptions might be cold environments as related to improved gripping power with some gloves for certain objects. The use of protective clothing may also lead to decreased work quality since error rates increase with the use of protective clothing.

For chemical protective and some fire resistant clothing there are some general guidelines that need to be considered concerning the inherent conflicts between worker comfort, efficiency, and protection. First, the thicker the barrier the better the protection. Increased thickness will increase the time to breakthrough or provides greater insulation for thermal protection. However, the thicker the barrier the more likely it will decrease ease of movement and user comfort. Thicker barriers also increase the potential for heat stress. Second, barriers with excellent chemical resistance tend to increase the level of worker discomfort and heat stress. This is because the barrier normally will also deter water vapor transmission, therefore reducing evaporative cooling through sweating. Third, the higher the overall protection of the clothing, the more time the job will take to accomplish and the more likely there will be work errors. There are also some jobs or tasks where use of protective clothing could increase the risk related to other hazards, such as when working around moving machinery, or when working in high temperature areas. While these situations are rare, they must be considered.

Other issues relate to the physical limitations imposed by using protective clothing. For example, a worker wearing a thick pair of gloves may not be able to perform tasks that require a high degree of dexterity and repetitive motions. As another example, a spray painter in a totally encapsulating suit usually will not be able to look to the side, up, or down since the respirator facepiece and suit visor typically restrict the field of vision. These are only some examples of the ergonomic restrictions created when wearing protective clothing and equipment.

One of the primary ergonomic constraints for chemically-resistant suits and ensembles is the issue of heat stress. Once the worker dons the suit, the microclimate quickly approaches 100% relative humidity. The body core temperature rises since the suits have good insulating properties and present a barrier to the evaporation of perspiration. The amount of heat retained within the suit and the level of perspiration will depend on the metabolic work load. Nevertheless, almost all suits that are chemically resistant and cover all or most of the body present heat stress challenges. Solutions to the problem include providing protection from radiant heat (shielding), cooling outside environments (air conditioning or early/late work), replacing fluids frequently, and using rest breaks. Additional controls can include the use of ice-containing body vests, portable and integrated cooling systems (most use circulating cool water in a body garment), and venturi (air-based) coolers where applicable. Regardless of the measures used, workers in heat stress situations should be closely monitored.

The work situation must always be considered in the selection of the protective clothing for the job. The optimum solution is to select the minimum level of protective clothing and equipment that is necessary to do the job safely.

Selection of Protective Clothing

In the U.S., OSHA regulations (29 CFR 1910.132) require that a hazard assessment for personal protective equipment be conducted before assignment.[36] In summary, the regulation requires the employer to assess the workplace to determine whether hazards are present or likely to be present, and if so, to select the appropriate protective equipment for the specific hazard(s) involved. It also requires the selection decision to be communicated to the affected employee, for the equipment to fit properly, and training of employees in the use and limitations of the equipment provided.

The overall approach to the selection of protective clothing for most situations can be illustrated using an eight-step process that incorporates the required OSHA hazard assessment. These steps are as follows:

1. Determine the type of hazard(s) most likely to occur.
2. Determine the adverse effects of unprotected exposure.
3. Determine whether other control options can be used instead of protective clothing.
4. Determine performance characteristics needed for protection.
5. Determine the need for decontamination (as applicable).
6. Determine the ergonomic constraints presented.
7. Determine the cost of the various options.
8. Make the selection.

Determining the Hazards and Their Potential Adverse Effects

The risk assessment process is fundamental to the practice of occupational hygiene. It is covered in detail in Chapter 8. Therefore, the discussion of this topic will be limited to how it might be applied to protective clothing. In this regard, chemical hazards will be used as the model. The process should begin with a determination of the chemical hazards of the process or work task, likely exposures and routes of exposure, and extent of exposure.

The best method to determine the likely worker exposures and potential routes of exposure is to actually inventory the chemicals used and observe the task or work assignment. A second, but less informative approach, is to have the work process described or to evaluate it from a written description. Coupled with knowledge of the chemicals used in the process including physical characteristics such as vapor pressure, physical state, etc., an assessment of the most likely routes of exposure can be made. Likewise, an assessment of the dermal hazards presented by the chemicals used can be obtained from the MSDS and other reference sources.

Once the evaluation of the likely exposures, route(s) of entry, and toxicity of the materials has been completed, an assessment of the extent of potential exposure needs to be determined. That is, what is the nature and extent of worker contact? For liquid chemicals, as an example, is the nature of potential contact simply from an inadvertent splash, or do workers become wet from contact with the chemical? For those scenarios where the material is highly hazardous (e.g., liquid sodium cyanide) although the likelihood of contact is remote, the worker must obviously be provided with the highest level of protection available. The level of protection does not need to be absolute when the exposure represents a very minimal risk (e.g., a nurse applying rubbing alcohol to a patient). This selection logic is based essentially on an estimate of the adverse effects of the material combined with an estimate of the likelihood of exposure.

Other Control Options

The first consideration should always be whether the job or task can be safely done without the use of protective clothing. It has long been the philosophy of NIOSH that personal protective clothing should not be used before consideration of other control options.[37] These include substitution of a less hazardous material, use of automated or mechanical means for accomplishing the task, and use of engineering controls (e.g., ventilation) or non-engineering controls (e.g., administrative controls such as working in the mornings or evenings for hot work). As stated earlier in the chapter, this is because protective clothing is the last line of defense and its efficacy depends heavily on proper use by the worker.

Eye and Face Protection

The eyes are easily damaged; therefore, they must be protected from flying particles, molten metal, aerosols, liquids, gases, vapors, infrared and ultraviolet radiation, and lasers. Safety glasses that comply with ANSI Z87–1989 are designed to protect the eyes from impact. Prescription glasses can be manufactured to meet the impact requirements. Most glasses manufactured to meet the ANSI impact requirements will have side shields; however, some glasses will not. To protect the eyes from side impacts, these glasses must have side shields that slide onto the temple bars of the glasses.

Eye protection for lasers and welding are designed to filter electromagnetic energy. Laser glasses and goggles must be selected to have the minimum optical density (OD) needed to protect the eyes from the specific wavelength of the laser being used. Welding helmets and goggles need to have the minimum shade specified by OSHA in 29 1910.133 for the type of welding, cutting, brazing, or soldering. See Chapter 25 (Nonionizing Radiation) for a more complete discussion of protective equipment for lasers and ultraviolet radiation.

Protecting the eyes from liquid splashes, vapors, gases and aerosols require goggles that seal to the face or shields that are an integral part of a respirator or a totally encapsulating chemical protective suit. Chemical protective goggles are very different from impact-resistant goggles in that they do not have open vents. Liquid splash hazards can be averted using non-vented goggles or goggles with valves that close due to the force of a liquid stream. Non-vented goggles protect against vapors, gases, and aerosols.

Non-sealing face shields protect the face from some chemical splashes and from impact, but they do not provide sufficient protection for the eyes. These open-sided face shields must be augmented by either chemical goggles or impact-resistant glasses to provide adequate eye protection.

Determining Performance Characteristics

The physical and chemical hazards of the job will define the necessary performance characteristics of the protective clothing. Often these performance characteristics will require compromise, since no single selection will meet all of the criteria. For example, there is no commercially available glove that provides both good chemical and thermal or fire resistance. In this case other approaches such as the wearing of a sacrificial insulating outer glove over a chemically resistant glove would need to be considered. This approach would require disposal of the outer glove if contaminated since the fiber-containing gloves would tend to retain the chemical contamination. As another example, the patient would not want a brain surgeon to select a glove with excellent cut and puncture resistance for protection against bloodborne pathogens if its characteristics resulted in poor dexterity. In these cases the desired performance characteristics must be rank-ordered so that the greatest risk is resolved before lesser risks. This approach may also be needed for selection of chemical protective clothing where the challenge material is a mixture that has not been specifically tested. Selection of the barrier that provides the best protection against the most hazardous component of the mixture and then consideration of other options such as double gloving using two different barriers. There are standardized tests for most of the performance characteristics desired as well as for other factors such as ergonomic issues. Many of these test methods have been developed by ASTM and others.(38) These can be quite helpful in comparing performance among manufacturers.

Special caution is required for latex rubber because some proteins in latex rubber can cause an allergic reaction. Although the amount of latex exposure needed to produce sensitization or an allergic reaction is unknown, increasing the exposure to latex proteins increases the risk of developing allergic symptoms. Sensitized people can exhibit symptoms within minutes or hours after an exposure. Mild reactions to latex include skin redness, rash, hives, or itching. More severe reactions can produce a runny nose, sneezing, itchy eyes, scratchy throat, difficult breathing, coughing spells, and wheezing. Shock can occur, but this reaction is rare and is seldom the first sign of latex allergy.

If latex gloves are selected, it is important to use only powder-free gloves with reduced protein content and to make sure those who wear the gloves do not use oil-based hand creams or lotions, which can cause glove deterioration. Hands must be washed with a mild soap and dried thoroughly after the gloves are removed. Areas and equipment contaminated with latex-containing dust must be kept clean. A person with a latex allergy must avoid contact with latex products and avoid areas where they might inhale the powder from latex gloves worn by other workers.(38)

Determining the Need for Decontamination

For protective clothing that is used with hazardous chemicals, decontamination must be considered even if the clothing is intended for a single use. This is because cross-contamination can occur with doffing of the protective clothing. Not all situations will require decontamination; however, there are many case histories of workers needlessly exposed as a result of contact with contaminated clothing. This is an especially important consideration if the work clothing is stored with street clothing, reused, taken home, or laundered with regular clothing.(39)

Determining the Ergonomic Constraints

The ergonomic constraints presented by the job or task need to be evaluated. In some cases it may be necessary to redesign the work tasks to ensure performance requirements can be met while protective clothing is worn. For some tasks it may even be concluded that the work cannot be efficiently or safely performed using protective clothing. In these cases a different approach to accomplishing the task must be developed.

Determining the Economic Impacts

The final factor is the cost of the options available. The financial impact of reuse, including the consideration of decontamination measures when applicable, versus single use should be evaluated along with the other costs of administering an effective protective clothing program and of determining the overall life cycle costs of the clothing (i.e., cost per use).

Finally, the selection can be made using all of the information gathered. From this section of the chapter, it should be fairly clear that the selection choice will usually be the result of the consideration of many factors and not simply a choice based on product literature or a guidebook.

Maintenance, Inspection, and Repair

The proper storage, inspection, cleaning, and repair of protective clothing is important to the overall protection provided by the products to the wearer.

Some protective clothing will have storage limitations. These limitations may include a prescribed shelf-life, requirements for protection from ultraviolet radiation (sunlight), ozone, moisture, temperature extremes, and issues related to product folding. For example, natural rubber products are usually susceptible to all of these environmental factors. Many of the encapsulating polymer suits can be damaged if folded rather than allowed to hang upright. The manufacturer or distributor should be consulted for any specific storage limitations its products may have.

Inspection of protective clothing should be performed frequently by the user (e.g., on receipt, prior to use, and after each use). Inspection by co-workers is another technique that may be used to ensure the integrity of the selected protective clothing. As a management policy, it is also advisable to have the worker's supervisor periodically inspect protective clothing items that are reused routinely (e.g., weekly). Inspection criteria will depend on the intended use of the protective clothing item. However, it would normally include examination for any obvious defects such as tears, holes, imperfections, and degradation. As one example of an inspection technique, clean polymer gloves used for protection against liquids can be inflated with exhaled air to check for integrity.

Cleaning of protective clothing for reuse must be performed with care. Natural fabrics can be cleaned with normal washing procedures as long as they are not contaminated with toxic materials. Synthetic fibers and materials commonly have cleaning procedure limitations. For example, some flame-resistant treatments will lose their effectiveness if the garments are not properly cleaned.[40] Clothing used for protection against non-water soluble chemicals cannot usually be decontaminated by simple water and soap washing. Tests performed on protective clothing used by pesticide applicators indicate that normal washing procedures are not effective for many pesticides.[41] Dry cleaning of some protective clothing is not recommended since it is commonly ineffective and can degrade or contaminate the product. It is important to consult the manufacturer or distributor of the product before attempting cleaning procedures that are not specifically recommended.

Most protective clothing is not repairable. Repairs can be made on some items, such as fully encapsulating polymer suits, depending on the materials of construction and the location of the damage. In all cases, the manufacturer should be consulted for the proper repair procedures.

Worker Education and Training

Adequate education and training for users of protective clothing is essential. Training and education should cover the following:

- The nature and extent of the hazard(s);
- When protective clothing should be worn;
- What protective clothing is necessary;
- Use and limitations of the protective clothing to be assigned;
- How to properly inspect, don, doff, adjust, and wear the protective clothing;
- Decontamination procedures, if necessary;
- Signs and symptoms of overexposure or clothing failure;
- First aid and emergency procedures; and
- The proper storage, useful life, care, and disposal of protective clothing.

Pertinent training areas not already provided to the worker through other programs should also be included. For those topical areas already provided to the worker, refresher training should be given to the clothing user. For example, if the signs and symptoms of overexposure have already been provided as part of the training for working with chemicals, symptoms that are a result of significant dermal exposures versus inhalation should be reemphasized. Finally, workers should have an opportunity to try out the protective clothing before a final selection decision is made and significant quantities ordered.

Knowledge of the hazards and limitations of the protective clothing not only reduces the risk to the worker but also provides the health and safety professional with a person capable of providing feedback on the effectiveness of the protective equipment.

Developing and Managing a Protective Clothing Program

A written protective clothing program can reduce the chance for error, increase worker protection, and establish a consistent approach to the selection and use of protective clothing. A model program could contain the following elements:

- An organization scheme and administrative plan
- A risk assessment methodology
- An evaluation of other control options to protect the worker;
- Performance criteria for the protective clothing
- Selection criteria and procedures to determine the optimum choice
- Purchasing specifications for the protective clothing
- A validation plan for the selection with medical surveillance, as appropriate
- Decontamination and reuse criteria, as applicable
- A user training program
- An auditing plan to assure that procedures are consistently followed
- A demonstration by each user of protective clothing of the ability to use the equipment properly
- Retraining for any worker who does not understand or have the skill needed to use the equipment properly

Misuse of protective clothing is commonly seen in industry. Misuse is usually the result of a lack of understanding of the limitations of protective clothing by management or workers, or both. An example is the use of protective clothing that is not resistant to flame by workers handling flammable solvents or working where open flames, burning coals, or molten metals are present. Some protective clothing made of polymeric materials such as polyethylene will support combustion and actually melt, causing a more severe burn.

Another common misuse is the reuse of protective clothing, especially gloves, where the chemical has contaminated the inside. This can result in increased worker exposure with each subsequent use. A common variation of this problem occurs when workers use natural fiber gloves or wear leather shoes to work with liquid chemicals. If the chemicals contact the natural fibers or leather, they may be retained for long periods of time and migrate to areas where they may contact the skin. This issue can result in the exposure of an entire family if contaminated work clothing is taken home and cleaned with other articles of family clothing.[42] Since many chemicals are not water soluble, they can be spread to other clothes simply by mechanical actions. There have been several examples of this occurring, especially in industries that manufacture or process pesticides and heavy metals (e.g., poisoning of the families of workers handling mercury and lead).

These are only a few of the more prominent examples of the misuse of protective clothing. Many of these problems can be overcome by simply making sure the wearer understands the proper use and limitations of the protective clothing.

Summary

Dermal hazards are a leading cause of occupational illness and injuries. They may be categorized as chemical, physical, and biological. Chemical exposures can result from direct contact or from the more subtle exposure after permeation, mass penetration, or degradation of protective barriers. Physical hazards include those that can produce direct trauma to the skin (e.g., cuts) and those of a thermal nature, vibration, and radiation. Biological hazards include human, animal, and environmental pathogens. Performance requirements for protective clothing will be determined by the nature and degree of the hazard.

Protective clothing can be obtained in a variety of configurations. Most typically these include gloves, boots, and garments. These range from fully encapsulating gas-tight suits to simple hand coverings. Protective clothing of all types typically present ergonomic constraints and may lead to increased stresses, such as heat stress and lower productivity.

Selection of protective clothing should be based on:

1. A determination of the hazard
2. Determination of the adverse effects of exposure
3. Examination of other applicable control measures
4. Determination of the performance requirements for the protective clothing

5. Determination of the need for decontamination
6. Determination of the ergonomic constraints presented
7. Determination of the cost benefit of selection options

All protective clothing requires a program for maintenance, inspection, and repair. Worker education is especially important to ensure that the protective clothing selected is properly used and the hazards of exposure are understood.

Development of a comprehensive program for the selection and use of protective clothing can enhance the level of protection afforded to workers. A model approach could contain the following key elements:

1. An organization scheme and administrative plan.
2. A risk assessment methodology.
3. An evaluation of other control methods to protect the worker.
4. Performance criteria for the protective clothing.
5. Selection criteria and procedures to determine the optimum choice.
6. Purchasing specifications for the protective clothing.
7. A validation plan for the selection with medical surveillance, as appropriate.
8. Decontamination and rescue criteria, as applicable.
9. A user training program.
10. An auditing plan to ensure procedures are followed consistently.

References

1. **National Institute for Occupational Safety and Health (NIOSH):** *Proposed National Strategies for the Prevention of Leading Work-Related Diseases and Injuries.* Atlanta, GA: NIOSH, 1988.
2. **Mansdorf, S.Z.:** Risk assessment of chemical exposure hazards in the use of protective clothing-an overview. In R.L. Baker and G.C. Coletta, editors, *Performance of Protective Clothing (ASTM STP 900).* Philadelphia, PA: American Society for Testing and Materials, 1986.
3. **Perkins, J.L.:** Chemical Protective Clothing, Vol. I. *J. Appl. Ind. Hyg. 2*:222–230 (1987).
4. **Mansdorf, S.Z.:** Industrial hygiene assessment for the use of protective gloves. In G.A. Melstrom, J.E. Wahlberg, and H.I. Maibach, editors, *Protective Gloves for Occupational Use.* Boca Raton, FL: CRC Press, 1994.
5. **Grandjean, P: Skin Penetration:** *Hazardous Chemicals at Work.* New York: Taylor & Francis, 1990.
6. **American Conference of Governmental Industrial Hygienists (ACGIH):** Dermal absorption. In *Documentation of Threshold Limit Values and Biological Exposure Indices.* Cincinnati, OH: ACGIH, 1992.
7. **Forsberg, K. and S.Z. Mansdorf:** *Quick Selection Guide to Chemical Protective Clothing, 5th edition.* New York: Van Nostrand Reinhold, 2007.
8. **Mansdorf, S.Z.:** Anhydrous hydrofluoric acid. *Am. Ind. Hyg. Assoc. J. 48*:7 (1987).
9. **Linch, L.L:** Protective Clothing. In *The CRC Handbook of Laboratory Safety.* Steere, N.V. (ed.). Boca Raton, FL: CRC Press, 1971.
10. **Sansone, E.B. and Y.B. Tewari:** The permeability of laboratory gloves to selected solvents. *Am. Ind. Hyg. Assoc. J. 39*:169–74 (1978).
11. **Johnson, J. and K. Anderson (eds.):** *Chemical Protective Clothing, Vol. II.* Fairfax, VA: American Industrial Hygiene Association, 1990.
12. **Perkins, J.L.:** Solvent-polymer interactions. In *Chemical Protective Clothing,* 2nd edition. Anna, D.H. (ed.). Fairfax, VA: American Industrial Hygiene Association, 2003.
13. **American Society for Testing and Materials (ASTM):** *Test Method for Permeation of Liquids and Gases through Protective Clothing Materials Under Conditions of Intermittent Contact (Method F1383).* West Conshohocken, PA: ASTM, 2007.
14. **Henry, N. and N. Schlatter:** Development of a standard method for evaluating chemical protective clothing to permeation of hazardous liquids. *Am. Ind. Hyg. Assoc. J. 42*:202–07 (1981).
15. **American Society for Testing and Materials (ASTM):** *Test Method for Permeation of Liquids and Gases through Protective Clothing Materials under Conditions of Continuous Contact (Method F739).* West Conshohocken, PA: ASTM, 2007.
16. **American Society for Testing and Materials (ASTM):** *Test Method for Resistance of Protective Clothing Materials to Liquid Permeation-Permeation Cup Method (Method F1407-99a).* West Conshohocken, PA: ASTM, 2006.
17. **Coletta, G.C., S.Z. Mansdorf, and S.P. Berardinelli:** Chemical protective clothing test method development: Part II. Degradation test method. *Am. Ind. Hyg. Assoc. J. 41*:26–33 (1980).
18. **Johnson, J., A. Schwope, R. Goydan, and D. Herman:** *Guidelines for the Selection of Chemical Protective Clothing, 1991 Update.* Springfield, VA: National Technical Information Service, 1992.

19. **Forsberg, K. and L. Keith:** *Chemical Protective Clothing Performance Index Book, 2nd edition.* New York: John Wiley & Sons, 1997.
20. **Mickelsen, R.L. and R. Hall:** A breakthrough time comparison of nitrile and neoprene glove materials produced by different manufactures. *Am. Ind. Hyg. Assoc. J. 48*:941–47 (1985).
21. **Mickelsen, R.L., M. Roder, and S.P. Berardinelli:** Permeation of chemical protective clothing by three binary solvent mixtures. *Am. Ind. Hyg. Assoc. J. 47*:189–94 (1986).
22. **Stull, J., M. Connor, and C. Heath:** Development of a combination thermal and chemical protective ensemble for U.S. Navy fire fighting applications. In *Performance of Protective Clothing, Vol. 5 (STP 1237).* Johnson, J.S. and S.Z. Mansdorf (eds.). West Conshohocken, PA: American Society for Testing and Materials, 1996.
23. **Day, M.:** A comparative evaluation of test methods and materials for thermal protective performance. In J.S. Johnson and S.Z. Mansdof, editors, *Performance of Protective Clothing (ASTM STP 989).* West Conshohocken, PA: American Society for Testing and Materials, 1988.
24. **Davies, J.:** Conductive clothing and materials. In S.Z. Mansdorf, R. Sager, and A.P. Nielson, editors, *Performance of Protective Clothing (ASTM STP 989).* West Conshohocken, PA: American Society for Testing and Materials, 1988.
25. **Plog, B.A. and J.B. Olishifski:** Overview of industrial hygiene. In B.A. Plog, editor, *Fundamentals of Industrial Hygiene, 3rd. edition.* Chicago: National Safety Council, 1988.
26. **Brown, P.L.:** Protective clothing for health care workers: liquid proofness versus microbiological resistance. In J. McBrierty and N. Henry, editors, *Performance of Protective Clothing (STP 1133*). West Conshohocken, PA: American Society for Testing and Materials, 1992.
27. **Miller, A. and C. Volk:** Biological hazards. In *Fundamentals of Industrial Hygiene, 3rd. edition.* Chicago: National Safety Council, 1988.
28. **American Society for Testing and Materials (ASTM):** *Test Method for Resistance of Materials Used in Protective Clothing to Penetration by Synthetic Blood (Method F1670-07).* West Conshohocken, PA, ASTM, 2007.
29. **American Society for Testing and Materials (ASTM):** *Test Method for Resistance of Materials Used in Protective Clothing to Penetration by Blood-Borne Pathogens Using Phi-X174 Bacteriophage Penetration as a Test System (Method F1671-07).* West Conshohocken, PA, ASTM, 2007.
30. **American Society for Testing and Materials (ASTM):** *Test Method for Resistance of Materials Used in Protective Clothing to Penetration by Synthetic Blood Using A Mechanical Pressure Technique (Method F1819-07).* West Conshohocken, PA, ASTM, 2007.
31. **Noonan, E.:** Spunbonding in the 1990s: a technology on the move. *Nonwovens Ind.* March 1991.
32. **Mansdorf, S.Z.:** The Role and Future of Nonwovens in Personal Protective Equipment. Paper presented at the International Nonwovens Symposium, Munich, Germany, 1992.
33. **Johnson, J.S. and J. Stull:** Measuring the Integrity of Totally Encapsulating Chemical Protective Suits. In S.Z. Mansdorf, R. Sager, and A.P. Nielson, editors, *Performance of Protective Clothing (ASTM STP 989).* West Conshohocken, PA: American Society for Testing and Materials, 1988.
34. **National Institute for Occupational Safety and Health (NIOSH), Occupational Safety and Health Administration, U.S. Coast Guard, and Environmental Protection Agency:** *Occupational Safety and Health Guidance Manual for Hazardous Waste Site Activities* (NIOSH pub. 85-115). Cincinnati, OH: NIOSH, 1985.
35. **Slater, K.:** Comfort or protection: the clothing dilemma. In J.S. Johnson and S.Z. Mansdorf, editors, *Performance of Protective Clothing, vol. 5 (STP 1237).* West Conshohocken, PA: American Society for Testing and Materials, 1996.
36. "General Industry Standards," *Code of Federal Regulations* Title 29, Part 1910.132.
37. **Roder, M.:** *A Guide for Evaluating the Performance of Chemical Protective Clothing (CPC)* (NIOSH pub. 90-109). Cincinnati, OH: National Institute for Occupational Safety and Health, 1990.
38. **Henry, N.:** Four decades of protective clothing standards development. American Chemical Society, *J. Chem. Health Safety,* Nov/Dec, 2007.
39. **National Institute for Occupational Safety and Health (NIOSH):** *Latex Allergy: A Prevention Guide* (Publication 98-113). Cincinnati, OH: NIOSH 1998.
40. **National Institute for Occupational Safety and Health (NIOSH):** *Report to Congress on Workers' Home Contamination Conducted Under the Workers Family Protection Act.* Cincinnati, OH: NIOSH, 1995.
41. **Makinen, H.:** *The effect of wear and laundering on flame-retardant fabrics. In Performance of Protective Clothing (STP 1133).* West Conshohocken, PA: American Society for Testing and Materials, 1992.

42. **Laughlin, L. and C. Nelson:** Decontaminating personal protective equipment of applicators: A synthesis of research results. In *Proceedings of Quality and Usage of Protective Clothing*, Kittila, Finland: NOKOBETEF IV, 1992.

Outcome Competencies

After completing this chapter, the reader should be able to:

1. Define underlined terms in this chapter.
2. Describe operating principles of the various types of respirators.
3. Select appropriate respiratory protection.
4. Design, implement, and evaluate a management program for respirator use.
5. Explain respirator capabilities and limitations.
6. Recall respirator selection for nonroutine uses.
7. Explain the training needs for respirator users.
8. Recognize the importance of fit-testing.

Prerequisite Knowledge

Prior to beginning this chapter, the user should review the following chapters:

Chapter Number	Chapter Topic
7	Principles of Evaluating Exposure Assessment
9	Comprehensive Exposure Assessment
10	Modeling Inhalation Exposure
46	Confined Spaces

Key Terms

air-line respirator • assigned protection factor (APF) • bitter aerosol fit-test • breakthrough time • catalysts • chemisorption • closed circuit SCBA • continuous flow respirators • demand respirators • diffusion • end-of-service life indicator (ESLI) • filter efficiency degradation • fit factor • fit-tested • full facepiece • half facepiece • hazard ratio (HR) • helmet • hood • IAA fit-test • immediately dangerous to life or health (IDLH) • impaction • interception • irritant smoke fit-test • loose-fitting facepiece • maximum use concentration (MUC) • mouth bit respirator • negative pressure device • open-circuit SCBA • physisorption • positive pressure device • powered air-purifying respirator (PAPR) • pressure demand respirators • program administrator •respiratory inlet covering • qualitative fit-test • quantitative fit-test • quarter facepiece • saccharin fit-test • self-contained breathing apparatus (SCBA) • service life • sorbents • tight-fitting hood • user seal check • wear time

Key Topics

I. Introduction
   A. Respiratory Protection Program
   B. Respiratory Hazards

II. Types of Respirators
   A. Air-Purifying Respirators
   B. Atmosphere-Supplying Respirators
   C. Combination Air-Purifying and Atmosphere-Supplying Respirators

III. Respirator Selection
   A. Routine Use
   B. Nonroutine Use
   C. Biological Agents

IV. Maintenance and Care of Respirators

V. Training
   A. Training Requirements
   B. Wear Time

VI. Respirator Fit-Testing
   A. Quantitative Fit-Tests (QNFTs)
   B. Qualitative Fit-Tests (QLFTs)
   C. Test Exercises
   D. Respirator Sealing Problems

VII. Standards
   A. Respirator Test Standards
   B. Respirator Use Standards

Respiratory Protection

40

By Craig E. Colton, CIH

Introduction

A primary objective of an occupational health program is the prevention of adverse health effects. When a material becomes airborne, or dangerous concentrations of gases and vapors are present, the primary means of preventing injury is through the use of engineering and work practice control measures. When these measures are not feasible, while controls are being installed or implemented and during emergencies, appropriate respirators should be worn by workers.

If respirators are to function as designed, they must be properly selected, fit-tested, maintained, and used by trained employees. Because of medical or psychological conditions everyone may not be able to wear a respirator. Respirators may interfere with vision or voice communications. They can be hot and cumbersome to wear. These difficulties make respirators the least satisfactory method of control.

Despite these difficulties, respirators in many cases are the only feasible protection. To use a respirator and have it perform effectively requires a well-managed, complete, and systematic program. Even with the best program and most efficient respirator, inhalation exposures are only reduced, not completely eliminated.

Respiratory Protection Program

Government agencies[1], consensus groups[2,3] and technical committees[4] have recognized that when respirators are used, a formal, effective, and complete program is required. The safe use of a respirator requires at a minimum that the following program elements be addressed.

- Program administration
- Written work site specific operating procedures
- Exposure assessment
- Medical evaluation of respirator wearers
- Proper selection of respiratory protective equipment
- Training
- Respirator fitting
- Cleaning, inspection, maintenance, and storage
- Program evaluation

The Occupational Safety and Health Administration (OSHA) respiratory protection standard requires that these elements be addressed within a respiratory protection program.[1] The American National Standard for Respiratory Protection (ANSI Z88.2-1992) is a voluntary consensus standard containing similar program recommendations.[2] Both the OSHA and ANSI standards should be consulted in developing the program. Although the 1992 version has been withdrawn for administrative reasons, it does contain useful information.

The most important person for implementing and assuring the quality of the respiratory protection program is the program administrator. Program administration should be assigned to a single individual who is given the authority and responsibility for the overall program. Others may assist, but final responsibility remains with the single individual, thereby ensuring that there is coordination and direction for the program.

The complexity of the administrator's task in supervising the program varies depending on the respiratory hazards present, types of respirators used, workers, and workplace. The administrator must have sufficient knowledge and must keep abreast of current issues, technological advances, and regulatory changes pertaining to respiratory protection.

The program administrator's responsibilities include the following.

- Conducting an exposure assessment by measuring, estimating, or reviewing information on the concentrations of airborne contaminants in the work area. This is done prior to respirator selection and periodically during respirator use to ensure that the proper type of respirator is being used.
- Selecting the appropriate type of respirator to provide adequate protection for all contaminants present or anticipated.
- Maintaining records and written procedures to document the respirator program and allow evaluation of the program's effectiveness.
  Evaluating the respiratory protection program's effectiveness through ongoing surveillance of the program and respirator use.

In addition to ongoing surveillance, the program must be audited periodically to ensure that the written procedures are being followed and that the requirements of applicable regulations and industry accepted standards are being met.

To aid objectivity, the audit should be conducted by a knowledgeable person not directly associated with the program rather than by the respiratory protection program administrator. An audit checklist should be prepared and updated as necessary. Any defects or shortcomings found during the audit should be documented, including plans to correct problem areas and target dates for completion.

When a respirator program is implemented, there is other required administrative information. This includes policies, procedures, and forms for recording the results of program activities. Record keeping is an essential part of the program including such things as the results of training, fit tests, and audits. Some records are mandated by standards.

Several policies that need to be addressed include when respirators should be used, voluntary use of respirators, employee-purchased respirators, medical disqualification, and facial hair prohibition. These policies require that groups such as the organization's human resources, medical, safety, occupational hygiene, legal, and management personnel agree on specific program elements.

Written work site specific procedures must document the entire program. These specify the activity that will occur, where it will be done, who will perform the activity, and how often. For example, a maintenance procedure for a half-facepiece respirator will specify whether the employee or a designated person is responsible for cleaning the respirator, how the employee or maintenance person is trained, the specific cleaning and inspection procedure, how often the respirator is to be cleaned, and where replacement parts are obtained.

Forms should be used to document the completion of required activities and their outcomes.

Respiratory Hazards

Respiratory hazards may be excessive airborne concentrations of gases, vapors, or aerosols or the reduced concentration or partial pressure of oxygen. The degree of the respiratory hazard present may be classified either as immediately dangerous to life or health (IDLH) or not IDLH. The degree and type of respiratory hazard are important factors for choosing the appropriate respirator type.

Types of Respirators

Respirators are designed to cover the entrances to the respiratory system—the nose and mouth. They vary widely in design and function and can be described in terms of the design of the respiratory inlet covering and by the mechanism used to provide protection. Respirators are tested in the United States by the National Institute for Occupational Safety and Health (NIOSH). Respirators that pass NIOSH test criteria published in the *Code of Federal Regulations* (CFR) are referred to as "approved" respirators.[5] The NIOSH classification and limitations are used as the examples for specific respirator descriptions given in this chapter.

Respiratory inlet coverings provide a barrier between the environment and the wearer's respiratory system. The inlet coverings also are used to hold the parts that make a functioning respirator and are classified as either tight-fitting or loose-fitting.

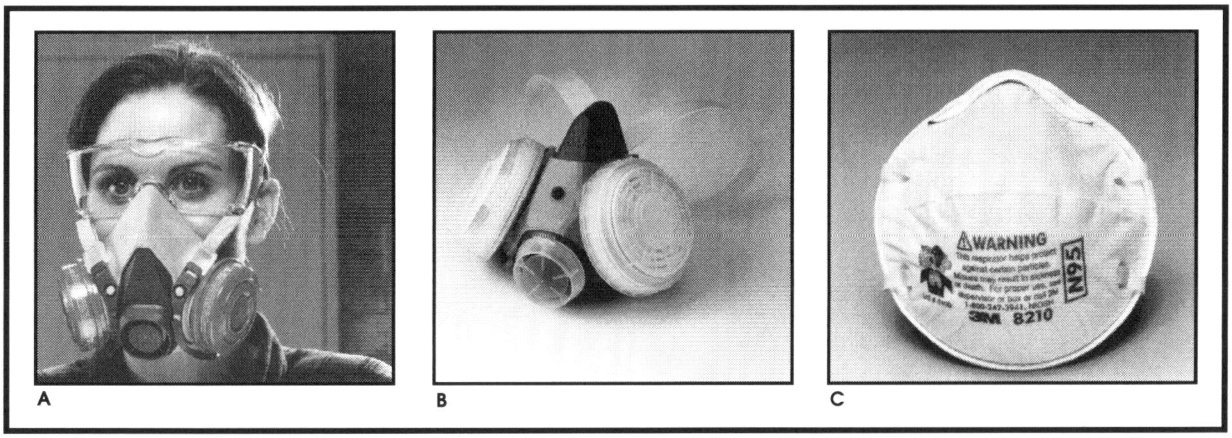

Figure 40.2 — Various half-mask respiratory inlet coverings. (A,B) Elastomeric dual cartridge half-masks made of two different materials; (C) N-95 filtering facepiece half mask (courtesy 3M, St. Paul, Minn.).

Tight-fitting respiratory inlet coverings take the following forms.

Mouth Bit Respirator. This respirator has a short tube designed to fit into the mouth and a nose clip to seal the nostrils. When the lips are closed over the mouth bit and the nose clip is used, the respiratory system is sealed. Mouth bits are used exclusively in escape-only type respirators.

Quarter Facepiece. This type covers the area of the face from above the nose to just under the lips and seals tight to the face. This type of respirator is not widely used (see Figure 40.1) in the United States, but is still used elsewhere.

Half Facepiece. This respirator (see Figures 40.2A, B, and C) covers the area from above the nose to underneath the chin.

Full Facepiece. This respirator (see Figure 40.3) covers from above the eyes to below the chin. The quarter, half, and full facepieces fit tight to the face. A full facepiece provides protection from eye irritants.

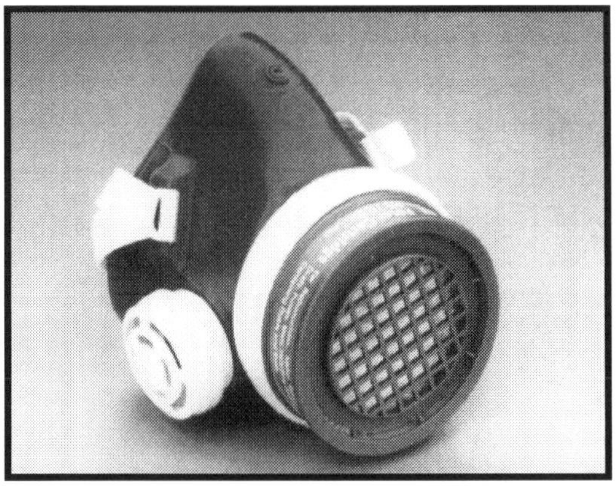

Figure 40.1 — Quarter-mask respiratory inlet covering (courtesy Aearo, Indianapolis, Ind.).

Tight-fitting Hood. This respirator covers the entire head and forms a complete seal. It often is referred to as a hood with a neck dam.

There are four types of loose-fitting respiratory inlet coverings.

- A hood covers the head and neck and may cover portions of the shoulders (see Figure 40.4A).
- A helmet is essentially a hood that offers head protection against impact and penetration (see Figure 40.4B) and has a bib that may cover the area down to the chest.
- A loose-fitting facepiece (see Figures 40.5A and B) covers the entire face but forms only a partial seal with the face. It does not cover the neck and

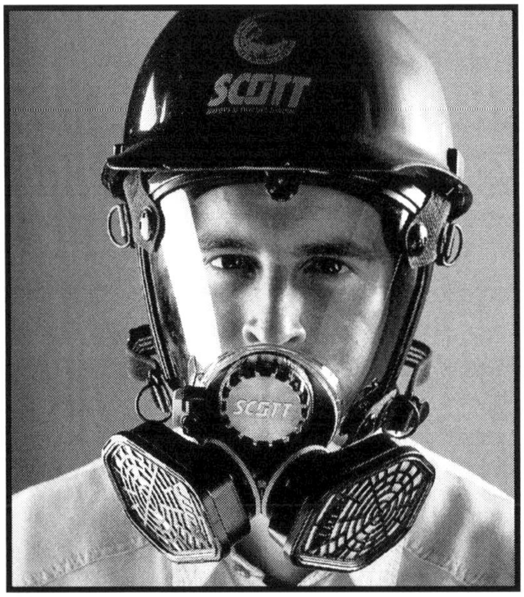

Figure 40.3 — Full-facepiece respiratory inlet covering (Scott Health and Safety, Monroe, N.C.).

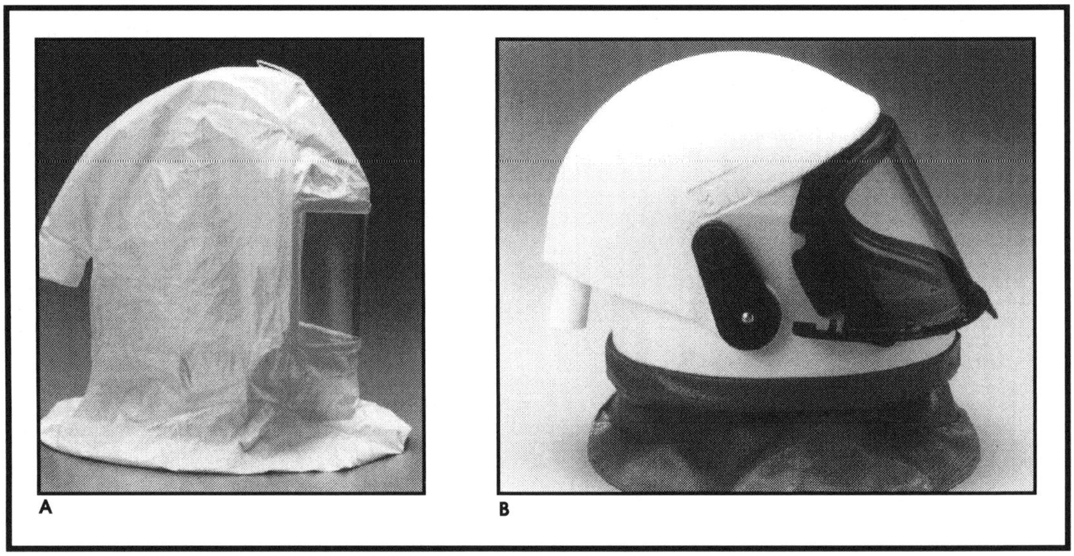

Figure 40.4 — Loose-fitting respiratory inlet coverings. (A) Hood; (B) helmet (courtesy 3M, St. Paul, Minn.).

shoulders and may not offer head protection against impact and penetration.

- A suit covers most of the body (e.g., from the head to the waist) or the entire body. It differs from a splash suit in that breathing air is supplied directly into the air suit. Splash suits and other body coverings are intended to be used with other types of respirators or no respirator at all.

For each type of inlet covering there are many variations in the materials of construction and individual design features. A half-facepiece respiratory inlet covering may be made of a variety of elastomers (e.g., rubber, silicone, thermoplastic; see Figures 40.2A and B) or made entirely of a filtering material (see Figure 40.2C). Full facepieces are also made of a variety of materials. Hoods and helmets may have wide viewing areas, provide face or eye protection, have neck dams for tight-fitting or have single or double bibs if loose-fitting, and may be made out of a variety of materials (e.g., coated fabrics, plastics). Loose-fitting facepieces may include head protection (see Figure 40.5A) and have rubber or fabric side-seals (see Figure 40.5B).

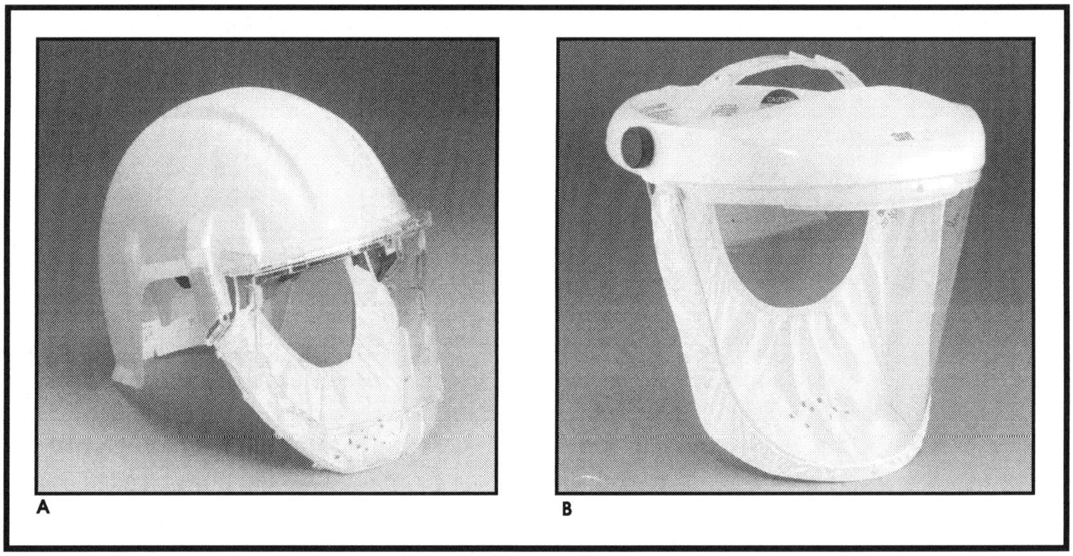

Figure 40.5 — Loose-fitting respiratory inlet coverings. (A) Loose-fitting facepiece with head protection against impact and penetration; (B) loose-fitting facepiece without head protection (courtesy 3M, St. Paul, Minn.).

The device providing respiratory protection can be described as either an air-purifying, atmosphere-supplying, or combination air-purifying and atmosphere-supplying respirator. Each is discussed in turn.

Air-Purifying Respirators

An air-purifying respirator cleanses a contaminated atmosphere. Ambient air passes through an air-purifying element that can remove specific gases and vapors, aerosols, or a combination of these contaminants. Particulate filters (commonly referred to as filters) are used to remove aerosols. Chemical filters (commonly referred to as chemical cartridges or canisters) are used to remove gases and vapors. Air-purifying respirators are classified as either powered or nonpowered. The nonpowered air-purifying respirator uses the person's breathing (inhalation) to draw air through the air-purifying element. The powered air-purifying respirator (PAPR) uses a blower to force air through the air-purifying element.[1] Several designs of PAPR exist with different styles of respiratory inlet coverings and placement of the blower in relation to the filter. Each design has its own advantages and disadvantages. Air-purifying respirators are limited to those environments in which there is sufficient oxygen to support life. The useful life of an air-purifying element is limited by the concentration of the air contaminants, the breathing rate of the wearer (air flow rate of a PAPR), temperature and humidity levels in the workplace, and the contaminant removal capacity of the air-purifying medium.

To be certified as a PAPR by NIOSH, the blower must provide at least 115 L/min (4 ft^3/min) of air to a tight-fitting facepiece (i.e., half facepiece or full facepiece) and at least 170 L/min (6 ft^3/min) to a loose-fitting facepiece, helmet, or hood.[5] The respirator manufacturers provide devices for verifying that the airflow exceeds these levels. These devices include flow meters, flow plates, and pressure gauges that can be attached to the respirator. The great advantage of the PAPR is that it usually supplies air at positive pressure, reducing inward leakage of contaminants when compared with the negative pressure (nonpowered) respirators. This is why PAPRs are generally assumed to provide a higher level of protection than their negative pressure counterpart. It is possible, however, at high work rates to create a negative pressure in the facepiece, thereby increasing the possibility of facepiece leakage. This concern is reduced by fit-testing tight-fitting PAPRs.

Aerosol Removing Respirators

Air-purifying respirators using filters provide respiratory protection against aerosols such as dusts, mists, fumes, and other particles, but do not protect against gases, vapors, or oxygen deficiency. Filters may be made of randomly laid nonwoven fiber materials, compressed natural wool, or synthetic fiber felt, or fibrous glass that may be loosely packed in a filter container or made into a flat sheet of filter material that is pleated and placed in a filter container. Pleating increases filter surface area, which can improve filter loading and efficiency and lower breathing resistance.

Removal Mechanisms. Aerosols can be removed by various mechanisms as they pass through the filter.[6] These filtration mechanisms include particle interception, sedimentation, impaction, and diffusion. In addition, some filters also use electrostatic attraction. As air moves through the filter, suspended particles flow with airstreams. As the airstreams approach a fiber lying perpendicular to their path, they split and compress to flow around the fiber. The airstreams rejoin on the other side of the fiber (see Figure 40.6).

In interception capture, the particles follow their original airstream. If the particle center comes within one particle radius of the fiber, it contacts the fiber surface and is captured. As particle size increases, the probability of interception increases.

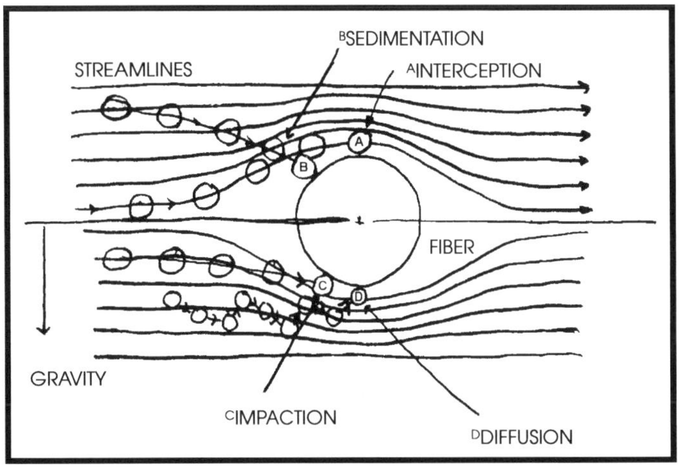

Figure 40.6 — Airflow pattern around a filter fiber showing four filtration mechanisms. (A) Interception; (B) sedimentation; (C) impaction; (D) diffusion.

Sedimentation capture works through the effect of gravity on the particle; therefore, the flow rate through the filter must be low. Particle settling in the filter results in contact with the fiber. It is most significant for large particles.

Particles with sufficient inertia cannot change direction sufficiently to avoid the fiber and therefore impact on it. As the airstreams split and change direction suddenly to go around the fiber, these particles are captured on the surface of the fiber because of impaction. A particle's size, density, speed, and shape determine its inertia.

Diffusion capture results from particle movement caused by air molecule bombardment (Brownian motion) and is important only for smaller particles. Particles randomly cross the airstreams and encounter a filter fiber. This random motion depends on particle size and temperature. For example, as particle size decreases, diffusive activity of the particle increases, which increases the chance of capture. A lower flow rate through the filter also increases the chance of capture because the particle spends more time in the area of the fiber.

Every respirator filter uses all of these filtration mechanisms to some degree, as the filter manufacturer attempts to make an efficient filter with low breathing resistance. The exact contribution of each mechanism depends on flow rate, filter solidity, fiber diameter, and particle size and density.

In addition to mechanical removal, attractive forces such as electrostatic attraction may augment filtration. Filters using both mechanical and electrical removal mechanisms are often referred to as electrostatic filters. In electrostatic capture the charged particles are attracted to filter fibers or regions of the filter fiber having the opposite charge. Uncharged particles may also be attracted depending on the level of charge imparted on the filter fiber. This removal process aids the other removal mechanisms, especially interception and diffusion. The advantage of using fibers with an electrical charge is that the filtration efficiency can be enhanced without making any contribution to airflow resistance. Two types of electrostatic materials used in respirator filters are referred to as resin wool and electrets.

The older version of the electrostatic filter is the resin wool filter. Local nonuniform electrostatic fields develop throughout the filter during manufacture. This type of filter no longer will meet U.S. criteria, but is still available in other places in the world.

Electret fibers are a recent development in filtration technology. These fibers have a strong electrostatic charge permanently embedded into their surface during processing. They maintain a positive charge on one side of the fiber and a negative charge of equal magnitude on the opposite side. Both charged and uncharged particles are attracted to electret fibers. Charged particles are attracted to the parts of the fiber that have an opposite charge. Uncharged particles have equal internal positive and negative charges. The strong electrostatic forces of the electret fibers polarize these charges, inducing a dipole within the particle, and the particle is then attracted to the fiber by a polarization force. Long-term environmental testing of resin wool electrostatic filters has indicated they are susceptible to filter efficiency degradation at high humidity and elevated temperature conditions.[7] Some electret filters are not affected by exposure to these same conditions.

Generally, large heavy particles are removed by impaction and interception, and large light particles are removed by diffusion and interception. Diffusion removes very small particles. When a single fiber is joined by other filter fibers to create a filter maze of certain average porosity and thickness, the different filtration mechanisms combine at different particle sizes to affect total filtration efficiency and breathing resistance. The capture mechanisms of sedimentation, interception, and inertial impaction combine effectively to remove nearly all particles larger than 0.6 μm. Also the low flow rates through respirator filters of only a few centimeters per second let diffusion play its part very effectively for particles below 0.1 μm.

However, in the region between these two particle sizes (i.e., 0.1–0.6 μm), diffusion and impaction are not as effective, and a minimum filtration efficiency exists, as shown in Figure 40.7. The lowest point on this curve is called the most penetrating particle size and can be determined empirically in the laboratory. The most penetrating size range can vary slightly with filter design and flow rate.[8] The addition of an electrostatic charge to the fibers can greatly improve the filtering ability for small particles.[9] Respirator filters made of fiberglass typically have a most penetrating particle size between 0.2 and 0.4 μm. This is the basis for the widely used dioctyl phthalate and sodium chloride filter tests using a 0.3-μm mass median aerodynamic diameter particle. For electret filters the most penetrating particle size occurs at a smaller size. NIOSH tests with aerosols equal to the 0.075 μm count median diameter (CMD) for sodium chloride aerosol and 0.185 μm CMD for dioctyl phthalate (DOP) aerosol. The test aerosols were chosen based on testing of both electret and mechanical filters.[8]

Filter Efficiency and Degradation. NIOSH and certification regulations of other countries allow for various levels of filter efficiency ranging from 80 to 99.97%. For example, NIOSH certifies three levels of efficiency: 95, 99, and 99.97%.[5] The efficiency of the filter in a given workplace depends on the conditions in that workplace.

Factors such as the particle size distribution, the nature of the aerosol, and work rate affect efficiency. Because NIOSH tests with a most penetrating particle size (as discussed above), the actual filter efficiency will be greater than that indicated by the approval. Because a respirator filter has measurable penetration of particles in the 0.2–0.4 μm range, it is easy to forget that anywhere else filtration efficiency is essentially 100%. It is especially important when considering the relatively large particle sizes found in the workplace.[10] While theory predicts that as the particle gets smaller than the most penetrating particle size, the filter efficiency increases, new concern has been raised with the introduction of engineered nanoparticles in the workplace. The theory has been shown to be true for particles in the 2–60 nm range.[11] A study conducted on NIOSH approved and CE approved filtering facepiece respirators showed particles below the most penetrating particle size showed a decrease in filter penetration levels with decreasing particle size as expected by single-fiber filtration theory.[12] The filters NIOSH certifies are listed in Table 40.1.

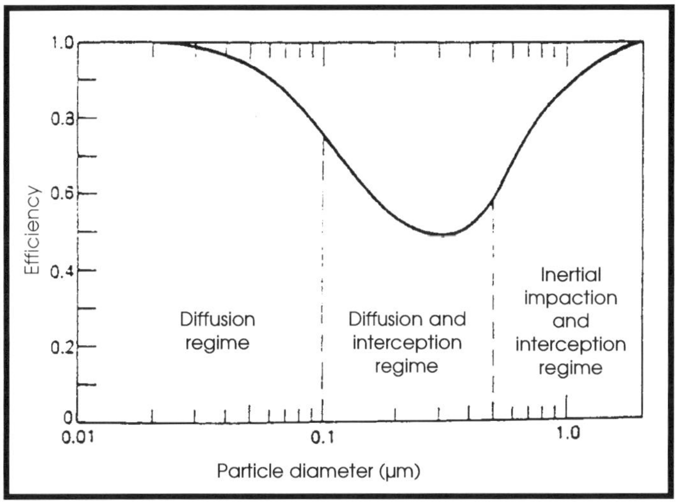

Figure 40.7 — Filter efficiency versus particle size schematic illustrating the different filtration regimes. (Source: K.W. Lee and B.Y.H. Liu, "On the Minimum Efficiency and the Most Penetrating Particle Size for Fibrous Filters" (*J. Air Pollution Control Assoc. 30*:377–381, 1980).

Table 40.1 — Description of Filter Classes Certified under 42 CFR 84

Filter Class (Test Agent)	*Minimum Efficiency (%)*	*Test Maximum Loading (mg)*	*Use*
N-series (NaCl[A])		200	Nonoil aerosols
N-100	99.97		
N-99	99		
N-95	95		
R-series (DOP oil[B])		200	oil and nonoil aerosols (time use restriction may apply[C])
R-100	99.97		
R-99	99		
R-95	95		
P-series (DOP oil[B])		stabilized efficiency	oil and nonoil aerosols
P-100[D]	99.97		
P-99	99		
P-95	95		

Source: Reference #5.
[A]NaCl = sodium chloride.
[B]DOP oil = dioctyl phthalate.
[C]In the presence of oil aerosols, service time may be limited to 8 hours of use or up until the total mass loading is less than 200 mg (100 mg/filter for dual filter respirators).
[D]The P-100 filter must be colored magenta.

Filter efficiency degradation is defined as a lowering of filter efficiency or a reduction in the ability of the filter to remove particles as a result of workplace exposure. Generally, solids and water-based aerosols do not reduce filter efficiency. Certain oils, such as dioctyl phthalate, have been shown to reduce filter efficiency of some filters for small particles. It may be due to the wetting of the filter fiber by the oil, masking the electrostatic charge. As a result, NIOSH has established the N-series of filters for nonoil aerosols and the R- and P-filter series for oil aerosols. The N-series filters are tested with a sodium chloride aerosol and are only intended for use with solids and non-oil (water or organic solvent such as most spray paints) based aerosols.

NIOSH test requirements assure that filter efficiency does not fall below the stated level with up to 200 mg of oil loaded on the respirator for R-series filters. The test is stopped at this point, so it is not known whether the filter efficiency decreases beyond the 200-mg load. It is recommended that R-series filters be limited to 8 hours of use or discarded when the respirator has collected 200 mg of oil (100 mg/filter for dual filter respirators).[11]

The NIOSH test requirements for P-series filters measures the filter efficiency until it stabilizes or is no longer decreasing. If filter efficiency is decreasing when the 200-mg point is reached, filter loading continues. When it stabilizes, the filter efficiency is determined. This ensures that the filter efficiency never goes below the stated efficiency level. NIOSH requires that the filter manufacturer state a time-use limitation recommendation for P-series filters when oil aerosols are present. P-series filters should only be used and reused in accordance with the manufacturer's time-use limitation.

For nonoil aerosols there is no time restriction on either N-, R-, or P-series filters because the nonoil aerosols are relatively nondegrading. Any decrease in filter efficiency can be offset by continual loading of the filter.[9] Aerosol filters generally become more efficient as particles are collected and plug the spaces between the filter fibers. Filters should be changed when users notice an increase in breathing resistance. Also, the filters should be changed when they are damaged or for hygiene reasons.

Gas/Vapor Removing Respirators

These air-purifying respirators protect against certain gases and vapors by using various chemical filters to purify the inhaled air. They differ from aerosol filters in that they use either cartridges or canisters containing sorbents or catalysts that remove or detoxify, respectively, harmful gases and vapors. Sorbents are usually granular porous materials that interact with the gas or vapor molecule to remove them from the air. Catalysts chemically react with harmful agents to form less toxic products; for example hopcalite converts carbon monoxide to carbon dioxide. The cartridges and canisters may be replaceable, or the entire respirator may be disposable.

Removal mechanisms typically involved are adsorption, or catalysis. In contrast to aerosol filters, which are effective to some degree no matter what the particle, cartridges and canisters are designed for protection against specific contaminants (e.g., ammonia gas or mercury vapor) or classes of contaminants (e.g., organic vapors).

Adsorption is the adherence of gas or vapor molecules to the surface of another substance called the adsorbent or sorbent either by physisorption (physical adsorption) or chemisorption. In physisorption the attractive force between the sorbent and the adsorbate molecule is small (on the molecular level) and is due to Van der Waal's forces of adhesion. Because only weak physical forces are involved, the process can be reversed.

Activated carbon is commonly used for removal of organic vapors via physisorption. For use in respirators, the surface area of carbon is greatly enhanced or "activated" using heat and an oxidizing process. The most common starting material for activated carbon is coconut or coal. Activated carbon has an extensive network of molecular-size internal pores and, consequently, large internal surface areas. The typical range of surface area is 1000–2000 m^2/g of carbon. In general, this material has a greater affinity for less volatile materials; the less volatile the organic chemical, the greater the amount of vapor adsorbed.[12] Generally, organic vapors of molecular weight greater than 50 or boiling points (BPs) greater than 70°C are effectively adsorbed by activated charcoal.[15] However, attempts to predict breakthrough time by relating it to a single property of a vapor have proved to be unrealistic.[14]

For gases and vapors that would otherwise be weakly adsorbed, sorbents (usually activated carbon) can be impregnated with chemical reagents to make them more selective. Chemical interaction occurring at the interface through the use of treated carbons is referred to as chemisorption.[14] Chemisorption refers to covalent or ionic bonding between the adsorbate and the impregnant. Chemisorption is usually irreversible. Examples are activated charcoal impregnated with iodine to remove mercury vapor or with metal salts such as nickel chloride to remove ammonia gas. Catalysts (e.g., hopcalite for converting carbon monoxide to carbon dioxide), which decompose and detoxify the contaminant by formation of relatively innocuous substances may be used in cartridges and canisters.[14]

These removal mechanisms are essentially 100% efficient until the sorbent's capacity is exhausted or the catalyst is poisoned, thus preventing its operation. At this point, breakthrough occurs as the contaminant passes through the cartridge or canister and into the respirator.

Canisters are very similar to cartridges. In the United States, the basic difference is the volume of sorbent rather than function for cartridges and canisters designed for the same chemicals. Canisters have the larger sorbent volume. They do not provide greater protection than cartridges; they just last longer than a chemical cartridge under identical conditions. In Europe, gas and vapor filters are more commonly called canisters.

Under NIOSH approval requirements "gas mask" is a term often used for a gas- or vapor-removing respirator that uses a canister. Although gas masks are limited by contaminant concentration for routine use, they can be used for escape only from IDLH atmospheres that contain adequate oxygen to support life (19.5% oxygen). They must never be used for entry into an IDLH atmosphere.

Breakthrough time of undamaged, new cartridges and canisters that have been stored properly depends on the following factors.

- Quality and amount of sorbent
- Packing uniformity and density
- Exposure conditions, including breathing rate of the wearer
- Relative humidity (RH)
- Temperature
- Contaminant concentration
- Allowable breakthrough concentration
- Affinity of the gas or vapor for the sorbent
- Presence of other gases and vapors

Generally, high concentrations, high breathing rate, and humid conditions adversely affect breakthrough time. Because exposure conditions are subject to wide variation, it is difficult to estimate the breakthrough time of canisters and cartridges, even when other conditions (e.g., temperature and RH) are constant. Table 40.2 shows various chemical cartridge breakthrough times for different organic gases and vapors.) While these tests were performed on cartridges and sorbents that are no longer commercially available, this table allows the comparison carbon capacity for different chemicals, under identical laboratory conditions. Breakthrough times in Table 40.2 are useful for comparison purposes only as performance of individual cartridge models varies. It is difficult to extrapolate these values from this table into meaningful workplace service times. The table shows that although the organic vapor cartridge is approved for organic vapors by testing against carbon tetrachloride, it may last longer (e.g., butanol) or much shorter (e.g., methanol) when compared with the test agent. Hence, an organic vapor cartridge may be recommended for use against butanol, but not for methanol (molecular weight <50; BP <70°C) even though both compounds are classified as organic vapors.

Most data reported for chemical cartridge breakthrough times have been for single contaminants. The evaluation of cartridges against mixtures of contaminants has received very little attention.[14] Cartridge breakthrough may occur earlier in the presence of mixtures than would have been predicted from data for a single chemical. Unfortunately, cartridge use for mixtures is more reflective of the real world. More recently study has been done to concentrate on this workplace reality resulting in better information for mixtures.[20]

Another concern when using cartridges or canisters is desorption of adsorbed compounds during respirator use against single contaminants or mixtures. A well-adsorbed vapor at a high concentration can cause

Table 40.2 — Selected Chemical and Physical Properties of Organic Chemicals Mentioned in this Chapter

Chemical	*Mol. Wt.*	*Boiling Point °C*	*Vapor Pressure torr (20°C)*	*IDLH*[14] *(ppm)*	*Threshold Limit Value*[15] *(ppm)*	*Geometric Mean Odor Threshold*[16] *(ppm)*	*Range Odor Threshold*[16] *(ppm)*[A,B]	*Laboratory Breakthrough Time*[17] *(min.)*[C]
Benzene	78.11	80.1	75	3000	0.5	61	34–119	88.6
Toluene	92.1	110.6	22	2000	50	1.6	0.16–37	114
m-Xylene	100.6	139.1	9	10,000	100	20	20	116
Methanol	32.04	64.7	97	25,000	200	160	4.2–5960	3.2
Ethanol	46.07	78.5	44	—	1000	180	49–716	45.3
Isopropanol	60.09	82.5	33	20,000	400	43	37–610	81.8
n-Butanol	74.12	117	6	8000	C 50	1.2	0.12–11	141
3-methyl-1-butanol	88.15	131.4	2.8	8000	100	121		
Methylene chloride	84.94	40.1	349	5000	50	160	160	15.8
Chloroform	119.4	61.3	160	1000	10	192	133–276	52.4
Methyl chloroform	133.4	74.1	100	1000	350	390	390	58.9
Trichloroethylene	131.4	87	58	1000	50	82	82	83
Carbon tetrachloride	153.8	76.75	91	300	5	252	140–584	90
Acetone	58.1	56.2	180	20,000	500	62	3.6–653	46
2-Butanone	72.1	79.6	77.5	3000	200	16	2-85	94.4
2-Pentanone	86.1	102.2	27	5000	200	7.7	7.7	12
4-Methyl-2-pentanone	100.2	115.8	16	—	50	0.88	0.1–7.8	
Pentane	72.15	36	426	5000	600	—	119–1147	71.3
n-Hexane	86.18	68.7	124	5000	50	—	65–248	64.6
Heptane	100.2	98.43	40	4250	400	230	230	89.8
Cylclohexane	84.16	80.74	78	10,000	300	780	780	82.3
Methyl acetate	74.08	56.9	173	10,000	200	180	46.5	
Ethyl acetate	88.12	77.06	73	10,000	400	18	6.4–50	84.7
n-Propyl acetate	102.13	101.6	25	8000	200	4.1	0.5–34	85.6
Butyl acetate	116.16	126.5	10	10,000	150	0.31	0.063–7.4	96.9
Isopentylacetate	130.19	145.6	4	3000	100	0.22	0.0034–209	88.3

[A]Range of acceptable values based on an evaluation of the studies.
[B]Single acceptable study, geometric mean is the single value.
[C]Tested at 22°C, 50% RH, at an airflow of 53.3 L/min. Test concentration: 1000 ppm; breakthrough concentration: 10 ppm.

early breakthrough of a poorly adsorbed vapor when both are present in the workplace either sequentially or simultaneously.[21,22] In general, organic compounds with low BPs have increased desorption properties. Another concern is whether desorption will take place if the cartridge is partially used and then reused after a short period (hours) without use (e.g., overnight). Organic vapors adsorbed on a used cartridge can also migrate through the carbon bed without airflow. Breakthrough could occur when the respirator is used next. This is most significant for the most volatile and poorly retained organic vapors (e.g., BP <65°C), especially low-boiling oxygenated compounds and low-boiling fluoro- and chlorofluorocarbons.

It has been recommended, especially for agents that desorb readily, the cartridge should not be worn intermittently because of desorption that can lead to hazardous concentrations during subsequent use, even in an uncontaminated work area.[14]

Combination Aerosol Filter/Gas or Vapor Removing Respirators

These respirators use aerosol-removing filters with a gas or vapor filter for exposure to multiple contaminants in different physical forms or a single chemical in more than one physical form (e.g., mist and vapor). The aerosol filter can be either permanently mounted or replaceable on the gas or vapor filter. Replaceable aerosol filters are sometimes used because the filter and chemical cartridge or canister are not exhausted at the same time. This allows for disposal of only the part that needs changing. Aerosol filters used in combination with gas and vapor filters must always be located on the inlet side of the cartridge or canister. This way, any gas or vapor adsorbed onto a filtered particle is captured by the sorbent as it evaporates or desorbs from the particle.

Atmosphere-Supplying Respirators

Atmosphere-supplying devices are the class of respirators that provide a respirable atmosphere to the wearer, independent of the ambient air. The breathing atmosphere is supplied from an uncontaminated source – either a compressor or cylinders filled with air, which must conform to certain purity levels. In the United States, Grade D air is required as specified in the OSHA respiratory protection standard 29 CFR 1910.134.[(1)] These are essentially the same requirements listed in the Compressed Gas Association standard, "Commodity Specification for Air."[(23)] Table 40.3 lists the air quality requirements for Grade D breathing air.

Compressors provide essentially an unlimited supply of air as long as the compressor is running where cylinders provide a finite amount of air depending on the number and size of cylinders in use. The use of cylinders practically eliminates the use of continuous flow supplied air respirators because of the limited air supply and the large volume of air required to operate continuous flow respirators.

Concerns when using a compressor include that it must:

- provide air at sufficient volume and pressure to meet the air requirements for the respirator model and number being used
- be constructed and situated so as to prevent entry of contaminated air into the air-supply system from outside sources such as vehicle emissions

Air compressors may or may not be oil-lubricated. For compressors that are not oil lubricated, it must be ensured that carbon monoxide levels in the breathing air do not exceed 10 ppm. When oil-lubricated compressors are used, carbon monoxide may be released into the air if the oil is overheated. Therefore, they must be continuously monitored for carbon monoxide with either a high temperature alarm or a carbon monoxide alarm. Whatever the air source, the air quality must be ensured that it meets the purity standards

Atmosphere-supplying respirators fall into three groups: air-line respirators, self-contained breathing apparatus (SCBA), and combination air-line and SCBA.

Table 40.3—Air Quality for Atmosphere-Supplying Respirators

Limiting Characteristics	Allowable Maxima
Percent O_2 balance is predominantly N_2	19.5–23.5
Water, ppm (v/v)[1]	
Oil (condensed) (mg/m^3 at NTP[2])	5 [3]
Carbon monoxide (ppm)	10 [4]
Carbon dioxide	1000[4,5]
Odor	None

Source: **Compressed Gas Association (CGA):** Commodity Specification for Air. Chantilly, VA: CGA, 2004.
Note: Grade D air (Quality Verification Level D)
[1]The water content of compressed air required for any particular verification level may vary from saturated to very dry. For breathing air in conjunction with SCBA in extreme cold, where moisture can condense and freeze causing the breathing apparatus to malfunction, a dew point not to exceed -50°F (63 ppm v/v) or 10° lower than the coldest temperature expected in the area is required. If a specific water limit is required, it should be specified as a limiting concentration in ppm (v/v) or dew point. Dew point is expressed in °F at one atmosphere pressure absolute, 101 kPa abs. (760 mmHg).
[2]NTP = normal temperature and pressure.
[3]Not required for synthesized air whose oxygen and nitrogen components are produced by air liquefaction.
[4] Not required for synthesized air when oxygen component was produced by air liquefaction and meets the United States Pharmacopeia (USP) specification.
[5] Not required for synthesized air when nitrogen component was previously analyzed and meets the National Formulary (NF) specification.

Air-Line Respirators

Air-line respirators, sometimes referred to as Type C or CE supplied-air respirators, deliver breathing air from either a compressor or compressed air cylinders through a supply hose connected to the respiratory inlet covering. A flow control valve, regulator, or orifice is provided to govern the rate of airflow to the worker. Depending on the NIOSH certification, up to 300 ft of air supply hose is allowable.[5] Hose supplied by the respirator manufacturer along with recommended hose lengths and operating pressures must be used. The maximum permissible inlet pressure is 125 psi.[5] The approved pressure range and hose length is noted on the certification label or operating instructions provided with each approved device.

Air-line respirators should be used only in non-IDLH atmospheres—or in other words, atmospheres in which the wearer can escape without the use of a respirator. This limitation is necessary because the air-line respirator depends entirely on an air supply that is not carried by the wearer of the respirator. If this air supply fails, the wearer may have to remove the respirator to escape from the area. Another limitation is that the air hose limits the wearer to a fixed distance from the air supply source.

Air-line respirators operate in three modes: demand, pressure demand, and continuous flow. The respirators are equipped with half facepieces, full facepieces, helmets, hoods, or loose-fitting facepieces.

Versions of these respirators may be designed for welding or abrasive blasting. Supplied-air respirators designed for abrasive blasting (Type CE) are equipped to protect the wearer from impact of the rebounding abrasive material. A special hood or shroud may be used to protect the wearer's head and neck, and shielding material may be used to protect the viewing windows of the head enclosures.

Demand. These air-line respirators are equipped with either half or full facepieces. The design of the regulator allows for airflow only on inhalation (i.e., the wearer demands air). These respirators are negative-pressure devices, meaning that a negative pressure with respect to the outside of the respirator is created in the facepiece on inhalation. Although these respirators can still be found on work sites, they are not recommended; the pressure demand air-line respirator is much more protective, and the cost differential between the two is negligible.

Pressure Demand. These respirators are very similar to the demand type but are designed so that the pressure inside the respirator is generally positive with respect to the air pressure outside the respirator during both inhalation and exhalation. This positive pressure means that when a leak develops in the face seal due to head movement, for example, the leakage of air would be outward.

The regulator generally has a small spring that forces the airflow valve open. In the facepiece the exhalation valve also has a small spring or another mechanism that forces the exhalation valve closed. Air flows into the facepiece until the air pressure inside the facepiece and the regulator are equal. This flow results in a small positive pressure inside the facepiece that remains positive during inhalation, provided airflow through the regulator is greater than the breathing rate.

Thus, <u>pressure demand respirators</u> provide a higher degree of protection to the user compared with <u>demand respirators</u>. Demand and pressure demand respirators are available only with tight-fitting respiratory inlet coverings. These respirators are used because <u>continuous flow respirators</u> generally exhaust a bottled air supply too quickly to be practical.

Continuous Flow. A continuous flow unit has a regulated amount of air delivered to the respiratory inlet covering and is normally used where there is an ample air supply, such as that provided by an air compressor. These devices may be equipped with either tight-fitting or loose-fitting respiratory inlet coverings.

NIOSH establishes airflow requirements.[5] Units equipped with tight-fitting enclosures, (i.e., a half or full facepiece) must provide at least 115 L/min (4 ft^3/min) measured at the facepiece. When loose-fitting helmets, hoods, or facepieces are used, the minimum amount of air to be delivered is 170 L/min (6 ft^3/min). In either case the maximum flow is not to exceed 450 L/min (15 ft^3/min). Also, the pressure requirements of the respirator must be compatible with the pressure ranges of the air source. Operating these respirators using the proper pressure, number of air hose sections, and lengths of air hose as identified in the operating instructions ensures proper airflow.

SCBA

SCBA provides respiratory protection against gases, vapors, particles, and an oxygen-deficient atmosphere. The wearer is more mobile than with an air-line respirator and independent of the surrounding atmosphere as the breathing gas is carried by the wearer. SCBA may be used in IDLH and oxygen-deficient atmospheres either as escape-only devices or for entry into and escape from these atmospheres.(5) A full facepiece is most commonly used with SCBAs, though half facepieces, hoods, and mouth bits are available on some units. There are two major types of SCBAs: closed circuit and open circuit.

Closed-Circuit SCBA. In closed-circuit SCBA all or a percentage of the exhaled gas is scrubbed and rebreathed. Closed-circuit units have the advantage of lower weight for the same use duration as open-circuit devices. Service life for the units ranges from 15 minutes to 4 hours. Disadvantages include increased complexity (e.g., a carbon dioxide scrubber is required in many of the units) and cost. In many of the devices the air supply can become quite warm because the exhaled air is breathed again. Closed circuit SCBA are available as both negative and positive pressure devices. The positive pressure devices with service lives greater than or equal to 30 minutes are recommended for entry into and escape from IDLH atmospheres.(1) They may be designed as stored oxygen or oxygen-generating systems.

Stored oxygen systems use compressed oxygen from cylinders or oxygen carried as a liquid. Oxygen is admitted to a breathing bag either in a continuous flow or controlled by a regulator governed by the pressure or degree of inflation of the bag. The wearer inhales from the bag and exhales into it. Exhaled breath is scrubbed of carbon dioxide by a chemical bed, usually a caustic such as sodium hydroxide.

Oxygen-generating systems rely on chemical reactions to provide the needed oxygen. Water vapor and carbon dioxide from the exhaled breath react with a solid chemical, usually potassium superoxide, in a canister-size container that releases oxygen. This reaction in the canister removes the carbon dioxide from the exhaled breath.

Open-Circuit SCBA. In an open-circuit SCBA the exhaled breath is released to the surrounding environment after use rather than being recirculated. The breathing gas is generally compressed air. They are typically designed to provide 30 to 60 minutes of service and are available in both demand (negative pressure) and pressure demand (positive pressure) styles. Because of the greater protection provided by pressure demand devices, they are recommended over negative pressure systems. Only the positive pressure devices with 30 minutes or longer of service life are recommended for entry into and escape from IDLH atmospheres.(1)

Escape SCBA. Some SCBAs are designed for escape only. They are similar in design to the types described above, but the use duration tends to be shorter, typically 5, 7, 10, or 15 minutes. Units approved as escape-only may not be used to enter a hazardous atmosphere.

Combination SCBA and Air-Line Respirators

These units are air-line respirators with an auxiliary self-contained air supply that can be used if the primary air supply fails. Because they have backup or escape provisions, these devices are usable in IDLH and oxygen-deficient atmospheres.

An advantage of these devices is that they can be used in IDLH situations requiring extended work periods when an SCBA alone does not provide sufficient time. Also, because the SCBA needs to supply only enough air for escape, the cylinder can be smaller compared with a 30-minute SCBA. The smaller SCBA cylinder on many of these units makes them particularly convenient for use in confined spaces. Operation in the air-line mode allows for longer service times than a fixed-duration SCBA.

The auxiliary SCBA may be NIOSH-approved either in the 3-, 5-, or 10-minute service time category or the 15 minutes or longer category.(5) If the SCBA portion is rated for a service life of 3, 5, or 10 minutes, the wearer must use the air-line during entry into a hazardous atmosphere, and the SCBA portion is used for emergency egress only.

When the SCBA is rated for service of 15 minutes or longer, the SCBA may be used for emergency entry into a hazardous atmosphere (e.g., to connect the air-line) when not more than 20% of the air supply's rated capacity is used during entry. This allows for enough air for egress when the warning device indicates a low air supply. These units must also have a gauge visible to the wearer and a low-air warning device.

The combination SCBA/air-line respirator may operate in demand, pressure demand, or continuous flow modes. These devices use the same principles as the respective air-line respirator. Demand mode is not recommended.

Combination Air-Purifying and Atmosphere-Supplying Respirators

Another type of respirator is a combination of an air-line respirator with an auxiliary air-purifying element attached, which if properly selected provides protection in the event the air supply fails. NIOSH has approved combination air-line and air-purifying respirators with the air-line operating in either continuous flow or pressure demand mode. These respirators can be used in either an air-purifying or atmosphere-supplying mode. The most popular versions have high efficiency filters such as an N-, R-, or P-100, but devices are available with complete arrays of chemical cartridges as well.

These respirators have additional limitations. They are not for use in IDLH atmospheres or in atmospheres containing less than 19.5% oxygen; only the hose lengths and pressure ranges specified on the approval label may be used; and they may be used only in atmospheres for which the air-purifying element is approved.

The approval label must be consulted for proper use of the respirator in the air-purifying mode. The restrictions can vary from manufacturer to manufacturer depending on the respirator design.

Respirator Selection

Routine Use

Selection of a particular respirator depends on a number of factors. The selection process includes an analysis of workplace hazards, the physical characteristics of the work area, the physical demands of the work, and the capabilities and limitations of the various types of respirators.

Workplace Hazards

An exposure assessment is one component of hazard analysis in the workplace. Other components include determining characteristics of the hazard such as the physical state of the contaminant, skin absorption and eye irritation potential, oxygen concentration, and warning properties for gases and vapors.

For respirators, an exposure assessment is usually limited to airborne hazards. Chapters 7 and 9 contain discussions of the information needed and methods used to conduct an assessment. For respirator selection the exposure assessment may be based on data collected by air sampling, by estimating or modeling exposures, or on the potential for exposure.

Chapter 10 discusses methods for modeling or estimating the magnitude of exposures.

Respirators are selected for routine use in two situations: documented overexposure or positive exposure assessment and potential exposure. For selection based on potential exposure, it is presumed that an exposure will occur even though prior experience indicates otherwise.

For example, in the chemical industry the use of a respirator is generally required for the first break into a closed system such as a pipe. Work practices and prior experience at such tasks may have shown that exposures do not occur. Yet, it is standard practice to require a full-facepiece pressure demand air-line respirator in many chemical plants on the chance that material may still be in the line being opened and a release may occur.

Another important step in evaluating the workplace hazard is determining the physical state of the airborne contaminant. Care is required in selecting air-purifying respirators for materials that exist as both particles and vapors. In the past, generalizations about the contaminant phase have been based on the listing of the American Conference of Governmental Industrial Hygienists' Threshold Limit Value (TLV®).[20] Materials with a TLV® indicating sampling for both aerosol and vapor can be expected to occur in both the particle and vapor phase requiring a chemical cartridge and particle filter. In addition to the guidance in the TLV® booklet[17] general guidelines have been developed for estimating the airborne phase for air sampling and can be applied to respirator selection.[24] Some respirator selection guides also will indicate when a contaminants existence in dual forms may occur.

Physical Characteristics of the Work Area

The area where the respirator will be used and its environmental conditions can affect respirator selection. The distance a person will have to travel to a location having respirable air also needs to be considered in selection. This includes planning for the escape of workers if an emergency occurs, for the entry of workers to perform maintenance duties, and for rescue operations. For example, an air-line respirator generally requires that the person enter and exit the work area the same way because the air hose limits the direction and distance a person can travel. In areas with moving equipment, such as a warehouse, hoses may get in the way or be run over.

Environmental conditions such as temperature can affect which respirator can be used. In hot humid conditions, use of lightweight respirators is one means to lessen the burden of respirator wear. Air-line respirators can be equipped with vortex heaters or coolers to condition the air. An air-line respirator also provides cooling because of the flow of air and adiabatic expansion of the compressed air.

Physical Demands of the Work

The work an employee will perform and other required personal protective equipment used while wearing a respirator needs to be considered. Factors such as work rate, work movements, noise levels, communication and vision requirements, the compatibility of the respirator with the other PPE, and length of time that the respirator will be worn affect selection. For jobs that demand physical effort, selecting the lightest and easier breathing respirator may reduce the burden. Respirators that facilitate communication or are compatible with communication devices may need to be selected so workers can talk clearly with each other. Full facepiece respirators may interfere with field of vision. (Glasses with temple bars cannot be worn with full-facepiece respirators.)

Respirator Capabilities and Limitations

In addition to the capabilities and limitations discussed in the description of respirator types, other limitations include the level of performance for a specific type of respirator (the assigned protection factor [APF]), the need for an independent supply of air, the efficiency of filters, the capacity of the cartridges and canisters, and any regulatory maximum use concentration.

APFs. The US Occupational Safety and Health Administration (OSHA) defines an APF as the workplace level of respiratory protection that a respirator or class of respirators is expected to provide to employees when the employer implements a continuing, effective respiratory protection program as specified in its respiratory protection standard.[1] Many groups have developed lists of APFs. The APFs listed by these groups are not the same in all cases because they were developed at different times using different types of respirator performance information and use restrictions. Table 40.4 lists the OSHA APFs. OSHA also lists APFs in the butadiene substance-specific standard. These APFs are specific for butadienel. Other lists of APFs can be found by other organization such as the Canadian Standards Association[3] NIOSH[26] and countries.[27] While the values may differ, their application for selecting respirators is essentially the same.

In selecting a specific respirator for use, the APF must be greater than the expected air contaminant concentration (Cair) divided by its exposure limit (TLV®).

$$APF \geq C_{air}/TLV \qquad (40\text{-}1)$$

For example, if the expected concentration is 30 ppm and the exposure limit is 2 ppm, a respirator with an APF of at least 15 must be used. This is also called the <u>hazard ratio</u> (HR) or APF needed, where the HR equals the concentration divided by the exposure limit. A similar selection concept used in OSHA regulations is the <u>maximum use concentration</u> (MUC). The MUC is the maximum atmospheric concentration of a hazardous substance from which an employee can be expected to be protected when wearing a respirator.[1] The respirator MUC for a given chemical is the APF of the respirator or class of respirators × the exposure limit of that chemical. Other factors affect the MUC.

The maximum use concentration of a respirator is based on several factors including the APF, IDLH concentrations, and regulatory limits. A respirator may not be used at a concentration greater than the exposure limit times the APF for the respirator. In addition, air-purifying and air-line respirators may not

Table 40.4 — OSHA Assigned Protection Factors(1)

Type of respirator [1,2]	Quarter mask	Half mask	Full facepiece	Helmet/ hood	Loose-fitting facepiece
1. Air-Purifying Respirator	5	[3]10	50	—	—
2. Powered Air-Purifying Respirator (PAPR)	—	50	1000	[4]25/1000	25
3. Supplied Air Respirator (SAR) or Airline Respirator					
Demand mode	—	10	50	—	—
Continuous flow mode	—	50	1000	[4]25/1000	25
Pressure-demand or other positive-pressure mode	—	50	1000	—	—
Self-Contained Breathing Apparatus (SCBA)					
Demand mode	—	10	50	50	
Pressure-demand or other positive-pressure mode (e.g.,open/closed circuit)	—		10,000	10,000	

Notes:

[1] Employers may select respirators assigned for use in higher workplace concentrations of a hazardous substance for use at lower concentrations of that substance, or when required respirator use is independent of concentration.

[2] The assigned protection factors in Table 36.4 are only effective when the employer implements a continuing, effective respirator program as required by this section (29 CFR 1910.134), including training, fit testing, maintenance, and use requirements.

[3] This APF category includes filtering facepieces, and half masks with elastomeric facepieces.

[4] The employer must have evidence provided by the respirator manufacturer that testing of these respirators demonstrates performance at a level of protection of 1,000 or greater to receive an APF of 1,000. This level of performance can best be demonstrated by performing a WPF or SWPF study or equivalent testing. Absent such testing, all other PAPRs and SARs with helmets/hoods are to be treated as loose-fitting facepiece respirators, and receive an APF of 25.

[5] These APFs do not apply to respirators used solely for escape. For escape respirators used in association with specific substances covered by 29 CFR 1910 subpart Z, employers must refer to the appropriate substance-specific standards in that subpart. Escape respirators for other IDLH atmospheres are specified by 29 CFR 1910.134 (d)(2)(ii).

be used at concentrations greater than the IDLH. Finally, respirator-use regulations may preclude the use of a respirator above specific limits such as levels that cause eye irritation.

Filter Selection. Filter selection is based on classification of the aerosol. For NIOSH-approved filters, if the aerosol is an oil mist or includes oil particles, only R- or P-series filters can be considered.(5,13) The decision to use an R- or P-series filter can be made after consideration of desired service time, applicable time use restrictions, breathing resistance, and cost differences. If no oil is present, then an N-series filter can be selected. The filter efficiency needed may be specified by an OSHA substance-specific standard. If not, a 95% filter normally is adequate. For PAPRs only filters with 99.97% efficiency are available.

Cartridges/Canisters. Unlike aerosol filters, cartridges have high removal efficiency initially and at some point become less efficient and lose the ability to trap the contaminant completely. Therefore, selection of an air-purifying respirator for gases and vapors must consider the service life of the cartridge or canister. To protect workers, the chemical cartridge or canister must be changed before significant breakthrough occurs. There are two ways to determine when to change the cartridge or canister needs to be replaced. These are to use a cartridge or canister with an end-of-service-life indicator (ESLI; not widely available), or to set a replacement schedule so that the cartridges or canisters are changed before significant breakthrough occurs. The reliance on warning properties to determine when breakthrough has occurred is no longer allowed under OSHA regulations. Warning properties still provide a useful backup for a change schedule if the material has adequate warning properties.

Warning properties of gases and vapors refer to an odor, taste, or irritation indicating the chemical's presence in the environment. Warning properties can be classified as adequate or poor. Poor warning properties are defined as an odor, taste, or irritation effect that is not detectable or persistent at concentrations at or below the occupational exposure limit (includes those with no warning properties).[2] Odor thresholds are the most commonly used warnings; irritation levels are second. Nose and throat irritation work for all respirators, but eye irritation is only useful for full-facepiece respirators.

Warning properties can provide some indication to the wearer that the cartridge or canister is reaching the end of its useful service life. Because they rely on human senses, they are not foolproof. Amoore and Hatula reported that "the ability of members of the population to detect a given odor is strongly influenced by the innate variability of different persons' olfactory powers, their prior experience with that odor, and by the degree of attention they accord to the matter."[28] It should be noted that odor threshold data reported in the literature differ considerably; commonly the values may range over four orders of magnitude for the same chemical.[18] Compilations of chemical lists with odor thresholds also exist.[18,29] Table 40.2 lists odor thresholds for some common chemicals.

Despite these limitations, warning properties can still provide valuable secondary information. Employees should be trained that if they detect a chemical prior to the ESLI turning or the established change schedule, they should leave the area, replace the cartridge and report to the program administrator that a problem occurred. This allows the evaluation of the change schedule to determine whether the ambient concentration or basis for the change schedule is adequate.

An ESLI is a system that warns the user when the chemical cartridge or canister is nearing the end of its service life. Currently, the ESLIs in use are passive devices, so the respirator user must periodically check the ESLI status to know when to replace the cartridge or canister. Most ESLIs use a color change indicator. When the indicator color matches the reference color corresponding to exhausted service life, the cartridge or canister must be changed. Commonly available ESLIs are used on cartridges and canisters for mercury vapor, ethylene oxide, and carbon monoxide gas.

When a respirator with an ESLI is not available, and an atmosphere-supplying respirator may be impractical because of lack of feasible air supply or need for worker mobility, the only method available for replacing cartridges or canisters before breakthrough is via a cartridge replacement or change schedule. This schedule must be based on cartridge breakthrough time data, desorption studies, expected concentrations, patterns of use, and duration of exposure.[2] If the cartridges are replaced daily or more frequently, desorption studies may not be necessary.

Cartridge service life is a function of sorbent characteristics, chemical concentration, environmental conditions, and work rate. Service life or the change time can be estimated using general guidelines, determined by testing cartridges in the laboratory or in the field, or calculated using breakthrough equations. Each is explained in the following paragraphs.

Following are guidelines for estimating change schedules for organic vapor cartridges.[15]

- If the organic vapor's BP is greater than 70°C and its concentration less than 200 ppm, the organic vapor cartridge should last 8 hours at a normal work rate (assuming normal breathing rate).
- Breakthrough time is inversely proportional to flow rate.
- If the concentration is reduced by a factor of 10, the breakthrough time will only increase by a factor of 5.
- Humidity greater than 85% generally reduces breakthrough time by 50% at high concentrations (e.g. 1000 ppm). Recent studies have shown that the effect may be greater for lower concentrations with more volatile chemicals.[30]

These guidelines are best used in conjunction with one of the other methods to set a change schedule.

Using these guidelines, one would expect an organic vapor cartridge to last at least 8 hours for n-butanol (BP >70°C) at a concentration of 200 ppm, 50% RH, and a normal work rate (30 L/min). At 20 ppm of n-butanol it would be expected to last at least 40 hours (8 hours at 200 ppm×5=40 hours at 20 ppm). At 200 ppm n-butanol, RH at 90%, and a breathing rate of 60 L/min, the guidelines would predict a breakthrough time of 2 hours (8 hours × 0.5 [50% reduction at 90% RH] ÷2=2 hours at 90% RH and work rate of 60 L/min).

In a laboratory test the time to breakthrough is measured at various concentrations and humidity chosen to represent the workplace. Many commercial labs are equipped to run tests for a fee. Breakthrough time studies have been reported in the literature.[19,31,32] Table 40.2 lists breakthrough data for several chemicals. Although this information is for single chemicals, it is possible to test more than one chemical simultaneously at concentrations and RH that mimic the work environment. When the testing conditions are not representative, it is more difficult to extrapolate to the workplace. The preceding guidelines can then be used to estimate the breakthrough time for workplace conditions that are different from the laboratory data. For example, toluene has a breakthrough time of 114 minutes when tested at 1000 ppm (Table 36.2). At 100 ppm, the estimated breakthrough time would be ~500 minutes (concentration reduced by 10, service life increases by a factor of 5).

In a field test the time to breakthrough is measured directly in the workplace. The cartridge or canister is connected to a high-flow pump to simulate breathing (~20 L/min is light work, ~40 L/min is moderate), and samples are collected downstream to determine the time to breakthrough. Two advantages of this testing are that no equipment is needed to reproduce the work environment, and the results are easier to extrapolate to the workplace. The disadvantages include the awkwardness and space limitations of setting up laboratory equipment (e.g., high flow pumps, detectors) in the workplace.

Another field test that can be performed is to sample behind the cartridge at the end of the use period. This method is particularly useful to verify the adequacy of the established change schedule. Several manufacturers make a fit-test adapter that sits between the facepiece and the air purifying element. A short tube is connected to the adapter that allows an air sample to be collected from behind the cartridge. Any air sample method with sufficient sensitivity can be used. The advantage of this method is that actual workplace conditions are used including employee work rate and exposure. If the concentration of the contaminant is less than the chosen criteria, the change schedule is adequate.

Procedures have been developed to estimate breakthrough time for organic vapor cartridges and canisters.[33,34] The most recent model allows for multiple vapors and different relative humidities and can be found on the NIOSH website (http://www.cdc.gov/niosh/npptl/multivapor/multivapor.html)[34] The calculation of breakthrough time depends on solvent variables, carbon variables, and ambient conditions. Most manufacturers have software or tables of breakthrough times for their cartridges and canisters. The software is similar; data on the contaminant, concentration, chemical cartridge, work rate, and environmental conditions are entered; the estimated breakthrough time is then given. For some materials that have variable compositions such as VM&P naphtha or gasoline, a surrogate can be used to get an estimated breakthrough time. Heptane would be a good surrogate for a petroleum distillate that had a boiling point near 100°C.

Once a breakthrough time is estimated or known, a change schedule needs to be set. In most cases a simple schedule is used, once every 4 hours, once a day or week. The schedule is set so that the estimated breakthrough time is longer than the change schedule.

In summary, cartridges and canisters should be replaced earlier than the change schedule indicates in any of the following situations.

- If the ESLI shows the specified color change
- If breakthrough is detected by smell or taste, or by eye, nose, or throat irritation
- If the shelf life is exceeded
- If an OSHA regulation specifies a disposal frequency (e.g., formaldehyde)

If a person is wearing a cartridge or canister that needs replacement, he or she should return to fresh air as quickly as possible. In addition, if uncomfortable heat in the inhaled air is detected or the wearer has a feeling of nausea, dizziness, or ill-health, it is imperative to return to fresh air. (A properly operating cartridge or canister may become warm on exposure to certain gases or vapors, but a device that becomes extremely hot indicates that concentrations greater than the device's limits have been reached.)

Nonroutine Use

Three types of hazardous atmospheres require careful consideration for respirator selection because of the unusual nature of the hazard. These are entries into confined spaces, oxygen-deficient atmospheres, and emergencies. Confined spaces and oxygen-deficient atmospheres may be IDLH.

IDLH

Numerous definitions have been presented for IDLH atmospheres. ANSI defines any atmosphere that poses an immediate hazard to life or poses immediate, irreversible debilitating effects on health as being IDLH.[2] The common theme in all the definitions is that IDLH atmospheres affect the worker acutely as opposed to chronically.

Thus, if the concentration is above IDLH levels, only highly reliable respiratory protective equipment is allowed. The only two devices that meet this requirement and provide escape provisions for the wearer are (1) pressure demand or other positive pressure SCBA rated for 30 minutes or longer or (2) combination type, pressure demand airline respirators with auxiliary self-contained air supply.

OSHA has not established IDLH limits. The most complete set of IDLH limits was established by NIOSH in its *NIOSH Pocket Guide to Chemical Hazards* for the purpose of respirator selection.[16] NIOSH revised the list in 1994; however, OSHA currently uses the IDLH values published in 1990 as a guide for enforcement.[35] Questions have been raised on the adequacy of the revised IDLH levels because some of them are equal to OSHA PELs. Two factors have been considered when establishing IDLH concentrations: (1) The worker must be able to escape within 30 minutes without losing his or her life or suffering permanent health damage; and (2) the worker must be able to escape without severe eye or respiratory irritation or other reactions that could inhibit escape.

A location is considered IDLH when an atmosphere is known or suspected to have chemical concentrations above the IDLH level. A confined space containing less than the normal 20.9% oxygen should also be considered IDLH, unless the reason for the reduced oxygen level is known.[2] Otherwise, according to OSHA, oxygen levels of less than 19.5% are IDLH.[1] OSHA makes an exception, however, if the oxygen content is known and maintained within specific ranges (Table 40.5). The IDLH level may be as low as 16% depending on altitude; any supplied air respirator may be used. When there is doubt about the oxygen content, the contaminants present, or their airborne levels, the situation should be treated as IDLH. If an error in respirator selection is made, it should be on the side of safety. Thus, in emergency situations, such as a spill when the chemical or its airborne concentration is unknown, one of the above two respirators must be selected.

When no IDLH concentration has been established, concentrations in excess of the lower explosive limit (LEL) are considered to be IDLH. Generally, entry into atmospheres exceeding the LEL is not recommended except for lifesaving rescues. For concentrations at or above the LEL, respirators must provide maximum protection.

Because fire fighting is also considered IDLH by NIOSH, the only practical device providing adequate protection for this activity is pressure demand SCBA.[26] In addition to being NIOSH-approved, the SCBA used for fire fighting should comply with the most current edition of the National Fire Protection Association (NFPA) standard, NFPA 1981.[36] The NFPA requirements exceed the NIOSH

Table 40.5 — Table of Exception to SCBA Requirement for Oxygen Deficient Atmospheres

Altitude (ft.)	*Oxygen Deficient Atmospheres (%Oxygen) for Which an Atmosphere Supplying Respirator Many Be Used*
Less than 3001	16.0–19.5
3001–4000	16.4–19.5
4001–5000	17.1–19.5
5001–6000	17.8–19.5
6001–7000	18.5–19.5
7001–8000	19.3–19.5

requirements in many areas such as flow rate, harness assembly, and fire and heat resistance. These SCBAs are required to have many more features that an SCBA that is strictly for industrial use. Detailed discussion of these devices are beyond the scope of this chapter and the NFPA 1981 standard should be consulted if these devices are being used.

Biological Agents

One of the more recent areas seeing increased respirator usage is for biological aerosols, predominantly in healthcare settings. Respiratory protective devices have been used or are being purchased to reduce exposure to bioaerosols (such as droplet nuclei containing *Mycobacterium tuberculosis* [TB], severe acute respiratory syndrome [SARS] and pandemic flu and anthrax spores). Particle removing respirators such as N95 filtering facepieces respirators and powered air purifying respirators have been recommended by the Centers for Disease Control and prevention (CDC) for these agents. This area presents many challenges including unknown safe levels of exposure for these agents or respirator efficacy for bioaerosols. Acceptable airborne levels have not been established for potentially infectious aerosols. NIOSH approved or certified respirators are not tested against bioaerosols such as TB.

This lack of information makes the respirator selection process difficult. Use of a properly selected respirator may reduce the risk due to exposure to these materials, but cannot guarantee protection. Respirators with high assigned protection factors should be expected to reduce risk to a lower level than respirators with lower assigned protection factors when used within a respirator program and worn properly and diligently by the worker. On the other hand, respirators with higher assigned protection factors are more complex, burdensome to the worker, and costly. The proper balance needs to be achieved. Filtering facepiece respirators mentioned earlier have been used in health care settings because of their simplicity, cost, and efficiency, and also because of the ease of disposal if they become contaminated. Reuse of a respirator or its disposal must also be consistent with the operating procedures of the infection-control program of the health care facility.

Related to concerns for biological agents is the concern for exposures to chemical warfare agents as a result of a terrorist activity. This concern has result in numerous approval categories for respiratory protection for chemical biological radiological nuclear (CBRN) materials. This is a specialized field of respiratory protection. More information can be found on these devices on the NIOSH website.

Emergency Procedures

In some industries in which the possibility of a chemical release, process upset, or the need to rescue someone during an emergency may require advance planning, a wide variety of possible conditions requiring the emergency or rescue use of respirators can be envisioned. An adequate emergency and rescue respirator response capability can be achieved through a serious effort to plan for the worst foreseeable consequences of particular malfunctions or mishaps.

Written work site specific procedures for the emergency and rescue uses of respirators can be developed by anticipating the likely processes, tasks, and materials that may lead to an emergency. The possible consequences of equipment or power failures, uncontrolled chemical reactions, fire, explosion, or human error should be evaluated.

Past occurrences requiring emergency or rescue uses of respirators, as well as conditions that resulted in such respirator applications, can be used to help determine what may be necessary. The procedure should be reviewed by someone thoroughly familiar with the particular process or operation, ensuring that appropriate types of respirators are selected; an adequate number is provided where they may be needed for emergency or rescue use; and the respirators are stored, maintained, and regularly inspected so that they are readily accessible and operational when needed.

Maintenance and Care of Respirators

Proper maintenance of respiratory protection is important so it is ready and functional. A maintenance program provides for the proper cleaning and disinfecting, storage, inspection, and repair of respirators.

The wearer must be provided with a respirator that is clean, sanitary, and in good working order. The respirator manufacturer's recommendations for cleaning and disinfecting should be followed. When a respirator is issued for the exclusive use of one employee they must be cleaned and disinfected as often as necessary to be maintained in a sanitary condition. Respirators issued to more than one employee must be cleaned and disinfected before being worn by different individuals. Respirators maintained for emergency use need to be cleaned and disinfected after each use.

It is important to ensure that the respirators are stored to protect them from damage, contamination, dust, sunlight, extreme temperatures, excessive moisture, and damaging chemicals. While being stored the deformation of the facepiece and exhalation valve must be prevented

Prior to use all respirators used in routine must be inspected before each use and during cleaning. All respirators maintained for use in emergency situations shall be inspected at least monthly and in accordance with the manufacturer's recommendations. These respirators used for emergency situations must be checked for proper function before and after each use. Emergency escape-only respirators need to be inspected before being carried into the workplace for use. The respirator manufacturer's instructions should be consulted for what needs to be inspected and how to inspect it. Self-contained breathing apparatus must be inspected monthly in addition to the above times. Air and oxygen cylinders must be maintained in a fully charged state and shall be recharged when the pressure falls to 90% of the manufacturer's recommended pressure level. It also must be determined that the regulator and warning devices function properly.

Respirators that fail an inspection or are otherwise found to be defective must be removed from service, and either discarded, repaired or adjusted in accordance with the respirator manufacturer's instructions using only the respirator manufacturer's NIOSH-approved parts designed for the respirator.

Training

Training is an important aspect of a respirator program. For the safe use of any respirator it is essential that the user be properly instructed in its operation. Supervisors as well as the person issuing respirators must be instructed by a qualified person who has knowledge of respiratory protection and workplace contaminants. Emergency and rescue teams must be given adequate training to ensure proper respirator use and covering other issues such as health hazards, work practices, use of other equipment on site, and medical surveillance requirements. All workers need to be trained on initial assignment of a respirator and kept current with annual training as a minimum.

Training Requirements

Each respirator wearer should be given training that includes the following.

- An explanation of the need for the respirator, including an explanation of the respiratory hazard and what happens if the respirator is not used properly
- Instructions to inform their supervisor of any problems related to respirator use
- A discussion of what engineering and administrative controls are being used and why respirators are still needed for protection
- An explanation of why a particular type of respirator has been selected
- A discussion of the function, capabilities, and limitations of the selected respirator
- Instruction in how to don the respirator and check its fit and operation
- Successful completion of either a qualitative fit-test (QLFT) or quantitative fit-test (QNFT)
- Instruction in respirator maintenance
- Instruction in emergency procedures and the use of emergency escape devices and regulations concerning respirator use

Training on donning the respirator must include an opportunity to handle the respirator, and it should provide instructions for each wearer in the proper fitting of the respirator, including demonstrations and practice in how the respirator must be worn, how to adjust it, and how to determine whether it fits properly. Respirator manufacturers can provide training materials that tell and show how the respirator is to be adjusted, donned, and worn. The training session must also allow time to practice. Hence, a lecture or just showing a videotape is not sufficient unless it is followed up with actual hands-on time. Close, frequent supervision can be useful to ensure that the workers continue to use the respirator in the correct manner. Supervisory personnel should periodically monitor the use of respirators to ensure they are worn properly.

As a minimum, written record of the names of those trained and the dates when the training occurred, who conducted the training, and what was covered must be kept.

Wear Time

Wear time is the percentage of time the respirator is worn during the time it is needed to prevent inhalation of a contaminant. Not wearing a respirator for short periods while it is needed can have a profound effect on overall protection. While a respirator is not worn, the protection factor it provides is 1; that is, the individual is exposed to the ambient contaminant concentration.

The effect of nonwear time can be calculated from the following equation.

Effective Protection Factor =
Work shift time in minutes ÷
(1/APF)(Wear time in minutes) +
Nonwear time in minutes (40-2)

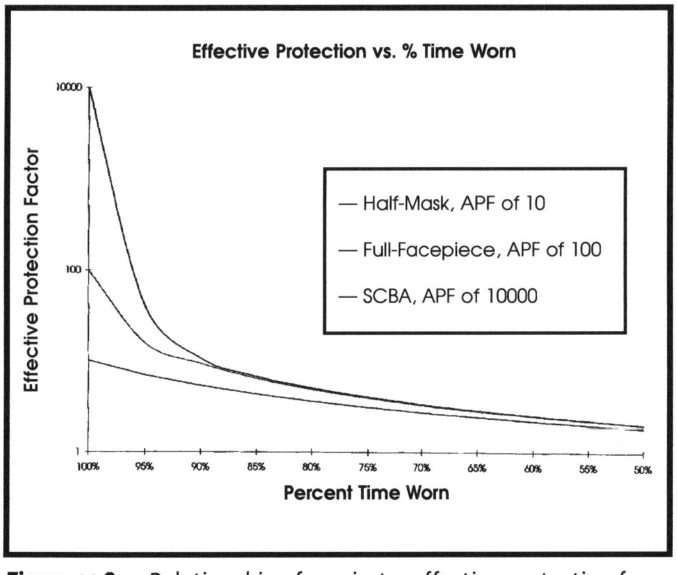

Figure 40.8 — Relationship of respirator effective protection factor to time worn.

Note: The exposure during wear time can be reduced by the APF or any assumed level of protection.

For example, if a person removes his or her respirator for 1 minute to talk during a task that takes 1 hour, the wear time is 98%. If the person uses a respirator with a level of protection of 1000, the effective level of protection actually achieved is 56, including this 1 minute nonwear time. In training it is important that people understand the effect of nonwear time on the level of performance that can be achieved. As nonwear time increases for any respirator, the protection levels for all respirators approach 1. When poor wear habits are practiced, the effective protection levels of an SCBA and a negative pressure half-facepiece respirator may be identical (see Figure 40.8).

Respirator Fit-Testing

Each respirator wearer of tight-fitting devices must be provided with a respirator that fits. To find the respirator that fits, the worker must be fit tested. Fit testing verifies that the selected make, model, and size of a tight-fitting respirator adequately fits the wearer. It also provides assurance that the wearer has learned to don the respirator properly. Fit testing is a critical component of a respirator training program. There are both QLFT and QNFT methods.

In addition, each respirator wearer must be required to check the seal of the respirator by appropriate means each time they don the respirator. Each respirator manufacturer provides instructions on how to perform these user seal checks. A user seal check is a test conducted by the wearer to determine whether the respirator is properly adjusted to the face. The procedures may vary slightly from one respirator to another because of differences in construction and design. In any case the employee is either checking for pressure or flow of air around the sealing surface.[37] User seal checks are not substitutes for QLFTs or QNFTs. Care must be taken in conducting user seal checks. Respirator wearers must be given thorough training in carrying out these checks and in how to recognize the endpoint.

Respirator fit-testing is conducted to determine whether a particular model and size of facepiece fits an individual's face.

Prior to the test the person should be trained on proper respirator use and donning and the purpose and procedures for the fit-test. Because respirator fit-testing is done to evaluate face-seal leakage only, the respirator must be equipped with the appropriate filters or cartridges to prevent penetration through the air-purifying element. Either QLFTs or QNFTs can be used[2]; each has its advantages and disadvantages.

QNFTs

In a QNFT either air leakage is determined [known as the controlled negative pressure technique[38]] or a test substance is measured both inside and outside the respirator while it is being worn. The test result can be reported as percent leakage or the ratio of test agent concentration outside the respirator (C_0) to the concentration inside (C_i). The ratio of C_0 to C_i is called a fit factor. A number of methods are available commercially that use oil mists[39], salt mists[40], or ambient particles[41] as test substances. The controlled negative pressure technique models the negative pressure generated inside the respirator at breathing rate identified by the fit tester and measures the amount of this air flow that comes through respirator leaks. This ratio results in the fit factor. Figure 40.9 shows schematics of the commercially available QNFT methods.

There are advantages and disadvantages associated with a QNFT. The advantages include a direct and objective measurement of fit and, with some methods, real-time documentation. The disadvantages include the cost of equipment needed (typically $4000-$13,000), maintenance, training in the operation of the sophisticated test equipment, and the need for specially probed respirators or adapters. OSHA accepted QNFT methods using test aerosols require high efficiency filters (N-, R-, or P-100). An aerosol QNFT method for fit testing respirators with non-high efficiency filters is on the market but has not been included in the OSHA standard as an accepted method. (OSHA allows non-high efficiency filters to be tested using the existing methods as long as a fit factor of 100 is found.) The non-high efficiency filter method uses the PortaCount® with the N95 Companion. The controlled negative pressure technique can only be used on respirators with replaceable filters.

The minimum fit factor required to pass a QNFT is a value 10 times the APF of the respirator.[2] For a half-facepiece respirator with an APF of 10, the minimum fit factor required is 100. The factor of 10 is used to account for differences in performance that occur when a respirator is actually used versus the measured performance during the fit-test. For negative pressure full facepiece respirators used for concentrations greater than ten

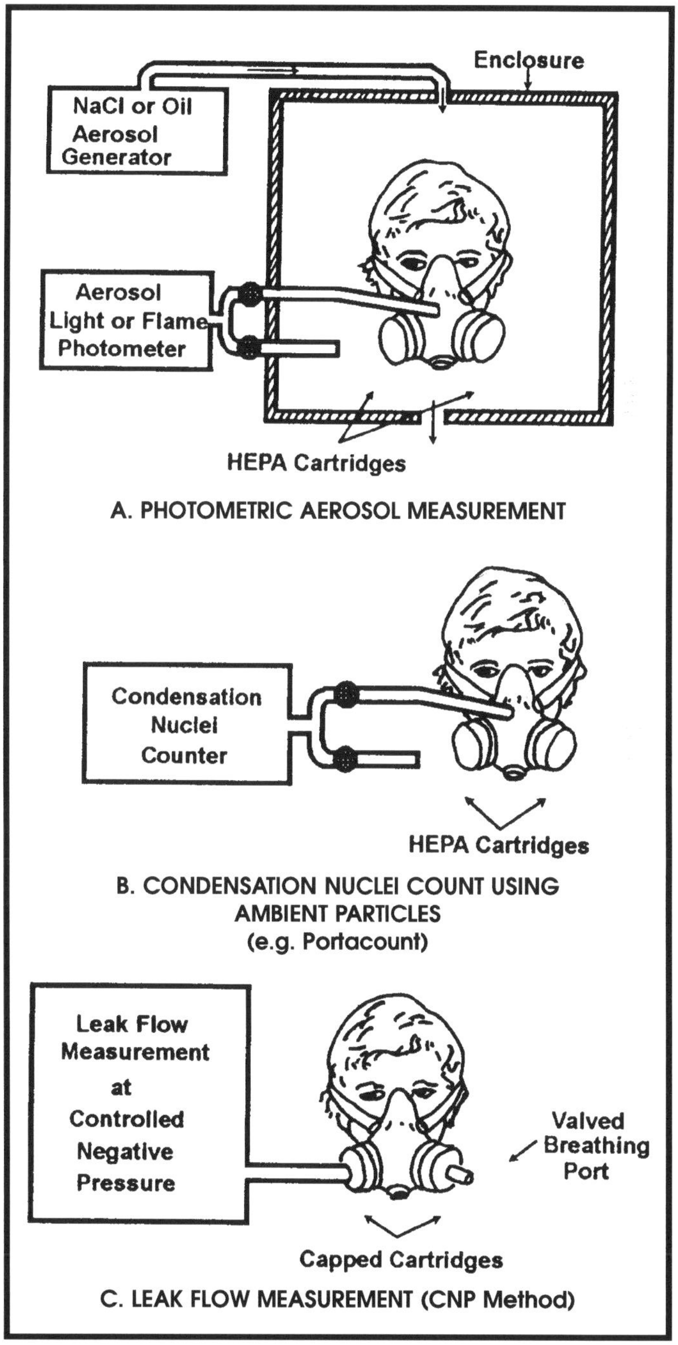

Figure 40.9 — Schematic representation of commercially available QNFTs (adapted from reference 37).

times the occupational exposure limit and less than or equal to fifty times the occupational exposure limit, QNFT must be used with a minimum required fit factor of 500.

QLFTs

In a QLFT a face-seal leakage evaluation similar to QNFT is made, but no direct measurements of the test and leak concentrations are made. A QLFT evaluates face-seal leakage using the person's sense of taste, smell, or irritation to detect unacceptable leakage. The respirator wearer is exposed to a challenge agent and must honestly report if the agent is detected at any time during the fit test. If the challenge agent is not detected the result is a pass. If the agent is detected the result is a fail. A test procedure is used to control the concentration outside the respirator. A threshold test of each person's ability to sense a very low concentration of the challenge agent is required prior to the fit-test to qualify them for the specific QLFT method. Persons who cannot detect the threshold concentration cannot be fit tested with that method. QLFTs are generally simple to perform, require only a few pieces of inexpensive equipment, and can be done in almost any location. The tests do not give a numerical indication of fit.

OSHA accepted QLFT methods use the following test agents: isoamyl acetate (banana-like odor), saccharin (sweet taste), Bitrex™ (bitter taste), and stannic chloride.[1] These QLFTs (summarized below) were carefully developed in the laboratory to facilitate tight control of the threshold and full-strength challenge agent concentrations. The methods were compared against QNFT to verify that passing the QLFT means the person has a fit factor of at least 100.[43–46]

IAA Fit-Test

The IAA fit-test protocol uses the sense of smell to detect the test agent so careful controls are necessary to prevent odor fatigue and to determine whether the test subject can smell low levels of the IAA. Because IAA is an organic vapor the respirator must be able to be fitted with a chemical cartridge capable for removing organic vapors.

Saccharin Fit-Test

A QLFT protocol has been developed using a saccharin mist. The saccharin fit-test can be used for any respirator equipped with any type particulate filter. A worker's own respirator can be used with no modification other than the addition of a prefilter for those respirators not equipped with aerosol filters. A person's ability to taste saccharin is used as the criterion to determine whether the fit is acceptable.

Irritant Smoke Fit-Test

The irritant smoke fit-test uses a ventilation smoke tube containing stannic chloride on pumice. When exposed to air, the metal chloride reacts with moisture to form a mixture of hydration products and hydrochloric acid. This fume is irritating and will cause people to sneeze, cough, or react in some fashion to the irritation. Some people have been found not to react to the material. A pump or a squeeze bulb delivering 200 mL/min is connected to the tube to generate a steady stream of smoke.[1] Few data on the concentrations generated during the testing or sensitivity check phase of the test have been published. In a health hazard evaluation, NIOSH found potential exposure to high concentrations of hydrochloric acid during the irritant smoke QLFT resulting in NIOSH not recommending this fit test method.[47]

Bitter Aerosol Fit-Test

A bitter aerosol fit-test QLFT has been developed using denatonium benzoate, commonly known as Bitrex™.[46] Bitrex has been used as a taste aversion agent in household liquids (to keep children from drinking them). The fit-test is based on the saccharin fit-test protocol. This test can be used for any respirator equipped with any type particulate filter.

Test Exercises

To mimic the movements of a person in the workplace, a series of test exercises is normally performed during a fit-test. The following seven exercises are required by OSHA: normal breathing, deep breathing, moving head side to side, moving head up and down, talking, bending over, or jogging in place, and normal breathing. For QNFT a grimace exercise is used to determine that if the seal is broken and that the respirator reseals on the face. Each exercise is performed for 60 seconds while standing.

Complete copies of the OSHA fit testing procedures are found in Appendix A of 29 CFr 1910.134.[1] For additional information on fit testing and fit test protocols see ANSI/AIHA® Z88.10.[48]

Respirator Sealing Problems

A respirator equipped with a facepiece (tight or loose-fitting) must not be worn if facial hair comes between the sealing periphery of the facepiece and the face, or if facial hair interferes with valve function. Both negative and positive pressure tight-fitting respirator performance has been shown to be reduced when the respirators are worn over facial hair.[49] Only respirators equipped with loose fitting hoods or helmets are acceptable with facial hair.[2]

In some industrial environments safety glasses or goggles must be worn to protect the eyes from flying objects. With a half-facepiece respirator, safety glasses, regular eyeglasses used to improve vision, or goggles can interfere with the fit of the respirator where it sits on the bridge of the nose. Wearing glasses with temple bars that pass through the sealing surface of a full facepiece respirator is not acceptable.

For half-facepiece respirators a fit-test is used to determine whether the respirator fits properly. The subject of the fit-test should wear any glasses, goggles, or other protective equipment normally used while wearing a respirator that may interfere with how the respirator fits. The fit-test is used to demonstrate that the glasses or other equipment do not interfere with the function of the respirator.

For full-facepiece respirators the options are to use contact lenses or spectacle kits that hold special eyeglasses that mount inside the facepiece. Most manufacturers supply a special spectacle kit that can be used. Research has shown that people can use contact lenses with respirators without difficulty.[50]

Standards

Respirator regulations fall into two categories: respirator testing or approval standards, and respirator use standards. Although they appear to address two different concerns, both types of standards affect the use of respirators and have implications for respiratory protection programs.

Respirator Test Standards

The primary objective of a respiratory protective equipment test standard or certification program is to assure users that a minimum level of performance is achieved by the respirator. This is important because this equipment is used to guard health or protect life. A second objective of the certification program is to supply the user with respirator use and limitation information. Many of the selection restrictions placed on the various respiratory protective devices are a result of performance levels established by the certification tests.

Many countries and standards organizations have established respirator testing standards. In addition, countries that do not have their own testing standards may recognize certified or approved respirators developed elsewhere. Table 40.6 lists some of the countries with respiratory protective device certification programs.

Respirator Use Standards

Various standards, regulations, and voluntary use standards exist for proper use of respirators. Most voluntary standards are consensus standards developed when a group of respirator experts met to establish a standard of practice. Table 40.7 lists some of the organizations with use standards. These organizations may also have established standards relating to other areas of respiratory protection. For example, the Canadian Standards Association developed a standard for compressed breathing air and systems[51], and ANSI established standards for medical evaluations of respirator wearers.[52]

In the United States, various government agencies have established respirator use regulations including OSHA[1], the Mine Safety and Health Administration[53–55], and the Nuclear Regulatory Commission.[56]

Summary

The proper selection and use of respiratory protection is essential to controlling exposures with respirators. A complete respiratory protection program must be established and implemented that is based on knowledge of the performance limitations and capabilities of the respirators and the appropriate standards and regulations for their use.

Table 40.6 — Countries with Respirator Testing Standards

Country	*Standard Name*	*Location*
Australia	AS/NZS 1716	Standards Australia, 1 The Crescent, Homebush NSW 2140 Australia.
Brazil	Several standards covering many types of respiratory protective devices	ABNT, Av. Treze de Maio, 13-28.o andar, CEP20003 – Caixa Postal 1680, Rio de Janeiro – RJ Brazil.
CEN[A]	Several standards covering all respiratory protective devices	CEN, Central secretariat, rue de Stassart,36 B-1050 Brussels, Belgium. For English: British Standards Institute, Linford Wood, Milton Keynes, MK14 6LE Tel:44-(0)1908 221166
China	Various standards	Division Chief, Bureau of Occupational Safety and Health Ministry of Labour, 12, Heipingli Zhongjie, Beijing 100716, P.R.C.
Japan	Standards for Dust Respirators Notification No. 19 of Ministry of Labor March 30, Showa 63-nen	Ministry of Labor 2-2, Kasumigaseki 1-chome Chiyoda-ku Tokyo 100, Japan
	Standards for Gas Masks Notification No.68 of MOL (September 26, Heisei 2-nen) Notification No. 1 of MOL (January 8,Heisei 8-nen Revised	Japanese Standards Association, 1-24, Akasaka 4-chome, Minato-ku, Tokyo 107 Japan
	Various standards	
Korea	Standard for Dust Respirators Notification No. 90–71 of Ministry	KISCO (Korea Industrial Safety Corp.), 34-4, Gusan-dong, Bupyong-gu, Inchon City, Zipcode: 403-120
	Corporation (Revised Dec. 28, 1990) Standard for Gas Masks Notification No.91–82 of Ministry of Labor (Dec. 7, 1991)	
	Standards for Supplied Air Respirators Notification No. 95–12 of Ministry of Labor (Jun. 17, 1995)	
Mexico	NOM–116–STPS	STPS, Secretaria "B", Direccion General de Seguridad e Higiene en el Trabajo, Direccion de Normalizacion e Investigacion, Avenida Azcapotzalco la Villa no. 209, Barrio de Santo Tomas, Delegacion Azcapotzalco, C.p. 02020 Mexico D.F.
New Zealand	AS/NZS 1716	Standards New Zealand, Standards House, 155 The Terrace, Wellington 6020, New Zealand
Russia	Various standards	Gosstandart of Russia, c/o Ms. N. Tinofeeva, 3, Electrichesky per., Moscow, 123856, Russia
South Africa	SABS 1455	Standard Specification Part I-IV South African Bureau of Standards, Private Bag X191, Pretoria, South Africa 0001
United States	42 CFR 84 Various statements of standards for CBRN equipment	NIOSH, Certification and Quality Assurance Branch, Division of Safety Research, 944 Chestnut Ridge Road, Morgantown, WV 26505
	NFPA 1981	NFPA, Quincy, MA

[A] Standards cannot be bought from CEN; they can only be purchased from the member associations in the language of the country. Committee for European Normalization members: Austria, Belgium, Denmark, Finland, France, Germany, Greece, Iceland, Ireland, Italy, Luxembourg, Netherlands, Norway, Portugal, Spain, Sweden, Switzerland, and United Kingdom.

Table 40.7 — Countries with Respirator Use Standards

Country	*Standard Name*	*Location*
Australia	AS/NZS 1715	Standards Australia, 1 The Crescent, Homebush NSW 2140 Australia
Brazil	Respiratory Protection Program — Selection and Use of Respirators	Fundacentro, Rua Capote Valente, 710, São, Paulo, Brazil
Canada	Selection, Use and Care of Respirators, Z94.4 Compressed Breathing Air and Systems, CAN3-Z180.1	Canadian Standards Association, 178 Rexdale Boulevard, Rexdale (Toronto), Ontario, Canada M9W 1R3,
CEN[A]	EN529 Respiratory protective devices — Recommendations for selection, use, care and maintenance — Guidance document	CEN, Central secretariat, rue de Stassart,36 B-1050 Brussels, Belgium. For English: British Standards Institute, Linford Wood, Milton Keynes, MK14 6LE Tel:44-(0)1908 221166
New Zealand	AS/NZS 1715:	Standards New Zealand, Standards House, 155 The Terrace, Wellington 6020, New Zealand
South Africa	SABA 0220:1988 Code of Practice, The Use, Care and Maintenance of Respiratory Protective Equipment	South African Bureau of Standards, Private Bag X191, Pretoria, South Africa 0001
United States	29 CFR 1910.134 ANSI Z88.2 ANSI Z88.6 ANSI Z88.10 NFPA 1500	OSHA, 200 Constitution Ave. NW, Washington, DC 20210 ANSI, 11 West 42nd Street, New York, NY 10036 NFPA, Quincy, MA
United Kingdom	HSE 282/28 Fit Testing of Respiratory Protective Equipment Facepieces	source:http://www.hse.gov.uk/
Venezuela	Covenin 1056/I	Norma Venezolana Covenin, Comision Venezolana de Normas Industriales, Ministerio de Fomento, Av. Andres Bello Edif. Torre Fondo Comun Piso 11, Caracas, Venezuela

[A] Standards cannot be bought from CEN; they can only be purchased from the member associations in the language of the country. Committee for European Normalization members: Austria, Belgium, Denmark, Finland, France, Germany, Greece, Iceland, Ireland, Italy, Luxembourg, Netherlands, Norway, Portugal, Spain, Sweden, Switzerland, and United Kingdom.

The information presented here is not intended to be all-inclusive in content or scope. A description of common respirators explains basic modes of operation. This is key information for proper selection of respirators. The information provided in Table 40.2 can be used to illustrate many of the selection principles discussed. A complete summary of the OSHA regulations was not attempted as they are not followed worldwide. For additional information the reader should consult the references and regulations and standard sources listed.

References

1. "Respiratory Protection," *Code of Federal Regulations* Title 29, Part 1910.134. 2008. pp. 419–445.
2. **American National Standards Institute:** *American National Standard for Respiratory Protection* (ANSI Z88.2). New York: American National Standards Institute, 1992.
3. **Canadian Standards Association:** *Selection, Use, and Care of Respirators* (Z94.4-02). Rexdale, Ontario, Canada: Canadian Standards Association, 2002.

4. **Colton, C.E., L.R. Birkner, and L.M. Brosseau (eds.):** *Respiratory Protection: A Manual and Guideline*, 3rd ed. Fairfax, Va.: American Industrial Hygiene Association, 2001.
5. "Approval of Respiratory Protective Devices," *Code of Federal Regulations* Title 42, Part 84. 1996. pp. 528–593.
6. **Japuntich, D.A.:** Respiratory particulate filtration. *J. Int. Resp. Prot. 2*:137–169 (1984).
7. **Ackley, M.W.:** Degradation of electrostatic filters at elevated temperature and humidity. In *World Filtration Congress III*, pp. 169–176. Croydon, England: Upland Press, 1982.
8. **Stevens, G.A., and E.S. Moyer:** "Worst case" aerosol testing parameters: I. Sodium chloride and dioctyl phthalate aerosol filter efficiency as a function of particle size and flow rate. *Am. Ind. Hyg. Assoc. J. 50*:257–264 (1989).
9. **Brown, R.C.:** Air Filtration. Oxford, England: Pergamon Press, 1993.
10. **Hinds, W.C., and P. Bellin:** Effect of facial-seal leaks on protection provided by half mask respirators. *Appl. Ind. Hyg. 3*:158–164 (1988).
11. **Kim, C.S. et al.:** "Filtration efficiency of a fibrous filter for nanoparticles", *Journal of Nanoparticle Research 8(2)*:215-221 (2006).
12. **Rengasamy, S., B.C. Eimer and R.E. Shaffer:** Comparison of Nanoparticle Filtration Performance of NIOSH-approved and CE-Marked Particulate Filtering Facepiece Respirators. *Ann. Occup. Hyg. 53*:117–128 (2009).
13. **National Institute for Occupational Safety and Health (NIOSH):** *NIOSH Guide to the Selection and Use of Particulate Respirators Certified Under 42 CFR 84* (DHHS/NIOSH Publication no. 96-100). Washington, D.C.: U.S. Department of Health and Human Services/NIOSH, 1996.
14. **Moyer, E.S.:** Review of influential factors affecting the performance of organic vapor air purifying respirator cartridges. *Am. Ind. Hyg. Assoc. J. 44*:46–51 (1983).
15. **Nelson, G.O.:** "Rules of Thumb for Cartridge Service Life." July 29, 1996. [Private communication]. Miller-Nelson Research, 8 Harris Court, Suite C-6, Monterey, CA 93940.
16. **National Institute for Occupational Safety and Health (NIOSH):** *NIOSH Pocket Guide to Chemical Hazards* (DHHS/NIOSH Publication no. 90-117). Washington, D.C.: U.S. Department of Health and Human Services/NIOSH, 1990.
17. **American Conference of Governmental Industrial Hygienists (ACGIH):** *Threshold Limit Values (TLVs) for Chemical Substances and Physical Agents and Biological Exposure Indices (BEIs).* Cincinnati: ACGIH, 2009.
18. **American Industrial Hygiene Association (AIHA):** *Odor Thresholds for Chemicals with Established Occupational Health Standards.* Fairfax, Va.: AIHA, 1989.
19. **Nelson, G.O., and C.A. Harder:** Respirator cartridge efficiency studies: VI. Effect of concentration. *Am. Ind. Hyg. Assoc. J. 37*:205–216 (1976).
20. **Wood, G., and Snyder, J.:** Estimating service lives of organic vapor cartridges III: multiple vapors at all humidities. *J. Occup. Environ. Hyg. 4*:363-374 (2007).
21. **Yoon, Y.H., J.H. Nelson, J. Lara, et al.:** Effect of solvent mixtures on service life. *Am. Ind. Hyg. Assoc. J. 52*:65–74 (1991).
22. **Lara, J., Y.H. Yoon, and J.H. Nelson:** The service life of respirator cartridges with binary mixtures of organic vapors. *J. Intl. Soc. Respir. Prot.11*:7-26 (1995).
23. **Compressed Gas Association:** *Commodity Specification for Air* (CGA G7.1). Arlington, Va.: Compressed Gas Association, 2004.
24. **Perez, C., and S.C. Soderholm:** Some chemicals requiring special consideration when deciding whether to sample the particle, vapor, or both phases of an atmosphere. *Appl. Occup. Environ. Hyg. 6*:859–864 (1991).
25. **Soderholm, S.C.:** Particle and gas phase interactions in air sampling. In *Air Sampling Instruments for Evaluation of Atmospheric Contaminants*, 8th ed., pp. 67–80. Cincinnati, Ohio: American Conference of Governmental Industrial Hygienists, 1995.
26. **Bollinger, N:** *Respirator Decision Logic* (DHHS/ NIOSH Publication no. 2005-100). Washington, D.C.: U.S. Department of Health and Human Services/NIOSH, 2004.
23. "Formaldehyde," *Code of Federal Regulations* Title 29, Part 1910.1048. 1994. pp. 411-443.
27. **Amoore, J.E., and E. Hautala:** Odor as an aid to chemical safety: odor thresholds compared with threshold limit values and volatilities for 214 industrial chemicals in air and water dilution. *J. Appl. Toxicol. 3*:272–290 (1983).
28. **Fazzalari, F.A. (ed.):** *Compilation of Odor and Taste Threshold Value Data.* Philadelphia: American Society for Testing and Materials, 1978.
29. **Lodewyckx, P., and E.F. Vansant:** The influence of humidity on the overall mass transfer coefficient of the Wheeler-Jonas equation. *AIHAJ 61*:461–468 (2000).
30. EN529 Respiratory protective devices — Recommendations for selection, use, care and maintenance — Guidance document. Brussels: European Committee for Standardization, 2005.
31. **Yoon, Y.H., and J.H. Nelson:** Breakthrough time and adsorption capacity of respirator cartridges. *Am. Ind. Hyg. Assoc. J. 53*:303–316 (1992).

32. **Henry, N.W., III, and R.S. Wilhelme:** An evaluation of respirator canisters to acrylonitrile vapors. *Am. Ind. Hyg. Assoc. J. 40*:1017–1022 (1979).
33. **Wood, G.O.:** Estimating service lives of organic vapor cartridges. *Am. Ind. Hyg. Assoc. J. 55*:11–15 (1994).
34. **Wood, G., and Snyder, J.:** "Estimating service lives of organic vapor cartridges III: multiple vapors at all humidities" *Journal of Occupational and Environmental Hygiene 4*:363-374 (2007).
35. **Occupational Safety and Health Administration (OSHA):** "Memorandum for Regional Administrators; OSHA Application of the NIOSH IDLH Values." J.B. Miles, OSHA, Washington, D.C. May 21, 1996. [Memo]
36. **National Fire Protection Association (NFPA):** *Open-Circuit Self-Contained Breathing Apparatus for Firefighters* (NFPA 1981). Quincy, Mass.: NFPA, 2007.
37. **Myers, W.R., M. Jaraiedi, and L. Hendricks:** Effectiveness of fit check methods on half mask respirators. *Appl. Occup. Environ. Hyg. 10*:934–942 (1995).
38. **Cruthchfield, C.D., M.P. Eroh, and M.D. VanErt:** A feasibility study of quantitative respiratory fit testing by controlled negative pressure. *Am. Ind. Hyg. Assoc. J. 52*:172–176 (1991).
39. **Hyatt, E.C., J.A. Pritchard, and C.P. Richards:** Respirator efficiency measurement using quantitative DOP man tests. *Am. Ind. Hyg. Assoc. J. 33*:635–643 (1972).
40. **Hounam, R.F., D.J. Morgan, D.T. O'Connor, and R.J. Sherwood:** The evaluation of protection provided by respirators. *Ann. Occup. Hyg. 7*:353–363 (1964).
41. **Willeke, K., H.E. Ayer, and J.D. Blanchard:** Methods for quantitative respirator fit testing with aerosols. *Am. Ind. Hyg. Assoc. J. 42*:121–125 (1981).
42. **Han, D.H., K. Willeke, and C.E. Colton:** Quantitative fit testing techniques and regulations for tight-fitting respirators: Current methods measuring aerosol or air leakage, and new developments. *Am. Ind. Hyg. Assoc. J. 58*:219–228 (1997).
43. **Nelson, T.J., O.T. Skredtvedt, J.L. Loschiavo, and S.W. Dixon:** Development of an improved qualitative fit test using isoamyl acetate. *J. Int. Soc. Resp. Prot. 2*:225–248 (1984).
44. "Qualitative Fit Testing Protocols Under the Lead Standard" (Posthearing data submission, docket no. H-049A). 3M, Box 33275, Building 275-6W-01, St. Paul, MN 55144. Oct. 23, 1981.
45. **Marsh J.L.:** Evaluation of irritant smoke qualitative fitting test for respirators. *Am. Ind. Hyg. Assoc. J. 45*:371–376 (1984).
46. **Mullins, H.E., S.G. Danisch, and A.R. Johnston:** Development of a new qualitative test for fit-testing respirators. *Am. Ind. Hyg. Assoc. J. 56*:1068–1073 (1995).
47. NIOSH Health Hazard Evaluation Report No. HETA-93-040-2315, Anchorage Fire Department, Anchorage, Alaska http://www.cdc.gov/niosh/hhe/reports/pdfs/1993-0040-2315.pdf
48. **American Industrial Hygiene Association (AIHA®):** *ANSI/AIHA® Z88.10-2010 Respirator Fit Testing Methods.* Fairfax, VA: AIHA®, 2010.
49. **Stobbe T.J., R.A. daRoza, and M.A. Watkins:** Facial hair and respirator fit: a review of the literature. *Am. Ind. Hyg. Assoc. J. 49*:199–204 (1988).
50. **Lawrence Livermore National Laboratory:** "Is it Safe to Wear Contact Lenses with a Full Facepiece Respirator?" by R.A. daRoza and C.S. Wearver (UCRL-53653). Livermore, Calif.: Lawrence Livermore National Laboratory, 1986.
51. **Canadian Standards Association:** *Compressed Breathing Air and Systems* (Z180.1-00). Rexdale, Ontario, Canada: Canadian Standards Association, 2000.
52. **American National Standards Institute:** *American National Standard for Respiratory Protection-Respirator Use-Physical Qualifications for Personnel* (ANSI Z88.6). New York: American National Standards Institute, 1984.
53. "Control of Exposure to Airborne Contaminants," *Code of Federal Regulations* Title 30, Part 56.5005. 1993. pp. 338.
54. "Control of Exposure to Airborne Contaminants," *Code of Federal Regulations* Title 30, Part 57.5005. 1993. pp. 409–410.
55. "Respiratory Equipment," *Code of Federal Regulations* Title 30, Subpart D. 1993. pp. 493–494.
56. "Use of Individual Respiratory Protection Equipment," *Code of Federal Regulations* Title 10, Part 20.1703. 2001. pp. 327–328.

Outcome Competencies

After completing this chapter, the reader should be able to:

1. Define underlined terms used in this chapter.
2. Explain total quality management (TQM).
3. List general components of TQM.
4. Discuss goal setting in occupational and environmental health.
5. Discuss the rules of accountability and measurability.
6. List total quality rules for communication.
7. Discuss kaizen or continuous improvement.

Prerequisite Knowledge

None

Key Terms

activity-based costing (ABC) • benchmark • brainstorming • catchball • continuous improvement • customer • cycle time • failure modes and effects analysis • fault tree analysis • flowchart • House of Quality • inspiring • integrated product development • (IPD) • interpreting • kaizen • mental models • milestones • mobilizing • operating plan • pareto analysis • personal mastery • policy deployment • process • quality function deployment (QFD) • queue time • reflective listening • rework • robust design • root cause • shaping • shared vision • strategic plan • supplier • systems thinking • Taguchi experiments • team learning • total quality • total quality control (TQC) • total quality environmental management (TQEM) • total quality management (TQM) • vision statements • what gets measured gets managed

Key Topics

I. Management Skills
   A. Integration into Organizational Priorities
   B. Program Planning
   C. Rationale for EHS Program Elements
   D. The Role of Management Skills in Occupational Hygiene
   E. Management from a Support Position
   F. Career Planning

II. Management Theory
   A. Organizational Structure
   B. Leadership

III. Management Practices and their Application to Occupational Hygiene
   A. Management Systems
   B. Total Quality
   C. Lean Manufacturing
   D. Integrated Product Development
   E. Benchmarking
   F. Policy Deployment
   G. Policy Management
   H. Resource Management
   I. Negotiation Skills
   J. Program planning
   K. Team Dynamics

Program Management

41

By Alan J. Leibowitz, CIH, CSP

Introduction

Occupational Hygiene is, at its core, a technical profession. Given this fundamental orientation, Occupational Hygiene has historically tended to focus on the sampling and analytical aspects of the profession. While appropriate for a profession charged with using environmental evaluations to protect life and environment, this technical focus has left many ill prepared for workplaces where interpersonal and managerial skills are as highly valued as technical prowess; where possession and transmission of technical information is not sufficient to ensure that concerns and recommendations are acted upon.

As occupational hygiene has evolved, team contributions and performance have eclipsed the value of the individual technical contributor. To successfully participate in this environment it is increasingly important that Occupational Hygienists, and more broadly Environmental Health and Safety (EHS) professionals, be capable of communication on many levels and to various audiences.

Whether they practice as outside consultants, educators or in industry occupational hygienists must understand their customer's organizational culture. A culture that includes the assumptions, values, norms and tangible signs (artifacts) of organization members and their behaviors.[1] Many programs do not succeed when the occupational hygienist fails to recognize how decisions are made in their organization and how change is initiated and managed.

Change comes only when the benefit to an organization can be clearly articulated and understood. The pace and magnitude of change in business is increasing at a rapid rate.[2] To participate in this process successful Occupational hygienists must function as "agents of change" to influence their customers and organizations toward the proper course in the protection of health and the environment. As Tom Peters stated in his book *Thriving On Chaos*[3], "Today, loving change, tumult, even chaos is a prerequisite for survival, let alone success."

Integration into Organizational Priorities

A key attribute of a successful EHS program is a high level of distribution of responsibility for program actions among functional departments. Where EHS professionals are solely responsible for the success or failure of all program elements it is much more difficult, if not impossible, to succeed. Every organization should have a clearly stated EHS policy which articulates the organization's commitment to EHS and clearly distributes responsibilities to appropriate functional areas within the organization. An example Corporate EHS Policy is provided in Appendix A. In order to ensure that all departments understand and accept their EHS responsibilities they must become a part of the company culture. The occupational hygienist must speak the language of the organization and participate in the important rituals that establish internal priorities and goals.

Each aspect of an EHS program requires integration with appropriate functional departments. Figure 41.1 illustrates an example of the relationship between the essential tools of EHS and the critical processes they

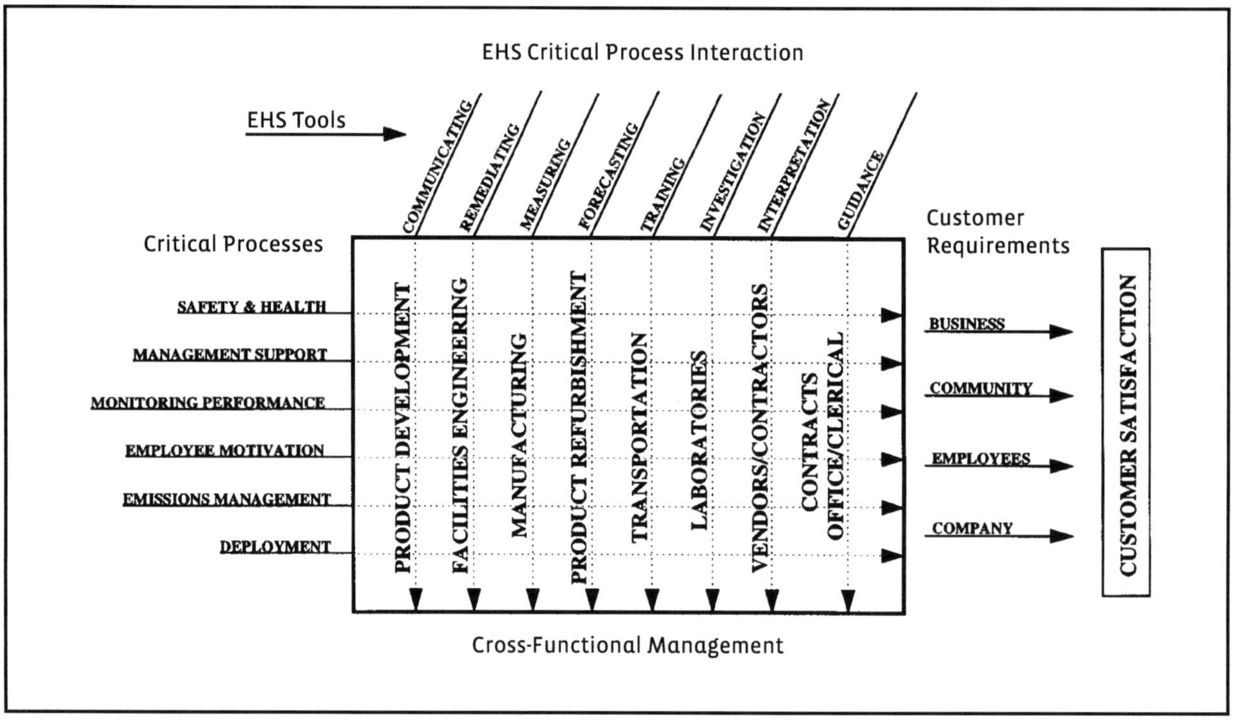

Figure 41.1 — Example Cross-Functional EHS Program Support Relationship Analysis (adapted from a matrix developed by D. Polzo, ITT Avionics).

support. For each tool a potential supporting function is identified. Involvement of all functional aspects of an organization is critical to an effective EHS program as measured by customer satisfaction.

An occupational hygienist's first goal should be to understand the larger organization. The professional must identify previously established priorities and how EHS issues fit into them. For example, if the organization's current goals include growth in international sales, the EHS department must understand regulations in the markets being explored. If this goal also includes an increase in production, then EHS must be prepared to review production plans for new equipment, facility modifications, training and sampling needs. Often the most critical aspect of production changes, from an EHS perspective, is the evaluation of new regulatory requirements that may be introduced. In some cases obtaining a permit can take many months and if the need is not properly anticipated this aspect can delay important programs. This does not endear the EHS department to the rest of the organization. Even development of appropriate personal protective equipment strategies can take time if sampling is required using a phased approach.

Program Planning

In order to avoid unacceptable delays or interference with global goals the occupational hygienist must be aware of the plans of the organization in specific detail where IH issues might exist. Later in this chapter a discussion of Integrated Product Development (IPD) will describe how IH issues can be included in specific process design planning. Before the specific detail of a particular process is established the occupational hygienist should participate in the goal setting process for the organization. Most often this takes the form of long-range or strategic planning and near-term or operations planning.

An organization's *strategic plan* generally describes where it would like to be in the next three to five years. As a general rule, strategic plans are likely to change each year as new information becomes available and the marketplace evolves. The dynamic nature of the organizational planning process requires constant vigilance to insure that EHS issues are included and kept up to date. This part of the planning process has a longer time horizon than development of an *operating plan*, which generally looks one to two years out. The longer viewpoint requires management to assess potential modifications to their current strategy in terms of opportunities or threats which might arise in the future. This planning includes an evaluation of future resource needs, particularly if there is a requirement to move the organization into new areas. The Occupational hygienist can be most valuable when the organization is evaluating entry into previously unexplored areas. EHS should provide input to the strategic plan based on their goals and current expectations of impacts on the organization from regulatory and technical trends. Some organizations include a section in their written strategic plans which focus on EHS trends and assumptions. Others simply include EHS issues as part of the body of their plans where principle strategic issues have EHS elements.

Operating plans establish the organization's specific short term goals. These plans are much more fixed than strategic plans and considerable resources are expended to ensure that the goals established have a strong chance of success. A company's operating plan usually focuses on significant opportunities and challenges faced in the near term. Resource intensive or high profile EHS activities should be included in the written plan.

The deployment of both Strategic and Operating Plan objectives throughout an organization is critical to its success. There are many different routes to help ensure that top level goals are aligned throughout an organization.[4] In larger organizations the procedure is often highly structured. Initial planning is first accomplished on the corporate level, then at business units and then in functional departments within the unit. At the corporate level broad initiatives are established which provide a direction for the rest of the organization. Business units must then look at what areas of their operations can potentially support the larger organization's goals. At the business unit detailed financial goals are established and action plans are developed delineating specific functional responsibilities. Finally each functional area must look at its plans and determine how its intended actions support the broader goals of the organization. On this base tier of the planning process, the nature and sequence of specific required actions are established.

While not every action of the EHS department must fit the global plan, it is important that the link between EHS and broad operational goals is clearly established throughout the organization. This linkage must be articulated in a manner which supports acceptance of EHS integration by all of management including members of the EHS department. EHS Managers must participate in planning and deployment to ensure that EHS issues are considered at all stages of the process. Since these documents become the bibles of the organization, it is also very helpful if specific EHS actions are included in the plans. This reminds the organization that EHS is part of their responsibilities to the business as a whole and is not an added responsibility to be managed when time permits. A Strategic Plan should include an evaluation of anticipated impacts for the plan period. These impacts might, for example, include new regulations or enforcement initiatives. Operating Plans can, by their nature, include more specific detail on what actions are to be taken during the life of the plan. It is

ACTION REGISTER						
LOCATION/PROGRAM: Plant C - East			**SUBJECT AREA:** Occupational Hygiene/Safety			**DATE:** 10/7/11
ITEM NO.	**ISSUE**	**DATE ASSIGNED**	**DATE DUE**	**STATUS**	**ASSIGNED TO**	**REMARKS/ACTION**
AJL-1.3	Wave solder pot cleaning IH sampling.	4/7/11	5/30/11	Complete	R. Kotick/ M. Sue	Above standard. Ventilation improvement required.
AJL-1.3 V1	Wave solder ventilation upgrade.	8/10/11	4/9/12	Duct work being fabricated.	J. Abel/ A. Samuel	
FM-95.1	Toxic gas handling training required.	9/18/11	2/10/12	Wafer lab complete.	M. Bezar	Additional SCBA on order.
APL -1e	No sprinkler - main aisle b15 - b23.	8/23/11	2/21/12	Design under development.	A. Polin/ J. Abel	

Figure 41.2 — Example Operating Plan Action Register.

appropriate to require that an action plan, such as is shown in Figure 41.2, be included for major items in each business unit's portion of the plan.

Rationale for EHS Program Elements

Early in the development of the program, every EHS Manager must provide management with a rationale for each of the areas where the program will focus. Maintaining a successful EHS program is not inexpensive, and it is important that management understand where their resources are being applied and why. The first step in establishing focus areas is an evaluation of the internal and external EHS issues which face the organization. Areas to explore include regulatory compliance history, marketing priorities, environmental exposure potential and internal initiatives.

Regulatory compliance history and challenges are important because they have impact on the magnitude of exposure to the organization and responsible management. An organization with a historically poor compliance record faces a higher level of fines for repeat violations. Previous compliance history also has bearing on the level of criminal liability under federal sentencing guidelines. Where an organization is in a heavily regulated area, pharmaceuticals for example, the potential for episodes of noncompliance are magnified by the sheer number of compliance issues. In such cases regulatory compliance will be a priority for the organization.

Marketing priorities have an impact based on intended customers and shareholder interests. As an example, a supplier of consumer goods, such as health and safety products, has a much greater potential impact on the bottom line from publicity regarding EHS issues, than does a manufacturer of heavy machinery for industrial use. The benefits of good publicity and the consequences of bad will be magnified in a company where the customer chooses its product based on a notion of the "goodness" of the organization from an ethical viewpoint. Shareholder initiatives may also provide incentive for participation in activities such as EHS Management Systems standards or other external, structured initiatives that might not otherwise be required in well managed EHS programs. Given that such initiatives generally require substantial resources including them as a priority must have sound business advantage.

The potential for environmental exposure to the organization based on its mode of operation or history can also have a bearing on priorities. If an organization is in an acquisition or divestiture mode, considerable resources will be required for *due diligence* activities, which evaluate the risks associated with the transaction. These risks can include noncompliance issues, improper hazardous materials use and possible contamination concerns.

The nature and location of operating locations is also an issue. If there are many older facilities, evaluation of the properties and remediation of historic issues will be a priority. Operating many smaller locations will require resources to support non-professional EHS coordinators at these locations. Foreign operations also can require different priorities, as other regulations must be evaluated and transaction times for all aspects of the program will be increased due to language and cultural barriers. It is important to understand how each of these issues is addressed in transaction documents including a clear recognition of who is responsible for what going forward.

Internal commitments developed by the organization must also be considered in establishing program priorities. If the organization has ESH leadership aspirations, resources must be dedicated to the programs which support this goal. For example, senior management might commit to elimination of a particular material, such as beryllium, from their processes. This effort may require considerable resources from EHS to evaluate process changes and potential substitute materials. Too often in a rush to meet commitments new materials are placed into use without proper scrutiny. These substitutes may present a greater employee hazards which could go unrecognized as users may feel that, since this is a replacement for a "bad" material, they have nothing to be concerned about.

When establishing the rationale for the EHS program for management each of these areas must be evaluated and inclusion of resources to address them clearly articulated. Since many companies today are data driven it may be helpful to use an evaluation methodology which evaluates each aspect of the EHS function semi-quantitatively and calculates the needed resources in a relatively objective fashion. Appendix B contains an example of a tool developed by ITT to assist in determining the level of resources required at each location. The tool can be easily modified to reflect the needs of any organization.

Except in consulting, organizations EHS is rarely a profit center, since most accomplishments are injury or cost avoidance based, it is difficult to quantify the benefits of program improvements. Using the Resource Evaluation tool provides a starting point for resource discussions with management. These discussions should follow an agenda, established prior to the meeting, which includes senior management support for agreed upon initiatives. A detailed proposal should be presented and specific actions and resource needs addressed. Once finalized, the program plan should serve as a guide to future actions and should be updated on a regular, at least annual, basis.

The Role of Management Skills in Occupational Hygiene

As a general rule, Occupational hygienists have limited formal authority to accomplish their job tasks. While they may have some positional authority the individuals required to support the ESH program rarely report to them. Their role is typically focused on obtaining the data necessary to determine what changes, if any, are required in a company's processes to ensure the protection of workers and other potentially exposed individuals. That data is then used to develop recommendations which can be communicated to the individuals responsible for the process in question. The success or failure of a facility's occupational hygiene program depends on the occupational hygienist's ability to convince those individuals able to change a process, of the value of their advice and the benefits of the required action. Effective occupational hygiene management must consider not only hazard control, but also any potential added value represented by the recommendations to the business. For example, installation of a dust collector to protect employees may also collect valuable product which can be recycled or reclaimed.

Most occupational hygienists practice not among their scientifically inclined peers, but in the greater business world where leaders are more likely to have a business education. In order to communicate with this decision making population, occupational hygienists must be able to convey necessary information in a manner that is comfortable for their audience. This requires an understanding of management philosophy, nomenclature and presentation norms. For example, most organizations have a method for presenting statistical data which is typically used for internal presentations. That style should be adopted for presenting occupational hygiene data.

It is also important that occupational hygienists be comfortable with making business presentations as their stature advances within the organization. As senior EHS managers advance they will more frequently be asked to participate in projects and meetings that are not specifically focused on EHS issues. Their participation will only be of value if they can understand the issues under discussion in sufficient detail to identify where EHS concerns might arise.

Management from a Support Position

Occupational hygienists typically function from a support position. This means that while they may exercise considerable influence over decisions they do not have the final say. In his book "Getting Things done When You are not in Charge" Geoffrey Bellman[5] identifies several characteristics of support positions that Occupational hygienists may recognize;

- More expertise than authority
- Important influence but not the final say
- Free access to the organization
- Regular interaction with people of greater authority
- Future planning is difficult
- Accused of not appreciating "the big picture" or the "bottom line"
- Important customers do not appreciate or understand the function
- Seen as a cost center to be at best tolerated
- Predecessor reputation may have an adverse effect

- Battles with other support professionals vying for limited resources

Given these characteristics, the support role brings some daunting challenges which are best addressed by focusing on those areas where change is required, and convincing those in authority to take required actions. This often requires the creation of a vision of a future state where the issues of concern have been addressed and the development of a plan to reach that goal. A *vision* statement identifies where you want to be in the future. In broad terms it establishes the end point for an improvement process and allows the development of a plan to move from an unacceptable present to a beneficial future.

The key to convincing others that your recommendations provide the most appropriate path for your organization is understanding customer motivations. In this case the *customer* is anyone who is potentially impacted by the information developed though sampling or other analysis of the work environment. These customers may be internal or external. Some examples of IH customers are regulatory agencies, employees, purchasers of services/products and company management

Career Planning

In management as in all other aspects of life the old adage "to thine own self be true" applies. If managers are to continue to be productive contributors to their organization they must develop and grow. Like most aspects of management behavior this growth occurs most efficiently when a clear plan is developed and followed.

Career planning for EHS professionals is not unlike that of most technical specialties except that the breadth of the profession offers a greater range of options than most. In most cases unless the individual is part of a large organization focused on EHS, career options are not obvious and development of a career plan requires careful deliberation. These plans are usually specific to the individual and only a few organizations provide assistance with their preparation. The following lists some basic steps to be considered when developing a career plan.

1. Develop a vision based on various career stages. What would you like to do next year, in five years or in ten years? Try not to limit options to what appears obvious. Seek assistance from associates, mentors and outside resources.
2. Evaluate each option in terms of requirements to meet the goal and the way each development step supports future goals. Asking someone who has achieved a level of success you admire, what was required can help clarify the steps you need to take.
3. Explore other functional areas or aspects of EHS, when the opportunity presents itself. This will help you evaluate what others do and avoid the "grass is always greener" phenomena.
4. Write down your plan and share it with others for comment as appropriate. Sharing the plan with your boss, if possible, can have significant advantages in ensuring that your ambitions are understood.
5. Readjust your plan on a regular basis.

Opportunities for growth should be considered both within and outside of the organization. Most companies recognize the need to develop their employees and to enhance the skills they bring to their jobs. A good company will continue to educate employees even where their education and experience exceed the needs of their present jobs. While this presents a possibility that the employee may leave for a more advanced position, smart organizations know that having the best person for the job entails some risk. In EHS, overqualified rather than under qualified is the preferred situation from an organizational perspective. If EHS Managers do not have the education their position requires, serious consequences could arise while they are learning on the job.

If the organization does not encourage individual growth and development employees may feel that they have nowhere to go. Morale and productivity will be reduced. Harvey Mackay[6] suggests an employee explore the following areas when they feel that their career is stagnating;

1. *Readjust your pace* — ensure that your expectations are realistic. See what other organizations offer.
2. *Analyze your competition* — How do you compare to others in the same

functional area in or out of the company? Get to know your value and options.
3. *Look for sideways growth* — If you have reached your limit in EHS, explore other functions such as engineering, marketing or product safety.
4. *Study the corporate culture* — Compare how you present yourself and your ideas to those who succeed in the organization.
5. *Take a look at your personal risk factor* — There are always ways to advance, but more drastic measures carry greater risk. Before you propose bold new ideas or take on difficult projects make sure you can accept the possibility of failure. Often the risk is worth it, but acceptance of risk should be a conscious decision, not a surprise.

A career is a lifetime pursuit made up of a series of jobs even within the same organization. Employees control their own careers by the choices they make, and only one thing is certain; mistakes will be made along the way. The true test of whether it is a career or a job is the ability to recover from the bumps in the road.

Management Theory

Ever since people organized into groups with common goals there has been a need to establish methods to manage the group to minimize duplication of efforts and to ensure completion of all tasks necessary for the group's survival. Management of these groups was often determined by leaders chosen for their physical characteristics such as strength or heredity. While history is replete with great civilizations flourishing under effective management there are also many examples of failure when inappropriate leaders were selected or developed. Where success occurred the techniques employed by the leaders were often not recorded and were lost to those who might later try to emulate the methods employed. In more recent times organizational and management theorists have tried to quantify what make successful leaders and organizations.

Organizational Structure

Organizations employ many different structures in their attempt to ensure that processes are conducted in the most efficient manner possible. Some of the theories describing such structure have been designated by letters Theory X, Theory Y and Theory Z.

Theory X directs a work-centered approach to organization. This theory as presented by Douglas McGregor in the early 1960s[7], rests on four assumptions: (1) Work is a chore; (2) People dislike work and will avoid it if possible; (3) People must be coerced or otherwise forced to put forth maximum effort; (4) People prefer to be led and to avoid responsibility.

Given these factors, there is little self-motivation possible, and an organization requires strong leaders and a rigid hierarchy to meet their goals. In a Theory X organization all decisions are made at the top where leaders use their authority to align the workers. In this application *authority* may be defined as the power to exact obedience. The organization is structured around a strict chain of command, with decision making at each level of the organization dependent on approval from the next higher level. This centralized structure makes communications very difficult, as access to the appropriate individual, both higher and lower in the organization, often requires passing through several intervening functions or individuals. In this type of structure it is most important that the EHS function be represented at the highest level of the organization. If not, the often difficult information that must be communicated in a good EHS program could be suppressed. Such circumstances can force the professional to balance career security against ethical conduct.

At the same time he discussed Theory X, McGregor presented an alternative designated Theory Y. People are at the center of a Theory Y organization. The assumptions of Theory Y are: (1) work is a normal part of life and is not inherently disliked; (2) people can exercise self control and do not necessarily require threats to work effectively; (3) people commit to objectives based on their perception of potential rewards; (4) people seek responsibility under appropriate circumstances; (5) most people can be innovative when given the opportunity; and (6) most people utilize a fraction of their intellectual potential in most jobs.

Taking these factors into account leads the Theory Y organization to seek a participative structure. In this arrangement, decision making is distributed throughout the organization. Objectives are achieved by persuading the group that a given direction is appropriate. In this type of organization, employees are organized into groups with significant interaction between them.

Both Theory X and Y are limited by the extremes of their perception of the organization. Theory Z attempts to address this deficiency by moving beyond simply considering work and people, to evaluation of such factors as organizational size, degree of interaction, personalities, alignment of goals, level of decision making and the state of the system. This type of analysis focuses on an organization's culture and how it would best reflect selected goals. The focus is on clear and open communications at all levels and a sense of collective responsibility for all members of the organization. This type of organization depends on team performance to meet its objectives and reflects the general trend in business today, to drive decisions and responsibility down into the organization where the actual work is performed. Decision making is participative, but an individual is responsible for the final decision. Even with the team focus that is so popular today, there is still a need for individuals to manage the process and make decisions. Team dynamics are discussed later in this chapter

In his book *Reengineering Management*, James Champy[8] recognizes the continued need for managers despite on-going flattening of organizations. He sees managers at four levels:

- *Self-managers*, who answer only for the quality of their work whether as individuals or as part of a team.
- *Process and people managers*, who answer for the work of others. In current team thinking this position often rotates as the project develops and the team requires different skills.
- *Expertise managers*, whose responsibility is for identifying future trends and needs.
- *Enterprise managers*, with profit and loss responsibilities.

While occupational hygienists might fall in any of these categories, they are most often expertise or self-managers. In most organizations they are valued for their abilities to help the organization avoid trouble and to act without specific direction.

All of these elements acting in concert allow a decentralized organization to work. This structure with distributed responsibility, greatly facilitates the function of an EHS program. When provided with a fair and open forum in which to make a case for EHS improvement, few proposals will be ignored. Whether proposals are approved or denied, decisions will be quicker and opportunities to revisit areas of concern will continue to exist.

Most current business publications exhort organizations to develop the ability to respond quickly to the rapidly changing global marketplace. Like Theories Y and Z, their advice leads to more decentralized organizations. In his book *The Fifth Discipline*, Peter Senge[9] discussed the need for an organization to be able to learn as a group. He sees this fundamental requirement as dependent on five "component technologies" or disciplines:

1. The ability to see all processes as a system of interrelated events. This *systems thinking* allows identification and correction of unacceptable patterns.
2. Employees' commitment to their own learning as demonstrated by a desire to focus their energies in continually aligning their personal growth activities with the needs of the organization. This *personal mastery* addresses the organization's need, on group and individual levels, to have a spiritual commitment to learning.
3. The ability to identify fundamental *mental models* or paradigms that limit the organizations ability to move forward. These ingrained assumptions about how the world works may limit the team's ability to move past obsolete practices and procedures.
4. Developing a *shared vision* of an appropriate future for the organization. This is a level beyond simply signing onto the personal vision of a charismatic leader. It is the ability to translate such a vision throughout the organization in a manner which fosters a genuine commitment.
5. Finally, and most importantly, is the concept of *team learning* where teams develop the ability to think as a group. As is discussed later in this chapter,

teams are the fundamental unit in many organizations today but, all too often patterns of defensive behavior limit their ability to achieve the collective insights that are not available to individuals. Teams must develop an atmosphere of open communications to allow these achievements to occur.

An organizational structure which focuses on learning, with an emphasis on teams, is ideal if change in the EHS program is required. EHS deficiencies are rarely the result of conscious decisions to violate the law or adversely affect employees. Rather these concerns arise from a lack of awareness of responsibilities and the basis for policy requirements. In a learning organization, with EHS representatives participating on teams, corrective education and training comes naturally. Concerns which arise can be dealt within the normal course of business, rather than as special events which cause resentment when they interrupt production processes.

Leadership

Leadership is the ability to mobilize available resources toward achieving the organization's vision and goals. These resources may be employees and their ideas, or the organization's physical assets. Leadership is most important when the organization is undergoing, or in need of, change. In their role of "agents of change" Occupational hygienists are often called upon to exercise their leadership abilities.

Many of the opportunities to exercise leadership in the workplace today come in the role of team leader. As is described later in this chapter, teams have become a critical part of the developmental process in industry today. The Evolution of leadership applications is described in the following table.[10]

Traditionally it was believed that leadership was not a learned ability but rather some inherent quality of individuals that made them stand out from the group. Current understanding is that leadership is more related to a given situation than an accident of birth. Each employee possesses a set of personality traits and abilities. Different situations require different skills in leaders. Leadership needs in the relatively stable past were quite different from those required today with fierce competition and a bewildering array of external requirements. Training and education can develop further skills which can be applied to leadership situations.

The Forum Institute[11] categorizes the tools necessary for leadership as abilities in four areas: Interpreting, Shaping, Mobilizing and Inspiring;

1. *Interpreting* — Data is available from many sources. Communication with external customers, peer organizations and information from regulatory sources can provide substantial data. Another source of information is inside the organization. Every group has information regarding its goals and the role of each function in meeting them. It is sometimes necessary to dig beneath surface policies and procedures to find the real expectations of the group. On a fundamental level, information and observations of the motivation and capabilities of the IH work group provides valuable information. Finally introspection is necessary to ensure understanding of personal motivation and capabilities to identify their effect on relationships and work. A leader must be able to obtain and utilize this information to identify the potential impact on the organization.

Table 41.1 — The Evolution of Leadership

Supervisory Leadership	*Participative Leadership*	*Team Leadership*
Direct people	Involve people	Build trust and inspire teamwork
Explain decisions	Get input for decisions	Facilitate and support team decisions
Train individuals	Develop individual performance	Expand team capabilities
Manage one-on-one	Coordinate group effort	Create a team identity
Contain conflict	Resolve conflict	Make the most of team differences
React to change	Implement change	Foresee and influence change

Interpretation of information from many different sources is a critical leadership skill. By using active communications skills, listening and asking questions, a leader is able to select that information which is most important to the organizations future.
2. *Shaping* — With this information leaders are able to *shape* a vision for the future which reflects the organization's values and goals. With the current pace of change many groups develop a sense that it is impossible to keep up with the present, let alone plan for the future. Good leaders can develop a strategy that seems both appropriate and achievable. They can elicit the support of their organizations by creating a meaningful picture of the future and the group's role in achieving it. Each step along the path is identified and measurable action plans developed.
3. *Mobilizing* — Achieving the organization's vision requires *mobilizing* available resources toward an identified goal. Leaders can focus in the required direction the efforts of a group comprised of individuals with varying motivations, abilities and ideas. This takes an ability to clearly communicate to all members of the group in a manner which ensures their understanding of the specific tasks they are expected to complete. This clear communication allows the leader to trust the team, and fosters the development of a supportive and cooperative work environment. In such an environment employees can contribute to the best of their abilities.
4. *Inspiring* — Finally, leaders can *inspire* their team to achieve success. By sharing authority and acknowledging the contributions of others, leaders enable others to feel and act like leaders. This sense of ownership by team members helps the group to achieve peak performance. Under strong leaders, team members are encouraged to develop their talents and to accept increasing levels of responsibility. Feeling that they have a stake in the results of their actions, and that their efforts will be recognized, encourages the entire work group to respond to the peaks and valleys of events in the workplace, with acceptance of the present and enthusiasm for future improvement.

Management Practices and their Application to Occupational Hygiene

Management Systems

A management system is the process an organization follows to achieve their goals. All of the procedures, policies, practices and functions of an organization comprise its management system. Whether they are aware of it or not every organization has a management system. It is the quality of that system that determines the success of their EHS program.

For example *ANSI/AIHA® Z10-2005, an Occupational Health and Safety Management Systems*[12] is designed to provide organizations with an effective tool for continual improvement of their occupational health and safety performance.

As described in the standard, "The OHSMS cycle entails an initial planning process, and implementation of the management system, followed by a process for checking the performance of these activities and taking appropriate corrective actions. The next step (management review) involves a review of the system for suitability, adequacy and effectiveness against its policy and this standard. The complete cycle is repeated, resulting in ongoing continual improvements in occupational health and safety. Improvements result from reducing hazards and risks in a systematic manner, a goal that is traditionally pursued through independent and often uncoordinated programs. In addition to the direct benefits of improved employee health and safety, a management system can also yield positive business outcomes, including enhanced productivity, financial performance, and employee satisfaction.

The management system approach is characterized by its emphasis on continual improvement and systematically eliminating the underlying or root causes of deficiencies. For example, in a system approach, if an inspection finds an unguarded machine, not only would the unguarded machine be fixed, but there would also be a systematic process in place to discover and eliminate

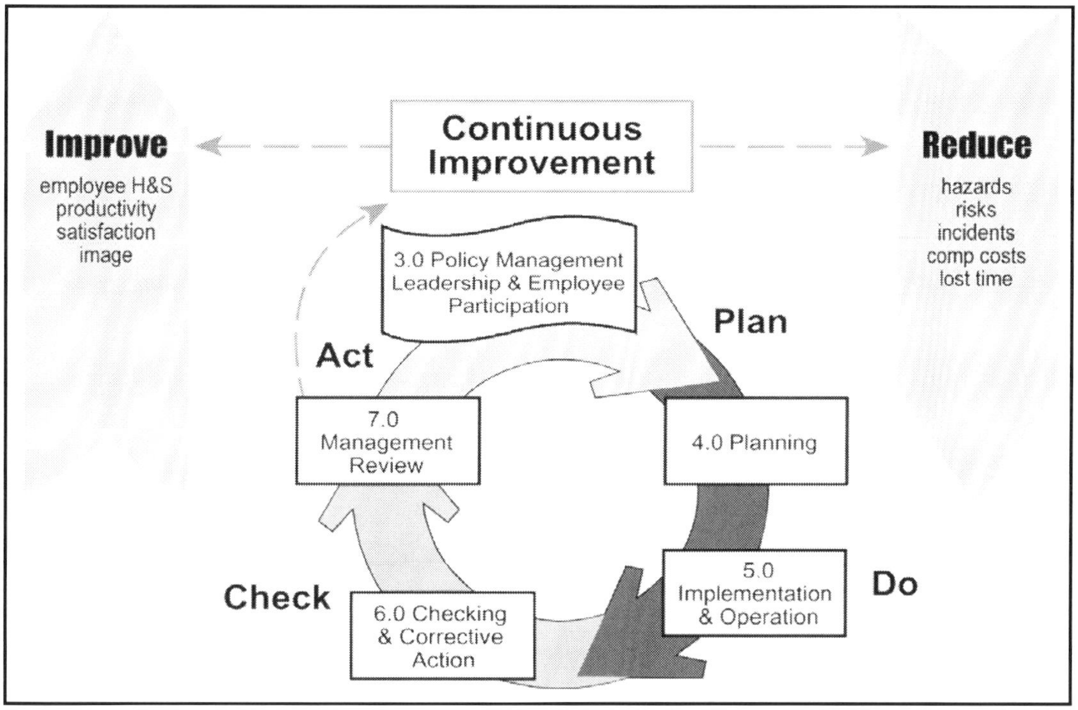

Figure 41.3 — ANSI/AIHA® Z10-2005 Management System incorporating the Deming Wheel.

the underlying reason for the deficiency. This process might then lead to the goal of replacing the guards with a more effective design, or to replacement of the machines themselves so that the hazard is eliminated. This systematic approach seeks a long-term solution rather than a one-time fix."(12)

Examples of ESH related management systems include:

- ISO 9001 Quality Management,
- ISO 14001 Environmental Management,
- ANSI/AIHA Z10, OHSAS 18001 Health and Safety Management,
- ISO 19011 Quality and Environmental Management Auditing

Total Quality

One of the key elements in the evolution of Management Systems was the concept of *total quality*. Total quality programs are often called Total Quality Management (TQM), Total Quality Control (TQC), or even Total Quality Environmental Management (TQEM). Total quality is a management methodology which emphasizes the improvement of the processes by which businesses operate and products are produced. The *process* includes all activities that produce an output for a *customer*. The provider of that output is the *supplier*. All aspects of business focus on supplier to customer relationships. The suppliers and customers may be internal or external to the organization. For example, customers of the EHS department might be regulators, management or employees. Suppliers might be regulators, consultants or internal departments such as purchasing.

Total quality initiatives involve all suppliers and customers and thus all employees in an organization. This type of management embraces the use of data and quantitative analysis over subjective processes such as the use of intuition or brute force. The methods used to improve processes center on the reduction of variability and the elimination of wasteful activities that often accompany processes developed without structured tools.

The philosophy of total quality requires a paradigm shift, away from a reluctance to tamper with processes that appear to be working, to one which states that all processes are imperfect and an organization must strive for continuous improvement. This philosophy of *continuous improvement* or *kaizen* ensures that the organization will never be satisfied with less than optimal performance in any of its processes. Kaizen indicates that every process can and should be continually evaluated and improved, in terms of time required, resources used, resultant quality and other aspects relevant to the process.

Many tools have been developed to facilitate the pursuit of total quality. Most of these tools focus on identifying, measuring, controlling, predicting and reducing waste. One of the fundamental tools used in this process is the Deming Wheel, named after W. Edwards Deming who introduced statistical process control to the Japanese in the 1950s. While the concepts he adapted from work by Shewhart and others at Bell Laboratories were largely ignored in his native United States, they were eagerly embraced by the Japanese. The unprecedented growth in Japanese economic power can largely be attributed to this single event.

The Deming Wheel is used to help solve problems by identifying weaknesses in processes. As is seen as part of Figure 41.3 the circuit consists of Plan, Do, Check and Act. The use of this tool, and others like it, usually entails the establishment of a team to evaluate a process or complete a project. The team members are trained in problem solving methodologies and team building. They are also provided technical support as required.

Since many of these evaluations are conducted on existing processes they would begin with the Check phase which looks at the past. This step is used to determine what has or has not been done in the past. This step most often begins by developing a *flow chart* of the process, which breaks it

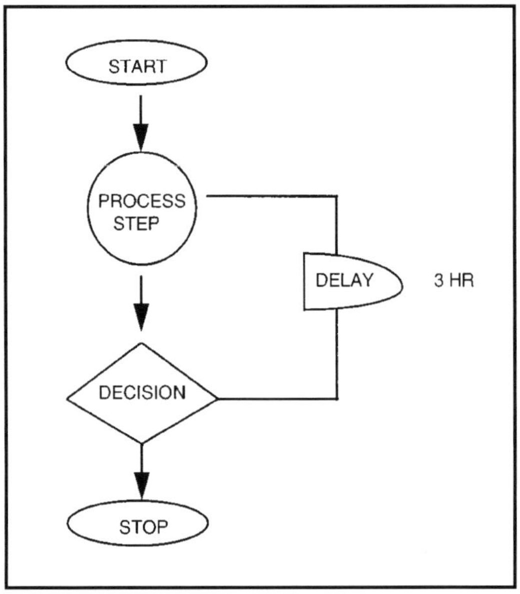

Figure 41.4 — The flow chart.

down into discrete steps. A properly constructed flow chart provides a pictorial representation of all steps in a given process.

A set of standard symbols is used to identify the type of action taking place in each step and the amount of time each step and the time between each step, or *queue time*, is clearly identified.

Each step in the process is then evaluated to determine if it adds value or is wasteful. Evaluation of the flow chart is also used to determine where bottlenecks exist and what actions are constraining optimal performance of the process. Data is gathered detailing performance in key areas of constraint or bottle neck and is then evaluated using process analysis tools such as *pareto analysis*. This tool was developed by Wifredo Pareto at the turn of the century. He looked at the distribution of wealth in the Italian states and discovered that 80% of the wealth was controlled by 20% of the population. This same ratio has been found in many other systems. Often 80% of the problems in a process are the result of only 20% of the potential causes. This 80/20 ratio is referred to in some areas of safety management as "The Principle of the Critical/ Vital Few."(13) Pareto analysis is used to isolate and identify areas of significant concern from a group of many potential concerns. Proper use of Pareto diagrams can help the team avoid using its limited resources to address a less important aspect of the problem.

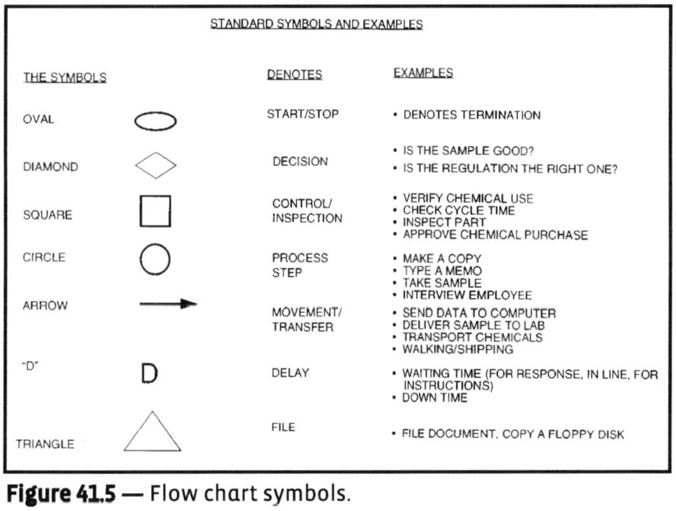

Figure 41.5 — Flow chart symbols.

As part of the Act step, Pareto Charts developed earlier are analyzed in an effort to establish cause and effect relationships for identified areas of concern. Solutions to the cause are then sought, often using *brainstorming* techniques. In brainstorming, groups are encouraged to think creatively about potential solutions. This process usually begins with unfiltered collection of potential solutions which are later analyzed to select the most likely answers. Potential quick solutions identified during this step are then implemented in an effort to contain the problem, while more targeted solutions to the *root cause* of the problem are identified, using more formal problem-solving tools. The root cause is the activity which if corrected or eliminated will eliminate the identified problem. Root causes might be identified using more advanced tools such as additional sublevel Paretos, Taguchi Experiments and Fault Tree Analyses.

Taguchi experiments provide a method for evaluating several different elements of a process at the same time as opposed to classic experimental design which focuses on time and resource consuming technical analysis of one factor at a time. This tool was designed by Genichi Taguchi as a cost effective way to improve processes under industrial conditions and limitations. Taguchi experiments use standard statistical tools to evaluate how much each selected cause contributes to the variation of the product. Using the Taguchi method insignificant factors are quickly eliminated allowing focused attention on the manipulation of those factors which increase the product's or process' robustness against variation. *Robust design* is a technique for making the utility of the final product insensitive to variations in the manufacturing process. In EHS terms this might mean that no matter how different the input chemicals are within a given range the final product will have no increased exposure potential from one batch to the next.

Fault Tree Analysis is a graphical method of performing a *Failure modes and Effects Analysis*. These techniques focus on relationships between data and not its quantification. They are useful in perfecting a process or design and in problem-solving.

The Plan step focuses on the development of a plan to eliminate the root cause of the problem. Central to any such plan is establishing accountability and a method to track the progress of necessary corrective actions. An Action Plan is often developed for this purpose. This plan identifies the problem and chosen corrective action, along with a schedule for completion and the person responsible for the action.

The Do portion of the wheel is the measurement step. Here the effect of the chosen action is measured to evaluate its impact on the root cause. Again, statistical measurement tools such as Pareto and trend charts along with histograms may be employed. Elimination of each root cause is analyzed in the context of its contribution to the overall problem. Most operational or EHS concerns have many root causes each of which have a different potential to address the initial concern. Finally, the Do step ends with an analysis to ensure that a permanent solution to the problem has been implemented. Again statistical process evaluation tools are employed in this process.

Then the wheel is "spun" again if the chosen solutions do not appear to have achieved final correction of the problem. Remember, continuous improvement demands that these processes continue until optimal solutions are found. In reality if at this stage the process has been significantly improved to an extent that other concerns have a higher priority for attention, it is preferable to address these greater concerns and then return to the initial problem when time and resources allow.

Lean Manufacturing

Lean is a systematic approach to identifying and eliminating non-value-added activities (waste or *Muda*) through continuous improvement and flow of the product or service by customer pull and in pursuit of perfection. Lean was first developed as the Toyota Production System and was developed as a means to increase production efficiency.[14] Developed at Toyota Automotive after World War II in an effort to smooth operating flow it evolved into a focus on maximizing *value added* activities which increase the market, form, or function of the product or service.

Lean focuses on identifying and eliminating the seven key areas of waste.

- Waste in Transportation
- Waste of Inventory

- Waste of Motion (Worker and Objects)
- Waste of Rework/Defects
- Waste of Processing (Too Fast, Too Slow)
- Waste of Waiting (Idle)
- Waste of Overproduction

Most organizations include ESH evaluation as part of the Lean process. This provides many potential improvement opportunities. Reduction in process steps and the material waste elimination associated with *just in time* production reduces exposure and injury opportunities. Ergonomic exposures can, in particular, be reduced if work flow improvements are properly designed. Safer more orderly work areas also result from using the *five S* process.

Five S is part of establishing a *Visual Workplace* that ensures that improvements in the workplace are clearly visible, readily understood and consistently followed. The Five S program focuses on having visual order, organization, cleanliness and standardization. A Five S program is comprised of the following elements.

- Sort — identify and eliminate nonessential process steps
- Set In Order — organize the work area for optimal workflow
- Shine — establish a routine cleaning and maintenance schedule

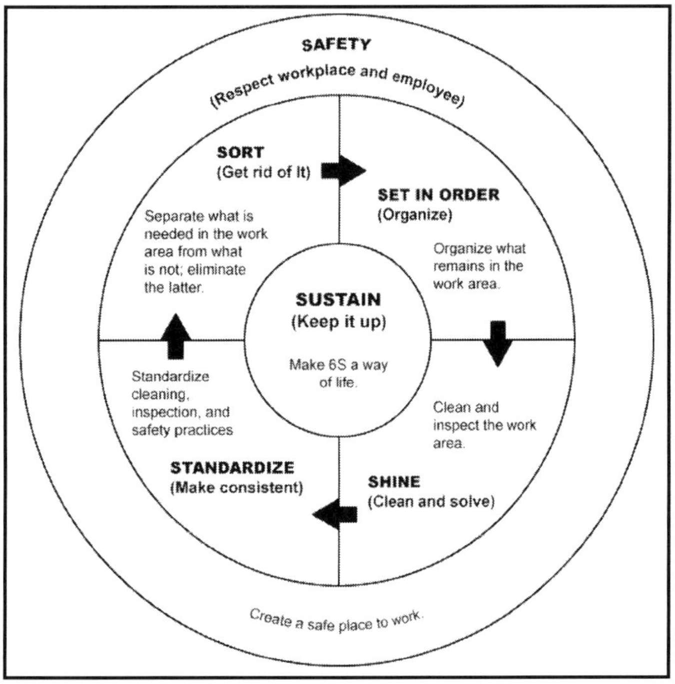

Figure 41.6 — 6S approach EPA Lean and Environment Toolkit 1-2006.

- Standardize — simplify and standardize the process to make it easy to maintain
- Sustain — maintain the improvements

As can be seen in Figure 41.6 below many organizations add a sixth S for safety.(15) This is primarily a reminder that safety should be considered in all 5S steps.

Care must however be taken to ensure that a focus on waste and minimization of the supply or process chain does not have adverse ESH impacts. For example lean can add risk if high hazard processes are brought in-house to shorten the supply chain. If an ESH professional is not involved in the Lean review process essential ESH protections such as personnel, machine guards and dedicated time can be inadvertently eliminated by those who do not understand their purpose. Lean resource optimization carried to extremes can also reduce an organization's ability to respond to unexpected events.

Integrated Product Development

Integrated Product Development (IPD) is a systematic approach to the multifunctional, concurrent design of products and their related processes. It includes manufacturing and support of the products through their life cycle. This multifunctional team approach is intended to decrease product development and deployment cycle time by addressing all elements of the product life cycle from conception through disposal, from the outset of the process. The multifunctional team includes representatives from all relevant internal functional areas and external members from customers and suppliers. Team members participate during appropriate phases of the project and are provided with the authority, responsibility and accountability necessary to meet customer requirements. An important aspect of continuous improvement is the reduction of the time it takes to bring a new product to market. This *cycle time* includes all elapsed time from the start of the of any process to its conclusion.

Process cycle time is reduced though open and rapid communications among all participants in the process. This helps ensure that major issues are not overlooked and problems are quickly surfaced and resolved. In a typical IPD process each phase of the project is managed by a team whose leaders

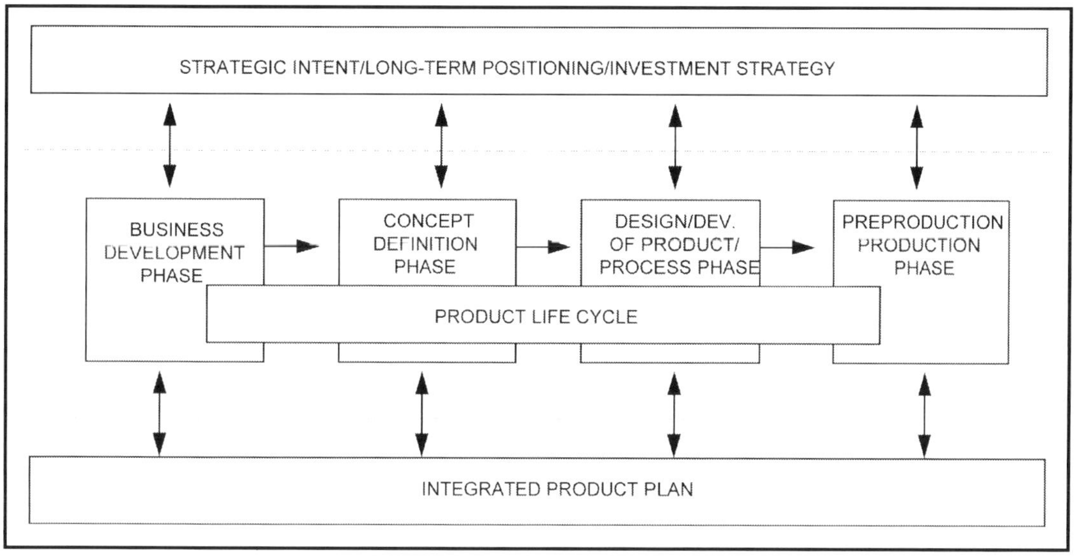

Figure 41.7 — IPD Process Overview.

and members vary as appropriate to the task at hand. Each phase has a thorough checklist which broadly identifies the major elements which must be dealt with at that time.

Process cycle time has become a critical indicator of a successful enterprise. Under current conditions, where the first-to-market company often has the greatest success, any wasted effort can have a significant impact on profit and survival. Every process consists of many cycle time elements. The cycle time is the length of time each discrete element of a process takes from initiation through completion. Individual elements can be added together to give a total process cycle time.

A typical method of measuring cycle time is to follow examples of the process' output from beginning to end. Issues which must be considered when measuring cycle time include whether or not to count time when people are not working, differences in the lengths of units of measure like months, and how to include *rework*. Rework is that portion of the output which must undergo additional processes to correct any unacceptable characteristics which were introduced during initial production.

Occupational hygienists can utilize the IPD process to ensure that EHS issues are raised earlier in the design process, to ensure that the overall program will not be delayed if IH concerns are uncovered too late. Like other functional experts IH professionals would typically not be a part of the core IPD team. Rather, a top level view of their issues would be included in the various checklists and they would be called in to participate with the team when issues in their area arise. Successful implementation of the IPD process and inclusion of EHS issues can help overcome one of the principle frustrations occupational hygienists face, getting other departments to identify IH issues in a timely fashion. This allows these issues to be properly addressed without the conflict that inappropriate process delays can create.

The IPD process consists of four phases; Business Development, Concept definition, Design/Development and Reproduction/ Production. In each phase EHS issues are considered where appropriate.

1. **Business Development:** Begins with identification of opportunities and ends with a decision to pursue or not. In this phase the effort is focused on determining the customer's actual requirements, the risks involved and the capability of the organization and/or partners to achieve the desired result. Occupational Hygiene issues at this stage might include new chemicals or processes to be introduced.

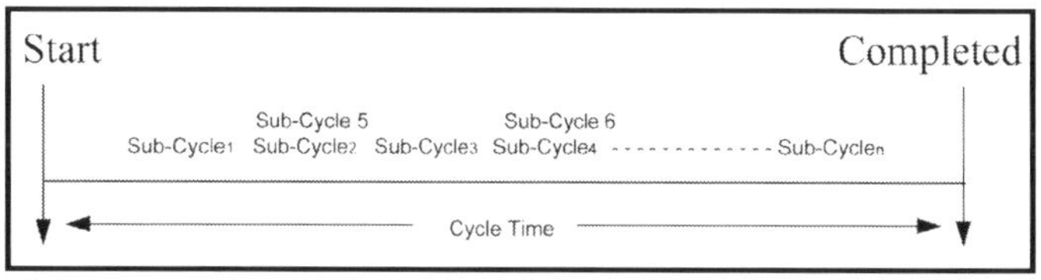

Figure 41.8 — Total Cycle Time is the sum of the cycle time of all process sub-elements.

2. **Concept Definition:** Further definition of requirements as part of the construction of a strategy to win the business. EHS input is necessary to ensure that internal EHS advantages are included and that all areas requiring additional EHS activities are identified.
3. **Design/Development:** Completion of detailed design along with validation of production readiness. EHS must insure that product safety issues have been addressed, and any required protective equipment has been included, and that necessary training has been identified. This phase is the most important from an accident prevention standpoint.
4. **Preproduction/Production:** Qualification of the process and production implementation. Once the actual manufacturing activity begins, a through EHS review is required to ensure that all hazards are as described during the development process, and that they have been adequately addressed. This phase also includes product life cycle maintenance through disposal.

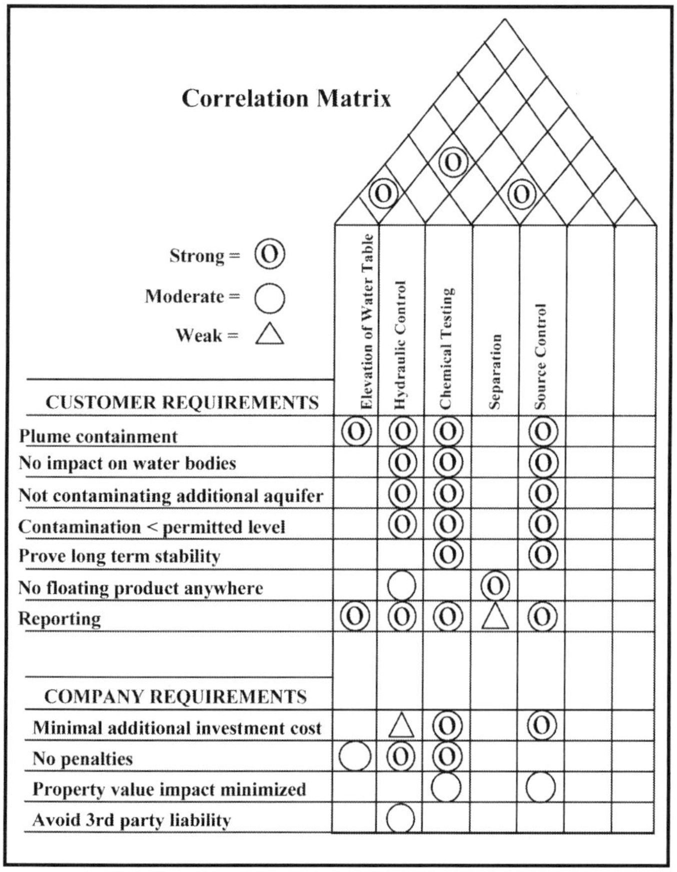

Figure 41.9 — Environmental Remediation House of Quality.

Quality Function Deployment

Quality Function Deployment (QFD) is a systematic means of ensuring that the demands of the customer are accurately translated into action within the supplier organization. The use of this tool must be carefully managed, since its output can be used in the development of operating and strategic plans. To effectively use QFD, substantial information on customer requirements is necessary. From the customer data, product and process requirements can be developed, including appropriate performance measurement tools.

A useful tool in correlating customer needs with process design requirements is known as "The House of Quality." As is seen in Figure 41.9, this matrix evaluates the "whats" of customer needs in terms of the "hows" or capabilities of the operation. This structure helps identify what priorities exist, based on the level of correlation between the hows and the whats.

This "House of Quality" correlates customer and company requirements against possible approaches. In this example, these requirements are the "whats", or what the company wants to accomplish. They are correlated in the body of the house with potential remedial approaches, the "hows", or specific actions which could be taken. For example, in the preceding figure, plume containment is strongly correlated with hydraulic control. The triangular correlation matrix, or roof, represents the correlation between each of the "hows." In this example, elevation of the water table is strongly correlated with hydraulic control. Such a tool can assist the user to quickly determine what actions will most satisfy the customer. In an occupational hygiene context, this approach might be used to evaluate regulatory and aesthetic requirements prior to an asbestos removal project.

Benchmarking

A benchmark is a standard of excellence or achievement against which other similar processes can be measured or judged. Use of benchmarks allows an occupational hygienist to compare their program to other world-class, operations to determine where areas of potential improvement exist. Benchmark facilities can also be used as a source of program ideas and for obtaining program examples to avoid reinventing what others have already accomplished. Environmental health and safety is typically treated as a noncompetitive area, and most companies will freely share or trade their programs.

Benchmarking is not simply a matter of comparing internal processes to the benchmark partners. It involves evaluating another organization to select those methodologies which provide a level of performance worth emulating. Selecting appropriate organizations to benchmark requires thought and consideration of the specific objectives of the project at hand. Rarely does a benchmark begin without a detailed plan of what will be evaluated and the anticipated results.

Most world-class organizations have only a few areas where they are truly exceptional. It is these areas where benchmarking efforts should be focused. It is also important to not limit yourself to only peer organizations. For example, even light manufacturing operations can often gain substantial useful information by benchmarking a major chemical manufacturer's chemical handling procedures.

Benchmarking is most effective when carried out by the employees who are responsible for the benchmarked activity within their own operation. Participation by the affected employees and departments ensures their support when changes are required. Once the team sees what could be accomplished its members will be more willing to accept challenging performance targets.

10 Step Model for Benchmarking

(adapted from Xerox model)

1. *Identify Benchmarking Subject* — Select an area of substantial impact to the organization where improvement would have real meaning to customer satisfaction.
2. *Identify Benchmarking Partners* — Look for the most productive examples for the issue in question. Do not restrict selections to your own industry.
3. *Determine Data Collection Method and Collect Data* — Develop a formal process and follow it.
4. *Determine Current Performance Gap* — Look for differences between the processes used by the benchmark partner and your own.
5. *Project Future Performance* — Evaluate the future impact of the integration of identified improvements.
6. *Communicate Findings and Gain Agreement* — Present results and analysis of improvements which could be adopted.
7. *Establish Functional Goals* — Develop specific goals to meet selected improvements.
8. *Develop Action Plan* — Establish a plan with measurable milestones and identified leaders to meet selected goals.
9. *Implement Plans and Monitor Progress* — Conduct periodic progress evaluations.
10. *Recalibrate Benchmark* — Determine if completed actions meet expectations, and look for further opportunities for improvement. This step may include a new round of benchmarking.

Resource Management

Every EHS program must support its organization's financial, as well as operational, goals. In order to evaluate performance against financial goals, all EHS-related costs must first be identified. For those costs directly associated with the function of the EHS department, a separate budget should be established which accounts for all anticipated expenditures required to manage the program. All costs to other departments should be determined and communicated prior to budgets being prepared. While it is common for unexpected costs to arise in EHS funds must be budgeted for known activities. Too often, EHS items will be left off initial budgets on the theory that they will have to be addressed anyway and the funds will be found somewhere. Omitting EHS items from the budgeting process is a classic example of a lack of control in company EHS management.

Many companies assign EHS costs to overhead and do not associate them with particular processes or products. This method assures that the costs are identified but does not encourage accountability from those areas generating the costs. As an example, suppose an operation has a goal to reduce the amount of solvent waste generated in its manufacturing process. There is little incentive for local supervision to meet that goal if all waste disposal costs are paid out of the EHS department. Where they are required to budget for their own waste costs departments will pay better attention to how they manage their wastes.

Cost Accounting

In an effort to address this issue, several organizations use *Activity-Based Costing* (ABC), to identify and allocate costs based on measurable activities.(16) ABC can be conducted on any aspect of the EHS program, and begins by identifying all costs associated with that portion of the program. There are two elements of ABC, activity analysis and cost object analysis. Activity analysis for all of EHS would be difficult, given its broad scope. For occupational hygiene the following are some examples of activities which should be included in this process:

- Sampling — planning, setup, on-site work, employee training, results review and presentation to employees.
- Regulatory — interaction with agencies, review of publications, communication to management and employees and any fines associated with noncompliance
- Chemical Issues — Material Safety Data Sheet review, evaluation of alternative products and processes, employee training and communication with customers and suppliers

Four types of resources are potentially expended on each identified activity: payroll costs, operating costs, capital expenditures and current and future liability costs.(16) The next phase of ABC extracts the costs in each resource area for each activity. The first three are relatively easy to identify, future liability costs are however difficult to quantify and can only be an estimate developed by experts in the given area.

Cost object analysis focuses on the activities required by products. For example if a product requires the use of a toxic solvent in its production, costs for monitoring and control might be assigned on a per product basis. This is an example of unit based activity. Other types of events that drive activities are batch-based, product-sustaining and facility-sustaining. Each case identifies specific required activities and the resources they consume. In this way the costs are distributed where they are actually used.

ABC provides a tool to identify what drives activities requiring corporate resources, and where those resources are used. Given this information, a management program could be developed to eliminate or reduce non-value-added activities. The distribution of costs also places accountability where it belongs, with the processes and departments which require the expenditure of resources. These departments are also much more able to manage and potentially reduce these costs since they control the processes involved.

Policy Deployment

Every EHS program has many policies and procedures designed to ensure that the organization understands the requirements which apply to the operations. These policies must be deployed to all affected employees, in a manner which ensures that they understand and accept their responsibilities.

The basic principles of *policy deployment* require a company to develop policies, including improvement targets, and deploy them throughout the organization. This deployment is performed in a manner which permits the operating organizations to establish supporting goals and targets, along with a method to measure performance. In the policy deployment process senior management evaluates the organizations' performance in a given area, and develops policies designed to correct any deficiencies. This policy moves through the organization, gaining supporting actions and associated measurements. The results of these measurements are fed back to senior management and the process begins anew. An important aspect of this process is continuing two-way communications at all levels of the deployment process, to evaluate lower level plans and the continuing utility of the original policies. The two-way communications required by this process is often referred to as *catchball*.

This same process is appropriate to deployment of EHS policies. The principle difficulty in ensuring that all appropriate individuals are aware of, and are following, EHS policies is the lack of feedback on how the process is working. If, when a policy is created, time is taken to work with the affected locations and functions to ensure their understanding, and to agree on appropriate measurement and reporting frequencies, there will be little doubt whether or not the process is working. For example, if the

EHS department determines that a policy to eliminate the use of all known human carcinogens from the process is appropriate, it would first develop a clear policy, working with the affected functions in its development. Affected individuals would then receive training in the application of the policy. Their adherence to the policy might then be measured by first requiring an inventory of all human carcinogens and specific action plans for their elimination developed. Performance against these plans could be measured on a monthly basis, with percent reductions displayed on bar charts for ease of understanding.

Policy Management

Policies cannot be static constructs. As organizations change their policies must also evolve. For example in a fledgling program policies focused on compliance and basic safety will be established. As time passes and a system of controls is established the policies will likely evolve into more management system focused documents.

Policies should be reviewed at least on an annual basis and adjusted for changing regulations and manufacturing processes. Each significant change should be reviewed and approved by senior leaders. Leadership participation and endorsement of the process is critical to its success.

Under a management system effective document control includes procedures to;

- Identify all ESH policies and procedures that must be used worldwide and establish procedures to control both electronic and hard copy versions of them, including historical revisions and revision numbering.
- Develop and keep up-to-date a distribution list for all policies and procedures.
- Establish procedures to notify affected parties of changes to the documents.
- Ensure that all documents are legible, dated (including dates of revision) and readily identifiable.
- Periodically review, and revise as appropriate, all ESH policies and procedures.
- Ensure that current versions of ESH policies and procedures are available to all involved in the ESH program.
- Ensure that obsolete documents are promptly removed from all points of use

Goal Setting

Most statistical measures of performance or metrics in EHS have zero as their ultimate goal. Depending on how the metrics for hazardous waste, employee exposures, accidents and the like are constructed, they generally improve as they decrease. The issue of goal setting arises in the time period between the identification of an area of concern and its elimination. Unless the concern can be eliminated in a short period of time, interim goals or *milestones* will be required to evaluate the success of the program. Beating or achieving the goal on an ongoing basis is an indication that the process is functioning acceptably, assuming the goal was properly chosen in the first place. It is important to remember that *what gets measured gets managed*. If the measurement criteria is not properly aligned with the goal, employees may find methods to meet the goal without addressing the problem. For example, if emergency response time has been a problem, a location might choose "average minutes to respond" as one of their metrics. If EHS starts sending inadequately trained personnel to the emergency because they are more available they will have reduced response time, but not addressed the root cause issue.

In establishing functional goals, it is important to keep some basic principles in mind. First limit the number of goals to those which are manageable, given the available resources, unless the consequences of such a limitation are unacceptable. If, for example, ten situations presenting an immediate threat to employees are uncovered the organization cannot choose to address only eight because the full project is not included in the budget. In most circumstances, however, a few appropriate goals which can be achieved are better than dozens of goals which scatter resources and make it unlikely that any will be satisfactorily achieved.

Second, goals should be aligned with the organization's long term plans. As is discussed earlier in this chapter, functional goals should flow from a company's strategic and operating plans. For example, if the organization has an aggressive acquisition strategy, the EHS department might have a goal to develop and implement a comprehensive due diligence policy and procedure.

Finally, at least some of the organization's goals should be very ambitious. As Champy stated in his book *Reengineering Management*, What companies actually require to thrive is rarely anything so "reasonable" and "realistic' as a 10 percent improvement in some performance measure or other. What we actually require is more often something like a 50 percent improvement or a 75 percent improvement."[8] Setting challenging goals encourages the organization to use its resources to their maximum potential. There is a risk, however, that, if unreasonable goals are established employees may become discouraged at continued failure, and operate at less that their best if they feel that even their best is not sufficient.

Negotiation Skills

EHS management has sometimes been called making seemingly unpleasant options palatable or even preferable. While many of the programs developed to protect health and environment have obvious positive result, often these results are the avoidance of a problem making identification of a specific contribution to a company's bottom line difficult. While these efforts may have a real effect on profitability it is often difficult to convince management to commit what may be considerable initial resources to projects with long term benefits. Unfortunately business works on an ever decreasing time horizon. What was once an inadequate two year planning cycle has continued to erode to the point where many operations focus on quarter by quarter, if not month by month, results. This can present a substantial obstacle to the occupational hygienist proposing a program to avoid chronic effects which might not appear for ten to twenty years. The fact that such programs are usually initiated is the result of successful negotiations.

Negotiation skills are an essential tool for the EHS professional. The skills required are generally the same as required by any salesperson. A set of eight appropriate points for selling your point of view are described by Chester Karass in his book *Give and Take*.[17]

1. *Talk less and listen more.* One key point in negotiations is to ensure that there is not already initial agreement. Too often, difficult negotiations end when the parties involved realize they had just misunderstood each others position.
2. *Don't interrupt.* Interruptions block communications and can irritate the other party.
3. *Don't be belligerent.* Raising the level of hostility in a negotiation is rarely a good tactic. Despite the success that may occur by forcing a decision through intimidation, it is usually short-lived. In most cases EHS negotiations will occur among people with long term relationships, that are likely to involve a series of such events. If a negotiation ends in a confrontation, the result is likely to adversely affect all future discussions.
4. *Don't be in a hurry to bring up your points.* If you listen to the other side's points, you may find many areas of common ground upon which to build a final agreement.
5. *Restate the other party's position and objectives as you understand them.* Many experts in communications suggest that practicing reflective listening, where you summarize and repeat the position of the other party, can aid in clear communications. Knowing that you will have to repeat the other parties position will also force you to listen better.
6. *Identify the key point and stick to it.* By focusing the discussion each element of the proposal can be evaluated. If there are several options involved in the proposal make it clear what can be modified an what must be implemented exactly as proposed.
7. *Don't digress from the key point and keep the other party from digressing.* There are three ways to avoid digression: agree to some non-essential point, agree to discuss it later or identify the intrusion as being somewhat off the point.
8. *Be "for" a point of view, not "against".* Accentuating the benefits of a proposal rather than deriding others viewpoints is usually the best tactic. While an opinion is often required make it clear that you respect the other parties efforts and viewpoint. There is rarely gratuitous opposition; the other side has a reason for its position.

Negotiations will not always succeed and when they do not the importance of the proposal must be evaluated in deciding what to do next. If the issue does not require immediate action to prevent irreparable harm a decision to delay or cancel the project can be accepted. In this case the proposal might be reevaluated and presented in a modified form at a later date when more data becomes available or conditions change. If, however, it appears there is an imminent danger or other ethically unacceptable concern, further action must be taken. This action must be prompt and could consist of gathering more data and re-presenting the proposal, elevation of the issue to a higher level in the organization, or involving external assistance. Each of these options are progressively more difficult and potentially costly to the professional. When taking these more drastic steps, facts must be checked and rechecked, and evaluation of the issue by another professional is appropriate.

Each of the EHS professions has its own code of ethics. The American Board of Industrial Hygiene (ABIH) has developed an enforceable Code of Ethics for all ABIH-certified professionals. The American Industrial Hygiene Association (AIHA®), AIHA's Academy of Industrial Hygiene (AIH), and ACGIH® have created a set of principles that complement the enforceable Code of Ethics. Chapter 2 Ethics, contains thorough discussion of professional ethics and its role in the practice of industrial hygiene.

Such codes leave little room to feel that one's duty has been discharged by simply notifying management or the client of a serious problem. Technical professionals must ensure that proper action is taken to correct situations of potential serious harm. In most cases those potentially affected will be unaware of the risk they face without such action.

Team Dynamics

The era of functional areas acting independently in an organization has passed. There is recognition that in order to work efficiently all parts of an organization must work together. Where formality is appropriate, this is often accomplished through the use of teams. Teamwork requires shared responsibility and accountability. Each participant of the team comes to rely on the other members to help insure the team's success. There is diminished emphasis on individual contributions, developed and presented in isolation.

Team members are selected based on their expertise and their potential contribution to solving the problem at hand. Each member's contribution is critical to team success and there must be a commitment on the part of the individual and management to seeing the process to completion. If a team is to be successful, all members must feel empowered to participate on an equal level with all other members, without regard to their rank outside of the team. Team dynamics will determine the success or failure of the team, as all products should be developed by consensus. The most useful decisions are developed by exploring all views and options and then reaching agreement.

An essay from Zenger Miller Incorporated[10] describes the required attributes of a successful team:

- A clear, articulated vision and sense of mission
- Strong, visible support from senior management
- Long-term, organization-wide commitment
- Sharing of information
- The transfer of real authority and decision-making power
- Skills training to support the assumption of new duties and new ways of interacting
- Continued coaching of teams and feedback from team leaders
- Systems that support teams

With the evolution of the work place from a top-down-directed structure to one where responsibility is distributed teams have become essential. Teams can only succeed when they clearly understand the boundaries of their authority and responsibility. This information can best be conveyed when the team is established. Senior management should work with the team to ensure that the limits the team faces and its mission are clearly understood. At this same time, training should be provided to the team members, and particularly the team leaders to prepare them for the interaction they can expect as members of a team.

References

1. **Burnes, B.:** *Managing Change*, 4th edition. Harlow, England: Pearson Education Limited, 2004.
2. **McGregor, J.:** There is No More Normal. Business Week Special Issue: Managing Smarter, Issue 4124:30–34 (2009).
3. **Peter, T.:** *Thriving on Chaos; Handbook for a Management Revolution.* New York: Alfred A. Knopf, Inc., 1988.
4. **Lorange, P.:** *Strategic Planning and Control: Issues in the Strategy Process.* Oxford, U.K.: Blackwell Publishers, 1993.
5. **Bellman, G.M.:** *Getting Things Done When You are Not in Charge: How to Succeed from a Support Position.* San Francisco, CA: Berrett-Koehler Publishers, Inc., 1992.
6. **Mackay, H.:** *Beware of the Naked Man Who Offers You his Shirt.* New York: William Morrow and Company, 1990.
7. **McGregor, D.:** *The Human Side of the Enterprise.* New York: McGraw-Hill Book Company, 1960.
8. **Champy, J.:** *Reengineering management: The Mandate for New Leadership.* New York: HarperCollins, 1995.
9. **Senge, P.M.:** *The Fifth Discipline: The Art and Practice of the Learning Organization.* New York: Doubleday Currency, 1990.
10. **Berrey, C., A. Klausner, and D. Russ-Eft:** "Highly Competitive Teams: The Key to Competitive Advantage", Essay, San Jose, CA: Zenger Miller, 1993.
11. **Forum Corporation:** *Individual Leadership.* Chicago, IL: Forum Corporation, 1995.
12. **American Industrial Hygiene Association® (AIHA®):** *ANSI/AIHA® Z10-2005 Occupational Health and Safety Management Systems.* Fairfax, VA: AIHA®, 2005.
13. **Bird, F.E.:** *Loss Control Leadership,* Loganville, GA.: International Loss Control Institute, Inc., 1985.
14. **Womack, J.:** *Lean Thinking: Banish Waste and Create Wealth in Your Corporation.* London, England: Simon and Schuster, 2003.
15. **U.S. Environmental Protection Agency (EPA):** *The Lean and Environmental Toolkit.* EPA-100-K-06-003. Washington, D.C.:, EPA, October 2007.
16. **Heller, M.:** Pay Attention Now or Pay Dollars Later. *Logistics Spectrum 30(2)*:7–13 (1996).
17. **Karrass, C.L.:** *Give and Take: The Complete Guide to Negotiating Strategies and Tactics.* New York: Thomas Y. Crowel Co., 1974.

Appendix A. Example Corporate EHS Policy

POLICY

The health and safety of our employees is a primary consideration in all Company operating decisions. The success of the Company Environmental Health and Safety Program is directly related to the level of management support it receives. Therefore, it is the firm and continuing policy of Company to:

- Conduct all operations in a manner which complies with applicable laws designed to ensure the protection of our employees, facilities, local community, and the environment.
- Hold management responsible for the compliance of their operations with applicable laws and requirements concerning the workplace health and safety of employees.

RESPONSIBILITIES

The President and Chief Executive Officer shall be responsible for:

1. Ensuring that each Unit is aware of its responsibilities under this program.
2. Including Environmental Health and Safety Program compliance in Unit performance reviews.
3. Approving Company Environmental Health and Safety policies.
4. Ensuring that sufficient funds are provided to allow proper operation of this program.

The Unit General Manager or a delegate shall be responsible for:

1. Including Environmental Health and Safety considerations in operating decisions and performance reviews.
2. Selecting a qualified Environmental Health and Safety Program Coordinator who has an appropriate background to implement and manage an effective EHS program.
3. Allocating sufficient resources to maintain an effective program.
4. Approving Unit Environmental Health and Safety policies.
5. Notifying the Company Director, Environmental Health and Safety during the same business day of an incident that involves a fatality or environmental, safety or health circumstance likely to subject the Company to adverse consequences.

The Company Director, Environmental Health and Safety shall be responsible for:

1. Guiding management in the establishment of a sound Environmental Health and Safety Program and for coordinating efforts in achieving stated EHS goals.
2. Visiting Company facilities to review Environmental Health and Safety performance.
3. Advising Company management of the compliance status and occurrences relating to the Environmental Health and Safety Program.
4. Providing consulting services to Company Units.
5. Receiving and reviewing Unit inputs and providing executive summaries for Company management.
6. Preparing and maintaining Company Environmental Health and Safety policies and reporting forms.
7. Administering ongoing EHS programs.
8. Reviewing facility lease, acquisition or divestiture plans and other capital requests to ensure that EHS issues have been properly considered.

Appendix B

EHS Resources Analysis Worksheet Instructions

Section 1: Task Details

1. In column 2 (Estimated Annual Workdays) indicate the estimated total number of annual workdays required to complete the task indicated in column 1. Use blanks in column 1 to describe tasks unique to your location or otherwise not listed on the form.
2. In column 3 (Cost excluding personnel) indicate the estimated cost of meeting the requirements of the task indicated in column 1.
   NOTE: Where data is available it should be used to make these estimates as accurate as possible. However, it is important to recognize that this process will only provide an estimate of a locations required resources. The results of this exercise should be used as a data point in discussions of needed resources.
3. Sum each column as indicated and transfer the data to the EHS Annual Workdays Estimate sheet. (NOTE: This transfer and subsequent calculations will be performed automatically when using the computer spreadsheet)

Section 2: EHS Annual Workdays Estimate

4. The summation data from each section should be entered in the appropriate 75% block.
5. The 75% data is then extrapolated to 100% using the following formula:

$$\frac{\text{75\% Sum}}{3} \times 4 = \text{100\% Estimate}$$

example:

$$\frac{\text{210 Safety days}}{3} \times 4 = \text{280 days at 100\%}$$

NOTE: This assumes that only 75% of an individual's time can be identified with specific tasks.

6. These days are then converted to individual employees using the following formula:

100% days = Number of required
250 full time equivalents

Example:
280 Days = 1.12 Full time safety
250 equivalents

Full time equivalent = Personnel resources equal to a full time employee

Section 3: Level Analysis

7. Complete the questionnaire by placing the indicated weighting score (column 2) in each box in column 3 (Score) which applies to your facility.
8. Determine the minimum level of personnel at your location requires by summing the Score column and comparing your Unit total to the following ranges.

Total Score	Qualification Level
0–3	Locally Developed EHS Coordinator
4–6	Technician Level
7 or greater	Professional Level

NOTE : Qualification Level indicates the minimum level for at least one of the site EHS personnel.

EHS Skill Competencies Required to Meet Corporate Commitment

Professional Level Skill Set (required by Units with Significant EHS Exposure)	1. Knowledgeable of all Federal, State and local regulations. 2. Knowledgeable of all corporate Policies, and requirements. 3. Able to function as a creditable resource to comment on pending legislation, as well as, an advisor within appropriate industry groups. 4. Familiar with up-coming trends in environmental. Legislation. 5. Knowledgeable of the various solutions to complex environmental problems. 6. Able to direct company policy to establish leading edge programs. 7. Key member of company's Senior management team. 8. Able to work effectively with line managers and plan employees at all levels. 9. Professional degree or equivalent experience required.
Technician Level Skill Set (required by Units with Moderate EHS Exposure)	1. Active role in the EHS management of a particular company. 2. Primary responsibility is EHS (little shared responsibility). 3. Strong commitment to corporate EHS program. 4. Able to work with line managers and plant employees. 5. Working knowledge of Fed, State, and local regulations and technical requirements. 6. Technician level degree or equivalent experience required.
Locally Developed EHS Coordinator (required by Units with Minimal EHS Exposure)	1. Familiar with corporate environmental and audit protocols. 2. May be shared responsibility with EHS and other disciplines outside of the environmental field. 3. Committed to corporate EHS program. 4. Able to work with line managers and plant employees. 5. Familiar with applicable regulatory requirements for a localized business.

TASK DETAILS WORKSHEET

GENERAL EHS	*Estimated Annual Workdays*	*Cost (excluding personnel)*
REPORTS		
EHS Self Evaluation		
Company Headquarters		
Metrics		
Other		
INSPECTIONS		
Qualitative Audit Program		
Consultant		
Company Staff		
Insurance		
Program		
State/Local		
Subcontractor/Vendor		
Other		
TRAINING/MEETING		
Coordinator Education		
Emergency Response		
Hazard Communications		
Supervisory		
Corporate		
Trade/Professional Associations		
Other		
PROGRAMS		
Department Meetings		
Management Presentations		
Procedure/Process Review		
Contract/Proposal Input		
Community/Regulator Relations		
Integrated Product Development		
Industry/Professional Groups		
Budgeting		
Due Diligence		
Other		
TOTAL GENERAL EHS	**0**	**0**

TASK DETAILS WORKSHEET

OCCUPATIONAL HYGIENE	*Estimated Annual Workdays*	*Cost (excluding personnel)*
REPORT		
Chemical Inventory		
Regulatory		
Other		
INSPECTIONS		
Regulatory		
Other		
TRAINING		
Hearing Conservation		
Respirator		
Indoor Air Quality		
Other		
PROGRAMS		
Asbestos		
Labeling		
Lasers		
MSDS Review/Management		
Radiation		
Ventilation		
Other		
MONITORING		
Atmospheric		
Noise		
Radiation		
Other		
TOTAL OCCUPATIONAL HYGIENE	**0**	**0**

TASK DETAILS WORKSHEET

ENVIRONMENTAL	*Estimated Annual Workdays*	*Cost (excluding personnel)*
REPORTS		
Waste Water Discharge		
Hazardous Waste Generator		
Hazardous Waste Manifests		
Emissions (i.e. SARA)		
Chemical Management (i.e. TSCA)		
PERMITTING/AUTHORIZATIONS		
Air		
Polychlorinated Biphenyls (PCBs)		
Sewer		
Hazardous Solid Waste		
Nonhazardous Solid Waste		
Storage Vessels (i.e. tanks)		
Groundwater\Surface Water		
Other		
INSPECTIONS		
Regulatory Agencies		
Subcontractor		
Waste Disposal Facilities		
Other		
TRAINING		
Waste Management/Handling		
Spill Prevention		
Chemical handling		
Waste Minimization		
Other		
PROGRAMS		
Remediation		
Hazardous/Special Waste Disposal		
Medical Waste Disposal		
Other		
MONITORING		
Air		
Water		
TOTAL ENVIRONMENTAL	0	0

TASK DETAILS WORKSHEET

SAFETY	*Estimated Annual Workdays*	*Cost (excluding personnel)*
REPORTS		
Accident		
Emergency Preparedness		
Loss Prevention/ Loss Control		
Liability		
Worker's Compensation		
Other		
INSPECTIONS		
Regulatory		
Fire Systems		
Departmental		
Other		
TRAINING		
Accident Investigation		
Job Safety Analysis		
Specific Operation		
Ergonomics		
Driver		
Fire Prevention		
Other		
PROGRAMS		
Department Meetings		
Purchase Review		
Safety Committees		
Product Safety		
Fire Prevention		
Other		
PERMITTING		
Building		
Hot Work		
Radiological		
Confined Space		
Other		
TOTAL SAFETY	**0**	**0**

TASK DETAILS WORKSHEET

MEDICAL	*Estimated Annual Workdays*	*Cost (excluding personnel)*
REPORTS		
Accident/Near Miss		
Records Management		
Absence Paperwork		
Worker's Compensation		
Other		
TRAINING		
Bloodborne Pathogens		
Medical Counseling		
Health Education		
Other		
PROGRAMS		
Consultations		
Examinations		
Emergencies		
Pre-\Post-placement Evaluation		
Other		
TOTAL MEDICAL	**0**	**0**
TOTAL EHS	**0**	**0**

NOTE
- Data is for scheduled activities which account for approximately 75% of the workload
- Data does not account for clerical assistance

EHS Annual Workdays Estimate

General EHS Workdays 75%	0
Extrapolated to 100%	0
Number of General EHS Employees	0
Safety Workdays 75%	0
Extrapolated to 100%	0
Number of Safety Employees	0
Occupational Hygiene 75%	0
Extrapolated to 100%	0
Number of IH Employees	0
Environmental 75%	0
Extrapolated to 100%	0
Number of Environmental Employees	0
Medical 75%	0
Extrapolated to 100%	0
Number of Medical Employees	0
Combined EHS 75%	0
Extrapolated to 100%	0
Number of EHS Employees	0
Current Staffing	
Full Time Equivalents Required	0

Level Analysis	Weighted Score	Score
Population		
less than 100 Employees	0	
100-300 employees	1	
300-500 employees	3	
500 or more employees	5	
Hazardous Chemical Use*		
Extremely Hazardous Substances	1	
Greater than 10,000 pounds per year	1	
Greater than 100,000 pounds per year	1	
Remedial Activities*		
Water	1	
Soil	1	
Processes*		
Plating	2	
Machine Shop	1	
Spray Coating	1	
Laser User	1	
Ionizing Radiation (x-ray, radioactive materials)	2	
Radiofrequency Sources	1	
Heavy Equipment Use	1	
Fleet Operations	1	
Construction	2	
Confined Spaces	1	
Cleaning Operations	1	
Other		
Human Factors*		
Ergonomic Issues	1	
Total Score		**0**

* = select all that apply

Outcome Competencies

After completing this chapter, the reader should be able to:

1. Differentiate occupational hygiene surveys from audits.
2. Differentiate between baseline and comprehensive surveys.
3. List the elements that comprise an occupational hygiene surveys and audits.
4. Know base competencies needed to conduct a survey or audit.
5. Participate on an occupational hygiene survey or audit team.

Prerequisite Knowledge

General occupational hygiene background.

Prior to beginning this chapter, the reader should review the following chapters:

Chapter Number	Chapter Topic
1	History of Industrial Hygiene
3	Legal Aspects of Industrial Hygiene
7	Principles of Evaluating Worker Exposure
8	Occupational and Environmental Health Risk Assessment / Risk Management
9	Comprehensive Exposure Assessment
41	Program Management

Key Terms

auditor competency • baseline survey • comprehensive survey • full-shift sampling • grab sampling • occupational hygiene audit • occupational hygiene survey • OHSMS audit • ISO 19001:2002

Key Topics

I. Occupational Hygiene Surveys
   A. Survey Types
   B. Survey Methods
   C. Survey Quality
   D. Survey Forms

II. Occupational Hygiene Audits
   A. Audit Philosophy
   B. Audit Scope
   C. Audit Types
   D. Preparing for an Audit
   E. The Audit Team
   F. Audit Logistics
   G. Audit Report
   H. Post-audit Actions
   I. Legal Concerns

III. Additional Reading

IV. Appendix A: Pre-Audit Questionnaire

Surveys and Audits

42

Charles F. Redinger, PhD, CIH and Nancy P. Orr, CIH, CSP

Conducting surveys and audits are central activities of occupational hygiene. These activities involve collecting information and data that is used to make decisions about worker safety and health. While similar in many ways, there is a difference between surveys and audits. Surveys deal with the characterization of hazards and risks whereas audits deal with the assessment of their control and management. Surveys can also be thought of as addressing nuts and bolts issues, whereas audits deal with larger programmatic and systematic issues. Surveys can be thought of as a necessary precursor to audits. For example, an occupational hygienist may conduct a noise survey to determine noise levels in an area, and then perform an audit of the overall noise program that is more comprehensive, including training and PPE considerations.

Activities associated with surveys date back to the origins of occupational hygiene. These activities include dust sampling, noise surveys, and exposure assessment. Auditing is newer with its use increasing in the 1970s, in the U.S. for example, with the formation of the Occupational Safety and Health Administration (OSHA) and increasing civil litigation dynamics. During the 1980s in the U.S., auditing frequently focused on evaluating a site's compliance with applicable health and safety regulatory requirements. With the advent of Occupational Health and Safety Management Systems (OHSMS) in the 1990s and 2000s, auditing practices developed in the quality assurance field began to be applied to occupational hygiene auditing.

Common issues of surveys and audits are: pre-visit preparation; surveyor or auditor competence; data quality (also referred to as precision/accuracy and reliability/validity); objectivity; field conduct; reporting methods; and finding follow-up and closure.

Occupational Hygiene Surveys

In a way, every field activity performed by occupational hygienists represents some form of a survey. An <u>occupational hygiene survey</u> is an activity carried out by a qualified individual to evaluate and measure various biological, chemical, ergonomic, and physical parameters in the workplace. The process involves collecting information about raw materials and process steps, observing work practices, evaluating engineering and other controls, and measuring various chemical, biologic or physical agents. Exposure assessments, whether qualitative or quantitative, represent a type of survey. The surveys result in an opinion or judgment concerning the extent of risk posed by the process or agent or the level of compliance with existing standards for acceptable exposure.

The goal of an occupational hygiene survey is to identify and prevent or control foreseeable workplace risks through a systematic evaluation process. Surveys should be conducted periodically to track known potential risks and also to detect new or missed ones. Within management system approaches, regular self-inspections, and preventive and corrective action activities are forms of a survey.

It is important to involve workers in surveys so that they can help ensure that all process steps are identified and understood by the occupational hygienist. Surveys also provide an excellent opportunity to communicate with workers about the nature and extent of workplace risks, the measures they can take to protect themselves, and the reasons for continued monitoring. These discussions can help the workers understand workplace risks and realize their own responsibilities in minimizing potential overexposures through proper work practices and use of personal protective equipment (PPE). The results of both quantitative and qualitative surveys should be shared with the impacted workforce.

Surveys are useful to detect not only outlying conditions, such as levels of contaminants that do not conform to regulatory standards or to internal facility requirements, but also to discover unsafe physical conditions or work practices that may adversely affect employee health and safety. Surveys may be done with a prescribed regularity and placed on a checklist or schedule as part of a routine monitoring program. They may also follow an irregular schedule and be conducted on an as-needed basis (e.g., new machine start-up, seldom-run operations, employee complaints, or one-time events, including spills). Though the initiating reasons may vary, the primary purpose of surveys – to evaluate and reduce risks – remains the same. Often this takes the form of a quantitative assessment with some instrumental device, ranging from a sampling pump with the appropriate sorbent collector to direct-reading instrumentation.

The importance of employing only qualified individuals to perform occupational hygiene surveys cannot be overemphasized, since the reduction of workplace risks can only be as effective as the experience and aptitude of the hygienist conducting the survey.

Before starting a survey, the hygienist should be clear on the survey goals and purpose. One should give consideration to how survey findings will be used and interpreted. For instance, are data going to be collected?

Survey Types

There are several types of occupational hygiene surveys, including baseline and comprehensive surveys. Surveys can be conducted as part of an accident investigation or during an emergency situation. They can also be initiated to resolve specific employee complaints or concerns, or in response to a regulatory agency site visit.

Baseline Survey

A baseline survey refers to the initial evaluation of a health and safety parameter that will be used as the basis for all future comparisons. A baseline survey may be the first evaluation of a process at start-up, or it may be the first recorded measurement of a long-standing process. The scope may focus on a single airborne contaminant or physical agent, or be expanded to include situations that have not been previously examined and documented. Baseline surveys may evaluate the following agents individually or in combination: hazardous dusts; chemical vapors and gases for which there are occupational exposure standards; physical hazards such as temperature extremes, noise, ionizing or non-ionizing radiation; vibration; lasers; and ergonomic exposures.

It is preferable to characterize a process or an operation at its inception to obtain an accurate understanding of the impact of a given activity; within an OHSMS framework, this initial characterization is required, it is not optional. However, if an initial assessment was not conducted at start-up, the first evaluation becomes the baseline for assessing the level of risk of potential exposure or injury. Also, the effectiveness of engineering or other controls to mitigate airborne contaminant or physical agent levels may be determined. From either a physical measurement or visual evaluation standpoint, the baseline survey represents the beginning or reference point against which future evaluations will be gauged.

The primary reason to conduct any type of survey must be worker protection through the assessment of the risk of injury or illness from working in a defined environment. When conducting surveys, the hygienist should think both in terms of identifying hazards and estimating associated risk. By considering the potential likelihood of adverse effect from the exposure and the severity of the outcome, the hygienist will be in a position to make the most effective recommendation to reduce subsequent risk to workers. In assessing the potential of injury and illness, the medical surveillance program may also need to be evaluated.

Another important reason to perform a survey is to determine the level of compliance with existing occupational hygiene and safety regulatory standards or internal facility standards. Surveys may also be conducted to ascertain standings compared with a particular national consensus standards. In the U.S., these may include the American National Standards Institute (ANSI), the American Society of Heating, Refrigerating and Air-Conditioning Engineers (AHSRAE), and the American Conference of Governmental Industrial Hygienists (ACGIH®).

Comprehensive Survey

A comprehensive survey is a multifaceted examination of all recognized health and safety hazards in a defined work environment to determine either regulatory compliance or conformance to internal or non-governmental standards. It encompasses a wall-to-wall evaluation of the health and safety factors that may place an employee at increased risk of developing an adverse effect from working in a specific setting. It is apt to include an evaluation of a wide range of chemical and physical agents as a result of a "walk around" inspection of the workplace for apparent and potential hazards. For example, a comprehensive occupational hygiene survey of a machine shop could include evaluation of the following issues or conducting the following sampling activities:

- noise levels;
- airborne oil mist levels;
- degreasing solvents used;
- metal fumes from welding operations;
- metal dusts from grinding operations;
- lighting levels;
- exhaust ventilation capture velocities at contaminant control points;
- presence of machine guarding and required clearances;
- shields to contain ultraviolet light from welding operations;
- secure storage of gas cylinders;
- separate storage areas for full and empty gas cylinders;
- job-required eye, respiratory, hearing, face, foot, skin, hand, and head protection;
- hazard labels on chemical containers;
- inventory of all hazardous chemical products and review material safety data sheets for these products;
- hand-washing and emergency shower facilities;
- general and emergency exits;
- labeled electrical panels;
- spill protection measures; and
- general housekeeping.

Survey Methods

With either baseline or comprehensive surveys, the measuring techniques used may determine the validity and applicability of the test results. Consideration needs to be given to the role that data collection will have in the application of survey findings. In some instances, qualitative assessments may suffice. In others, sampling may be needed to provide quantitative information. The occupational hygienist needs to understand the pros and cons of different sampling strategies.

Grab Sampling and Short Term Observation

Grab sampling employs a short measurement period for quantifying the level of airborne contaminant or physical agent present. It is often associated with a direct-reading instrument or colorimetric detector tube. While the grab sample approach takes the least time to conduct, it is difficult, if not impossible to characterize the full-shift exposure based solely on short-term sampling.

In like fashion, with qualitative assessments that involve observing work practices, consideration needs to be given to variations there may be between workers and shifts. It may be the case that different work practices take place on different shifts or with different workers.

Full-shift Sampling and Multiple Observations

Full-shift sampling collects survey information over the course of a full shift to determine the actual 8-hour time-weighted average exposure concentration. Attention must also be paid to quantifying potential exposures associated with extended shifts. Full-shift sampling is preferred for accurately characterizing potential exposures associated with an operation during baseline and on-going monitoring, as well as for documenting regulatory compliance. Even though regulatory agencies may have adopted short-term exposure limits (STELs) for many chemicals, compliance determinations for hundreds of agents are routinely based on personal sampling results that cover the entire work shift and provide an average of the fluctuations that normally occur during the shift.

With qualitative assessments that include use of observation of work practices, consideration should be given to conducting observations throughout a work shift. With facilities with multiple shifts, efforts should be taken to observe all shifts.

Survey Quality

The accuracy of occupational hygiene surveys depends on several factors, including:

- the use of proper equipment;
- calibration of the equipment before and after sampling;
- specifying the correct analytical method;
- comparing results to the proper standard;
- issuing appropriate recommendations to minimize employee exposures and risk; and
- accurate and complete record keeping of all pertinent survey information.

It is especially important to calibrate and operate equipment according to the manufacturer's instructions and to use only supplies and repair centers that are approved by the equipment maker to maintain operational validity. When sampling is conducted, it is useful to communicate with the analyzing laboratory beforehand to discuss sample handling and collection methods.

Another important aspect to recognize when conducting a survey is the variability inherent in contaminant levels in the workplace as well as workplace practices themselves. Whether conducting sampling to assess the extent of a chemical concentration in air, or to measure the level of a physical agent such as noise or heat, a reading or result represents what was present or happening at the time the sample was collected and may not represent what will happen the next hour, day or week. Variability is an inherent aspect of the measurement process that must be examined in light of random occurrences, process or operational fluctuations, and seasonal effects. The concept of statistical distributions, confidence intervals, and confidence levels can be seen as playing an important role in the quantification and assessment of worker exposures to the agents of interest. It is much more meaningful to state that the measured level is 14 ppm with a standard deviation of ± 0.7 at the 95% confidence level, than to simply indicate that the level is 14 ppm.

Survey Forms

Before beginning a planned survey, the method in which data and information will be captured needs to be considered. Uniform means of collecting data and information during surveys should be used. To increase the credibility and cohesiveness of a survey, the occupational hygienist needs to have clear field notes. Survey forms are one way to do this. Another is to use a bound field notebook.

Survey forms are quite useful as a type of checklist to ensure that various pieces of information are collected about the process steps, raw materials, worker activities, sampling parameters and workplace controls. The actual categories of information vary according to the kind of survey being conducted.

Occupational Hygiene Audits

An occupational hygiene audit is a multi-disciplinary, systematic process that uses objective evidence to evaluate the existence and the effectiveness of health and safety program elements and OHS management systems. An audit is a key tool in determining the adequacy of the practices, procedures, management systems and controls necessary to achieve an organization's internal and external goals. Audits provide opportunities to learn about deficiencies in existing programs and systems, and to engage workers in continual improvement activities.

Audits have traditionally been performed to determine regulatory compliance or in response to civil litigation concerns. They are also conducted to assess conformance with internal organizational standards, and standards developed by non-governmental bodies, such as the International Organization for Standardization (ISO) and the International Labour Office.

Determining conformance with international standards such as OHSAS 18001 or ISO 14001 are common audit activities.

The audit function is a sub-set of a larger activity called conformity assessment. A detailed discussion of conformity assessment schemes is beyond the scope of this book. These schemes are complex and address issues such as certification of management systems and lead auditors, as well as the accreditation of certifying bodies.

A key concept in auditing is the collection of objective evidence by competent personnel. There are typically three types of evidence used to make audit assessments: visual observations, interviews with workers and managers, and documentation. For a given issue, the extent that there is confluence between these three types of evidence, leads to strength in the findings. Defining auditor competency is not straight forward, with a range of views on how to define "competency." At a minimum, auditors should have technical expertise in the areas that they are auditing and should have training in auditing itself. The skill set needed to perform audits goes beyond the core quantitative training of occupational hygiene to include more qualitative survey research and communication skills.

An audit will usually determine if the facility has anticipated all the health and safety requirements and risks associated with its operation, has developed the workplace controls and procedures to address these requirements and risks, and whether these measures are adequate. The audit can also provide useful information as to whether the distribution and type of resources available at the site to deal with these health and safety requirements are sufficient and appropriate. In the end, the most valuable outcome from a well-executed audit should be a clear road map for the site to reach regulatory compliance or conformance with internal or management system standards.

Audit Philosophy

Successful audits require a significant amount of preparation and activity prior to conducting the actual audit. Pre-audit preparation starts with garnering support from senior management. It is important that an organization's leadership values the process, and recognizes the advantages of determining the status of key issues in advance of regulatory discovery or other system failures. It should be emphasized that an audit should not be undertaken without a strong commitment to correct identified inadequacies and to effectively resolve the issues raised during the course of the audit. Without this commitment, the audit will at best be a frustrating waste of resources or, even worse, evidence of noncompliance that regulators could use to demonstrate previous knowledge of uncorrected hazards. It could also lead to failure to obtain certification to an OHSMS such as ANSI/AIHA Z10-2005 or OHSAS 18001.

The whole purpose of an audit revolves around evaluating risk. This involves the risk assessment, risk management, and risk reduction processes, which, in turn, seek to protect workers and increase organizational effectiveness.

The audit process represents a systematic approach to the comprehensive examination of OHS programs or management system elements. At the conclusion of a successful audit, the organization should have a clear understanding of the performance gaps and regulatory deficiencies that exist and be able to develop a strategy to close these gaps. Once this list is compiled, the next phase involves following up on findings, with clear assignments of responsibility and dates for completion, and documentation of appropriate closure.

An audit can be a tremendous learning experience for personnel. When the audit team is comprised of members internal to the organization, it can also be an effective method of expanding their technical and leadership skills. An additional outcome of a well-structured audit can include a clear delineation of areas of responsibility, which results in an effective mechanism for covering the wide range of regulatory requirements. Actions to be taken at the conclusion of an audit can be aptly paraphrased using the *Five W's*: who, what, when, where, and why.

- What are we supposed to do?
- Why do we need to do it?
- When (or how often) do we need to do it?
- Who is responsible for doing it and what is the expected timeframe for completion?

An audit can also be an opportunity for management to appreciate the multitude of OHS regulations and the resources needed to comply with them. An audit should not be viewed as a one-time event. Rather, it should be thought of as a program unto itself just as noise sampling is conducted within an overall hearing conservation program. Auditing of program or system elements should be repeated at some defined interval to ensure continual improvement. It is common for audit intervals to range between one to three years. A typical strategy is to audit one-third of all programs or the overall management system each year, so that all program and system elements are assessed every three years.

No audit is capable of detecting all of the deficiencies within the wide spectrum of occupational hygiene. Therefore, different approaches may be undertaken to systematically review the program to ensure that the continually expanding arena of applicable health and safety issues is addressed. One such approach is to focus on a few major compliance issues at a time, perhaps those recognized as posing the most risk. The choice of areas to examine in the first round of visits will be determined in large part by the business nature and complexity of the site. However, after a few audit rounds have been completed, many major risk areas will have been systematically identified and addressed. An audit should be thought of more as a financial investment, or as insurance, rather than as an expenditure with no benefits. Then, it will be considered as one forward step in a series of efforts toward continual quality improvement. Just as audits are conducted to ensure quality issues are addressed within an organization for the purposes of customer satisfaction, so should EHS audits be considered a business function to ensure excellent health and safety performance. In addition, implementing corrective actions identified in a comprehensive audit can reduce potential reputational risks and increase stakeholder value in an organization.

Audit Scope

It is important to be clear on the audit scope prior to initiating the audit. The scope of an audit may be limited to one regulatory area, a series of regulatory areas, or a more comprehensive review of all regulations that apply, or of all systems. In addition, the scope may be expanded to address various non-regulatory consensus standards, as well as internal corporate requirements or, when no other measure exists, practices that are recognized as "best industry practices." Another consideration is the physical boundary or functional area(s) of the audit. Is just one location covered? Or are there multiple locations, such as warehouses and other ancillary operations covered? An evolving area of audit scope deals with telecommuting and home offices. This is an example of the subtle nuances that should be considered when establishing audit scope. In any case, the scope of the audit must be clear to the team and the organization prior to the start of on-site activities.

Due to the large number and complexity of regulations that may apply to a site, a comprehensive regulatory audit may not be feasible. Ranking approaches may be used to focus the audit scope on the issues that represent the greatest risk. These factors may include the size of the site, the nature of its operations, the length of time since its last audit, the number of regulatory programs to which it is subject, the jurisdiction in which it is located, and recent modifications to its processes. If there are limited resources, audit activities may need to be directed to the issues with the highest risk or the programs that can best reflect the site's overall OHS performance.

A related topic to audit philosophy and scope relates to whether an audit is either a quantitative audit or ISO-based audit. Quantitative audits use detailed scoring schemes to summarize audit findings. In quantitative approaches, there is rarely a "show-stopper" function were one major fault, deficiencies, or finding can lead to overall audit failure. This is opposed to the ISO-audit philosophy where a major non-conformance finding can lead to certification failure. In either case, quantitative or ISO-based, consideration needs to be given to how audit findings will be used and to ensure that the proper type of auditing method is selected to meet an organization's needs.

Audit Types

There are two dimensions upon which audit types can be characterized. The first dimension deals with who performs the audit.

There are typically three types of audits on this dimension: first-, second-, and third-party audits. The second dimension deals with what is being audited. There are also typically three types of audits on this dimension: compliance to regulations; conformance to a management system; or conformance to non-governmental standards or guidelines to which the organization subscribes. There are also hybrid models where audit teams contain both external and internal auditors, and where compliance and management system audits are conducted at the same time.

First Party — Internal Audits

First-party audits refer to audits that are conducted internally within an organization by members of the organization. Many companies have robust internal audit programs that assess both regulatory compliance and conformance with non-governmental standards or management systems.

Internal audits should be conducted by personnel who are technically competent, have audit training, and are capable of making unbiased and independent assessments. Internal auditors should not have direct responsibility for activities at the site being audited. This is essential in order to maintain audit integrity and independence. An internal audit will generally assemble several individuals who are experienced within their respective disciplines and who may even know the facility and its operations. The audit team should be sufficiently large and broad to adequately address all the anticipated issues. When working with teams drawn from internal sources only, this can sometimes be difficult to achieve. Every audit also requires deft team leadership and communication, skills that may be difficult for an internal person to obtain or keep current if they do not audit on a regular basis. Lead auditors should have training in leading audits. Governmental bodies and for-profit organizations are a source for compliance and management system auditing training.

There are distinct advantages to the organization for using an internal audit team. The out-of-pocket costs associated with an internal program can be lower than an external program, though the time commitment internal auditors must make to the program does have a significant impact for the organization. Participating on audits provides an excellent way to upgrade regulatory knowledge, and technical and leadership skills. Robust audit programs allow for the development and sharing of best practices amongst sites. Once auditors have completed their work, they return to their respective sites and, hopefully, implement best practices or program improvements they have recently seen on an audit. However, unless the organization empowers the internal auditing function with the authority to clearly identify all issues, and sets the expectation that senior management will respond to these issues, some internal programs may lack the impact of an externally-run program.

Second- and Third-Party External Audits

These audits are conducted by personnel who are not members of the organization that is being audited. In the case of second-party audits, within a supply-chain, a customer performs an audit of a supplier. Second-party audits are common in the quality management circles (e.g. ISO 9001), but are not as common in the occupational hygiene area. Third-party audits refer to audits performed by people independent of the organization being audited. These are typically performed by consultants, and in the management system arena, by what are called, third-party-registrars. Third-party audits are common in the management system arena.

There are several advantages to using external auditors. First, because the audit will be based on a consulting contract, it should provide access to highly qualified individuals best suited to evaluate the site and its unique operations. Secondly, there should be fewer time and resource issues that plague internal audit programs because auditors are not being pulled off an already full work schedule. Finally, a report from an unbiased outside firm has the advantage of being perceived as presenting the true picture as it lacks any local biases.

Organized labor concerns about external auditors, if any, need to be addressed. A concern that can surface is the potential bias that external auditors may have to not report bad findings for fear of losing future work with the organization. This concern can be addressed by using credible third-party auditors who hold themselves to a high level of ethical conduct.

Compliance Audits

Compliance audits are performed to determine compliance with governmental regulations. These are typically very technical and detailed; they often use quantitative scoring schemes. Auditors need to have an excellent understanding of the regulations that the site is being audited against. The use of checklists are often helpful when performing compliance audits.

These types of audits involve issues for which many occupational hygienists have a good understanding and knowledge. On comprehensive compliance audits an extremely broad range of regulations may apply and an auditor may need to become familiar with new requirements prior to the initiation of the audit.

Management System Audits

Management system auditing has evolved since the late 1990s with the issuance of ISO 9001, ISO 14001, and a range of OHS management systems. These audits are more qualitative than traditional compliance audits. It is important that personnel performing management system audits have training in this type of auditing since it requires an expanded skill-set from compliance auditing. For example, there is greater emphasis on conducting interviews and interpretation of documents that require the auditor to make assessments and judgments that go beyond simply following a checklist.

At the time of this book's publication, the primary OHS management system standards in use were OHSAS 18001:2005, ANSI Z10:2005, and the ILO OHSMS:2001. These standards are periodically updated, so it is important that auditors understand which version of a particular management system standard is being used by a site. It is common for sites to have an integrated management system that includes both OHS and environmental management elements. When defining the audit scope, it is important to understand if a stand-alone OHSMS or an integrated EHSMS is being audited.

Hybrid Approaches

Audit programs in some organizations use hybrid audit teams that include both internal-company representatives and external consultants. This approach yields benefits with deep organizational understanding from the internal team members and auditing and external expertise from the consultant. An increasing trend has also been to combine compliance and management system audit functions, thus auditing both at the same time. Caution should be taken to ensure that neither is diluted when combined.

Preparing for an Audit

Thorough preparation before the audit will lead to more effective audit results. Pre-audit preparations include gaining an understanding of:

- activities, processes, and risks;
- previous audit findings and OHS performance history;
- physical layout and location of buildings and areas of interest;
- the organizational structure and OHS accountabilities;
- recent construction, modifications or organizational changes;
- the use of contractors;
- pertinent regulatory agency activity for the site;
- security and clearance needs for site access;
- the need to have company representatives escort team members;
- unique hazards and subsequent PPE requirements; and,
- OHS policies and procedures relevant to the audit scope.

When the audit process is initiated, the lead auditor should have a meeting or phone call with the site representative who is the lead coordinator for the site. In addition to overall audit logistics, such as audit dates, the lead auditor can begin to understand the above site-specific issues. This information will also help the lead auditor understand the expertise he or she will need on the audit team. At this time, the lead auditor should make sure that there is a mutual understanding about the audit scope. Any discrepancies in understanding of the scope need to be resolved before proceeding any further.

The part of pre-audit activities involved with reviewing site policies and procedures before the official site-visit is called the "desk review." This is where documents relevant to the audit scope are reviewed by the lead auditor and team members to determine initial compliance or conformance with regulations or standards against which the site is being audited. In management systems audits, when non-conformances are found during the desk review, it is common for the lead auditor to suggest that the site bring these areas into conformance before making the official site-visit.

A valuable component of pre-audit preparation is the use of a pre-audit questionnaire (an example is shown in Appendix A) to be completed by the site in advance of the site visit. The purpose of the questionnaire is to provide the lead auditor with necessary background information that will help her or him plan the audit in the most effective manner. Pre-audit questionnaires help lower costs by decreasing the time that the audit team must spend on-site gathering background information. It is effective to identify an on-site coordinator who will act as the key liaison between the facility and the audit team and can facilitate scheduling and logistics for the team.

The pre-audit questionnaire also serves an important internal function. The act of collecting data, gathering policies and procedures, and completing pre-audit forms is an educational process for both the on-site coordinator and the individuals gathering the documents. Even before the audit team arrives on site, the coordinator will usually have a good estimate of the facility's overall compliance or conformance with the areas or issues within the audit scope, from examining the general pattern of responses to items on the questionnaire, there is value in seeing this at the early stages of the audit. The pre-audit questionnaire also provides the opportunity for senior management to see what may be ultimately included in the final report. Finally, for issues with significant risks, this provides an opportunity to take immediate action.

A memo from senior management to the key site personnel prior to the audit emphasizing their need to cooperate and participate can help make the on-site activities proceed smoothly.

During pre-audit activities, the lead auditor should ask the site contact to ensure that sufficient on-site working space and resources are provided for the audit team. This includes a conference room or office of sufficient size, telephone, internet access, photocopying support, and document access. For remote locations, consideration of bringing in food for lunch should be considered to increase efficiencies.

The method(s) of information and data collection during the audit should be determined before the site-visit. This typically includes the preparation of forms and even audit notebooks that contain the forms. The forms should be designed to capture information from interviews, document reviews, visual observations. With management system audits, a typical form is called a "non-conformance" or "corrective action" form. These are used to capture the various types of objective evidence upon which an audit finding is based.

The Audit Team

It is the lead auditor's responsibility to assemble an audit team with personnel whose technical expertise match the anticipated audit scope needs. The audit team should include qualified individuals experienced in the investigation process, and most importantly in the areas they will be examining. Individuals should have a complete and deep understanding of the areas to which they are assigned. This means that they should be current with regulations and various agency interpretations of regulatory compliance approaches, and of course, they should have excellent knowledge of the standard. In like fashion, with management system audits, auditors need to understand the standards and interpretation nuances.

Within the U.S., credentials in various technical fields, such as Certified Industrial Hygienist, Certified Safety Professional, Certified Hazardous Material Manager, Certified Professional Environmental Auditor, or Professional Engineer may be useful, but even more germane is broad, practical experience in the field and excellent auditing skills. Auditing skills can be honed through week-long trainings provided on ISO 14001 and OHSAS 18001 auditing.

ISO 19001 provides guidelines for auditing quality and environmental management systems. Section 7 of 19001:2002 provides guidance on auditor competence and evaluation criteria for auditors. Personal attributes suggested are that auditors should be:

- Ethical, i.e. fair, truthful, sincere, honest, and discrete;
- Open-minded, i.e. willing to consider alternative ideas or points of view;
- Diplomatic, i.e. tactful in dealing with people;
- Observant, i.e. actively aware of physical surroundings and activities;
- Perceptive, i.e. instinctively aware of and able to understand situations;
- Versatile, i.e. adjusts readily to different situations;
- Tenacious, i.e. persistent, focused on achieving objectives;
- Decisive, i.e. reaches timely conclusions based on logical reasoning and analysis; and
- Self-reliant, i.e. acts and functions independently while interacting effectively with others.

The audit team size is based upon the size and complexity of operations, the number of issues under study, and the site's health and safety performance history. One auditor assigned to a 3,000-employee facility to conduct a comprehensive safety, health and environmental audit is an obvious mismatch of resources to scope. Six auditors conducting an examination of health and safety issues at a 250-employee plant does not represent the optimal use of resources either. If the audit team is too small for the facility and the issues involved, then the process is likely to be lengthy and lose momentum. Conversely, if the team is too large, it will not operate efficiently due to an inadequate number of facility employees available to interface with the audit team and supply needed information. Typical OHS audit teams range in size from two to five team members.

Audit Logistics

Opening Meeting

An audit normally commences with an opening meeting during which the audit team presents details of the on-site and post-audit activities, including the intended scope, time frame, progress report/meeting frequency, format of draft and final report, and method of delivery. This is also an excellent opportunity for the team to raise any issues from the pre-audit questionnaire that need further clarification. Methods of communication and preferred communication channels are typically reviewed at the opening meeting.

Typically, the site management takes this opportunity to provide an overview to the site's operation and describe any aspects of the programs and systems that may not have been included in the pre-audit questionnaire or pre-audit discussions. The opening meeting is frequently followed by a preliminary tour of the facility, often led by operations and site health and safety personnel. The tour enables the auditor(s) to ask any additional questions in light of the pre-audit questionnaire and the opening conference, as well as identify areas to which they want to return later in greater depth. At the conclusion of the tour, the audit team usually meets alone, briefly, to draw up a specific plan for how the scope of the audit will be covered in the time specified. If a company representative is needed to escort audit team members, ensure that there are enough representatives to manage a large audit team.

It is important at this time to work with site personnel to identify key individuals the team is interested in interviewing in depth to ensure these personnel will be available.

During the Audit

The remainder of the on-site activities of the audit involves interviewing site personnel, reviewing documentation and records, and re-visiting site areas to verify what the audit team is learning. Many audit teams chose to conduct daily briefings to update site personnel of their observations and provide a forum to resolve any misinterpretations immediately. These daily gatherings help to make the official close-out meeting run smoothly.

During the audit, auditors should immediately bring to the attention of the site coordinator any observed life-threatening or high risk issues.

An important component of an audit is conducting interviews with site personnel. Auditors should have training in how to conduct effective interviews. Interviews should be structured so that the interviewee can be open and honest without concern about potential retribution. The audit team should be involved with the selection of who will be interviewed to make sure that there is no potential bias. Beyond key managers and persons with OHS accountabilities, selection of interviewees should be done randomly. Interviews are typically conducted alone between the an auditor and interviewee, management representative participation should be discouraged.

At the conclusion of each day, the audit team should meet to discuss findings and the observations of each team member. Collaboration of objective evidence happens at this point. Each day, the lead auditor should assemble the audit finding from that day. This will help avoid a rush of work on the last day on site, and allows for discussion with site personnel about findings as they come up. As issues that come up on a daily basis that maybe out of a team member's area of expertise, the issue should be re-examined the next day by a qualified team member.

Closing Meeting

At the conclusion of the audit, a closing meeting is typically scheduled to discuss the audit findings and to answer any unresolved questions or issues. This meeting should be chaired by the lead auditor. Ideally, the most senior manager of the site should be present at this meeting to ensure the findings are presented to the individual most able to affect change. During the closing meeting, a date should be determined for the delivery of the draft and final reports. The closing meeting should be structured to provide upper management with a concise summary of critical issues that require immediate action. When the major items are presented in an abbreviated and prioritized format, senior management can make important resource allocation decisions well in advance of receiving a written report.

A key goal for the audit team should be that there are "no surprises" at the closing meeting and hence in the written final report. Audit observations that lead to audit findings should be reviewed daily with site personnel when they arise. The closing meeting and written report should serve to recapitulate what was itemized in the closing conference.

Audit Report

While all audit team members have input into the audit report, the final report should be written by the lead auditor. The report should include the audit objective and scope, and list the site areas included. It may be appropriate to include the initial audit plan and lists of people who attended opening and closing meetings.

The format of the audit report will vary depending on the culture of the organization being audited and the type of management reports already prevalent in the organization. One approach may be to structure the report to list only the deficiencies. These items may be grouped by severity to facilitate prioritizing corrective actions. This report style has the advantage of being concise and to the point; however, it does not acknowledge the good work being done. Morale can be affected if the only newsworthy material is negative in nature.

A different report style can list both the elements that were found to be in compliance and the deficient areas. This format can alert management to all of the problems, while at the same time providing information on the positive aspects that are being handled well by the employees. Therefore, areas in need of attention are denoted at the same time that recognition is given for items that do reduce risks. This type of report can provide senior management with a good overall perspective of facility status.

Still another report type may state only a recommended course of action based on the observations made during the facility visit. Recommendations can be generic or specific and serve to point a facility in a certain direction (e.g., replace verbal procedures and agreements with written documentation) or assign responsibility (e.g., for material safety data sheet collection and storage) to one person.

Finally, an opinion report can provide the relative degree to which compliance is met by subject area, and include phrases indicating that the facility is "wholly," "substantially," or "minimally" in compliance.

It is often helpful to include a one-page executive summary at the beginning of the report to apprise upper management of the overall status of the facility and any significant recommendations. It is common for the audit report to be delivered in draft form to ensure that the information is accurate and that the format and style are consistent with past agreements. Once the draft has been revised by the audit team, a final report is issued. Whatever format is chosen for the final report, it should be clearly stated prior to the initiation of the audit.

Post-Audit Actions

Following the audit, a plan of action to address any deficient areas must be established. It is increasingly common for the audit findings to be entered into a tracking system that will facilitate the resolution. The action plan for audit findings resolution should include identification of the person accountable for resolution and the expected completion date. For complex issues, a detailed action plan may be needed with numerous components that include consideration of necessary resources, both financial and personnel. When a robust tracking system is used, it can keep the original spirit of the audit alive by permitting periodic status reports to be forwarded to management. Statistics detailing percent of serious deficiencies corrected and remaining items sorted by priority and deadline provide a tangible measuring stick for facility administrators.

When management systems are audited, the post-audit period provides an opportunity to evaluate potential deficiencies in the overall system. There is value in performing a root cause analysis of each audit finding to see if the finding occurred from a deficiency in some part of the system. A nice process for handling audit findings is included in ANSI/AIHA Z10–2005, Section 6.5, where audit findings, along with findings from incident investigations, and corrective and preventative actions are fed back into the planning process. By examining these issues through the planning process lens, risk assessment considerations can be made that may impact OHS objectives, targets, and operational controls. It may be found that improvements are needed in training and communicating elements of the management system.

Legal Concerns

Confidentiality, security and legal concerns should be discussed before the audit is conducted. There may be legal concerns regarding the confidentiality of audit findings. Another concern is the potential discussion of trade secrets or material that may address sensitive issues. If these are important matters, then legal counsel should be sought prior to initiating the audit to determine the distribution and access to the audit report.

An understanding should be gained about the potential for audit reports to become available to regulatory agencies, thereby increasing a facility's vulnerability. It should be acknowledged and understood that the audit report forms a paper trail that can conclusively document that the facility had prior knowledge of violations. Therefore, if a compliance inspection finds these same violations noted in the audit report, they may be viewed as willful violations, which carry a much higher monetary penalty and possibly increased liabilities. This perspective is heightened if a facility chooses to conduct an audit but does not adequately correct the deficiencies that are identified. Should these concerns persist, legal counsel should be consulted to determine whether the audit findings may be sheltered from public or regulatory scrutiny under an attorney/client privilege or other legal mechanisms. In the United States, for instance, some states and the EPA have adopted policies that provide a certain amount of protection if an audit is conducted for the purpose of finding and correcting any compliance deficiencies. However, a self-disclosure of audit findings, along with an aggressive compliance strategy and timetable, sent to the appropriate regulatory agency prior to any inspection activity at that facility, may be required to receive this audit privilege protection.

Additional Reading

American Industrial Hygiene Association (AIHA®): *ANSI/AIHA Z10-2005 Occupational Health and Safety Management Systems.* Fairfax, VA: AIHA®, 2005.

British Standards Institute: *Occupational Health & Safety Management Systems - Specification*; OHSAS 18001:2007. London: BSI, 2007.

DiNardi, S.R.: *Calculation Methods for Industrial Hygiene.* New York: Van Nostrand Reinhold, 1995. pp. 124–164.

Huey, M.A.: The Industrial Hygiene Program. In *Fundamentals of Industrial Hygiene*, 4th edition. Itasca, IL: National Safety Council, 1996. pp. 749-758.

Leibowitz, A.J. (ed.): *Industrial Hygiene Auditing: A Manual for Practice*. Fairfax, VA: AIHA, 1995.

International Organization for Standardization: *Guidelines for Quality and/or Environmental Management System Auditing*. ISO 19001:2002. Geneva, Switzerland: ISO, 2002.

International Labour Office: *Guidelines on Occupational Safety and Health Management Systems*. ILO-OSH 2001." SafeWork - ILO InFocus Programme on Safety and Health at Work and the Environment. Geneva, Switzerland: ILO, 2001.

Rice, P.B.: The Safety Professional. In *Fundamentals of Industrial Hygiene*, 4th edition. Itasca, IL: National Safety Council, 1996. pp. 675–699.

Appendix A.

Pre-Audit Questionnaire[1]

This questionnaire is extremely extensive and may be burdensome for some facilities, such as a smaller site, to complete. Some of the more detailed information requested in the survey can and should be developed during the course of the on-site activities of the audit itself. Although it is provided as an example, a more concise questionnaire may develop a more complete list of useful information for auditors.

Please fill out this questionnaire as completely as possible. The background information about your facility's operations will be used to tailor the scope of the audit and select suitable audit team members.

1.0 GENERAL INFORMATION

1.1 Identifying Information:

- Unit/Site Name: ____________________
- This questionnaire completed by: NAME: ____________________
- Date: ______/______/______ PHONE: ____________________

1.2 Location:

- Mailing Address (Administrative Office): ____________________
- Shipping Address: ____________________
- City: ____________________
- County: ____________________
- State/Province: ____________________
- Zip Code/Country Mail Code: ____________________
- Telephone Number: ____________________
- Telefax Number: ____________________

1.3 Facility Personnel: Phone

- General Manager: ____________________
- Site/Facility Manager: ____________________
- Operations or Production Manager: ____________________
- E/S Coordinator: ____________________
- Total number of employees at facility: ____________________
- How many work shifts are operated? ____________________

[1] From Industrial Hygiene Auditing-A Manual for Practice, edited by Alan J. Leibowitz, CIH, CSP, AIHA Press, 1994.

1.4 Facility Size:

- Facility floor space in square feet (include multiple floors in calculations): ____________

____

- If unit/facility includes more than one building (at different address), please list all buildings and itemize their floor space in square feet. ____________

____

- Site size in acres: ____________

1.5 Facility Activities:

- Type of activities/processes at site (check all that apply and give approximate number of employees engaged in each).

YES	NO		NUMBER OF EMPLOYEES
____	____	Abrasive blasting	________
____	____	Acid/alkali cleaning	________
____	____	Adhesive bonding	________
____	____	Administrative/office work	________
____	____	Anodizing	________
____	____	Assembly operations	________
____	____	Casting of metal parts	________
____	____	Coating/painting	________
____	____	Degreasing/solvent cleaning	________
____	____	Drilling/machining	________
____	____	Glass/ceramic production	________
____	____	Grinding/polishing/buffing	________
____	____	Heat treating	________
____	____	Ionizing radiation (e.g., X-rays)	________
____	____	Lasers	________
____	____	Metal machining	________
____	____	Metal forging/stamping/forming	________
____	____	Packaging	________
____	____	Plastic formulation/extrusion/blow molding	________
____	____	Plating	________
____	____	Printing	________
____	____	RF/Microwave heating	________
____	____	Shipping/Receiving	________
____	____	Soldering/brazing	________
____	____	Wastewater treatment	________
____	____	Welding	________
____	____	Woodworking	________
____	____	Other activities of concern (specify)	________

- Is facility owned or leased:

Owned by: ____________ Leased from: ____________

• Standard Industrial Classification (SIC) Codes under which the facility operates: ___________

____

____

____

____

____

____

2.0 EMPLOYEE SAFETY/OCCUPATIONAL HYGIENE

2.1 Exposures/Controls:

	YES	NO	N/A
• Do you have any potential worker exposure to physical agents such as noise, radiation, heat, etc.?	_____	_____	_____
• Do you have any potential worker exposure to chemical agents?	_____	_____	_____
• Do you have any automatic monitoring or automatic alarm systems to detect hazardous materials?	_____	_____	_____
• Do you routinely or regularly measure air contaminant levels for any particular substances?	_____	_____	_____
• Have employees been informed of their exposure levels?	_____	_____	_____
• Are exposure records kept in a way that lets you estimate exposures for job categories?	_____	_____	_____
• Are all exposures within established limits for chemical and physical • agents (e.g., ACGIH TLVs, OSHA PELs)?	_____	_____	_____
• Are any areas designated as limited access "regulated" areas?	_____	_____	_____
• Are any areas posted with hazard warning signs such as "high noise • area," "respirators required," or "carcinogen area"?	_____	_____	_____
• Are any ventilation systems used to control hazardous materials exposures?	_____	_____	_____
• Do ventilation systems have:			
- Routine maintenance programs?	_____	_____	_____
- Regular airflow rate tests?	_____	_____	_____
- Regular filter changes?	_____	_____	_____
• Were ventilation systems designed or approved by a qualified engineer or occupational hygienist?	_____	_____	_____
• Are any other engineering controls used for control of hazards (e.g., noise enclosures, controlled-atmosphere control rooms)?	_____	_____	_____
• Are any administrative measures used to limit employee exposures to hazards (e.g., job rotation, temporary job reassignments)?	_____	_____	_____
• Does your facility have an Analytical or Quality Control Laboratory?	_____	_____	_____
• Are any types of personal protective equipment (e.g., gloves, glasses respirators) available?	_____	_____	_____
• Is there a written respirator program at the facility?	_____	_____	_____
• Are there training programs related to hazardous materials?	_____	_____	_____
• Is there a medical surveillance program including preemployment exams and periodic follow-up exams?	_____	_____	_____
• Is there a hearing conservation program that includes everyone exposed to noise in excess of 85 dBA?	_____	_____	_____

		YES	NO	N/A
2.2	**Safety:**			
	• Has the facility been reviewed within the past 2 years by OSHA or other internal or external reviewers?	____	____	____
	• Does the facility have a safety manual or safety guidelines?	____	____	____
	• Is there an up-to-date facility emergency response plan?	____	____	____
	• Are records maintained on work-related injuries and illnesses?			
	- OSHA record keeping?	____	____	____
	- Corporate/division reporting?	____	____	____
	- Incident reporting?	____	____	____
	- Motor vehicle accident reporting?	____	____	____
	- Dispensary log?	____	____	____
	• Does your facility operate a motor fleet?	____	____	____
	• Is there a written program for motor fleet safety?	____	____	____
2.3	**Emergency Response:**	YES	NO	N/A
	• Does the facility have an emergency response team (ERT) or fire brigade (FB)?			
	- Is there formal ERT or FB training?	____	____	____
	- Are there routine evacuation/fire drills?	____	____	____
	• Are there formal programs in place to provide for emergency care of the injured?	____	____	____
	• Are there any off-site facilities that fall under your direct control?	____	____	____
	• Please specify. ____			
	____			
	• Do you have programs in place for regular inspection of:			
	- Fire detection systems?	____	____	____
	- Sprinkler control valves?	____	____	____
	- Water flow test on sprinkler system?	____	____	____
	- Fire pumps?	____	____	____
	- Fixed fire extinguishing systems?	____	____	____
	- Fire extinguishers?	____	____	____
	- Alarm systems?	____	____	____

3.0 E/S PROGRAM DOCUMENTATION

		YES	NO	N/A
3.1	**Employee Safety/Occupational Hygiene:**			
	• Does the facility have any of its own specific policies, procedures, standards, or guidelines pertaining to:			
	- Evaluating work exposures (i.e., chemical, noise, radiation)?	____	____	____
	- Calibrating, testing, and maintaining occupational hygiene sampling equipment?	____	____	____
	- Quality assurance for analysis of occupational hygiene samples?	____	____	____
	- Informing employees of occupational hygiene monitoring results?	____	____	____
	- Review of material safety data sheets or other hazard communication information?	____	____	____
	- Safety training program?	____	____	____
	- Hazardous work permits (i.e., hot work, confined space entry, electrical lockout)?	____	____	____
	- Use and maintenance of personal protective equipment other than respirators?	____	____	____
	- Contractor on-site safety?	____	____	____
	- Testing and maintenance of fire protection equipment?	____	____	____
	- Injury, illness, and accident reporting investigation?	____	____	____
	- Motor fleet safety?	____	____	____
	- Any additional written health and safety procedures that are not required by law?	____	____	____

3.2 Documentation Practices:

• Describe the facility's documentation practices regarding the following:

Governmental EHS inspections ______________________________

____

____

Ongoing correspondence with governmental agencies and personnel concerning regulatory interpretations, permit renewals, other compliance-related guidance sought ______________

____

____

• Is the information received orally from governmental agencies confirmed with them via written correspondence? ______________________________

____

____

4.0 E/S PROGRAM MANAGEMENT

4.1 Environment & Safety Coordinator:

• Is there a designated ES coordinator(s)? ______________________________

• What is his or her name and title (other than ES coordinator)? ______________

____

• To whom does he or she report (name and title)? ______________________________

____

• Is the ES coordinator(s)' position full time? ______________________________

If not, what percentage of time is actually spent on ES-related activities:______________

____

• Does the coordinator(s)' job description include current ES responsibilities?

____

• What type of training has the ES coordinator(s) completed to execute his or her responsibilities?

____

• Have the ES coordinator(s)' responsibilities been clearly defined and communicated by management to site personnel?

____

• Is the ES coordinator(s)' performance evaluation influenced by the execution of ES responsibilities? ______________________________

- How does the coordinator(s) keep up with regulatory developments and company ES policies?

- How is this information shared with other facility personnel who undertake ES program activities?

4.2 Supervisors, Managers, and Site Personnel:

- Have the responsibilities for ES within each department been clearly defined and communicated by top management to supervisors, managers, and site personnel?

- Has training been conducted for department supervisors and managers for their roles and responsibilities for ES?

4.3 Performance Reviews:

- Describe the facility's overall system for reviewing the performance of its ES programs (e.g., facility audits or inspections, ES self-evaluation, review of records and reports) and for identifying departures from established standards and policies (governmental and company).

- Have specific performance goals and measurements for ES been established for all staff and site personnel?

4.4 Project Review:

- Who completes safety project reviews when new products or operational changes are anticipated?

- When is their review undertaken (e.g., several months prior to project initiation, the week before)?

- What criteria are used to determine when this review should be performed?

4.5 Communication and Awareness:

- How are facility and company management kept informed of ongoing ES activities?
- What mechanisms are used?

Who is notified? ______

______

Is all ES program activity communicated to management? If not, what is communicated?

______

How often do these communications take place? ______

______

Who is responsible for communicating this information? ______

______

- How are facility and company management made aware of ES problems or incidents (e.g., reportable releases, increase in employee accidents/injuries)? What mechanisms are used?

______

Who is notified? ______

______

What criteria are used for communicating this information? (Are all ES problems communicated to management? If not, what is communicated?) ______

______

How often do these communications take place? ______

______

Who is responsible for communicating this information? ______

______

4.6 Risk Management:

- To obtain an understanding of the facility's risk management system, specifically, what are the facility's systems and mechanics for the identification of hazards, determining risk acceptability, developing and implementing risk control systems, and providing for periodic risk review?

______

______

______

______

______

______

5.0 E/S PROGRAM ADMINISTRATION

What person or persons at the facility are responsible for development, implementation, and administration of programs for compliance with applicable governmental and company requirements for each of the following functional areas on a day-to-day basis?

NOTE: Include training and experience level of these staff members for each area of the Environment & Safety (ES) Program. Indicate those ES areas that do not apply to this facility.

5.1 Equipment Safety:

	Training Degree Courses, etc.	Experience (# of Years)
Overall responsibility		
______________________	__________	__________
Identification and evaluation of machine guarding needs		
______________________	__________	__________
Maintenance of equipment guards		
______________________	__________	__________
Hoist maintenance (i.e., testing, labeling)		
______________________	__________	__________

5.2 Administrative Control Programs (i.e., hazardous work permits, confined entry procedures):

Overall responsibility

______________________ __________ __________

Development of procedures

______________________ __________ __________

Issuance of work permits, lock-out tags

______________________ __________ __________

5.3 Injury, Illness, and Accident Reporting:

Overall responsibility

______________________ __________ __________

Development of investigation guidelines

______________________ __________ __________

Determining and recording reportable injuries

______________________ __________ __________

Coordinating medical services on-site and off-site

______________________ __________ __________

	Training Degree Courses, etc.	Experience (# of Years)
5.4 Employee Safety Training and Awareness:		
Overall responsibility		
____________________	________	________
Job safety and training programs		
____________________	________	________
First aid training		
____________________	________	________
CPR training		
____________________	________	________
Supervisor, safety training		
____________________	________	________
5.5 Fire Prevention and Life Safety:		
Overall responsibility		
____________________	________	________
Testing and maintaining fire prevention equipment		
____________________	________	________
Managing flammable storage areas		
____________________	________	________
Developing and overseeing emergency plans		
____________________	________	________
5.6 Hazard Communications:		
Overall responsibility		
____________________	________	________
Training		
____________________	________	________
Review of MSDS		
____________________	________	________
Distribution and maintenance of MSDS		
____________________	________	________

5.7 **Occupational Hygiene:**	Training Degree Courses, etc.	Experience (# of Years)
Overall responsibility		
______________________________	__________	__________
Identification of physical and chemical exposures in the workplace		
______________________________	__________	__________
Measurement of ventilation performance		
______________________________	__________	__________
Calibration of occupational hygiene monitoring devices		
______________________________	__________	__________

chapter 43

Outcome Competencies

After completing this chapter, the reader should be able to:

1. Define underlined terms used in this chapter.
2. Summarize the role of hazard communication in a workplace safety and health program.
3. Describe the three major components of a hazard communication program.
4. Prepare a simple written hazard communication program.
5. Describe the international approach to hazard communication.

Key Terms

chemical • employee • exposure • hazard statement • hazard warnings • health hazard • identity • pictogram • physical hazard • precautionary statement • responsible party • signal word

Prerequisite Knowledge

General occupational hygiene background.

Key Topics

I. Introduction
   A. Role of Hazard Communication in the Workplace
   B. History of the Development of Legal Requirements for Hazard Communication

II. The Federal Hazard Communication Standard
   A. Overview of the Approach
   B. Detailed Description of the Requirements

III. The Globally Harmonized System for Classification and Labelling of Chemicals (GHS)
   A. The Proposed Modifications

IV. Hazard Determination vs. Hazard Classification
   A. Labeling Specifications
   B. Safety Data Sheets
   C. Other Provisions

V. Summary

VI. References

Hazard Communication

43

By Jennifer C. Silk

Introduction

Role of Hazard Communication in the Workplace

Occupational hygienists trying to protect exposed workers from hazardous chemicals before the 1980s had to spend a considerable amount of time researching the hazards of the chemicals in the workplaces under their control. While some chemical manufacturers voluntarily transmitted information about their products through labels and material safety data sheets (MSDSs), it was more often the case that the occupational hygienist or other health and safety professional had to conduct a scavenger hunt to obtain the most basic information about the products of concern, particularly if they were proprietary mixtures.

This changed with the advent of the worker right-to-know movement in the 1980s. Worker representatives successfully lobbied state and federal government authorities to ensure that workers exposed to chemicals are apprised of their potential hazards and appropriate precautionary measures. Provisions that implemented this important right for workers had the additional benefit of informing occupational hygienists and other health and safety professionals about hazardous chemicals in the workplaces they are responsible for, thus easing their tasks and improving overall protection.

Today there is increasing evidence that the most beneficial approach to worker safety and health in a workplace is a systematically developed comprehensive safety and health management program. Effective hazard communication is a cornerstone of that comprehensive approach. Without adequate information about the chemicals in use, it is not possible for an occupational hygienist or other professional to design or implement an appropriate protective program for exposed employees.

Providing information to employees as well as to health and safety professionals serves to empower employees to be active participants in an employer's safety and health program. For example, workers who understand why a respirator must be worn when working with a particular chemical are more likely to wear it when needed and to ensure that it is worn properly.

Together, the actions of employers and employees who have the necessary information about the chemicals in their workplaces will reduce the potential for chemical source illnesses and injuries-thus accomplishing the underlying purpose of the federal hazard communication standard (HCS).

History of the Development of Legal Requirements for Hazard Communication

It has been suggested that the first attempts at communicating hazards to users of chemicals can be found in the hieroglyphics in Egyptian tombs.[1] Some of these markings have been interpreted as information about various herbal preparations or medicinal materials. They provided precautions for safe use as well as other information that users of these preparations and materials would find helpful.

Development and transmittal of information about chemical products continued to evolve throughout the centuries that followed. By the 19th century, chemists often provided users with notes regarding chemical properties and safety considerations. Early in the 20th century these became more prevalent and standardized. Labels have been accepted business practice in the chemical industry for many years, including the development of voluntary industry consensus standards on the subject more than 50 years ago. MSDSs have also been in use for some time-the Manufacturing Chemists' Association (predecessor to the American Chemistry Council) made them available as early as 1949.[2]

These activities to provide information about hazardous chemicals were voluntary on the part of manufacturers until the late 1960s. At that time the Bureau of Labor Standards adopted requirements for MSDSs in the maritime industries. These standards were adopted by the Occupational Safety and Health Administration (OSHA) in the early 1970s. OSHA developed a two-page format (the OSHA Form 20) that was used for many years to provide MSDS information in the maritime industries.

Coverage of other industries was a long-term project for OSHA. The agency adopted the HCS in 1983. This was the culmination of nearly 10 years of rulemaking activity. The implementing legislation for OSHA, the Occupational Safety and Health (OSH) Act of 1970[3], included provisions that addressed labeling of chemicals in the rulemaking authority for the agency. Under Section 6(b)(7) OSHA was required to include in any substance-specific standard addressing toxic substances provisions to prescribe "the use of labels or other appropriate forms of warning as are necessary to insure that employees are apprised of all hazards to which they are exposed, relevant symptoms and appropriate emergency treatment, and proper conditions and precautions of safe use."

OSHA took this substance-specific approach to labeling, including provisions in health standards when promulgated as anticipated under the provisions of the act. It soon became clear, however, that this time-consuming and laborious process was not adequately apprising employees. OSHA's rulemaking process is slow and deliberative, often taking years to complete each individual standard for a chemical substance. However, the number of chemicals in the workplace that pose potential hazards to exposed employees is large. OSHA has estimated that there are about 880,000 hazardous chemical products in American workplaces. Ultimately, OSHA decided that the lack of information about hazardous chemicals in the workplace was a significant risk to workers and that a way to address them generically needed to be developed.

Thus, in 1974 the agency formed a standards advisory committee to make recommendations to OSHA on how to proceed in developing a standard that addressed labeling and provision of information. This committee, formed under the requirements of the OSH Act, was comprised of members of the public, labor representatives, and management representatives. They completed their report in 1975 and suggested that OSHA needed a standard with requirements for classifying chemicals as to their hazards, labels, MSDSs, and training.[4]

Also in 1975, the National Institute for Occupational Safety and Health (NIOSH) provided a criteria document to OSHA that included similar recommendations. They advised OSHA that a standard including hazard classification, labels, MSDSs, and training was needed to provide employers and employees with information about chemicals.[5]

While these recommendations appear straightforward and were based on the practices of progressive employers, there were many complicated issues involved in implementing them in a mandatory standard. These included which hazards to cover; how to define them; whether the requirements should be performance- or specification-oriented; what chemicals to cover; what employers to cover; and how to address the confidentiality of trade secrets. OSHA had to develop regulatory provisions for these issues to propose a standard. An advance notice of proposed rulemaking was published in 1977 to elicit public comments on these issues. After several years of considering various options, a proposed standard titled Hazards Identification was published in January 1981 by the outgoing Carter administration.

This 1981 proposal diverged from the recommendations OSHA had previously received, since it addressed only hazard classification and labeling. There were no requirements for either MSDSs or training. The chemical industry objected to many of the proposed requirements, and the new Reagan administration withdrew the proposal in February 1981 for further consideration of regulatory alternatives.

In the meantime, employee representatives grew tired of waiting for a federal standard to address worker right-to-know and began lobbying state governments for standards. This was a successful endeavor, and soon it appeared there would be a number of varying requirements for shipping chemicals around the United States. The state standards covered different chemicals, different employers, and had divergent requirements for disclosing information. The specter of 50 different state standards elicited considerable support for a harmonized federal approach.

Thus, OSHA introduced a new proposed standard in March 1982 and completed rulemaking by issuing a final standard in November 1983.[6] It was comprehensive in its coverage of chemicals and hazards but was limited to the manufacturing sector of industry. This scope was immediately challenged in court by worker representatives, and in 1987 OSHA was ordered to expand the scope to cover all employers. OSHA published a new final rule in August 1987 to comply with this order.[7] As a result of various legal and administrative challenges, and the agency's desire to clarify some of the provisions, a third final rule with relatively minor modifications was published in February 1994.[8] The preambles to each of these final rules provide a more detailed history of the proceedings, as well as a summary and explanation of the requirements. These should be consulted for additional information.

The HCS is codified in the Code of Federal Regulations (CFR) in several places. The general industry standard can be found at 29 CFR 1910.1200. The construction, maritime, and agriculture industries are also covered in provisions that are identical to the general industry standard, but are found at 29 CFR 1915.1200, 1917.28, 1918.90, 1926.59, and 1928.21. While this chapter describes the provisions of the HCS, it is not intended to be a substitute for consulting the actual regulatory requirements when designing a program for purposes of compliance. In addition to being in the CFR, OSHA maintains a home page where the regulations can be accessed, as well as a database of interpretations that can be searched and the compliance instructions given to OSHA compliance safety and health officers to guide them when enforcing the standard.

In addition to the worker right-to-know provisions of the HCS, the U.S. Environmental Protection Agency (EPA) implements community right-to-know provisions under requirements of theEmergency Planning and Community Right-to-Know Act (EPCRA). Chemicals required to have MSDSs under OSHA provisions are subject to the requirements of EPCRA Sections 311 and 312 for reporting information to communities. See the Solid Waste and Emergency Response/Emergency Management section of the EPA website for more information.

The Federal Hazard Communication Standard

Overview of the Approach

The HCS is unique among OSHA regulations in a number of respects. It covers more workers than any other single health standard-about 40 million of them exposed to hazardous chemicals in over 5 million establishments. It includes requirements for evaluating the hazards of all chemicals, preparing written hazard communication programs, labeling containers, providing MSDSs, and training employees. Before examining the specifics of these requirements, it may be helpful to understand the overall design of the standard and the unique characteristics of OSHA's approach to hazard communication.

The HCS covers all industries and all sizes of facilities that fall under OSHA's jurisdiction. The information OSHA collected during its rulemaking process indicated that chemical exposures occur in all types of workplaces and all sizes of facilities. Since the HCS is an information-transmittal standard rather than a standard that establishes specific control measures for a chemical, it appeared that its provisions were also feasible in all types of workplaces and that exposed workers have an equal need for information regardless of the type of work they are performing or the size of their workplace. Unlike some other standards that have different requirements in various industries (e.g., asbestos in construction), OSHA determined that industry-specific differences under the HCS could be reasonably accommodated through flexible implementation and did not require differing provisions. (Note: The Mine Safety and Health Administration (MSHA) published a final standard for hazard communication in the mining sector in 2002. Information about the requirements, which are very similar to OSHA's standard and guidance for compliance can be found on the MSHA website.

The HCS is a performance-based standard, establishing goals for compliance but providing minimal specifications for how employers are to reach those goals. This requires employers to use professional judgment to comply and OSHA's enforcement staff to use the same type of judgment to enforce the rule. To regulate all types of workplaces and all sizes of facilities, OSHA determined that it should maintain provisions that are performance-oriented to allow employers the flexibility to implement them in a manner suitable to that particular workplace. There are certain specification aspects in the requirements that help to ensure a consistent approach, however, such as the hazard determination provisions. But each employer is given significant latitude in determining the best way to establish a hazard communication program in his or her workplace. For example, the manner in which training is to be delivered and the amount of time to be spent on training are not specified. Employers may choose from a wide variety of options including toolbox talks, videos, and interactive computer programs. The choices made will depend on the needs of the particular work force, the availability of equipment, and the number of hazardous chemicals being addressed.

The HCS is a generic standard, covering 880,000 hazardous chemical products. Hazards are defined, not listed by product, so the scope increases as new products that meet the definition of hazard are developed. During the HCS rulemaking OSHA considered promulgating a list of chemicals to define the scope of coverage for the standard. However, the agency found that (1) there is no list that captures all of the chemicals of concern; and (2) requiring employers to consult a list is an additional burden. Furthermore, a list is fixed in time and does not allow the standard to remain current with actual workplace conditions as products change and new products develop. The criteria-driven approach incorporated in the HCS allows it to remain up-to-date without changing the rule itself.

The HCS includes a downstream flow of information (i.e., chemical manufacturers are required to prepare and provide information about their products to employers using them). In designing the standard, OSHA determined that one of the key problems for employers using chemicals was obtaining information about them. If their suppliers did not provide it voluntarily, it was difficult for employers using the chemicals in their workplaces to ascertain what was in the product and obtain information from some other source. Thus, it appeared clear to the agency that the standard had to take the unique approach of requiring the producers or suppliers to provide the data to their customers. The assessed burdens of the standard showed that this was a much more cost-effective approach overall than to have numerous customers attempting to obtain or develop information about the same product.

It addresses controversial and unique issues, such as preemption of state laws in states that do not have their own plans and trade secret protection. While preemption provisions in the OSH Act address this issue for all standards, it has never been such a key concern in a rulemaking as it was when the HCS was initially promulgated. For suppliers of chemicals, uniformity in requirements for labels and MSDSs was the primary reason for supporting a federal hazard communication standard that preempted requirements in existing state standards that posed a burden on interstate commerce. It should be noted, however, that there are some states that have right-to-know requirements that differ in some respects from the federal approach. These requirements may be intended to protect the public or emergency response personnel, and thus are not preempted by the federal standard.

In the area of trade secrets, another key concern of suppliers involved divulging confidential business information to people outside of their firms. This is also an issue that is covered in the OSH Act, but the provisions in the HCS itself were the result of extensive comment in the rulemaking and much negotiation and discussion. The key issue was to balance the needs of workers to be protected with the desire of suppliers to protect their legitimate trade secret concerns.

The HCS depends on people modifying their behavior when they receive information. Employers must use the information to provide better employee protection. Employees must use the information to participate in the protective programs. Together, these actions will result in a decrease of chemically related illnesses and injuries. While the HCS requires the transmittal of information, its sphere of influence on safety and health in the workplace is much broader than the simple receipt of that information. The successful functioning of the standard requires people to act on the information they receive to improve conditions in the workplace — an active process of using the information, not a passive paper trail.

To help ensure that this active process is achieved, the agency examined the communication aspects of existing workplace programs to determine what worked in this regard. As a result, the information transmitted under the standard comes in three forms: labels, MSDSs, and training. The label is a simple snapshot of the hazards- a quick and abbreviated information source that reminds workers and other users that there are hazards and more information is available. The MSDSs provide the comprehensive information available about a chemical and associated precautionary measures. These are reference documents, and in addition to being accessible to workers, they provide the information that health and safety professionals need to design protective programs for exposed workers, as well as information important to employees responsible for emergency response. And last, employee training is required. It is in this setting that the information can be explained and related to the specific workplace situation. Training helps make the labels and MSDSs effective. These three aspects of the standard are thus interdependent, and effective information transmittal requires all three to work.

The scope of the HCS determined the scope of EPA's community right-to-know requirements under EPCRA. This greatly expanded the target audience for the information - in particular, the already extensive audience for MSDS information - to community emergency responders and local planning authorities.

The HCS was thus a departure for OSHA and the regulated community in many respects. Its implications and impact on worker safety and health are broad, and the standard was written to ensure that the requirements remain current and active as time passes. This appears to have been successful. The HCS is still frequently addressed and challenged in many different fora, particularly in Congress and small business lobbies.(9) However, it also appears to continue to have a significant impact in the workplace and on expectations regarding the information that can and should be made available to chemical users.

Detailed Description of the Requirements

Paragraph (a): Purpose

The stated purpose of the HCS is to ensure that the hazards of all chemicals produced or imported are evaluated and information concerning their hazards is transmitted to employers and employees. The standard further states that this is to be accomplished by means of comprehensive hazard communication programs, including labels, MSDSs, and training. In addition, OSHA also included a paragraph specifically addressing the preemptive authority and intent in this area.

The underlying purpose of the standard is to reduce the incidence of chemical source illnesses and injuries. While providing the right-to-know is an important goal, the use of the information for protection makes the transmittal effective. Working with chemicals without knowing what the hazards are puts the workers at significant risk of developing an adverse health effect. Since these chemicals may have the potential to cause severe acute effects as well as long-term, cumulative damage, it is important to ensure that everyone handling them has information about their hazards and the appropriate precautionary measures to implement.

Paragraph (b): Scope and Application

The scope and application paragraph of any OSHA health standard indicates who and what are covered by the standard. In the case of hazard communication, it describes not only what is covered but provides exemptions for items that are either not covered or are covered in a limited fashion.

First, the standard requires all chemical manufacturers or importers to assess the hazards of chemicals they produce or import. Second, all employers are required to provide exposed employees with information about hazardous chemicals in their workplaces. And third, distributors are required to transmit information to their downstream customers.

The HCS applies to "any chemical which is known to be present in the workplace in such a manner that employees may be exposed under normal conditions of use or in a foreseeable emergency." This is a particularly important part of the scope and application of the standard. It establishes that all chemicals present in the workplace are potentially included in the scope and thus require evaluation (such as byproducts or intermediates of a process). It also indicates that any exposure triggers coverage of the standard; it is not in any way related to exposure above a permissible exposure limit. This includes potential exposure as well as actual exposure, and foreseeable emergencies must be addressed (such as ruptured pipes or containers). However, if there is no potential for exposure (i.e., the chemical is inextricably bound or in a physical state where exposure is not possible) the chemical is not covered. This provision is thus key to determining which chemicals in a workplace fall under the scope of the HCS.

The HCS includes a series of exemptions or situations of limited coverage. These are based on considerations of special handling circumstances, limited exposure or risk, or coverage by other federal standards.

Laboratory operations and operations where employees handle only chemicals in sealed containers (such as warehousing) have limited coverage. In these work operations, labels on incoming containers must not be removed or defaced, employees must be trained, and MSDSs must be provided on employee request. Written hazard communication programs are not required and employers do not have to ensure there is an MSDS available for every hazardous chemical in the workplace.

A number of federal standards require labeling of various chemical products. Where such labeling requirements are already in place, OSHA is preempted from requiring additional labeling even if the existing labeling does not have all of the information OSHA would require under the HCS. The products currently subject to labeling under other agencies include pesticides, some toxic substances, food, food additives, drugs, cosmetics, medical or veterinary devices, distilled spirits, consumer products or hazardous substances for consumer use, and agricultural or vegetable seeds treated with pesticides. The HCS should be consulted for the specific terms of these labeling exemptions.

There are also a number of situations in which OSHA has determined that application of the HCS is not warranted, either because the chemicals are already regulated elsewhere by another federal agency or their hazards occur outside the workplace. These include chemicals that are already regulated as hazardous wastes; tobacco or tobacco products; wood or wood products in terms of flammability or combustibility; articles (where chemicals are bound and are not available for exposure); food or alcoholic beverages in a retail establishment or consumed by workers in the workplace; drugs in solid, final form, packaged for sale to consumers or intended for personal use by employees; cosmetics packaged for sale to consumers or intended for personal consumption by workers; consumer products when used as a consumer would use them with similar exposures; nuisance particulates that pose no physical or health hazards to employees; ionizing and nonionizing radiation; and biological hazards.

It is important to refer to the actual language in the HCS when determining if any of these exemptions applies to specific products or the products in use in specific workplaces. When in doubt, the best rule of thumb is to assume the product is covered if it is hazardous. The exemptions are intended to avoid duplicative coverage or coverage of products where the risk is small and addressed through other means. However, this is an area where OSHA has received many questions, and there are extensive interpretations regarding the extent of coverage in a number of these areas.

Paragraph (c): Definitions

This paragraph of the HCS includes definitions of a number of key terms in the standard. OSHA defines terms used in the standard for a particular purpose and it is important to proper understanding and interpretation to consult these terms when implementing the HCS in the workplace.

The terms include a number of definitions that help define the scope of coverage: chemical manufacturer, chemical, employee, employer, and workplace are examples of terms used that are defined for purposes of this standard. Employee, for example, is defined as "a worker who may be exposed to hazardous chemicals under normal operating conditions or in foreseeable emergencies. Workers such as office workers or bank tellers who encounter hazardous chemicals only in non-routine, isolated instances are not covered."[10]

Thus, this definition includes an important interpretation of the scope of the standard as applied to certain types of employees. Similarly, the term "exposure" means that an employee is subjected in the course of employment to a chemical that is a physical or health hazard, and includes potential (e.g., accidental or possible) exposure. "Subjected" in terms of health hazards includes any route of entry (e.g., inhalation, ingestion, skin contact or absorption).[10]

This is key to determining which employees and which chemicals are covered by the standard.

Scope questions regarding chemicals covered are addressed in a number of definitions addressing chemical properties, such as health hazard, physical hazard, explosive, oxidizer, etc. These are to be used by chemical manufacturers and importers when evaluating the hazards of their products.

Paragraph (d): Hazard Determination

Under the requirements of the HCS, chemical manufacturers and importers are responsible for evaluating the hazards of the chemicals they produce or import. The producers of the chemicals are in the best position to know what is in the product, the characteristics of the product, the hazards associated with it, and what precautionary measures are appropriate to deal with these hazards. Thus, the standard requires them to generate such information, put it on labels and MSDSs, and provide it automatically to downstream users of the product. Employers who use chemicals are permitted under the HCS to rely on the hazard evaluations performed by their suppliers.

While hazard determination is an area that requires extensive professional judgment in the identification and evaluation of the scientific literature, OSHA decided that certain parameters needed to be established to ensure consistency in approaches. These are described in the hazard determination paragraph, as well as in two mandatory appendices to the standard, Appendix A (Health Hazard Definitions) and Appendix B (Hazard Determination). In addition, OSHA included a nonmandatory appendix describing available sources for information to perform a hazard determination (Appendix C, Information Sources).

The determination of physical hazard potential under the standard is relatively straightforward. Definitions of physical hazards such as flammability tend to be based on objective, measurable criteria (e.g., the flashpoint). Chemical manufacturers and importers generally test for such effects when establishing the characteristics of their products.

The more difficult hazard determinations involve health hazard potential. Chemicals are not generally tested for the full range of health effects, and testing is particularly deficient in the area of chronic effects. Furthermore, there are often disagreements about the interpretation of available data and its applicability to human exposures. This paucity of data and difficulty of interpretation is further complicated by the fact that few employees are exposed to chemical substances; most are exposed to mixtures of those substances. The large majority of hazardous chemical products in a workplace are mixtures unique to a single manufacturer. Few such mixtures have been tested, so a system must be devised to project the hazards of a mixture based on the hazards of its components.

OSHA believes that the threshold data requirements for transmittal of information vs. establishment of specific control measures should be relatively low to ensure that downstream employers and employees get as much information as possible on which to base decisions about protective measures. Thus, OSHA requires chemical manufacturers and importers to consider the existence of one good study to be a sufficient level of evidence for purposes of communicating hazard information. The study must be conducted according to scientific principles and have statistically significant results that indicate the potential for adverse effects. Both human and animal evidence must be evaluated to determine whether the chemical meets the standard's definition of a health hazard.

OSHA anticipated that despite this guidance, there would be differences of opinion regarding the coverage of the standard. Thus, the agency established a "floor list" of chemicals that are to be considered hazardous under the rule in all situations. This list includes all chemicals for which OSHA has adopted a permissible exposure limit (PEL), as well as all those for which the American Conference of Governmental Industrial Hygienists (ACGIH®) has adopted a threshold limit value (TLV®). In addition, OSHA was aware that the definition of carcinogenicity would be likely to generate the most controversy under the hazard determination provisions of the rule. To establish a consistent approach, the agency indicated that any chemical found by the National Toxicology Program (NTP) or the International Agency for Research on Cancer (IARC) to be a carcinogen or potential carcinogen was to be considered as such for hazard communication purposes. In addition, any chemical for which there is one good study indicating potential carcinogenicity is to be considered carcinogenic for purposes of the standard.

In the area of mixtures, OSHA specified that where a chemical has been tested as a whole to determine its hazards, that information shall be used for purposes of hazard communication. Where such testing has not been done, the rule basically requires the chemical manufacturer or importer to consider the mixture to have the same health hazards as its components. If a health hazard is present in concentrations of 1% or greater, the mixture is presumed to have the same hazard. The exception is for carcinogens, which render the mixture hazardous when present in concentrations of one-tenth of a percent or greater. The rule also has a backup provision for situations where these cutoffs are too high to protect employees. If the component can still exceed the PEL or TLV® in those concentrations, or still present a health risk to employees, the mixture is covered when the component is present in the smaller concentrations as well.

The chemical manufacturer or importer is required to document the hazard determination procedures used. While it is not necessary to document each individual hazard determination for a chemical, many producers do so to ensure they can duplicate the decision-making process if questions arise.

Paragraph (e): Written Hazard Communication Program

Employers with hazardous chemicals in their workplaces are required to develop, implement, and maintain a written hazard communication program. The purpose of the written program is to coordinate the hazard communication activities in the workplace and ensure that they are addressed in a comprehensive and consistent manner. It is intended to be a blueprint for action, indicating what's covered, how, and who is responsible for the various components. The program does not need to be lengthy or complicated to accomplish this intent, but anyone reading it should be able to determine how the program works in that facility.

The provisions requiring a written hazard communication program have been cited more than any other requirement of the standard. This often leads people to the conclusion that the cited employers have implemented the other requirements of the standard, and have simply found the written program requirements to be too burdensome, difficult, or unnecessary and have chosen not to comply with them. This conclusion is not accurate, however, since for many years OSHA told its compliance officers to cite the lack of a written program in cases where an employer had done nothing to comply with hazard communication. It is believed to be very unusual for an employer to have complied with all of the other provisions without having a written program.

The written program is required to describe how the employer plans to meet the requirements for labels, MSDSs, and training. It must also include a list of the hazardous chemicals in the workplace. The list may be compiled by work area or for the workplace as a whole. The names used for the list may be common or chemical names, as long as the identity used also appears on the labels for the chemical product and the MSDS. The identity can thus be used to link these three sources of information together.

The written hazard communication program must also include the methods the employers will use to inform employees of the hazards of unusual tasks. During the rulemaking, OSHA received comments that employees are sometimes asked to do tasks that have not been addressed in the training they receive on normal workplace activities. Cleaning out reactor vessels occasionally might be an example of such a task. In this type of situation, the employer must ensure that there is a plan to inform employees of the hazards of this special task and associated protective measures.

Another issue discussed during the rulemaking involves the hazards associated with chemicals contained in unlabeled pipes in workplaces. At one point, OSHA considered requiring that labels be placed on pipes at some regular interval. Manufacturing employers presented information indicating that this approach would be very burdensome, and in many cases employees are stationed in control rooms and only enter the plant areas for specific maintenance or quality control checks. In these situations they can be apprised of the hazards in some other way and achieve the same purpose. OSHA has allowed this to be done, as long as the method is addressed in the written program.

Another issue raised during rulemaking discussions involves protection on multiemployer work sites. An employer may have developed and implemented an adequate program to protect employees from the hazards of the chemicals used by the employer, but if the work takes place on a site where other employers operate, this may not be enough. While construction sites are usually considered the primary example of this situation, nearly every workplace is multiemployer at one time or another. Frequently, employers have contractor employees on site to perform certain tasks like maintenance work. Other repair or service personnel may also be required to work on site, sometimes for long periods of time. Where this occurs, both employers have a responsibility to ensure information is exchanged or made available so the employees are protected from all hazardous chemicals to which they are exposed, not just those generated by their own employer. On a construction site, for example, this may mean that each subcontractor provides a copy of the MSDSs for the chemicals they may bring on site and leaves them in the site trailer. Or perhaps their MSDSs will be accessible from a laptop computer on site. The written program must indicate how this issue will be addressed, but does not specify how the employer must accomplish this. The requirements are flexible so the particular situation in the workplace may be taken into consideration.

The written program is to be made available on request to employees, their designated representatives, OSHA, and NIOSH. Where employees travel between workplaces during a shift, an employer may satisfy the obligation to make the written program available by keeping it at the primary workplace location.

Preparation and implementation of a written hazard communication program should not be viewed as a paperwork exercise. If done right, it ensures that the hazard communication program pieces are properly integrated and produce an effective program. It also serves as a checklist to ensure all the parts have been addressed. The list of chemicals is essentially an inventory of what MSDSs are needed to be in compliance. The written program can thus be an important tool to gauge completeness and compliance and can be part of an employer's assessment of the effectiveness of the approach implemented in a given workplace.

Paragraph (f): Labels and Other Forms of Warning

The HCS transmits hazard information to employees and employers through three communication mechanisms: labels on containers, MSDSs, and training. At one time, the agency considered simply requiring labeling as the only form of information transmittal. However, there were several drawbacks to this approach. A label can convey only a limited amount of information. Besides space considerations, some labels are on containers that are moving and thus only convey the message for a brief period. There is also evidence to indicate that the more information there is on a label, the less likely it is that people will read and act on it. Thus, OSHA determined that while labels have an important role to play in the overall scheme, they do not function well in most situations as the only source of information. Under the HCS, labels are an abbreviated source of information about hazards. More information is available through MSDSs, and both label and MSDS information is reinforced by training.

The HCS requires chemical manufacturers, importers, and distributors to ensure that shipped containers of hazardous chemicals are labeled with the identity of the material, appropriate hazard warnings, and the name and address of the chemical manufacturer, importer, or other responsible party.

As previously described, the identity can be either a chemical or common name, as long as it also appears on the list of hazardous chemicals and the MSDS. The MSDS also contains a list of hazardous ingredients and thus is the primary source for the specific chemical components of a mixture.

Hazard warnings convey the physical or health hazard of the chemical. For example, "potential carcinogen" or "causes lung damage" would be considered appropriate hazard warning statements. Where available, health hazard warnings must convey the target organ effect. It is not considered sufficient to indicate that a chemical is harmful if inhaled, for example. The effect when inhaled is the appropriate hazard warning.

Labels on shipped containers often include other information than that required by OSHA, such as first aid information or precautionary measures. The agency was aware of that when the HCS was adopted and decided to focus on those items that were less frequently present but were nevertheless necessary to worker protection. Other information may be included. There is a voluntary industry consensus standard that provides guidance for label preparation (ANSI Z129.1-2006), including statements that can be used to convey information.[11]

Unfortunately, many labels in the workplace today are not designed to communicate information effectively to exposed workers or the employer. They are written to satisfy legal requirements and become cluttered with details that often are not assimilated by the user. Simple labels with direct, easily understood warnings are the most likely to have the desired effect (i.e., workers will modify their behavior to follow safe work practices for the chemical).

Labels or other forms of warning are also required on containers in the workplace. Those containers that are used simply as received with the label from the supplier do not require additional labels. Other containers do require preparation of labels. As with the shipped containers, an identity must be on the label. The workplace labels must also have an appropriate hazard warning. The HCS is a bit more flexible in the warnings permitted on these internal workplace containers. Many different types of in-plant labeling systems have been developed that use numerical rating systems, colors, symbols, and other unique ways of conveying hazards. While they may not provide specific information in some respects, in the context of the overall hazard communication program they can be effective. Employers can use these types of systems as long as the specific information is available immediately in some form in the workplace, and workers are trained to recognize the components of the system.

The HCS also allows alternative forms of warning to suffice in lieu of an actual label for stationary process containers. These may include signs, placards, batch tickets, and similar means of conveying the information in writing, as long as the information is readily accessible and clearly identifies the containers to which it applies.

The standard also contains provisions requiring labels to be prominently displayed and legible. With regard to language requirements, the information must be in English, but may also be in other languages if appropriate for the employee audience.

Paragraph (g): MSDSs

While the label serves as a quick reminder of the hazards and the need for appropriate precautionary measures, the MSDS is a detailed reference source that includes all of the pertinent information on a chemical, its characteristics, and ways to handle it safely. These documents may be referred to by exposed employees when they need additional information. But they also serve as reference documents for the employer and for a host of health and safety professionals who provide services to the employee and the employer. Emergency responders, physicians, occupational health nurses, safety engineers, and occupational hygienists all use this document to obtain information to perform their work.

Chemical manufacturers and importers bear the primary responsibility for the development and dissemination of MSDSs.

Employers are required to have one for each hazardous chemical in the workplace. The standard is designed to have a downstream flow of information from the producers of the chemical, through the distributors, to the ultimate user.

The HCS does not specify the format in which information is to be disseminated. At the time of the OSHA rulemaking on the HCS, many chemical manufacturers testified that they already prepared and distributed MSDSs for their products and had developed formats they found suitable and appropriate for that purpose. Thus, they supported performance-oriented requirements in the OSHA standard-specification of what information is required, but no particular format. This was the approach OSHA adopted in the final rule.

An MSDS is required to include the following information:

- Identity information, including chemical and common names of hazardous ingredients;
- Physical and chemical characteristics (such as vapor pressure);
- Physical hazards;
- Health hazards, including signs and symptoms of exposure, and medical conditions that may be aggravated by exposure;
- Primary route(s) of entry;
- Exposure limits;
- Carcinogenicity;
- Precautions for safe handling and use, including hygienic practices, protective measures during repair and maintenance, and spill and leak procedures;
- Control measures, such as appropriate engineering controls, work practices, or personal protective equipment;
- Emergency and first aid procedures;
- The date of preparation of the MSDS, or the last change to it; and
- The name, address, and telephone number of a responsible party who can provide additional information or emergency procedures.

MSDSs are to be readily accessible to employees when they are in their work areas during the work shift. This means they are able to consult the MSDS for necessary information at any time during the workday. Many employers are managing their MSDSs electronically and allow access to them through terminals in the work areas or similar electronic means. Electronic access is permitted as long as there is no barrier to obtaining the information.

Many of the users of MSDSs have argued for a standard format to facilitate accessing the information. This has been a particular concern of the emergency responder community, but it is relevant to employees and other users as well. Under the performance-oriented system, the information may appear in a different order and on different pages depending on the manufacturer producing the MSDS. This makes it difficult to find the particular data of concern and may add to the time necessary to obtain information in an emergency.

In response to these types of comments from users, the American Chemistry Council sponsored development of an American National Standards Institute (ANSI) voluntary industry consensus standard on preparation of MSDSs.[12] Designated as ANSI Z400.1–2004, the MSDS standard outlines a preferred 16-section order of information, as well as providing guidance to preparers on how to design the form to communicate effectively and how to fill in the various sections. Many chemical manufacturers are now using this approach. There is also an international standard using the same approach, ISO 11014–1, Safety Data Sheet for Chemical Products. Standardization of the format makes electronic storage and transmission of MSDS information easier and facilitates management of MSDS collections, as well as improving the utility of the sheets themselves.

Paragraph (h): Employee Information and Training

The final communication component of the HCS is employee information and training. Without training, communication of the information via labels and MSDSs is not likely to be effective. Training ensures that employees understand the information presented to them in written form, have an opportunity to clarify it, and know where they can obtain additional information if necessary. The training requirements in the HCS are performance-oriented. The employer is free to choose the method of delivery (e.g., lecture, interactive computer, or videotape). It is unlikely, however, that a purchased program would meet all of the training requirements. Employers who use such programs must supplement them with site-specific information. No training records are required to document individual employee participation in training, although for purposes of internal program management, documentation is encouraged.

Many occupational hygienists are tasked with conducting worker training but have not been trained themselves to do so. This is a serious deficiency, since many people who are technically competent in the subject areas addressed by the training do not have the skills necessary to adequately transmit the information to others. Effective training requires knowledge of appropriate training techniques in addition to familiarity with the subject of the training.The HCS requirements are divided into two parts. The first deals with the simple presentation of information, rather than training. Under these requirements, the employer must inform employees of the requirements of the HCS, the location of hazardous chemicals in their work areas, and the location and availability of the written hazard communication program and MSDSs. Such information transmittal is passive.

Training should be a more active process designed to ensure that the employee knows and understands the information being transmitted. Under the HCS, employees are to be trained on how they can detect the presence of hazardous chemicals in their workplace, the physical and health hazards of the chemicals, the measures they can take to protect themselves, and the details of the employer's hazard communication program.

It is important to note that the intent of this training is not to have each employee memorize and be able to repeat all of the information presented. There are written materials available for reference for that purpose. Rather, the training heightens awareness about the existence of hazards in the workplace, the need to handle them appropriately, and how to obtain and use the information available about the hazards, protective measures, and emergency procedures. Employees will be faced with different kinds of labels and forms of MSDSs; the training helps to coordinate these sources of information in a form usable to the worker.

Paragraph (i): Trade Secrets

The HCS requires disclosure of the identity of all hazardous chemicals on the MSDS. However, in some limited circumstances the specific chemical identity of such a chemical may be withheld if it is a bona fide trade secret.

At the time the HCS was promulgated, when MSDSs were being prepared and disseminated voluntarily, trade secret claims for identity information were common. A major issue in the rulemaking process was the question of what constitutes a legitimate trade secret and under what circumstances it can be withheld to protect its secrecy. A special rulemaking just to address this issue followed later.

As a result the HCS includes an appendix that provides a detailed explanation of the types of characteristics that qualify a hazardous chemical identity as a trade secret. An employer must be able to show, for example, that research or extensive developmental processes were required to discover the product or its uses; that extraordinary means have been undertaken to keep the identity secret; and that it would not be a simple analytical process for someone wishing to reverse engineer the product and determine the secret.

The specific chemical identity may only be maintained as a trade secret under the HCS if it meets the tests specified in common law for establishing a trade secret.

Nevertheless, even when a chemical identity is a trade secret, protection of exposed workers must be the ultimate concern. Therefore, the HCS requires disclosure of the identity when there is an occupational health need for the information, such as to conduct or assess sampling of the workplace atmosphere to determine employee exposure levels.

In these circumstances the holder of the secret may require the requestor to sign a confidentiality agreement. The HCS specifies the legal constraints for the agreement and a process of adjudication should there be a difference of opinion on the need or the ability to maintain confidentiality.

A considerable amount of the rulemaking process was devoted to this issue, but there have been few complaints about violations of the approach during implementation of the standard. The trade secret provisions have rarely been cited, and as a general rule trade secret claims are rarely seen on MSDSs.

Paragraph (j): Record Keeping

There are no long-term record keeping provisions in the HCS. The written program must be kept current; outdated or changed programs need not be kept. MSDSs must be present in the workplace for those chemicals that are also present. One common misconception about the HCS is that it requires MSDSs to be maintained for 30 years. The Access to Employee Exposure and Medical Records regulation[13], requires MSDSs to be kept for 30 years if there is no other record of exposure. Where the employer has actual exposure monitoring or generates a record with lists of chemicals, locations, etc., the MSDSs need not be maintained.

Appendices

The provisions of the HCS are accompanied by five appendices that provide additional information. As discussed above, Appendices A and B are related to defining health hazards and making a hazard determination. These are mandatory. Appendix C lists possible references to be consulted when preparing a hazard determination. It is advisory. Appendix D defines a trade secret. And Appendix E walks the reader through the requirements of the standard in lay (nonlegal) language. It is intended to assist the small employer who uses rather than produces chemicals.

Other Issues

This discussion is an abbreviated explanation of the requirements of the HCS. To properly implement the standard in a workplace, the requirements of the rule itself should be reviewed. In addition, there are other sources that provide more detailed guidance for compliance.[14]

The HCS has now been in effect since 1983. OSHA has reported that acute illnesses and injuries due to chemical exposures have dropped approximately 42% since the standard was first promulgated.[15] However, the need for effective hazard communication continues to be important given the ever increasing number of chemicals that may be encountered in workplaces (there are now 50 million chemicals that have Chemical Abstracts Service (CAS) Registry Numbers)[16], and new technologies that are developed to use them (such as nanomaterials). In 2004, OSHA examined implementation issues related to the HCS, and wrote a report on hazard communication in the 21st century[17] that gave the Agency's analyses of the issues and ideas for the future. Key among the concepts raised involved development of an internationally harmonized approach to hazard communication.

The Globally Harmonized System for Classification and Labelling of Chemicals (GHS)

The widespread distribution and use of chemicals in the workplace as well as in other sectors has led many national, regional, and international authorities to require the dissemination of information about them. There is no way that any regulatory authority could address each hazardous chemical individually in terms of specifying control procedures. However, requiring the dissemination of information about the hazards and associated protective measures helps to ensure that the chemicals are used in a way that reduces the potential for harm. It gives the user the ability to take steps to minimize or eliminate exposures, and thus prevent the occurrence of adverse effects.

In the U.S. regulatory system, information dissemination is key to requirements under the U.S. Department of Transportation's (DOT) hazardous materials regulations; the U.S. Environmental Protection Agency's (EPA) pesticides' rules; and the Consumer Product Safety Commission's (CPSC) standards for chemicals in consumer products in addition to OSHA's HCS. Domestically, each of these agencies has addressed how hazards are defined, and how they are communicated on labels or placards. While similar, these requirements vary enough that the same chemical may be treated differently in terms of hazards and other information depending on what it is used for, or what stage of the life cycle is being addressed.

These domestic differences are magnified when examined internationally. In addition to the U.S., the European Union has label and MSDS requirements for chemicals, as do other U.S. trading partners such as Canada, Japan, and Mexico, and many other countries. Thus chemical producers in the U.S. that ship to these other countries must often prepare multiple labels and MSDSs to satisfy the requirements of the importing countries. This may result in barriers to trade, particularly for smaller companies that aren't able to deal with the multitude of laws governing these types of requirements.

The development and maintenance of hazard classification and communication systems requires a significant infrastructure that may not exist in some countries. For these nations, it is difficult to implement chemical safety and health management programs to protect those exposed because they cannot develop and maintain a regulatory approach to establish the information base for such programs. Thus these countries look to the relevant international organizations for assistance in obtaining the necessary information.

In 1992, the United Nations Conference on Environment and Development (UNCED) adopted an international mandate to address the concerns of both developed and developing countries by harmonizing existing requirements to establish a globally harmonized system of hazard classification and labeling:

> "A globally harmonised hazard classification and compatible labelling system, including material safety data sheets and easily understandable symbols, should be available, if feasible, by the year 2000."

Implementation of this mandate required multiple international organizations, many countries, representatives of non-governmental organizations, and extensive work for many years. The technical work for the Globally Harmonized System of Classification and Labelling of Chemicals (GHS) was completed in 2001, and adopted by the United Nations Economic and Social Council in 2003 when it was also made available to countries for adoption. The international goal for such adoption was 2008. While this seems like a long period of time, it was actually quite ambitious. For developed countries with existing systems, the difficulty was in changing well-established regulatory approaches to something new and different. For developing countries, the difficulty was in establishing an appropriate infrastructure, and educating people on the need for the system as well as the means to implement it. In 2010, implementation is still a work in progress, but many countries have either adopted the GHS or are in the process of doing so.

A United Nations' Subcommittee of Experts on the GHS meets twice a year to maintain the system, update it as necessary, and oversee implementation around the world. The United States is an active participant in the work of this Subcommittee and its parent committee. The UN published the third revised edition of the GHS (commonly referred to as The Purple Book) in 2009.[18]

The GHS includes harmonized criteria for health, physical and environmental hazards. These criteria provide the processes to be followed to review data available on a substance, and determine what type of hazard it poses as well as the degree of severity of the hazardous effect. The criteria also address how mixtures will be evaluated to determine if they pose the same hazardous effect as the substance. The harmonized criteria were developed by international experts in these areas, and will be updated when scientific developments require modifications.

In addition to hazard criteria, the GHS specifies the label elements to be included to convey the hazards to users, as well as information on safe handling and use. These include a signal word, symbol, and harmonized hazard statement for each hazard class and category. In addition, precautionary statements are also recommended. Thus once a hazard has been classified, the GHS provides the exact information required to be on a label for the substance.

The GHS also includes requirements for safety data sheets (SDSs). It specifies a 16-section order of information for the SDSs, as well as indicating what information should be addressed in these sections. The GHS SDS is comparable to the ANSI MSDS in the U.S., which is also a 16-section approach.

OSHA published an advance notice of proposed rulemaking (ANPR) regarding their plans to revise the HCS to align it with the GHS in 2006.[19] The ANPR provided background regarding the history of the development of the GHS, as well as information about the provisions of the harmonized system and what parts of it OSHA expected to adopt. More than 100 commenters submitted responses.

On September 30, 2009, OSHA published a notice of proposed rulemaking (NPRM).[20] This document provides the intended modifications to the HCS to align it with the GHS. The rulemaking process will likely take 18 months to two years to complete a final rule. This will be followed by a phase-in period of compliance that has yet to be determined but OSHA proposed three years.

The Proposed Modifications

The rulemaking to revise the HCS is unique in a number of respects. First, the agency has never taken part in an international effort to harmonize safety and health requirements before. In fact, it is believed that development of the GHS is the only such effort to have taken place in this field. This can be explained in part by the trade aspects of these types of requirements. Other safety and health rules do not have an effect on companies or workers in other countries. However, given the extensive nature of international trade in chemicals, the requirements of a country for hazard communication definitely affect what information is developed on chemicals produced there, as well as what information may be transmitted when the products are shipped across borders.

The international interest in pursuing development of a global approach is also related to the need for comprehensive information on chemicals in order to establish effective chemical safety and health management programs. Continuing international efforts to control chemical exposures around the world depend on the ready availability of chemical identities, hazard information, and recommendations for precautionary measures.

The HCS, as described above, is a performance-oriented approach. This means that the agency has specified what the employer needs to do (for example, put a label on a container), and what information is required (e.g., a hazard warning), but does not specify how to do it (for example, provide the language of the hazard warning). This approach does not lend itself to being harmonized, or ensuring that the same information is presented on a chemical by multiple suppliers. Therefore, the GHS is a specification approach. Once a chemical is classified according to the criteria outlined, it specifies exactly what must be put on a label for the chemical. Adoption of the GHS will therefore change the underlying approach to hazard communication in the U.S. from a performance orientation to more of a specification standard.

In addition to this change, the agency has outlined other assumptions that were used to develop the proposal. First, as supported by commenters to the ANPR, only those provisions of the HCS that are impacted by the GHS are being revised. Other provisions that are not directly affected will remain the same. The proposal is a modification of the current HCS, and not a completely new standard.

OSHA is also proposing to minimize any country-specific deviations from the GHS provisions so as to be as harmonized as possible. The greatest benefits of the GHS will be achieved if countries follow this principle. As suggested by stakeholders, OSHA has also examined what its major trading partners have done in terms of adopting the GHS, and tried to be consistent where appropriate. The trading partner of most significant concern in this regard is the European Union, which has already adopted the GHS.[21]

Unlike other rulemakings, OSHA cannot change many of the proposed provisions in the final rule because to do so would mean the rule would not be harmonized with the GHS. While there are some aspects that are to be determined by the competent authority, most must be consistent with the GHS to be considered harmonized. The following is a summary of the major revisions that have been proposed.

Hazard Determination vs. Hazard Classification

While the overall scope of chemicals covered by the HCS, as well as the hazards addressed, will remain the same, the details of how such hazards are evaluated and conveyed will change significantly under the proposed modifications.

The current rule defines twenty-three types of health and physical hazards that are covered, and provides the methods to determine whether a chemical presents these hazards in paragraph (d) (hazard determination). This is supplemented by hazard definitions in paragraph (c) (definitions) and Appendix A. Appendix B provides additional parameters for the evaluations. The definitions generally do not include any indication of severity, i.e., either a chemical is a carcinogen or it is not.

The proposed modifications change the process from a determination to hazard classification. Under hazard classification, the data are used to establish that there is a potential hazard, as well as to characterize the potential severity of the effect. So the hazard class is identified (e.g., carcinogen) but the relative severity is also determined by assigning the chemical to a hazard category within that class based on the weight of evidence (e.g., Category 2 based on limited evidence of carcinogenicity in animals).

The criteria for hazard classification are much more detailed and specific than the definitions and principles used in the current standard. Each health and physical hazard class has a chapter in the GHS that outlines how data are to be evaluated to place the chemical in the appropriate hazard class and category. OSHA has similarly provided these detailed criteria in new Appendices A (Health Hazards) and B (Physical Hazards). Chemicals will have to be reassessed to ensure they are classified appropriately under the HCS when it is modified.

Labeling Specifications

Under the current HCS, the label requirements are perhaps the most performance-oriented part of the rule. Chemical manufacturers and importers are required to provide identity and hazard information on labels, but may use any format, language, or tools such as symbols that they deem appropriate. This means that workers are seeing little consistency in labels on containers, which may impact the comprehensibility of the information provided.

The GHS, and thus the proposed modifications to the HCS, take a completely different approach. Once a chemical is classified (i.e., its hazard class and category have been determined), the proposed rule indicates exactly what will be required on the label for the chemical—including the following label elements:

Signal Word: A word used to indicate the relative level of severity of hazard and alert the reader to a potential hazard on the label. The signal words used are "danger" and "warning." "Danger" is used for the more severe hazards, while "warning" is used for the less severe.

Pictogram: Composition that may include a symbol plus other graphic elements, such as a border, background pattern, or color, that is intended to convey specific information about the hazards of a chemical. The pictograms for GHS are a black symbol on a white background in a red diamond-shaped frame.

Hazard Statement: A statement assigned to a hazard class and category that describes the nature of the hazards of a chemical, including, where appropriate, the degree of hazard. An example of a hazard statement is: Causes eye damage.

Precautionary Statement: A phrase that describes recommended measures that should be taken to minimize or prevent adverse effects resulting from exposure to a hazardous chemical or improper storage or handling. An example of a precautionary statement is: Wear protective gloves.

The NPRM includes a new Appendix C which includes the label elements for each hazard class and category covered. If the chemical is a Category 2 carcinogen, for example, Appendix C will provide the appropriate signal word, pictogram, hazard statement, and precautionary statements to include on the label for that substance.

Table 43.1 is taken from Appendix C of the proposal, and illustrates the symbols included in the document. The use of symbols is one of the most significant aspects of the proposed modifications in terms of impact on HCS labels since most labels in use under the current rule do not include graphic representations of the hazards. However, their inclusion should be beneficial where employees have limited literacy or where English is not their first language. This is one of the reasons symbols are often used in other countries' hazard communication standards, and are thus part of the GHS.

Safety Data Sheets

OSHA is proposing the 16-section safety data sheet (SDS) provisions in the GHS. Since many U.S. chemical manufacturers already

Table 43.1 — Hazard Symbols and Classes

Flame	*Flame Over Circle*	*Exclamation Mark*	*Exploding Bomb*
		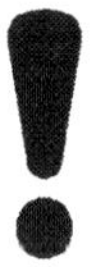	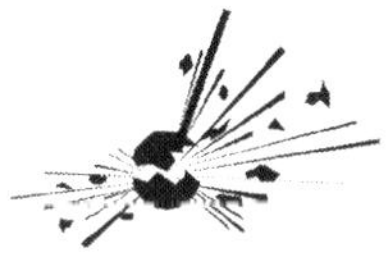
Flammables Self Reactives Pyrophorics Self-heating Emits Flammable Gas Organic Peroxides	Oxidizers	Irritant Dermal Sensitizer Acute Toxicity (harmful) Narcotic Effects Respiratory Tract Irritation	Explosives Self Reactives Organic Peroxides
Corrosion	*Gas Cylinder*	*Health Hazard*	*Skull and Crossbones*
		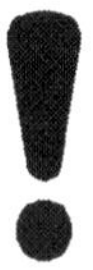	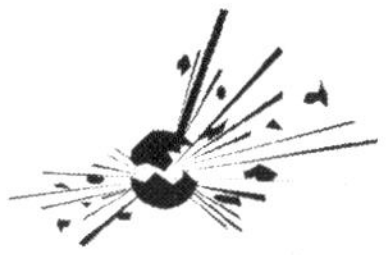
Corrosives	Gases Under Pressure	Carcinogen Respiratory Sensitizer Reproductive Toxicity Target Organ Toxicity Mutagenicity Aspiration Toxicity	Acute Toxicity (severe)

follow the 16-section format in the ANSI MSDS standard(12), this will be familiar to many workers. However, several of the sections address areas of information that are outside OSHA's jurisdiction (e.g., transport and environmental information). OSHA has indicated that it will not be enforcing these sections.(12–15) A new Appendix D addresses what information should be included in the sections of the SDS.

Other Provisions

OSHA has indicated that training on the new label and SDS formats would be required for all workers. Other provisions of the rule such as the scope and application, written hazard communication program, and trade secrets, would remain essentially the same as the current HCS under the proposed modifications.

Summary

A properly implemented hazard communication program can form the basis for a comprehensive safety and health program in the workplace. It provides the information needed to design appropriate protective measures and to give workers what they need to take steps to protect themselves. Each employer with hazardous chemicals in the workplace must have a written hazard communication program. Containers of such chemicals must be labeled, MSDSs must be available for each hazardous chemical in the workplace, and employees must be trained about the hazards and how to obtain and use the hazard information. OSHA has proposed to modify and refine these protections by adopting the GHS, and including more detailed specifications for hazard classification and labeling in the HCS. The agency expects these changes to increase the comprehensibility of information provided to workers, and thus lead to additional reductions in chemical source illnesses and injuries in the workplace.

References

1. **Kaplan, S.A.:** "Development of Material Safety Data Sheets." Paper presented at American Chemical Society meeting, April 1986.
2. "Chemical Safety Data Sheets Available Through Manufacturing Chemists' Association." Ind. Hyg. Quart., March 1949, p. 22.
3. "Occupational Safety and Health Act," Pub. Law 91-596, Section 2193. 91st Congress, Dec. 29, 1970; as amended, Pub. Law 101-552, Section 3101, Nov. 5, 1990.
4. **Standards Advisory Committee on Hazardous Materials Labeling:** "Report to the Assistant Secretary for Occupational Safety and Health, U.S. Department of Labor." June 6, 1975.
5. **National Institute for Occupational Safety and Health (NIOSH):** A Recommended Standard-An Identification System for Occupationally Hazardous Materials. (NIOSH Pub. No. 75-126). Cincinnati, OH: NIOSH, 1975.
6. "Final Rule: Hazard Communication," Federal Register 48:53280 (November 1983).
7. "Final Rule: Hazard Communication," Federal Register 52:31852 (August 1987).
8. "Final Rule: Hazard Communication," Federal Register 59:6126 (February 1994).
9. National Advisory Committee on Occupational Safety and Health: "Report to OSHA on Hazard Communication." September 1996.
10. "Hazard Communication Standard," Code of Federal Regulations Title 29, Section 1910.1200.
11. **American National Standards Institute (ANSI):** *American National Standard for Hazardous Industrial Chemicals-Precautionary Labeling (ANSI Z129.1–2006).* New York: ANSI, 2006.
12. **American National Standards Institute (ANSI):** *American National Standard for Hazardous Industrial Chemicals-Material Safety Data Sheets-Preparation (ANSI Z400.1–2004).* New York: ANSI, 2004.
13. "Access to Employee Exposure and Medical Records," Code of Federal Regulations Title 29, Section 1910.1020.
14. **Silk, J.C., and M.B. Kent (eds.):** *Hazard Communication Compliance Manual.* Washington, DC: The Bureau of National Affairs, Inc., 1995.
15. **Occupational Safety and Health Administration (OSHA):** OSHA Press Release/Conference To Announce a Proposal to Modify the Hazard Communication Standard to align with the Globally Harmonized System of Classification and Labeling of Chemicals (September 29, 2009)(available at www.osha.gov)
16. Chemical Abstracts Service (CAS) Registry Press Release, September 9, 2009 (available on their web page at www.cas.org)
17. **Occupational Safety and Health Administration (OSHA):** Hazard Communication in the 21st Century Workplace — Final Report, March 2004 (available at www.osha.gov)
18. **United Nations:** *Globally Harmonized System of Classification and Labelling of Chemicals (GHS),* Third Revised Edition, United Nations, Sales No. E.09.11.E.10, New York and Geneva, 2009.
19. Hazard Communication Advance Notice of Proposed Rulemaking, 71 FR 53617 (September 12, 2006).
20. Hazard Communication Notice of Proposed Rulemaking, 74 FR 50280 (September 30, 2009).
21. Regulation (EC) No 1272/2008 of the European Parliament and of the Council of 16 December 2008 on classification, labeling and packaging of substances and mixtures, amending and repealing Directives 67/548/EEC and 1999/45/EC, and amending Regulation (EC) No 1907/2006. OJ L353 of December 31, 2008 at p. 4.

Outcome Competencies

After completing this chapter, the reader should be able to:

1. Define underlined terms used in this chapter.
2. List the benefits of developing an emergency response plan.
3. Describe a cross-functional team and its role in emergency planning.
4. Describe the role of the occupational hygienist in emergency response.
5. Describe the process of hazard risk assessment.
6. List the essential elements of an emergency response plan.
7. Design a basic emergency response plan for a familiar facility.
8. Identify and describe community services chartered for emergency response.
9. Describe the benefits of emergency response drills and mock emergencies.
10. Justify emergency readiness for a specific scenario from minimal to ultimate response plan.

Key Terms

Acute Exposure Guideline Levels (AEGLs) • bioterrorism • Clean Air Act • codes • consensus standards • Continuous Exposure Guidance Levels (CEGLs) • covert act • credible scenarios • crisis • crisis management • cross-functional teams • emergency planning • emergency response • Emergency Exposure Guidance Levels (EEGLs) • Emergency Response Planning Guidelines (ERPGs) • emergency response plan • fail-safe • Hazard Index • HazMat • HAZWOPER • IDLH • index of suspicion • levels of concern (LOCs) • line diagrams • medical surveillance program • nonmandatory guidelines • quarantine • risk • risk assessment • EPA's Risk Management Program • root cause investigations • Subcommittee on Consequence Assessment on Protective Actions (SCAPA) • standards • shelter in place • Temporary Emergency Exposure Limits (TEELs) • terrorism • threshold concentration

Prerequisite Knowledge

Prior to beginning this chapter, the user should review the following chapters:

Chapter Number	Chapter Topic
3	Legal Aspects of Industrial Hygiene
8	Occupational and Environmental Health Risk Assessment/Risk Management
9	Comprehensive Exposure Assessment
11	Sampling of Gases and Vapors
15	Principles and Instrumentation for Calibrating Air Sampling Equipment
17	Direct-Reading Instruments for Determining Concentrations of Gases, Vapors, and Aerosols
34	Prevention and Mitigation of Accidental Chemical Releases
39	Personal Protective Clothing
40	Respiratory Protection
45	Risk Communication
50	Developing an Occupational Health Program
52	Occupational Safety

Key Topics

I. Requirements for Development of ERPs

II. National Fire Protection Association

III. Hazard and Risk Assessment for Emergency Response Planning
   A. Business or Facility Type
   B. Emergency Types
   C. Incident Command System for Emergency Response
   D. ERP Development
   E. ERP Drills and Preparedness

IV. Occupational Hygienist Roles in Emergency Response
   A. Roles in ERP Development
   B. Roles During Emergency Response

V. Audits of ERPs
   A. General Audit
   B. Occupational Hygiene Aspects of the ERP Audit

Emergency Planning and Crisis Management in the Workplace

44

By Susan D. Ripple, MS, CIH

Introduction

Emergencies can happen in any organization. The extent of anticipation and recognition of risks, coupled with planning and practice before an emergency or crisis occurs, can determine how serious the impact will be. This chapter provides a general overview of emergency planning essentials and describes the role of the occupational hygienist in developing a reasonable response plan. It also addresses actions during emergency response to keep the personal, community, and business impacts to a predictable, manageable level. Preparedness is the most important aspect of assuring that an unplanned event or an emergency has minimal impact on the enterprise, its workers, the environment, and the surrounding community. Occupational hygienists are an integral part of emergency response, using their knowledge and experience to aid cross-functional teams in the planning of appropriate responses required for unplanned events. The emergency response plan (ERP) is the basis for identifying and assessing the risks associated with potential emergencies, planning for appropriate response and recovery, and training those who would be involved or affected should the emergency occur. Facilities that depend solely on the local community fire, police, and emergency medical services to handle an emergency without including them in emergency response planning may later find an increase in injuries, deaths, and economic losses because time is lost struggling to determine the proper course of action. An ERP provides knowledge to everyone affected so that they may react and respond quickly and safely.

Another important benefit of emergency response planning is the prevention of unplanned events, because the potential risks are recognized. As credible scenarios are identified, preventive measures to lessen their impact or prevent their occurrence are of significant value. Many preventive maintenance procedures are put in place as a result of ERPs.

In the United States, emergency response programs are driven by several Occupational Health and Safety Administration (OSHA) and by the Environmental Protection Agency (EPA) regulations, as well as by state and local regulations. Generally, if the ERP is written to protect facility employees, company assets, community neighbors, and the environment, the regulatory requirements will likely be met.

It is essential for company management who want to keep emergency impacts minimal to allocate resources to ensure that adequate safety measures and emergency response planning are in place prior to an emergency event. This quality and extent of preparedness for unplanned events is predicated on the risk acceptance level of top management. A cross-functional team comprised of personnel designated by the facility's management best accomplishes the ERP. The team should include representatives from maintenance, safety, fire, medical, and occupational hygiene groups, who should then interact with and train community emergency response teams. Depending on the nature of the potential catastrophes, representatives from environmental, security, and public affairs could be included in the planning. The occupational hygienist can provide many skills to this team related to evaluation of health risks, developing credible scenarios, personal protective equipment (PPE) selection and planning, scene management, training, drills, and audits of the ERP, as well as providing assistance during actual emergencies.

A number of excellent resources are available (listed under the Additional Sources section of this chapter) that treat the subject of emergency response planning with more detail and explanation, while providing templates for the ERP based on applicability.

Requirements for Development of ERPs

Numerous OSHA and EPA standards require an ERP for emergency and crisis planning and management. Table 44.1 is a limited list of federal standards that may be applicable to facility emergency response planning. All employers with more than 10 employees are required to develop a written ERP covering those designated actions that employers and employees must take to ensure employee safety from fire and other emergencies that could occur at the facility. The written plan must be kept at the workplace and the provisions for emergencies communicated to the employees and made available for employee review. Employers with 10 or fewer employees may communicate their plans to employees orally and do not need to maintain a written ERP.[1] Several of the OSHA chemical-specific standards in *Code of Federal Regulations* (CFR) Title 29, Part 1910, Subpart Z have reporting requirements for chemical spills or vapor releases, whether or not exposures occur.[2] In addition to federal regulations, state regulations and local requirements add to the complexity of developing an effective ERP.

National Fire Protection Association

The National Fire Protection Association (NFPA) produces consensus standards as national fire codes. There are 275 codes and standards, which are used in almost every building, process, service, design, and installation.[3] OSHA standards for fire protection (29 CFR 1910.156 through .165) reference many of these national consensus standards as nonmandatory guidelines that would be considered acceptable in complying with requirements of Title 29, Part 1910, Subpart L.[4] Table 44.2 lists some of the NFPA standards that may be used in emergency planning and response.

Hazard and Risk Assessment for Emergency Response Planning

Business or Facility Type

The nature and location of the business or agency governs, to a significant extent, whether an emergency will affect customers

Table 44.1 — Limited List of Federal Regulations Requiring Emergency Planning or Reporting

Employee Emergency Action Plans	29 CFR 1910.38
Employee Alarm Systems	29 CFR 1910.165
Hazardous Waste Operations and Emergency Response (HAZWOPER)	29 CFR 1910.120
Process Safety Management of Highly Hazardous Substances	29 CFR 1910.119
Toxic and Hazardous Substances	29 CFR 1910, Subpart Z
Risk Management Programs for Chemical Accident Release Prevention	40 CFR Part 68
Spill Prevention Control and Countermeasures Plan	40 CFR Part 112
Contingency Plan and Emergency Procedures	40 CFR 264.50-264.56, Subpart D
Response Plans for Onshore Oil Pipelines	49 CFR Part 194
Oil Pollution Act of 1990 (OPA)	
Superfund Amendments and Reauthorization Act (SARA)	
Title III Emergency Planning and Community Right-to-Know Act of 1986	

Table 44.2 — Limited List of NFPA Standards for Use in Emergency Planning or Response

Recommended Practice for Responding to Hazardous Materials Incidents	NFPA 471
Recommended Practice for Disaster Management NFPA 1600	
Standard for Professional Competence of Responders to Hazardous Materials Incidents	NFPA 472
Standard on Industrial Fire Brigades	NFPA 600
Standard on Fire Department Incident Management System	NFPA 1561

or the community beyond the physical bounds of the facility itself. Facilities that involve hazardous activities and agents such as chemicals, radiation sources, infectious agents, high-energy equipment, or temperature critical processes have greater probability for unplanned incidents than do commercial offices. Virtually every building, process, service, or installation has the potential for an emergency. The first planning team effort should focus on identification of potential site-specific emergencies. A generic or laundry list pulled from a safety manual may omit critical issues at that particular facility because of the unique nature of the business, its location, outside resources, or staffing level.

The business activities, materials involved in production, degree of fire protection, and degree of emergency preparedness training should be considered when assessing hazards. The emergency response planning team relies on the occupational hygienist to recognize the workplace hazards present in that facility and to anticipate the risks to human health and safety should an unplanned event occur. Emergency response planning should include any potential health and safety concerns for neighboring residences and businesses as well as the possibility for transportation incidents and customer emergencies.

Emergency Types

A variety of hazards that could cause emergency situations may be present for any type of business or facility. The risk management (or containment) capability of even the best-prepared emergency plan can be taxed, depending on whether the emergency condition originates from within or outside the facility. Table 44.3 lists five categories of emergency—natural disasters, human error, process error, equipment failure, and terrorism—and includes several examples for each classification. This table is intended as a starting point in the planning process. Site-specific items should be considered in addition to these examples.

Natural disasters, including severe weather, can halt operations without warning, creating as much risk of an emergency as can an explosion. Geographic location governs to what extent natural disasters should be included in the emergency plan. Risk assessment guidance may be obtained from federal, state, county, and city emergency management offices. Hurricanes may be endemic to coastal areas, whereas tornadoes, floods, and winter storms might be more prevalent in other locations. Warnings for these potential weather situations are the responsibility of the National Weather Service. Some facilities must consider earthquakes, avalanches, and volcanic eruptions in their planning. The Federal Emergency Management Agency can assist the ERP team in assessing the risk of these disasters for a facility in the United States.

Natural disasters have the associated risk of utility outages and interruption of essential services that may cause unsafe conditions to develop, thereby necessitating fail-safe or redundant engineering design for loss prevention. Timely evacuations and process shutdowns can prevent injury and health risks to employees when adequate natural disaster warnings are available. Some facilities may be linked to services such as natural gas, electrical utilities, or pipeline feedstock from off-site suppliers and may be affected by their equipment or process failures. Regardless of the cause of the service interruption (e.g., traffic accident involving a critical utility pole, severe weather, provider equipment failure), the potential detrimental effect could result in a chain of uncontrollable emergency events such as fires, explosions, or chemical releases. The timing required to replace or repair the service interruption can determine the impact

Table 44.3 — Categories of Emergency for Emergency Response Planning

Natural Disasters	*Human Error*	*Process Error*	*Equipment Failure*	*Terrorism*
severe weather	vehicle impact	process overheat	utility outages	bioterrorism
floods	confined space entry	process overflow	valve leaks	chemical terrorism
earthquakes	aircraft crashes	vapor release	chemical spills	sabotage threats
avalanches	packaging failures	explosions	fires	radiation terrorism
volcanic eruptions	public/civil disturbances		community noise	radiation accidents

Note: In reviewing the examples, realize that any of these events may cause personal injuries and illness.

on the facility operations, and appropriate preplanning should account for the risks associated with these outages.

Fires, explosions, radiation exposures, and chemical spills or releases are obvious hazards with high risk potential in some businesses. Although some facilities may plan to evacuate for some of these scenarios, others may determine that the appropriate action would be to "shelter in place" in their building with air intake equipment to the building turned off.

The occupational hygienist can provide vital insight into the health risks associated with these scenarios to achieve the safest emergency response actions for everyone. Emergency planning is necessary to direct emergency responders in remote locations regarding viable response actions. Emergency responders might also have the potential to respond to high visibility or controversial community complaints about excessive noise, environmental spills, or odors. Transportation and shipping accidents can occur anywhere between the manufacturer and its destination. Rail cars, tank trucks, cargo planes, marine vessels, and mail services that handle products may be the unintentional cause or target of an accidental spill or release involving human health risks or environmental damage. Where there is a community health concern, businesses usually rely on their occupational hygiene, medical, toxicology, and public relations personnel to interface with the media and the public to explain the associated health risks of the emergency. Anticipation of these situations may not preclude their occurrence, but certainly will make community explanations more credible if appropriate emergency responses are predetermined.

Biological hazards for responders and nearby workers may exist from contact with body fluids (e.g., blood, vomit, saliva) from injured victims, biotechnology releases, or sick personnel. Although the safety and health of injured victims is the first priority in emergency response, consideration for the health of emergency responders is also important. Recognition of this potential, anticipation of the correct protective clothing (along with proper donning, doffing, decontamination, and disposal), and training are the responsibilities of the occupational hygienist and medical personnel. The ERP team should consider the provisions required in OSHA's Bloodborne Pathogens standard (29 CFR 1910.1030) and any guidelines available from the Centers for Disease Control and Prevention for protection from infectious diseases (including those spread by bioterrorism), which outline specific procedures for emergency medical technicians and other medical providers to use to protect themselves from occupational exposure to blood or other potentially infectious materials (e.g., AIDS, tuberculosis, hepatitis, bioterrorism agents).[5,6]

A discussion of potential emergencies would not be complete without mention of emergencies caused intentionally by individuals. This type of emergency may involve personnel health concerns from accidental injury, illness, or life-threatening situations such as terrorism. Emergency response planning for risks associated with terrorism, workplace violence, sabotage, bomb threats, strikes, and civil unrest must be considered. No one expects these scenarios to happen in the workplace, but adequate thought and planning could reduce the risk—or better yet, the occurrence—of injury and economic loss if they do. In listing the types and nature of potential emergencies for the organization, an assessment can be made of impacts affecting the health and safety of people or those events with purely economic consequences (crisis management of a facility shutdown due to terrorism, sabotage, or equipment failure). Management must determine the level of risk acceptance for strictly property-impact events. Cost and speed of recovery for the lost or damaged resources will be a factor. Customer consequences also must be considered by management in setting risk acceptance. Damage limited to finished deliverables may be more acceptable to management than impacts on production equipment or creation of long lead-times of the raw material inventory. When planning for an emergency response, business interruption is also an essential emergency planning issue.

Crisis management planning should consider the impact that a community or facility biological, chemical, or radiation terrorism act would incur. Consideration of the safe shutdown of processes and the financial impact of impaired commerce are the initial focuses of planning should there be terrorist acts. Because terrorism can be covert, an index of suspicion (knowledge of the signs and symptoms of the agents of a covert act) should be considered in planning for these emergencies. Special consideration for the impacts of mass quarantines and mass illness, not to mention the panic and fear associated with these attacks, is essential in emergency and crisis planning, because the resources needed to continue work processes may not be available. Workers may be too ill, quarantined, or be too afraid to come to work. There are many helpful publications on planning and responding to terrorism acts, and the hygienist should prepare himself or herself for response to this type of incident. The Centers for Disease Control and Prevention and the World Health Organization, among other agencies and organizations, have assessed the various potential terrorism scenarios and provide risk assessments, scenario planning, and guidance. These resources are continually updated and available from a variety of published sources, including the Internet.[6,7]

Incident Command System for Emergency Response

OSHA's hazardous waste operations and emergency response (HAZWOPER) standard (29 CFR 1910.120) specifies requirements for the establishment and implementation of the ERP when there is potential for the accidental release of hazardous agents. The standard also defines the process for establishing the incident command system (ICS); designation and training of incident commanders, first responders, and HazMat teams; and definition of personnel roles, lines of authority, and communication.[8] It is very important to avoid having too many "commanders" and not enough "responders." Whether the HAZWOPER standard applies to the facilities of interest, the provisions serve as a model for planning for any facility. There must be very clear lines of command, communication, and responsibility. During the planning phase of each scenario establish agreement on who will be the incident commander and the details of an ICS for either site response or response by outside agencies.

The senior emergency response official responding to an emergency should be designated as the individual in charge of a site-specific ICS. All emergency responders and their communications are coordinated and controlled through the individual in charge of the ICS assisted by the senior official present from management of the facility. The senior official at an emergency response is the most senior official on the site who has the responsibility for controlling the operations at the site. Initially, it is the senior officer on the first piece of responding emergency apparatus to arrive on the incident scene. As more senior officers arrive (e.g., battalion chief, fire chief, state law enforcement official, site coordinator) the position is passed up the line of authority, which has been previously established.

The individual in charge of the ICS should identify, to the extent possible, all hazardous substances or conditions present and address, as appropriate, site analysis; use of engineering controls; emergency response guidelines; exposure limits; hazardous substance handling procedures; and use of any new technologies. The incident commander should limit the number of emergency response personnel at the emergency site in areas of potential or actual exposure to those who are actively performing emergency operations. Back-up personnel should be standing by with equipment ready to provide assistance or rescue at the direction of the incident commander. Qualified basic life support personnel, as a minimum, should also be nearby with medical equipment and transportation capability. The incident commander should designate a safety officer, knowledgeable in the operations being implemented at the emergency response site, with the responsibility to identify and evaluate hazards and to provide direction with respect to the safety of operations for the emergency at hand.[8]

ERP Development

The development and practice of the ERP should include representatives from all operating areas of the business or commercial entity, including environmental, health, safety, and occupational hygiene. To be effective the ERP needs to be well understood and known by all on the property. This includes contractors and other on-site visitors.

The hazard and risk assessment provides internal guidance and good emergency management practices to the organization and should provide the foundation for the development of the ERP. Emergency response planning requires site response teamwork with outside services (e.g., local HazMat teams, fire brigades, hospitals, and police). The appropriate ERP team members, including community responders, should be determined based on the types of potential risks for the facility.

Emergency management in this general context includes chemical, biological, and radiation inventories; hazard analysis; consequence assessment; and development of emergency plans (including protective actions) for workers, uninvolved workers, and the general public. Once the risks are prioritized based on probability of occurrence and impact on workers, community, and environment, credible scenarios should be developed. For example, hurricanes can have devastating impacts on a facility, but if the business location is not in a coastal area, priority for emergency response planning for hurricanes would be less than that for fires or evacuations. When there is equal probability of risks occurring, then the planning priority should be higher for those with the most impact on the health of workers or community residents, and secondarily for economic losses.

An effective ERP depends on proper coordination between the emergency responders and the assignment of responsibilities.[9] The incident command organization and role assignments should be determined and documented during the emergency planning phase, especially for scenarios that involve response from more than one organization or agency. The ERP should document all aspects of an emergency response for each of the various scenarios, including assignment of responsibilities; coordination with outside agencies; procedures to alert employees; escape routes and procedures for accounting for all evacuees; emergency equipment available; and location and training of response personnel. In assigning responsibilities in the plan, keep in mind that variable scheduling, vacations, illness days, and holidays create special demands on response effectiveness. Each risk should be evaluated to determine whether the facility and outside responders have the ability to react adequately.

In looking at the risk assessment list, realize that any of the events may result in chemical, biological, or radiological exposures or personal injuries and illness. The location of the effected site governs the extent to which the facility establishes internal first aid capability. In an urban location with ample local medical and ambulance services a telephone call to 911 may be the only emergency action needed. In a rural setting well-trained emergency medical technicians and first aid supplies become more critical within the facility. This resource is a valuable consideration in any emergency plan, because outside response may be unreliable depending on the community impact of the emergency. Consider in the development of an ERP the types of medical emergencies that are most probable, may be possible, or are unlikely to occur. A combination of events, including inclement weather and a train derailment, should be well thought out as part of the ERP. Could a nearby fire, traffic accident, or blocked intersection prevent emergency responders from reaching the facility? Could such an event block the only access driveway from the property? In a situation known to the authors the only community hospital for three towns was located on the fence line of a major chemical company comprised of 87 different manufacturing plants at that location. After assessing the risks imposed by the plant on the hospital staff, patients, and their ability to respond in the event of a major emergency, the company donated land for the relocation of the hospital away from the risks associated with being located near the plant.

Site security during emergencies is an additional concern that should be part of the ERP. This starts with directing evacuees, responders, curious spectators, and the news media to a safe location well clear of emergency control activities.

The plan should also name an assigned spokesperson to answer questions from community leaders, the public, and the news media. Other personnel should defer all outside questions to the designated individual or spokesperson. Some firms make this a function of the legal staff, public relations, or senior management.

Communication capabilities during emergency response are crucial. Once evacuated from a building, telephones are of no value. Cellular phones, commercial two-way radios, or portable megaphones allow directions to be communicated to the many people involved. One drawback of this technology is that community members can monitor and misinterpret what is said during emergencies unless messages are scrambled or encoded. In addition to communicating during an emergency, provision for summoning emergency responders should be made in case facility telephones cease working. Pagers worn by on-call emergency responders make response time much quicker than in the past, when the city siren was the summoning device.

It may be prudent for a company to help public responders by providing facility tours and a copy of the emergency plan. Familiarity with the site, its operations, and its materials may help ensure a proper response should it become necessary. Such cooperation with the emergency response community helps assure reliable, competent emergency event handling while also building good will.

Interview-based templates for ERP development are available from a number of publishers in a variety of formats (hard copy versus electronic) but are too numerous to list in the Additional Sources section. These templates may not include all the potential scenarios for a facility, but they provide a strong basis for the most common emergency risks. The written ERP can be divided into sections that address emergency plans within the various categories of emergencies, as well as sections for community, transportation, and customer-related emergencies. The ERP also should include maps of the facility and its exit routes, line diagrams of utilities and process lines, locations of shut-off valves, and a list of hazardous agents inside the facility. The written ERP must be accessible to all employees at all times and should be stored for easy retrieval should an emergency arise. Its storage near the likely source of an emergency would be imprudent, because the emergency response team might need to use it for guidance during an unplanned event.

ERP Drills and Preparedness

Once the ERP is complete, the effectiveness of the plan should be tested regularly through drills and mock emergencies (e.g., annually or quarterly), and, when possible, should include outside responders. Practice through drills provides two important facets to the preparedness for an emergency. First, a drill or mock emergency provides a training opportunity, so all participants know exactly what their responses should be for a given situation and can practice their assigned responsibilities. It is much easier to remember what is expected, and panic is less likely, if one has gone through the drill before the emergency occurs. The second point of value is the opportunity to assess the emergency drill for improvements to the ERP. Visitors to the facility may not know what to do, or a key responsibility or need may have been overlooked. Perhaps the training of community responders was inadequate, equipment was unavailable or inaccessible, or perhaps an important aspect of the emergency response was not performed because someone was on vacation or designated as injured in the drill. In the latter situation, a primary and two levels of trained alternate responders may be needed. Whatever deficiencies are identified, take the opportunity to find a solution so that they will not be repeated during the real emergency. Once the drill or mock emergency has been evaluated, the ERP should be reviewed and updated with all of the corrective actions and recommendations documented. Also, if anything was learned that might help prevent future unplanned events, this might be an opportunity to develop a preventive response plan or facility safe operating procedures such as sign-in books or on-call responders.

Occupational Hygienist Roles in Emergency Response

Roles in ERP Development

The occupational hygienist is expected to aid in the development of the ERP by identifying health hazards that might arise in an emergency based on possible scenarios. Familiarity with material safety data sheets (MSDSs) and the likely routes of chemical exposure in each emergency situation help determine whether to evacuate the premises, shelter in place, or remain to mitigate the emergency. MSDSs provide a wealth of information regarding the potential health effects of exposures, the type of PPE to be worn by responders, physical and chemical properties of the substance, and the regulations and requirements that might apply to the facility during an emergency. Some MSDSs also include proper decontamination and disposal procedures for PPE.

Occupational hygienists may be asked to train emergency responders on aspects of the ERP, such as HAZWOPER, health hazards and risks, odor thresholds, or the National Institute for Occupational Safety and Health's (NIOSH's) immediately-dangerous-to-life-and-health guidelines (IDLH),[10] and proper PPE for response. The hygienist should identify emergency responders in the facility who are required to be in a medical surveillance program, directing the content, frequency, and adequacy of examinations and physicals for compliance purposes. The hygienist should identify personnel who must wear respiratory protection during emergency response so that medical certification, respirator training, and respirator fit testing are conducted according to 29 CFR 1910.134 requirements. The emergency responders must be medically fit to wear a respirator as certified by specific tests run by a physician, must be clean shaven, be respirator fit-tested every 2 years for the specific type of SCBA they will wear, and must be trained in the safe use, limitations, and maintenance of the respirator they will wear.

Community Exposure Guidelines

Hygienists also provide expertise in estimating health effects of exposures to workers, community members, or responders with the aid of various community guidelines for acute exposure. A variety of concentration-limit guidelines may be used in emergency planning for various chemicals. Preference should be given to guidelines developed specifically for use in emergency exposure conditions and planning, and specifically to those that have been peer-reviewed and published for that purpose. The American Industrial Hygiene Association's (AIHA®) Emergency Response Planning Guidelines (ERPGs)[11] or EPA's Acute Exposure Guideline Levels (AEGLs)[12] are developed based on an assessment of the health risks in extensive peer-review processes and are published regularly. ERPGs are available annually from AIHA® in the *ERPG/WEEL Handbook*. AEGLs, available from EPA, are published in the United States *Federal Register*. Supporting technical documents for each ERPG or AEGL are also published and should be reviewed by the hygienist during the consultation process. These are available from AIHA and EPA, respectively.

The number of approved ERPGs and AEGLs is extremely limited compared with the number of chemicals for which values are needed for emergency planning. The Department of Energy (DOE) Subcommittee on Consequence Assessment on Protective Actions developed Temporary Emergency Exposure Limits (TEELs)[13,14] to fill the gaps where there are no ERPGs or AEGLs. In fact, some of the chemicals for which the TEELs are developed may be too obscure to ever be on a priority list for community exposure limit development. Although TEELs are not peer-reviewed, the methodology for their development is consistent with health-based criteria for setting ERPGs and AEGLs.

The main distinction between the ERPGs, AEGLs, and TEELs is the exposure time component, and this must be factored into the risk assessment planning and actual emergency response. ERPG levels 1, 2, and 3 are based on a 1-hour exposure time for a total of 3 values. AEGL levels 1, 2, and 3 have 10-minute; 30-minute; and 1-, 4-, and 8-hour values for a total of 15 values. The four levels of TEEL values are based on a 15-minute time-weighted average (similar to a short-term exposure limit) for a total of 4 values. All of these guidelines are estimates of concentration ranges above which acute exposure would be expected to lead to adverse health effects of increasing severity for concentrations at levels 1, 2, and 3. The level 3 values for ERPGs, AEGLs, and TEELs are the estimated threshold concentrations above which deaths could occur.[14,15] Level 2 values are the estimated threshold above which severe, irreversible health effects would occur, and when individuals would have difficulty in their efforts to escape the emergency. Level 1 values are threshold concentrations below which nearly all individuals could be exposed without experiencing other than mild, transient, adverse health effects or perceiving a clearly defined objectionable odor. The TEELs incorporate a fourth level of "0," which is "a threshold below which most people will experience no appreciable risk of health effects."[14]

Other guideline values have been set by EPA, the National Academy of Sciences Committee on Toxicology (NAS/COT), U.S.

Federal Emergency Management Agency (FEMA), and the U.S. Department of Transportation (DOT). Emergency Exposure Guidance Levels (EEGL), set by NAS, and levels of concern (LOCs), set by EPA, FEMA, and DOT, were developed specifically for emergency exposure conditions, but the documentation supporting those values is not published. NAS also developed Continuous Exposure Guidance Levels (CEGLs) and five short-term exposure guidance levels (SPEGLs).[16–18] The CEGLs are not appropriate for the typical emergency exposure times, and therefore are not recommended for use in emergency planning. SPEGLs may be used for this purpose, but exist for only five chemicals.[18]

ERPG and AEGL values should be used as the primary guidelines for chemical emergency planning. When ERPGs and AEGLs are not available, it is recommend that an alternative exposure limit parameter hierarchy be followed (Table 44.4).[18]

The hygienist should compare these values with the published odor threshold values to ensure that planning for community recognition of an annoying odor would be appropriately considered. An odor that is below the detection limit of our equipment or the level 1 of the community exposure guidelines can result in hospitalization of a member of the public, as "perception is reality to those who perceive it." Hygienists can obtain further clarification on use and planning from the respective organizations setting these values. Hygienists should keep in mind that occupational exposure limits are not applicable to members of the general public (including children, elderly, sick, etc.), and conversely, community exposure limits are not applicable to the occupational setting.

DOE recommends that in emergency cases when there is a release or spill of a mixture of chemicals, hygienists should consider additive, synergistic, or antagonistic health effects. It is recommended that a hazardiIndex ($HI_i=C_i/ERPG_i$, where C_i is the concentration of chemical i) be calculated for each chemical, and unless sufficient toxicological knowledge is available to indicate otherwise, that they be summed. That is:

$$\sum_{i=1}^{n}, \text{ where } HI_i = HI_1 + HI_2 + \ldots + HI_n \qquad (44\text{-}1)$$

A sum of 1.0 or less means the limits have not been exceeded.[19]

Table 44.4 — Recommended Hierarchy of Emergency Planning Guidelines

Primary Guideline	*Hierarchy of Alternative Guidelines*	*Source of Exposure-Limit Concentration (†)*
ERPG-3 or AEGL-3[11,12]		AIHA or EPA
	TEEL-3[13,14]	DOE (SCAPA)[A]
	EEGL (30-min)[16,17]	NAS (COT)
	IDLH(10)	NIOSH
ERPG-2 or AEGL-2[10,11]		
	TEEL-2[13,14]	DOE (SCAPA)
	EEGL (60-min)[16,17]	NAS (COT)
	LOC[21,22]	EPA; FEMA;[B] DOT[C]
	$PEL_{Ceiling}$[2]	OSHA
	$TLV_{Ceiling}$[23]	ACGIH[D]
	TLV_{TWA} X 5[23]	ACGIH
ERPG-1 or AEGL-1[10,11]		
	TEEL-1[13,14]	DOE (SCAPA)
	PEL_{STEL}[2]	OSHA
	TLV_{STEL}[23]	ACGIH
	TLV_{TWA} X 3[23]	ACGIH

Source: Reference 13.
Note: PEL = permissible exposure limit; TLV® = threshold limit value; STEL = short-term exposure limit.
[A]DOE = U.S. Department of Energy (Subcommittee on Consequence Assessment on Protective Actions (SCAPA)
[B]FEMA = Federal Emergency Management Agency
[C]DOT = U.S. Department of Transportation
[D]ACGIH = American Conference of Governmental Industrial Hygienists

Globally, governments now require facilities that may affect the community through spills and releases to communicate the hazards, risks, and the zones of impact to those potentially affected. EPA's Risk Management Program rule (40 CFR Part 68) requires community exposure risk assessments and hazard communication, specifying the process and required outcomes.[20] Hygienists should assist management or incident command in planning the community alert and response process and should assist in the determination of when it is "safe" to return to the area. The hygienist should also be familiar with any computerized modeling equipment (e.g., ALOHA, Daisy Mae, or MIDAS) used by the facility to model, predict, or measure chemical release concentrations at various locations within or outside the facility boundaries. These models utilize ERPGs, AEGLs, or TEELs as the basis for predicting what actions should be taken at predicted concentrations in a particular release scenario.

The hygienist is also responsible for anticipating the proper PPE for reentry into a mitigated emergency either by direct measurement of remaining concentrations or by the use of dilution ventilation calculations. The prepared occupational hygienist will ascertain and obtain the proper chemical or radiation monitoring equipment and be familiar with its use and limitations prior to emergencies. If the equipment is not available, documenting chemical-specific dilution calculations ahead of time ensures that the needed data is available if an emergency occurs.

Planned communication procedures used during emergencies should include the hygienist so that constant consultation is available as the emergency unfolds.

Roles During Emergency Response

The occupational hygienist is part of the emergency scene management team once an emergency situation occurs and is consulted by management or the incident commander throughout. Based on the roles and responsibilities assigned in the ERP for the ICS, the hygienist's role during emergency response may include performing initial health risk assessments at the scene using direct measurement equipment or vapor concentration calculations. Health risks to community members may be provided to the incident commander or management based on predicted movement of a vapor release. Consultations on proper PPE for unplanned events might be needed, as well as reminders of the need for a buddy system when entering an emergency situation if the concentrations of vapor or smoke are not known. The hygienist might be assigned the duty of actually donning appropriate PPE and entering the emergency scene to evaluate the identity or concentration of a chemical in a release situation or to determine whether decontamination and cleanup can be performed. Frequently this means using direct-reading equipment or media to measure concentrations of chemical vapors, explosive atmospheres, or low-oxygen situations. Other response situations may require that the hygienist suit up properly and evaluate fence-line concentrations to verify computerized models of vapor releases for community alerts. These measured concentration values are important in validation of "predicted" concentrations and can be used in agency reporting or analysis of scenario planning. Medical providers will need to consult with the hygienist during triage of those injured in the emergency to determine what exposures, if any, might have occurred so that proper treatment can be given.

Once the emergency is over, the hygienist may need to identify workers, responders, or community members affected by the emergency for medical evaluation. If a chemical release or spill has occurred, there may be reporting requirements to federal and state organizations such as OSHA and EPA, whether or not there have been exposures. This is often the responsibility of the occupational hygienist.

Root cause investigations and assessments of the emergency response from the hygienist's perspective are required as follow-up. There is always educational value in revisiting the emergency to determine what went right, went wrong, and should be anticipated for the next situation. A review and update of the ERP should include any educational experiences from the actual response. Applying these lessons to other emergency scenarios is appropriate and may help identify ways to prevent unplanned events in the future.

Audits of ERPs

General Audit

Audits of the ERP should be made regularly (e.g., annually or more frequent) to reassess whether it is current. The audit should be made on all aspects of the plan and should include the planning process; the risk assessment; assignment of responder responsibilities; training; drills; reviews; and updates. An audit of community responder facilities may be appropriate to ensure that their availability, proximity, and plans coincide with the facility's expectations as outlined in the ERP. First aid supplies and emergency equipment needed by the responders should be quickly accessible, ready to use, and adequate to meet expectations.[8] There are ERP audit checklists available in the listed resources at the end of this chapter. Regardless of the audit checklist used, the most important aspect of the process is the follow-up with corrective actions and recommendations. These are opportunities to review the ERP with a third party who can provide another perspective on the plan. Documentation of the follow-up completed in response to deficiencies is important to show that the ERP is part of the continuous improvement process.

Occupational Hygiene Aspects of the ERP Audit

The occupational hygiene section of the ERP audit should evaluate the health risk assessment plans, training of workers and responders on health risks, medical surveillance, and PPE elements of emergency planning. Because training is vital to the success of the actual emergency response, it is the most important aspect of the occupational hygiene audit of an ERP. Auditors should determine whether the exact training needs of all applicable regulations have been met (e.g., HAZWOPER training requires 8 to 40 hours). Although training documentation and sign-in sheets may prove that training has been done, the audit should use interviews with responders and facility personnel to evaluate whether the training program was effective.

Another aspect of the occupational hygiene audit should focus on the PPE for the emergency responders to assure that it is appropriate for the hazards that might be encountered. Equipment used for emergency response must be inspected periodically and documented to ensure that it is still available in the designated location, effective, clean, and ready to use. The storage locations must be assessed to determine whether they are accessible during emergency situations or whether they are too close to an identified risk area.[8]

Medical surveillance of emergency responders should be up to date, and health exams, medical approval for respirator use, and fit testing should be documented. The content of the physicals should be assessed during the audit to determine the quality of the medical examinations. The names of employees for whom medical limitations (e.g., respirators or weight limits) have been determined during medical surveillance should be noted to prevent responder emergencies occurring from unrealistic expectations of their abilities. Remember that medical records are confidential.

Summary

Emergency response preparedness is most effectively achieved through extensive emergency risk assessment, development of the ERP, and subsequent drills and audits. Emergency response teams are limited in their action by the severity of the unplanned event, emergency preparedness, and adequacy of training. The role of the occupational hygienist in this process is to provide insight in the area of health risk and exposure assessment. Particular areas of expertise are health regulations and requirements, PPE, air monitoring, training, and auditing of the ERP. Occupational hygienists may be called on in community emergencies to anticipate the potential exposures and impacts of the emergency on the community. Hygienists should keep in mind that occupational exposure limits are not applicable to members of the general public (including children, elderly, sick, etc.), and conversely, community exposure limits are not applicable to the occupational setting. Knowing limitations—and knowing what, with whom, where, when, and how to proceed during emergency response—should significantly lower the impacts of unplanned events on the health of employees and the community and also should reduce financial losses.

Additional Sources

Centers for Disease Control and Prevention website: www.cdc.gov

U.S. Department of Energy (DOE SCAPA) website for TEELs: www.bnl.gov/scapa/

American Industrial Hygiene Association (AIHA): *AIHA 2001 Emergency Response Planning Guidelines and Workplace Environmental Exposure Level Guides Handbook.* Fairfax, Va.: AIHA Press, 2001.

American Industrial Hygiene Association (AIHA): *Documentation of ERPG Values.* Fairfax, Va.: AIHA Press, 2001.

American Society for Testing and Materials (ASTM): *Safe Handling of Hazardous Materials Accidents,* 2nd ed. Philadelphia: ASTM, 1990.

L.P. Andrews: *Emergency Responder Training Manual for the Hazardous Materials Technician.* New York: Van Nostrand Reinhold, 1992.

W.A. Burgess: *Recognition of Health Hazards in Industry: A Review of Materials and Processes,* 2nd ed. New York: John Wiley & Sons, 1995.

T.A. Burke (ed.): *Regulating Risk: The Science and Politics of Risk.* Washington, D.C.: International Life Sciences Institute, 1993.

R.G. Campbell and R.E. Langford: *Introduction to Hazardous Materials Incidents.* Boca Raton, Fla,: Lewis Publishers, 1991.

N.P. Cheremisinoff: *Handbook of Emergency Response and Toxic Chemical Releases: A Guide to Compliance.* Morganville, N.J.: SciTech Publishers, 1995.

T.S. Ferry: *Modern Accident Investigation and Analysis,* 2nd ed. New York: John Wiley & Sons, 1988.

J.W. Hosty: *A Practical Guide to Chemical Spill Response.* New York: Van Nostrand Reinhold, 1992.

R.B. Kelley: *Industrial Emergency Preparedness.* New York: Van Nostrand Reinhold, 1989.

J.D. Kipp and M.E. Loflin: *Emergency Incident Risk Management: A Safety & Health Perspective.* New York: Van Nostrand Reinhold, 1996.

T. Kletz: *What Went Wrong? Case Histories of Process Plant Disasters.* Houston: Gulf Publishing, 1998.

J.P. Kohn, M.A. Friend, and C.A. Winterberger: *Fundamentals of Occupational Safety and Health.* Rockville, Md.: Government Institutes, 1996.

P.A. Michaud: *Accident Prevention and OSHA Compliance.* Boca Raton, Fla.: Lewis Publishers, 1995.

National Institute for Occupational Safety and Health (NIOSH): *NIOSH Pocket Guide to Chemical Hazards.* Cincinnati, Ohio: NIOSH, 1994.

National Safety Council (NSC): *Accident Investigation.* Itasca, Ill.: NSC, 1995.

National Safety Council (NSC): *Accident Prevention Manual for Business and Industry: Engineering and Technology,* vol. 2, 10 ed. Itasca, Ill.: NSC, 1996.

National Safety Council (NSC): *Guide for Identifying Causal Factors and Corrective Actions.* Itasca, Ill.: NSC, 1996.

National Safety Council (NSC): *Study Guide: Accident Prevention manual for Business and Industry,* 10th ed. Itasca, Ill.: NSC, 1996.

G.M. Rusch: The history and development of emergency response planning guidelines. *J. Haz. Mat. 33*:192–202 (1993).

T.D. Schneid: *Fire Law: The Liabilities and Rights of the Fire Service.* New York: Van Nostrand Reinhold, 1995.

L. Theodore: *Accident and Emergency Management.* New York: John Wiley & Sons, 1989.

U.S. Environmental Protection Agency (EPA): *EPA Training Manual: Emergency Response to Hazardous Material Incidents* (Manual 165.15). Washington, D.C.: EPA, 1995.

J.W. Vincoli: *Basic Guide to Accident Investigation and Loss Control.* New York: Van Nostrand Reinhold, 1994.

Transport Canada, U.S. Department of Transportation, and the Secretariat of Communications and Transportation of Mexico: *2000 North American Emergency Response Guidebook.* Available at http://hazmat.dot.gov/erg2000/erg2000.pdf (2000).

References

1. "Employee Emergency Plans and Fire Prevention Plans." *Code of Federal Regulations* Title 29, Part 1938 (2003).
2. "Toxic and Hazardous Substances." *Code of Federal Regulations* Title 29, Part 1910 Subpart Z (2003).
3. **Stringfield, W.H.:** *Emergency Planning and Management: Ensuring Your Company's Survival in the Event of a Disaster.* Rockville, Md.: Government Institutes, 1996.
4. "Fire Protection." *Code of Federal Regulations* Title 29, Part 1910, Subpart L, Appendix B (2003).
5. "Bloodborne Pathogens." *Code of Federal Regulations* Title 29, Part 1910, Subpart Z, 1910.1030 (2003).
6. **Centers for Disease Control and Prevention:** "CDC Public Health Emergency Preparedness & Response Site." Available at www.cdc.gov (Accessed February 2003).
7. **World Health Organization:** *Health Aspects of Chemical and Biological Weapons.* Upton, N.Y.: Brookhaven National Laboratories, Associated Universities, 2002.

8. "Occupational Safety and Health Administration: Hazardous Waste Operations and Emergency Response. *Code of Federal Regulations* Title 29, Part 1910.120 (2003).
9. **Leibowitz, A.J.:** *Industrial Hygiene Auditing, A Manual for Practice.* Fairfax, Va.: American Industrial Hygiene Association, 1995.
10. **National Institute for Occupational Safety and Health (NIOSH):** *NIOSH Pocket Guide to Chemical Hazards.* Washington, D.C.: NIOSH, 1997.
11. **American Industrial Hygiene Association (AIHA):** *Emergency Response Planning Guidelines and Workplace Environmental Exposure Level Guides.* Fairfax, Va.: AIHA, 2003.
12. "Establishment of a National Advisory Committee for Acute Exposure Guideline Levels (AEGLs) for Hazardous Substances." *Federal Register* 60:55376-55377 (31 Oct. 1995).
13. **Department of Energy Subcommittee on Consequence Assessment on Protective Actions:** *TEEL Revision/Update Status and TEEL List.* Available at www.bnl.gov/scapa/. (Accessed February 2003).
14. **Craig, D.K., J.S. Davis, D.J. Hansen, and A.J. Petrocchi:** Derivation of temporary emergency exposure limits (TEELs). *J. Appl. Toxicol. 20*:11–20 (2000).
15. **AIHA ERPG Committee:** *Concepts and Procedures for the Development of Emergency Response Planning Guidelines (ERPGs).* Fairfax, Va.: American Industrial Hygiene Association, 1989.
16. **National Academy of Sciences:** *Criteria and Methods for Preparing Emergency Exposure Guidance Level (EEGL), Short-Term Public Emergency Guidance Level (SPEGL), and Continuous Exposure Guidance Level (CEGL) Documents.* Washington, D.C.: National Academy Press, 1986.
17. **Committee on Toxicology, Board on Environmental Studies and Toxicology, National Academy of Sciences:** *Emergency and Continuous Exposure Guidance Levels for Selected Airborne Contaminants,* vols. 1–7. Washington, D.C.: National Academy Press, 1985.
18. **Craig, D.K., J.S. Davis, R. Devore, D.J. Hansen, A.J. Petrocchi, and T.J. Powell:** Alternative guideline limits for chemicals without Environmental Response Planning Guidelines. *Am. Ind. Hyg. Assoc. J. 56*:919–925 (1995).
19. **Craig, D.K., R.L. Baskett, J.S. Davis, et al.:** Recommended default methodology for analysis of airborne exposures to mixtures of chemicals in emergencies. *Appl. Occup. Environ. Hyg. 14*:609–617 (1999).
20. "Accidental Release Prevention Requirements: Risk Management Programs Under the Clean Air Act, Section 112(r)(7); List of Regulated Substances and Thresholds for Accidental Release Prevention, Stay of Effectiveness; and Accidental Release Prevention Programs Under Section 112 (r) (7) of the Clean Air Act as Amended, Guidelines; Final Rules and Notice." *Code of Federal Regulations* Title 40, Part 68 (2002).
21. **U.S. Department of Transportation (DOT):** *Documentation for the Health Criteria Used to Derive U.S. DOT Initial Isolation and Evacuation Zones.* Washington, D.C.: DOT Research and Special Programs Administration, 1995.
22. **U.S. Environmental Protection Agency, Federal Emergency Management Agency, and U.S. Department of Transportation:** *Technical Guidance for Hazards Analysis. Emergency Planning for Extremely Hazardous Substances* (EPA-OSWER-88-0001). Washington D.C.: U.S. Government Printing Office, 1991.
23. **American Conference of Governmental Industrial Hygienists (ACGIH):** *2002 TLV®s and BEI®s. Threshold Limit Values for Chemical Substances and Physical Agents; Biological Exposure Indices.* Cincinnati, Ohio: ACGIH, 2002.

Outcome Competencies

After completing this chapter, the reader should be able to:

1. Define underlined terms used in this chapter.
2. Become familiar with the laws that mandate risk communication.
3. Distinguish between types of and approaches to risk communication.
4. Explain the principles on which risk communication is based.
5. Describe an effective risk communication plan.
6. Recognize the importance of crisis communication and the media.

Key Terms

hazard • perceived risk • risk • risk assessment • risk communication • risk management • risk managers • stakeholder

Prerequisite Knowledge

Prior to beginning this chapter, the user should review the following chapters:

Chapter Number	Chapter Topic
1	History of Industrial Hygiene
3	Legal Aspects of Industrial Hygiene
7	Principles of Evaluating Worker Exposure
8	Occupational and Environmental Health Risk Assessment
9	Comprehensive Exposure Assessment
33	Occupational Health Psychology
41	Program Management
43	Hazard Communication

Key Topics

I. Historical View of Risk Communication

II. Regulatory Basis for Conducting RC
   A. EPA Regulations and Websites
   B. Occupational Safety and Health Administration (OSHA) Regulations and Websites

III. RC Models: Approaches, Applications Challenges, and Guidelines
   A. National Research Council
   B. Mental Models Approach
   C. Risk = Hazard + Outrage Approach
   D. Trust and Credibility Approach
   E. Crisis Communication
   F. RC Challenges
   G. Basic RC Guidelines
   H. Summary

IV. The News Media and Risk Issues: Five Key Steps You Need to Know
   A. Step 1: Fully Understand the Issue
   B. Step 2: Media Relationships
   C. Step 3: What Is Your Message?
   D. Step 4: Anticipation, Practice, and Performance
   E. Step 5: Become a Student of Media Relations

V. Developing an RC Plan
   A. The RC Team
   B. The RC Plan
   C. The RC Process

Risk Communication

45

By Paul B. Gillooly, PhD; Terry Flynn, MS, APR; Heidi E. Maupin, MS, PE ; Mary Ann Simmons, BS, CHMM; and Sarah M. Forrest, BS

Introduction

In recent years the public has become more aware of issues regarding environmental, health, and safety risks and less willing to accept these risks without both information to understand the cause and a chance to provide input into the management and handling of the risks. Whether it is communicating with plant workers on issues such as a cancer cluster in their workplace, or a cancer cluster in the community perceived to be caused by plant activities or hazardous waste disposal practices, the ability to communicate effectively may have a profound impact on stakeholder safety and health, and ultimately, the plant's success. Skill and competency in risk communication (RC) principles are required when these issues become emotional, high stress, and low trust.

Occupational hygienists are called on more and more by management to serve as credible and knowledgeable spokespersons on health risk issues that involve a larger audience than just the workers at the plant. Dealing with the public or other groups on emotional, high-stress, and low trust issues requires specialized communication skills to ensure that the message is heard and understood by all and does not damage the company's reputation and standing in the community. This chapter was written for the occupational hygienist whose responsibilities might include communicating environmental, safety, and occupational health risks and therefore needs good RC skills.

At its most fundamental level, RC is the research-based approach to communicating risk to affected stakeholders. Two key terms that must be defined before any discussion of RC are *risk* and *stakeholder*. Risk, in general, can be defined as the likelihood that injury, damage, or loss will occur as a result of a given hazard. The damage or loss is not always health based and can include anything that is valued such as legal, economic, or political considerations. Similarly, hazard can be defined as a situation with a potential for injury, damage to property, or damage to the environment. A stakeholder is anyone who might be affected by a risk or a decision based on a risk, whether real or perceived. The type of risk determines who the stakeholders are and may include groups such as workers, worker's families, management, local community, the general public, the media, and other scientists.

RC differs from the usual communication of technical or scientific information in that it most often involves two-way communication between the organization managing the risk and the affected stakeholders. In many cases the stakeholders participate in the decision-making process regarding the management of the risk. It requires specialized skills, because simply disseminating information without regard for communicating the complexities and uncertainties of risk is typically not effective when addressing concerns and questions from upset, angry, or distrustful stakeholders. Effective RC is a skill that takes planning, practice, and experience. As the National Research Council stated, "Many decisions can be better informed and their information base can be more credible if the interested and affected parties are appropriately and effectively involved in deliberation."[1]

RC differs from hazard communication, which is a more traditional one-way communication targeted to workers regarding the chemicals (and the physical hazards) they are exposed to in the workplace. OSHA has estimated that more than 32 million workers are exposed to 650,000 hazardous chemical products in more than 3 million American workplaces.[2] The OSHA Hazard Communication Standard requires this to be accomplished by establishing workplace hazard communication programs to include labeling, material safety data sheets, and training. The basic goal of a workplace hazard communication program is to ensure that employers and employees know about work hazards and how to protect themselves so that the incidence of chemical illnesses and injuries can be reduced.

A desired outcome of effective RC is agreement among stakeholders on what is an acceptable level of risk, resulting in an appropriate action or reaction. Effective RC may result in alerting stakeholders to a scientifically determined risk or calming them in the absence of a scientifically determined risk.[3] When risks are perceived to be unacceptable despite the absence of scientifically determined risk evidence, effective RC will calm stakeholders. It can also eliminate the needless spending of resources on actions to make people safe when, in fact, they are already safe.

Some of the goals of RC include the following:

- Establishing, maintaining, and/or increasing trust and credibility
- Allowing affected stakeholders to participate
- Raising awareness of potential hazards
- Educating stakeholders about a risk
- Reaching agreement on how to address a risk
- Informing and improving decision-making
- Fostering understanding and a cceptance of decisions made
- Motivating action

RC is also part of the science of risk assessment and risk management. Risk assessment is the scientific process that characterizes risk, either qualitatively or quantitatively, and determines its probability and outcome. For example, a risk assessment might quantify the number of potential serious side effects from receiving a vaccine. It might also quantify the potential risk to a community of implementing a cleanup remedy of a nearby hazardous waste site.

Risk management use information from the risk assessment and integrates it with other information such as political, social, and economic considerations to make decisions regarding what to do about the risk. These decisions and the process by which they are made are usually communicated to the stakeholders. Frequently, stakeholders participate in the decision-making process.

Communication among stakeholders (including risk managers) can occur using one or a combination of several forms of RC distinguished along functional lines such as care communication, consensus communication, and crisis communication. As with other forms of communication, such as hazard communication, there can be overlap, but each risk issue usually requires a different approach to be effective (see Figure 45.1).

Care communication concerns traditional health and safety risks such as in occupational hygiene and hazard communication. Care communication involves informing and training the worker about hazards to motivate participation in the protective programs (e.g., respiratory protection). Recently, however, this type of communication also has begun to emphasize health care communication or health promotion activities designed to inform employees about health risks such as stress management, nutrition, tobacco cessation, sexual health and responsibility, fitness, and so forth.

Consensus communication seeks to encourage and promote cooperation of stakeholder groups to reach a common ground on how a particular risk will be managed. An example is the community involvement required by Superfund during the cleanup of hazardous waste sites, which requires greater citizen participation, a community relations plan, and methods to alert the community of opportunities for involvement such as fact sheets and media releases.

Crisis communication has taken on particular significance since the terrorist attacks on the World Trade Center and the Pentagon on "9/11," and the subsequent passage of the Homeland Security Act of 2002. To be sure, the list of environmental, safety, and occupational health crises is a long one and includes Three Mile Island, Bhopal (Union Carbide), Tylenol (Johnson & Johnson), Exxon Valdez, Firestone/Bridgestone, and the anthrax attacks to name a few.

When an organization simply responds to an external crisis such as an explosion or accident, the communication goal is usually straightforward, such as instructions to motivate employees to move to a safer location. When an organization is the cause of the crisis, the objective is to effectively communicate ongoing information to employees and key stakeholders. This is usually much more complicated than the previous situation and will have highly complex goals that involve reestablishing trust and credibility, increasing key stakeholders' support, and enhancing the organization's reputation. To successfully weather a crisis requires planning, building precrisis relationships, and a leadership mindset in the organization that allows such preparation to occur.

The remainder of this chapter gives an overview of basic RC research and theory. It includes a brief summary of the history of RC and the regulatory basis, a discussion of several RC models, and general guidelines to follow when dealing with the media and when developing an RC plan. As stated previously, RC is a skill that requires training and practice to be truly effective.

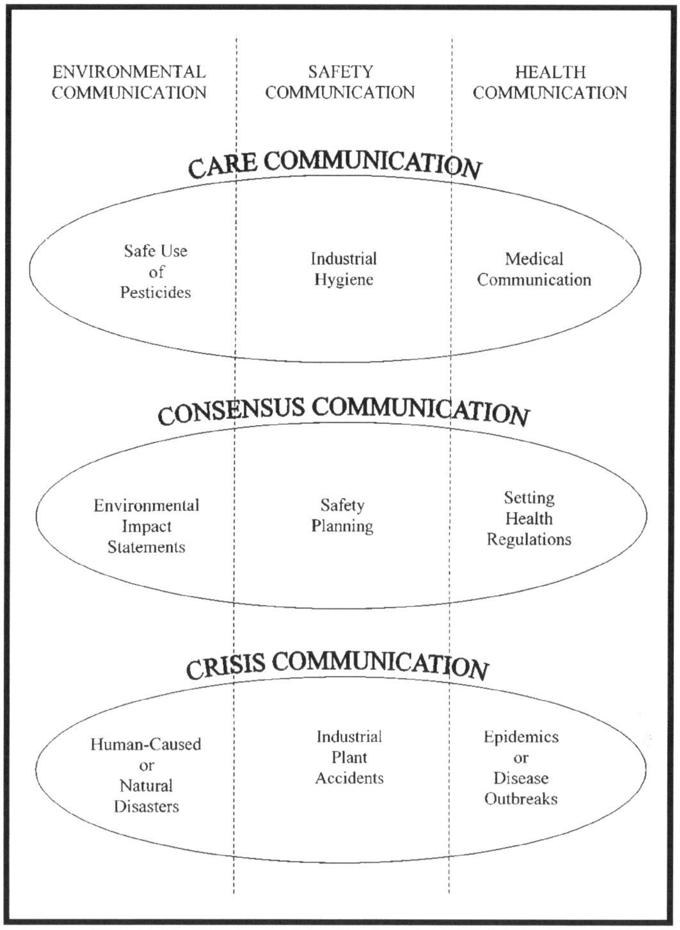

Figure 45.1 — Examples of various types of risk communication. (Adapted from Reference 7.)

Historical View of RC

The history of RC goes back nearly 30 years and is rooted in the environmental movement to educate the public about risks. Public perceptions of risk strongly affect congressional and regulatory actions, such as passage of the Comprehensive Environmental Response, Compensation and Liability Act of 1980 following the 1978 disclosures of problems in Love Canal, N.Y. William Leiss described three phases in the evolution of RC, each emerging in response to the earlier phases.[4]

Phase I emphasized the quantitative expression of risk estimates to the public and argued that regulatory actions and the public's perception of risks should be based on comparison of risk estimates. The use of technical risk-based decision-making by the experts and their contempt for the public's perception of risk was not effective and indeed alienated the public from this approach.

Phase II then sought to use persuasion to convince the public about the correctness of a certain viewpoint. This approach used modern marketing practices that acknowledged the characteristics of the audiences and the legitimacy of their perception of the risk. Although this approach enjoyed some success with personal health risk issues such as smoking and drinking, it still had difficulty reducing the gap between technical risk assessments for risk issues such as nuclear waste and public perceptions of that risk. This approach failed largely due to issues of lack of trust and credibility between the public and the institutions behind the messages.

The third and current phase of RC acknowledges lack of trust is inherent in risk issues and that the focus must not be solely on technical risk assessments or persuasive communication. RC today seeks to emphasize two-way communication between the public and risk managers with the objective of building mutual trust. This has the effect of making the public a partner in the shared attempt to manage risks.

Communicating occupational health and safety risks to employees in the workplace has a different history. Although unacceptable today, historically occupational hygienists were advised against communicating with employees. Frank Patty illustrated this point in his second edition of Patty's Industrial Hygiene and Toxicology, which was in use up until the mid-1970s:

> It is unpardonable conduct on the part of an [occupational hygienist] to ask an employee a suggestive question such as: "Do you feel all right? Do you get sick often? Does breathing this atmosphere cause you any discomfort or irritation?" The psychological effects of such questioning, which is only one step short of suggesting to a workman that he is ill, are obvious and undesirable. To some workmen the mere fact that tests for airborne toxic materials are being made may indicate that dangerous conditions exist, and careless remarks of the investigator may grow to dire proportions and cause needless alarm among the workers.
>
> Although management often finds it advantageous to inform employees in advance of the purpose of an industrial hygiene survey, discussion with employees should be avoided by the industrial hygienist and left to the foreman or other representatives of management. ... To the direct question "What are you doing?" or "What does that instrument do?" a disarming reply should be given. The industrial hygienist might say that he is making routine tests, determining ventilation requirements, studying the efficiency of the exhaust system, measuring solvent loss, or he may make some other similar statement of fact. Any remark about measuring the toxic vapors here would be an ill-considered, and possibly alarming reply. It is not that the workman should be deceived but rather that he should not be alarmed about something that he probably would not fully understand.[5]

Today occupational hygienists recognize that workers have a fundamental right to know about all hazards in the workplace and whether they present a risk to human health. The occupational hygienist accomplishes this by involving the worker as an active participant to ensure that all hazards are evaluated and control measures are in place where necessary.

Regulatory Basis for Conducting RC

A growing number of organizations (private and government) acknowledge RC is a necessary and demanded activity and that it makes good business sense to keep workers, their families, communities, and other stakeholders aware of the potential risks related to their activities. This section provides an overview of the major legal drivers in the United States that require organizations to conduct RC with all interested stakeholders during certain activities such as cleanup of hazardous wastes sites or introduction of a new chemical into the workplace. These laws are usually a part of the risk assessment and risk management process. These legal requirements for RC can be found in environmental and health and safety standards.

The information here is not intended to be comprehensive nor to make the reader a regulatory expert. Rather, its purpose is to inform the reader sufficiently about relevant regulations to show why organizations must conduct RC activities. You must be sufficiently aware of these requirements to:

- provide justification for funding from your organization to conduct "required" RC activities versus optional activities;
- avoid legal actions against your organization by stakeholders for failure to comply; and
- avoid fines and criminal prosecution for failure to comply.

Christine Todd Whitman, administrator, U.S. Environmental Protection Agency (EPA), from January 2001 to June 2003, stated that "Communicating the results of our work in a clear manner will lead to a better understanding of environmental risks and how best to manage those risks. As citizens become better acquainted with the scientific basis for EPA's actions, they can make more informed decisions concerning the environment, their health, and the health of their families."[6]

Incorporating good RC is an integral part of every environmental, health, and safety program. Open communication with all interested stakeholders is required by federal regulations. Several federal laws and regulations include public involvement requirements, which mandate RC programs and efforts. For example, within the federal government, program areas requiring risk assessment and RC activities include the pollution prevention program, occupational health programs, and hazardous waste cleanup efforts. This section lists the federal regulations requiring stakeholder involvement in environmental restoration activities, risk assessment, risk management, and occupational safety and health. Because many states have enacted similar legislation, which may or may not be more stringent, be sure to check these before you begin planning your RC activities. The following is a partial list of regulations that identify and discuss stakeholder involvement.

EPA Regulations and Websites

National Environmental Policy Act (NEPA)

NEPA (40 CFR Parts 1500–1508), as implemented by the Council on Environmental Quality Regulations, requires public involvement in the environmental impact statement process.

Comprehensive Environmental Response, Compensation and Liability Act of 1980 (CERCLA)

CERCLA or Superfund (U.S. House of Representatives, U.S. Code, Title 42, chap. 103) provides broad federal authority to respond directly to releases or threatened releases of hazardous substances that may endanger public health or the environment.

Superfund Amendments and Reauthorization Act (SARA)

SARA (U.S. House of Representatives, U.S. Code, Title 42, chap. 103) amended CERCLA on October 17, 1986. EPA's experiences in administering the complex Superfund program during its first 6 years resulted in SARA, which made important changes and additions to the specific procedures required to assess the release of hazardous substances at inactive waste sites. Those changes mandate the addition of "community relations" in the evaluation process. Specifically, the RC changes increased state involvement in every phase of the Superfund program; encouraged greater citizen participation in making decisions on how sites should be cleaned up; called for development of community relations plans; and mandated a transparent process, such as fact sheets and media releases, for alerting the community to opportunities for involvement.

National Oil and Hazardous Substance Pollution Contingency Plan (NCP)

The National Oil and Hazardous Substance Pollution Contingency Plan (NCP) is the regulation that implements CERCLA. The NCP (40 CFR 300) is the federal government's blueprint for responding to oil spills and hazardous substance releases. The NCP establishes the overall approach for determining appropriate remedial action at Superfund sites. It identifies nine separate criteria for evaluating alternatives for acceptable remedial actions. Two of the "Modifying Criteria," state acceptance and community acceptance, emphasize the importance of establishing "public involvement" early and throughout the process. The following are examples of the NCP RC requirements.

Section 300.155, Public information and community relations. This section requires that the public be given prompt and accurate information on the nature of an incident, and the actions to mitigate.

Section 300.415 (n), Community relations in removal actions. This section states that you must:

- designate a spokesperson;
- publish notice of availability of administrative record and allow public comment;
- respond to comments;

- conduct interviews with local officials, residents, and groups to solicit their concerns and needs and find out how they would like to be involved;
- establish a local information repository; and
- prepare a formal community relations plan.

Safe Drinking Water Act (SDWA)

The SDWA (U.S. House of Representative, U.S. Code, Title 42, chap. 300) requires public notices for failure to comply with the maximum contaminant levels of the SDWA and "public notification" regarding the level of contaminants in drinking water as required by the SDWA.

Clean Air Act (CAA)

The CAA (42 U.S.C. s/s 7401 et seq.; 1970) is the comprehensive federal law that regulates air emissions from area, stationary, and mobile sources. This law authorizes the EPA to establish National Ambient Air Quality Standards to protect public health and the environment.

Public participation is a very important part of the 1990 CAA. Throughout the act the public is given opportunities to take part in determining how the law will be carried out. For instance, you can take part in hearings on the state and local plans for cleaning up air pollution. You can sue the government or a source's owner or operator to get action when EPA or your state has not enforced the CAA. You can request action by the state or EPA against violators.

The reports required by the CAA are public documents. A great deal of information will be collected on just how much pollution is being released; these monitoring (measuring) data will be available to the public. The 1990 CAA ordered EPA to set up clearinghouses to collect and give out technical information. Typically, these clearinghouses serve the public as well as state and other air pollution control agencies.

Title V of the CAA amendments of 1990; Permits Sec. 502. Permits allow recording in one document all of the air pollution control requirements that apply to the source. This gives members of the public, regulators, and the source a clear picture of the air pollution control requirements that apply to the source and what the facility is required to do to keep its air pollution under the legal limits. Specifically it provides for the following:

- Requiring the source to make regular reports on how it is tracking its emissions of pollution and the controls it is using to limit its emissions. These reports are public information, and you can get them from the permitting authority.
- Adding monitoring, testing, or record keeping requirements where needed to assure that the source complies with its emission limits or other pollution control requirements.
- Requiring the source to certify each year whether it has met the air pollution requirements in its Title V permit. These certifications are public information.
- Making the terms of the Title V permit federally enforceable. This means that EPA and the public can enforce the terms of the permit, along with the state.

Community Environmental Response Facilitation Act (CERFA)

Congress enacted CERFA (Pub. L. 102-426) on October 19, 1992. CERFA amends CERCLA to facilitate the rapid identification and return to local communities of clean properties identified in the Federal Base Realignment and Closure process. CERFA requires "appropriate consultation with the public and coordinating and concurring with regulatory agencies" to make property available for reuse in a timely manner.

Emergency Planning and Community Right to Know Act (EPCRA)

In 1984 a deadly cloud of methyl isocyanate killed thousands of people in Bhopal, India. Shortly thereafter, there was a serious chemical release at a sister plant in West Virginia. These incidents underscored demands by industrial workers and communities in several states for information on hazardous materials. Public interest and environmental organizations around the country accelerated demands for information on toxic chemicals being released "beyond the fence line"—outside of the facility. Against this background, EPCRA (42 U.S.C.11001 et seq.) was enacted in 1986.

Also known as Title III of SARA, EPCRA was enacted by Congress as the national legislation on community safety. This law was designated to help local communities protect public health, safety, and the environment in regard to chemical hazards. The regulations contain provisions for reporting both accidental and deliberate releases of certain toxic chemicals. EPCRA requires that facilities collect information to assess the dangers of hazardous chemicals present within their jurisdictions, to develop emergency response plans, to train emergency response personnel, and to better respond to chemical spills. EPCRA mandates that the public be informed about the chemicals present in communities and establishes emergency and notification actions should a release occur.

Local emergency planning committees. The standard also requires state emergency response commissions to appoint members of a local emergency planning committee for each emergency planning district. Each committee includes, at a minimum, representatives from each of the following groups or organizations: elected state and local officials; law enforcement, civil defense, fire fighting, first aid, health, local environmental, hospital, and transportation personnel; broadcast and print media; community groups; and owners and operators of facilities subject to the requirements of this law. Committees appoint a chairperson and establish rules by which the committee functions. Such rules include provisions for public notification of committee activities, public meetings to discuss the emergency plan, public comments, response to such comments by the committee, and distribution of the emergency plan.

Toxic Release Inventory (TRI). TRI is a publicly available EPA database that contains information on toxic chemical releases and other waste management activities reported annually by certain covered industry groups and federal facilities. This inventory was established under the EPCRA. It was expanded by the Pollution Prevention Act of 1990, which required that additional data on waste management and source reduction activities be reported under TRI. The goal of TRI is to empower citizens, through information, to hold companies and local governments accountable in terms of how toxic chemicals are managed.

Occupational Safety and Health Administration (OSHA) Regulations and Websites

Occupational Safety and Health Act (OSH Act) Hazardous Waste Operations and Emergency Response (HAZWOPER) Standard

HAZWOPER (29 CFR 1910.120) requires that all employees, supervisors, and management working on a hazardous waste site and exposed to hazardous substances be informed of and trained about their health hazards or safety hazards before they are permitted to engage in hazardous waste operations.

Occupational Safety and Health Act (OSH Act) Hazard Communication Standard (HAZCOM)

HAZCOM (29 CFR 1910.1200) contains provisions for communicating information concerning hazards of specific chemicals and appropriate protective measures to employees who use them. HAZCOM requires that the hazards of all chemicals produced or imported are evaluated, and that the information concerning their hazards is transmitted to employees and employers. This is to be accomplished by a comprehensive hazard communication program, which is to include container labeling and other forms of warning, material safety data sheets, and employee training.

OSH Act Access to Employee Exposure and Medical Records Standard

This standard (29 CFR 1910.1020) provides right of access to relevant exposure and medical records to employees, their representatives, and the assistant secretary of labor and applies to general industry, maritime, and the construction industry where workers exposed to toxic substances or harmful physical agents are employed.

The following are a few examples of OSHA standards having RC requirements for notification of employees when monitoring for exposures has occurred.

OSH Act; Asbestos (29 CFR 1910.1001)

29 CFR 1910.1001 (d)(7)(i)). Employee notification of monitoring results: The employer shall, within 15 working days after the receipt of the results of any monitoring performed under the standard, notify the affected employees of these results in writing either individually or by posting of results in an appropriate location that is accessible to affected employees.

1910.1001(d)(7)(ii). The written notification required by paragraph (d)(7)(i) of this section shall contain the corrective action being taken by the employer to reduce employee exposure to or below the TWA [time-weighted average] and/or excursion limit, wherever monitoring results indicated that the TWA and/or excursion limit had been exceeded.

OSH Act; Lead (29 CFR 1910.1025)

1910.1025(d)(8). Employee notification.

1910.1025(d)(8)(i). Within 5 working days after the receipt of monitoring results, the employer shall notify each employee in writing of the results which represent that employee's exposure.

1910.1025(d)(8)(ii). Whenever the results indicate that the representative employee exposure, without regard to respirators, exceeds the permissible exposure limit, the employer shall include in the written notice a statement that the permissible exposure limit was exceeded and a description of the corrective action taken or to be taken to reduce exposure to or below the permissible exposure limit.

OSH Act Process Safety Management of Highly Hazardous Chemicals

This standard (29 CFR 1910.119) requires employee participation and that employers develop a written plan of action regarding the implementation of the employee participation as required by the standard. Employers are required to consult with employees and their representatives on the conduct and development of process hazards analyses and on the development of the other elements of process safety management in this standard. Employers are also required to provide employees and their representatives access to process hazard analyses and to all other information required to be developed under this standard.

Force Health Protection

Presidential Review Directive 5 (PRD-5): A National Obligation. Planning for Health Preparedness for and Readjustment of the Military, Veterans, and Their Families After Future Deployments, November 8 1997. PRD-5 established broad goals for achieving progress in the area of military health and deployment and RC, otherwise known as Force Health Protection. On Veterans Day 1998 the president directed the creation of the Military and Veterans Health Coordinating Board (MVHCB) with the specific task of focusing on issues associated with deployment health, research, and communications regarding health risks. Creation of the MVHCB satisfied the specific Presidential Advisory Committee Special Report recommendation that the Department of Defense (DoD), the Veterans Administration, and the Department of Health and Human Services should complete the comprehensive RC program for Gulf War veterans, as well as for forces deployed in the future, and that community-based outreach should receive particular focus.

PRD-5 requirements are implemented through the following DoD guidance documents:

- DoD Instruction 6490.3 (August 7, 1997) – Implementation and Application of Joint Medical Surveillance
- DoD Directive 6490.2 (August 30, 1997) – Joint Medical Surveillance
- Joint Chiefs of Staff Memorandum MCM-0006-02 (February 1, 2002) – Updated Procedures for Deployment Health Surveillance and Readiness

RC as defined by DoD is the "process of adequately and accurately communicating the magnitude and nature of potential environmental and occupational health risks to commanders and to Service members" (DoD Instruction 6490.3, August 7, 1997; Implementation and Application of Joint Medical Surveillance). DoD now requires service members be made aware of significant health threats and corresponding medical prophylaxis, immunization, and other unit and individual countermeasures. It also requires that commanders be kept informed before, during, and after deployments of the health of the force, health threats, stressors, risks, and available countermeasures using appropriate RC. And finally, it requires that the commanders establish an RC plan addressing the occupational and environmental risks in understandable terms for the commanders, operational planners, and deploying personnel.

The Deployment Health Support Directorate has taken over for the MVHCB and now serves as the focal point for the many activities and programs required by PRD-5 ongoing within DoD, Veterans Administration, and the Department of Health and Human Services.

Additional Information

An excellent source of information on the laws that mandate RC is Chapter 3 of *Risk Communication—A Handbook for Communicating Environmental, Safety, and Health Risks*, by Regina E. Lundgren and Andrea H. McMakin.[7] Table 45.1 is adapted from this reference and provides an overview of the regulations applying in care, consensus, and crisis communication.

RC Models: Approaches, Applications, Challenges, and Guidelines

At one time, the primary (if not only) communication model used was one-way communication. The technical experts provided as much information as they deemed necessary and expected the audience to be satisfied. In some circles this is referred to as the "DAD" model—decide, announce, defend. The field of RC has grown dramatically over the past 30 years, primarily in union with the environmental movement. As the public demanded increased protection for resources—health, safety, and environmental—they also clearly made known that they wanted to be included in the process and decision-making.

To assist the RC practitioner, a number of approaches for RC have been developed. Some of the more common approaches, as well as their applications, are discussed in the following sections.

National Research Council

Due to growing concern, in 1989 the National Research Council (NRC) commissioned an extensive project to try to find ways to improve RC. A committee of experts representing a cross-section of experience and disciplines concluded that "many participants in the process lack fundamental understanding of the important points that form the basis for successful risk communication." The committee viewed RC as "an interactive process of exchange of information and opinion among individuals, groups, and institutions."[8] They further described successful RC occurring when it "raises the level of understanding of relevant issues or actions for those involved and satisfies them that they are adequately informed within the limits of available knowledge."[8] The document published as a result of the committee's work, *Improving Risk*

Table 45.1 — Applicability of Laws and Regulations to Risk Communication

Type of Risk Communication	CERCLA	CERFA	EPCRA	EO12898	EO13045	NCP	NEPA	NRDA	OSHA	PRD 5	RCRA	RMP	SDWA
Care Communication													
Health communication					✔				✔	✔			✔
Occupational hygiene									✔	✔			
Worker notification									✔	✔			
Consensus Communication													
Hazardous waste	✔	✔		✔	✔	✔			✔	✔	✔	✔	✔
Solid waste				✔	✔					✔	✔		
Environmental issues	✔	✔		✔	✔	✔	✔	✔	✔	✔	✔	✔	✔
Crisis Communication													
Emergency planning			✔		✔	✔				✔		✔	
Actual crisis						✔		✔		✔			

Abbreviations not defined in text: EO = executive order; NRDA = Natural Resources and Damage Assessment; RCRA = Resource Conservation and Recovery Act ; RMP = Risk Management Program Rule; SDWA = Safe Drinking Water Act (Adapted from Reference 7.)

Communication, is a seminal work in this field. A key theme from the NRC's work is the necessity of two-way (interactive) communication. Anyone who communicates risk must incorporate an "exchange of information and opinions."

Mental Models Approach

The mental model approach examines how people view and understand various phenomena. Its underlying premise is that to effectively communicate risk information, the risk communicator must first understand what the audience already believes about the risk issue. After the intended audience is recognized, representatives are interviewed to obtain information on how the risk is viewed. The information gained from the interviews is used to form a "mental model" of how the audience perceives the risk. This mental model is then compared to the "expert model," or how the scientists perceive the risk. Appropriate RC messages can then be prepared that address misperceptions or information gaps. The intent is to provide the audience information to help them make an informed decision. The mental model approach largely originated from researchers at Carnegie-Mellon University.(9)

Risk = Hazard + Outrage Approach

The RC approach likely to be most familiar to the occupational hygiene world is from Dr. Peter Sandman. This approach is largely based on research conducted by Dr. Paul Slovic and Dr. Baruch Fischhoff. Sandman asserts that the person's perception of risk depends on both the hazard and a variety of outrage factors.(10) A stakeholder's perception of risk is not necessarily the same as the risk assessor's determination. The risk assessor tends to focus only on the hazard and often neglects the emotional component. Although it is important to ensure the stakeholders' knowledge and understanding of the hazard, neglecting the outrage component that affects a stakeholders' perception of risk will make the RC process inadequate. Dr. Sandman's book, Responding to Community Outrage, lists potential outrage components.(3) Some of the possible outrage components of note follow:

Is the risk voluntary or coerced; do people have a choice about being exposed to the hazard?

Is the risk natural in origin or industrial? Hazards that arise from natural causes are perceived to be less risky than those that arise from human activities.

Is the risk familiar or exotic (not familiar)? This can be an especially challenging outrage component to overcome in the occupational arena, where employees are familiar with their surroundings and can easily become complacent.

Does the stakeholder perceive him- or herself to be in control of the events that may affect him? An example would be the difference in perception of control associated with driving a car and being a passenger.

Is there dread associated with the risk? Cancer and nuclear waste are examples of dreaded outcomes of a risk, increasing a person's perception of the magnitude of a risk assessor's quantitatively determined risk.

Is there a sense of fairness regarding costs and benefits? When stakeholders are asked to take all the potential costs of a risk without a share in the benefits, outrage can be increased.

Is the risk communicator trusted? Gaining trust based on consistent and genuine actions can reduce potential for outrage, hence reducing perceived risk.

An important implication of Dr. Sandman's work is that the act of simply presenting facts does not likely equate to successful RC. Success entails acknowledging and addressing the stakeholders' emotional needs.

Trust and Credibility Approach

Stemming from the aforementioned research, the risk perception components of trust and credibility of the risk communicators by stakeholders warrants separate discussion. Effective RC occurs only in the presence of trust by the stakeholders.(11) Regardless of the presence or absence of the other risk perception factors, if trust is lacking, acceptance of risk will be difficult at best. An important goal for effective risk communicators to achieve is to establish and maintain trust and credibility. Several characteristics that determine whether a stakeholder perceives a communicator as trusted and credible are empathy and caring, honesty and openness, dedication and commitment, and competence and expertise. Of these characteristics the qualities of empathy and caring are by far the most important in establishing trust and credibility.[12,13] An effective communicator will likely be perceived by stakeholders to have these four characteristics building stakeholder trust.

Slovik illustrates the fact that the presence or lack of trust influences a stakeholder's interpretation of an event in the following example of the incident that occurred at Three Mile Island.

> "Persons who trusted the nuclear power industry saw the events at Three Mile Island as demonstrating the soundness of the "defense in depth" principle, noting that the multiple-safety systems shut the plant down and contained most of its radiation. Persons who distrusted nuclear power prior to the accident took an entirely different message from the same events, perceiving that those in charge did not understand what was wrong or how to fix it and that catastrophe was averted only by sheer luck."[14]

Hence, trust is a crucial element in effective RC. One effective method in increasing trust is to have a third-party credible source agree with your message. A communicator can take on the trust and credibility of a bolstering third-party source.[12] Besides achieving trust from third-party credible sources, the establishment of trust can be achieved only through trustworthy actions, and once achieved must be maintained and/or enhanced. Once lost, trust is very difficult to regain.

Crisis Communication

A crisis is an untimely event that may prevent management from accomplishing its efforts to create the understanding and satisfaction between the organization and interested parties needed to negotiate the mutually beneficial exchange of stakes.[15] If unattended or poorly managed, the crisis can prevent the organization from making satisfactory progress toward achieving its mission. Crises vary in degree and probability, but all share the threat of causing damage to companies that can be measured in terms of harm to the corporate image and actual financial losses.[16] Furthermore, a crisis threatens the physical system of an organization.[17] To incorporate crisis communication into a strategic framework, a number of researchers categorize this function as crisis management. Table 45.2 describes the crisis leadership approach to crisis communication.

Approaches to crisis communication generally address why various techniques and strategies work or do not work; whether the techniques and strategies could apply to other crisis situations; and suggestions for what needs to be done to make improvements. Well-planned and well-executed crisis RC can give the organization the critical edge necessary to ensure that limited resources are available to best respond during the crisis situation, and determine the success or failure of how the crisis is handled.

The term "crisis communication" is most often used to describe an organization facing a crisis and the need to communicate about that crisis to stakeholders and the public. Typically, a crisis is an event that occurs unexpectedly, may not be in the organization's control, and may cause harm to the organization's reputation or viability. An example of an organization facing a crisis is

Table 45.2 — The Crisis Leadership Approach

1. Your senior management team has the vision and the leadership to anticipate crises within and outside your organization.
2. Your team has identified the most likely threats and challenges to your organization's operations and you have written and tested effective response plans.
3. Your organization has a multidisciplinary crisis management team established and ready to respond.
4. Your primary goal during a crisis is to attend to the immediate needs of the organization and your key stakeholders and resolving the crisis in the interests of your organization and the public.
5. Your public relations staff/consultants have the necessary resources to manage a crisis today.
6. Your senior management team has delegated the authority to your crisis management team to make the critical organizational decisions during a crisis.
7. You have identified your key stakeholders (employees, neighbors, shareholders, suppliers, customers) and have the means to communicate with them during a crisis.
8. Your organization is committed to open, ethical, and timely communication with the public during a crisis.
9. You are part of a learning organization and have already put in place a "lessons learned" process for your next crisis.
10. You understand that effective crisis communication and management is a long-term commitment.

the occurrence of an industrial explosion, especially if it results in fatalities and/or extensive environmental damage. In most instances the organization faces some legal or moral culpability for the crisis, and stakeholders and the public judge the organization's response to the crisis.

An important facet of crisis communication is media communication. This often is the avenue in which the risk communicator can most effectively get his message out to the stakeholders. Techniques for dealing with the media are addressed in a later section of this chapter.

RC Challenges

Covello and Sandman[18] identified four obstacles to effective RC:

(1) Inappropriate risk messages. For the most part, risk information is complex and fraught with uncertainty. There are large information gaps, which lead to the inability to provide definite information or answers.[18]

(2) Distrust in the information source. There are many reasons for a lack of trust, such as lack of coordination between organizations, disagreement between experts, insensitivity, lack of knowledge of basic guidelines for effectively communicating risk, a history of distortion, and so on.

(3) Selective reporting by the media. The general public depends strongly on the media for risk information. However, research has shown that journalists are highly selective in reporting risk issues and tend to report on issues involving people in unusual or sensational situations. Many stories may omit important information or present distorted, inaccurate, or oversimplified information. Often reporters do not have the training or background necessary to accurately report the scientific or technical information.

(4) Psychological and social factors that affect how information is processed. Seven factors are identified: (a) heuristics (mental short cuts)—the tendency to form biased opinions or base opinions on partial information; (b) apathy—often people are not interested in learning about a risk; (c) overconfidence and unrealistic optimism—people believe that "it won't happen to me," leading them to ignore or dismiss risk information; (d) difficulty in understanding probabilistic information; (e) demands for scientific certainty—people expect the experts to have factual information and have difficulty dealing with uncertainty or unknowns; (f) reluctance to change strongly held beliefs and willingness to ignore evidence that contradicts them—once formed, strong beliefs are very difficult to change; and (g) misjudging the magnitude of risk—the "outrage" factors that form risk perceptions (voluntariness, controllability, familiarity, fairness, benefits, and so on).

Basic RC Guidelines

In 1988 EPA published a document called *Seven Cardinal Rules of Risk Communication*. The material provides sound "how to" RC advice and is provided in Table 45.3.[19]

Summary

Approaches to RC have evolved and become more complex over the past 30 years. Factors such as psychological, social, cultural, economic, and political factors are being studied and added to the list of things that need to be considered to effectively communicate risk issues. For more information about these approaches as well as others, see Reference 5.

The News Media and Risk Issues: Five Key Steps You Need To Know

The news media are a powerful and important force within society. Some researchers have called the media the world's main source of information and knowledge; others see the media as agents of social control; still others view them as champions of social problems.[20-22] Overall, the media are in a pivotal place to prompt social change either through helping to set the political agenda or by keeping issues and groups out of the public discussion. Because the media are the channels through which information from environmental organizations pass to their key audiences, it is essential that your organization become a recognized and

Table 45.3 — Seven Cardinal Rules of Risk Communication

Rule 1: Accept and Involve the Public as a Legitimate Partner.

A basic tenet of risk communication in a democracy is that people and communities have a right to participate in decisions that affect their lives, their property, and the things they value.

Guidelines: Demonstrate respect for the public and underscore the sincerity of your effort by involving the public early before important decisions are made. Involve all parties that have an interest or a stake in the issues under consideration. If you are a government employee, remember that you work for the public. If you do not work for the government, the public still holds you accountable.

Rule 2: Plan Carefully and Evaluate Your Efforts.

Risk communication will be successful only if carefully planned.

Guidelines: Begin with clear, explicit risk communication objectives-such as providing information to the public, motivating individuals to act, stimulating response to emergencies, or contributing to the resolution of conflict. Evaluate the information you have about the risk and know its strengths and weaknesses. Classify and segment the various groups in your audience. Aim your communications at specific subgroups in your audience. Recruit spokespeople who are good at presentation and interaction. Train your staff-including technical staff-in communication skills; reward outstanding performance. Whenever possible, pretest your messages. Carefully evaluate your efforts and learn from your mistakes.

Rule 3: Listen to the Public's Specific Concerns.

If you do not listen to people, you cannot expect them to listen to you. Communication is a two-way activity.

Guidelines: Do not make assumptions about what people know, think, or want done about risks. Take the time to find out what people are thinking: use techniques such as interviews, focus groups, and surveys. Let all parties that have an interest or a stake in the issue be heard. Identify with your audience and try to put yourself in their place. Recognize people's emotions. Let people know that you understand what they said, addressing their concerns as well as yours. Recognize the "hidden agenda," symbolic meanings, and broader economic or political considerations that often underlie and complicate the task of risk communication.

Rule 4: Be Honest, Frank, and Open.

In communicating risk information, trust and credibility are your most precious assets.

Guidelines: State your credentials; but do not ask or expect to be trusted by the public. If you do not know an answer or are uncertain, say so. Get back to people with answers. Admit mistakes. Disclose risk information as soon as possible (emphasizing any reservations about reliability). Do not minimize or exaggerate the level of risk. Speculate only with great caution. If in doubt, lean toward sharing more information, not less-or people may think you are hiding something. Discuss data uncertainties, strengths, and weaknesses-including the ones identified by other credible sources. Identify worst-case estimates as such, and cite ranges of risk estimates when appropriate.

Rule 5: Coordinate and Collaborate with Other Credible Sources.

Allies can be effective in helping you communicate risk information.

Guidelines: Take time to coordinate all inter- and intraorganizational communications. Devote effort and resources to the slow, hard work of building bridges with other organizations. Use credible and authoritative intermediaries. Consult with others to determine who is best able to answer questions about risk. Try to issue communications jointly with other trustworthy sources (for example, credible university scientists, physicians, or trusted local officials). If you are a government employee, remember that you work for the public. If you do not work for the government, the public still holds you accountable.

Rule 6: Meet the Needs of the Media.

The media are prime transmitters of information on risk; they play a critical role in setting agendas and in determining outcomes.

Guidelines: Be open with and accessible to reporters. Respect their deadlines. Provide risk information tailored to the needs of each type of media (for example, graphics and other visual aids for television). Prepare in advance and provide background material on complex risk issues. Do not hesitate to follow up on stories with praise or criticism, as warranted. Try to establish long-term relationships of trust with specific editors and reporters.

Rule 7: Speak Clearly and with Compassion.

Technical language and jargon are useful as professional shorthand. But they are barriers to successful communication with the public.

Guidelines: Use simple, nontechnical language. Be sensitive to local norms, such as speech and dress. Use vivid, concrete images that communicate on a personal level. Use examples and anecdotes that make technical risk data come alive. Avoid distant, abstract, unfeeling language about deaths, injuries, and illnesses. Acknowledge and respond (both in words and with actions) to emotions that people express, such as anxiety, fear, anger, outrage, and helplessness. Acknowledge and respond to the distinctions that the public views as important in evaluating risks, for example, voluntariness, controllability, familiarity, dread, origin (natural or man-made), benefits, fairness, and catastrophic potential. Use risk comparisons to help put risks in perspective, but avoid comparisons that ignore distinctions that people consider important. Always try to include a discussion of actions that are underway or can be taken. Tell people what you cannot do. Promise only what you can do, and be sure to do what you promise.

(Adapted from Reference 19.)

dependable force in promoting your views on risk issues. According to Shoemaker, interested groups can do this by becoming a formidable force in the gatekeeping process, providing information and messages as a regular part of the media routine, and as a result becoming a credible source of ongoing information for the media.[23]

The media can greatly influence the nature, development, and ultimate success of an environmental risk issue. Interested groups need the media more than the media need them. Even with the explosion of the Internet, a more direct method of communicating with environmental stakeholders and policy makers, the mass media remain "the primary link between the public and the political system."[24]

Given that "most Americans know what they know about the environment from watching television news and reading newspapers," and furthermore, that much of what most people discuss about risk issues comes from the media, it is important for us to learn how to work with the media to bring risk information to the public.[25–27] The following discussion provides the five key steps that you need to know before interacting with the media.

Step 1: Fully Understand the Issue

A primary challenge during risk controversies is to distill a complex technical issue into a manageable and meaningful media message. Environmental and health risk issues that have been managed effectively in the public arena have often been the result of a detailed, strategic, media relations approach. The first step for any successful media campaign is to be prepared—to understand how the issue fits within the current political and public landscape. The easiest way to achieve this understanding is to perform an external issues analysis by conducting "top-line" research with a systematic sample of key stakeholder groups and target media outlets. What kind of information are they looking for? How would they like to receive information? What other issues are competing for their attention? The purpose of this step is to begin to frame the issue in the eyes and ears of the stakeholders. This is your opportunity to begin to develop a message in a way that will be acceptable and ultimately received by those groups that could eventually determine the success or failure of your campaign. Remember, this takes time, and starting this program well in advance of the public release of your message is critical—think months and weeks and not days and hours and you will establish a solid issue foundation.

Step 2: Media Relationships

The media have a constitutionally guaranteed role to play in all political and risk issues. The company may not like the job they are doing or believe that they are well equipped to communicate about risk issues, but in reality, they are here to stay. It is a basic tenant of human relations, but it is one that is sometimes overlooked about during risk controversies: the public and the media will believe you and see you as a credible source, if they know you and have an ongoing relationship with you. Obviously this is a difficult and somewhat challenging step, but in today's 24/7 media world, you have something that the media needs...information. Think of it as a quid pro quo type of system. You need them to carry your message to the public, and they need your information. But they need that information in a manner, style, and at a time that best suits their needs. Your objective is to develop, as best as you can, working relationships with those journalists who may cover your issue: local, regional, national, broadcast, print, and electronic. It takes time and research to find them and develop relationships with them, but in the end, when your issue is hitting the public arena, it is better to systematically deliver your message to reporters who have a working knowledge of your issue and know where they can reach you for comment.

Step 3: What Is Your Message?

Researchers tell us that the average consumer is inundated by more than 3000 different messages each day. From television commercials, to newspaper ads, to political messages, to personal "to do's," people are bombarded by products, services, and family members that want to capture an individuals attention and thoughts. In this competitive environment your message needs to be able to break through the clutter to frame your position and set the agenda for the media and the public. Refining your message into an easily understandable headline is difficult and complex. What is your objective: awareness—creating a cognitive linkage between your message and the public as a way of increasing knowledge of your issue; appreciation—although your audience may be aware of your position, do they understand it, and are they ready to form an opinion about your message? Finally, are you attempting to create an action or change a behavior through your message? Your message can focus on only one of these objectives. And if you want your audience to do something with your message, then first, they need to be aware of your position, and second, they must have an appreciation for your message in relation to all the other messages that are bombarding them. These two steps are critical before anyone will eventually decide to act on your message.

Step 4: Anticipation, Practice, and Performance

The media's ability to broadcast a disaster or an issue from any part of the world in a relatively short period of time magnifies the need to always be ready. The media's satellite technology can beam images and comments to millions of television sets in just minutes. Therefore, you and your organization must be prepared to deal with a potential media blitz. You need to establish a media management system, so that you are ready for the onslaught of journalists whether you are in control of the announcement or reacting to a crisis event. Identify the most capable spokespeople and regularly train them on your key messages. Train them also to respond to what at times seems like an unruly mob. Your spokesperson should be able to communicate your message effectively in a confident, credible, and empathetic manner. Unfortunately, their credibility and the credibility of your organization will be judged by their performance under the spotlight.

Step 5: Become a Student of Media Relations

There are literally thousands of books, videotapes, websites, and consultants to keep you up to date on the "do's and don'ts" of effective media relations. Better yet, there are hundreds of minutes of daily newscasts that can provide you with the ability to critique, review, and assess the most effective media performances on television. Look, listen, and think about the spokespeople that you see on the news. What are their messages? How well were they able to articulate the messages? How did they respond to difficult questions? Were they prepared for the media interview? If you were in their shoes, what would you do differently?

Furthermore, visit any bookstore—in person or on the web—and search for books on media training skills. Read them and take their advice to heart. Unfortunately, it will not be as easy as the books imply. Effective media relations take time, practice, and skill to implement. If you want a more hands-on approach to skills building, hire a media-training specialist, someone who has worked with risk issues, and have them train you and your team. Using outside experts is a cost-effective approach to building the critical skills that enable organizations to effectively and efficiently manage risk issues in the media.

When all is said and done, you and your organization must be comfortable participants in the media arena. You need to develop the media relations plan that best meets your goals and objectives while ensuring that you are prepared to successfully manage the outcome.

Developing an RC Plan

Issues about risk to personal health or the environment are often complex and involve numerous stakeholder groups with different concerns that need to be addressed individually. Addressing these concerns requires time-consuming research, planning, and outreach efforts that typically are not accomplished by one person working alone. For most significant risk issues you need to form an RC team, and this team needs a plan to follow to engage and exchange information effectively with stakeholders. This section contains guidance on how to organize a team, what components to include in a typical RC plan, and how to effectively implement the RC process.[28]

The RC Team

Occupational hygienists are called on routinely to explain environmental, safety, and health issues to personnel and management. This explanation can be as limited as a one-on-one conversation about how to use personal protective equipment, or it can be as involved as communicating with large groups of people about a catastrophe, emergency, or a perceived risk such as a cancer cluster among workers at a plant. In the first example the task is more straightforward, and the RC team would likely include just the occupational hygienist or possibly the occupational hygienist, his or her supervisor, and the employee's supervisor. But in crises or other situations that involve many people with mixed perceptions of risk or a risk that is causing unnecessary fear or concern among stakeholders, a larger team is needed to coordinate the RC process.

For big or crisis issues an effective RC team could easily include 10 or more people from various departments or groups within an organization. The goal in organizing this team is to have all of the information sources on the issue represented, so that as management makes decisions or takes action the team can quickly and efficiently determine how best to share that information to address the needs of the stakeholders. To meet this goal, virtually all RC teams need to include three standard members:

(1) a management representative with the authority to make decisions about information to be released,
(2) a public relations or public affairs expert to release information through the media and provide guidance on how to deal with the media, and
(3) an occupational hygienist or another medical expert to provide information on health issues.

The remainder of the team will vary based on the issue or the response that the organization has developed. For example, issues that involve a catastrophic accident such as a major explosion or hazardous chemical spill would require team members who can provide information on why or how the accident happened, what is being done to control the situation or clean up the spill, and how the company will prevent this from happening again in the future. These team members might include representatives from various engineering and maintenance departments within the company, someone from accounting to be aware of and provide guidance on money or funding issues, and the company's legal representative, environmental program manager, and safety program manager (if this person is not already represented by the occupational hygienist). Regardless of what the issue is, keep in mind that the team members should be selected to provide or have access to all of the corporate knowledge that is needed to explain what happened, the company's current actions, and plans for future action. Once a team is formed that is designed to provide this corporate knowledge, then the members need to work together to develop a plan of action known as an RC plan.

The RC Plan

Most RC plans are organized around a particular care, consensus, or crisis communication goal such as encouraging the use of protective equipment to avoid chemical exposures in a given workspace, obtaining regulatory and community approval on a waste incinerator permit, or explaining possible health effects of a hazardous substance spill and the subsequent cleanup and future spill prevention efforts. To be comprehensive a plan must include strategies to communicate with each of the various stakeholder groups concerned with the issue in ways that will both address their concerns and meet your goals at the same time. As a result, an RC plan for complex issues with multiple stakeholder groups can be quite lengthy and detailed.

Because of the time involved in dealing with many RC issues, the question may arise, "Why would anyone want to take the additional time to write a formal plan?" There are many reasons to formalize an RC plan. The following are just a few:

- All roles and responsibilities are formally acknowledged in a plan to help prevent internal miscommunication. This hopefully cuts down on the number of times potentially disastrous statements like "I thought he/she was doing that" or "That's not what we agreed to do" are made.
- A formal plan that has been accepted by management can help when setting priorities and seeking approval and funding for planned activities.
- A comprehensive plan is a great defense in the almost inevitable event

that someone from inside or outside the organization challenges the methods or approach.

It is easier to evaluate the communication efforts if there is a formal plan to help relate results directly back to the purpose and objectives, schedule, and audience.[7]

These reasons apply to both routine and complex issues that involve both large and small RC teams. Because of this, it is a good idea for occupational hygienists to develop a generic RC plan to cover hazard communication or other care- or consensus-type RC efforts you might routinely perform. It would also be wise to review your company's crisis management plan to ensure it includes a component on RC. Both the RC plan and the crisis management plan can be drawn on when dealing with more complex or high visibility issues. Regardless of the issue or the size of the team, there are typical elements that should be included in all RC plans. Figure 45.2 is an outline for a typical RC plan.

The difficult work begins once the RC team has an outline for the plan and is ready to build and execute the various elements. As listed in Figure 45.2, the first section of a typical plan is the introduction. It should be developed by the RC team to provide background information on the issue along with the purpose of the plan, the purpose of the RC effort, and the company's objectives for these efforts. The second section of the plan should be devoted to information on the stakeholders. This information must be gathered before the team develops the plan, because it drives the selection and development of RC strategies. The work that goes into researching, planning, and executing the stakeholder profile and RC strategies sections is the start of the real RC process.

The RC Process

The RC process in a simplified form involves four main steps.

(1) Research: Getting to know the stakeholders and their concerns and gathering corporate knowledge about the issue and the company's plan of action
(2) Developing information or messages that are designed to address stakeholders' concerns and meet the company's purpose and goals, as described in the RC plan
(3) Sharing and discussing information and messages with the stakeholders
(4) Evaluating the effectiveness of the communication efforts

Profiling the community is a term used by RC practitioners to describe the process of getting to know stakeholders and their concerns for a given issue. The first step in getting to know stakeholders is identifying who they are. You can identify stakeholder groups in various ways, such as brainstorming among the RC team, talking with colleagues and other employees not included in the team, reviewing media coverage, reviewing telephone call-in logs for the company,

Risk Communication Plan Outline

Introduction
- Purpose of the plan
- Scope of the plan
- Background on the risk
  - What is the risk?
  - Who is affected by it?
- Authority
  - Under what authority (law or organizational mandate) is the risk being communicated?
- Purpose of the risk communication effort
- Specific objectives

Stakeholder Profile
- How was stakeholder information gathered?
- Who are the stakeholders?
- What are their issues or concerns?

Risk Communication Strategies

Evaluation Strategies

Schedule and Resources
- General explanation of RC Team with roles and responsibilities
- Detailed schedule that identifies tasks and people responsible for completing them
- Estimated Budget
- Other resources to be used (equipment, meeting rooms, etc.)

Internal Communication
- How progress will be documented
- Approval needed

Signoff Page
Names, job titles, and signatures of key staff members acknowledging that they have read and concur with the plan

*Additional elements may be required for specific plans depending on the issue.
Adapted from Lundgren and McMakin (1998)

Figure 45.2 — Risk communication plan outline. (Adapted from Reference 7.)

Questions to Help Identify Key Stakeholders

1. Which groups have been previously involved in this issue?
2. Which groups are likely to be affected directly or to think they are affected directly by the company's action?
3. Which groups are likely to be angry if they are not consulted or alerted to the issue?
4. Which groups would be helpful for you to consult with because they might have important information, ideas, or opinions?
5. Which groups should you involve to ensure that the company has communicated with a balanced range of opinion on the issue?
6. Which groups will others seek out for their opinions on the company's action (you don't want them to be blindsided or ill-informed)?
7. Which groups have responsibility relevant to the company's action (e.g. firefighters, regulators)?
   Which groups may not especially want input, but do need to know what your company is doing?

Figure 45.3 — Questions to help identify key stakeholders. (Adapted from Reference 29.)

Potential Stakeholders

(This list is not all-inclusive. It is meant to trigger your thinking)

1. **Government** — Federal, state, county, and municipal agencies and elected officials; legislative committees; quasi-government agencies such as sewage authorities, regional planning commissions, and environmental commissions; emergency responders such as police and fire fighters.
2. **Employees** — And their families. Also retirees.
3. **Geographical Neighbors** — Local residents and businesses.
4. **Environmental Groups** — National, state-wide, and local groups; specific issue groups such as Superfund or siting groups; conservation groups dealing with watersheds, hiking, fishing, and natural features; groups with specific functions, such as legal, lobbying, research, or organizing.
5. **Civic Organizations** — League of Women Voters; associations such as Kiwanis, Rotary, etc.; associations of senior citizens; ethnic groups.
6. **Professional and Trade Associations** — Health professionals (doctors, nurses); technical people (sanitarians, water purveyors, consultants, planners); business organizations (realtors, chambers of commerce, industrial and agricultural groups).
7. **Educational and Academic Organizations** — Colleges; agricultural extensions; public and private schools; academic experts in field relevant to the company's action.
8. **Community Organizations** — Social service groups, etc.
9. **Religious Organizations** — Churches, community ministries.

Figure 45.4 — Potential stakeholders. (Adapted from Reference 29.)

and talking with local government officials and other respected community members. Figures 45.3 and 45.4 list some questions that might help identify and prioritize stakeholder groups and also give a list of some typical or potential stakeholder groups when issues deal with environment, safety, and health.[29] Remember that the general public is typically not a stakeholder group. There are some exceptions to this, as when dealing with some crisis communications situations. Usually this large group must be broken down into smaller groups to effectively identify which concerns or issues are most important to be addressed.

Once the stakeholders are identified, their questions, concerns, and perceptions need to be identified. The best and most efficient way to get to know stakeholders and their concerns is through direct methods such as face-to-face meetings, conducting surveys, and hosting focus groups. Unfortunately, these methods often are not used during the planning process because of time constraints or because the audience is hostile and refuses to associate with anyone connected with the risk issue. If direct methods to meet and profile stakeholders are unfeasible, then there are less direct methods available to gather information. Note that these efforts are based on assumptions and extrapolations that may be wrong and may impact the effectiveness of the RC effort.

Two indirect methods to learn about stakeholders are to use surrogate groups or consult existing sources of information. Surrogate groups are people who are easily accessible and seem to approximate the stakeholders. Figure 45.5 gives a list of some existing information sources that may be useful in learning about your stakeholders.[7]

The second and third steps in the RC process involve developing messages and presenting and discussing this information with the stakeholders. The results of these steps combine to form the RC strategies section of the plan. These strategies are made up of the 3 Ms of RC: message, messenger, and media.

Message Development

A major component of any communication process is to exchange information or to convey a message. Developing this message is the first component of an RC strategy. Because RC is founded on a two-way exchange of information, effective messages are developed to meet the goals of the company's communication effort while at the same time addressing stakeholders concerns and their perceptions of the risk. Most important, messages should relay information that will help establish and/or maintain the stakeholder's trust in the communicator. Well-crafted messages alone typically do not overcome established beliefs or perceptions about your company or the risk at hand, nor do they build trust where there was none. But when good messages are combined with the proper spokesperson or representative who is perceived as caring, competent, and dedicated, then building trust or rebuilding lost trust is possible. The following information is a short summary of the most important points to remember when developing risk messages for crisis, care, or consensus communication on environmental, health, and safety issues.

Effective messages contain a balanced amount of information. They do not give people so much data and technical information that they are overwhelmed, and they do not oversimplify information so much that important information is not received. To reach this balance, careful consideration must be given to the content and organization of the message.[28] There are three initial message development questions to use when sorting through the information and determining what is key or crucial to convey. They are:

- What are the three most important things the company or risk manager wants to convey to the stakeholders?
- What three things would the stakeholders most like to know?
- What are the three points the stakeholders are most likely to get wrong unless they are emphasized?

The answers to these questions are what should be packaged into key messages. When dealing with angry, upset, or distrustful people, these messages need to be as short and to the point as possible. They should focus on the positive efforts and plans that the company or risk manager has made and not be a defensive response to allegations. There are three general guidelines that help when laying out key messages:

- Provide verbal and nonverbal messages that convey empathy/caring, honesty/openness, and dedication/commitment
- Avoid messages that convey only technical facts and information
- Recognize the impact of credible third-party sources

Most people with a scientific or engineering background have a hard time creating messages based on the first two bullets. Their training is based in fact and science and this seems the easiest, most logical way to present the necessary information. So when trying to explain the relative risk or safety of an action or event in "nontechnical language," people naturally try to compare the risk to something that is familiar to everyone to make it easier for the audience to understand the information or put it into perspective. Comparing risks can be very powerful when used skillfully and in the right application. But these risk comparisons (e.g., the risk of breathing particulates and gases from a nearby smokestack is 100 times less than the risk of smoking 1 cigarette a day for 10 years)[30] are often damaging as part of an RC message because they do not take risk perception factors into consideration. Thus, it is best to avoid making risk comparisons.

When choosing information to include in an RC message, try to consider the stakeholders' perceptions of the risk and the factors that effect this perception. Four of these factors (trust, benefit, control, and familiarity) are very important in developing RC messages. A person's perception of the magnitude or danger of a risk is generally lowered as their feeling of trust in the message/messenger goes up, as they recognize potential benefits from the risk producing action, as they feel they have more control over the action or risk, and as they become more familiar with or better understand what is causing the risk. Messages that are developed and presented in a manner to help stakeholders understand and become familiar with the issues while increasing trust and emphasizing any benefits and areas for control will be the most successful in overcoming established risk perceptions.

Selecting a messenger is the second component of an RC strategy. RC efforts typically involve explaining scientific or other complex information to a mixed audience. In many instances people are upset or distrustful because of their risk perceptions or past experiences. When explaining complex risk issues to distrustful, upset stakeholders, selecting the right messenger becomes a critical part of the communication strategy. The right messenger can help a company establish or rebuild trust and credibility with stakeholders, whereas the wrong messenger can make a bad situation worse. Typically, a good spokesperson is comfortable and effective as a public speaker and is perceived by the stakeholders as open, caring, competent, and dedicated.

The third component of an RC strategy is the media used to convey or share information and hopefully encourage dialogue with the stakeholders. There are many different ways to share information, ranging from one-on-one meetings; to full-scale public meetings involving presentations, posters, and other written material; to strictly written material such as a press release, newsletter article, or a fact sheet. Typically, one information medium will not meet the needs of all stakeholders.

Stakeholders' needs may differ based on their personal beliefs, preferences, or time constraints or based on the goal of the RC strategy. Understand-ing the stakeholders preferences and needs is part of the community profiling discussed earlier.

Table 45.4 provides a good summary of how to use knowledge about stakeholders to develop effective messages, select a good messenger, and choose the appropriate media.[7]

Information Sources on Community Stakeholders and Their Concerns

- *Environmental Documents Available for Public Review* — Several environmental laws require public involvement or studies that consider impacts on people and the environment. Documentation of this work can provide a good insight into the local community and their typical concerns. The National Environmental Policy Act (NEPA) requires Environmental Impact Statements that often incorporate information about the local communities and economy. In addition, sites covered by the Comprehensive Environmental Response, Compensation, and Liability Act (CERCLA or Superfund) are required to have a community relations plan. US EPA or your state's official environmental management office keeps a listing of work done under either of these laws. Documents on both NEPA and CERCLA work are open to the public for review. Check local libraries or government document repositories for copies of the documents.
- *Local Media Advertising Profiles* — The media needs to know their audience to attract advertising and viewers, listeners, or readers.
- *State or Local Elected Officials or Political Groups* — These organizations need to know their constituents to be reelected. They may be willing to share this information if you explain why you need it. In smaller communities the local mayor and his/her staff can be a very valuable resource because they personally know a large segment of the population and are likely aware of community concerns.
- *Health care agencies and cancer centers* — Public affairs or communication groups within larger health care agencies often have to communicate to large groups and will have developed community profiles.
- *Chambers of Commerce or other community economic development organizations* — These groups also conduct community research to provide information that might attract new businesses to the area.
- *Letters to the editor in the local newspaper and local media coverage* — These will tell you or elude to what the local concerns are and which groups are most vocal.
- *Related Information Materials* — Other organizations besides yours may be communicating about the risk or may have done so in the past. Look at the focus of their materials and the information they are providing for insight into typical concerns.

Figure 45.5 — Information sources on community stakeholders and their concerns. (Adapted from Reference 7.)

Conclusion

RC differs from the usual communication of technical or scientific information in that it most often involves two-way communication between the organization managing the risk and the affected stakeholders. It requires specialized skills because simply disseminating information without regard for communicating the complexities and uncertainties of risk is typically not effective when addressing concerns and questions from upset, angry, or distrustful stakeholders. For diverse stakeholders the pure mathematics of risk calculations are typically insufficient to address all facets of risk and risk perceptions. When engaging in RC activities, the total spectrum of risk must be considered; emotion-laden factors cannot be eliminated simply because they are subjective or difficult to measure. In any population these factors include legal, political, ethical, social, economic, cultural, and in some cases operational factors. Understanding the importance of these factors that affect risk perceptions, and establishing trust and credibility, is of utmost importance and must be considered when developing and implementing an RC activity.

Table 45.4 — Developing Effective Messages

Information Learned	*How to Tailor the Strategy*
Stakeholders unaware	Use graphic method-high color, compelling visuals, and theme.
Stakeholders apathetic (or feel like victims)	Open risk assessment and management process to allow stakeholder participation; show where past interactions have made a difference; provide choices.
Stakeholders well informed	Build on past information.
Stakeholders hostile	Acknowledge concerns and feelings; identify common ground; open risk assessment and management process to allow stakeholder participation.
Stakeholders highly educated	Use more sophisticated language and structure.
Stakeholders not highly educated	Use less sophisticated language and structure. Make structure highly visible, not subtle.
Stakeholders of mixed education level or upset or hostile	Use less sophisticated language and layer your information. Start with the most basic or to-the-point messages and move to the more complex.
Who the stakeholders trusts	Use that person to present risk information.
Where the stakeholders feel comfortable	Hold meetings in that location.
The method by which the stakeholders get most of their information	Use that method to convey your message
How the stakeholders want to be involved in the risk assessment or management of the issue	If at all possible, given time, funding, and organizational constraints, involve the audience in the way they want to be involved.
Misconceptions of risk or process	Find facts from sources the audience trusts (credible third-party sources) to fill gaps in knowledge and help correct false impressions.
Stakeholder concerns	Acknowledge concerns and provide relevant facts.

(Adapted from Reference 7.)

References

1. **National Research Council:** *Understanding Risk.* Washington, D.C.: National Academy Press, 1996.
2. **Occupational Safety and Health Administration:** Safety and Health Topics: Hazard Communication. [Online] Available at www.osha.gov/SLTC/hazardcommunications/index.html. (Accessed April 2003).
3. **Sandman, P.M:** *Responding to Community Outrage: Strategies for Effective Risk Communication.* Fairfax, Va.: AIHA Press, 1993.
4. **Liess, W.:** Three phases in the evolution of risk communication practice. *Ann. Am. Acad. Pol. Soc. Sci. 545*:85–94(1996).
5. **Patty, F.A.:** The industrial hygiene survey and personnel. In *Industrial Hygiene and Toxicology,* vol. 1, 2nd ed., p. 45. New York: John Wiley & Sons, 1948.
6. **Whitman, C.T.:** "Remarks of Governor Christine Todd Whitman, administrator of the U.S. Environmental Protection Agency." Presented at the EPA Science Forum, Washington, D.C., May 1, 2002.
7. **Lundgren, R., and A. McMakin:** *Risk Communication—A Handbook for Communicating Environmental, Safety, and Health Risks,* 2nd ed. Columbus, Ohio: Battelle Press, 1998.
8. **National Research Council:** *Improving Risk Communication.* Washington, D.C.: National Academy Press, 1989.
9. **Morgan, B., B. Fischoff, A. Bostrom, L. Lave, and C.J. Atman:** Communicating risk to the public. *Environ. Sci. Technol. 26*:2048–2056 (1992).
10. **Sandman, P.:** Risk communication: Facing public outrage. *EPA J. 13(9)*:21–22 (1987).
11. **Peters, R.G., V.T. Covello, and D.B. McCallum:** The determinants of trust and credibility in environmental risk communication: An empirical study. *Risk Anal. 17*: 43–54 (1997).
12. **Covello, V.T.:** Trust and credibility in risk communication. *Health Environ. Dig. 6(1)*:1–3 (1992).
13. **Covello, V.T.:** Risk communication and occupational medicine. *J. Occup. Med. 35*:18–19 (1993).
14. **Slovic, P.:** *The Perception of Risk.* London: Earthscan Publications, 2000.

15. **Heath, R.L.:** *Strategic Issues Management: Organizations and Public Policy Challenges.* Thousand Oaks, Calif.: Sage Publications, 1997.
16. **Williams, D.E., and B. A. Olaniran:** Expanding the crisis planning function: Introducing elements of risk communication to crisis communication practices. *Pub. Rel. Rev. 24*:387–400 (1998).
17. **Pauchant, T.C., and I.I. Mitroff:** *Transforming the Crisis-Prone Organization: Preventing Individual, Organizational, and Environmental Tragedies.* San Francisco, Calif.: Jossey-Bass, 1992.
18. **Covello, V., and P. Sandman:** Risk communication: Evolution and revolution. In A. Walbarst, editor, *Solutions to an Environment in Peril*, pp. 164–178. Baltimore, Md.: John Hopkins University Press, 2001.
19. **Environmental Protection Agency (EPA):** *EPA Superfund Community Involvement Toolkit—Risk Communication.* [Online] Available at www.epa.gov/superfund/tools/pdfs/37riskcom.pdf (Accessed April 25, 2003).
20. **Rogers, E.M.:** The field of health communication today: An up-to-date report. *J. Health Comm. 1*:15–23 (1996).
21. **Shoemaker, P.J.:** Media treatment of deviant political groups. *Journalism Q. 61*:66–75 (1984).
22. **Yanovitzky, I., and C. Bennett:** Media attention, institutional response and health behavior change. *Comm. Res. 26*:429–453 (1999).
23. **Shoemaker, P.J.:** *Gatekeeping.* Newbury, Calif.: Sage, 1991.
24. **Ball-Rokeach, S.J., Power, G.J., Guthrie, K.K., and H.R. Waring:** Value-framing abortion in the United States: An application of media system dependency theory. *Int. J. Pub. Opin. Res. 2*:249–273 (1990).
25. **Salome, K.L., M.R. Greenberg, P.M. Sandman,** & **D.B. Sachsman:** A question of quality: How journalists and news sources evaluate coverage of environmental risk. *J. Comm. 40*:117 (1990).
26. **Shanahan, J., M. Morgan, and M. Stenbjerre:** Green or brown? Television and the cultivation of environmental concern. *J. Broadcast. Elect. Media 41*:305–323 (1997).
27. **Archibald, E.:** Problems with environmental reporting: Perspectives of daily newspaper reporters. *J. Environ. Edu. 30*:27–32 (1999).
28. **Navy Environmental Health Center (NEHC):** *Risk Communication Primer,* 2nd ed. Norfolk, Va.: NEHC, 2002.
29. **Hance, B., C. Chess, and P. Sandman:** *Industry Risk Communication Manual—Improving Dialogue with Communities.* Boca Raton, Fla.: Lewis Publishers, 1990.
30. **Covello, V.T., P.M. Sandman, and P. Slovic:** *Risk Communication, Risk Statistics, and Risk Comparisons: A Manual For Plant Managers.* Washington, D.C.: Chemical Manufacturers Association, 1988.

Outcome Competencies

After completing this chapter, the reader should be able to:

1. Define underlined terms used in this chapter.
2. Recognize confined spaces.
3. Distinguish between types of confined spaces.
4. Recognize confined-space hazards.
5. Evaluate confined-space hazards.
6. Assess appropriate methods for elimination and control of confined-space hazards.
7. Design confined spaces to eliminate the need for entry and/or hazards.

Key Terms

attendant • confined spaces • entrants • entry • entry personnel • entry supervisor • horizontal entry • lower explosive limit • lower flannable limit • oxygen deficient atmospheres • oxygen enriched atmosphere • permit required confined spaces •upper flammable limit • vertical entry

Prerequisite Knowledge

College chemistry and physics.

Prior to beginning this chapter, the user should review the following chapters:

Chapter Number	Chapter Topic
1	History of Industrial Hygiene
4	Occupational Exposure Limits
5	Occupational Toxicology
7	Principles of Evaluating Worker Exposure
9	Comprehensive Exposure Limits
10	Modeling Inhalation Exposure
11	Sampling of Gases and Vapors
14	Sampling and sizing of Airborne Particles
15	Principles and Instrumentation for Calibrating Air Sampling Equipment
16	Preparation of Known Concentrations of Air Contaminants
17	Direct-Reading Instruments for Determining Concentrations of Gases, Vapors, and Aerosols
34	Prevention and Mitigation of Accidental Chemical Releases
35	General Methods for the Control of Airborne Hazards
37	Local Exhaust Ventilation
40	Respiratory Protection
41	Program Management
43	Hazard Communication
45	Risk Communication

Key Topics

I. Introduction
II. Why Are Confined Spaces a Concern?
III. Identifying and Classifying Confined Spaces
   A. Non-Permit Confined Spaces
   B. Permit-Required Confined Spaces
IV. Examples of Confined Space Types
V. Hazards Associated with Confined Spaces
   A. Atmospheric Hazards
   B. Hazards Originating in Adjacent Areas
   C. Perspectives on Industry-Specific Hazards
VI. Elements of a Confined Space Program
VII. Hazard Control Options
   A. Project Planning and Oversight
   B. Cleaning the Confined Space Surface to Reduce Hazards
   C. Ventilation to Reduce Hazards
   D. Why Ventilate Confined Spaces?
   E. Other Benefits of Ventilation
   F. Atmospheric Testing and Personal Air Monitoring While Ventilating
   G. Atmospheric Monitoring Process
   H. Air Moving Devices
VIII. Isolation of Hazardous Energy (Lockout-Tagout or LOTO)
   A. Lockout versus Tagout
   B. Elements of a Lockout/Tagout Program
   C. Energy Control Equipment
   D. Lighting
IX. Confined Space Design and Reducing Risk
X. References

Confined Space Entry

46

By Michael K. Harris, PhD, CIH

Introduction

The fundamental hazards of work in confined space workplace are, in most cases, essentially the same as they are in open work environments. However, work in confined spaces is typified by restricted access and egress as well as diminished natural ventilation. Because of these characteristics, work in confined spaces often increases risk of overexposure to atmospheric hazards due to compromised diffusion of airborne contaminants. Furthermore, work in confined spaces may be associated with physical hazards which are difficult to escape due to restricted egress.

Review of accident data by the National Institute for Occupational Safety and Health (NIOSH) and the Occupational Safety and Health Administration (OSHA) indicates that the primary hazards associated with confined-space entries can be grouped into five categories: (1) asphyxiation; (2) elevated concentration of toxic contaminants; (3) increased risk of fire or explosion; (4) entrapment and/or engulfment; and (5) other mechanical hazards such as crushing or electrocution.

Starting from this list of hazards, developing a confined space program is, in essence, nothing more than an exercise in applied industrial hygiene. A summary of the requirements of ANSI Z-117.1 outlines what is required:

- Identify permit-required confined spaces.
- Inform employees of the hazards posed by unauthorized entry.
- Establish procedures for identifying and controlling hazards associated with authorized entries into confined spaces.
- Develop a written confined space entry program.
- Complete a written confined space entry permit before entry.
- Establish a means for ensuring appropriate atmospheric monitoring, physical and chemical hazard isolation and ventilation.
- Designate employees who will be actively involved in the entry. These include entrants, attendants and those with supervisory responsibilities.
- Develop and emergency response plan.
- Establish a means for ensuring that those are involved in confined space entries are adequately trained and qualified.

It is evident that this process is a combination of anticipation, recognition, evaluation and control of hazards in the workplace, hazard communication, emergency planning and training. These skill sets are expected areas of competency for industrial hygienists who are frequently in leadership positions in developing these programs. This chapter provides insights into the application of the IH profession in the circumstances associated with confined space entries.

Why Are Confined Spaces A Concern?

Although there are other definitions of a "confined space," for the purposes of this chapter, a confined space can be described as exhibiting the following characteristics:

- An enclosed or partially enclosed workspace
- Limited means of entry and exit
- Subject to the accumulation of toxic and flammable contaminants
- May develop an oxygen deficiency or other atmospheric hazard
- Not intended for continuous employee occupancy.

Note that these characteristics focus primarily on development or accumulation of atmospheric hazards. Work in some confined spaces may involve possible exposure to physical hazards as well. Work in confined spaces may necessitate addressing sources of hazardous energy that may be unintentionally released, possibly leading to injury or death of workers in the space. Examples of physical hazard include:

- Engulfment by the contents of the space, as has happened in grain elevators.
- Drowning in liquids introduced into the space by workers inadvertently opening a valve.
- Electrocution by contact with compromised electrical equipment.
- Maiming by mixers which are energized while entrants are in the space.

A few summaries may illustrate the kinds of events that have resulted in death or injury in confined spaces:

> Two men were working outside a bin that was being emptied of grain. Believing that the bin was completely empty, one of the workers entered the bin through the bottom access door. Once inside, he was buried by material that suddenly broke loose from the sides of the bin. The worker was unable to find the access door, and the other worker could not locate him in time to save him.[1]
>
> Two workers were cleaning a wheat storage bin by using an auger to remove the grain. One worker was caught in the flowing grain created by the auger and was not able to free himself, even with the assistance of the other worker in the bin. The second worker was unable to communicate with workers outside the bin or to exit from the bin in time to get help and save the trapped worker.[1]
>
> On December 5, 1984, a 22-year-old worker died inside a toluene storage tank that was 10 feet in diameter and 20 feet high while attempting to clean the tank. The worker entered the tank through the 16 inch diameter top opening using a 1/2 inch rope for descent. Although a self-contained breathing apparatus was present, the worker was not wearing it when he entered the tank. The worker was overcome and collapsed onto the floor the tank. In an attempt to rescue the worker, fire department personnel began cutting an opening into the side of the tank. The tank exploded, killing a 32-year-old firefighter and injuring 15 others.[2]
>
> On July 2, 1985, a crew foreman became ill and was hospitalized after using an epoxy coating, which contained 2-nitropropane and coal tar pitch, to coat a valve on an underground waterline. The valve was located in an enclosed service vault (12' x 15' x 15'). The worker was released from the hospital on July 3, 1985, but was readmitted on July 6, 1985. He lapsed into a coma and died on July 12, 1985, as a result of acute liver failure induced by inhalation of 2-nitropropane and coal tar pitch vapors. A co-worker was also hospitalized, but did not die.[2]

Failure to anticipate, recognize, evaluate, and control these hazards has resulted in an incredible number of preventable deaths and injuries resulting from inappropriate confined-space entries. Some perspective on the magnitude of the problem maybe gained from a frequently referenced review of 28,450 accident reports from a 3-year period from 1974 to 1977. This work, sponsored by NIOSH, reported 276 confined-space entry incidents that resulted in 193 deaths and 234 injuries.(5) Underreporting of industrial accidents was no less a problem 30 years ago than it is today, and this data almost certainly underreports the true number of incidents, particularly injuries.

In the absence of a formal Confined Space Program and concomitant training,

Personnel preparing to enter confined spaces may not recognize the hazards that confront them. In many cases, previous entries into the work area may have been made without any adverse effects, reducing the perception of the extent or intensity of the hazards. Many confined-space entry death and injury reports state that spaces in question have been entered previously with no adverse effects, or at least none reported. This inconsistency reflects the experience that hazards may not develop (at least to the same extent) every time a space is entered. This variability in hazard expression or development may be a function of a number of factors that vary from one entry to the next. Some of these might include:

- Previous contents of the space,
- Length of time since previous entry,
- Work to be conducted in the space, and
- Ventilation of the space prior to an during the entry.

Since the hazards associated with confined spaces may not be immediately evident to personnel who are about to enter the spaces, a Confined Space Program is a useful tool for identifying and mitigating these hazards.

Industrial hygienists working with confined space issues in the U.S. are directed by federal and state standards. It must be emphasized that this chapter is not intended as a guideline for compliance with these standards. However, the definitions and requirements listed therein offer valuable information for Confined Space Program development and federal standards are listed below for ease of reference. Bear in mind that, since the publishing of this text, standards could have been added, changed, or deleted.

- 29 CFR 1910.146 — Permit Required Confined Spaces
- 29 CFR 1910.147 — Control of Hazardous Energy
- 29 CFR 1910.146 — Permit Required Confined Spaces
- 29 CFR 1910.147 — Control of Hazardous Energy
- CFR 1910.119 — Process Safety Management of Highly Hazardous Chemicals
- 29 CFR 1910.134 — Respiratory Protection
- 29 CFR 1910.253 — Welding, Cutting and Brazing
- 29 CFR 1910.94(d) — Open Surface Tanks
- 29 CFR 1910.268 — Telecommunications
- 29 CFR 1910.269 — Electric Power, Generation, Transmission and Distribution
- 29 CFR 1910.272 — Grain Handling Facilities
- 9 CFR 1915 Subpart B — Shipyard Employment
- 29 CFR 1926.21(6) — Safety Education and Training
- 29 CFR 1926.352(g) — Fire Prevention

Also, the following texts provide valuable perspective for planning or confronting work in a confined space.

- **American Industrial Hygiene Association (AIHA®):** *Confined Space Entry, An AIHA Protocol Guide*. Chambers, G. (ed.). Fairfax, VA: AIHA®, 2001.
- **McManus, N.:** *Safety and Health in Confined Spaces*. Boca Raton, FL: Lewis Publishers, 1999.
- **Rekus, J.F.:** *Complete Confined Space Handbook*. Boca Raton, FL: Lewis Publishers, 1994.
- **Finkel, M.H.:** *Guidelines for Hot Work in Confined Spaces*. Des Plaines, IL: American Society of Safety Engineers, 2000.

The reader is encouraged to keep the following two questions in mind while contemplating work in a confined space:

1. Is it absolutely necessary to enter the space? If there is some other reasonable way to do the proposed work without a confined-space entry, that option should be investigated.
2. If there is no alternative to entering the space, is there a means of eliminating the hazards prior to entry, rather than simply dealing with them as they are?

If possible, the first choice in controlling confined-space hazards is to avoid entry.

Identifying and Classifying Confined Spaces

A widely accepted definition of a confined space is outlined in the OSHA Permit-Required Confined Space Standard, 29 CFR 1910.146. This federal standard states that a confined space meets all three of the following criteria:

(1) It is large enough and so configured that an employee can bodily enter the space and perform her/his assigned work;
(2) it has limited or restricted means for entry or exit, and
(3) it is not designed for continuous human occupancy.

It is important to realize that confined spaces meeting the above criteria are not necessarily extraordinarily hazardous work environments. Generally speaking, the primary concern in these cases is that limited or restricted means of entry and exit (e.g., obstructions within the space or excessive distances between the work area and the entrance) may make rescue difficult in the event of an injury or sudden illness, such as a broken limb or heart attack. In the absence of any other hazards, one may regard such spaces generally as non-permit confined spaces.

Non-permit Confined Spaces

The term "non-permit confined spaces" refers to confined spaces that do not contain, or do not have the potential to contain, any hazard capable of causing death or serious physical harm. In most cases this determination is based on the absence of atmospheric hazards, although other considerations such as engulfment, drowning, crushing and release of hazardous energy must be taken into account. Examples of non-permit confined spaces would include areas above dropped ceilings or vented electrical vaults. If a confined space is classified as a non-permit confined space, it is necessary to specify what conditions and precautions must be in place to allow for an entry without a permit. Further, it must be made clear that non-permit spaces may be re-classified as permit-required confined spaces if work to be conducted in the space may change the hazards associated with entry.

Permit-Required Confined Spaces

The physical restrictions and reduced dilution ventilation associated with confined spaces requires one to determine whether there are health or safety hazards either (1) present in the space or (2) associated with the work to be conducted in the confined space. If a confined space exhibits any of the following characteristics one may anticipate that illness, injury, and/or death may be outcomes of careless entry into the space.

- The space contains a hazardous atmosphere or may have the reasonable potential to contain a hazardous atmosphere.
- The space contains a material that may engulf an entrant. (People entering confined spaces are called entrants.)
- The space has an internal configuration with inwardly sloping walls or a tapering cross-section that may allow the entrant to become trapped or asphyxiated.
- The space contains any other serious health or safety hazard.

Recognizing the need to identify and control these hazards, confined spaces that exhibit any of these characteristics are defined as permit-required confined spaces. Examples of such spaces that should be investigated to determine whether they meet the above criteria include but are by no means limited to storage tanks; process vessels; silos; boilers/fire boxes; open surface tanks; storm drains; pits beneath equipment; storage drums; manholes; cooking vessels; railroad tank cars; and furnaces. It should be emphasized that in the absence of the existence of hazards noted above, a permit may not be required to enter a confined space. However, the tasks to be performed in the confined space must also be carefully evaluated to ascertain whether they may create atmospheric or physical hazards in the confined space.

When possible, it is best practice to eliminate the hazards prior to entry. This reduces risk and may allow the space to be classified as non-permit required.

Examples of Confined Space Types

A few examples of confined space configurations are offered here along with comments regarding the hazards that may be specific or typical for those spaces. Among the characteristics that affect the hazards associated with a confined space are its physical characteristics (e.g., configuration) and atmospheric characteristics (e.g. oxygen deficiency or presence of toxins).

The comments provided here are not to be regarded as all-inclusive or as an exhaustive list. Rather, this discussion is intended to provide a starting point for questions during the Facility Survey noted below. The physical layout of the space will affect entry accessibility, ventilation options and rescue access. The effects of configuration cannot be isolated from the effects of the activity to be conducted in the space and comments regarding work activities are included in this section for purposes of illustration.

Some examples of various physical characteristics include:

- Vertical axis dominant
- Horizontal axis dominant
- Internal structures
- Presence of entryways
- Piping associated
- Mixers associated
- Electrical energy associated
- Mechanical energy associated
- Pressurized energy source associated
- Engulfment hazards
- Below grade
- Behind embankments

As an example, the fractionation towers in Figure 46.1 are vertical axis dominant. These shapes are conducive to vertical airflow for dilution ventilation. Process piping can be disconnected from the sides, tops and/or bottoms of these towers for purposes of isolating the towers from chemical processes prior to entry. The flanges from which the piping has been disconnected can be used for access to the internal spaces of the towers (Figure 46.2). These flanges may also serve as locations for attaching ventilation equipment and for make-up air entry. Fractionation towers also have internal structures associated with their operation. The internal structures may be called trays, riser supporters or distributors, among other terms. In some instances, these internal structures may be used as working platforms by entrants or, in other cases, they may be the components to be removed and replaced by entrants. In either case these structures are likely to affect the flow of dilution ventilation through the tower.

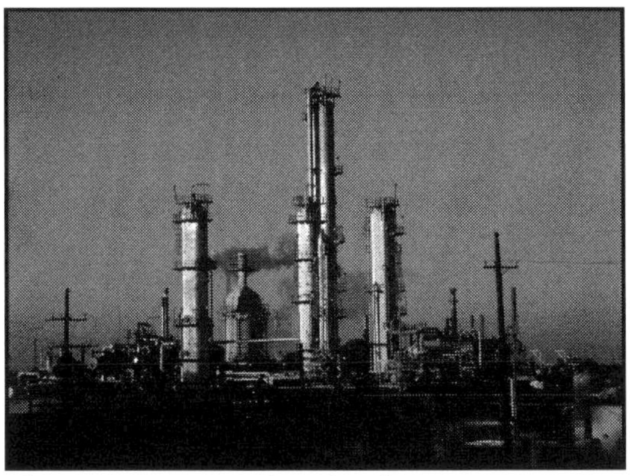

Figure 46.1 — Vertical confined spaces.

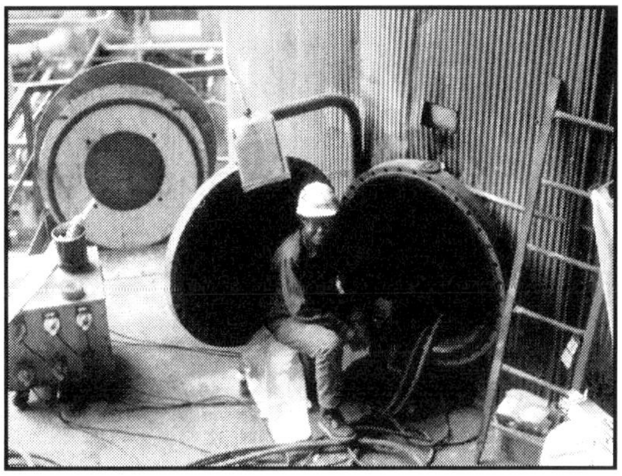

Figure 46.2 — Process piping connections used as entry manways.

Internal structures may also be, in themselves, confined spaces. Figure 46.3 illustrates an item of petrochemical process equipment that has been taken out of service. Note that this tower, now resting on its side, consists of two concentric tubular spaces. The inner space is a "confined space with a confined space." When conducting a facility survey, this characteristic may not be evident upon visual inspection. Reference to engineering drawings and/or interviews with site personnel may be necessary to identify this characteristic.

Horizontal axis dominant confined spaces may be illustrated by the rotary kiln illustrated in Figures 46.4 and 46.5.

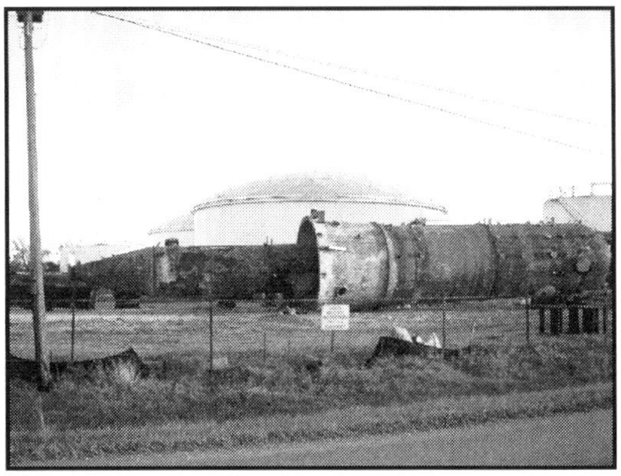

Figure 46.3 — Confined space within a confined space.

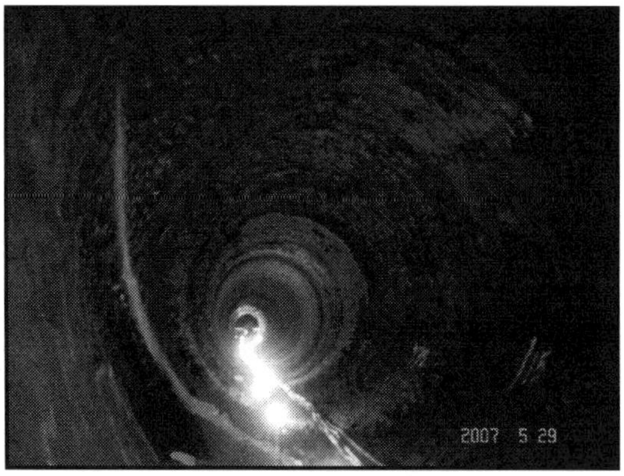

Figure 46.4 — Horizontal confined space.

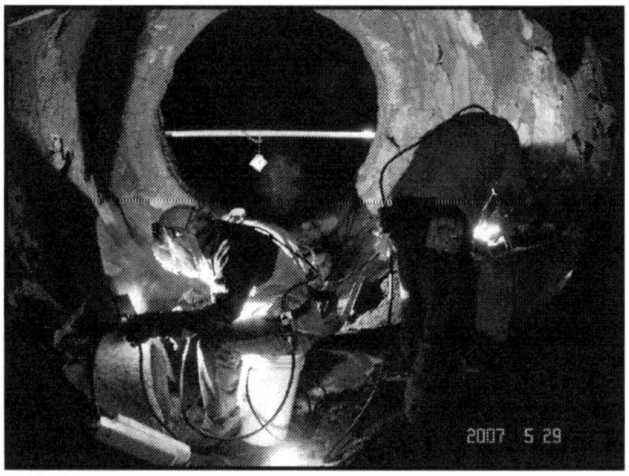

Figure 46.5 — Welding inside a horizontal confined space.

Horizontal spaces often offer easier access and movement within the space. However, scaffolding may be necessary to allow access to the upper portions of the interior of the equipment cannot be rotated. Examples of horizontal axis dominant spaces include highway chemical trailers, rail cars and petrochemical plant equipment. One of the more common confined spaces exhibiting a horizontal axis is a pipeline. When certain corrosion resistant metals are welded, the section of the pipeline being welded must be purged of oxygen. This process may involve the following sequence: 1) placing temporary dams in the pipeline on either side of the area to be welded, 2) connecting a source of inter gas, such as argon, to the space defined by the dams, 3) purging the section to be welded of oxygen 4), testing to confirm lack of oxygen, 5) welding the pipeline and 6) venting the pipeline so that it can be inspected from the inside.

On April 29, 1994, a welder's helper performed an unauthorized entry into a 30" diameter stainless steel pipeline in Alaska. The purpose of the unauthorized entry was to inspect a temporary dam which was believed to have shifted from its correct location. This unauthorized entry was performed before the pipeline had been ventilated to remove the argon and restore the atmosphere to a breathable condition. When the crew working on the job had completed ventilating the pipeline they sought the welder's helper to inform him that entry was now possible. When the crew noticed the hard hat belonging to the welder's helper at the entrance to the pipeline, they entered and found the helper unconscious. He was removed from the space and attempts were made to revive him but they were unsuccessful.

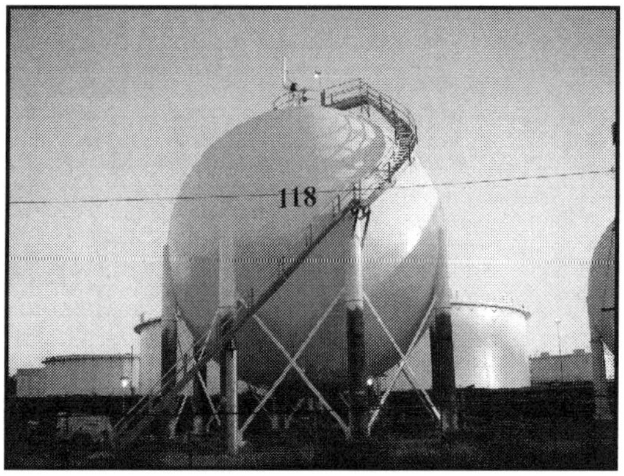

Figure 46.6 — Spherical confined space.

Spherical confined spaces, like those illustrated in Figure 46.6, are often devoid of any internal structures. Work within these spherical storage vessels may include removing old coatings, applying new coatings and/or replacing metal that has been compromised by corrosion. Spherical storage vessels may have very little piping connected to them, limiting entry and ventilation options. In addition, any work on the walls of the spherical storage vessel will require erection of scaffolding to allow access to these walls. Scaffolding is also commonly used in vertical towers. Use of scaffolding may generate an increased potential for fall hazards within the confined space.

Other physical characteristics to be targeted for investigation include piping that passes through the confined space or is connected to the confined space when it is on normal operation. High pressure steam, nitrogen, and other compressed gasses present hazards to entrants if those pressurized gases are released.

When the confined space includes mixers, blenders, grinders, shredders or other components that can injure entrants if energized, these components must be isolated from their sources of energy. These sources may include electrical, hydraulic, mechanical or pneumatic power. Isolation of these energy sources are addressed by OSHA in 29 CFR 1910.147.

Work below grade or within embankments is worthy of analysis for possible hazards. Engulfment by unstable soil is a sufficiently common hazard to warrant a specific OSHA Standard (29 CFR 1926.651). Work locations below grade may also be work locations which exhibit poor natural ventilation. As an example, NIOSH reports the 1989 deaths of two brothers who entered a manure pit on a dairy farm.[3] The pit was approximately 12 feet square and 4½ feet deep. A waste pump line was clogged and one brother entered the pit to clear the blockage. This person soon collapsed and his brother entered the pit to retrieve him. The second brother was also overcome by a concentration of gases in the pit believed to include hydrogen sulfide, carbon dioxide and methane. Both men, who were in their 30s and had worked at the farm since they were teenagers, died. In view of this event, and others like it, subgrade locations or areas behind embankments that are subject to accumulations of heavier-than-air chemical asphyxiants, physical asphyxiants or toxins should be treated as confined spaces.

Hazards Associated With Confined Spaces

Although there are innumerable lists of confined space hazards it may be most convenient to remain with the basic list below derived from the General Industry Confined Space Standard and offer some examples that illustrate and expand on these hazards.

- The space has been identified as containing a hazardous atmosphere prior to commencing work.
- The space may have the reasonable potential to contain a hazardous atmosphere.
- The work to be conducted in the space may generate an atmospheric hazard.
- The space contains a material that may engulf a person entering the space.
- The space has an internal configuration with inwardly sloping walls or a tapering cross-section that may allow the entrant to become trapped or asphyxiated.
- The space contains any other serious health or safety hazard.

Atmospheric Hazards

There are two fundamental facets of the atmospheric hazard identification process:

- Identify the characteristics of the atmosphere before work begins (pre-entry atmosphere). The pre-entry atmosphere must be characterized prior to commencing work in the confined space. A thorough knowledge of the history and use of the confined space is necessary to anticipate and recognize possible atmospheric hazards that may exist prior to entry.
- Prior to beginning work, determine if the work to be performed in the space will affect the atmosphere as the work progresses (work atmosphere). In order to plan for potential hazards associated with the work atmosphere, one must become familiar with the tasks and work practices to be followed while working in the confined space.

Evaluation of either the pre-entry atmosphere or the work atmosphere requires measuring several atmospheric constituents. Some facilities use the term "atmosphere testing" and others may employ the term "gas testing" for this evaluation. Whatever the procedure is called, a number of aspects are commonly addressed:

- Oxygen content.
- Presence of flammable gases, vapors, mists, fibers or dusts
- Presence of toxic gases, vapors, mists, smoke, fibers or dusts
- Less often, airborne biological contaminants may be addressed.

Once work has begun in the confined space, frequent air monitoring may be necessary to track possible changes in the workplace atmosphere due to the tasks being performed. A brief discussion of these potential atmospheric hazards may help illustrate the importance of evaluating each of these factors.

Oxygen Deficiency

Oxygen deficiency is among the most common atmospheric hazards associated with confined space entry. Individuals who enter the space, either for preliminary inspection or with the intent of performing work, without first performing atmospheric testing for oxygen, are at risk of experiencing oxygen deficiency. The acute adverse effects of oxygen deficiency can present with astonishing rapidity and the general working population does not seem to be well versed in the symptoms of oxygen deficiency. McManus has summarized the acute symptoms of oxygen deficiency as follows[4]:

- At concentrations of less than 16% at standard temperature and pressure (STP) or less than 122 mmHg partial pressure: Increased heart rate, increased breathing rate, some decrease in coordination, increased breathing volume, impaired attention and impaired thought processes.
- At concentrations of less than 14% at standard temperature and pressure (STP) or less than 107 mmHg partial pressure: Abnormal fatigue upon exertion, emotional upset, faulty coordination, impaired judgement
- At concentrations of less than 12% at standard temperature and pressure (STP) or less than 91 mmHg partial pressure: Very poor judgement and coordination, impaired respiration, tunnel vision
- At concentrations of less than 10% at standard temperature and pressure (STP) or less than 76 mmHg partial pressure: Nausea, vomiting, lethargy, inability to perform vigorous movements, possible unconsciousness followed by death.
- At concentrations of less than 6% at standard temperature and pressure (STP) or less than 46 mmHg partial pressure: Convulsions, shortness of breath, cardiac standstill, spasmodic breathing, death in minutes.
- At concentrations of less than 4% at standard temperature and pressure (STP) or less than 30 mmHg partial pressure: Unconsciousness within 1 or 2 breaths followed by death.

The onset of symptoms is affected by a number of factors, including:

- breathing rate
- work rate
- temperature
- emotional stress
- age
- individual susceptibility[4]

A minimum value of 19.5% oxygen has been widely accepted as an acceptable criterion for identifying a space as oxygen deficient. However, the reader is cautioned that the human body responds to the aveolar partial pressure of oxygen rather than the percent of oxygen in respired air and that there remains substantial lack of agreement as to what actually constitutes an oxygen deficient atmosphere. A number of factors may easily result in oxygen alveolar partial pressures less than that equivalent to an atmosphere containing 20.9% oxygen at STP.[4] These factors may include work at higher elevations (above 2,000 feet msl), work in spaces containing low levels of chemical asphyxiants such as carbon monoxide or methylene chloride or vigorous work that reduces the dwell time of the hemoglobin at the alveoli with consequent reduced oxygen uptake. Reduced oxygen uptake may result in reduced aveolar partial pressure of oxygen.

It is more prudent to use 20.9% as an acceptable value for oxygen content simply because it is a rare set of circumstances that will reliably and consistently provide workers with some oxygen content other than 20.9%. If a confined space atmosphere does not measure 20.9% oxygen, there is something happening in the space that must be identified, evaluated and controlled. If the reason for a non-standard oxygen content cannot be identified and controlled, the justification for entry with respiratory protection other than an air line supplied air respirator or self-contained breathing apparatus with an escape pack should be re-evaluated.

Oxygen deficiency may be caused by the displacement of the normal atmosphere by simple asphyxiants such as acetylene, argon, ethane, ethylene, helium, hydrogen, methane, nitrogen, neon, propane and propylene. Acetylene, argon, helium, hydrogen, propane and propylene are gases which may be employed in welding and cutting processes. Leaking hoses or fittings may release these gases to the confined space atmosphere. However, the most common source of these gases may be simple failure to turn the torch valves off fully when exiting the space for breaks.

Biological process may also cause oxygen deficiency by consuming oxygen through bacterial metabolism. This may be exacerbated by production of methane (a simple asphyxiant) as product of the microorganism's metabolism. This set of conditions is frequently associated with sewers and subgrade electrical vaults (manholes).

A fairly common cause of oxygen deficiency is rusting of steel surfaces; oxidation of the steel removes oxygen form the confined space atmosphere as the oxygen is combined with iron in the steel. Also, the use of an internal combustion engine within the space (for example, a portable engine-driven pump) may consume the available oxygen within the space.

Oxygen Enrichment

Oxygen enrichment is less common than oxygen deficiency but may be found in deep mines or when working in caissons. Oxygen enrichment may also develop in confined spaces if a welding torch is allowed to leak oxygen into the workplace atmosphere. Elevated aveolar partial pressure of oxygen may result in respiratory irritation, throat irritation, tracheal irritation, tingling of fingers and toes, visual impairment, hallucinations, and other central nervous system disorders.

An oxygen enriched atmosphere (generally defined as greater than 23.5% oxygen) also introduces increased flammability hazards. Less thermal energy is required for ignition and the rate of flame travel is greater in an oxygen enriched atmosphere. Oxygen enriched atmospheres must be regarded as highly hazardous environments. As an illustration, in the heat of the so-called "Space Race", the three man crew of Apollo One was burned alive on January 27, 1967 on the launch pad at Cape Kennedy in a pure oxygen atmosphere while testing their spacecraft.[1] This event caused NASA to halt further manned use of the Command Module for approximately a year. During this period, NASA and the contractor who had built the spacecraft redesigned it to eliminate possible causes of ignition and to allow the spacecraft to operate with a normal earth atmosphere of 20.9% oxygen.

Use of Inert Gasses

Many industrial processes require a non-oxidizing atmosphere in the process vessel. These non-oxidizing atmospheres are referred to as "inert" even though the "inerting gas" is usually nitrogen, which is far from inert. Frequently, the requirement for a non-oxidizing atmosphere is driven by the use of pyrophors in the process or by the generation of pyrophors during the process. Iron sulfide is a commonly found pyrophor in certain petroleum refining processes. When it is necessary to enter these process vessels, it may not be possible to remove all of the pyrophors prior to entry. As a consequence, the confined space may remain intentionally "inerted." Entries into these confined spaces are, of course, conducted in supplied air breathing apparatus with an escape pack.

When it is possible to remove the pyrophors from the process vessel prior to entry, entries are usually allowed without supplied air. Herein lies the possibility that the wrong valve may be turned by an uninformed person and nitrogen or other gasses may be introduced into the vessel. Consequently, strict controls of the means of introducing inert gases into confined spaces are considered an integral part of most corporate confined space programs. In many cases, simply padlocking two valves in the inert gas supply line in the closed position is deemed adequate. In other cases, the more conservative decision is made to disconnect the inert gas line from the vessel or to insert a blanking or blinding plate into the line at one of the valve flanges. This procedure may also be incorporated in a "Lock Out, Tag Out" program that compliments the Confined Space Entry program.

Flammable Gases, Vapors, Mists, Fibers or Dusts

A fire in an open environment is bad enough. A fire or explosion in a confined space brings about consequences for the entrants that are beyond adequate verbal description. Possible sources of flammable gases, vapors, mists or fibers may include:

- Contents of confined spaces used for storage or processing; e.g., silos, petroleum storage tanks, refinery process vessels and ship cargo holds.

1 The three U.S. Astronauts were Gus Grissom, Ed White and Roger Chaffee.

- Coatings on the internal surfaces of the space; e.g., paint and insulation.
- Residue from incomplete cleaning of the internal surfaces of the space; e.g., petroleum products in corners of tanks or in the void spaces between vessel liners and the vessel shell.
- Airborne materials evolving from tasks or procedures taking place inside the space; e.g., welding gases, gases evolving from sludge removal, dusts generated by disturbing silo contents.

In order to begin the process of anticipating the flammability hazards that may be associated with work in a confined space, it is imperative that the occupational hygienist, with responsibility for confined space entries, review the Material Safety Data Sheets (MSDSs) for:

1. The material stored or processed in a space;
2. Coatings which may have been applied to internal surfaces of the space, and
3. Materials which will be introduced into the space during the entry (welding gases, solvents, cleaning solutions).

All flammable vapors and gases have a lower and an upper flammable limit, which together set the boundaries of the flammable or explosive range. A generally accepted safe level for flammable gases or vapors is 10% of the lower explosive limit (LEL). This concept is illustrated Figure 46.7 using the data for gasoline vapors as an example. These vapors are ignitable only within the flammable range. If an ignition source were introduced into a concentration of vapors below the lower flammable limit, the mixture of gasoline vapors and air would not burn. Below the lower flammable limit the mixture is too lean; not enough fuel vapors are present. The mixture would not ignite above the upper flammable limit because it is too rich, having too many fuel vapors compared with the oxygen in the air. The target for controlling potentially flammable atmospheres is to maintain an environment below 10% of the lower flammable limit . This allows a 90% safety margin before the bottom of the flammable range is reached. The Fire Protection Handbook and the National Fire Code® set contains detailed information on the characteristics of combustible dusts and their appropriate handling.

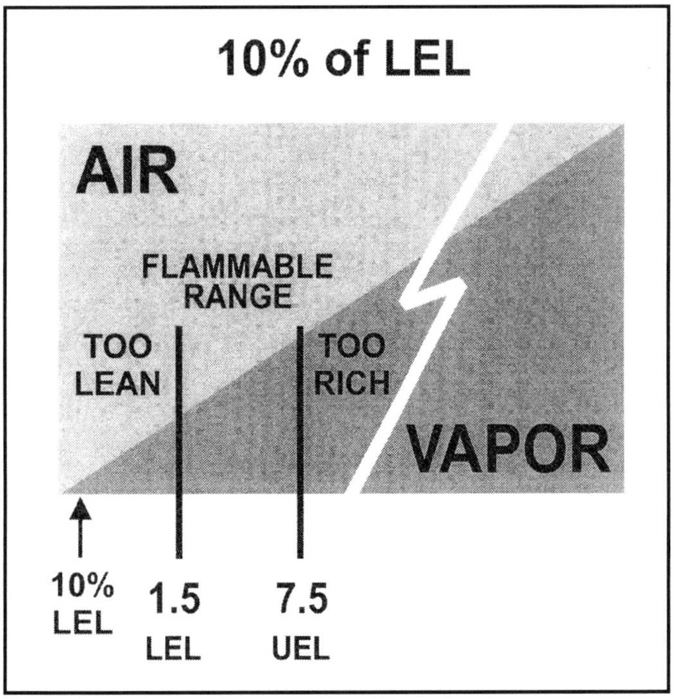

Figure 46.7 — Target range for controlling flammable atmospheres.

Presence of Toxic Gases, Vapors, Mists, Smoke, Fibers or Dusts

In order to determine if a potential for overexposure to toxins exist, one must first identify:

- What was in the space during operations or use;
- What is in the space right now (including cleaning compounds or residue as well as inerting or purging gases);
- What chemicals or materials will be taken into the space to perform the required work, and
- What tasks will be performed in the space.

The occupational hygienist must therefore be thoroughly familiar with all phases of the work to anticipate possible overexposures. In addition, review of the pertinent MSDSs is required to identify the health hazards from overexposure to recognized toxins that may be associated with a confined space entry. Many of the chapters in this text address human response to a variety of toxins. Conducting work in a confined space neither increases nor decreases the adverse health effects of overexposure to these toxins. In terms of toxins, the differences between work in a confined space and work in an open area lie primarily in reduced air movement, and increased chances of excessive skin contact with agents affecting the skin.

Reduced air movement in most confined spaces results in:

- *Increased airborne concentrations of volatile compounds which may out-gas from the inner surfaces of the space or from the contents of the space.* This may affect the pre-entry atmosphere.
- *Accumulation of atmospheric contaminants which may be generated by biological process.* Again, this affects the pre-entry atmosphere.
- *Concentration of contaminants generated by work being performed during the entry.* Welding fumes, paint and solvent vapors and grinding dust as well as volatile compounds evolving from sludge clean-out are examples of sources of these contaminants. Heating of the surfaces of metal storage surfaces that have contained leaded gasoline or sour petroleum products in known to release tetraethyl lead and sulfur dioxide, respectively, into the confined space atmosphere.

  Another example involves personnel removing ash and boiler scale accumulations from fuel-oil-fired electrical power plant fire boxes. The dimensions of these fireboxes dimensions are measured in tens of meters. These workers have been overexposed to vanadium pentoxide even when the vanadium concentrations in the fuel oil is less than 200 parts per million. The presence of the vanadium in the fuel oil was NOT determined from the MSDS as this metal was present in amounts less than the 1% reporting threshold for non-carcinogens. Indeed, at 200 ppm in the boiler ash, the vanadium concentrations did not meet the criterion in 29 CFR 1910.1200 of 0.1% for carcinogens. This metal was detected during laboratory analysis of the fuel oil by the power plant Quality Assurance Lab personnel. Personal breathing zone monitoring of workers removing the ash showed overexposures an order of magnitude above the TLV®-TWA of 0.05 mg/m^3 for vanadium pentoxide dust or fume. Workers who had been removing boiler scale without respiratory protection had previously complained of upper respiratory tract and skin irritation. Had the Quality Assurance Lab personnel failed to note the presence of traces of vanadium pentoxide in the boiler scale, the source of this complaint may have remained unidentified and unresolved. In this case, the matter was addressed with a water mist during removal to reduce dust concentrations as well as use of skin and respiratory protection.
- *Concentration of contaminants produced by decomposition or reaction of materials within the space.* Examples include: evolution of lead from burned paint and decomposition of chlorinated hydrocarbon degreasers into phosgene and hydrochloric acid when heated. The MSDS review must therefore include reference to the "Hazardous Products of Decomposition" and "Reactivity" sections of the MSDS.

These concerns regarding accumulation or generation of toxins are most often addressed via mechanically powered ventilation systems which force uncontaminated air through the space, providing dilution ventilation. Recommendations for confined space ventilation are found later in this chapter.

Possible Engulfment

Identification of possible engulfment hazards may be more readily amenable to visual examination than atmospheric hazards. Silos, hoppers, bins and similar storage spaces contain materials that are expected to flow freely under normal circumstances. Some materials, such as shredded wood or bark are fibrous in nature and may temporarily lock together, forming a "bridge" in a silo or hopper. If the wood fibers stop flowing from the bottom of the silo or hopper, workers may enter to investigate. If they attempt to walk on upper surface of the wood strands, their weight may cause the "bridge" to collapse and the entrant(s) may become engulfed in the shredded wood and bark. The weight of the surrounding material may make expansion of thoracic cavity impossible and the entrant(s) may suffocate. Similar circumstances may apply for grain, damp sand or cement, or any other material stored in silos bins or hoppers.

Large storage spaces may exhibit sloping accumulations of loose materials that can cascade or avalanche down carrying entrants with the moving materials. The effect is similar to that experienced by skiers caught in a snow avalanche. Stairs, flooring and temporary scaffolding (for repair or construction) may not be structurally sound or may become damaged or weakened by corrosion. Consequent structural failure may lead to personnel being dumped into the loose material below. Fall protection becomes an important element of a confined space entry program when possible engulfment and, as noted below, unfavorable internal configurations are identified.

The space has an internal configuration with inwardly sloping walls or a tapering cross-section that may allow the entrant to become trapped or asphyxiated.

Removing the contents from silos, hoppers, bins and similar storage spaces may not remove all possible hazards. Entrants have become wedged in the tapering, funnel-like, bottoms of cyclones and storage spaces. This concern may be exacerbated by slippery surfaces. In some cases, this has resulted in asphyxiation due to restriction of the thoracic cavity.

The space contains any other serious health or safety hazard.

Other possible serious health or safety hazards may seem almost innumerable. A partial listing, much of which is summarized from *Confined Space Entry, An AIHA® Protocol Guide*, is offered below. The mere presence of these hazards does not automatically mean that an entry permit is required prior to entry. However, these potential hazards are certainly worthy of investigation and an evaluation of potential for injury or death.

- Noise hazards

  Elevated sound pressure levels (e.g., from ventilation fans) may require the use of hearing protection. The internal surfaces of many confined spaces are hard and smooth and provide excellent sound reflection properties. These confined spaces may be reverberant fields which provide little sound attenuation. These factors may complicate communications between the entrants and attendant, resulting in increased risk for the entrant. Extreme noise conditions may present hazards from vibration.
- Animals such as rodents, pigeons, snakes, skunks, and many others pose hazards from bites, scratches, and in the case of skunks, getting sprayed. Animal waste and dead animals may create atmospheric problems in the space.
- Insects may present a nuisance or an actual hazard. They can be quite bothersome even when not dangerous, but many insects do bite or sting, and some are poisonous. Particular care is required if a nest of insects is present.
- Disease organisms may be present in human waste and other biological materials. Proper protection of entry personnel is essential in these situations.
- Ignition sources within the confined space.

  Examples may include; grinding, welding, cutting, burning, brazing, space heaters, hand tools, power tools, exposed light bulbs and potential sources of static electricity discharge (e.g., synthetic clothing or the transfer of liquids and gases through lines that are not electrically bonded or grounded).
- Skin contact with irritant or corrosive agents.

  Prior to entry, many industrial process vessels are chemically cleaned. Either the chemical cleaner or the material to be removed may be associated with dermal insults. This can be a concern during work in confined spaces, particularly in awkward spaces. Anyone who has worked in a petroleum refinery "turn-around" or a power plant "shut-down" can attest that skin contact with the interior walls will occur during entry. Skin contact issues are covered elsewhere in this text (see Chapters 20 and 21)
- Surface temperature extremes create a contact hazard.
- This may be a particular problem with metal tanks. Consider items such as steam or cryogenic lines within the space. Furnaces and ovens are good examples of common confined spaces where surface temperatures will be high.
- Fluid Levels.

  Fluid levels within a confined space pose two primary challenges to entrants: 1) the liquid itself may be hazardous or 2) even nonhazardous fluids such as water distort a worker's ability to detect surface changes in the bottom of the space. Rapidly changing fluid levels may also present a hazard. For example, entries into open storm sewer lines expose personnel to the risk of rapid flooding of the confined space.

- Potential for falls from heights.
  Many permit-required confined spaces are tall fractionation towers with internal pans or trays. Portions of these trays are removed during maintenance procedures and the resultant openings present potential fall hazards. This concern may be exacerbated by slippery surfaces.
- Falling objects.
  Examples include; tools, debris and structural materials.
- Movement of confined spaces that are not adequately secured prior to entry, e.g.,
  — Ships and barges not tied up
  — Railcars and tank trucks not chocked or blocked
  — Shifting or falling of tank trucks lacing a cab or jack stand
- Process material lines, if open or leaking, may introduce materials which exhibit the following hazards into the confined space:
  — Toxic
  — Flammable
  — Oxidizing
  — Corrosive
  — Chemical or physical asphyxiation
  — Thermal hazards from heated or chilled materials (e.g., steam or liquefied petroleum gases)
- Hazardous energy sources.
  This suite of hazards is of sufficient concern that OSHA has promulgated a separate standard to address them. 29 CFR 1910.147, Isolation of Hazardous Energy, requires employers to develop a formal program with procedures for identifying and controlling hazardous energy sources that may impact workers. This standard applies to the entire workplace, not just confined spaces. However, the potential for serious injury or death may be increased in confined spaces. All potential energy sources that could pose a risk to entry personnel must be identified and eliminated or controlled prior to entering the space. Potential hazards of concern include:
  — Moving mechanical equipment:
  Examples include: agitators, tumblers, crushers, mixing blades, screw conveyors and shakers.
  — Electrical power sources:
  Examples include: transmission and distribution lines, junction boxes and transformers.
  — Electrically, hydraulically or pneumatically powered equipment which may be: 1) taken into the space by workers or 2) permanently installed in the space as part of the facility. **These items of equipment are particularly hazardous if they can be remotely started or operated.** Little imagination is required to envision the consequences of being inside a vessel with mixing blades when the equipment is energized.
  — Pressurized lines must be depressurized prior to entry.
  Examples include: steam, hydraulic, pneumatic, fuel and other gases and water lines.
  — Radiation sources inside confined spaces may include: 1)ionizing radiation sources (frequently used as level gauges) and 2) nonionizing sources such a ultraviolet lamps (for curing polymers) or lasers.
- Limited lighting is associated with at least two concerns:
  — Difficulty in work safely due to reduced vision.
  — Apprehension and claustrophobia may increase in poor lighting conditions.
- Temperature extremes may be associated with work in metal spaces due to the high thermal conductivity of metal. These places tend to be quite hot in the summer an cold in the winter. Thermal environmental stresses may be exacerbated by:
  — PPE such as welding leather or nomex clothing.
  — Thermal emissions from repair and maintenance tasks being performed in the confined space.
  — Heated or chilled process material lines passing through the space.
  — Radiant heat from adjacent process vessels.

Hazards Originating in Adjacent Areas

Use of mechanical ventilation to control atmospheric hazards by dilution is common in confined space work. The fundamental assumption in using this engineering control is that the replacement air is cleaner than the air in the confined space. Unfortunately, this assumption may not hold true. Common sources of contaminated make-up air include:

- Other maintenance and repair operations near the air intake to the confined space such as:
  - Welding, cutting and burning
  - Abatement of lead-containing paint
  - Abatement of asbestos-containing materials (ACM)
  - Abrasive blasting
- Exhaust or flue gases from:
  - Operating process furnaces
  - Portable air compressors and generators
  - Exhausts from adjacent ventilated confined spaces
- Leaks or releases of process chemicals from valves, vents and pumps.

In addition, processes in close proximity to a confined space entry can pose physical contact hazards or provide sources of ignition for flammable vapors or gases. Machinery and equipment may also leak contaminants that could enter the space. For example, a propane-powered lift truck with a slight leak at a fitting could introduce propane to the space. The potential for these items to present sources of ignition should the atmosphere within the space be flammable cannot be overlooked. NIOSH statistics reveal that in over half of the fatalities involving fires and explosions, the source of ignition was outside the confined space.

Perspectives on Industry-Specific Hazards

The reader is cautioned that the outlines and synopses above are focused on the suite of industries identified by OSHA as "general industry" and are, of necessity, rather broad in nature. In practice, there are often specialized definitions and/or particular hazards associated with specific industries. As examples, three industries are briefly noted here: 1) welding, 2) construction excavation and 3) shipyard work,

Welding

A welding site in a restricted area requiring special attention to ventilation is defined by the American Welding Society (AWS) and OSHA [29 CFR 1910.252 (c)(2) by any of the of the following characteristics:

- Less than 10,000 cubic feet of volume per welder
- A ceiling height of less than 16 feet
- Other obstructions to dilution ventilation.

Such a location may or may not be a confined space in the sense defined by the definitions noted above. However, welding and thermal cutting processes are capable of generating substantial amounts of fume in a short period of time. This specific definition reflects a number of atmospheric hazards identified with welding and allied processes that may be exacerbated by the restricted ventilation associated with many confined spaces. One may note that a welding shop encompassing less than 1250 ft^2 of floor area (with an 8-ft ceiling) would meet the first criterion. Also, there are also many light industrial complexes, wherein welding is conducted, with ceiling heights of less than 16 ft. Mechanical ventilation is required for welding operations to be conducted in accordance with the OSHA standard [29 CFR 1910.252 (c)(2)] in these facilities.

Construction Excavation

The construction industry standards provide examples of work sites often considered confined spaces that are not specifically addressed in the General Industry Confined Space standard. Specifically, the Construction Industry Excavation standard [29 CFR 1926.650, subpart P, paragraph (g)] identifies any excavation more than 4 ft deep as a work site requiring atmosphere testing prior to beginning work. The required atmospheric testing is essentially the same as that required by the Confined Space standard. Due to this similarity and a number of other parallels in administering work performed in excavation entries and confined-space entries, many facilities include entries into any subgrade work site in a facility's con-fined-space entry program for the sake of administrative convenience.

Shipyard Work

Shipyard work is addressed in 29 CFR 1915, subpart B. This work is sufficiently specialized (and certainly adequately hazardous) that an entire class of professionals, marine chemists, has been established to address the hazards associated with this work. The marine chemist is responsible for anticipating, recognizing, evaluating, and controlling hazards associated with work conducted inside and on the hulls of ships. It is not unreasonable to consider a ship, particularly a tankship, as a conglomeration of confined spaces such as cargo tanks or holds; ballast tanks; certain engine room spaces; bow thruster rooms; some pump rooms; and some generator rooms. Consider the consequences of performing a welding operation on the walls (these are called bulkheads on a ship) of a pump room. Perhaps the goal of the work is to simply weld a bracket on the bulkhead to support a new piece of hardware. If a welder were to heat the bulkhead sufficiently to allow welding to take place, what would be the outcome if the other side of the bulkhead were a cargo tank that had recently contained gasoline? The outcome would almost certainly be catastrophic. The marine chemist is tasked with preventing this outcome from taking place. Planning ahead to consider the possible outcomes of welding tasks on a ship is an example of the forward thinking required when working in a confined space

As noted earlier, it is not feasible to address every conceivable circumstance in regulations and standards. It is more useful to view the various confined space standards as starting places to address the specific hazards of specialized tasks to be performed in such spaces, with regulatory compliance being regarded as the first step, rather than the end point, of the OEHS effort.

Elements of a Confined Space Program

If there are no reasonable alternatives to entry into a confined space, then it is prudent (and, in the U.S., required by federal regulation) to develop appropriate programs and procedures to guide facility management in mitigating the hazards prior to entry. It must be recognized that programs and procedures do not, in themselves, reduce the frequency or severity of hazards in the workplace. Rather, it is the concentrated and concerted efforts of management and all affected employees that achieves this goal. Programs and procedures provide a framework and guidelines that facilitate this effort. Confined space programs and procedures formalize the process of hazard evaluation and hazard control from each confined space at a site. Complete support by the top levels of management is fundamental to the success of this endeavor. The industrial hygienist should not labor under the impression that he or she is solely responsible for development of an appropriate confined-space entry program. This is a team effort that requires full cooperation of safety professionals, plant managers, and operators of affected equipment to be successful.

Two excellent resources for the OEHS professional addressing confined space program development, revision, are:

- Confined Space Entry, An AIHA Protocol Guide.[5]
- ANSI Z-117.1 Safety Requirements for Confined Spaces.[6]

Much of the information in this section has been condensed from these sources. It must be emphasized that there are other approaches to constructing and implementing a confined space entry program.

In addition to defining the scope of the program and the responsibilities of affected personnel, the confined-space entry program should include the following elements.

Survey and Inventory All Confined Spaces at the Facility. This is the initial step in developing a confined-space entry program, and the result should identify the confined spaces within a facility. This task amounts to an Industrial Hygiene Walk-Through with an emphasis on identifying confined spaces. Record the following for each confined space:

- Name of the confined space (e.g., wood chip silo, tower T-6, F-13 furnace)
- Type or description of the confined space (e.g., subgrade electrical vault, hydraulic press pit)

- Location of the confined space (e.g., hydrocracker unit, steam plant desalinization plant); location of access points (e.g., manway at 3rd level)
- The "owner" or manager of the area in which the confined space is located.
- Dimensions
- Date of inventory
- Other useful information as deemed desirable by the investigation team.

Classify the Confined Spaces. Each confined space must be identified as either non-permit required or as permit-required. It is essential to be clear in determining whether this a permit-required confined space or not. In some instances, the distinction may be based on the activity to be conducted in the space, rather than on the hazards presented by the space itself. See the previous section, Identifying and Classifying Confined Spaces. It is worth repeating that, when possible, the best practice is to eliminate the hazards prior to entry. This reduces risk and allows the space to be classified as non-permit required.

Perform an Initial Hazard Assessment. For each confined space, identify the chemical, biological, mechanical and physical hazards associated with entry. Note again that the hazards may be originate from the activity to be conducted on the space, rather than on the hazards presented by the space itself. Consider the following factors:

- How many workers will be affected?
- What trades will be affected?
- What are the probable hazards that will be associated with the activities of these trades?
- What is the magnitude of the hazard? (e.g., chemical toxicity, amount of energy that could be released, possible fall distance)
- What is the likelihood of occurrence?
- What are the consequences if the hazard is allowed to impact workers? (e.g., eye irritation, chemical overexposure, electrocution, engulfment, death)
- Are conditions expected to change during entry? (e.g., welding, sand blasting, or shoveling sludge can be expected to release contaminants to the confined space atmosphere)
- What techniques/strategies are available to mitigate or eliminate the hazards? The preferred sequence is familiar: eliminate, substitute, isolate, engineering controls, administrative and work practice controls and PPE.
- What is the impact on Emergency Responders? Rescue from horizontal spaces (e.g. ship double bottoms) can be a challenge.

Hazards are addressed in more detail in the section "Hazards Associated with Confined Spaces."

Establish Procedures for Working with Contractors. It is common practice for the facility operators who have confined spaces onsite to arrange for outside firms (contractors) to work in confined spaces. Specialty tasks such as blasting, painting, welding, structural inspection and scaffold erection are examples of these tasks which are often performed by contractors. Prior to beginning work, the facility operator or prime contractor should be certain the contractors who are to work in the confined space have the appropriate training, expertise and qualifications for accomplishing the contracted tasks within confined spaces. One means for achieving this is to interview the contractor and go over the contractor's Confined Space Program in the context of the work to be performed. It is vital that contractors whose employees will enter the confined space are, at a minimum, informed of the following:

- The classification of the space (permit required or non permit required).
- Hazards that have been identified with entry into the space. (see Initial Hazard Assessment, above).
- Other operations that are to take place within or near the confined space during the contractor's entry and the hazards associated with those operations.
- Previous experience with entering the confined space. (A brief history of earlier work in the confined space may allow the contractor to anticipate conditions to be encountered during the upcoming entry.)
- Precautions and procedures that have been implemented for protection of workers in and around the confined space.

The most common means of assuring that this communication takes place is an effective Confined Space Entry Permit System or Program.

<u>Develop a Confined Space Entry Permit System.</u> The importance of an effective Confined Space Entry Permit System or Program can scarcely be over-emphasized. The entry permit is a communication tool and that communication is a two-way street. The permit system should facilitate communication of hazards associated with the space to the entrants and the procedures for mitigating those hazards. The entrants are expected to communicate the hazards associated with their work to the facility operator. If multiple groups of entrants are to work in the space, the permit system is the means by which each set of entrants is informed of the hazards associated with each other's work.

The facility operator is, in most cases, the permit-issuer. Depending on the size of the job, the permit-issuer may the prime contractor. In either case, the permit-issuer assumes responsibility for deconfliction, or assuring that the work of one group of entrants will not cause an elevated hazard for other entrants or trades. Examples of work that would create hazards for other trades may include:

- Carbon Arc Cutting (hazards include carbon monoxide, metal fumes, UV exposures and noise);
- Abrasive blasting (hazards include noise and airborne particulate), and
- Scaffold erection (hazards include work overhead and associated falling object hazards).

Information on the permit should include:

- Name of the confined space (e.g., wood chip silo, tower T-6, F-13 furnace);
- Type or description of the confined space (e.g., subgrade electrical vault, hydraulic press pit);
- Location of the confined space (e.g., hydrocracker unit, steam plant desalinization plant);
- Date and time of entry;
- Names of permit issuer and permit accepter;
- Signature lines for permit issuer and permit accepter;
- Type of work to be performed;
- Hazards to be controlled or eliminated prior to entry;
- Hazards to be expected during entry;
- Engineering controls, PPE, work practices and other precautions required to perform the work;
- Names of entrants (this may be incorporated in a sign-in/sign-out sheet rather than the permit itself);
- Type of atmospheric tests required prior to entry and the results of those tests;
- If atmospheric test are to be required during entry, the type of atmospheric tests required and the results of those tests should also be entered o the permit;
- Arrangements for confined space rescue, and
- Duration of the permit (usually for no longer than a single work shift or half-shift).

Simply filling out a Confined Space Entry Permit prior to entry is NOT sufficient to ensure that hazards are communicated to the extent possible. The permit must be completed before each entry and the information on the permit communicated to each entrant. That communication may simply take the form of a "tool-box or tail-gate safety meeting" but regardless of the level of formality, the communication must be recorded.

One should also anticipate that conditions in the confined space may change as the work progresses. New hazards may be introduced as additional trades enter the space. If the new hazards are not addressed in the original permit, or if atmospheric or other entry conditions are compromised, the permit must be revoked and entrants must exit the space until the new conditions are mitigated or the work-associated hazards are addressed.

<u>Establish the Roles Involved in Confined Space Entries.</u> Defining the roles and responsibilities of affected personnel clarifies what is expected of each employee and what actions are allowed and what actions are not allowed.

- <u>Authorized Entrants</u> are personnel who are trained in the hazards of working in confined spaces and have specific duties to be performed in the confined space. These individuals are required to sign in on the Confined Space Entry Permit immediately prior to entering to perform their duties. They are also required to sign out on the Confined

Space Entry Permit upon leaving the confined space. Authorized Entrants are also expected to be able to recognize the hazards associated with their work inside the confined space, to monitor those hazards and maintain communication with the other entrants and the Authorized Attendant

- The Authorized Attendant is assigned responsibility for:
  - — Maintaining communication with the Entrants,
  - — Monitoring conditions in and around the confined space that may affect conditions within the confined space,
  - — Tracking the activities of the Entrants
  - — Ensuring the Entrants sign in and sign out on the Confined Space Entry Permit and
  - — Summoning rescue services if required.

  Clearly, these are weighty responsibilities to be entrusted to a person who recognizes these responsibilities and is trained in the execution thereof.
- The Entry Supervisor responsible for oversight of the entry operation. Responsibilities include:
  - — Checking permits for accuracy and completion. Note that is not a "paper exercise." On-site and Hands-on supervision is required to execute this assignment.
  - — Verifying the entry conditions are acceptable and meet the requirements listed on the permit.
  - — Verifying the rescue services are available and there are appropriate means for contacting these services.
  - — Authorizing entry by signing or initialing the permit
  - — Removing Entrants from the space when the work is completed or entry conditions change.
  - — Terminating the permit at the end of the job.

Training. The occupational hygienist may anticipate a central role in this aspect of confined-space hazard control. The role here is twofold:

- Inform affected workers of the health hazards associated with the work: All of the hazards associated with work in confined spaces are not necessarily health hazards, and occupational hygienists should not expect themselves to be expert in all aspects of all hazards. However, the occupational hygienist is uniquely qualified to summarize the health hazards and present that information in a way that is comprehensible and useful to the intelligent lay person. (Course work in public speaking may provide experience to make such presentations easier. Students should realize that communication skills are increasingly important to playing an effective role on the OEHS team and are well worth the effort required to develop them.)
- Educate supervisors: Change the supervisors' and workers' perceptions of hazards from "Well, it'll probably be OK" to "If I'm not really sure about this, I'm going to ask someone who knows!"

Training records from prework meetings and "tail-gate safety meetings" provide a means of auditing the knowledge base of program administrators, entrants, attendants, entry supervisors, and in-house rescuers. Occupational hygienists usually are expected to provide the "health" part of the content for these meetings and are often required to present that content.

Using the Confined-space hazard Analysis Form from *Confined Space Entry, An AIHA Protocol Guide*, is likely to be a productive means of identifying training topics. If the hazards are checked off on the form, they are worth communicating to the affected workers. An outline of training requirements should include:

1) Training should be sufficient so that all employees whose work is associated with confined spaces acquire the understanding, knowledge and skills necessary for safe performance of those duties.
2) Training shall be provided to each affected employee
   a) Before the employee is first assigned
   b) Before there is a change in duties
   c) Whenevr a change in the confined space operations that presents a hazard about which the emplotyee has yetbeen trained

d) When ever there is reason to believe that there have been changes in, or deviations from, the confined space procedures or if there are inadequacies in the employee's knowledge or use of those procedures.

3) Training shall establish employee proficiency in the duties required of each affected employee.

4) The employer shall establish and maintain written certification of the training, deviations from, the confined space procedures or if there are inadequacies in the employee's knowledge or use of those procedures.

Hazard Elimination versus Hazard Control. Earlier in this chapter, in the section, "Perform an Initial Hazard Assessment," it was noted:

> "What techniques/strategies are available to mitigate or eliminate the hazards? The preferred sequence is familiar: eliminate, substitute, isolate, engineering controls, administrative and work practice controls and PPE."

Given all this information on hazard control or mitigation, it may be easy to overlook the preferred approach; hazard elimination. When planning a confined space entry, it is worth asking if the entry really is absolutely necessary. In many cases, the task to be performed has been done before and "That's the way we've always done it." Perhaps so, but that may not be the only way to do the job. A few examples are offered as food for thought:

- If the work involves fabrication of a confined space can the work sequence be modified to re-schedule closing out the confined spaces in the fabricated item until a later stages in the work? Examples of fabricated items might include ships, petrochemical equipment, rail cars or highway chemical trailers. Re-scheduling closing out the spaces may result in decreased fabrication time due to avoiding the delays associated with confined space entries.
- If the space has been classified as permit-required confined space due to the presence of process residue in the space, is there a more effective way to clean the space prior to entry? Flushing petrochemical vessels with sodium hydroxide followed by flushing, steaming and re-flushing is a common procedure in refineries and chemical plants. Would a similar procedure work for the confined space in question?
- If an atmospheric hazard is responsible for classifying a space as permit-required, would better ventilation or a longer period of ventilation eliminate the hazard and allow for re-classification as a non-permit space?
- If the work to be performed will result in partial or total dismantling of the space, will opening the space to the atmosphere earlier in the process eliminate the need for some or all of the entries?

Repeating for the sake of emphasis from an earlier section in this chapter: "Why Are Confined Spaces a Concern?," the IH should again ask:

- Is it absolutely necessary to enter the space? If there is some other reasonable way to do the proposed work without a confined-space entry, that option should be investigated.
- If there is no alternative to entering the space, is there a means of eliminating the hazards prior to entry, rather than simply dealing with them as they are?

If possible, the first choice in controlling confined-space hazards is to avoid entry.

Hazard Control Options

Project Planning and Oversight

At the risk of being excessively repetitive, at the first stage of project planning, one must always ask:

- "Must people enter this space?
- Are there alternatives to a confined space entry?"

Ideally, hazards should be eliminated. If this is not possible, they should be controlled to a level of acceptable risk. Clearly, the most reliable means of controlling the risk is to avoid entry. The reader is reminded that not all confined spaces exhibit the hazards associated with permit-required confined spaces. A careful hazard evaluation may indicate that many entries may be conducted as a routine activity. It is most prudent to assume that a confined space is a permit-required confined space until a hazard evaluation indicates otherwise.

At the beginning of the project a meeting should be conducted with the contractor and all in-house personnel who may have roles in the confined space work. Effective planning can minimize the opportunity for unexpected occurrences during the project. This planning should include clear communications about the scope of the project and the project schedule. The project planning effort must also address foreseeable health and safety hazards and the means by which these hazards will be minimized and controlled. The project schedule should be designed to minimize the number of entries needed and their duration. Part of the planning process should ensure that all items such as tools, supplies, and equipment required during the confined space entry are available prior to starting the work. This may not be possible on an emergency repair but should be done whenever possible.

On the first day of the job, it may be worthwhile to visit the job site and discuss health and safety issues with contractor personnel. Repeat visits should be part of the job oversight or monitoring process. Contractor performance and hazards of the work will determine the timing. If the contractor is performing as agreed, fewer visits will be necessary. If health and safety performance seems less than expected, more frequent visits may be needed to ensure that safety issues are properly addressed.

Plan to visit the job site during any operations that involve significantly increased risk. For example, if part of the project will involve cutting operations in the confined space, a visit during the beginning of that phase would be prudent. During job site visits, talk with the contractor supervisor and employees to determine that the project is progressing as planned from a safety perspective. Observe operations to ensure that the agreed on health and safety procedures are in fact being used. Review the permit during each visit and compare it to actual operations. Observe the condition of PPE. With the exception of minor soiling on coveralls, the PPE should be in "as new" condition as possible to provide the level of protection published by the manufacturer.

It may be worthwhile to tactfully question the contractor about any discrepancies noted and listen carefully to their responses. The IH should ask about working conditions inside the confined space including topics such as ventilation, lighting, surface contaminants, build-up of construction or demolition debris, heat or cold stress and other worker complaints.

Plan for Emergencies

It must be assumed that emergencies will occur. Any variance from acceptable entry conditions as established by the entry permit may constitute an emergency. Even a situation such as a battery failure on atmospheric monitoring equipment may be considered an emergency. Efforts to prevent emergencies need to be constant, but there is a good chance that eventually an emergency will have to be handled. If the entry crew is prepared, it may be handled without a problem. If preparations are not adequate, the emergency may turn into a fatality.

At a minimum the plan should include a briefing of the entire crew on how each individual is expected to respond if an emergency occurs. This briefing must emphasize that the attendant is not to enter the space. The attendant should never enter the space to attempt rescue. The attendant's role is to summon emergency help and use retrieval devices if available. Confined space accident statistics clearly indicate that rescue attempts often lead to additional fatalities. Rescue is not a hazard on control option but planning for hazards associated with rescue is certainly necessary.

Plan for Effective Communication

Effective communications allow entrants to deal effectively with potential emergencies in confined spaces and just tugging on a rope is not a particularly effective means of communication. Voice communication alone is easiest if it is effective. Where distance or noise make this impossible, other methods must be used. In situations where the entrant and attendant can maintain visual contact, signals may be sufficient for communications. Other options include radios or hard-wired communications systems. To call for emergency help, a radio, telephone, or cellular phone is the best option.

If flammable hazards exist, all communication equipment must be intrinsically safe. It's essential that personnel be familiar with the operation of any communication equipment that may be used. Equipment should be tested prior to entry and immediately after entering the space. Failure of communication equipment is an emergency and should be handled accordingly by evacuating the space.

Cleaning the Confined Space Surface to Reduce Hazards

Some confined spaces are tanks, drums, towers, rail cars or highway trailers that have been used for transporting, processing or storing materials that may pose a health or safety risk. In these instances it is prudent to ensure that the space has been cleaned as much as possible prior to opening the access openings (e.g., tanks tops or manways) for atmosphere testing and/or entry. As an example, petrochem process vessels are generally drained in procedures called "oil-out" and the piping serving these vessels is designed to allow the vessels to drain reasonably well. Subsequent cleaning steps often entail alternating cycles of flooding the vessel with sodium hydroxide (called "caustic" in the plants) followed by draining the sodium hydroxide solution and injecting live steam into the vessel to remove the sodium hydroxide This procedure is repeated as necessary until the vessel is deemed "clean." The number of cleaning cycles is usually dictated by previous experience with the confined space under consideration. Interiors of vessels that have been properly treated in this manner are remarkably clean. However, it is not unusual to find traces of residue around bolt heads. If the vessel has been used for processing or storage of petroleum substances that contain hydrogen sulfide (H_2S), even these small traces of petroleum can present a health hazard if the they are heated. If the bolts (or other parts of the vessel with residue) are to be cut with carbon arc cutting or oxy-acetylene cutting torches, one may anticipate rapid evolution of sulfur dioxide (SO_2). Sulfur dioxide is a severe irritant to the upper respiratory tract and eyes. Rapidly increasing concentrations of sulfur dioxide can therefore result in hasty evacuation of the confined space. Haste in a confined space is not a good thing as unduly quick action may lead to a slip, trip or fall injury. The point being that while these vessels may be adequately clean for entry for inspection, they may not be adequately clean for hotwork[2]. When the OEHS professional is asked "How clean do I have to get this thing before you'll let my people go in?" the answer should include reference to just what the people are going to be doing in the confined space. Will it be just for inspection or will other activities (e.g., welding, cutting, abrasive blasting, sanding, grinding) take place that may require the affected surfaces to be particularly clean?

Pre-entry cleaning of confined spaces is not always possible. Again using the petrochem industry as an example, equipment used to process petroleum is occasionally shut down without "oiling out." This may happen when the equipment is found to be operating outside if accepted parameters and is shut down as a precautionary measure. Under these circumstances the cleaning procedure may resemble the work practices of the early part of the 20th Century, e.g., shovels, buckets, muck, sludge, oil, carbon build-up, broken parts, compromised structural components, unpredictable airborne hydrocarbon concentrations as the sludge is shoveled out, substantial probably of gross skin contact, etc. Each time the confined space contents are disturbed (i.e., each shovel full) there is a potential for release of hydrocarbon vapor. Continuous real-time monitoring of substances with high vapor pressures, oxygen and LEL is prudent as well as continuous observations of work practices. A decontamination station may be worthwhile in order to control the spread of material from the confined space to the rest of the facility. The OEHS professional should be aware that, if this confined space cleanout is associated with an unplanned release

[2] The term "Hotwork" as used here includes all forms of thermal joining and cutting processes as well as other processes, such as grinding, that may produce sources of ignition. These processes and the health hazards associated with them are described in *Welding Health and Safety: A Field Guide for OEHS Professionals* (AIHA®, 2002.)

of substantial quantities of material, the provisions of the Hazardous Waste Operations Standard (29 CFR 1910.120) may apply for work conducted in the U.S.

There are also occasions when cleaning of a confined space may require both cleaning prior to entry and final cleaning by entrants. Examples would include cleaning barge or ship cargo tanks, rail car or highway trailer tanks or process/storage vessels that have been shut down without cleaning. For instance, ships that carry crude petroleum accumulate heavy oil fractions (sludge) in the cargo tanks. This sludge includes sand, silt and clay carried over from the ground from which the oil was pumped. Before the ship enters the shipyard for scheduled maintenance, these cargo tanks must be cleaned to avoid fire and explosion hazards from welding or cutting tasks that may performed on the vessel in the shipyard. Although the tanks must eventually be cleaned using water it is more effective to first use a method known as Crude Oil Washing to remove these deposits. The ship's tanks are plumbed with high-pressure wash lines and nozzles through which crude oil is sprayed on the tank surfaces. Crude Oil Washing is usually done as the vessel discharges its cargo so that the deposits, which would normally remain in the tank. are discharged with the cargo. If done on a regular basis (i.e. several tanks each time the ship discharges) it will prevent the build up of excess deposits thus making it easier to clean when the tanks are entered. The Crude Oil Wash is followed by washing the tanks with water. Since saltwater is found in abundance around the ship, saltwater is commonly used for this procedure. The water wash may be hot or cold. In many instances, the structural members of the ship (baffles, bulkheads, stringers, etc.) will interfere with the high-pressure blast from the fixed nozzles and "shadows" of waxy residue remain on the tank walls. The ship's crew will address this from outside the cargo tank by opening hatches (called "Butterworth Hatches") and lower portable high pressure washing equipment (called "Butterworth machines") into the tank from above. These portable machines allow the crew to complete a more thorough water wash. Before any washing takes place (Crude Oil Wash or Water Wash) the atmosphere in each tank to be washed must be checked for oxygen content. For most tank washing situations it should not exceed 8% by volume. The ship is equipped with a system to flood the tanks with "Inert Gas." That is, a combination of gases having a low oxygen content, formed from the combustion of the ships' fuel or from an Inert Gas Generator. Most crude oil ships use the flue gas from the ship's stack.. After water washing the hydrocarbon rich atmosphere in the tank must be removed. This is done by "purging" the tank with inert gas. When the hydrocarbon level in the tank has been reduced to acceptable level (less than 2% by volume) the venting (gas freeing) process can begin. Venting is necessary to make the tank atmosphere safe for entry. The deck plates are removed and fresh air is introduced, often by means of portable air or water driven fans. The cleaning stages from outside the tanks are followed by additional atmosphere testing prior to allowing the ship's crew to enter for inspection of the cargo tanks (which are about the size of a high school basketball gym) and or mucking (using shovels and buckets to shovel the sludge from the bottom of the cargo tanks). Routine crude oil washing reduces and sometimes eliminates the need for this labor intensive, potentially dangerous task.

Railcar and highway trailers frequently require cleaning after unloading a consignment and before loading new commodities. This procedure generally takes place at break-in-bulk terminals. Railcars and highway trailers rarely, if ever, are equipped with the washing mechanisms described above for ships. As a consequence, confined space entry into tanks that have been drained but not cleaned is the rule rather than the exception. In these cases the entrants may be working with a wide variety of substances and the health and safety hazards may not be adequately addressed. There may concerns regarding frequent and substantial skin contact with the residue on the walls and bottom of the tanks cars, as many chemical substances transported in this manner (e.g., amines) are to some degree skin irritants or may be corrosive. Unusual hazards have been produced by common substances in these settings. Among the more interesting but, unfortunately, fatal events involves pig blood which was transported in a highway trailer. After the trailer was unloaded, two people were sent in to clean the trailer with buckets and mops. The possibility of an oxygen-deficient atmosphere was not addressed by atmosphere testing prior to entry. Pig blood contains hemoglobin, which effectively placed a large biological oxygen demand (B.O.D.) on the tank atmosphere. The entrants were asphyxiated.

In all cases that require personnel to enter a confined space for cleaning, it's good practice to limit the number of entrants to those personnel necessary to do job. This limits the number of potentially exposed personnel to a minimum until the confined space is clean enough for the planned work to proceed.

Ventilation to Reduce Hazards

Resources

A number of detailed treatments of ventilation principles are readily available which offer the information necessary for thorough evaluation and design of scores of ventilation applications. The most widely known, *Industrial Ventilation, A Manual of Recommended Practice* is published by ACGIH®. This book is now in the 27th edition and covers a wide variety of ventilation topics. This text is generally written for specialists who design permanent ventilation systems for manufacturing facilities. Two other volumes of interest for non-specialists faced with the need to implement successful temporary ventilation of confined spaces are noted below. By comparison with ACGIH® *Manual of Recommend Practice* these volumes focus on a very specific and field-oriented aspect of on-the-job applications of ventilation principles for temporary entry into confined spaces.

- Portable Ventilation Systems Handbook(8)
- Field Guidelines for Temporary Ventilation of Confined Spaces(9)

Much of this ventilation section is derived and condensed from the latter volume.

Why Ventilate Confined Spaces?

Normally confined spaces are not designed for convenient ventilation but are designed to allow periodic entry for inspection, cleaning maintenance and/or repair. Steps must be taken to ensure the air inside a confined space is breathable before it is entered and to maintain acceptable air quality inside the confined space. Temporary ventilation of confined spaces is often used to control atmospheric hazards by removing contaminated air and replacing it with fresh air. For effective ventilation of most confined spaces, mechanical ventilation must be provided by fans or eductors (often called "air movers" in the field).

The reader is cautioned that it is not always possible to provide a healthful confined space atmosphere by means of ventilation alone. In some circumstances, such as arc gouging in small confined spaces or working with particularly toxic metals, supplied air respirators are the only means of assuring that workers are adequately protected. In all cases it must be noted that **makeup air quality remains of primary importance whether ventilation is natural or if ventilation is mechanically assisted**.

Mechanical ventilation, once installed and working properly, can reduce respiratory protection requirements or may eliminate the need for respiratory protection altogether. Effectiveness of an engineering control is generally much less dependant on minute-by-minute worker attention to personal protection than is the case with respiratory protection. Also, the effectiveness of engineering controls may be easier to validate in the field. Finally, the OSHA Respiratory Protection Standard specifies that engineering controls must be used rather than respirators when effective controls are feasible [(29 CFR 1910.134(a)].

There are a number of reasons to ventilate a confined space. Ventilating a confined space may be of benefit whenever the atmosphere in the space:

- May not contain sufficient oxygen or is too rich in oxygen
- Contains flammable dusts or vapors
- Contains hazardous or toxic vapors, mists, fumes, gases or fibers
- May be subject to activities that may generate hazardous mists, vapors, fumes or gases or that may create an oxygen deficiency (or oxygen excess)
- Introduces heat stress on workers

As an alternative to ventilation in a confined space, supplied air respiratory protection may be specified as Personal Protective Equipment (PPE) (29 CFR 1910.252 and 29 CFR 1926.353) if hotwork is being performed. However, most people resist wearing this

PPE and the tangle of supplied air hoses in a presents a hazard that can be avoided in many cases with adequate mechanical ventilation.

Other Benefits of Ventilation

Ventilation of confined spaces provides a number of additional benefits. When air contaminants are removed, workers frequently experience less irritation and work more productively. Also, illnesses which may be caused by overexposure to welding fumes and gases will be avoided and the need for respiratory protection can be reduced. In hot weather, the air temperature may be reduced, potentially increasing productivity and reducing the likelihood of heat-related illnesses.

Atmospheric Testing and Personal Air Monitoring While Ventilating

There are some hazards which cannot be completely eliminated by using mechanical ventilation alone. Ventilation, by itself, may not be sufficient during activities such as arc gouging or plasma arc cutting, especially when elevated concentrations of toxic metals may be present. Atmospheric testing and/or personal air monitoring is strongly recommended to ensure that the ventilation application is effective. Ultimately, whether respiratory protection is required in addition to mechanical ventilation will be determined by the results of atmospheric testing and/or personal air monitoring for the contaminants of concern while the work is progressing in the confined space.

There are considerable variations in vapor density among contaminants that may be found in a confined space. Vapor density is a comparative measure, with air equal to 1. Substances with a vapor density greater than 1 are heavier than air and would tend to sink in air. Substances exhibiting a vapor density less than 1 are lighter than air and would tend to rise in air. This characteristic affects the vertical distribution of gases and vapors in a confined space. In some instances, (e.g., out of service petrochem equipment) confined spaces may exhibit little or no air movement and consequent mixing of gases. This may result in density stratification within the confined space. For example, if there are gases or vapors with a density greater than air (e.g., hydrogen sulfide, vapor density = 1.189) in the confined space, it is not unusual to find that density stratification will result in greater concentrations of the more dense gases or vapors at the lower levels of the confined space. Conversely if methane (vapor density = 0.6) is present one would anticipate that methane would accumulate in the upper portions of the space. The possibility of density stratification within a confined space requires one to engage in more detailed confined space atmosphere testing than may otherwise seem necessary. This may require using an extension hose/probe and testing the confined space atmosphere at various levels to verify that the confined space atmosphere is acceptable for entry (or that additional cleaning and/or ventilation is required before entry). McManus notes the NIOSH finding that "two out of three explosions involving confined spaces occur at the time the space is first disturbed.[7] This statistic argues for exercising caution when opening confined space for atmosphere testing. Clearly it is prudent to attempt to obtain small samples for testing via existing holes or valves or by cautiously opening a hatch just enough to obtain a sample. Simply throwing the hatch open and thrusting a direct reading instrument into the confined space at the interface between the confined space (with a potentially ignitable gas or vapor) and the surrounding air (which may provide the correct amount of oxygen for ignition) may create needless risks. In addition, this shortsighted practice may fail to identify relevant atmospheric hazards in other locations in the confined space.

Atmospheric Monitoring Process

In confined space entry operations there will always be a need for atmospheric monitoring. The sequence for atmosphere testing is:

- Oxygen first
- Flammability second
- Toxics third

Oxygen is always checked first, followed by flammability. This is because nearly all flammability (or "LEL") sensors employ a Wheatstone Bridge which requires normal oxygen content to yield accurate readings. The oxygen sensor may be used in many operating environments without specific identification of other gases that may be present. There are some gases, however, that "poison: oxygen sensors. Prior to use, refer to the manufacturer's literature to determine if the gases known to be in the confined space may adversely affect the oxygen sensor

Flammability sensors are typically broad range instruments that detect flammability problems without specifically identifying the flammable substance involved. Usually, there are response factors that must be taken into consideration since the calibration gas is often not the same as the flammable gas or vapors in the confined space.

Toxic sensors are most often chemical specific. This requires that potential toxic contaminants be specifically identified prior to selecting the appropriate monitoring equipment. See Chapter 7, Principles of Evaluating Worker Exposure or Chapter 17, Direct Reading Instruments for Determining Concentrations of Gases, Vapors, and Aerosols for additional insights into these processes.

If problems were discovered during atmospheric monitoring, correct the problem when possible. If the problem cannot be corrected, forbid entry or protect personnel with respiratory protection equipment.

Remote Sampling

Remote sampling equipment includes pumps, hand aspirating bulbs, tubing, and probes. These accessories are commonly available in a wide variety of specific configurations.

Maximum draw distance and draw rates vary among manufacturers. Maximum tubing allowed is typically 100 feet or less. Draw rates average 1 ft/sec. Filtration devices are also available for avoiding the intake of dust and fluids.

A dilution tube is a specialty accessory for sampling flammable atmospheres in areas of reduced oxygen concentration with a catalytic bead sensor. The dilution tube allows air, containing oxygen, into the sample stream in measured amounts allowing accurate flammable readings to be obtained using a conversion factor.

Horizontal Entry Situations

Atmospheric monitoring should begin outside the entryway prior to opening the confined space. This allows assessment of any hazards in the area that may have nothing to do with the confined space but may have an impact on the internal atmosphere once the entryway is opened. This technique is also useful for identifying a hazardous atmosphere that may be seeping through the confined space opening.

After determining that it is safe to remove the cover to the opening, initial monitoring inside the space is done with a probe. Use of a rigid probe allows sampling farther into the space. Extend the probe up and down as far as reach allows, assessing as much of the space as possible from outside. Monitoring throughout the space will need to be completed as well. Based on knowledge of the space and results of initial atmospheric monitoring, assess the potential for a hazardous atmosphere within the space. Entry for the remainder of the initial test may need to be completed by an individual using respiratory protection.

Vertical Entry Situations

For vertical entries also monitor outside the space prior to opening the cover. If the cover has an access hole the probe may be used for initial monitoring inside the space. When there is no hole the cover must be removed, and monitoring will begin at the opening.

When this technique is used the tubing must be lowered slowly into the space to allow sampling at all levels. If the sample tube is lowered more rapidly than the draw rate of the sample pump, areas may not be effectively measured.

Low-level obstructions may interfere with monitoring. In this situation if the tubing cannot be placed on the other side of the obstruction from outside the space the monitoring will need to be completed after entry. Divisions of this type within a confined space are relatively common. This situation may be present in a confined space with a depressed drain area or a sump pit.

Air Moving Devices

These are two types of widely used air moving devices for ventilating confined spaces: fans and venturi-type eductors. Fans may be either air or steam driven or electrically powered. The author's experience with fans used for ventilating confined spaces has been primarily with air-driven and this section focuses on this equipment. However, some comments are offered regarding use of electrically-driven equipment.

Air-driven fan diameters usually range from 18" to 24." Eductors (sometimes referred to as "air horns" or "air movers") are always air powered and rely on venturi-effects to move air. Eductor diameters commonly are from 6" to 10" in diameter. The air moving devices are bolted to an opening in the vessel and are often oriented to pull air out of the vessel. Because the air moving devices reduce the air pressure in the vessel, surrounding air enters the vessel through the openings that are not occupied by the air movers. This incoming air is called "makeup air". The rationale behind using air-driven fans and eductors in the "pull" mode rather than the "push" mode is based on incidents wherein the air-driven devices were connected to plant nitrogen lines instead of plant compressed air lines[3]. The discharge of almost all air-driven devices is into the throat of the fan or eductor. This air is driven into the confined space along with the air delivered by the action of the fan or the venturi effect of the eductor. Conse-quently, the nitrogen displaces the air in the confined space and asphyxiation may result. When one is working in an environment where the only source of compressed gas is compressed air, this potential hazard does not exist.

The application of air moving devices to pull air through a confined space is by no means universal. In many applications the air moving devices are oriented so that they push air into a space. The use of "Positive Pressure Ventilation" has been documented for use by firefighters and tunnel ventilation as described in Appendices, B and C of McManus's work noted above.

Fans and eductors are rated according to several criteria:

- The quantity of air (usually in cfm) they will move with no air flow restriction, often referred to as "free air delivery". This quantity of air is expressed in cfm and is the highest number on the "Fan Rating Curve" included on the Specification Sheet for most air moving equipment. The labels on some brands of equipment may state this as the "Free Air Delivery Capacity in CFM."
- The quantity of air they will move while overcoming obstacles to air flow. The amount of restriction to air flow is generally labeled as "inches of static pressure"[4] on the rating curves supplied by the fan or eductor manufacturer. The greater the "inches of static pressure", the less air will be moved. The labels on some brands of equipment may call this the "Effective Blower Capacity" when used with specific elbows and/or specific lengths of flexible ducting.
- The quantity of air (SCFM) and air pressure (psi) required to operate air-driven devices at their rated capacities.
- The quantity of air (SCFM) and electrical power requirements (expressed as watts or a volts and amps) required to operate air-driven devices at their rated capacities.

Factors Reducing Air Moving Device Performance

In the real world, fans and eductors used for dilution ventilation must overcome a multitude of obstacles while moving air through a confined space. The more restrictions an air moving device must overcome, the less air is moved. If the air will not move as fast as the fan blades, the blades operate inefficiently, resulting in a circumstance similar to cavitation of a boat propeller.

[3] Plant compressed gas connections are typically color-coded to reduce the likelihood of this occurrence. It also common practice to use non-compatible fittings on each type of compressed gas line to obviate the possibility of connecting to the wrong compressed gas line. However, a creative mechanic faced with a tight schedule can overcome these minor annoyances and succeed in connecting the wrong line to the air-moving device.

[4] Strictly speaking, static pressure is the air pressure in a duct that tends to collapse or burst the duct. If a fan or eductor is moving enough air that it is trying to collapse or burst duct to any significant extent, then the fan is expending some of its energy in changing the density of the air, rather than in moving air. Similarly, if a fan or eductor must overcome static pressure to move air, the air moving device must overcome some restrictions to airflow in addition to moving air through the confined space.

Causes or examples of airflow restrictions in confined spaces may include the following:

- Equipment components in the confined space; e.g., brackets, trays, pipes.
- Maintenance/construction materials erected in the confined space; e.g., tube and clamp scaffolds, scaffold boards, fire blankets.
- Obstructions in the makeup air manway; e.g., Attendant's (hole watch's) body, weather enclosures around manways, local exhaust ducts, welding cables, and load-in and load-out operations.
- Insufficient number of makeup air manways. If possible, it is best to have at least one makeup air manway for each air moving device. Of course, if positive pressure mode is used, then one would hope to have at least one exhaust for each positive pressure ventilation device.

An additional factor that will reduce performance of air driven fans and eductors is a reduction in air pressure and volume delivered to these air moving devices. These devices are often driven from the plant compressed air system. During the course of the maintenance or construction activities of which the hotwork in a confined space is a part, many workers are using air-powered equipment, reducing the pressure available to operate the air moving equipment. Also, the air hoses supplying the fans or eductors may be excessively long. Measurements of plant air pressure during petrochem turnarounds has shown that these factors can result in reducing air pressure at the air moving devices by as much a 50%.

On-site airflow measurements have shown that the net effect of the above performance-inhibiting factors is to reduce the effectiveness of a 20" air-turbine-driven axial flow fan from a free-air rating of over 10,000 cfm to 3,000 to 3,500 cfm on the job site. The fan rating curves for these fans indicates that this performance would be expected for fans operating against approximately 3–4" static pressure.

Increasing Air Moving Device Performance

While little can be done to reduce internal restrictions to airflow in a confined space, at least three techniques are available to maintain airflow though a confined space.

- When using air-driven equipment, plant air pressure may be less than the air moving device manufacturer's recommendations. In this circumstance, a supplemental air compressor that is dedicated to the air moving devices only can be effective.
- Supplemental air compressors can also be connected to local plant air system to provide air for air tools as well as air moving devices.
- Eliminate "Short Circuiting" of airflow around the fans or eductors.

Electrically-Driven Centrifugal Fans

As noted above, airflow restrictions in confined spaces lead to increased static pressure burdens and reduced fan effectiveness, particularly with axial flow fans. Centrifugal fans, which are generally electrically-driven, are designed to overcome higher static pressures than axial flow fans.

Electrically-driven fans are not subject to the above air supply concerns. However, electrical current of the correct type (single phase or three phase), voltage (usually 220 vac but may be 110 vac or 440 vac) with adequate circuit protection (circuit breakers and ground-fault interrupters) and conductor capacity (wire size) must be available.

Other considerations regarding electrically-driven centrifugal fans include:

- Electrically-driven fans are usually heavier than air-driven equipment. This can make them more difficult to use in high, distant or awkward locations. Consequently, these units are often placed the ground and connected to the vessel with duct work. See the following section (Local Exhaust) regarding ductwork pitfalls.
- If centrifugal fans are used remotely, an advantage is reduced noise levels in the confined spaces, particularly when compared to air-turbine-driven axial flow fans with similar free-air ratings.
- If centrifugal fans are placed on the ground, it is prudent to arrange a guard to keep large debris from restricting the fan intake.
- Due to high exit velocities and the ability to move large particles, it may be prudent to place a screen/filter/diverter at the outlet of centrifugal fans.

Local Exhaust

Dilution ventilation cannot be expected to be appropriate for every operation in every confined space. In these instances, local exhaust ventilation may be a suitable means of controlling contaminant concentrations. Local exhaust devices ("smoke suckers") are lengths of flexible ducting connected to an air moving device. Local exhaust devices may be connected to commercially available fans made for the purpose or may be connected to an eductor or fan by a locally made adapter. Circumstances in which local exhaust would be appropriate include:

- Single manway confined spaces; or confined spaces that have multiple manways, but only one manway has been opened for the hotwork operations.
- Confined spaces with interior obstructions that may decrease ventilation effectiveness or create "dead spots."
- Confined spaces which do not offer feasible way to attach an air moving device in a way that will produce controlled air flow though the space.
- Work with metals such as nickel, chromium, zinc, lead, beryllium, or cadmium. Note that this **not** an exhaustive list. One should carefully examine the MSDSs for the base metal and the filler metal for any hotwork process.

Although the tangle of numerous air lines for supplied air respirators is to be avoided if feasible, bear in mind that there remain circumstances when supplied air respiratory protection may be the only practical solution.

Makeup Air Quality

Mechanical ventilation pulls air in from the areas surrounding the makeup air manways or pushes air in from the areas surrounding the air moving devices. **It is critical to ensure that these areas are not sources of airborne contaminants.** A number of sources of contamination have been noted earlier in this chapter (Section E. Hazards originating in adjacent areas). Review these potential sources of contaminated air when contemplating ventilation of confined spaces. Also, it is important to ensure that air exhausted from one portion of the vessel is not drawn into the vessel through another opening. Also, avoid blowing contaminated from the vessel toward other workers outside the vessel.

Isolation of Hazardous Energy (Lockout-Tagout or LOTO)

The purpose of a Lockout-Tagout program is to provide a set of procedures that guard against employee injury or death due to unintentional and/or unexpected releases of hazardous energy from machinery or equipment. Sources of hazardous energy may include mechanical, hydraulic, pneumatic, chemical, thermal or other energy, such as high intensity electromagnetic fields. In confined spaces, the consequences of being adversely impacted by release of such energy are often fatal. However, the mere existence of this energy is not necessarily considered a hazard[5]. The hazard lies in the unexpected or unintentional release of the energy. Injuries due to these energy releases are most commonly associated with servicing and maintenance operations performed on equipment that contains energy that may be unexpectedly released. The OSHA Lockout/Tagout standard (29 CFR 1910.147) is a performance standard[6] requires employers to establish programs and procedures to prevent unexpected energization, start-up or release of stored energy in order to prevent injuries to employees. Specific procedures are required for each type of equipment at a facility. Lockout/Tagout Programs may work in conjunction with Confined Space Entry Programs, particularly when entries into potentially energized equipment is planned.

Lockout Versus Tagout

The OSHA standard states that if the energy isolation device can be locked out, lockout is required rather than tagout. An exception is

[5] Occupational Safety and Health Administration (OSHA) Control of Hazardous Energy (Lockout/Tagout) standard (29 CFR 1910.147).

[6] OSHA Instruction STD 1-7.3, Subject : 29 CFR 1910.147, The Control of Hazardous Energy (Lockout/Tagout) — Inspection Procedures and Interpretive Guidance dated September 11, 1990, notes that this a performance standard that provides ample latitude for an employer to develop an appropriate program specific to that employer's needs.

allowed if the employer can demonstrate that tagout is just as effective as lockout in providing full protection to the employee. Generally, tagout is used only when the equipment has not been designed to accommodate lockout. Since lockout provides a positive means of preventing an energy release, it is inherently more secure than tagout, which only provides a warning.

Since January 2, 1990, energy isolation devices for equipment that is undergoing replacement, major repair, renovation or modification must be modified or designed to accommodate lockout. However, many facilities still have equipment that has not been modified or designed to accommodate lockout devices.

"Energy isolating devices" are mechanical devices that physically prevents the transmission or release of energy. This may include an electrical circuit breaker that can be removed or locked, but NOT a switch. Unless specifically designed to accommodate a lockout device. Local valves and bolted-in line blocks are also included. "Lockout devices" use a positive means to hold an energy isolating device in a safe (blocking) position. The positive means may include combination locks, keyed locks, blank or blind flanges, and slip flanges. "Locking out" refers to the action of placing a lockout device on an energy isolating device. That is, locking a valve or placing a blind flange in a line. This must be done in accordance with the an established procedure. Lockout ensures that the equipment being controlled cannot be operated until the lockout device is removed.

A "Tagout" device is a prominent warning which can be securely fastened to an energy isolating device. Typically, this is a weather-resistant tag attached by a wire or plastic strap to the valve, switch or other energy isolating device. Verbiage on the tag prohibits operation of the energy isolating device until the tag is removed.

Elements of A Lockout/Tagout Program

The Lockout/Tagout Program is a written program describing:

- energy control procedures,
- energy control equipment
- periodic inspections and
- employee training.

The purpose of the Lockout/Tagout program is to ensure that equipment has been isolated from the energy source and rendered inoperative prior to worker contact with the point of potential hazard. In order to be truly effective, the program should require at least the following"

- Lockout\Tagout devices should be applied only by the authorized employees who are performing the servicing or maintenance.
- All affected employees should be notified when energy control devices are applied or removed.
- Periodic inspections of energy control procedures are generally conducted at the beginning of each shift and include the following requirements:
  - — Periodic inspections must be performed by an authorized person other than those using the isolated equipment.
  - — Periodic inspections are conducted to identify and correct any deviations from established procedures or energy isolation inadequacies.
  - — Periodic inspections must include a review between the inspector and the employee who applied the lockout/tagout device(s) of the employees responsibilities. If tagout devices are used, the limitations of tags must be discussed with each employee who may be affected by the energy source isolated by the tagout device.
  - — Some facilities have elected to use a daily sign-in/sign-out list to document this requirement

Energy Control Equipment

Lockout/Tagout equipment requirements are as follows:

- The employer is responsible for providing the necessary hardware to allow for energy isolation.
- Lockout/Tagout devices may be locks, chains, tags, wedges, blocks, blind flanges or any other suitable equipment.
- Lockout devices must be substantial enough to resist removal unless metal cutting tools are used.
- Tagout devices must be sufficiently durable to withstand the environment

to which they are exposed and substantial enough to resist inadvertent removal.

- Tagout devices shall be at least equal to an all-environment-tolerant nylon cable tie and have release strength of at least 50 pounds.
- Tagout devices shall carry warning language such as "DO NOT START" or "DO NOT OPERATE", etc.
- The Lockout/Tagout devices must be labeled for exclusive use in the energy isolation program and shall not be used for other purposes.
- Lockout\Tagout devices shall be standardized throughout the client's facility.
- Lockout\Tagout devices shall indicate the identity of the employee who applied the device.
- Electrical Energy Isolation

  Electrical equipment hazards involve both equipment operation and the electric current present. Switches and circuit controls should be easily identified and well designed for the placement of lockout devices. With few exceptions, a switch will isolate a circuit. However, it may be difficult to lockout a switch unless it has been specifically designed for lock out. All switches and controls may not be in the immediate area of the device being isolated. Electrical systems generally do not have the capability to store energy, though a few exceptions need to be considered. Systems with capacitors in the circuit must be isolated between the work area and the capacitor. A capacitor may store electricity for a long period, and anything creating a short circuit across the capacitor will cause it to discharge. Systems involving batteries, particularly battery backup power, may be more difficult to identify and isolate. Emergency generators present similar challenges. Also consider any automatic controls such as restart units, level sensors, and pressure sensors.
- Hydraulic and Pneumatic Energy Isolation

  Hydraulic and pneumatic systems also pose the hazard of inadvertent equipment operation and residual pressure on the system. These systems may be more difficult to secure because it is frequently not as easy to identify the appropriate shut-off devices. Many of these systems may be of a loop design that allows flow toward the device from at least two directions. This requires isolation to be established at multiple points for a single system. These devices may also be equipped with internal backup systems, low-pressure sensors, and automatic start-up systems that must be identified and secured. Control of valves, pumps, and compressors is not enough. These systems may hold pressures for an extended period of time and must be bled off. "Double block and bleed" procedures are employed by many facilities to ensure that chemical, thermal hydraulic and pneumatic hazards are isolated from the confined spaces of concern.
- Mechanical Energy Isolation

  Mechanical equipment and systems offer the risk of physical injury due to operation of the system or shifting within the system. Mechanical stored energy includes springs that are compressed or stretched and heavy objects held at height. Mechanical potential energy is the most difficult to identify in many cases. Careful evaluation is required to ensure that this hazard is properly assessed. Usually there are no clearly identified points to secure this energy, which adds to the difficulty.
- Thermal energy considerations

  Sufficient time must be allowed for interior surfaces to reach reasonably ambient temperatures prior to entering the space. Freezers and refrigeration units should be allowed to warm prior to work to reduce the potential for cold contact injuries. If sufficient time to allow for temperature changes is not available, personnel will need proper protective equipment to work around these surface temperature extremes.

Lighting

Adequate lighting must be provided for the exterior and interior areas of the confined space. Lighting is essential for safe performance and reduces psychological stress for entrants. A backup lighting option should always be available for immediate use inside the confined space. There are several types of lighting equipment that may be used in confined space work. The most common categories include conventional electrical powered, low voltage, battery operated, and chemical. Conventional 110-volt lighting may be a useful option when an outlet is readily available and facility procedures allow their use in confined spaces. This type of equipment is usually the best choice when there are no hazards such as wet operating environments that would prevent it. Ground fault circuit interrupters must always be used. Low-voltage systems, usually either 12 or 24 volt, the preferred selection when shock hazards are a concern. This would include use in metal tanks and wet areas. Battery-operated flashlights and hand lights are an option for primary lighting if neither of the previous options is practical. Battery-operated devices are also an excellent option for backup lighting. Chemical light sticks should never be used as the primary lighting but make an excellent backup light source.

Placement of lighting should not obstruct access to the confined space or create hazards such as cords that can be tripped over. Ideally, the interior lighting should be placed close to the work area within the space. Trying to light the interior with lighting placed at the opening can create hazards and is generally not as effective. Another disadvantage of this placement is that entrants cannot see back to the opening well because they are looking directly into the light.

If hazards warrant, all lighting equipment must be intrinsically safe. This means that the lighting equipment itself will not contribute to the ignition of a flammable gas, vapor, or dust. Rated equipment is tested to ensure compliance with standards. In the United States the most common testing organizations are Underwriters Laboratories and Factory Mutual. The U.S. Mine Safety and Health Administration standards are some of the most aggressive, and approval under these guidelines is required for items used in mines.

Confined Space Design and Reducing Risk

Once again, the best way to eliminate the potential for confined space injuries and fatalities is to eliminate the need to enter confined spaces. While this may not be a practical short-term solution, this is the desired objective. Two primary approaches are to either 1) eliminate the confined space, or 2) eliminate the need to enter the space. The first option amounts to designing the "confined" out of the space.

Redesigning the work area to eliminate the characteristics that make it a confined space is the ideal approach. This approach will not work for all, and arguably not even most, confined spaces. However, it is possible for some, and the effort should be made to find and use these opportunities. For example, an area containing a tank in a below-grade vault was redesigned to eliminate the features that make it a confined space. Fixed stairs replaced ladder access. Installed ventilation to provide 20 air-changes per hour was built into the vault and fixed lighting was added. Access and potential atmospheric hazards were the only initial issues. The redesign eliminated both of these problems.

The second option, eliminating the need to enter the space, is sometimes easier to apply. Changes in the design of the space may be made that allow personnel to perform functions such as inspection, cleaning, and maintenance from outside the space.

Examples include:

- access ports placed to allow scraping and cleaning to be accomplished from outside the space
- pullout sensor panels that allow sensors to be removed from the space for maintenance or replacement; and
- pull-up pumps that can be raised from outside the space for maintenance or repair.

When complete elimination is not practical, or even possible, the risk may be minimized by reducing the number of entries, their duration, and the number of people needed in the space.

Reducing the number of entries may be accomplished by grouping inspection and preventive maintenance activities within the space into one work project. This is particularly easy to do with a computerized maintenance scheduling system. Start by identifying all the tasks that require entry and then schedule them to come up on the maintenance calendar at the same time.

Reducing the duration of entries is primarily a function of effective planning of the job. Make sure that all of the required items such as tools, parts, and supplies are available and ready before the work crew enters the space.

Reducing the number of people in the space can be a double-edged sword. Fewer people in the space means fewer people at risk, which is good. But reducing the number by too many can overtax the people doing the work. Strike an effective balance between having enough people to do the work safely and eliminating extra people in the space. In most cases keeping the number in the space at any one time as low as possible and rotating crews regularly is the best method. This keeps the number of people small so that if something goes wrong fewer people will need assistance. It also avoids overtaxing a few individuals because crew rotation allows individuals to refresh themselves between work periods. This technique can be particularly useful when heat stress is a concern. Difficult access spaces present the most challenges for this operational method. When access to the work area within the space is difficult, and getting into position to do the work requires a great deal of time and effort, crew rotation will not be an effective technique.

Design improvements can also be made to reduce the opportunity for problems within the space. An example of this approach is using larger and better-positioned openings. Safety features such as installed ventilation and improved isolation designs can also be built in.

Small vertical openings are usually the most challenging, followed closely by small horizontal openings. Vertical entries through a larger opening are usually more difficult than horizontal entries through a larger opening. Modified openings offer an opportunity to reduce the chance of problems during entry by improving the ability of personnel to enter and leave the space easily. However, changing the design of openings is not always possible with current technology. For example, pressure vessel requirements limit the practical size of some openings. Needs of the process may work against larger or better positioned openings in some process vessels. There is, however, much opportunity for improvement within the limits of performance requirements, and safety and health professionals should take advantage of every opportunity.

An excellent example of looking for opportunities to reduce risk by changing a design occurred in a water company. The company had numerous below-grade vaults in its distribution system. Each was equipped with an instrument to monitor chlorine levels. An employee checked each instrument weekly. Initially, this required entry into each below-grade vault. This job was done by one individual (no attendant). Radio contact was used to keep track of the employee's location and to monitor the time spent in the vault, but had a problem occurred there would have been a significant delay before help could be sent. This situation created a potential for many things to go wrong. The piping and instrumentation system was changed to relocate the instruments to grade level above the vaults. This simple design change completely eliminated the need for routine entries into these vaults.

These suggestions cannot be applied to all situations. There is no magic solution. Progress can be made, however, if opportunities are constantly sought. The IH should strive to eliminate the confined spaces by design, eliminate the need to enter those areas that must remain confined spaces, and reduce the risk of those entries that must be made.

References

1. **National Institute for Occupational Safety and Health (NIOSH):** Preventing Entrapment and Suffocation Caused by the Unstable Surfaces of Stored Grain and Other Materials. DHHS (NIOSH) Publication No. 88-102. Cincinnati, OH, NIOSH, 1987.
2. **National Institute for Occupational Safety and Health (NIOSH):** Confined Spaces NIOSH ALERT: DHHS (NIOSH) Publication No. 86-110. Cincinnati, OH: NIOSH, 1986.
3. **National Institute for Occupational Safety and Health (NIOSH):** WORKER DEATHS IN CONFINED SPACES, A Summary of NIOSH Surveillance and Investigative Findings. DHHS (NIOSH) Publication No. 94-103. Cincinnati, OH: NIOSH, 1994.
4. **McManus, N.:** *Safety and Health in Confined Spaces.* New York: Lewis Publishers, 1999.
5. **American Industrial Hygiene Association (AIHA®):** *Confined Space Entry, An AIHA Protocol Guide.* Chambers, G. (ed.). Fairfax, VA: AIHA®, 2001.

6. **American Society of Safety Engineers (ASSE):** ANSI/ASSE Z117.1 – 2003 Safety Requirements for Confined Spaces. Des Plaines, IL: ASSE, 2003.
7. **National Institute for Occupational Safety and Health (NIOSH):** Worker Deaths in Confined Spaces (DHHS/PHS/CDC/NIOSH Pub No. 80-106) Cincinnati, OH: NIOSH, 1979.
8. **McManus, N.:** *Portable Ventilation Systems Handbook.* New York: Taylor & Francis, 2000.
9. **Harris, M.K., Carter, S.R., and L.E. Booher:** *Field Guidelines for the Temporary Ventilation of Confined Spaces with an Emphasis on Hotwork.* Fairfax, VA: AIHA®, 1996.

Outcome Competencies

After completing this chapter, the reader should be able to:

1. Describe how construction differs from other sectors with regard to occupational exposures and disease.
2. Summarize types of construction.
3. Identify chemical, biological, and physical exposures of concern that may be present in various construction processes and tasks.
4. Recognize how exposure assessment strategies in construction may be similar to, or differ from, those in other settings, and the importance of obtaining both qualitative and descriptive data.
5. Explain examples of engineering, administrative, and personal protective equipment controls in construction, and the potential advantages and disadvantages of each.
6. Understand the basic tiers of management involved in typical construction projects.
7. Discuss the importance of training to construction hygiene and safety.
8. Develop an understanding of how construction hazards are regulated.
9. Recognize the value of prevention through design (P+D).

Key Terms

Abrasive blasting • apprenticeship • arsenic • asbestos • beryllium • bricklayer • cadmium • cement • concrete • confined space • contractor • dermal • dust • epoxies • ergonomics • fibers • fume • grinding • hazard communication • hearing loss • hexavalent chromium • ironworker • lead • local exhaust ventilation • manganese • masonry • metals • mold • noise-induced • nonionizing radiation • OSHA • painting • pipefitter • plumber • sawing • silica • solvents • subcontractor • substitution • task • terrazzo • vibration • welding • worker rotation

Note to readers: There are additional key terms underlined within the chapter.

Prerequisite Knowledge

Basic biology, basic chemistry, basic math, basic physics, introductory industrial hygiene, introductory knowledge of industrial/construction processes and tools, basic safety management

The user is also referred to the following chapters:

Chapter Number	Chapter Topic
18	Indoor Air Quality
24	Noise, Vibration, and Ultrasound
30	Ergonomics
39	Personal Protective Clothing
46	Confined Spaces

Key Topics

I. What Makes Construction Different for the Practicing Industrial/Occupational Hygienist
II. Types of Construction
III. Anticipating Health Hazards by Construction Occupations and Trades
IV. Construction Health Hazard Recognition
    A. Chemical Hazards — Metal Fumes and Dust
    B. Silica, Asbestos, and Man-made Mineral Fibers
    C. Solvents
    D. Skin Hazards
    E. Physical Agents
    F. Biological Hazards
    G. Confined Spaces in Construction
V. Exposure Assessment in Construction: Challenges and Alternative Approaches
VI. Controlling Construction Health Hazards
VII. Management, Communication, and Training
    A. Incorporating Health and Safety Requirements into Construction Contracts
    B. Prevention through Design (PtD): Health and Safety During the Design and Pre-Construction Phases
    C. A Word about Maintenance and Rehabilitation Work in Industrial Settings
    D. Integrating Hazard Analysis and Prevention into Skills Training
VII. Regulatory Perspective

Industrial Hygiene Issues in Construction

47

By Barbara L. Epstien, MPH, CIH; John D. Meeker, ScD, CIH; Pam Susi, MSPH; C. Jason McInnis, MHSc, ROH, CRSP and James W. Platner, PhD, CIH

What Makes Construction Different for the Practicing Industrial / Occupational Hygienist?

Introduction

Construction is change. There are no continuous production processes or assembly lines subject to routine exposure monitoring, incremental improvements and regular verification of control effectiveness. Every structure or project is unique, and the workforce and tasks being performed often change daily, if not hour by hour. Many of the tasks and the occupational health hazards found on construction sites are similar to those found in general industry, including exposures to welding fumes, solvent vapors, noise, and ergonomic concerns. However, employment is transient, so workers may be employed by a large number of employers over the course of their career, if not in a single year. This constantly changing and mobile nature of construction work presents numerous, unique challenges when it comes to anticipating, recognizing, evaluating, and controlling associated occupational health hazards.

Construction involves complex and dynamic multi-employer organizational structures that pose challenges to communication and occupational safety and health management systems. Organization of work, safety culture and management systems are largely built from scratch with each project. Multi-tiered subcontracting relationships also complicate communication between employers and can muddy the lines of responsibility for controlling hazards or shift liability to lower-tier subcontractors who may fail to adequately control risk. This, along with often complex scheduling and the sequential process of multiple subcontractors and crafts involved in each phase of the job, translates into numerous different trades working in close proximity at any given time, which necessitates the additional consideration of bystander exposures. This can extend beyond the various other subcontractors on a jobsite and may involve those in nearby buildings or adjacent occupied spaces within a building being renovated and even to the general public. Exposures to hazardous chemical and physical agents are often brief, intermittent, and may be extremely high or variable, making it difficult to accurately characterize exposures.[1,2] Add to that the variability of jobsite settings, from work performed outdoors in the open (e.g., exposure to extremes in temperature as well as to biological hazards such as those from animals, insects, and allergic reactions to poisonous plants), to working in enclosed, restricted, or confined spaces. This diversity additionally challenges the traditional approach to the development and implementation of effective controls. Still other concerns are found in renovation, repair, and demolition work, where managing worker exposures requires consideration of existing materials, coatings, structural constraints, and process hazards.

This chapter is dedicated to the unique challenges of construction. While other chapters in this book provide detailed discussion on the wide variety of subjects germane to the profession, this chapter focuses on application of the principles of health hazard anticipation, recognition, evaluation, and control in construction. The chapter starts with an overview of the construction industry, then provides examples of different construction occupations, work settings, and/or tasks to illustrate where the industrial hygienist might encounter certain hazards. The special needs of exposure assessment and control in construction are explored and the pragmatic adaptations to traditional approaches in evaluating and managing hazardous exposures are discussed. For example, there is increasing evidence that intermittent high-peak exposures associated with a relatively small number of tasks may contribute a significant portion of a construction worker's full shift time-weighted average exposure. In addition, more research has focused on identifying important task variables or exposure determinants in estimating exposure risk and targeting control technologies. Logically, then, task-based intervention and control measures can be an effective approach to mitigating hazards.

Magnitude of the Problem

The construction industry bears a disproportionate number of work-related deaths resulting from work related injuries. In 2005, although construction accounted for only 8% of the overall workforce, it experienced approximately 22% of the total number of occupational fatalities.[3] This trend continues even though recent safety initiatives have emphasized prevention of fatal falls and electrocutions in very high risk occupations like structural steel erectors (ironworkers) and electrical power line installers (power installers). Construction workers also bear a disproportionate burden for occupational illnesses such as asbestosis and silicosis and are consistently over-represented among elevated lead levels in state blood lead registries. While some construction tasks such as sand blasting or asbestos removal have been recognized as hazardous for many years, recognition of many other occupational health hazards has fallen behind in the awareness of safety hazards in construction. As a result, occupational hygiene in construction is a relatively fresh arena and industrial hygiene professionals are a rare presence on most jobsites.

For a variety of reasons industrial hygiene practice and the application of engineering control measures in the construction industry has lagged behind general industry. Construction is dominated by small employers; approximately 80% have less than 10 employees, nearly one quarter of the workforce is self employed, and an unknown fraction works for cash in a growing informal sector that is often made up of undocumented workers. However, the majority of construction *workers* are still employed by somewhat larger contractors, with 61% of employees working for contractors with 20 or more employees.[3]

Although occupational disease remains poorly characterized in this population, there is a substantial amount of evidence that many construction workers face a higher risk of occupational disease and cancers than in other industry sectors.[1,2,4–16] Elevated occupational exposures, and to a lesser extent, the efficacy and feasibility of various control options, are increasingly well documented in construction.[1,4] Journal articles on hazards and controls for general construction have been published along with sector and hazard specific information for highway construction[5,6], ceiling and wall texturing[7], crystalline silica from concrete[8–14], welding and thermal cutting fumes[2], vitreous fibers[15], chromated copper arsenate (CCA) treated wood dust[17], tunneling dust and gas[18], lead[19,20], isocyanates in polyurethanes[21,22], in residential construction[16], construction site clean-up[23], water-based paints[24], organic solvents[25] and other agents and tasks. Translation of these and similar findings into changes in work site practices and materials across the industry presents significant challenges.

Implementation of control strategies in construction can be more difficult than in other industries and there may be an over reliance on respiratory protection and other personal protective technologies as a result. The Bureau of Labor Statistics (BLS) and National Institute for Occupational Safety and Health (NIOSH) reported that in 2001 nearly 10% of construction workers used respirators as part of employer-required programs over a 12-month period, second only to mining and compared to about half of that (4.8%) among manufacturing employers. Figure 47.1 illustrates this practice, showing the most common hazards for which respirators were used in construction in 2001. However, the development and implementation of effective respiratory

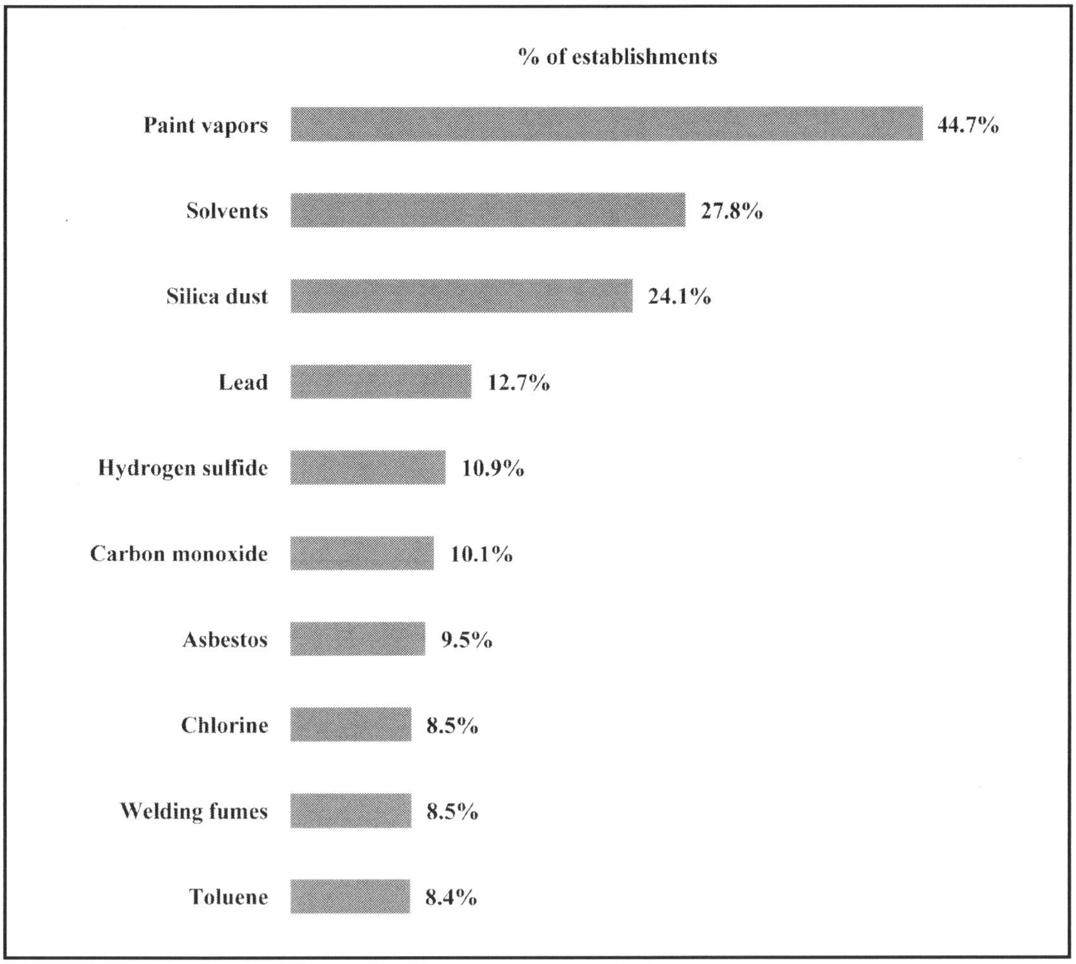

Figure 47.1 — Common hazards Identified with respirator use, by construction establishments, 2001 (BLS/NIOSH, 2003).

protection programs is lacking, with only one-half of those employers providing training as mandated by the Occupational Safety and Health Administration (OSHA).[26] Understandably, managing respirator programs for a transient workforce presents its own challenges.

Types of Construction

Construction is a large, dynamic, complex industry and an important segment of the economy. Construction workers build roads, homes, schools, and workplaces. They also build, repair, renovate, and maintain the structures and facilities that generate power, process chemicals, refine oil, and produce consumer goods, as well as the buildings where people go to shop, eat, and transact everyday business. The goal of this chapter is not to provide an in-depth description of the entire construction sector, but rather provide a brief overview of the types of construction worksites and work activities an industrial hygienist might encounter, the various occupations involved, and the health hazards to which those workers may be exposed.

Rarely is there only one employer on a construction jobsite; the typical multi-employer organizational structure is one of the complicating factors that make exposure assessment and control so challenging. On a construction project of any size or duration there are typically many tiers of management. Starting at the top is the owner or client who wishes to build, renovate, maintain, or demolish a structure; he or she then contracts with a general contractor or project manager who in turn may contract with multiple sub-contractors. While management activities may occur at a fixed place of business, for many contractors there are typically multiple, concurrent project sites underway at any given time. Given the decentralized nature of construction, workers and employers further down the communication chain may or may not receive effective hazard communication regarding prevention efforts that may have been initiated at the top. Project durations vary, which presents an additional challenge to industrial hygienists. Larger construction projects may last for a number of years, but many more are measured in months and some may be as short as a few days.

While new construction presents many opportunities for exposures to chemical and physical agents, renovation and demolition of existing structures and facilities introduces added concerns about existing materials, coatings, and structural constraints such as, enclosed, restricted, or confined spaces with minimal or no ventilation. While new construction has trended away from the use or installation of some legacy hazards, such as asbestos and lead-based paint, these materials still present a significant concern when demolishing, renovating or maintaining older buildings and structures. The removal and handling of hazardous materials and waste as part of remediation or abatement work requires special precautionary work practices and protective equipment. As in new construction, multiple trades are involved in renovation and maintenance work, and often work side by side. In addition, some renovation and maintenance work in occupied buildings also may present concerns for building occupants. Finally, working in operational industrial facilities introduces construction workers to process hazards of the host facility.

For purposes of characterizing economic activity, the construction sector has historically been divided into three major categories.[27][1]

Construction of Buildings

The building construction sub-sector may encompass new work, additions, alterations, maintenance, and repairs and includes residential and nonresidential (industrial, commercial, institutional) buildings. Typically this work is performed by a number of subcontractors who may be coordinated by a general contractor or project manager.

Heavy and Civil Engineering Construction

This sub-sector primarily is engaged in the construction of large engineered projects, often public works such as highways and other roadways, bridges, tunnels, and dams. It also encompasses private utilities and pipelines. A large variety of trades will work on these projects; however, much of the work involves basic trades such as laborers, carpenters, and operating engineers engaged in earth moving, foundation and form work, and steel erection.

Specialty Trade Contractors

This sub-sector is comprised of a variety of specialized, skilled trades who perform a wide array of construction and renovation activities involving both interior and exterior building components. Specialty trade contractors are usually subcontracted by general contractors or project managers, but may also be hired directly by the property owner (especially in remodeling or repair work). Most of their work is performed on the jobsite although some prefabrication work may be performed in a shop and then transported to the site. This is often the case with sheet metal work, for example.

Anticipating Health Hazards by Construction Occupations and Trades

There are dozens of trades that make up the building construction workforce, from the highly visible carpenter framing homes in suburbia to the less evident boilermaker bolting or welding pressure vessel structures together in industrial facilities. A list of

[1] These categories correspond to the major construction groups or sub-sectors as described by both the Standard Industrial Classification (SIC) system, which was developed in the 1930s and used for more than 60 years with numerous revisions throughout that time, and the North American Industry Classification System (NAICS), which was developed in the 1990s through a collaborative effort by the United States, Canada, and Mexico and adopted in 1997. In 2002, the SIC system was retired and replaced by NAICS, which more accurately represents new and emerging industries as well as changing definitions within industries. While the transition poses some challenges for researchers, the NAICS use of a strictly production-oriented framework and a six-digit structure versus the four-digit structure of the SIC allows for greater flexibility.

construction occupations as defined by the U.S. Department of Labor appears in Table 47.1. The industrial hygienist may find it useful to group some of the various construction trades together in certain settings for the purpose of anticipating and assessing the types of hazards that might be encountered during different stages of the con struction process. While building schedules and skill requirements may vary substantially from one job to another, at the start of any new construction project, workers sometimes referred to as the "basic trades" will make up the bulk of the workforce. These include the carpenters, laborers, operating engineers, cement masons, and ironworkers, who are involved in site preparation, grading, concrete form and building foundations work, loading and unloading materials, tying rebar, and steel erection. Other major trade groups involved in various stages of construction include the welding trades, (pipefitters, boilermakers, sheet metal workers, and structural and ornamental ironworkers) and the trowel trades (cement masons, plasterers, and brickmasons).

Construction Health Hazard Recognition

The principles of hazard recognition and control familiar to the industrial hygienist and described in other chapters of this book apply in construction as well. However, as illustrated throughout this chapter, there are certain characteristics of construction that present additional challenges to the industrial hygienist when adapting those principles to construction work environments.

In addition to the transient nature of construction work along with the varied and complex workforce and employment relationships, the industrial hygienist should consider the changing nature of building materials over time that represent new potential hazards. The roofer who may have been concerned more about asphalt fumes and coal tar in the past, for example, may now need to be aware of the hazards posed by isocyanates used in single ply roofing systems. Further, that roofer may be working in extreme temperatures on a black top roof remote from soap, hand-washing water, shade, and facilities to clean and maintain respiratory protection equipment. Yet another consideration for the roofer performing repair work on an existing building might be exposure to *Legionella* if working in close proximity to a cooling tower.

How Are Hazards Generated?

Anticipating and recognizing health hazards in construction starts with an understanding of how they are generated. There are three general ways in which construction workers may be exposed to health hazards:

- From the tasks they perform, which can be generated from materials being used (e.g., solvents, paints) or from in place materials (e.g., asbestos, lead);
- From hazards present on site or at a host facility (e.g., process chemicals); or
- From hazards generated by a nearby craft or sub-contractor (e.g., welding, cutting).

Despite the challenges, anticipating and recognizing hazards in construction is possible and ideally involves workers familiar with their trade. More so than in many other industries, building trades unions are instrumental in training the workforce and thus are familiar with the skills and/or tasks carried out by the trades they represent and the materials and conditions that might give rise to health hazards the industrial hygienist needs to be able to recognize. Consequently, building trades unions and training programs are an important resource for the industrial hygienist seeking to better understand the work processes and hazards of a given construction occupation.

Some examples of construction processes and tasks associated with various chemical, physical, and/or biological exposure agents are described below. This discussion is not intended to be an exhaustive listing of every health hazard that might be encountered by construction workers (nor would such an attempt be feasible). However, the following will illustrate some of the diverse exposure hazards found in construction to help prepare the industrial hygienist for working in those settings.

Chemical Hazards — Metal Fumes and Dusts

Construction workers are commonly exposed to particulate matter in the form of dust and fume. Exposures to dusts and metal fumes

Table 47.1 — Construction Trades and Occupations[2]

Trade/Occupation	*Description*
Boilermakers	Fabricate, assemble, install, test, maintain, and repair boilers, pressure vessels, tanks, vats, towers, heat exchangers, and other heavy metal structures. Inspect, repair or replace defective pressure vessel parts.
Brickmasons and Blockmasons	Lay and bind building materials, such as brick, structural tile, concrete block, cinder block, glass block, and terra-cotta block, with mortar and other substances to construct or repair walls, partitions, arches, chimneys, smokestacks, sewers, and other structures. May also restore, clean, or coat existing brick structures, and line or reline furnaces and boilers.
Carpenters	Construct, erect, install, repair, or maintain structures and fixtures made of wood, such as concrete forms; building frameworks, including partitions, joists, studding, and rafters; wood stairways, window and door frames, and hardwood floors and flooring assemblies. May also install cabinets, siding, drywall, and batt or roll insulation.
Construction Carpenters	Construct, erect, install, and repair structures and fixtures of wood, plywood, and wallboard.
Rough carpenters	Build rough wooden structures, such as concrete forms, scaffolds, tunnel, bridge, or sewer supports, billboard signs, and temporary frame shelters, according to sketches, blueprints, or oral instructions.
Carpet Installers	Lay and install carpet from rolls or blocks on floors. Install padding and trim flooring materials.
Cement Masons and Concrete Finishers	Smooth and finish surfaces of poured concrete, such as floors, walks, sidewalks, roads, patios, or curbs using a variety of hand and power tools. Align forms for sidewalks, curbs, or gutters; patch voids; use saws to cut expansion joints; operate power vibrators to compress and/or distribute concrete; apply hardening and sealing compounds to cure concrete surfaces; install anchor bolts, steel plates, and other fixtures in freshly poured concrete.
Construction Laborers	Perform tasks involving physical labor at building, highway, and heavy construction projects, tunnel and shaft excavations, and demolition sites. May operate hand and power tools of all types. May clean and prepare sites, dig trenches, set braces to support the sides of excavations, erect scaffolding, clean up rubble and debris, and remove asbestos, lead, and other hazardous waste materials.
Drywall and Ceiling Tile Installers	Apply plasterboard or other wallboard to ceilings or interior walls of buildings. Apply or mount acoustical tiles or blocks, strips, or sheets of shock-absorbing materials to ceilings and walls of buildings to reduce or reflect sound. Materials may be of decorative quality.
Electricians	Install, maintain, and repair electrical wiring, equipment, and fixtures in all types of buildings and structures. Ensure that work is in accordance with relevant codes. May install or service street lights, intercom and other communications systems, or electrical control systems.
Floor Layers, Except Carpet, Wood, and Hard Tiles	Apply blocks, strips, or sheets of shock-absorbing, sound-deadening, or decorative coverings to floors.
Floor Sanders and Finishers	Scrape and sand wooden floors to smooth surfaces using floor scraper and floor sanding machine, and apply coats of finish.
Glaziers	Cut, fit, install, and replace glass in windows, skylights, store fronts, and display cases, or on surfaces, such as building fronts, interior walls, ceilings, and tabletops.
Insulation Workers, Floor, Ceiling, and Wall	Line and cover structures with insulating materials. May work with batt, roll, or blown insulation materials. May also remove old insulation from buildings such as during renovations.
Insulation Workers, Mechanical	Apply insulating materials to pipes or ductwork, or other mechanical systems (heating, cooling, refrigeration) in order to help control and maintain temperature. May also remove old insulation from mechanical system components such as during repairs or renovations.

(continued on next page.)

[2] Adapted from http://online.onetcenter.org/find/family?f=47&g=Go, the Occupational Information Network (O*NET) is sponsored by the U.S. Department of Labor/Employment and Training Administration (USDOL/ETA) through a grant to the North Carolina Employment Security Commission.

Table 47.1 — Construction Trades and Occupations (cont.)[2]

Trade/Occupation	*Description*
Operating Engineers and Other Construction Equipment Operators	Operate one or several types of power construction equipment, such as motor graders, bulldozers, scrapers, compressors, pumps, derricks, shovels, tractors, or front-end loaders to excavate, move, and grade earth, erect structures, or pour concrete or other hard surface pavement.
Painters, Construction and Maintenance	Paint interior and exterior walls, equipment, buildings, bridges, and other structural surfaces. May remove old paint to prepare surface prior to painting. Use brushes, rollers, or spray equipment.
Paperhangers	Cover interior walls and ceilings of rooms with decorative wallpaper or fabric, or attach advertising posters on surfaces, such as walls and billboards. May also remove old materials from surface to be papered.
Paving, Surfacing, and Tamping Equipment Operators	Operate equipment used for applying concrete, asphalt, or other materials to road beds, parking lots, or airport runways and taxiways, or for tamping gravel, dirt, or other materials.
Pile-driver Operators	Operate pile driving rigs mounted on skids, barges, crawler treads, or locomotive cranes to drive pilings for retaining walls, bulkheads, and foundations of structures, such as buildings, bridges, and piers.
Pipefitters and Steamfitters	Lay out, assemble, install, and maintain pipe systems, pipe supports, and related hydraulic and pneumatic equipment for steam, hot water, heating, cooling, lubricating, sprinkling, and industrial production and processing systems.
Pipelayers	Lay pipe for storm or sanitation sewers, drains, and water mains. Grade trenches or culverts, position pipe, or seal joints.
Plasterers and Stucco Masons	Apply interior or exterior plaster, cement, stucco, or similar materials to finish, maintain, or restore these materials on walls, ceilings, and building partitions. May also set ornamental plaster. Work involves leveling, smoothing, cleaning, and preparing surfaces.
Plumbers	Assemble, install, and repair pipes, fittings, and fixtures of heating, water, and drainage systems, according to specifications and plumbing codes.
Plumbers, Pipefitters, and Steamfitters	Lay out, fabricate, assemble, install, alter, maintain, and repair pipelines or pipe systems that carry water, steam, air, or other liquids or gases. May install heating and cooling equipment and mechanical control systems. Work involves welding, cutting, cleaning, pipe bending, and use of hand and power tools.
Reinforcing Iron and Rebar Workers	Position and secure steel bars or mesh in concrete forms in order to reinforce concrete. Use a variety of fasteners, rod-bending machines, oxy-acetylene cutting torches, blowtorches, and hand tools.
Roofers	Cover roofs of structures with shingles, slate, asphalt, aluminum, wood, gravel, and related materials. May spray and/or otherwise install materials to bind, seal, insulate, waterproof, or soundproof sections of roof and/or siding structures. Install, repair, and replace single-ply roofing systems using waterproof sheet materials such as modified plastics, elastomeric, or other asphaltic compositions.
Sheet Metal Workers	Fabricate, assemble, install, and repair sheet metal products and equipment, such as ducts, control boxes, drainpipes, and furnace casings.
Stonemasons	Build stone structures, such as piers, walls, and abutments. Lay walks, curbstones, or special types of masonry for vats, tanks, and floors.
Structural Iron and Steel Workers	Raise, place, and unite iron or steel girders, columns, and other structural members to form completed structures or structural frameworks.
Tapers	Mix, spread, smooth, and sand sealing compound to seal joints between plasterboard or other wallboard to prepare wall surface for painting or papering.
Terrazzo Workers and Finishers	Apply a mixture of cement, sand, pigment, or marble chips to floors, stairways, walls, and cabinet fixtures to fashion durable and decorative surfaces using various mixing, grouting, grinding, cleaning, and polishing procedures.
Tile and Marble Setters	Cut, shape, polish, and install tile and/or marble to walls, floors, ceilings, and roof decks. Use hand and power tools to cut and fit tiles and mix and apply cement, mastic, plaster, or other adhesives.

come from a variety of sources. Some of the more common sources are pigments in paints and alloys used in steels and in abrasive media. Hexavalent chromium is likely to be present in Portland cement, which presents dermal exposure risks when wet, and though less well documented, may pose inhalation hazards when dry. Construction workers employed in industrial rehabilitation and maintenance projects may be exposed to a variety of metals including those found in fly ash generated by coal-power plants and metals associated with smelting such as arsenic from copper smelting. Vanadium exposure has been seen in boilermakers involved in overhaul of oil power plants.

Welding. One of the most important sources of metal fume exposure in construction comes from hot work tasks, namely welding, brazing and thermal cutting. Estimates on the number of workers exposed to welding fumes range from 410,000 full-time welders to over 1 million who weld intermittently.[28] Welding is an important skill in construction and trades that perform welding are among those expected to see the largest gains in future job growth. Sheet metal workers and pipefitter/plumbers are expected to see employment growth of 22.8% and 22.5%, respectively.[29] Welding is used on structural steel in buildings, bridges and other structures; for piping used in heating and ventilation systems; and for industrial process piping, duct work, laboratory hoods, tanks, boilers and vessels. Welding may also be used for ornamental purposes such as hand rails or other non-structural applications. Thermal cutting, which also generates metal fumes, is common in construction for demolition and for cutting steel rebar and other materials. The primary welding trades in construction are pipefitters, ironworkers, boilermakers and sheet metal workers. Employment for these trades is estimated at 444,000 plumbers/pipefitters; 48,000 ironworkers; 7,000 boilermakers; and 77,000 sheet metal workers. In addition, 103,000 construction workers are classified as "welders."[3]

Welding often occurs in confined spaces such as tanks or boilers or other poorly ventilated settings. Local exhaust ventilation to reduce welding fume exposures is rare on most construction sites. Given the potential for poorly controlled metal fume exposures, workers may be at increased risk for a variety of preventable occupational illness such as lung cancer and occupational asthma from hexavalent chromium and nickel or neurological illnesses associated with manganese.

While construction welding trades share similar skills, their specific job descriptions differ. Boilermakers fabricate, install and repair boilers, vats and other vessels. Often they are employed in power plants and industrial settings such as refineries. The nature of their work involves regular entry into enclosed or confined spaces. Pipefitters install and repair piping used in power plants, industrial and manufacturing facilities, and in heating and cooling systems. Sheet metal workers fabricate and install heating and ventilation system components, duct work, laboratory hoods, restaurant equipment, and countertops, and test and balance air conditioning and ventilation systems. Ironworkers erect steel columns and girders that make up the structural framework of buildings, bridges and other large structures such as water towers. Welding is involved in the majority of tasks described above.

Commonly used welding processes may differ among trades. Shielded metal arc welding (SMAW) or "stick" welding is likely the most common welding process in construction. However, other welding processes including gas metal arc (or metal inert gas, MIG) welding (GMAW), gas tungsten arc (or tungsten inert gas, TIG) welding (GTAW), and flux-cored arc welding (FCAW) may generate very high fume levels as well. The welding process along with the materials used are important determinants of the fume composition and generation rate, which, together with ventilation patterns and other worksite characteristics will govern the exposure.[30]

While there is interest in hexavalent chromium exposures from welding as a result of an OSHA standard (29 CFR 1926.1126) that was promulgated in 2006, there is typically significant nickel content along with chromium in high alloy and stainless steel metals and electrodes.[31] Health effects associated with nickel include increased risk of lung, nasal and larynx cancer; respiratory irritation, increased respiratory infection, pulmonary fibrosis, bronchial asthma, and allergic contact dermatitis.[32]

Significant exposures to welding fume have also been reported in the construction industry during excavation work.[33] Personal breathing zone samples meeting or exceeding American Conference of Governmental Industrial Hygienists (ACGIH®) threshold limit values (TLVs®) for total fume, fluoride, and manganese were found. Verma et al.[4] also reported excessive total fume exposures from arc welding, gouging, soldering, and thermal cutting in the construction trades especially among ironworkers, laborers, plumbers and pipe fitters. Exposures as high as 28.3 milligrams per cubic meter (mg/m^3) total fume and 17.3 mg/m^3 inhalable fraction were reported. A study of construction worker welding fume exposure conducted by the Center for Construction Research and Training (CPWR) found elevated exposures for total fume, manganese, nickel, and hexavalent chromium.[2,34] With respect to manganese, 72% of boilermaker exposures exceeded the ACGIH® TLV®. Among ironworkers and pipefitters, 15% and 7%, respectively, of the sampled exposures were above the TLV®. The mean hexavalent chromium exposure exceeded the current OSHA permissible exposure limit (PEL) of 5 $\mu g/m^3$. Zinc oxide fumes are also generated from welding galvanized metal which can cause metal fume fever.

Abrasive blasting. Abrasive blasting is another important source of metal exposures in construction. Painters and other trades that perform abrasive blasting on painted steel or concrete surfaces encounter a mixture of metal exposures generated not only from the paint, but in many cases, from the abrasive. Meeker et al.[35] reported on a three-year field comparison of the following alternative abrasives: specular hematite, coal slag, and steel grit. Paint from all three years contained a high percentage of quartz (5.9–9.6%) and high concentrations of lead, chromium, manganese and titanium. Clean steel grit contained higher concentrations of cadmium, chromium, lead, manganese, and nickel than the other two abrasives, while coal slag contained more beryllium and titanium. Results of personal breathing zone sampling showed steel grit to be associated with higher exposures to cadmium, chromium, manganese, and nickel than specular hematite and coal slag; this was consistent with results from the clean abrasive bulk samples. In addition to total and respirable particulate, coal slag was associated with higher exposures to beryllium and titanium compared to both specular hematite and steel grit, and higher exposure to vanadium compared to specular hematite. For beryllium and titanium, the higher exposures associated with coal slag were consistent with clean abrasive bulk sample results.

Lead. Lead is likely the most pervasive non-ferrous metal encountered in construction. Lead paint covers miles and miles of steel surfaces in industrial facilities, on bridges and on other structures such as water towers. It is also commonly found in commercial and residential buildings constructed before 1978. Lead is widely used in plastics and can be found in electrical wiring insulation and vinyl products. Although PVC pipe now dominates the plumbing industry, lead pipe still abounds in older plumbing.

When the abrasive blaster propels sand, grit or shot at 100 pounds per square inch (psi) on lead painted steel or the ironworker or demolition worker uses his or her oxy-acetylene torch to cut painted steel surfaces, extremely high lead exposures are generated, which can result in acute lead poisoning if not well controlled. Carpenters and painters who disturb lead paint during commercial and residential renovation may also experience elevated lead exposures albeit to a lesser degree than their counterparts employed in industrial settings. Lead is also used for shielding in nuclear reactors and pipefitters who specialize in that work may be exposed to lead fume during thermal processes.

Lead targets a number of biological processes and organs including blood formation, the kidneys, the central and peripheral nervous systems and may result in reproductive disorders. Lead is also associated with gastrointestinal symptoms, joint pain and elevated blood pressure.[36]

Manganese. The neurotoxicity of manganese has been well known for decades, particularly in the case of manganism, a more overt condition resulting from very high exposure and often seen among miners. However, more current research has shown an association between manganese fume generated from welding and a neurological condition very similar to Parkinson's disease, often referred to as manganese induced Parkinsonism (MIP). Researchers have also identified pre-clinical neurobehavioral effects from manganese exposures using tests that measure motor function, fine motor coordination and cognitive effects.[37] The exposure concentrations at which these symptoms occur remain controversial. The ACGIH® TLV® has been lowered progressively from 6 mg/m³ in 1948 to 0.2 mg/m³ where it has remained since 1992. In 2010, ACGIH® published a Notice of Intended Change to lower the TLV® to 0.02 mg/m³ for respirable particulate to prevent neurobehavioral and neuro-psychological changes.[38]

Given the prevalence of welding in construction and of manganese in steel, the potential for manganese exposure among the welding trades is of particular concern. An analysis of three large welding fume exposure data sets found that mean manganese exposure among arc welders were consistently over one-half the TLV® and in some cases exceeded the TLV®. This was the case for data collected among boilermakers by CPWR, which showed a mean exposure of 0.26 mg/m³.[38] The same study documents statistically significant reductions in manganese and total fume exposures with use of mechanical and LEV. However, there was some evidence that mechanical ventilation alone did not always provide adequate exposure reductions.

Arsenic. The International Agency for Research on Cancer (IARC) classifies arsenic as a Group 1 human carcinogen. Target sites for cancer are the lung, skin and probably the liver.[37] Arsenic may be used in special solders, arsenite sulfides have been used in paint pigments, and arsenates have been used as a wood preservative. Arsenic also occurs as an impurity in copper ores and can be found in coal fly ash. Construction workers employed in maintenance and/or rehabilitation of copper smelters and coal power plants are at risk of arsenic exposure. Abrasive blasting of surfaces coated with paints containing arsenic compounds and/or use of copper slag abrasive media may result in elevated arsenic exposures.

Cadmium. Cadmium is used in pigments and as an alloy material. It occurs naturally with zinc and to a lesser extent with lead; therefore, cadmium fume may be generated during smelting operations. It has a low boiling point which facilitates relatively rapid generation of fumes during hot work involving cadmium containing materials.[36] As described above, the study comparing abrasive blasting media (specular hematite, coal slag, and steel grit) found concentrations of cadmium were elevated in bulk samples of clean steel grit abrasive and in personal breathing zones of abrasive blasters using steel grit.

Beryllium. The three major health outcomes of beryllium are acute beryllium disease from short duration/high exposure concentrations; chronic beryllium disease (CBD) and lung cancer. The latency period for CBD ranges from a few weeks to several years.[39] Beryllium was not used commercially until the late 1920s. During World War II beryllium was used in nuclear weapons production and it is also used in nuclear reactors including those used in power generation. Use of beryllium for defense applications has subsided along with decreased nuclear weapons production.[40] However, an abundance of beryllium dust residue is still present on the U.S. Department of Energy (DOE) sites which made up the U.S. weapons complex during the Cold War era. Ironworkers, pipefitters and other trades may encounter beryllium dust exposure in these facilities when working above old piping and steel beams where dust may have accumulated over the years. According to a study of U.S. industries where beryllium exposure may occur, seventeen DOE facilities have "actual or potential" exposure among a workforce that includes both DOE and contract workers.[40] Beryllium is also used in alloys and has been increasingly used for consumer products such as personal computers and mobile phones.

In the previously described study there were thirteen construction SIC codes represented among industries with beryllium exposures greater than or equal to 0.1 µg/m³. Two of the five SIC codes that comprised 44% of all those industries with positive beryllium exposures were 1721 (painting and paper hanging); and 1799 (special trade contractors not elsewhere classified). Construction trades with elevated beryllium exposure included laborers, welders, carpenters, abrasive blasters, painters, electricians, cutters, burners and operators involved in demolition work; insulation and abatement workers. Beryllium exposure also occurs in paper mills and primary and secondary metal industries. Workers involved in renovation and demolition work on existing facilities within these industries may be at risk of beryllium exposure if poorly controlled.

Silica, Asbestos, and Man-made Mineral Fibers

Construction is a dusty industry and construction workers experience elevated disease rates from fibrotic lung disease and other respiratory disorders. A study of death certificates in selected states from 1991–1993 showed that a number of trades had a 25% higher risk of death from "pneumoconiosis and other respiratory diseases."[(41)] Pneumoconioses are a group of interstitial lung diseases caused by inhalation of particulate matter, especially mineral or metallic dusts.

Asbestos and silica are well recognized hazards in construction and are associated with fibrotic lung disease and lung cancer. However, despite the prevalence of these exposure risks, the occurrence of these diseases are believed to be underreported.[(3)] A study of death certificates from New Jersey residents occupationally exposed to silica whose cause of death was reported as "chronic obstructive pulmonary disease, tuberculosis, or cor pulmonale" used radiographic evidence to show that silicosis was present in 8.5% of this population and asbestosis showed evidence of 10.7%. These results suggest that approximately 20% (19.2%) of these deaths involved silicosis and asbestosis that were previously undetected and under-counted.[(42)]

Silica. Silicosis, a fibrotic disease of the lungs, is irreversible, often progressive (even after exposure has ceased), and potentially fatal. Because no effective treatment currently exists, prevention through exposure control is essential. Silica has also been classified by IARC as a Group 1 human carcinogen. In a study of death certificates of white males under age 65, construction workers experienced a three-fold increased risk of death from silicosis based on proportionate mortality ratios (PMRs).[(43)] More than a third of people who died with silicosis from 1990 through 1999 worked in the construction and mining industries.[(44)] Lyons et al.[(45)] described the case of a 30-year-old mason who presented with silicoproteinosis following six months of work involving cutting and grinding masonry with a demolition saw and grinder.

NIOSH reported that 215,754 workers in construction were potentially exposed to respirable crystalline silica in 1986.[(46)] Many construction tasks have been associated with overexposure to crystalline silica.[(11,33,47–49)] Among these tasks are tuckpointing, concrete cutting, concrete grinding, and abrasive blasting[(9,10,38,48,50–53)], where time-weighted-average worker exposures can routinely exceed concentrations that are 20 to 100 times higher than recommended limits.[(9,51)] CPWR has documented high probabilities of exceeding recommended exposure limits for silica among sampled trades including bricklayers, painters, operating engineers and laborers. Linch[(10)] found elevated exposures to silica during abrasive blasting of concrete surfaces, drilling concrete highway pavement, concrete grinding, concrete sawing, and milling of asphalt from concrete highway pavement. Akbar-Khanzadeh et al.[(54)] have described crystalline silica dust exposures associated with concrete grinding activities and lists concrete finishers, brick masons, and laborers as trades likely to perform this task.

Linch et al.[(55)] estimated that 13,800 masonry and plastering workers were exposed to concentrations of respirable crystalline silica that were at least 10 times the NIOSH Recommended Exposure Limits (REL). Bricklayers are routinely exposed to silica during mortar mixing, cutting brick, block and other masonry material and during masonry restoration work. There were approximately 213,000 bricklayers employed in the construction industry in 2005.[(3)] A proportionate mortality study of deceased members of the International Union of Bricklayers and Allied Crafts (IUBAC) found significantly elevated PMRs for cancers of the digestive organs and peritoneum, respiratory system, and cancers of other unspecified sites. Proportionate mortality ratios were also elevated for silicosis (PMR = 322) but the lower confidence level included 100.[(56)] A study of deceased members of the IUBAC in Ontario found significantly elevated rates of lung cancer (Standard Mortality Ratios [SMRs] of 158; 130–190) and stomach cancer (SMR = 235; 140–370).[(57)]

OSHA's guidance document, *Controlling Silica Exposures in Construction*, states that exposures associated with tuckpointing are among the highest seen.[(58)] Tuckpointers are a specialized craft within the masonry trades that replaces old mortar between masonry units. This involves a great deal of continuous grinding of mortar joints. Based

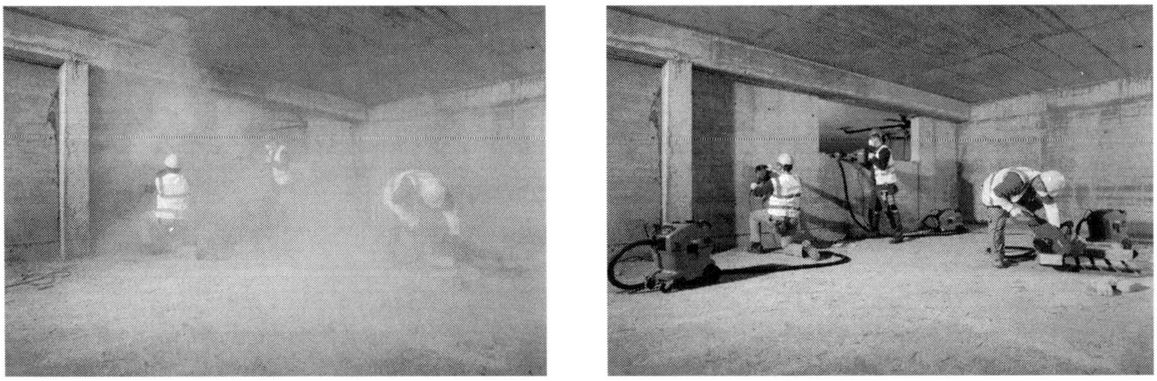

Figure 47.2 — Concrete cutting and grinding with and without LEV controls. (Courtesy of Hilti, Inc.)

on OSHA case files, more than half of exposure measurements collected while tuckpointing were greater than twice the NIOSH REL for respirable silica. Drawing on a small number of case studies (three) using engineering controls, the document reports vacuum dust controls to be generally effective but rarely used. In one such case, workers initially had difficulty using the vacuum shroud, which reduced its effectiveness in reducing exposure levels.[58]

Despite evidence of elevated exposure to silica the use of engineering controls for silica remains limited in construction. The absence of regulatory pressure, perceived costs and logistical drawbacks, and limited awareness within the industry of the dangers of silica and available controls serve as barriers to their widespread use. A general discussion providing some examples of engineering controls may be found elsewhere in this chapter; however, some silica-specific examples are discussed here. The OSHA document provides guidance on controls for nine different tools / tasks associated with elevated silica exposure, including stationary masonry saws; handheld masonry saws; hand-operated grinders; tuckpointing/mortar removal; jackhammers; rotary hammers and similar tools, vehicle-mounted rock drilling rigs; drywall finishing; and housekeeping and dust control through use of dust suppressants. An example of LEV used to reduce exposures is shown in Figure 47.2. Nash and Williams[9] evaluated a shroud on a grinder with a hose attachment leading to a collection bag, was capable of a nearly 93% reduction in respirable silica exposure. In another study, respirable quartz exposures were reduced by about 98% when an angle grinder with a vacuum shroud was used for tuckpointing.[51] Thorpe et al.[14] described silica exposure reductions of at least 90% for cutting concrete slabs with cut-off saws using water to suppress dust and cutting concrete slabs with a grinder using LEV. Croteau et al.[52] examined the use of LEV for reducing exposures from several construction tasks, including tuckpointing and block cutting, with exposure reductions ranging from 80% to 95% at the higher of two ventilation rates tested. Meeker et al.[59] compared exposures with and without use of LEV with no exposure control during block and brick cutting and found that a portable LEV unit significantly reduced mean respirable quartz exposures by 96 and 91 percent, respectively ($p < 0.01$). The use of stationary wet saws was also associated with 91% reductions in exposure ($p<0.01$). For tuckpointing, the reductions in mean respirable quartz concentrations were between 91 and 93 percent with the LEV controls ($p<0.05$). Laboratory studies have suggested that because of the large amount of dust generated by tuckpointing, it is necessary to maintain an airflow rate above 80 to 85 CFM to adequately control respirable silica exposures during tuckpointing.[53]

Although research on control effectiveness has begun to emerge, improvement of available controls is needed as is instruction on correct operation and maintenance. Research on engineering controls for silica is among the 2009 National Occupational Research Agenda (NORA) priorities.[60]

Asbestos. Most newly manufactured

building materials in the U.S. no longer contain asbestos, although some uses of new asbestos continue. However, the use of asbestos in numerous building materials including insulation, floor tiles, roofing, and acoustical materials, has left a legacy of potential exposure risks for trades who are working in older buildings where asbestos is still present, such as during demolition, renovation, decommissioning, or maintenance. In addition, asbestos-containing materials can still be found in brake and clutch plate components for cranes and heavy equipment. In some cases asbestos containing material will surface for the first time as renovation is underway and walls and ceilings are removed. Asbestos-containing building materials were used predominantly during the 1950s through the 1980s. When renovation or maintenance work is performed in facilities built during this timeframe, the owner should exercise due diligence in communicating where asbestos may be present (and/or the contractor should ask). Removal of and/or maintenance or repair work on these materials must be done in such a way as to protect workers, as well as nearby building occupants, from any resultant exposure to elevated levels of airborne fibers.

The U.S. Environmental Protection Agency (USEPA) began publishing detailed regulatory standards and guidelines in the 1970s specifically to address demolition and renovation work involving handling previously installed asbestos-containing materials in buildings. OSHA progressively lowered the asbestos PEL during its early years, and then in 1986 published one of its first expanded health standards for the construction industry. For the first time, this rulemaking (originally 29 CFR 1926.58, later revised and recodified to 1926.1101) grouped together not only demolition and removal, but also maintenance and repair involving previously installed asbestos-containing materials into a single, comprehensive standard with specific provisions for construction activities.[61,62]

Man-made mineral fibers (MMMF). Man-made mineral fibers are amorphous fibers made from rock, ceramic, slag, or glass. Short-term exposure effects of these agents are mostly skin related and involve itching, rashes, or burning. MMMFs may also irritate the upper respiratory system (nose and throat) and may result in bronchitis. Long term effects involve scarring of the lung. Studies involving MMMF production workers have shown some elevated rates in lung cancer.[63]

In addition to the materials already discussed, there are numerous other particulate hazards in construction including asphalt and diesel fumes, wood dust, and drywall dust. In addition, activities such as dry sweeping, sanding, and use of powered tools for cutting, grinding and abrading may result in very high dust and particulate airborne concentrations.

Solvents

Solvents can be found in a wide range of products common to construction including adhesives, glues, cleaning fluids, contact cement, epoxy resins, plastics, paints, paint thinners, and primers. Solvents have a wide range of applications within the construction industry such as:

- dissolving grease, oil and paints (e.g. to clean tools);
- thinning or mixing pigments, paints, glues, pesticides and epoxy resins;
- removing paint and other materials from surfaces (e.g. to prepare welding surfaces);
- fiber-reinforced plastic (FRP) welding;
- release agents used in prefabrication of concrete elements; and
- coatings on metallic vessels and tanks.

Primary routes of exposure to solvents include inhalation, dermal exposure, and to a lesser extent ingestion. Depending on the degree of exposure and solvent(s) involved, some common health effects from overexposure to organic solvents can range from local effects (such as skin irritation/rash, irritated eyes/nose/throat, dermatitis, burns, blistering); to systemic effects (such as headaches/dizziness, nausea, stomach pains), to more serious biological damage of the kidneys, nervous system, respiratory system and heart. Many organic solvents are recognized by NIOSH as carcinogens, reproductive hazards, and neurotoxins.

In a recent study of 1,000 construction painters and carpenters, risk factors for respiratory symptoms and chronic bronchitis were linked to the use of epoxy, glue, and urethane products. Water-based paints were not identified as a common cause of symptoms in this study.[64] While industry as a whole has trended away from organic solvents and toward the use of water-based solvent products since the 1970s, organic solvents still comprise a significant occupational health hazard due to their common use.

Exposures to solvents in construction can be controlled much like other hazards through improved work processes and procedures (e.g., safe handling of solvents, proper hygiene, appropriate PPE (e.g. respirator, gloves), engineering controls (e.g., adequate ventilation, substitution of less harmful solvents where feasible) and worker education. Some useful points to consider in any occupational risk management strategy involving solvents include:

- the identification of the specific solvent(s) of interest for a given work site or work activity, e.g. material safety data sheet (MSDS) or safety data sheet (SDS), supplier or manufacturer specifications and/or labels, worker/employer interviews;
- whether or not you are handling a single solvent compound or a mixture of chemicals (more common). If in mixture, consider the type of combined toxicity (e.g. additive, synergistic, antagonistic);
- understanding solvent route(s) of exposure and acute/chronic health effects (how is the chemical used, work patterns, duration of exposure, temperature, evaporation rate, airflow, exposed solvent surface area, etc);
- potential secondary chemical exposures (e.g. welding in the presence of chlorinated solvents) and variations in source solvent vapor concentration as a result of welding on materials recently cleaned using solvents (especially in enclosed, restricted, or confined spaces); and
- consideration of both inhalation and skin absorption routes.

A number of solvent TLVs® have skin notations indicating the dermal exposure route as a potentially major contributor to overall exposure. In these cases, careful consideration should be given to using biological exposure monitoring as a part of an overall exposure monitoring strategy. Resources such as ACGIH® TLV®-BEIs® Documentation and/or Lauwerys and Hoet[65] may be for further guidance on biological monitoring.

Other Chemical Hazard Concerns. Construction workers are exposed to a myriad of other chemical hazards beyond those described here. Temporary heaters and gasoline-powered tools present a risk of elevated carbon monoxide exposure. Wood dusts, especially in the residential construction sector, present a concern. Diesel exhaust and asphalt fumes are also present on many jobsites. Isocyanates can be produced during spraying of polyurethane foam. Benzene and other process chemicals present exposure risks during industrial maintenance or turnarounds. Elevated exposures to mercury, nitrogen dioxide, and sulfur dioxide (among other chemical agents) have been observed during maintenance, construction, and cleaning in pulp and paper industries.[4] Inorganic mercury has been used as a pigment, and organic mercury compounds have been used for their biocidal properties, and were added as antifouling agents to paints and as slimicides to paper pulp. It should be readily apparent that if the industrial hygienist was under the impression that there existed some finite listing of potential chemical exposure concerns in construction, that impression has now been vastly revised.

Skin Hazards

The industrial hygienist should be aware of a number of construction materials that can cause contact dermatitis. These include specific solvents such as alcohols, toluene, xylene, and turpentine; adhesives, epoxy resins, and some paints; also wet cement and some cement dusts; lime; metalworking fluids; and pitch and coal tar, which can also cause skin cancer.[66]

When selecting gloves to prevent skin exposure to solvents, it is important to consider the characteristics of the glove material. Common glove materials have limited protective properties and do not protect against all hazards. For example, some solvents, degreasers and other liquids can penetrate and/or dissolve rubber, neoprene or PVC.[67] The suitability of a glove type for a particular chemical is dependent on permeation rates, breakthrough time, and the degradation characteristics of the selected glove material associated with the chemical in question. Other factors such as work tasks and physical requirements (e.g.

abrasion protection, wet grip, dexterity) should also be considered when selecting protective gloves. Table 47.2 lists some glove materials suggested by the Construction Safety Association of Ontario for protection against a number of chemicals that may be encountered in construction work.[67] In addition, glove materials such as ethyl vinyl alcohol laminate (EVAL), butyl rubber, nitrile butyl rubber (NBR), and neoprene are protective for epoxy resins.[66] This type of information may provide a useful guide when the MSDS or SDS does not specify the type of glove to be worn.

Table 47.2 — Recommended Glove Material for Selected Chemicals

Chemical Name	*Glove Selection*
Acetone	Butyl Rubber
Cellosolve	PVA, PVC, Neoprene
Cellosolve Acetate	PVA, PVC
Cyclohexane	NBR, Viton®
Hexane	Neoprene, NBR, PVA
Methyl Alcohol	Neoprene, Rubber, NBR
Methyl Chloroform	PVA, Viton®
Methylene Chloride	PVA, Viton®
Methyl Ethyl Ketone	Butyl Rubber
Methyl Isobutyl Ketone	Butyl Rubber, PVA
Mineral Spirits	Neoprene
Naphtha	NBR, PVA
Perchloroethylene	NBR, PVA, Viton®
Stoddard Solvent	PVA, NBR, Rubber
Toluene	PVA, Viton®
Turpentine	PVA, NBR
Trichloroethylene	PVA, Viton®
1,1,1 Trichloroethane	PVA, Viton®
1,1,2 Trichloroethane	PVA, Viton®
Xylene	PVA, Viton®

PVA = Polyvinyl Alcohol
PVC = Polyvinyl Chloride
NBR = Nitrile Butyl Rubber
Viton® = Dupont tradename product

Source: CSAO, 2007.

Epoxies. Epoxy resin systems are two-part chemical mixtures that contain an epoxy resin and a curing agent or hardener. The most common epoxy resins are glycidyl ethers of alcohols; curing agents commonly contain amines. Both of these chemical classes are potent skin irritants. Dermal exposure effects can range from mild skin irritation to severe allergic reactions. In addition, inhalation exposure during mixing of epoxy resin systems can cause upper respiratory irritation and asthma. Cutting, sanding, or burning finished, hardened epoxies can produce exposure to irritant dusts. Exposure consideration should also be given to additives such as plasticizers, solvents, fillers, and pigments. Solvents such as acetone, methyl ethyl ketone, toluene, xylene, glycol ethers, and alcohols may be found either in the epoxy resin system itself or may be used where epoxies are handled, to clean up equipment and spills. Fillers may include glass fiber, calcium carbonate, powdered metals, pigments, and sand.

Epoxy resin systems are used in concrete bonding, epoxy flooring, marble laminate products, durable paints, plumbing sealants, and waterproof coatings. The following is a partial listing of construction occupations that commonly handle epoxy resin-containing materials and some examples of pertinent tasks or materials:

- Cement masons and concrete finishers: cement mixtures, coatings, and bonding materials
- Brickmasons: waterproof coatings for structures requiring corrosion protection
- Terrazzo workers and finishers; floor sanders and finishers: applying paints, liquid pastes, or mortars
- Tile and marble setters: epoxy resin-treated marble strips for decorative or strengthening purposes; epoxy adhesives and grouts
- Painters: paints and coatings that contain epoxy resins for surfaces requiring toughness and durability (steel structures, bridges)
- Plumbers: leak-proof sealants for piping; bonding adhesives[68]

Cement. In addition to epoxy resins, construction workers may encounter skin irritation and allergic dermatitis from working with the extremely alkaline Portland cement, found in plaster and concrete mixes. In addition, wet plaster contains slaked lime, or calcium hydroxide, which is even more caustic. Portland cement often contain trace amounts of hexavalent chromium, which is a strong sensitizing agent responsible for allergic dermatitis in cement workers.

Physical Agents

Noise. Hazardous levels of noise are commonly encountered in construction. According to recent data, overexposure to noise is routinely experienced by operating engineers, bricklayers (and allied craftworkers), carpenters, ironworkers, boilermakers, laborers, and other construction trades.[69–71] Not surprisingly, these trades also have the highest prevalence of noise-induced hearing loss (NIHL), with well over 50% of workers experiencing NIHL within some of these trades.[3] NIHL results in decreased quality of life and problems communicating, which can further lead to increased risk of accidents and injuries. In addition to NIHL, excessive noise exposure can cause stress, hormone disturbances, and cardiovascular effects.[72] Noise exposure and associated health effects among residents living near loud construction work is also receiving increased attention[73] and increasingly stringent public noise ordinances.

Besides trade designation, noise exposure is also related to construction method, stage of construction, and work task and tools.[70] Most noise overexposure in the construction industry is machine-generated, which in some instances can be exacerbated by vibrating work surfaces (e.g. cutting, punching, driving or drilling sheet metal) and/or through reverberation when working in enclosed spaces. Heavy machinery, such as front-end loaders and other earth-moving equipment, as well as compressors, generators, and power tools, are common sources of noise exposure in construction. Task-weighted noise exposure levels can range from 75 dB from an electrician's drill press to over 110 dB from a jackhammer, whereas impact noise levels can reach 140–160 dB from bolt guns and other pneumatic construction tools.[74,75]

A discussion of the various engineering, administrative, and personal protective equipment approaches to controlling exposure to noise and other construction hazards appears later in this chapter. Chapter 24 (Noise, Vibration, and Ultrasound) includes a more in-depth discussion of the fundamentals of noise exposure recognition, evaluation, and control. For a more comprehensive overview of the health effects, recognition and control of noise in the construction industry specifically, the reader is directed to the review by Suter.[71]

Vibration. Exposure to segmental (hand-arm) or whole-body vibration is also common in construction. Overexposure to hand-arm vibration, which can lead to vibration-induced white finger (VWF), sensorineural impairment of the fingers, and carpal tunnel syndrome, was found to be most prevalent among individuals employed in construction work , and more specifically bricklayers, masons, carpenters, joiners, electricians, and builders/building contractors, in a national survey conducted in Great Britain.[76] A follow-up study conducted among a subset of men from the study found that, based on self-reports, the risk of finger blanching and other sensory symptoms in the fingers were significantly higher among men working in construction (builders, carpenters and joiners, and laborers), specifically among men working with hand-guided concrete breakers, chain saws, jig saws, and other vibratory tools.[77] Additional tools used in construction associated with exposure to hand-arm vibration include jackhammers, pneumatic chipping hammers, hammer drills, impact drills, and handheld grinders, among many others.[74,75]

Overexposure to whole body vibration is associated with muscle fatigue, low-back pain, spinal degeneration, and other systemic effects. The extensive use of heavy machinery in construction, and especially among operating engineers who experience increased rates of injuries and disorders of the low back[78], results in widespread exposure to whole body vibration throughout the construction workforce at the frequencies (i.e. 4–8 Hz) that are most likely to impact the vertebral column. Mobile machinery is associated with higher levels of vibration than stationary machinery, and types of equipment that have been documented to have vibration levels exceeding recommended values (International Standards Organization [ISO] 2631) include wheel loaders, off-road dump trucks, scrapers, skid steer vehicles, back-hoes, bulldozers, crawler loaders, and concrete trowel vehicles.[74,79]

Other Physical Hazards. Construction work often times takes place outdoors, which can result in exposures to other physical hazards such as temperature extremes and UV radiation. Exposure to extreme cold can lead to hypothermia, trench foot, and frostbite, as well as increased risks of falling due to icy or slippery surfaces. In addition, if workers are required to wear added insulation and clothing to protect against extreme cold it can contribute to reduced performance and increased error rates and risk of injury. Overexposure to extreme heat can result in heat rash, syncope, heat exhaustion, dehydration, and, depending on individual susceptibility factors, heat stroke which can be fatal. Outdoor construction was recently found to account for the majority of heat-related illness workers' compensation claims in the state of Washington(80), and it has been estimated that heat exhaustion is likely a leading cause of all claims within the construction industry.(75) Like extreme cold, heat stress can also result in increased error rates and risk of injury.

Exposure to UV radiation can have positive (e.g. vitamin D) and negative (e.g. erythema and skin cancers) impacts on human health, and is inherent in outdoor work. Construction workers are among the most highly exposed to UV radiation, and proper sun protection is rarely instituted in construction and other outdoor occupations.(81) Among construction workers, UV exposure can vary widely by individual and task-related factors. For example, exposure is related to sun position, altitude, clothing, posture and orientation of the work.(82) In addition to UV radiation, outdoor work may be associated with exposure to other forms of nonionizing radiation. For example, maintenance work on telecommunications towers and work in close proximity to roof top transmitters can result in shocks, burns, and potential subsequent falls from exposure to high levels of radio frequencies.(83)

Aside from outdoor work, exposure to UV and other types of non-ionizing radiation (i.e. infrared, intense visible light) is also present in welding and other hot work tasks. Likewise, scenarios where significant heat stress can arise are common in construction activities that do not take place outdoors. For example, work in buildings located in hot climates that do not have operational air conditioning, work that involves high levels of physical activity, operations where heavy attire or personal protective equipment is worn that facilitates heat build-up, and/or hot-work tasks that involve working in close proximity to high temperature sources can also lead to worker heat stress and strain.

Ergonomics

A high prevalence of work-related musculoskeletal disorders (WMSDs) have been reported among construction workers.(84) Certainly a combination of physical force and repetitive motion, awkward and/or or static body positions, heavy lifting of materials, contact stress, vibration, extreme temperatures, and the physically demanding, fast pace of construction work are all contributing factors. In 2005, for example, strains and sprains accounted for nearly 35% of all nonfatal injuries and illnesses accounting for days away from work in the construction industry. Overexertion is the key risk factor for WMSDs in construction, with overexertion in lifting accounting for 42% of all WMSDs with reported days away from work, and an additional 34% caused by other types of overexertion such as pushing, pulling, and carrying.(3) A U.S. Bureau of Labor Statistics study showed certain construction trades to be more affected than others by overexertion injuries, including laborers; carpenters; electricians; plumbers, pipefitters, and steamfitters; helpers; roofers; drywall installers; and construction supervisors.(85)

The prevalence of WMSDs in construction is not surprising when one considers that much of construction work is done overhead and/or at floor level, which, by definition, presents ergonomic hazards. Overhead work such as drilling, driving fasteners, or finishing drywall, involves reaching up with one or both arms raised above shoulders and may involve tilting the head back, thus placing stress on the shoulders and neck and leading to muscle and joint injuries. The risk is increased when these motions are performed repetitively and/or force is applied, such as when lifting, holding, or positioning heavy or bulky objects. Some general solutions may include tools modified by use of extensions that allow the tool to be held at waist or shoulder height rather than above the head, use of mechanical lifts to raise and position building materials in place rather than by manually lifting them, or use of lifts to bring the worker closer to the work itself.

Floor-level work often involves repeated stooping, bending (causing fatigue and puts stress on the lower back), and kneeling, which can put direct pressure on the knee as

Table 47.3 — Examples of Ergonomic Risk Factors in New Construction[a]

Task	*Awkward Posture*	*Force*	*Weight*	*Repetition*	*Hand Tools*	*Static Position*	*Vibration*
Excavation / Foundation Work							
Surveying	X						
Grading with heavy equipment	X					X	X
Trenching by hand	X	X	X		X	X	
Setting forms	X	X	X		X		X
Compacting soil	X	X	X		X		X
Sinking elevator shafts	X						
Masonry							
Laying blocks	X		X		X		
Reinforcing - pouring cement in wall cavities	X		X				
Formwork							
Cut with worm-drive saw	X	X	X		X	X	X
Use sawhorses	X						
Lifting and bracing forms	X	X	X		X	X	
Shovel concrete after blowouts	X	X	X		X		
Dismantle forms	X	X	X		X		
Steel Erection							
Climbing and connecting	X	X			X		
Fastening, tighten bolts	X			X	X	X	
Welding	X				X	X	
Crane operation	X						
Concrete Work							
Rod tying	X	X	X	X	X	X	
Pouring concrete	X	X					X
Hand finishing	X	X			X		
Mechnical finishing	X	X	X				X
Removing set concrete with jackhammers	X		X		X		X
Work on Structure							
Spray fireproofing	X	X	X			X	
Duct work	X		X		X	X	
Plumbing	X		X		X	X	
Electrical work	X	X	X		X	X	
Elevator installation	X	X	X		X	X	
Roofing							
carrying buckets			X		X		
mopping	X	X					X
installing insulation board	X						X
kettle work		X	X				
Building Interior							
Scaffold erection	X	X	X			X	
Handling drywall	X	X	X		X	X	
Drywall finishing	X	X		X	X		
Flooring							
glue spreading	X				X	X	
carpet laying	X	X	X		X	X	
material handling	X		X	X	X		
tile/terrazzo work	X					X	
Ceiling fixtures	X		X		X	X	
Painting	X			X	X	X	
Trim work	X				X		
Door installation	X		X		X		

(continued on next page.)

Table 47.3 — Examples of Ergonomic Risk Factors in New Construction (cont.)[a]

Task	*Awkward Posture*	*Force*	*Weight*	*Repetition*	*Hand Tools*	*Static Position*	*Vibration*
Building Exterior							
Sheet cladding	X	X	X		X	X	
Stone, granite cladding	X	X	X		X	X	
Sand blasting	X		X			X	X
Window installation	X	X	X		X	X	
Work Outside of Building							
Trowel wall	X	X			X		
Setting sidewalk							
cutting	X	X	X		X		X
setting	X		X				
Asphalt paving							
raking	X	X			X		
riding							X
hand-held paver	X	X			X		X
Other							
Materials handling	X	X	X				
Clean-up	X		X		X		

[a] adapted from Schneider, S. and Susi, P., 1994

Table 47.4 — Examples of Possible Solutions to Ergonomic Problems in New Construction[a]

Task	*Solutions*
Heavy equipment operator vibration	Better seat design
Laying masonry blocks	Better handle design Adjustable scaffolds Keep brick stack at proper height Pump mortar to point of application Limit weight of blocks Redesign blocks with hand holds
Carrying buckets of cement	Better handle design
Formwork	Adjustable height saw horses Bent handle hammer design New forms that are easier to dismantle Use of smaller form components
Crane operation	Enclosed cabs, better seat design
Concrete floor work	Tool for tying rods from standing height Straight edge handle Welded fabric nets
Chipping hammer vibration	Vibration / noise dampened equipment Lighter-weight models
Spraying fireproofing	Attachment of sprayer to belt for support
Installation of ductwork	Use of hoist to crank ductwork to proper height
Plumbing installation	Install on side wall rather than overhead in utility tunnels
Electrical work - screwdriving	Better handle design Use of powered screwdrivers Use of TORX head screws Micropauses during continuous work

(continued on next page.)

Table 47.4 — Examples of Possible Solutions to Ergonomic Problems in New Construction (cont.)[a]

Task	*Solutions*
Drywall installation	Use of drill stand or bolt gun waist belt for overhead work Use of dollies or carts to transport boards Use of narrower boards (e.g., 90 cm) Use of handles, proper training Use of swivel-head screw guns Plasterboard lifts
Elevator construction	Use of dollies, carts, lifting hooks, and better planning
Roofing	Use of cranes, dollies Smaller tubes of asphalt Better bucket handles Use of asphalt tanker rather than kettle New tool for fastening roof from standing height
Building exterior	Use of motorized scaffold Use of sheet clad storage device Mechanical window installation device
Scaffold erection	Use of hoists Use of newer scaffolds that are easier to carry and assemble
Painting	Flange on painter's handle and neck pillow for overhead work Redesign of bucket handle and bucket Materials in smaller packages with handles
Ceiling grid installation	Use of better hand tools, powered screwdrivers
Flooring floor glue spreading carpetlaying	 Use of standing spreading tool Use of power stretchers instead of knee kicker Dollies for carpet rolls
Work at floor level	Use of wheeled stools with tool bins Combination knee pad / seat for kneeling work Border drills
Door installation	Foot levers Mechanical door installer
Setting paving stones	Dollie for setting stones
Asphalt paving	Better machines with less vibration

[a] adapted from Schneider, S. and Susi, P., 1994

well as stress on tendons, ligaments, and cartilage of the knee joints. The use of extension handles or storing materials above floor level can also help alleviate the amount of stooping or kneeling necessary.[86] While establishment of ergonomic injury and illness as work related historically has presented some challenges in both general industry and construction, some WMSDs among construction workers are well documented in the literature. A well-known example is "carpet-layer's knee", which is attributed to use of a knee kicker as well as kneeling for extended periods of time. Carpet layers comprise less than 0.06% of the workforce in the U.S.; however, 6.2% of all workers' compensation claims for knee injuries were submitted by carpet layers. Switching to use of power stretchers where possible has been recommended by NIOSH to reduce this risk.[85]

While floor work cannot be eliminated from construction, the industrial hygienist should recognize when some work is done on the floor simply because it is the only large, flat work area available. For example, when assembling sheet metal duct work, providing a workbench or using tables and sawhorses to raise the work to waist height can allow the task to be performed standing up.[86]

In addition to working overhead and at floor level, construction involves a great deal of hand-intensive work. Construction workers grip tools for extended periods of time, placing stress on the hand, wrist, and/or elbow. Gripping or bending the wrist with force, moving the wrist rapidly or repeatedly, frequent use of vibrating tools, and/or tool handles that are hard or sharp and press into the hand, wrist, or arm, can lead to serious muscle or joint injury. Sometimes a power tool may be substituted for a hand tool to reduce the amount of force needed and number of repeated movements (e.g. twisting motions). Use of extension handles, or use of ergonomically improved tools, such as those with a power grip or offset handles can also reduce ergonomic stress.

When it is not possible to modify work processes or materials, adjustment of work schedules and training provide options for ergonomic solutions. For example, limiting the amount time spent performing repeated tasks or taking even brief breaks during continuous hand-intensive work, can help reduce ergonomic injury. Worker involvement to evaluate feasibility and effective training are always essential components in implementing any of these solutions.

Table 47.3 presents some examples of ergonomic risk factors associated with specific construction tasks. Table 47.4 presents some examples of successful solutions that have been implemented for a variety of construction tasks.(87)

Biological Hazards

General Concerns. Since much construction work is performed outdoors, construction workers frequently may be exposed to biological hazards in addition to chemical and/or physical agents. A variety of potential hazards exist in this category, with routes of exposures including both inhalation and dermal. Construction workers may need to contend with creatures that live outdoors. Depending on the locale these may range from animal (rabid dogs) and/or insect bites (West Nile virus from disease-carrying mosquitoes) to allergic reactions from contact with certain plants (e.g., poison oak, poison sumac). Contact with contaminated soil, water, and/or sewerage can also present a health risk. Also consider biological exposure risks to construction and renovation or repair workers that may be present in hospitals and other healthcare settings.

Rodent-Borne Disease Risks During Demolition and Renovation Work. A number of potential rodent-borne disease hazards may be present during demolition or rehab of existing buildings, particularly those that have been closed up or vacant for long periods of time. Some examples are briefly discussed here.

Histoplasmosis. During renovation and demolition work inhalation of aerosolized dusts contaminated with bird manure or bat droppings presents a concern. Serious illness and death can result from occupationally acquired histoplasmosis, a disease caused by inhalation of the fungus, *Histoplasma capsulatum*. This fungus grows in soils worldwide. While prevalent throughout the U.S., the proportion of people infected by *H. capsulatum* is higher in central and eastern states. The fungus appears to grow best in soils having a high nitrogen content, which is often enhanced by the presence of bird and/or bat droppings. Dusts containing *H. capsulatum* spores can become aerosolized during construction, excavation, or demolition activities, which puts those workers at higher risk. In addition to demolition contractors, roofers, renovation contractors restoring old buildings, mechanical contractors installing or servicing HVAC equipment, and bridge inspectors or painters may encounter exposure sources. Bystanders also may be at risk because wind currents can transport the airborne spores readily over some distance. Most preventive measures to prohibit bird manure or bat droppings from accumulating in buildings in the first place are usually beyond the control of the construction or demolition worker. Further, there are limited commercially available methods for detecting these fungal agents in soil or dust samples, and no numerical exposure guideline exists for *H. capsulatum*. Therefore, to reduce the risk of infection and resultant disease development, appropriate exposure precautions and dust control measures to minimize dust generation are important where accumulations of bird manure or bat droppings are found. These may include water sprays or other dust suppression techniques, and containerizing resultant debris for prompt disposal. Shoveling or dry sweeping should be avoided. In some cases, removal using an industrial vacuum cleaner equipped with a high-efficiency particulate air (HEPA) filter for contaminated dusts may be appropriate. In some situations pre-demolition removal of these accumulations may be necessary. Quantity and locations of the material, structural soundness of the building, weather conditions, and proximity to other buildings occupied by susceptible populations are factors to be considered. Appropriate personal protective equipment for affected workers should be considered as well.[88]

Hantavirus pulmonary syndrome. Certain rodents are known to be carriers of hantaviruses causing hantavirbus pulmonary syndrome (HPS) in humans. The known rodent carriers in the U.S. are deer mice, cotton and rice rats (in the southeast), and the white-footed mouse (in the northeast), with the deer mouse being the primary reservoir. HPS is transmitted to humans through inhalation of fresh aerosolized excretia (urine, droppings, saliva, or nesting materials) from these rodents and their nests; therefore, when these are encountered, such as during renovation or demolition of an abandoned building, dry sweeping, vacuuming, or other dust-generating activity should be avoided. Although rare, HPS is potentially deadly. Since the viability of infectious hantavirus is measured in terms of hours or days, however, only active infestations present conditions that are likely to lead to human infection.[89] Nonetheless, awareness training and field sanitation are essential for appropriate hygiene and decontamination when such situations may be encountered.

Molds and Bacteria. While Chapter 18 (Indoor Air Quality) provides a detailed discussion of microbial concerns from an indoor environmental quality building investigation perspective, the purpose of this section is to acquaint the industrial hygienist with some construction and/or renovation scenarios where such potential exposures may exist for construction workers.

Moldy Buildings. Certain construction occupations, during certain tasks or activities both in new construction and renovation work, may be exposed to molds in varying degrees if handling or working around moldy building materials. Construction workers' exposures to molds range from minimal, for example, for the carpenter working outdoors framing a home using lumber that contains some minor mold spots, to more substantial exposures encountered by a remediation contractor removing heavily mold colonized gypsum wallboard (drywall) from a building following a flood. Drywall installers, painters, and paper hangers should be aware of working with moldy materials during both renovation and new construction. For example, even new drywall may become water damaged and thus subject to mold growth if not adequately protected during transit to the construction site or while stored on site. During renovation work in buildings that have a history of moisture damage the construction worker is likely to encounter moldy building materials. Precautions such as dust suppression and isolation should be taken to minimize disturbance of the material that may result in substantial release of spores.

Legionella. An outbreak of Legionnaires' disease is both an occupational and public health concern. The risk of infection is greater for older individuals or those with a compromised immune system. However, construction workers may also be at risk because of another risk factor, cigarette smoking, with nearly 38% of construction trades workers reported to be current smokers in 2005.[3] There are two clinically recognized types of legionellosis (diseases caused by *Legionella* bacteria): Legionnaires' disease, the more serious of the two, a multi-system disease that can include pneumonia and has a fatality rate of about 15%; and the milder, flu-like Pontiac Fever. The primary route of exposure is inhalation into the deep lungs. The bacteria are typically carried in an aerosolized mist of contaminated water, and there must be a sufficient number of virulent bacteria to cause disease. Although the infectious dose has not yet been determined, a general dose-response relationship exists.[90]

All sources of misting water may be potential sources of transmission of the bacteria, although well-maintained systems are less likely to be colonized with Legionellae than those that are poorly maintained. Cooling towers and other water systems may become contaminated through the make-up water.[90] Unfortunately, the condition of a building's water systems is beyond the control of the construction worker performing work in an existing building. Thus, while the risk for most workers is very low, awareness of potential sources and prudent practices are helpful. Some potential sources of Legionellae-contaminated water to which construction workers such as plumbers, roofers, and others may be exposed include:

- Cooling towers
- Evaporative condensers
- Humidifiers
- Potable water heaters and holding tanks
- Pipes containing stagnant warm water
- Shower heads and faucet aerators
- Decorative fountains
- Mister reservoirs
- Stagnant water in fire sprinkler systems, eyewash stations, and first-aid showers

Further, since water mist can travel with the wind, construction workers on a rooftop near a cooling tower should be vigilant about exposure.(91) Some precautionary measures include:

- Worker awareness
- Avoiding aerosolizing standing or stagnant water
- Ensuring availability of fresh water for work that uses water and creates mist (e.g. to cool saws or for dust control)
- Draining and flushing plumbing systems that may contain stagnant water before putting them back into service

Confined Spaces in Construction

A detailed description of hazards and controls associated with working in confined and/or enclosed spaces is provided in Chapter 46 of this book. Key hazards such as oxygen deficiency, atmospheres containing airborne concentrations of contaminants that are immediately dangerous to life and health (IDLH), and inadequate planning for and/or protection and training of rescue workers are common to all confined space work, whether performed by industrial or construction workers.

It is notable that as of 2011 OSHA has not published a construction industry-specific standard on confined spaces, although at least three existing construction standards contain some provisions for work performed in confined and/or enclosed spaces. These include: safety training and education [29 CFR 1926.21(b)(6)]; fire prevention [29 CFR 1926.352(g)]; and ventilation during welding, cutting, and heating [29 CFR 1926.353(b) and (c)]. In the absence of more specific regulatory requirements, the industrial hygienist working with industrial facility owners should recommend that contract documents address applicable requirements for repair and/or maintenance work such as in vessels, storage tanks, furnaces, boilers, ductwork, and others.

Whether using mechanical or natural ventilation, it is critical to maintain the quality of make-up air. Be aware of and address any airborne contaminant sources that may be drawn in from the surrounding area. Also be aware that confined and/or enclosed spaces, especially those having complex internal configurations, present additional challenges regarding use of respiratory protection.(92)

Exposure Assessment in Construction: Challenges and Alternative Approaches

Reasons for Exposure Assessment

The degree to which workers are at risk of occupationally-related disease and premature death is dependent on their exposure to hazardous agents. Exposure in turn is dependent on a number of factors including:

- the route through which a hazardous substance enters the body (e.g. inhalation, ingestion or skin absorption);
- the concentration of the agent in the air for inhalation hazards and on surfaces for those hazardous agents for which ingestion is a viable route of exposure; and
- the duration of time in which a worker comes into contact with a hazard.

These principles apply to construction just as they do to other industries. However, because work is performed on non-fixed work sites and workers move from job to job and employer to employer, special consideration must be given to how to characterize exposures in construction. First, exposures are likely to be highly variable between workers and on any given day, in part driven by the intermittency of tasks generating exposure hazards. Second, because work is performed from a non-fixed location, environmental conditions can be extreme. Construction workers seldom have the benefit of plumbed toilets and soap and warm running water with which to wash their hands. Given this context, ingestion and dermal routes of exposure are important to consider when determining overall risk, in addition to exposure via inhalation. Third, it is not uncommon for work to be underway in enclosed, poorly ventilated spaces such as process tanks at refineries or boilers and scrubbers in power plants. As such, exposures can be extremely high and quickly become immediately dangerous to life and health (IDLH). Finally, some trades routinely work extended work-shifts such as boilermakers engaged in turnaround work where 60 hour work weeks are common. When evaluating exposures relative to occupational exposure limits (OELs) based on 8-hour time-weighted averages (TWAs), adjustments should be made to reflect those extended periods of exposure.

While a comprehensive discussion of the principles of exposure assessment strategies may be found in Ignatio and Bullock[93], the purpose of exposure assessment generally falls into one (or a combination) of the following three categories:

Compliance. The most common reason for exposure assessment in the U.S. is to determine whether or not an employer is in compliance with OSHA standards. However, failure to conduct air monitoring is a common cause for OSHA citations in construction. For compliance, the primary question is whether or not an employee's 8-hour TWA exposure exceeds a PEL. Employers will commonly seek to determine the "worst-case" exposure as a means to ensure that all workers are exposed at levels lower than the PEL.

Health Hazard Surveillance or Exposure Characterization. Epidemiology studies and risk assessment depend heavily on accurate characterization of exposures to populations of workers. Ideally, exposure data are collected in such a way that exposure distributions for similarly exposed groups can be accurately characterized. The biggest obstacles to accomplishing this are: 1) biased sampling methods such as "worst-case" sampling campaigns as described above; 2) insufficient exposure measurements to capture the full range of exposure variability within a given group; and 3) the failure to record descriptive information associated with work processes and environmental conditions necessary to adequately group workers into similarly exposed groups and determine key exposure variables. The inherent statistical nature of exposure assessment and hence the importance of collecting exposure data in an unbiased manner has been described by Rappaport and others.[11,94,95] An exposure assessment strategy can be designed that meets the needs of both compliance and health surveillance, provided that collected data are representative of the full range of exposures within a population of workers and incorporate sufficient descriptive information with which to analyze variables that effect exposure.

Evaluation of Control Technologies. A very important but underutilized purpose of exposure assessment is evaluation of control technologies. As discussed in this chapter, employers have a legal obligation to design work processes to minimize occupational health hazards. In the case of engineering control evaluation, monitoring with direct reading instruments provides a quick and easy means to get preliminary information on how well a particular engineering control is working. Using direct reading instruments during the implementation of a control and as part of a regular maintenance program is particularly useful. Direct reading instruments are also useful in determining what elements of tasks or work processes generate the greatest exposure for targeting control strategies. Traditional integrated sampling methods can also be used for control technology evaluation as will be discussed later in this chapter.

Creating an Exposure Profile in Construction

What Must be Considered? Given all of the industry characteristics described thus far, characterizing exposures in construction requires an approach that considers the hazards generated by the tasks workers perform, exposures generated by other trades working near by, and hazards created by the host facility such as those common to industrial facilities. Typically, the combination of hazards resulting from each of these sources will change for workers over the life of their career in the trades. However, what remains relatively constant and is shared by several trades are the skills, or common tasks, which form the basis of their trades. A number of tasks in construction are associated with chemical hazards; examples include:

- welding fumes and gases generated from hot work tasks;
- asphalt fumes associated with roofing and paving;
- man-made mineral fibers released during insulation work;
- respirable silica associated with concrete drilling, grinding, cutting and masonry tasks;
- metals and silica from abrasive blasting; and
- solvent exposure from painting and waterproofing.

These and other hazardous chemical agents were monitored or observed on just one new construction project alone.[96]

Task-based Approaches and Sample Averaging Times. For the reasons outlined above, many industrial hygiene practitioners in construction have relied on task-based approaches to exposure assessment and control. For example, since 1993, CPWR has developed and used T-BEAM (Task-Based Exposure Assessment Model) for collecting both quantitative and qualitative silica and welding fume exposure data among seven trades (boilermakers, bricklayers, operating engineers, laborers, painters, ironworkers, and pipefitters). This approach has been used on 31 projects, 14 of which employed welding trades exposed to metal fumes and 17 of which employed bricklayers, laborers, operating engineers or painters engaged in tasks associated with silica exposure.

The T-BEAM approach involves journeymen construction workers in the exposure assessment process and emphasizes use and evaluation of engineering controls. Workers who are sampled as part of T-BEAM are selected in an unbiased manner (neither "best" nor "worst" case exposures are sought out) and detailed, standardized survey instruments are used to document a large number of task variables. Examples of documented variables include environmental conditions, such as whether work is done indoors or outdoors, whether and what type of ventilation is used, tool and process variables, and information on the intermittency of work. A *Task Variable Set Form* used for welding appears as Figure 47.3.

However, the term "task-based" means different things to different people and is not always clearly defined. For many, the term is used loosely to refer to a personal air monitoring strategy that only captures exposures associated with a particular task over the duration of time that the task is performed. In this context, "task-based" refers to *task TWA sampling* versus 8-hour time-weighted averages TWAs that would be derived not only from the tasks of interest but also whatever other exposures occurred during the full shift sampling period.

In the case of T-BEAM and other similar approaches, tasks are used as the central organizing principle for collecting large amounts of sampling data at multiple job sites, however, full shift sampling is performed *and* observational information is recorded on task duration and intermittency among other things. Statistical analysis is used subsequent to sampling campaigns to determine exposure distributions and the relative impact of a number of task variables, which includes categorical estimates of time engaged in a particular task, and considers exposure variation associated with the degree of enclosure where the task is performed, e.g. from open air to confined space. So perhaps a better descriptor of this approach is "task-centered".

There are a number of reasons for this approach. First, from a health surveillance point of view, the TWA exposure of the entire work shift is the most relevant measure, since it is likely to be more representative of exposures over long periods of time, which for many chronic adverse health effects may be more important than peak exposures. Second, as a practical matter, workers often perform a given task such as welding frequently and intermittently, starting and stopping the task under study to perform other activities. On a construction site where workers move around a great deal, and often work in hard-to-reach places, starting and stopping sampling pumps only when the worker was engaged in a particular task would be difficult, if not impossible, and certainly viewed as interfering with production. Third, full shift sampling is required to determine compliance with OSHA in most cases unless there is a Short Term Exposure Limit (STEL); however, even then, many regulated substances may have both an 8-hour TWA and a STEL. Fourth, statistical analysis of exposure data is complicated when using short and varying sampling times, which result in more "noise" in the data and poorly reflect the smoothing effect that longer sampling times have on measured exposure levels.

Welding, Brazing & Thermal Cutting Task Variable Set Form

PROCESS RELATED

THW-Type of hot work

1. welding
2. burning
3. brazing
4. thermal cutting

CI-Continuous or intermittent
Actual hot work time comprises what percentage of task observation time.

1. less than 25%
2. 25%-50%
3. 50%-75%
4. 75%-100%

CG-Contaminant generation
Number of other workers on average generating dust or fumes within 10' radius of sampled worker

WP-Welding process

1. sheilded or manual metal arc welding(SMA or MMA)
2. flux core
3. gas metal arc(MIG)
4. gas tungsten arc(TIG)
5. plasmaarc
6. resistance
7. not elsewhere classified (describe)

AMPS-Welding machine amperage setting

AT - Arc Time in minutes

MATERIALS or ELECTRODES

BMTL-Base metal
1. structural steel
2. mild steel
3. carbon steel
4. stainless steel
5. other (describe)

C-Consumable(describe e.g. 7010, etc.)

RS-Rod size diameter in inches
1. 3/32"
2. 1/8"
3. 5/32"
4. 3/16"
5. >3/16"

ENVIRONMENTAL CONDITION/VENTILATION

V-Ventilation

1. local exhaust ventilation
2. mechanical
3. natural
4. none

I/O-Indoors or outdoors

1. Indoors or within an enclosure
2. Outdoors

DC-Degree of confinement
Is enclosure a small compartment with very little air movement?

1. Yes
2. No

Recorder's Last Name:________________ **Date:**__________

***Employee's Last Name:**________________ **Worker ID:** _ _ _ _

Where applicable, choose among the selected task variable codes at the left of this form to describe the specific task you are observing. If the listed code is not applicable to the task you are observing, write "NA" for Not Applicable.

Process Related		Material or Electrodes (describe)		Environmental conditions/Ventilation	
THW	______	BMTL	______	V	______
CI	______	C	______	I/O	______
CG	______	RS	______	DC	______
WP	______				
AMPS	______				
AT	______				

Describe other variables you think may be important to exposure levels:

____

____

Describe placement of ventilation hood including number of inches from the weld:

____

____

Are there additional obvious sources of exposure?
__Yes __No
If yes, please describe:______________________________

____

Are any special work practices being used to minimize exposure?
__Yes __No
If yes, please describe:______________________________

____

(OVER)

Figure 47.3 — Welding, Brazing, and Thermal Cutting Task Variable Set Form.

SCHEMATIC

Key
X = worker performing task
☐ = barriers/walls/enclosures
o = source of fume
V = Mechanical Ventilation (use arrows for air flow in relation to worker)
N = Natural Ventilation (use arrows for air flow in relation to worker)

If work is done indoors or in an enclosure, describe the configuration:

____

____

Define approximate dimensions of the enclosure in feet:
If a square or rectangle: **L**______ft x **W**______ft x **H**______ft = ______ft^3

If a circular structure: **Diameter:** __________ft **Height:** __________ft

Figure 47.3 — Welding, Brazing, and Thermal Cutting Task Variable Set Form.

However, for purposes of engineering control studies, particularly at the early stages of equipment design and evaluation, a task-based approach, (e.g. collecting multiple samples with use of various engineering controls only over the period of time for which that task is performed) makes sense. Or, as described elsewhere in this chapter, when the objective is a diagnostic analysis to determine what elements of a process or task generate the highest exposure, task TWAs may be desirable.

This approach has been used to evaluate local exhaust ventilation (LEV) for both welding and masonry tasks, first in a controlled setting then followed by implementation and evaluation of the same controls in real-world settings. For example, in an off-site study using paired trials of portable LEV control versus no control for reduction of manganese fume generated from welding, use of LEV resulted in a 75% reduction in manganese exposure. Sample times were relatively short for the "controlled" evaluations with trials of 50 to 60 minutes with LEV and trials of 25 to 32 minutes when LEV was not used. In the field, the same LEV unit was tested; however, full shift time-weighted average exposures were used to measure manganese on days when LEV was in use versus those when it was not in use. In the field setting, the LEV reduced geometric mean manganese exposures by 53%. Although the reduction on the job was less than that seen in the controlled randomized trials, manganese exposure was appreciably lowered by the use of LEV in both cases.(97) Testing controls using a task-based approach initially to determine their relative effectiveness is advantageous to the contractor whose dual goal of making a profit, largely dependent on worker productivity, and remaining in compliance with OSHA, leaves little room for experimentation. Similar studies of LEV for grinders used by tuckpointers have shown a greater than 90% reduction in silica exposure.(59,98) Field studies conducted by CPWR measuring personal exposure to silica among tuckpointers using the same equipment tested in an experimental setting showed similar results.

Can exposures be determined absent a fixed site? In addition to determining: 1) what task variables, or exposure determinants, have the greatest impact on exposure; and 2) the impact of engineering controls in reducing exposure, the fundamental objective of T-BEAM was to see if a standardized approach to exposure assessment in construction could be used to establish exposures distributions among sampled groups of workers absent a fixed work site.

The answer to this question is yes and no. If exposure data are collected in an unbiased manner and sufficient data are gathered to accurately estimate exposure variance within a given population it is possible to estimate exposures to workers absent a fixed work site, at least theoretically. However, exposures for individual workers may vary from day to day, between workers and between job sites. Consequently, there is an enormous amount of variation which complicates good estimates of exposure in construction. An analysis of almost 200 measurements of personal exposure to manganese fumes associated with welding collected by CPWR among boilermakers, ironworkers and pipefitters is summarized in Table 47.5. These data were collected from a total of 11 job sites, with multiple sites for boilermakers and pipefitters, but only one site in the case of ironworkers. Predictably, since only one job was sampled for ironworkers, many of the variables that influence exposure remained constant (e.g. materials, type of hot work, degree of ventilation, etc.) and the highest exposure was only 16 times the lowest exposure. However, for boilermakers and pipefitters, where numerous jobs were sampled, the range of exposures was enormous. Highest exposures were 218 and 1474 times the lowest exposures among boilermakers and pipefitters, respectively. Because of the wide variability in construction exposures, typically, the more data collected (i.e. the more different jobs and scenarios sampled), the larger the variance will be, as demonstrated by these data.

Thus, although exposure distributions from multiple sites can be constructed, the degree to which those estimates adequately reflect actual exposure is influenced by the following: first, whether or not enough data have been collected from multiple sites in order to capture the full magnitude of variance for a given trade/task/exposure; and second, the degree to which exposures are well controlled. Using engineering controls such as LEV reduces both the mean and variance of exposures among sampled workers.

Table 47.5 — Manganese Welding Exposure Data (1995 - 2008), mg/m³ *

Trade	No. of samples	Range	Range fold	Mean	Mean/TLV (0.2 mg/m³)
Boilermakers	46	0.006–1.31	218	0.18	89%
Ironworkers	23	0.022–0.358	16.3	0.15	73%
pipefitters	122	0.0005–0.737	1474	0.08	39%

* mg/m³ = milligrams per cubic meter

This effect is extremely useful for employers who must ensure that the upper range of employee exposures never exceeds permissible exposure levels.

The above discussion is not intended to discourage the industrial hygienist from conducting personal air monitoring and estimating worker exposure to hazardous agents. Rather, the purpose is to encourage industrial hygienists to: 1) be strategic about sampling and control strategies with emphasis on those tasks which are most likely to generate hazardous exposure; 2) work towards the goal of identifying and verifying the effectiveness of engineering controls for the task/exposures being sampled; 3) collect sufficient data in an unbiased manner to arrive at a reasonable estimate of exposure distribution parameters (e.g. means and variance); 4) document exposure variables likely to affect exposure, including trade, materials, and environmental conditions, so as to enable interpretation and comparison of exposure measurements collected from multiple sites; and 5) involve workers in the exposure assessment and control strategy, as they have the best understanding of the tasks and work processes being evaluated and will assist in determining which controls are most likely to be viewed favorably by workers being asked to use them. Ultimately, an industrial hygienist should look at available exposure data as a useful starting point for making a priori judgments about the likelihood of over-exposure and needed controls. However, collection of additional data is necessary to confirm those assumptions and strengthen the exposure estimates over time, keeping in mind that the understanding of exposures may affect the health of workers.

Importance of Worker Involvement. Consulting with workers to better understand a work process is not a new concept for industrial hygienists. However, for construction, worker involvement is especially critical. On any construction project of any size, there are dozens, if not hundreds, of workers scattered throughout a job site and they seldom stay in one place. Within this group of workers are a number of trades, most of which have completed 3-5 year apprenticeship programs that ground them in the fundamental skills of their craft. For someone unfamiliar with construction and/or a particular job, even distinguishing an ironworker from a pipefitter may be difficult, not to mention finding them at the start of the sampling shift and throughout the day as they move about the nooks and crannies of a large job. Therefore, partnering with the trades who engage in the work or tasks for which exposure assessment is underway is an extremely valuable strategy. They know the material, the tools, and their typical work conditions. Finally, they are used to making things work under difficult conditions; the industrial hygienist working in this industry shares this plight.

As previously described, one of the central aspects of the T-BEAM approach used by CPWR was the involvement of journeymen trade workers in the collection of both quantitative and descriptive data. CPWR trained journeymen from the trades being sampled in air monitoring techniques and in use of survey instruments and then partnered them with industrial hygienists. Using this approach enabled collection of much more data than would have been obtained by relying on industrial hygienists alone for data collection. In addition, the quality of the descriptive data was particularly strong given their knowledge of the work. Partnering with workers in this fashion also increased the comfort and trust level of workers being surveyed, which in itself is important in collecting quality data in an unbiased manner.

In addition to exposure arising from specific tasks, as has been previously described, there are also the hazards associated with the environment where work is being performed. For example, an operating engineer working in a refinery rehabilitation or maintenance project may have concerns about benzene exposure associated with the host facility and perhaps silica or metal dust generated by painters working nearby who are involved in abrasive blasting. These hazards and the approach to controlling them have to be an ongoing and "real-time" effort. Involving workers, ideally through joint labor-management safety committees, is necessary to identify these hazards as they occur and to develop strategies for preventing excess exposure.

Controlling Construction Health Hazards

For elevated exposures to most chemical, biological, and physical agents, one should prioritize control options by first considering strategies that reduce generation of the agent at the source, then those that reduce the transfer of the agent in the pathway between the source and the receiver (i.e. worker), and finally those that reduce exposure levels at the receiver. As with other industries and settings, this translates into the following hierarchy of controls: 1) substitution, 2) engineering controls, 3) administrative controls, and 4) personal protective equipment (PPE). Note that classifications and definitions of the control hierarchy may vary slightly — for example, some consider substitution to be one form of engineering control, along with automation, ventilation, and isolation. Since elevated exposure levels to a number of hazardous agents are experienced by workers in many construction tasks, and in some instances relatively archaic processes and tools are used, the introduction of appropriate exposure controls can result in significant reductions in the prevalence and magnitude of worker overexposures.

However, due to some of the characteristics unique to construction described previously (e.g. mobility of work, transient workforce, small business employers, complex organizational structure, irregular scheduling and sequencing of work, and variable job settings that range from working outdoors in the open to working in enclosed spaces), the use of exposure controls can be somewhat challenging. While adherence to the traditional hierarchy of exposure controls should always be the ultimate goal, the use of respiratory protection as an interim measure may sometimes be necessary to supplement engineering controls until the latter had been effectively implemented or for exposures that are not adequately reduced by engineering controls alone. However, as later described, implementation of an effective respiratory protection program can be at least equally as challenging as setting up adequate engineering controls. Thought must also be given to mixed exposures and the impact controlling one hazard may have in creating or exacerbating another (sometimes referred to as "hazard shifting"). For example, moving a noisy cutting task from indoors to outdoors on a construction job to reduce dust and noise exposures that were being elevated in part by the enclosed space in which the task was being performed may expose the worker to increased heat and UV radiation depending on climate and season. Given the diversity of construction types, projects, settings, conditions, trades, tasks, tools, and exposures, it is not possible to provide a comprehensive description of all possible control options in construction here. Rather, examples are used to illustrate the various control approaches that may be applied to reduce worker exposures in construction.

Substitution

Perhaps the most desirable solution to preventing worker overexposure is one that allows for the elimination of the primary sources or contributing factors of exposure without compromising work quality and productivity. This may involve changing the processes, materials, or tools being used for a particular task to reduce or eliminate the generation of a hazardous agent. Since exposure reduction or elimination takes place at the source and not at the receiver, substitution does not rely on proper use and maintenance by the worker, as do other approaches. Substitution can also lead to reductions in bystander exposures, which can be important in construction where many workers may be working closely together on a site and, at times, in enclosed spaces.

There are numerous examples of process substitution opportunities to reduce worker exposures to various agents. This may include substituting manual welding with automated welding, or perhaps the selection of a welding process that generates less fume when joining two pieces of metal. For example, gas tungsten arc (or tungsten inert gas, TIG) welding generates considerably less fume than shielded metal arc welding (SMAW) (also referred to as manual metal arc [MMA] welding or "stick" welding), which is commonly encountered in construction. Abrasive blasting is a very common surface preparation technique used in construction often associated with extremely high worker exposures to lead, respirable silica, noise, and other agents. Alternatives to abrasive blasting may include water jetting, etching or mechanical scraping, chemical stripping, or automated techniques alone or in combination. Unfortunately, these methods are not yet widely used, in part because of cost and productivity concerns.[99] Isocyanates are often applied in roofing and other construction activities, and exposure may be reduced through changes in method of application (e.g. rolling instead of spray application). In work requiring pieces of stone, concrete, or masonry to be reduced in size, the use of a process to break the material (e.g. a guillotine) instead of sawing or grinding techniques may greatly reduce the generation of respirable silica dust. Many process substitution opportunities may also exist for reducing exposure to physical hazards as well, such as the selection of one process over another based on lower noise generation.

Examples of material substitution to reduce worker exposures in construction are also available. Historically, sand has been commonly used in abrasive blasting because it is readily available, cheap, and produces a desirable surface profile. However, because it results in extremely high exposures to respirable crystalline silica, many state and federal agencies have banned the use of sand in abrasive blasting and the availability and use of alternatives has been on the rise. In the isocyanate example given above, the need for isocyanates may be eliminated by instead using mechanical fasteners and ballast to fasten roofing material. In construction painting, the use of lead-based paints has been largely (though not completely) discontinued in lieu of safer alternatives, and efforts have been made in recent years to reduce the use of pigments containing hexavalent chromium. There also may be opportunities to replace toxic solvents such as toluene, xylene and methyl ethyl ketone with less toxic substitutes.

There are also many opportunities to control hazardous exposures through the substitution of tools and equipment. The replacement of older heavy construction equipment involved in the movement and manipulation of earth and other silica-containing materials with more modern versions equipped with enclosed cabs that are properly pressurized with filtration systems can greatly reduce worker exposures to silica dust.[11,100] For noise exposure, replacing a noisy tool with one that has a lower sound power level can reduce worker exposure. The National Institute for Occupational Safety and Health (NIOSH) has compiled a database of common commercially-available power tools that helps the user determine the "real-world" noise level of power tools as they are used on the job by including data on sound power level, sound pressure level, actual worker time-weighted average exposure data, and other information.[101] For ergonomic hazards in construction, NIOSH has also been working with CPWR to compile a database of proven, commercially available tools that are lighter and reduce or eliminate the need for bending, kneeling, reaching, and other awkward positions.[82,100]

While substitution has great potential to reduce worker exposures to a broad range of hazardous agents in a diverse array of tasks, there may be limitations with regard to feasibility, cost, and productivity. Another potential negative aspect to the use of substitution as a means of reducing exposure to an agent is the possibility of introducing new health and safety hazards. For example, in the case of alternative abrasive blasting agents, coal slag is a common alternative to silica. While coal slag may reduce worker exposures to silica it may also increase worker exposures to beryllium and other heavy metals.[35]

Engineering Controls

Engineering controls can be implemented to reduce worker exposure at the source of generation (e.g. local exhaust ventilation, water suppression, noise mufflers or silencers), in the pathway between generation source and the worker (e.g. sound barriers, mechanical or general dilution ventilation), or at the worker (e.g. isolation booths). As described earlier, the goal is to control the exposure as close to the source as possible. Like substitution, engineering controls not only reduce harmful exposures to the worker directly performing the task, but also eliminate or reduce exposures among others on site (sometimes referred to as "bystander exposures").

Local exhaust ventilation (LEV) is an effective way to reduce exposure to airborne agents as they are being generated. LEV has been demonstrated to be effective in controlling worker exposures to heavy metals and organic compounds in fume generated from welding(97) and asphalt paving(103), respectively. For welding, LEV may be in the form of a built-in system found in fabrication shops, portable trunk units, or the more highly portable high-vacuum/low-flow "shop-vac" units. Other specialized LEV systems may also be available in specific environments. For example, in power plant overhauls where many workers are welding simultaneously in varying and sometimes tight locations, a system which is gaining popularity involves a large and powerful central fan/scrubber unit with numerous bifurcating and flexible ducts and hoods that can be moved and placed by the individual welders as they change locations. Alternatively, for certain types of welding such as MIG, TIG, and FCAW, welding equipment with LEV incorporated into the design ("fume-extraction guns") may be available.(104) For any welding task, the selection of an appropriate LEV system and worker training on hood placement are vital to ensure maximum effectiveness. In asphalt paving, LEV added to the paving machines have proven effective at reducing exposures to organic particulate matter which can include polycyclic aromatic hydrocarbons and other carcinogens.(103,105)

LEV has also been shown to be effective in controlling respirable silica exposures during tasks involving concrete and masonry work that generate high levels of dust. These systems usually involve the incorporation of an exhaust hood right at the tool, either through factory design or as a retrofit. Significant reductions in worker silica exposure with the use of LEV has been reported for concrete surface grinding(52,54), with the use of concrete-cutting hammer drills(106), and during masonry cutting and tuckpointing (the cutting/grinding of mortar between bricks).(53,59) For certain tasks a reduction in exposure of over 90% has been achieved; however, the design of the LEV system needs to be carefully considered. One limitation in many of the LEV systems tested to date is the use of bags to collect dust, which for many tasks like tuckpointing results in a rapid loss of airflow and LEV effectiveness. In addition, episodic high exposure to silica can be experienced by workers when changing out full bags. New designs that include a cyclone pre-separator hold promise for mitigating some of these limitations.(53)

Other engineering controls may also be effective at controlling harmful exposures at the source of generation. The use of water for dust suppression has been applied in several construction tasks, including chipping, grinding, and cutting of concrete, masonry or stone, and in abrasive blasting operations.(11,54,107) For example, use of a low-flow water-spray attachment to suppress dust created during pavement breaking with jackhammers was found to reduce exposure to respirable dust by 70–90%.(108,109) In masonry tasks, reductions in respirable silica exposure of greater than 90% were achieved when cutting brick and concrete block with the use of a stationary wet saw compared to similar dry-cutting tasks.(59) The use of wet abrasive blasting for concrete surface preparation resulted in significantly lower concentrations of respirable silica than reported for dry blasting operations elsewhere in the literature.(110,111) While potentially effective, limitations of water dust suppression need to be considered. These may include the need for sources of water on remote construction sites, infeasibility in cold climates due to freezing, the introduction of electrocution hazards from using power tools in close proximity to water, and the presence of slipping hazards with the creation of wet surfaces.

Modification of a process or tool used in construction, without actually substituting the tool or process, can also reduce exposures in some situations. Examples include the selection of welding parameters associated with reduced fume generation (e.g. selection of voltage, current, wire feed rate, along with electrodes or filler wire containing less harmful constituents(112), the selection of blades used for sawing or grinding that produce less dust (e.g. the use of dual blades in tuckpointing), and modification of the application methods when using harmful materials in construction tasks (e.g. modifying application rates and nozzle pressures to reduce exposure to isocyanates during spray applications). Proper equipment maintenance is also an effective and inexpensive effort that can help reduce unnecessary exposures.

Administrative Controls

Administrative approaches are likely most appropriate for controlling worker exposures when used in conjunction with other control strategies such as engineering controls. To be used as a control strategy they require detailed knowledge of the hazards present during a task and work shift, as well as continuous oversight. One form of administrative control is through careful planning and manipulation of work and shift schedules to limit worker exposures to a particular hazard. For example, at construction sites where heat stress and high UV exposure from sunlight are a concern, work shifts are often modified to start much earlier in the day to minimize exposure to heat during the hottest part of the day. Another example may be the scheduling of tasks that generate high levels of dust throughout a site to take place when workers in other trades are not working in the area to reduce bystander exposures. However, the feasibility of this approach in construction is many times limited due to deadlines and project flow needs, long work shifts that span 12 or more hours, the uncertainty in specifying a "safe" or "acceptable" level and duration of exposure, and other factors. The use of worker rotation is another form of administrative control. For example, in the drywall finishing trade, some crews may have dedicated tapers who apply the joint compound and tape joints between wall boards and another set of workers dedicated to sanding drywall joints when dry. In such a scenario the latter set of workers are exposed to very high dust levels continuously. On the other hand, the authors have encountered drywall finishing crews where everybody tapes and everyone sands, so that the sanding process is done more quickly and exposures throughout the crew are shorter in duration. However, when using rotation as a means of exposure control, the industrial hygienist should be aware that extremely high exposures often occur in construction over short spans of time. Thus, even with the use of worker rotation, occupational exposure limits may be exceeded. Exposures are also highly variable. In such an environment, worker rotation would be ineffective in the absence of a continuous dosimetry indicator for the hazard in question over the course of the shift. In addition, construction tasks are often performed by skilled trades, thus limiting the number of workers who could be rotated around appropriately to finish a particular task. Finally, the use of worker rotation may not be desirable since it serves to expose more workers to the hazard, an important consideration in both construction and general industry.

The use of improved work practices is another common form of administrative control. This can involve worker training on overall safety, health and hygiene (e.g. housekeeping) principles, as well as specific work practices. Some examples of settings in which work practices may aid in the reduction of harmful exposures in construction include proper worker positioning (e.g. a welder who makes sure his or her breathing zone is kept out of the rising plume of welding fume), proper use of tools (e.g. maintaining a seal between a grinder shroud and the grinding surface during tuckpointing tasks to reduce the amount of dust thrown directly into the worker's breathing zone), and proper utilization of exposure controls (e.g. positioning an LEV capture hood as close to the weld as possible to ensure maximum fume collection). For exposure to noise and vibration, the use of minimal power required for a given task and proper equipment maintenance (e.g. lubrication, sharpening blades, correcting imbalances, etc) may result in reduced exposures. Proper hygiene practices and good housekeeping on site can also be extremely important in reducing not only a worker's exposure to harmful agents, but also the worker's family through take-home exposures on clothing and other articles.[113]

Personal Protective Equipment

While PPE should not be the first line of defense against occupational hazards, it is many times a necessity in construction. For example, PPE to protect against acute injuries, such as hardhats, eye protection, steel-toed boots, and fall protection harnesses are commonplace on construction sites.

Even in the presence of engineering controls, elevated exposures requiring the use of added hearing or respiratory protection are commonly encountered in construction. However, there are a number of disadvantages to relying heavily on PPE to reduce worker exposures in construction. First, the effectiveness PPE relies on proper use and maintenance by the worker, which may be difficult to achieve. A well-studied example of this is the use of hearing protective devices (HPDs). Although HPDs are proven to be effective at reducing one's exposure to noise, their use remains low in construction.(69,114,115) Even if use was high in high-noise construction tasks, HPDs also have other limitations such as improper fit or selection, potential over-attenuation (and compromised ability to communicate), and uncertainty about real-world noise reduction ratings. Another example is the use of respiratory protection, which requires a respiratory protection program involving worker training, medical evaluations, fit testing, effectiveness surveillance, maintenance, storage, inspections, and recordkeeping (29 CFR 1910.134, which also applies to construction). Many of the requirements outlined in the OSHA standard may be cumbersome and/or challenging in construction given the transient workforce and oversight needed for effective compliance. In addition, a number of tasks often encountered in construction, such as welding by pipefitters and boilermakers that requires work in hot environments and tight spaces, are not conducive to the use of hot, bulky forms of respiratory protection.

Another limitation to the use of PPE in construction is the possibility that the PPE selected may not offer enough protection in extreme exposure tasks. For example, the dry abrasive blasting of lead paint from a bridge, which generates large amounts of dust in an enclosed space, was recently reported to result in personal exposure levels that approach or exceed the highest attainable assigned protection factors.(35) Finally, as opposed to substitution or engineering controls, PPE does not serve to reduce bystander exposures. This is extremely important on construction projects that involve many workers performing a wide variety of tasks at the same site. Finally, as mentioned above, PPE does not reduce the amount of contaminant in the workspace which can lead to contamination of PPE, work clothing, lunch boxes, automobiles, and other items resulting in significant take-home exposures.(113)

Use and Adoption of Controls in Construction

Despite a vast range of opportunities to reduce worker exposures to hazardous agents in construction, their use in the industry lags due to a number of barriers, many of which may be problem of perception rather than reality. The barriers (real or perceived) most often cited for not incorporating more exposure controls in construction involve high cost, lack of technical feasibility or effectiveness, loss in job/product quality, and reductions in productivity. However, there are numerous success stories involving well-developed ideas that not only reduced worker exposures but also improved the bottom line, resulting in a win-win situation. For example, based on anecdotal reports from workers, reduction of dusts and fumes using LEV may increase productivity since working in a relatively dust-free environment minimizes time needed to clean the work area, improves visibility, and, in the view of some workers, results in feeling less fatigued over the course of the work day.

A number of approaches may aid in increased awareness and adoption of exposure controls in construction. These may include market forces such as increased consumer demand, which would likely increase the visibility and use of health and safety as a competitive advantage by equipment manufacturers, vendors and rental companies. This would provide increased availability of exposure controls and competition which would drive down costs. As construction continues to migrate toward "green building" and increased sustainability efforts, the control of worker exposures should receive more attention at the project design stage as well as during equipment design and procurement. An example of this are "buy quiet" programs being implemented by organizations that outline specific protocols for equipment procurement based on noise generation characteristics. Another way to increase the use of exposure controls on construction jobs is to have them written into contract specifications by the owners at the bidding stage. Finally, increased health and safety regulation and enforcement, such as more stringent regulations on exposure to respirable silica and increased citations involving worker overexposures to welding fume components like manganese and hexavalent chromium at the federal, state and local levels would likely result in increased use of exposure controls.

Management, Communication, and Training

General Management and Hazard Communication Issues

The structure of construction contracts, project organization, the design team and developer, owner, and project managers all play a role in driving health and safety during a construction project. Since the owner or client specifies the work to be carried out and the requirements contractors must meet to pre-qualify as bidders and be awarded contracts, they have the power to require contractors to build health and safety programs into the scope of work.

General contractors and project managers play a major role in scheduling and sequencing of work, which can also have an impact on safety and health. For example, if insulators apply spray-on fireproofing to steel beams and interior ceilings before ironworkers and electricians have completed their work, that material will be disturbed by the ironworker still welding on steel columns and/or the electrician installing wiring above the ceiling. In the former case, the insulation materials would likely be heated to very high temperatures causing thermal reactions that can generate release of unknown chemicals. Ideally, this can be prevented by scheduling the insulation contractor after the other trades have completed their work.

The multi-tiered subcontracting relationships in construction, along with the fact that the mix of subcontractors will change over different phases of a project, can make communication of health and safety information more challenging than in many other work settings. OSHA's Hazard Communication standard consistently has been cited among the top ten (indeed, often in the top five) violations throughout its existence, in both general industry and construction sectors.

While tracking the use of chemicals on a jobsite and coordination among sub-contractors spanning multiple trades is often challenging, such communications are essential to controlling health hazards given the dozens of trades that may be working side by side on most construction projects. While regulatory compliance alone should not be the driving factor, useful guidance is provided by OSHA in its multi-employer worksite policy on the roles and responsibilities of the different tiers of contractors and subcontractors in generating and mitigating a health hazard on a given jobsite.[116] Clearly, these roles are not mutually exclusive and overlap is common.

- The *creating* employer is one who causes a hazardous condition;
- The *exposing* employer is one whose own employees are exposed to a hazard (regardless of who generated the hazard);
- The *correcting* employer is responsible for correcting a hazard, e.g. responsible for installation and/or maintenance of a particular protective device or equipment; and
- The *controlling* employer, who has general supervisory authority over the worksite, including the power to correct health and safety violations or to require others to correct them. Control may be established by contract provisions, or even in the absence of explicit contract language, the party who in actual practice exercises broad control over subcontractors on site.

What this means is that for any given hazardous condition(s) on a construction site that violates an OSHA standard, multiple contractors/employers are at risk for receiving OSHA citations. Again, OSHA compliance should not be the driving factor behind health and safety controls and communications; however, reduction of regulatory liability ultimately should also mean reduction in hazardous exposures.

Incorporating Health and Safety Requirements into Construction Contracts

Prudent contractors usually include the cost of supplying safety equipment and employee training in their bids. Consequently, their bids may be higher, causing owners to look elsewhere. In other words, some effective health and safety programs often go unrewarded. Owners can change this paradigm by making health and safety considerations an integral part of their contract requirements and project management. Health and safety requirements should be objectively stated to avoid ambiguity and interpretation issues. The project team should work with legal and contract specialists to formulate project safety specifications.(117)

Health and safety contract specifications vary from company-to-company and often from project-to-project. A useful resource for facility / site owners and operators as well as for occupational hygiene and safety professionals is the AIHA® guideline *Health and Safety Requirements in Construction Contract Documents*.(118) This AIHA® guideline provides information on incorporating safety and health provisions in contract documents, including specification language, design phase considerations, and contract administration. These efforts help to proactively establish health and safety criteria, which, if enforced appropriately and through adequate communication, can greatly enhance the health and safety performance on the job.

Prevention through Design (PtD): Health and Safety During the Design and Pre-construction Phases

Integrating injury and illness prevention in the design and preconstruction planning phases can also have a significant impact in reducing injuries and illnesses that may occur during the construction phase of the project. The goal is to "design out' or minimize hazards and risks early in the design process. This is consistent with the important concept of Prevention through Design (PtD), defined by NIOSH as "addressing occupational safety and health needs in the design process to prevent or minimize the work-related hazards associated with the construction, manufacture, use, maintenance, and disposal of facilities, materials, and equipment."(119)

Health and safety considerations not addressed during the initial design phase often cost significantly more to retrofit or otherwise correct after the project is completed or even during the construction phase of the project. Constructability reviews by the architectural or design firm, construction manager and/or the general contractor during the design phase are also valuable. Ideally constructability reviews should involve the occupational health and safety professional, who can conduct a preliminary hazard assessment during the preconstruction phase to proactively identify high risk hazards early on so that safer and healthier alternative methods and materials can be used to construct the project, or to provide engineering solutions to effectively control hazards during the construction phase. Some examples of how health and safety issues may be addressed during the design and planning phase include specifying that temporary decking be installed as soon as possible to prevent injury from falling; designing permanent stairways and walkways to be constructed first so that the use of temporary scaffolding is minimized; removing or relocating utilities, and/or specifying less toxic products and materials to be used on the project.(117)

A Word about Maintenance and Rehabilitation Work in Industrial Settings

Throughout this chapter renovation and repair work and its impact on health hazard anticipation, recognition, evaluation, and control for construction workers has been discussed. It is important to recognize that construction hazards in industrial settings can be significantly greater than those confronted by production workers at the same facility as a result of process changes, line breaking, vessel entry, and other atypical tasks. Consider, too, the diversity of workplace environments that may employ industrial maintenance and rehabilitation construction contractors on a project-by-project basis, as well as the potentially highly mobile nature of this work. Obviously, then, industry-specific and site-specific factors must be considered in any exposure assessment of these workers in addition to their own work processes and materials. The need for effective hazard communication cannot be overemphasized here. Certainly, inadequately controlled hazards faced by the construction worker in this setting may also similarly endanger facility operations employees and property, and may threaten production and quality.[120] The promulgation of the OSHA process safety management (PSM) standard (29 CFR 1910.119) has made facility owners, especially those in the petrochemical industry, more diligent in prequalifying contractors based on injury and illness history, safety program elements, and various other safety and health criteria.

Integrating Hazard Analysis and Prevention into Skills Training

Construction employment is generally temporary and very often lasts for the duration of a particular project or project phase. This may vary from months (e.g. a form carpenter on a large project) to a few days, so most workers have several employers in any given year. In addition, construction workers often may find themselves working over large geographical areas from project to project. The construction workforce has a history of unionization at rates higher than general industry, starting in the 1890s. Nationwide, about 1,600 multi-employer Taft-Hartley trusts are jointly administered with unions to provide transferable pensions, health insurance and training in an inherently unstable employment setting where projects are short lived. By training a shared pool of workers, these multi-employer trusts help overcome employer concerns that training expenditures will be lost as trained employees are hired by their competitors. They also reduce barriers to training and job mobility by providing training, often on unpaid time, through common apprenticeship training and certifications based on the skills that are necessary for a given trade. Journeymen may work with several employers on multiple projects each year. Thus, as construction tradespersons carry their skills with them from job to job they often rely on their union as the principle source of continuity throughout their careers. Because much of what a tradesperson knows is cultivated during their apprenticeship program and the trades often work independently, these joint training programs are an important resource for integrating hazard analysis and prevention into skills standard operating procedures. One such example is the Mobilization, Optimization, Stabilization, and Training (MOST) joint labor trust fund established by the National Association of Construction Boilermaker Employers (NACBE) and the International Brotherhood of Boilermakers to maintain a skilled workforce in both current skills and new technologies and to instruct and teach safe work habits.

In the authors' experience, successes have been found by incorporating health and safety training and hazard recognition into apprenticeship and even pre-apprenticeship programs; this provides an excellent opportunity for reducing work-related injuries and illnesses, especially among young workers. One example is *WorkSmart*, a comprehensive introduction to the boilermaker trade founded by Local 146 (Edmonton, Alberta) of the International Brotherhood of Boilermakers. This two-week program exposes pre-apprentices to industry environments and safety and workplace culture by blending theory and hands-on skills training (e.g. welding, cutting, steel fabrication, rigging, and other skills essential to the boilermaker trade) with hazard identification, jobsite and safety culture, and applied safe practices and controls. Union training centers and colleges have also been exploring, developing, and implementing "virtual campuses" that employ interactive e-learning tools to enhance an organization's ability to deliver integrated skills and hazard prevention and control training.

The OSHA Outreach Training Program provides another important resource for the construction trades through its 10-hour and 30-hour courses in construction safety and health hazard recognition and prevention. There are more than 40 authorized OSHA Training Institute Education Centers across the U.S. Among those, working with CPWR, the Building and Construction Trades Department of the AFL-CIO and its affiliated unions provide this OSHA training through its Smart-Mark program, which encompasses a network of more than 5,000 authorized outreach instructors nationwide who have trained more than 175,000 workers since 1998. OSHA completion cards are issued to employees who complete the training, providing tangible evidence that a worker has received basic health and safety training.[121]

It should be apparent, then, that not only is worker involvement essential to help the industrial hygienist better understand the work processes and design and implement effective exposure assessment strategies in construction (as mentioned earlier in this chapter), but it is also extremely important for the development and delivery of effective health and safety training.

Regulatory Perspective

Construction in the U.S. has long been subject to parallel sets of occupational safety and health regulation (29 CFR 1926) that often lag behind general industry standards (29 CFR 1910). The OSHA standard on lead exposure in construction was published in 1993, well over a decade after the general industry lead standard, for example, and during that interim, the PEL for construction workers was four times that applied in general industry. Other examples include disparities between the silica PEL for construction and general industry standards and different or lacking standards in construction for confined space entry. Further, although hearing loss is pervasive among construction workers, the construction sector lacks a comprehensive noise standard as has been in place in general industry for many years. That said, however, there are currently at least 25 comprehensive, substance-specific OSHA health standards for construction work that require exposure assessments through initial and periodic monitoring as well as provisions for training, medical surveillance, and controlled or "regulated" work areas including specified engineering controls, housekeeping, and/or work practice requirements.

However, a significant driver for improved health and safety conditions in construction is its inclusion in job specifications and contracts. As mentioned earlier, construction is commonly subject to contractual, in addition to regulatory, requirements related to safety practices on larger projects and government contracts. These requirements predate the Occupational Safety and Health Act going back to the federal Walsh-Healey Public Contracts Act (1936) which imposed safety requirements in federal contracts over $10,000 (later increased to $100,000) and also promulgated more detailed safety regulations in 1960. This process of defining mandatory safety and health requirements in contracts and evaluating past safety performance and safety capabilities as a part of pre-qualifying bidders is now widely used in the private sector where project owner/customer involvement creates perhaps the most compelling motivation for improving safety and health performance. The remedy for nonconformance of contract specifications can include withdrawal of the contract, stopping work, withholding payment, or removal from future bid lists, rather than citations. When the Construction Safety Act passed in 1969, it built on this contractual foundation, because unlike the many state labor safety and health regulations that federal OSHA pre-empted, public and private contracting practices were not affected.

Several U.S. federal agencies have comprehensive safety and health contract language for construction including the Army Corps of Engineers, National Aeronautical and Space Administration, Environmental Protection Agency, Department of Transportation (which regulates construction of interstate gasoline and natural gas pipelines), and others.

State workers' compensation laws, along with local building, fire, and health codes, and local ordinances related to nuisance dust and noise can have important indirect impacts on worker health. These can have both positive (e.g., to reduce noise at the fence line, quieter tools or noise barriers may also reduce worker exposure) or negative (e.g., environmental enclosure during abrasive blasting of a lead painted bridge may elevate worker exposures) impacts on worker exposures. Local codes, permits, licensing, and enforcement may also serve to increase a small employer's or a worker's awareness that a hazard exists and that feasible controls are available. Although the language of the OSH Act assures that federal regulations pre-empt state and local regulations that are not part of an OSHA approved state plan, to the extent that construction occurs in proximity to the public, some significant impacts can occur.

Looking ahead, a number of emerging issues likely will also play a role in the anticipation, recognition, evaluation, and control of construction health hazards. One is the continued growth of "green" and sustainable building construction. While the benefits of moving to a green economy are many, there are many challenges as well. Green jobs are broadly defined as those that help to improve the environment; yet, attention must be paid to making sure that worker health and safety are not overlooked in the process. For example, in green building construction, the increased use of insulation products and recycled or alternative materials may introduce some new exposure hazards to consider for the workers who process or handle them. Although there is a fairly well-established history in the U.S. of designing safety for the general public, there has been less attention paid to integrating worker health and safety into the design, re-design, and retrofit of new and existing buildings, tools and equipment, and work processes.(119) This presents another important opportunity for the industrial hygiene profession to contribute its essential expertise.

Acknowledgements

The authors gratefully acknowledge Jerome Spear, CIH, CSP (J.E. Spear Consulting, LLC) for his insightful contribution to the Management, Communications, and Training section of this chapter. The authors are also indebted to Sherri Wilson-Kinard (Program Assistant, CPWR) for her assistance in assembling tables, figures, and references.

References

1. **Susi, P. and S. Schneider:** Chemical Exposures on a New Construction Site. *Appl. Occup. Environ. Hyg. 10(2)*:100–03 (1995).
2. **Susi P., M. Goldberg, P. Barnes, and E. Stafford:** The use of a task-based exposure assessment model (T-BEAM) for assessment of metal fume exposures during welding and thermal cutting. *Appl. Occup. Env. Hyg. 15*:26–38 (2000).
3. **Dong, X.:** *The Construction Chart Book: The U.S. Construction Industry and Its Workers, Fourth Edition.* Silver Spring, MD: CPWR - The Center for Construction Research and Training, 2007.
4. **Verma D.K., L. Kurtz, D. Sahai, and M.M. Finkelstein:** Current Chemical Exposures Among Ontario Construction Workers. *Appl. Occup. Environ. Hyg. 18*:1031–47 (2003).
5. **Blute, N.A., S. Woski, and C.A. Greenspan:** Exposure Characterization for Highway Construction. Part I. Cut and Cover and Tunnel Finish Stages. *Appl. Occup. Env. Hyg. 14*:632–41 (1999).
6. **Greenspan C.A, R. Moure-Eraso, D.H. Wegman, and L.C. Oliver:** Occupational hygiene characterization of a highway construction project: a pilot study. *Appl. Occup. Environ. Hyg. 10*:50–58 (1995).
7. **Verma, D.K., and C.G. Middleton:** Occupational Exposure to Asbestos in the Ceiling and Wall Texture Process. *J. Occup. Health Safety. 50*:21–24 (1981).
8. **Echt, A. and W.K. Sieber: Control of Silica Exposure from Hand Tools in Construction:** Grinding Concrete. *Appl. Occup. Env. Hyg. 17*:457–61 (2002).
9. **Nash, N.T. and D.R. Williams:** Occupational exposure to crystalline silica during tuck pointing and the use of engineering controls. *Appl. Occup. Env. Hyg. 15*:8–10 (2000).
10. **Linch, K.D:** Respirable concrete dust - silicosis hazard in the construction industry. *Appl. Occup. Environ. Hyg. 17*:209–21 (2002).
11. **Rappaport S.M., M. Goldberg, P. Susi, and R.F. Herrick:** Excessive exposure to silica in the U.S. construction industry. *Ann. Occup. Hyg. 47(2)*:111–22 (2003).
12. **Lumens, M.E. and T. Spee:** Determinants of exposure to respirable quartz dust in the construction industry. *Ann. Occup. Hyg. 45*:585–95 (2001).
13. **Ontario Ministry of Labour:** Lead and silica during tuckpointing and grinding at the Ontario legislative buildings. Ottawa, ON, Canada: Ministry of Labour, 1995.
14. **Thorpe, A., A.S. Ritchie, M.J. Gibson, and R.C. Brown:** Measurements of the effectiveness of dust control on cut-off saws used in the construction industry. *Ann. Occup. Hyg. 43(7)*:443–56 (1999).
15. **Breysse, P.N., et.al.:** End-User Exposures to Synthetic Vitreous Fibers: II. Fabrication and Installation Fabrication of Commercial Products. *Appl. Occup. Env. Hyg. 16(4)*:464–70 (2001).
16. **Methner, M.M., J.L. McKernan, and J.L. Dennison:** Task-based exposure assessment of hazards associated with new residential construction. *Appl. Occup. Env. Hyg. 15*:811–19 (2000).
17. **Decker, P., B. Cohen, and J.H. Butala:** Exposure to Wood Dust and Heavy Metals in Workers Using CCA Pressure-Treated Wood. *Am. Ind. Hyg. Assoc. J. 63*:166–71 (2002).
18. **Bakke, B., et al.:** Dust and Gas Exposure in Tunnel Construction Work. *Am. Ind. Hyg. Assoc. J. 62*:457–65 (2001).
19. **Goldberg, M., et al.:** A task-based approach to assessing lead exposure among iron workers engaged in bridge rehabilitation. *Am. J. Ind. Med. 31*:310–18 (1997).
20. **Sen, D., H. Wolfson, and M. Dilworth:** Lead exposure in scaffolders during refurbishment construction activity — an observational study. *Occup. Med. 52*:49-54 (2002).
21. **Bilan, R.A., W.O. Haflidson, and D.J. McVittie:** Assessment of Isocyanate Exposure During the Spray Application of Polyurethane Foam. *Am. Ind. Hyg. Assoc. J. 50*:303-306 (1989).

22. **Crespo, J and J. Galan:** Exposure to MDI during the process of insulating buildings with sprayed polyurethane foam. *Ann. Occup. Hyg. 43*:415–19 (1999).
23. **Riala, R.:** Dust and Quartz Exposure of Finnish Construction Site Cleaners. *Ann. Occup. Hyg. 32*:215–20 (1998).
24. **Wieslander, G., D. Norback, and C. Edling:** Occupational exposure to water-based paint and symptoms from the skin and eyes. *Occup. Environ. Med. 51*:181–86 (1994).
25. **Riala, R., et al.:** Solvent Exposure in Construction and Maintenance Painting. *Scand. J. Work Env. Hea. 10*:263–66 (1984).
26. **U.S. Department of Labor – Bureau of Labor Statistics (BLS) and National Institute for Occupational Safety and Health (NIOSH):** Respirator Usage in Private Sector Firms, 2001. In *The Construction Chart Book: The U.S. Construction Industry and Its Workers, Fourth Edition.* Silver Spring, MD: CPWR – The Center for Construction Research and Training, 2007.
27. **U.S. Department of Labor – Bureau of Labor Statistics (BLS):** *Occupational Outlook Handbook, Construction Trades and Related Workers, 2008–09 edition.* Washington, D.C.: BLS, 2009.
28. **Antonini, J.:** Health Effects of Welding. *Crit. Rev. Toxicol. 33(1)*:61–103 (2003).
29. **FMI Corporation:** *The 2005–2006 U.S. Markets Construction Overview.* Raleigh, NC: FMI, 2005.
30. **Burgess, W.A.:** *Recognition of Health Hazards in Industry: A Review of Materials and Processes, 2nd edition.* New York: J. Wiley & Sons, 1995.
31. **O'Brien, R.L. (ed.):** *Jefferson's Welding Encyclopedia, 18th edition.* Miami, FL: American Welding Society, 1997.
32. **American Conference of Governmental Industrial Hygienists (ACGIH®):** *Documentation of the Threshold Limit Values® and Biological Exposure Indices, 7th edition. Nickel and Inorganic Compounds including Nickel Sulfide.* Cincinnati, OH: ACGIH®, 2001. (TLV® updated in 2008).
33. **Woskie S.R., et al.:** Exposures to quartz, diesel, dust, and welding fumes during heavy and highway construction. *Am. Ind. Hyg. Assoc. J. 63*:447–57 (2002).
34. **Rappaport S.M., M. Weaver, D. Taylor, L. Kupper, and P. Susi:** Application of mixed models to assess exposures monitored by construction workers during hot processes. *Ann. Occup. Hyg. 43(7)*:457–69 (1999).
35. **Meeker J.D., P. Susi, and A. Pellegrino:** Comparison of occupational exposures among painters using three alternative blasting abrasives. *J. Occup. Environ. Hyg. 3*:D80–D84 (2006).
36. **Rom, W.N.:** *Environmental and Occupational Medicine, 2nd edition,* Boston, MA: Little, Brown & Company, 1992.
37. **Alessio, L., M. Campagna, and R. Lucchini:** Historical perspectives from lead to manganese through mercury: mythology, science, and lessons for prevention. *Am. J. Ind. Med. 50(11)*:779–87 (2007).
38. **Flynn, M.R. and P. Susi:** Manganese, iron, and total particulate exposures to welders. *J. Occup. Environ. Hyg. 7(2)*:115–26 (2010).
39. **American Conference of Governmental Industrial Hygienists® (ACGIH®):** *Documentation of the Threshold Limit Values® and Biological Exposure Indices®,* 7th edition. Cincinnati, OH: ACGIH®, 2001.
40. **Henneberger P.K., S.K. Goe, W.E. Miller, and D.W. Groce:** Industries in the United States with airborne beryllium exposure and the numbers of workers potentially exposed. *J. Occup. Env. Hyg. 1*:648–59 (2004).
41. **Dong, X.:** *The Construction Chart Book: The U.S. Construction Industry and Its Workers, 3rd Edition.* Silver Spring, MD: CPWR — The Center for Construction Research and Training, 2003.
42. **Goodwin, S., M. Stanbury, M.L. Wang, E. Silbergeld, and J.E. Parker:** Previously undetected silicosis in New Jersey decedents. *Am. J. Ind. Med. 44*:304–11 (2003).
43. **Robinson C., et al.:** Assessment of mortality in the construction industry in the United States, 1984–1986. *Am. J. Ind. Med. 28*:49–70 (1995).
44. **National Institute for Occupational Safety and Health (NIOSH):** *The Work-Related Lung Disease Surveillance Report,* 2002. Publication No. 2003-111. Cincinnati, OH: NIOSH, 2003.
45. **Lyons J.J.,et al.:** Case presentation: a breathless builder. *Breathe. 3*:386–90 (2007).
46. **National Institute for Occupational Safety and Health (NIOSH):** *NIOSH Hazard Review: Health Effects of Occupational Exposure to Respirable Crystalline Silica.* Cincinnati, OH: NIOSH, 2002.
47. **Chisholm J.:** Respirable dust and respirable silica concentrations from construction activities. *Indoor Built Environ. 8*:94-106 (1999).
48. **Flanagan M.E., N. Seixas, M. Majar, J. Camp, and M. Morgan:** Silica dust exposures during selected construction activities. *Am. Ind. Hyg. Assoc. J. 64*:319–28 (2003).
49. **Valiante D.J, D.P. Schill, K.D. Rosenman, and E. Socie:** Highway repair: a new silicosis threat. *Am. J. Public Health. 94*:876–80 (2004).
50. **Glindmeyer H.W. and Y.Y. Hammad:** Contributing factors to sandblasters' silicosis: inadequate respiratory protection equipment and standards. *J. Occup. Med. 30*:917–21 (1988).

51. **Yasui S., P. Susi, M. McClean, and M. Flynn:** Assessment of silica exposure and engineering controls during tuckpointing. *Appl. Occup. Environ. Hyg.18*:977–84 (2003).
52. **Croteau, G.A., M.E. Flanagan, J.E. Camp, and N.S. Seixas:** The efficacy of local exhaust ventilation for controlling dust exposures during concrete surface grinding. *Ann. Occup. Hyg. 48(6)*: 509–18 (2004).
53. **Collingwood, S and W.A. Heitbrink:** Field evaluation of an engineering control for respirable crystalline silica exposures during mortar removal. *J. Occup. Environ. Hyg. 4*:875–87 (2007).
54. **Akbar-Khanzadeh, F., et al.:** Crystalline Silica Dust and Respirable Particulate Matter During Indoor Concrete Grinding — Wet Grinding and Ventilated Grinding Compared with Uncontrolled Conventional Grinding. *J. Occup. Environ. Hyg. 4*:770–79 (2007).
55. **Linch K.D., W.E. Miller, R.B. Althouse, D.W. Groce, and J.M. Hale:** Surveillance of respirable crystalline silica dust using OSHA compliance data (1979–1995). *Am. J. Ind. Med. 34*:547–58 (1998).
56. **Salg, J. and T. Alterman:** A proportionate mortality study of bricklayers and allied craftworkers. *Am. J. Ind. Med. 47*:10–19 (2005).
57. **Finkelstein M.M. and D.K. Verma:** Mortality among Ontario members of the international union of bricklayers and allied craftworkers. *Am. J. Ind. Med. 47*:4–9 (2005).
58. **Occupational Safety and Health Administration (OSHA):** *Controlling Silica Exposures in Construction.* OSHA Publication 3362-04. Washington, D.C.: U.S. Department of Labor, 2009.
59. **Meeker, J.D., M. Cooper, D. Lefrowitz, and P. Susi:** Engineering control technologies to reduce occupational silica exposures in masonry cutting and tuckpointing. *Pub. Health Rep. 124(1)*:101–11 (2009).
60. **National Institute for Occupational Safety and Health (NIOSH):** *Mixed Exposures Research Agenda: A Report by the NORA Mixed Exposures Team.* NIOSH Publication No. 2005-106. Cincinnati, OH: NIOSH Publications Group, 2004.
61. **Epstien, B. and W. Spain:** Federal asbestos guidance and regulation: a chronology. *Environ. Choices. 5(1)*:3–10 (1996).
62. **Martonik, J.F., E. Nash, and E. Grossman:** The history of OSHA's asbestos rulemakings and some distinctive approaches that they introduced for regulating occupational exposure to toxic substances. *Am. Ind. Hyg. Assoc. J. 62*:208–17 (2001).
63. **National Institute for Occupational Safety and Health (NIOSH):** Morris Bean & Company, Yellow Springs, Ohio — Health Hazard Evaluation Report No. 86-038 (HETA 86-038-1807), Cincinnati, OH: NIOSH Publications Group, 1987.
64. **Kaukainen, A., R. Martikainen, R. Riala, K. Reijula, and L. Tammilehto:** Work Tasks, Chemical Exposure and Respiratory Health in Construction Painting. *Am. J. Ind. Med. 51*:1–8 (2008).
65. **Lauwerys, R.R. and P. Hoet:** *Industrial Chemical Exposure: Guidelines for Biological Monitoring, Third Edition.* Boca Raton, FL: Lewis Publishers, CRC Press, 2001.
66. **The Center to Protect Workers' Rights:** *Skin Problems in Construction — Hazard Alert,* Silver Spring, MD: CWPR, 2003.
67. **Construction Safety Association of Ontario (CSAO):** *Construction Multi-Trades Health and Safety Manual.* Etobicoke, ON: CSAO, 2007.
68. **CPWR — The Center for Construction Research and Training:** *Working with Epoxy Resin Systems in Construction: Best Practices Guide to Skin Protection,* Silver Spring, MD: CWPR, 2008.
69. **Neitzel, R. and N. Seixas:** The effectiveness of hearing protection among construction workers. *J. Occup. Environ. Hyg. 2(4)*:227–38 (2005).
70. **Neitzel, R., N.S. Seixas, J. Camp, and M. Yost:** An assessment of occupational noise exposures in four construction trades. *Am. Ind. Hyg. Assoc. J. 60*:807–17 (1999).
71. **Suter, A.H.:** Construction noise: exposure, effects and the potential for remediation: a review and analysis. *Am. Ind. Hyg. Assoc. J. 63*:768–89 (2002).
72. **Ward, W.D., J.D. Royster, and L.H. Royster:** Auditory and Nonauditory Effects of Noise (Chapter 5). In *The Noise Manual, 5th edition.* Berger, E.H., et al. (eds). Fairfax, VA: AIHA, 2003. pp. 123–144.
73. **Brugge, D., A. Dhar:** Residential health near major construction projects: unexplored hazards. *Rev. Environ. Health. 23(1)*:75–81 (2008).
74. **Schneider, S.E., E. Johanning, J.L. Belard, and G. Engholm:** Noise, vibration, and heat and cold. *Occup. Med. 10(2)*:363–83 (1995).
75. **Schneider, S. and P. Susi:** *An Investigation of Health Hazards on a New Construction Site. Center to Protect Worker's Rights (CPWR),* Report No. OSH1-93. Silver Spring, MD: CWPR, 1993.
76. **Palmer, K.T., M.J. Griffin, H. Bendall, B. Pannett, and D. Coggon:** Prevalence and pattern of occupational exposure to hand transmitted vibration in Great Britain: findings from a national survey. *Occup. Env. Med. 57*:218–28 (2000).
77. **Palmer, K.T., et al.:** Risk of hand-arm vibration syndrome according to occupation and sources of exposure to hand-transmitted vibration: a national survey. *Am. J. Ind. Med. 39*:389–96 (2001).

78. **Kittusamy, N.K. and B. Buchholz:** Whole-body vibration and postural stress among operators of construction equipment: a literature review. *J. Safety Res. 35(3)*:255–61 (2004).
79. **Cann, A.P., A.W. Salmoni, P. Vi, and T.R. Eger:** An exploratory study of whole-body vibration exposure and dose while operating heavy equipment in the construction industry. *Appl. Occup. Environ. Hyg. 18* :999–1005 (2003).
80. **Bonauto, D., Anderson, R., Rauser, E., and Burke, B.** Occupational heat illness in Washington State, 1995–2005. *Am. J. Ind. Med. 50(12)*:940–50 (2007).
81. **Glanz, K., D.B. Buller, and M. Saraiya:** Reducing ultraviolet radiation exposure among outdoor workers: state of the evidence and recommendations. *Env. Health. 6*:22 (2007).
82. **Antoine, M., S. Pierre-Edouard, B. Jean-Luc, and V. David:** Effective exposure to solar UV in building workers: influence of local and individual factors. *J. Expo. Sci. Env. Epi. 17(1)*:58–68 (2007).
83. **Banas, D.:** Employee exposure to high-level radio frequency radiation. *Appl. Occup. Envrion. Hyg. 17(3)*:154–56 (2002).
84. **Engholm, G. and E. Holmström:** Dose-response associations between musculoskeletal disorders and physical and psychosocial factors among construction workers. *Scand. J. Work Environ. Health 31(2)*:57–67 (2005).
85. **Schneider, S.** Musculoskeletal injuries in construction: a review of the literature. *Appl. Occup. Environ. Hyg. 16(11)*:1056–64 (2001).
86. **National Institute for Occupational Safety and Health (NIOSH):** *Simple Solutions: Ergonomics for Construction Workers.* DHHS (NIOSH) Publication No. 2007-122. Cincinnati, OH: NIOSH, 2007.
87. **Schneider, S. and P. Susi.** Ergonomics and Construction: A Review of Potential Hazards in New Construction. *Am. Ind. Hyg. Assoc. J. 56(7)*:635–49 (1994).
88. **National Institute for Occupational Safety and Health (NIOSH):** *Histoplasmosis: Protecting Workers at Risk.* Publication No. 2005-109. Cincinnati, OH: NIOSH, 2004.
89. **National Institute for Occupational Safety and Health (NIOSH):** *Hantavirus Pulmonary Syndrome — United States: Updated Recommendations for Risk Reduction. MMWR, 51(RR09)*; 1-2. Cincinnati, OH: NIOSH, 2002.
90. **Morris, G.K. and B.G. Shelton:** *Legionella bacteria in environmental samples: hazard analysis and suggested remedial actions; Technical Bulletin 1.5.* Norcross, GA: Pathcon Laboratories, 1998.
91. **Construction Safety Association of Ontario (CSAO):** [Online] *Legionellosis — Cause and Controls.* Ottawa, ON, Canada: Ministry of Labour, 2008. Available at http://www.csao.org/UploadFiles/Alerts/legionellosis_2008.pdf [Accessed January 2011.]
92. **Harris, M.K., L.E. Booher, and S. Carter:** *Field Guidelines for Temporary Ventilation of Confined Space.* Fairfax, VA: AIHA®, 1996.
93. **Ignatio, J.S. and W.H. Bullock:** *A Strategy for Assessing and Managing Occupational Exposures, 3rd edition.* Fairfax, VA: AIHA®, 2006.
94. **Rappaport S.M.:** Assessment of long-term exposures to toxic substances in air. *Ann. Occup. Hyg. 35(1)*:61–121 (1991).
95. **Rappaport, S.M. and L. Kupper:** *Quantitative Exposure Assessment.* El Cerrito, CA: Stephen Rappaport, 2008.
96. **Susi, P. and S. Schneider:** Database Needs for a Task-Based Exposure Assessment Model for Construction. *Appl. Occup. Env. Hyg. 10(4)*:394–99 (1995).
97. **Meeker, J.D.; P. Susi, and M.R. Flynn:** Manganese and Welding Fume Exposure and Control in Construction. *J. Occup. Env. Hyg. 4(12)*:943-951 (2007).
98. **Echt A., et al.:** *In-depth survey of dust control technology for cutting concrete block and tuckpointing brick at The International Masonry Institute Bordentown Training Center, Bordentown, NJ.* National Institute for Occupational Safety and Health (NIOSH), Report No. EPHB 282-13 (2007). Cincinnati, OH: NIOSH, 2007.
99. **Flynn, M. R. and P. Susi:** A Review of Engineering Control Technology for Exposures Generated During Abrasive Blasting Operations. *J. Occup. Environ. Hyg. 1*:680–87 (2004).
100. **Cecala, A.B., et al.:** Reducing enclosed cab drill operator's respirable dust exposure with effective filtration and pressurization techniques. *J. Occup. Environ. Hyg. 2(1)*:54–63 (2005).
101. **National Institute for Occupational Safety and Health (NIOSH):** [Online] *NIOSH Power Tools Database.* Available at http://wwwn.cdc.gov/niosh-sound-vibration/ [Accessed January 2011].
102. **CPWR — The Center for Construction Research and Training:** [Online] *Construction Solutions. Available at* http://www.cpwrconstructionsolutions.org. [Accessed January 2011].
103. **Mickelsen, R.L., S.A. Shulman, A.J. Kriech, L.V. Osborn, and A.P. Redman:** Status of worker exposure to asphalt paving fumes with the use of engineering controls. *Environ. Sci. Technol. 40(10)*:5661-5667 (2006).
104. **Wallace, M., S. Shulman, and J. Sheehy:** Comparing exposure levels by type of welding operation and evaluating the effectiveness of fume extraction guns. *Appl. Occup. Env. Hyg. 16(8)*:771–79 (2001).

105. **Herrick, R.F., M.D. McClean, J.D. Meeker, L. Zwack, and K. Hanley:** Physical and chemical characterization of asphalt (bitumen) paving exposures. *J. Occup. Environ. Hyg. Suppl 1*:209–16 (2007).
106. **Shepherd, S., S.R. Woskie, C. Holcroft, and M. Ellenbecker:** Reducing silica and dust exposures in construction during use of powered concrete-cutting hand tools: efficacy of local exhaust ventilation on hammer drills. *J. Occup. Environ. Hyg. 6*:42–51 (2009).
107. **Flynn, M.R. and P. Susi:** Engineering Controls for Selected Silica and Dust Exposures in the Construction Industry: A Review. *Appl. Occup. Environ. Hyg. 18*:268–77 (2003).
108. **Echt, A., et al.:** Control of respirable dust and crystalline silica from breaking concrete with a jackhammer. *Appl. Occup. Environ. Hyg. 18(7)*:491–95 (2003).
109. **National Institute for Occupational Safety and Health (NIOSH):** "Water Spray Control of Hazardous Dust When Breaking Concrete with a Jackhammer." NIOSH Publication No. 2008-127 (2008).
110. **Golla, V. and W. Heitbrink:** Control technology for crystalline silica exposures in construction: wet abrasive blasting. *J. Occup. Env. Hyg. 1(3)*:D26–D32 (2004).
111. **Old, L.T. and W.A. Heitbrink:** Wet abrasive blasting with a WIN nozzle: a case study. *J. Occup. Environ. Hyg. 4(6)*:D55–D59 (2007).
112. **Hewitt, P.J. and A.A. Hirst:** A Systems Approach to the Control of Welding Fumes at Source. *Ann. Occup. Hyg. 37(3)*:297–306 (1993).
113. **Virji, M.A., S.R. Woskie, and L.D. Pepper:** Skin and surface lead contamination, hygiene programs, and work practices of bridge surface preparation and painting contractors. *J. Occup. Environ. Hyg. 6*:131–42 (2009).
114. **Lusk, S.L., D.L. Ronis, and M.M. Hogan:** Test of the health promotion model as a causal model of construction workers' use of hearing protection. *Res. Nurs. Health, 20*:183–94 (1997).
115. **Lusk, S.L., M.J. Kerr, and S.A. Kauffman:** Use of hearing protection and perceptions of noise exposure and hearing loss among construction workers. *Am. Ind. Hyg. Assn. J. 59*:466–70 (1998).
116. **Occupational Safety and Health Administration (OSHA):** *Multi-employer citation policy*, OSHA Instruction CPL 2-0.124, 1999.
117. **Spear, J.:** Improving Contractor Performance. *The Synergist.* (September 2005).
118. **American Industrial Hygiene Association (AIHA®):** *Health and Safety Requirements in Construction Contract Documents — AIHA Guideline 4-2005.* Fairfax, VA: AIHA, 2005.
119. **National Institute for Occupational Safety and Health (NIOSH):** "NIOSH Program: Prevention through Design" (2009). Available at http://www.cdc.gov/niosh/programs/PtDesign/ [Accessed January 14, 2011].
120 **Murawski, J.A., P. Susi, and J. Platner:** Industrial maintenance and rehabilitation: construction in the pulp and paper industry. *Appl. Occup. Environ. Hyg. 17(8)*:534–35 (2000).
121 **Sokas R.K., L. Nickels, K. Rankin, J.L. Gittleman, and C. Trahan:** Trainer Evaluation of a Union-based, 10-hour Safety and Health Hazard Awareness Program for U.S. Construction Workers. *Int. J. Occup. Env. Health. 13*:56–63 (2007).

Outcome Competencies

After completing this chapter, the reader should be able to:

1. Define underlined terms used in this chapter.
2. Discuss the differences between the regulatory and generic definitions of hazardous wastes.
3. Summarize major federal legislative acts and amendments pertaining to hazardous wastes.
4. Classify hazardous wastes based on characteristics.
5. Draw a schematic diagram of the major phases of hazardous waste management.
6. Classify and summarize major methods for storage, treatment, and disposal of hazardous wastes.
7. Identify contributing factors and potential adverse health effects associated with exposure to hazardous wastes.
8. Identify the role and contrast the phases of occupational hygiene in relation to hazardous waste management.
9. Describe the measures for controlling exposures of workers on hazardous waste sites.

Prerequisite Knowledge

Prior to beginning this chapter, the user should review the following chapters:

Chapter Number	**Chapter Topic**
5	Occupational Toxicology
6	Occupational Epidemiology
7	Principles of Evaluating Worker Exposure
9	Occupational and Environmental Health Risk Assessment/Risk Management
11	Sampling of Gases and Vapors
14	Sampling and Sizing of Airborne Particles
17	Direct-Reading Instrumental Methods for Determining Concentrations of Gases, Vapors, and Aerosols
19	Biological Monitoring
20	The Skin and the Work Environment
21	The Development of Occupational Skin Disease
22	Biohazards and Associated Issues
26	Ionizing Radiation
34	Prevention and Mitigation of Accidental Chemical Releases
39	Personal Protective Clothing
39	Risk Communication
40	Respiratory Protection
42	Surveys and Audits
43	Hazard Communication
44	Emergency Planning and Crisis Management in the Workplace

Key Terms

biological wastes • chemical wastes • corrosive wastes • decontamination • disposal • flammable wastes • generator • hazardous • hazardous wastes • management • mismanagement • occupational hygiene • radiological wastes • reactive wastes • site control • Site Health and Safety Plan • storage • toxic wastes • treatment • waste reduction • wastes

Key Topics

I. Management vs. Mismanagement
II. Major Applicable Federal Legislative Acts
III. Definitions of Hazardous Wastes
V. Major Phases and Program Elements of Hazardous Waste Management
VI. Methods for Treatment of Hazardous Wastes
VII. Methods for Long-Term Storage and Disposal of Hazardous Wastes
VIII. Adverse Human Health Impact Due to Hazardous Waste Exposure
IX. The Role of Occupational Hygiene in Hazardous Waste Management
X. Measures for Controlling Exposures of Workers on Hazardous Waste Sites

Hazardous Waste Management

48

By William E. Luttrell, PhD, CIH; Michael S. Bisesi, PhD, CIH and Christine A. Bisesi, CIH, CHMM

Introduction

For as long as humans have existed, waste materials have been generated and mismanaged. Early problems were mainly associated with human and animal biological wastes. Management of these wastes was not an immediate problem, since population densities were low and land area for disposal was vast. Disposal of waste materials in soil and water were likely the earliest practices of waste management.(1)

The primitive management practices were perhaps examples of the adages, "Out of sight, out of mind," and, "The solution to pollution is dilution." In retrospect, however, it is clear that the disposal practices reflected mismanagement rather than management, although this was not realized at the time. As population densities increased, communicable infectious diseases often were correlated with the discharge of human feces on soils used as fields for growing edible crops and into waterways used as sources of drinking and bathing water.(2) The environment eventually demonstrated early signs of intolerance for excessive indiscriminate disposal of wastes.

The generation of chemical wastes in the United States became more prevalent following the initiation of industrialization during the nineteenth century. As industrialization rapidly increased and spread, manufacturing industries were so engrossed in output of product that little attention was focused on the generation of chemical wastes.(3) During the same period, radiological wastes were generated in increasing amounts from military, medical, and research sources.

Although indications of adverse environmental and public health impact were present earlier, it was not until the mid- to late-20th century that it became apparent that the environment had a threshold for the quantity of wastes that could be tolerated. After years of indiscriminate disposal of wastes into the environment, the quality of the air, water, and soil qualitatively and quantitatively exhibited signs of deterioration. In turn, the adverse impacts on the environment and public health were recognized and considered more seriously.

Management vs. Mismanagement

Management of hazardous wastes, regardless of sources, implies controlled and environmentally sound handling during the phases of generation, storage, processing for recovery or reuse, transporting, treating, and discharging into the air and water or discarding onto the soil. The concept of mismanagement, in turn, infers uncontrolled and environmentally unsound or indiscriminate handling of hazardous wastes, whether intentionally or unintentionally.

Several common denominators are essential for ensuring proper hazardous waste management. These include 1) defining and identifying hazardous wastes; 2) listing substances that meet the defined characteristics; 3) anticipating quantities and maintaining inventories; 4) determining appropriate methods for handling; 5) establishing plans for emergency response; and 6) accepting responsibility and liability. Only relatively recently, through enacted and amended legislative acts, have these practices and other factors been considered part of hazardous waste management.

Major Applicable Federal Legislative Acts

Legislative Responses to Mismanagement of Hazardous Wastes

In response to increased awareness of hazardous waste mismanagement, the regulatory framework was overhauled substantially during the 1970s. Environmental legislation was designated a priority and, accordingly, the regulatory framework was strengthened and new federal agencies such as the U.S. Environmental Protection Agency (EPA) and the Occupational Safety and Health Administration (OSHA) were established. Previously, environmental controls were loosely regulated mainly at state and local levels. At present, more than 20 federal acts[4–6] exist that address some aspect of hazardous wastes (Table 48.1). The statutes require state and local governments to be the primary implementers of the regulatory standards, though federal implementation and authority are permitted where and when deemed necessary.

The focus on environmental issues and legislation has resulted in the development of a prosperous and legitimate waste

Table 48.1 — Major U.S. Federal Legislative Acts Applicable to Hazardous Waste Management

Act and Citation	*Summary of Major Components*
Federal Insecticide, Fungicide and Rodenticide Act (1947 as amended 1988; 7 USCA 136 et seq.)	Regulates registration, sale, use, and disposal of pesticides
Clean Air Act (1955 as amended 1966, 1970, 1977 and 1990; 42 USCA 7401 et seq.)	Regulates air emissions from new and existing stationary and mobile sources; in 1990 established primary standards to protect health and secondary standards to protect welfare of the environment
Solid Waste Disposal Act (1965 as amended 1980; 42 USCA 3251 et seq.; 6901 et seq.)	Regulates wastes legally classified as solid wastes; foundation for regulation that defined hazardous wastes; amended as the Resource Conservation and Recovery Act of 1976
National Environmental Policy Act (1969; 42 USCA 4331 et seq.)	Requires federal agencies to prepare an environmental impact statement for any major federal action significantly affecting the quality of the human environment
Occupational Safety and Health Act (1970; 29 USCA 651 et seq.)	Regulates worker health and safety for general, construction, and maritime industries; established several standards including provisions for workers involved with hazardous waste and emergency activities
Clean Water Act (1972 as amended 1977; 33 USCA 1251 et seq.)	Originally the Federal Water Pollution Control Act of 1948 as amended 1961, 1972, and 1977 to the Clean Water Act; regulates point and nonpoint discharges into surface waters; established discharge standards and a permit system for generators discharging directly into surface waters (National Pollutant Discharge Elimination System); technology and water quality-based effluent limitations; new source performance standards
Marine Protection, Research and Sanctuaries Act (1972; 33 USCA 1401 et seq.)	Regulates the discharge of wastes into the ocean
Safe Drinking Water Act (1974 as amended 1986; 42 USCA 300f et seq.)	Regulates contaminant levels in public water systems used as potable systems; established standards to prevent contamination of groundwater due to disposal activities such as deep-well injection
Hazardous Materials Transportation Act (1975 as amended 1976, 1994; 49 USCA 1801 et seq.)	Regulates the transport of hazardous materials; established provisions for packaging, labeling, placarding, manifesting, and shipping

Table 48.1 — Major U.S. Federal Legislative Acts Applicable to Hazardous Waste Management (cont.)

Toxic Substances Control Act (1976; 15 USCA 2601 et seq.)	Regulates manufacture and registration of chemical products; requires data regarding intended use, potential toxicity to humans, and potential toxicity to environment
Resource Conservation and Recovery Act (1976; 42 USCA 6901et seq.)	Regulates wastes legally classified as solid and hazardous wastes; established criteria and lists for classification; permit and manifest to track wastes from initial source to ultimate disposal; identifies toxic flammable, corrosive, and reactive wastes as hazardous waste and pathogenic (medical) wastes as solid waste
Surface Mining Control and Reclamation Act (1977; 30 USCA 1201 et seq.)	Regulates surface coal mining operations and associated wastes; established management practices to minimize environmental impact
Uranium Mill Tailings Radiation Control Act (1978 as amended 1988; 42 USCA 7901 et seq.)	Regulates disposal of mill tailings from uranium mining and processing; addresses health and environmental impact, technology
Low-Level Radioactive Waste Policy Act (1980 as amended 1985; 42 USCA 2021b et seq.)	Regulates disposal of low-level radioactive wastes; established standards of performance
Comprehensive Environmental Response, Compensation, and Liability Act (Superfund; 1980; 42 USCA 9601 et seq.)	Regulates activities involving uncontrolled releases of hazardous substances into the environment; established provisions for response investigation and remediation of waste sites
Nuclear Waste Policy Act (1982 as amended 1987; 42 USCA 10101 et seq.)	Regulates the disposal/storage of high-level radioactive wastes; established standards of performance and engineering design for geologic repositories used for storage
Hazardous and Solid Waste Amendments (1984; 42 USCA 6901 et seq.)	Amendment to RCRA to include corrective action for releases of hazardous substances from RCRA permitted facilities; established schedule to minimize use of land as disposal sites and address underground storage tanks
Superfund Amendments Reauthorization Act (1986; 42 USCA 9601 et seq.)	Amendment to CERCLA (Superfund); established provisions for remediation activities, schedules, and protecting hazardous waste workers; provisions for inventory and storage of hazardous substances; Title III addresses Community Right-to-Know
Medical Waste Tracking Act (1988; 42 USCA6992 et seq.)	Amendment to RCRA to address medical wastes, including pathogenic or infectious wastes
Oil Pollution Act (OPA)(1990; 33 USCA 2701 et seq.) shorelines	Regulates oil pollution prevention and control; includes broadened provisions for the cleanup of oil spills on navigable waters and
Hazardous Materials Transportation Uniform Safety Act (1990; 49 USCA)	Requires the Secretary of Transportation to promulgate regulations concerning the safe transport of hazardous materials in intrastate, interstate, and foreign commerce; helps to clarify conflicting state, local, and federal regulations
Pollution Prevention Act (1990; 42 USCA 13101 et seq.)	Emphasizes prevention of waste through recycling, source reduction, elimination of toxic materials, and other methods to attain environmentally conscious manufacturing
Federal Facility Compliance Act (1992; 42 USCA 6961 et seq.)	Broadens the waiver of sovereign immunity under RCRA and provides for state fines against the federal government for RCRA violations; speaks specifically to mixed wastes and requires the federal government to prepare an inventory of mixed wastes, an inventory of treatment methods, and a plan for managing and disposing of mixed wastes

management industry, a need for increased public awareness, and an increased demand for environmental and occupational health professionals. Although major changes have been observed, legislative efforts should continue to focus on policies and practices for decreasing the generation and disposal of hazardous wastes.[7] To do so effectively, however, may require additional regulatory and economic incentives for waste reduction. For example, regulatory programs offering less complicated multimedia operating permits could ease the burden of generators implementing changes to reduce waste emissions and discharges.[8] In addition, waste reduction involving recovery and reuse could result in cost reductions for manufacturing and other facilities.[9]

Major Federal Enactments and Amendments

Prior to the changes in the 1970s, hazardous waste impact was connected predominantly with protecting water resources (i.e., Federal Water Pollution Control Act of 1948, as amended to Clean Water Act of 1972) and the air (i.e., Clean Air Act of 1955, as amended 1977). Water protection regulations were expanded with the Marine Protection, Research, and Sanctuaries Act of 1972 and the Safe Drinking Water Act of 1974.

Regulatory controls placed on discharging wastes into the air and water resulted in 1) generators directing wastes to land disposal sites instead; 2) new waste streams as a result of pretreatment requirements for existing waste streams; and 3) construction of municipal treatment facilities, such as wastewater treatment facilities that treated sewage and generated biological sludges.

The Solid Waste Disposal Act of 1965 addressed land disposal, but the regulation was weak in respect to industrial wastes that contributed significantly to the generation of hazardous wastes. The act was later amended via the Resource Conservation and Recovery Act (RCRA) of 1976, which, in turn, was amended via the Hazardous and Solid Waste Amendments of 1984.

The addition of RCRA to the existing regulatory framework strengthened the controls on hazardous wastes discharged to air, water, and soil. Subtitle C of RCRA established a federal program to manage hazardous wastes from cradle to grave. The objective of the Subtitle C program is to ensure that hazardous waste is handled in a manner that protects human health and the environment. Therefore, there are Subtitle C regulations for the generation, transportation, and treatment, storage, or disposal of hazardous wastes. This means regulating a large number of hazardous waste handlers. EPA has on record thousands of treatment, storage, and disposal (TSD) facilities, transporters, and large quantity generators. There are regulations identifying the criteria to determine which solid wastes are hazardous; regulations for the three categories of hazardous waste handlers: generators, transporters, and TSD facilities. Subtitle C regulations set technical standards for the design and safe operation of TSD facilities. These standards are to minimize the release of hazardous waste into the environment. These regulations serve as the basis for developing and issuing permits required by RCRA for each facility. It is through the permitting process that EPA or a state applies the technical standards to TSD facilities. Subtitle C regulates only hazardous waste, which is a subset of solid waste. Subtitle D of RCRA manages nonhazardous solid waste.[10]

RCRA is augmented by additional regulations such as the Surface Mining Control and Reclamation Act of 1977 to address mining run-off; the Uranium Mill Tailings Radiation Control Act of 1978; the Low-Level Radioactive Waste Policy Act of 1980 and the Nuclear Waste Policy Act of 1982 to address radioactive wastes; and the Medical Waste Tracking Act of 1988 (an amendment to RCRA) to address infectious wastes. In addition, to address the production and use of raw materials that may contribute to the generation of hazardous wastes, the Toxic Substance Control Act of 1976 was enacted and the Federal Insecticide, Fungicide, and Rodenticide Act of 1947 was amended.

The Hazardous Material Transportation Act (HMTA) of 1975 was enacted to address issues of transportation of hazardous materials. The objective of the HMTA was to protect the public against risks to life and property from the transportation of hazardous materials in commerce. The Secretary of the Department of Transportation (DOT) can designate as hazardous material any quantity or form of a material that may create an unreasonable risk to health and safety or property. The enforcement of the HMTA is shared by each of the following administrations with DOT: Research and Special Programs Administration (RSPA) for container manufacturers; Federal Highway Administration (FHA) for motor carriers; Federal Railroad Administration (FRA) for rail carriers; Federal Aviation Administration (FAA) for air carriers; and the Coast Guard for shipments by water. The Hazardous Materials Table in 49 CFR Part 172.101 designates specific materials as hazardous for the purpose of transportation. It also classifies each material and specifies requirements pertaining to its packaging, labeling, and transportation.

The Comprehensive Environmental Response, Compensation, and Liability Act (CERCLA, "Superfund") of 1980 was enacted to regulate the remediation of past and future environmental releases of hazardous materials. This law created a tax on the chemical and petroleum industries and provided broad federal authority to respond directly to releases or threatened releases of hazardous substances that may endanger public health or the environment. CERCLA established prohibitions and requirements concerning closed and abandoned hazardous waste sites, liability of parties responsible for releases of hazardous waste at these sites, and a trust fund to provide for cleanup when no responsible party could be identified. The law authorizes short-term removals and long-term remedial responses.

CERCLA was later amended via the Superfund Amendments and Reauthorization Act (SARA) of 1986. This law took into account the experiences of the EPA in administering the complex Superfund program during its first six years, and as a result, made several important changes and additions to the program. SARA stressed the importance of permanent remedies and innovative treatment technologies in cleaning up hazardous waste sites; required Superfund actions to consider the standards and requirements found in other state and federal environmental laws and regulations; provided new enforcement authorities and settlement tools; increased state involvement in every phase of the Superfund program; increased focus on human health problems potentially created by hazardous waste sites; encouraged greater citizen participation in making decisions on how sites should be cleaned up; and increased the size of the clean up trust fund to $8.5 billion. SARA also required EPA to revise the hazard ranking system (HRS) to ensure that it accurately assessed the relative degree of risk to human health and the environment posed by hazardous waste sites being proposed for placement on the National Priorities List (NPL). Sites are to be listed on the NPL based on their HRS score and public comments.

Although the Occupational Safety and Health Act of 1970 addressed worker health and safety for general, maritime, and construction industries, provisions specific to hazardous waste operations were not mandated until Superfund was amended. Thus, the OSHA standard known as Hazardous Waste Operations and Emergency Response (HAZWOPER), defined in 29 CFR 1910.120 and repeated in 29 CFR 1926.65, was promulgated in 1987, to cover workers on hazardous waste sites. The HAZWOPER standard requires site managers to develop a site-specific health and safety plan (HASP) to address all anticipated health and safety hazards and to include methods for employee protection.

A key OSHA rule is the Hazard Communication Standard of 1986, defined in 29 CFR 1910.1200. It requires training employees about the hazards associated with chemicals in the workplace; availability of material safety data sheets; and the labeling of chemical containers. The Occupational Exposure to Hazardous Chemicals in Laboratories Standard of 1992, defined in 29 CFR 1910.1450, sets forth requirements pertaining to hazardous chemicals exposures in laboratories. The Standard for Process Safety Management of Highly Hazardous Chemicals of 1992, defined in 29 CFR 1910.119, lists over 100 highly hazardous chemicals and threshold quantities of these chemicals when a process hazard analysis is required. The Personal Protective Equipment Enhanced Standard of 1994, defined in 29 CFR 1910, Subpart I, provides requirements pertaining to personal protective equipment for workers on hazardous waste sites.

Definitions of Hazardous Wastes

Regulatory Definition

Prior to the enactment of RCRA, hazardous wastes in the form of air, water, and soil pollutants were regulated mainly by the Clean Air, Clean Water, and Solid Waste Disposal

Acts, respectively. RCRA was the first act, however, in which a definition for "hazardous waste" was provided. The term was defined by Congress as follows and appears in Subpart C of RCRA:

> Solid waste, or a combination of solid wastes, which because of its quantity, concentration or physical, chemical, or infectious characteristics may: (i) cause or significantly contribute to an increase in mortality or an increase in serious irreversible, or incapacitating reversible, illness; or (ii) pose a substantial present or potential hazard to human health or the environment when improperly treated, stored, transported, disposed or otherwise managed.(11)

EPA was subsequently mandated to establish the regulations by which hazardous wastes would be identified. The regulatory definition, although more specific, appears somewhat narrower in scope than that of Congress. For example, the original definition included "physical, chemical, or infectious" wastes, whereas the EPA definition focuses only on "chemical" wastes:

> Solid wastes, including solid, semi-solid, liquid, and gaseous materials, which (i) contain or are materials listed in the regulations; (ii) exhibit defined characteristics of toxicity, ignitability, corrosivity, or reactivity; or (iii) is not excluded from regulation as a hazardous waste.(12)

Due to the specificity and exclusions, the RCRA hazardous waste regulations can fail to address waste streams as complete systems that may be hazardous whether classified as chemical, radiological, or biological. Furthermore, one could state that from the regulatory perspective not all wastes that are potentially or actually hazardous are specifically classified as such. Thus, there are "hazardous wastes" and there are "hazardous wastes as per RCRA."

It should not be inferred at this point that many hazardous waste streams are ignored from a regulatory perspective because the RCRA regulations are too narrow. Instead, it should be understood that there are numerous applicable federal acts that address wastes, but only one, RCRA, specifically defines and designates them as hazardous wastes. The intentions of the other acts, nonetheless, are to regulate wastes that are hazardous.

Generic Definition

The generic definition of hazardous wastes is intended to encompass all of the regulated wastes and more. From a more generic perspective, hazardous wastes must be defined in more literal contexts and as complete systems. This is accomplished best by considering the two terms, "hazardous" and "wastes."

The term "<u>hazardous</u>" can be defined in this context as the potential or real tendency—due to toxicity, flammability, corrosiveness, reactivity, radioactivity, or infectivity—to directly or indirectly contaminate and damage the environment and/or cause injury or illness among the inhabitants. The term "<u>wastes</u>" can refer to unused and used solid, semisolid, liquid, or gaseous materials, including by-products, residuals, and fugitive emissions, subject to both intentional and unintentional discharge without regard for recovery or reuse. Waste materials meant for recovery or reuse would be more appropriately labeled "used." Wastes include materials intentionally and unintentionally discarded, discharged, recovered, or reused.

Thus, the definition of hazardous wastes can imply a different meaning depending on regulatory (e.g., RCRA) or generic usage. The issue of considering wastes hazardous or nonhazardous involves more than simple semantics. Indeed, the issue influences the ability to compile an accurate qualitative and quantitative assessment of the inventory of total hazardous waste generation in the United States and elsewhere.

Classification and Sources of Hazardous Wastes

Classes of Wastes

Hazardous wastes are commonly divided into three classes: chemical, radiological, and biological (see Table 48.2).

Chemical Wastes

<u>Chemical wastes</u> can be either organic (hydrocarbons or substituted hydrocarbons) or inorganic (metallic or nonmetallic elements) and often are a mixture of the two.

The hydrocarbons are composed solely of carbon and hydrogen; substituted hydrocarbons also include functional groups composed of elements such as chlorine, nitrogen, phosphorous, sulfur, or oxygen. Inorganic waste materials are typically in the form of salts, hydrides, and oxides. The hazards associated with mixtures of organic compounds and the fate of the compounds in the environment depends mainly on their chemical compositions and associated physical properties.

Chemicals of greatest concern include volatile organics, polyaromatic hydrocarbons, organochlorines, heavy metals, and several nonmetallic radicals, such as cyanides, sulfides, nitrates, and phosphates. Chemical wastes are hazardous if they exhibit a single characteristic or combination of characteristics described as toxic, flammable, corrosive, and reactive.

Although distinctions are made among the subclasses of chemical wastes, it should be noted that a waste consisting of even a single chemical component may exhibit a combination of characteristics. Indeed, because any chemical is toxic at a specific dose or concentration, then all flammable, corrosive, and reactive wastes, as well as radiological and some biological wastes, are also toxic. The reverse, however, is not necessarily true. That is, all toxic wastes do not exhibit other hazardous characteristics.

Toxic wastes are those discarded or used materials that may induce biochemical and physiological changes in human systems following either systemic contact via absorption into blood and tissues, or local contact. The changes may be ultimately manifested as adverse effects such as morphological and functional abnormalities, illnesses, and premature deaths among those exposed or their offspring. As suggested above, toxicity is inherent in all compounds. The toxicity of a given agent, however, may be directly attributable to an original parent compound or indirectly attributable to an active metabolite formed via biotransformation in a human system. Secondary toxicants can be generated by flammable, corrosive, and reactive wastes in the form of toxic by-products released from reactions, fires, and explosions.

Flammable wastes include materials that serve as fuels (reducing agents) that can ignite and sustain a chain reaction when combined in a suitable ratio with oxygen (oxidizing agent) in the presence of an ignition source (heat, spark). Flammable wastes consist mainly of contaminated organic solvents, oils, pesticides, plasticizers, and complex organic sludges. Flammable materials are characterized in 29 CFR 1910.106(a) as having a low flash point (i.e., <38°C or 100°F), which is usually inversely related to vapor pressure. A flash point of less than 60°C (closed cup) is the criterion used by the EPA to determine if a chemical is hazardous by ignitibility. DOT classifies materials with flash points less than 60°C as flammable. In general, organic compounds vaporize at relatively lower temperatures and are much more sensitive to heat than inorganic compounds. Flammable wastes pose an obvious hazard due to potential burns to human tissue. Indirectly during combustion, however, flammable wastes can contribute to the formation of toxic atmospheres due to generation of by-products such as strong irritants and chemical asphyxiants, as well as by consumption of molecular oxygen during combustion.

Table 48.2 — Generic Classification of Hazardous Wastes

Class of Hazardous Waste	*Hazardous Characteristics*
Chemical	Toxicity Flammability Corrosivity Reactivity
Radiological	Radioactivity
Biological	Infectivity

Corrosive wastes include those materials that can induce severe irritation and destruction of human tissue on contact due to accelerated dehydration reactions. Corrosive wastes also include materials that can dissolve metal in a relatively short period of time. Typical examples of corrosives are organic and inorganic acids and bases. The strengths of acids and bases and the extremes of pH (i.e., <pH 2 and >pH 12.5, respectively) are directly correlated to the degree of corrosiveness.

Reactive wastes consist of chemically unstable materials typically characterized as either strong oxidizing or reducing agents. Chemical instability results in increased sensitivity to violent reactions, which may result in extremely rapid generation of heat and gases. In turn, this may culminate in ignition, explosion, or emission of toxic by-products. Some unstable wastes can react with air or water. Other wastes react if the pH of the medium they are in is altered. For example, wastes containing either cyanides or sulfides are more likely to react if the pH is increased above 2 or decreased below 12, resulting in generation of toxic hydrogen cyanide or hydrogen sulfide gases.

Radiological Wastes

Radiological wastes consist of radioactive components that emit ionizing radiation. The radioactive components are chemical elements or compounds that are electrochemically unstable due to an imbalance of protons (p^+) or neutrons (n^o) in the atomic nuclei. The elements and compounds undergo natural reactions to achieve stability by emanation of atomic energy in the form of particulates and electromagnetic photons. The particles and photons impart energy in excess of 30 electron volts to the matter with which they interact, resulting in ionization.

Ionizing particulate radiation consists of alpha particles ($2\ n^o + 2\ p^+$ in the form of a charged helium nucleus, ${}^4_2He^{+2}$); beta particles (negatron as e- and positron as e^+); and neutron particles (n^o). Ionizing electromagnetic radiation consists of X-rays and gamma rays. The particulate and electromagnetic forms of ionizing radiation can interact by direct or indirect ionization of macromolecular or cellular components of the human body. Ionizing radiation may induce adverse biochemical and physiological changes manifested as abnormalities, illnesses, or premature deaths among those exposed or their offspring.

Radiological wastes often are designated as high-level or low-level based on the intensity and type of ionizing radiation emitted. Spent nuclear fuels are examples of high-level radioactive wastes. Radioisotopes, such as those used in scientific research and medical diagnostics, like cobalt-60, are examples of low-level radioactive wastes.

Biological Wastes

Biological wastes are commonly referred to as pathogenic or infectious wastes. There are at least 193 identified pathogenic biologic agents that may be encountered in the environment.(13) They consist of agents that, if introduced into the human body, may disrupt biochemical and physiological function through infectivity or toxicity. The disruption can result in illness and death if the immune system cannot destroy the biological agents. Infectivity is related to the virulence and the population density of organisms present at a given target site. Toxicity can be induced by biological agents that synthesize and release a chemical toxin. Examples of pathogenic agents include bacteria, rickettsia, fungi, protozoans, helminths, nematodes, viruses, plants, and insects. Unlike radiological and chemical substances, all biological agents except viruses are examples of biotic or living organisms. Viruses are extremely simple microorganisms composed of biochemicals (i.e., proteins and nucleic acids) that may insert themselves into human cells, multiple, cause disruption, and then disease.

Sources and Estimating Amounts of Hazardous Waste

The traditional concept of hazardous waste generation often considered only chemical wastes from industrial manufacturing sources. A more complete view, however, includes the classes of radiological and biological wastes, as well as additional sources, such as from clinical, research, agricultural, business, and household settings.

A variety of statistics are available estimating the volume or mass of hazardous wastes. Many are based on the RCRA definition of hazardous wastes, and so do not include several waste streams such as radioactive and infectious wastes. Several factors that influence the ability to accurately estimate the total volume and mass of hazardous wastes generated domestically and internationally(14) include 1) variation in the scope of the estimates; 2) variation in the definitions of hazardous waste; 3) variation in measures for estimating the amount of waste generated or the capacity for storage, treatment, or disposal; and 4) errors due to poor data-collection techniques. Nonetheless, calculations based on one report,(15) assuming a population of 250 million, estimated that approximately 5.67×10^9 metric tons of gaseous, liquid, and solid wastes are generated annually in the United States.

Major Phases and Program Elements of Hazardous Waste Management

Overview

The major phases of hazardous waste management consist of generation; processing for recovery and reuse; transportation; treatment; storage; and disposal (as shown schematically in Figure 48.1). Inherent to the management scheme are auxiliary program elements that include organized occupational hygiene activities and preparedness for emergency response to environmental releases.

Generation

The source or generator of waste materials produces waste streams at a particular facility or site. Generators must qualitatively identify and quantitatively inventory their waste streams[16] to determine whether the wastes are 1) classified as chemical, radiological, or biological; 2) characterized as toxic, corrosive, flammable, reactive, radioactive, or infectious; 3) generically classified as hazardous or nonhazardous; and 4) legislatively classified as hazardous or nonhazardous. In addition, it is essential that generators account for the hazardous waste management process, including 1) on-site discharges to air, water, and land; 2) treatment, reuse, or disposal on site; and 3) transportation for treatment, reuse, or disposal off site.

Depending on the nature of the facility and the wastes generated, the wastes may be managed on site. From an economic perspective, on-site recovery, treatment, and disposal is favored because it leaves less waste to transport to off-site facilities.[17] Increased expense of managing generated wastes and the related risk of liability for wastes produced have shifted the emphasis toward reduction of waste production. Process modification and use of less hazardous chemicals[18,19] are two approaches to achieve waste reduction, but several other strategies have been suggested[20], including on-site recycling of household, office, and industrial wastes.

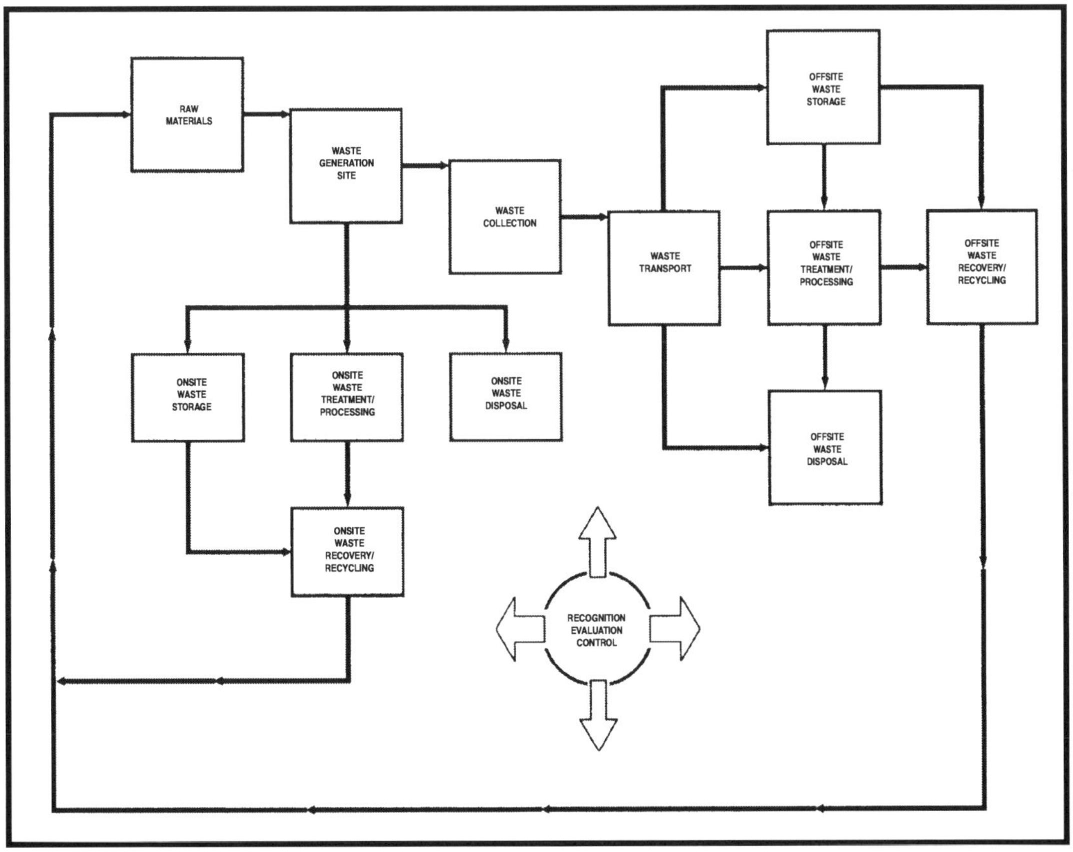

Figure 48.1 — Schematic diagram of the hazardous waste management process.

Short-Term Storage

"Short-term" implies temporary storage by generators during the interim between generation and processing on site or transporting off site to another facility. Storage practices and strategies must focus on 1) the nature of the wastes; 2) use of appropriate containers; 3) isolation of incompatible materials; 4) labeling of containers; 5) containment of material and releases; 6) duration of storage; and 7) overall storage safety.[21] These factors must be considered by generators on site as well as the off-site facilities that store wastes prior to processing, treating, disposing, or long-term storing. Numerous containers are used for stationary and mobile storage (see Table 48.3).[22]

Selection of storage containers involves consideration of a number of factors to ensure that applicable regulations are met.[23]

Transportation

An alternative to on-site processing is to have pretreated and treated wastes transported off site. Wastes may be transported off site on land using vehicles (see Table 48.4), though this may increase the risk of accidental release of hazardous materials into the environment. Wastes are typically contained in high-volume bulk storage tanks or low-volume storage drums during vehicular transport. The storage containers must be labeled and transport vehicles placarded during transit.

Table 48.3 — Summary of Major Container Types for Storing Hazardous Wastes

Container Type	*Description*	*Chemicals Stored*
Nonbulk Containers	May consist of single or multiple packaging	Transport liquid and dry chemical products (not gaseous)
Bags	Flexible packaging typically used for solid materials containing up to 100 lb.	Cement, fertilizers, and pesticides
Bottles	Glass, plastic, metal, or ceramic jugs or jars typically shipped in ounces up to 20 gallons	Antifreeze, laboratory reagents, corrosive liquids
Boxes	Rigid outside packaging for nonbulk packages for aerosol containers, bottles, and cans	Designed to carry variety of hazardous chemicals already containerized
Multicell packaging	Form-fitting box with one or more bottles	Specialty chemicals (e.g., hydrochloric and sulfuric acids or solvents)
Carboys	Glass or plastic bottles encased in outer packaging of polystyrene boxes, wooden crates, or plywood drums	Sulfuric acid, hydrochloric acid, ammonium hydroxide, or potable water
Drums	Metal, plastic, fiberboard, or other suitable material; capacity up to 55 gallons. Drums have removable "open" or nonremovable "closed" heads. Open heads attached to drum by ring or lugs. Closed/tight head contains two openings called "bungs" with 2-inch or ¾-inch diameters; may have liners or linings	Solid materials commonly found in open drums and liquid materials in those with closed/tight heads; containers carry a variety of contents depending on chemical characteristics.
Jerricans	Metal or plastic packaging with rectangular or polygonal cross-section	Antifreeze and other specialty products
Wooden barrels	Commonly called "kegs"; made of wood with steel, iron, or hardwood hoops	Distilled spirits

(continued on the next page.)

Some waste streams and by-products of processed waste streams are transported off site via emission into the atmosphere and discharge into surface waters and sewer systems. These are not always considered transport processes. The quality and quantity of wastes generated directly into the air and water must comply with the applicable air and water pollution control regulations.

Changes in treatment technology are constantly seen in response to environmental issues, regulatory controls, and legal

Table 48.3 — Summary of Major Container Types for Storing Hazardous Wastes (cont.)

Container Type	*Description*	*Chemicals Stored*
Bulk Containers	Cargo tanks (i.e., tank wagons, tank trucks, tank trailers, or tankers) are bulk transport vehicles	Transport liquid, dry, and gaseous chemical products
Nonpressure tanks	Usually uninsulated, bottom-unloaded, oval-shaped cargo tanks with cable-operated valve assembly, emergency shut-off system, and safety relief valve (<4 psig); often compartmentalized to carry multiple contents	Designed to carry flammable or combustible liquids (e.g., diesel, gasoline)
Low-pressure tanks	Usually bottom-unloaded, round-shaped cargo tanks with hydraulic-operated valve assembly, emergency shut-off system, fusible links, and safety relief valve (> 25 psig); often compartmentalized to carry multiple contents	Designed to carry poisons, certain volatile flammable/combustible liquids, and mild corrosives
Medium-pressure tanks	Usually top rear-unloaded, round-shaped cargo tanks with rear external ring stiffeners that carry a smaller capacity; design pressure may range from 35 to100 psig.	Designed to carry highly corrosive products (e.g., sulfuric acid, sodium hydroxide)
High-pressure tanks	Usually cylindrical with elliptical ends; usually bottom-unloaded; pressure > 500 psig	Designed to carry compressed gases (anhydrous ammonia or liquefied petroleum gases (LPG)) and hazardous liquids
Intermodal containers "Iso-tanks"	Bulk containers generally used in international transport; consist of a single noncompartmentalized vessel held by frame for lifting with cranes; most designed as pressure vessels	Designed to carry a variety of hazardous chemicals

Table 48.4 — Major Vehicles for Land Transport of Hazardous Wastes

Vehicle Type	*Description*	*Chemicals Transported*
General service tank cars	Nonpressure tank (pressures <100 psig) equipped with rupture disk or relief valves mounted in the car body	Designed to carry a variety of hazardous materials
Pressure tank cars	Designed to handle tank pressures >100 psig and <600 psig; have fittings mounted on top of car with protective housing	Designed to carry hazardous materials with high vapor pressures (e.g., ethylene oxide, LPG, anhydrous ammonia, chlorine)
Cryogenic tank cars	Very low tank temperatures	Designed to handle cryogenic materials, such as liquefied natural gas
High-pressure tube cars	Tank pressures >600 psig	Designed to carry high-pressure materials

liabilities.[24] Related to these changes is the development of a major waste transportation, off-site treatment, and storage industry and frequent public concern regarding the siting of treatment, storage, and disposal (TSD) facilities.[25]

Treatment, Long-Term Storage, and Disposal

Treatment alters a waste stream or contaminated waste site to reduce, eliminate, or immobilize hazardous constituents. Numerous treatment technologies are presently available and in development.[19,26–28] Treatment typically precedes long-term storage and disposal to stabilize the waste streams and reduce the volume and mass, if feasible. Some waste streams, however, may not be amenable to treatment and are stored or disposed as they are.

The purpose of long-term storage and disposal is to segregate waste streams from the environmental surroundings. Long-term storage implies quasi-permanent containment until the hazardous characteristic dissipates or technology is developed to eliminate the hazard. Disposal, however, implies disregard for return and, thus, is considered to be permanent storage or release.

Methods for Treatment of Hazardous Wastes

Concepts

Waste reduction can occur through source segregation, process modification, end-product substitution, and waste recovery and recycling.[29] Source segregation involves separating the hazardous from the relatively nonhazardous components to reduce the volume of a waste. Process modifications can reduce wastes by changing operational parameters, using less hazardous or smaller amounts of raw materials, or making use of newer, more efficient equipment. End-product substitution focuses on production of commodities that will result in decreased hazardous waste generation during manufacture and a less hazardous product. The concept of waste recovery and recycling reflects the idea that one generator's waste may be another's raw material. For instance, recovered wastes can be used in manufacturing processes and as supplemental fuels. Emphasis is placed on minimizing processing and, accordingly, determining which wastes can be used in their original state.

In general, waste streams should be subjected to some type of treatment prior to reuse or disposal. Those not recoverable or reusable should be destroyed or sequestered in some safe manner. In either situation, various treatment methods are applied.

The treatment of hazardous wastes focuses on three major concepts: 1) separation of a hazardous component from a waste stream to reduce the quantity of hazardous waste; 2) elimination of the hazardous component via destruction and/or detoxification of molecules to yield less hazardous compounds; and 3) segregation of an entire hazardous waste stream or contaminated area from noncontaminated areas by immobilization and containment.[30] Many treatment processes result in the generation of residuals and by-products in the form of airborne particulates/aerosols, gases, and vapors; chemical and biological sludges; saturated sorbents; and ashes. These warrant additional precautions as well as treatment and disposal.[16] Treatment methods are classified as thermal, physical, biological, or chemical processes.

Thermal Treatment

Thermal treatment processes involve destruction of hazardous organic components through elevated temperatures with concomitant reduction in volume (see Table 48.5). Common thermal methods include incineration and pyrolysis.[31] Some innovative technologies involving a combination of elevated temperature and pressure also have emerged, including volume reduction via supercritical water oxidation.[32]

Thermal processes such as incineration typically generate airborne emissions and residual solids. The composition of these residues depends on the composition of the waste input. Typical residues include carbon dioxide, water, sulfur dioxide, nitrogen oxides, hydrochloric acid, particulates, and ash. Hazardous residues are collected and subjected to additional treatment or disposal.

Physical Treatment

Physical treatment involves nonthermal processes that separate a hazardous component from a waste stream or segregate a hazardous waste stream from a

Table 48.5— Major Methods for Thermal Treatment of Hazardous Wastes

Process	*Treatment Methods and Summary of Concepts*
Incineration	Hazardous organic components are oxidized via high-oxygen combustion at temperatures ranging from 425 to 1650°C. Efficiency depends on duration of incineration (time), mixing and oxygenation (turbulence), and thermal conditions (temperature). **Rotary kiln incinerators:** Hazardous solid, liquid, and gaseous wastes (particularly solids and semisolids such as contaminated soils and sludges, respectively) are placed in a rotating cylinder that increases exposure of surface area and, in turn, oxygenation and heat transfer. **Multiple hearth incinerators:** Wastes enter at the top of the unit, which consists of a series of alternating shelves (or hearths) and a vertical rotating cylinder. Wastes descend from hearth to hearth as combustion occurs, permitting longer residence time in the incinerator. **Fluidized bed incinerators:** Wastes are injected into the unit and collide with hot, inert granules suspended via forced aeration from a perforated section at the base of the incinerator. Thermal interaction is enhanced via conduction of heat from granules to waste. Circulating bed combustion is an alternative for which increased efficiency is achieved via a higher operation velocity and use of fewer and finer granules. **Liquid injection incinerators:** Liquid wastes are atomized via a nozzle as they enter the incinerator, resulting in enhanced treatment efficiency via increased exposure of surface area to elevated temperatures and oxygen.
Pyrolysis	A form of incineration in which combustion occurs in an atmosphere deficient in molecular oxygen. The unit consists of a pyrolyzing chamber operated at 537 to 926°C and a secondary fume incinerator operated at 982 to 1648°C. The advantage of pyrolysis over conventional incineration is that inorganic components are not volatilized, so fewer corrosive air contaminants are generated.
Boilers and furnaces	Wastes such as flammable petroleum-based solvents are burned in industrial-scale boilers and furnaces as a supplemental fuel.
Molten salt reactors	Liquid, solid, or gaseous wastes are mixed with a molten bath of sodium carbonate or calcium carbonate salt heated to 815 to 980°C. Wastes are degraded via combustion, and corrosive residual acids (e.g., HCl) are neutralized. Residuals include ash plus numerous salts.
Plasma arc reactors	Wastes are exposed to an electrically conductive ionized gas (plasma) heated to temperatures above 28,000°C. Hazardous components are atomized, ionized, and eventually destroyed. An alternative is the microwave plasma reactor in which microwave energy is used as the source of electrons to produce a plasma.
Wet oxidation	Non-halogenated organic components are destroyed via combustion under highly oxidized conditions in a liquid state. Combustion reactions occur at temperatures ranging from 175 to 349°C and pressures of 68 to 136 atm. It is applicable for waste streams too dilute for efficient incineration and too toxic for biological treatment.
Supercritical water oxidation	Organic components are oxidized and degraded when a waste stream is mixed with highly oxygenated water maintained at temperatures exceeding 374°C and pressures exceeding 218 atm.
Vitrification	An in situ process in which soil contaminated with inorganic (including radioactive) components is exposed to intense electrical current. The soil initially melts and subsequently cools into a glass-like (vitrified) solid, immobilizing and thus segregating the contaminates from the surrounding area. Vitrified soil is either left in place or excavated for off-site disposal or storage. The process is also used for other applications such as combining a waste stream with borosilicate glass. The mixture is vitrified and the solid product stored or disposed.
Pasteurization	Wastes containing pathogenic organisms are heated to temperatures in excess of 70°C for a given time period to destroy pathogens.

noncontaminated area (see Table 48.6). Thus, theoretically, a hazardous waste stream is converted into separated and more concentrated hazardous and nonhazardous components. The concentrated hazardous component has less volume or mass than the original combined waste stream and is subjected to additional treatment, long-term storage, or permanent disposal.

Biological Treatment

Biological treatment processes use living organisms to accelerate the decomposition of organic wastes (see Table 48.7). The processes can be conducted under aerobic or anaerobic conditions depending on the type of organisms used as the biotic catalysts.[33] The methods use natural[30] and bioengineered species[34] of microbes as sources of enzymes to catalyze transformational reactions; accordingly, the process could be referred to as biochemical treatment. Although use of aerobic microorganisms is more common, the broad range of applications for anaerobic organisms is receiving increased attention.[35] In situ bioremediation of media such as contaminated soil and groundwater is rapidly increasing.[36] Studies also suggest that combining mixed communities of biological organisms, dynamically fluctuated temperatures, and geochemical catalysts accelerates biodegradation.[37]

Chemical Treatment

Chemical treatment degrades or separates hazardous components through the interaction of a chemical reagent and a waste stream (see Table 48.8). The principle is

Table 48.6 — Major Methods for Physical Treatment of Hazardous Wastes

Process	*Treatment Methods and Summary of Concepts*
Flocculation and sedimentation/ filtration	Colloidal solids within a waste stream interact and aggregate (flocculate). Flocculated solids are separated from the waste stream via sedimentation or filtration.
Dissolved air flotation	Insoluble components are separated from a liquid waste stream by aeration under high pressure and subsequent exposure to conditions at atmospheric pressure. Bubbles containing the insoluble components rise to the surface, where they are removed by skimming.
Carbon adsorption	Liquid or gaseous waste streams are passed though beds of porous activated carbon (charcoal) granules. Various organic and inorganic components adsorb to the carbon and are separated from the waste stream.
Resin adsorption/ ion exchange	Liquid or gaseous waste streams are passed through beds of ionized, porous, inert, resin granules. Organic and inorganic ionic components exchange with innocuous ions on the resins and are separated from the waste stream.
Liquid absorption	Gaseous waste streams are scrubbed as they pass through or interact with liquid reagents that absorb specific gaseous components.
Stripping	Volatile components are separated from solid or liquid waste either by the passage of air or steam or aeration/atomization, respectively.
Distillation/ condensation	Volatile components are separated from a waste stream via evaporation of the material and subsequent condensation and fractional collection of distillate.
Evaporation	Nonvolatile components are separated from a liquid waste stream by evaporation of the liquid phase via boiling to leave a solid nonvolatile residue.
Reverse osmosis	Liquid waste streams are passed at high pressure through a semipermeable membrane, thus separating hazardous inorganic and organic compounds from the waste stream by filtration.
Electrolysis	Organic and inorganic ions (e.g., metals) are separated from a waste stream by the addition of an electric current that causes the attraction of negatively and positively charged ions to oppositely charged electrodes.
Electrodialysis	Hazardous ions are separated from a waste stream via electrically enhanced differential diffusion across a semipermeable membrane.
Photolysis	Organic components in a waste stream are exposed to ultraviolet (UV) light to catalyze the destruction of chemical bonds via lysis.
Beta/gamma/UV irradiation	Wastes containing pathogenic organisms are irradiated with ionizing or nonionizing radiation to destroy the pathogens.

similar to biological treatment in that an exogenous substance is combined with a waste stream to enhance separation via adsorption or degradation via catalysis. However, biological treatment involves biotic agents (i.e., living organisms) while chemical treatment involves use of abiotic reagents (i.e., synthetic chemicals). Mixing chemicals with wastes separates hazardous components by coagulation, flocculation, and demulsification of solids and organics.[38] Solvents can be used to extract hazardous components from waste streams such as process sludges.[39] Chemical catalysts such as iron have been added to accelerate degradation of toxic substances.[40] Hydrogenation technology is emerging as an approach to chemically detoxify organics in liquid waste streams.[41]

Methods for Long-Term Storage and Disposal of Hazardous Wastes

Concepts

Hazardous waste treatment processes typically reduce the quantity of waste and render it less hazardous. Regardless of treatment processes, however, residuals and by-products (e.g., airborne emissions, incinerator ash, chemical and biological sludges, saturated sorbents) are generated. In addition, many hazardous wastes are not amenable to recovery, reuse, and treatment and therefore must be managed in their original states. The options at this phase of the hazardous waste management scheme consist of disposal or long-term storage of non-treated wastes, residuals, and by-products.

Long-term storage is a quasi-permanent method of confining wastes in special structures, geologic repositories, or surface impoundments until the hazards dissipate or treatment and disposal are developed. Long-term storage is a common option for handling radiological wastes.[42] Disposal typically involves a more permanent discharging and discarding of wastes without concern for additional or subsequent handling. Table 48.9 shows the major methods of storage and disposal.

Disposal Into Air

Wastes are discharged into the air via both mobile and stationary sources. Discharges can occur via direct emission from stacks and indirect emissions from volatile compounds.

Table 48.7 – Major Methods for Biological Treatment of Hazardous Wastes

Process	*Treatment Methods and Summary of Concepts*
Activated sludge	An aerobic process in which wastewater is pumped through an aeration tank where a suspended community of microorganisms consume and degrade the organic components.
Trickling filter	An aerobic process in which wastewater is sprayed over a fixed medium inhabited by a community of microorganisms that consume and degrade the organic components.
Rotating biological contact	An aerobic process in which wastewater is pumped through a chamber containing a series of continuously rotating disks inhabited by a community of microorganisms that consume and degrade the organic components.
Stabilization pond	A combined aerobic and anaerobic process in which wastewater is pumped into an anthropogenic reservoir where suspended and settled microorganisms consume and degrade the organic components.
Composting	A combined aerobic and anaerobic process suitable for semisolid waste streams such as sludges. Sludges are typically mixed with wood chips and arranged in windrows or piles, where microorganisms consume and degrade the organic components.
Anaerobic digestion	An anaerobic process suitable for semisolid waste streams such as sludges. The waste stream is placed under anaerobic conditions where a community of anaerobic microorganisms consume and degrade organic components.
Aerobic digestion	An aerobic process suitable for semisolid waste streams such as sludges. The process is similar to the activated sludge process but waste streams are subjected to extended retention time.
In situ bioremediation	Populations of microorganisms, either natural and/or bioengineered species, are introduced to a contaminated soil or groundwater site to consume and degrade hazardous organic components.

Table 48.8 — Major Methods for Chemical Treatment of Hazardous Wastes

Process	*Treatment Methods and Summary of Concepts*
Neutralization	The pH of an acidic or alkaline waste is adjusted to control corrosivity or maintain metallic components in a soluble state via the addition of an acidic or basic reagent.
Precipitation	Addition of a reagent to a waste stream to separate a soluble inorganic component by its conversion to an insoluble precipitate.
Hydrolysis	Addition of enzymatic reagents into a waste stream to catalyze the destruction of hazardous organic components via insertion of water molecules and subsequent lysis of chemical bonds.
Chemical oxidation	Addition of oxidizing reagents (e.g., air, hydrogen peroxide, ozone, perchloric acid, potassium permanganate) to enhance destruction of hazardous organic components via oxidation reactions. Reactions are accelerated via catalysts (e.g., iron, cobalt, UV light).
Chemical reduction	Addition of reducing reagents (e.g., alkalies) into a waste stream to enhance destruction of certain hazardous organic and inorganic components via reduction reactions.
Solvent extraction	Addition of a solvent to a waste stream to separate/remove a hazardous solid or liquid component.
Chemical solidification/ fixation/calcining/ grouting	Addition of reagents (e.g., Portland cement, silicates, fly ash, clay, calcium oxide, asphalt, polyethylene) to a waste stream to induce solidification and immobilize hazardous organic and inorganic components.

Discharge of hazardous emissions into the air can be considered a combination of disposal and treatment because the wastes are simultaneously discarded and diluted to some extent. The practice of incinerating wastes at sea is another example of this concept. Nonetheless, since wastes disposed into the air can also be transported to other destinations, concerns regarding widespread environmental contamination are justified.

Disposal Into Water

Wastes are discharged into the water via both point (specific) and nonpoint (nonspecific) sources. As with air dispersal, the waste stream is both discharged and diluted. The practice, including dumping wastes into the oceans, is highly debated due to the obvious risks of adverse environmental and public health impact following widespread transport of contaminants.

Disposal and Long-Term Storage in Soil

Although long-term storage and disposal on land for hazardous wastes is discouraged and even banned to some extent (as per the Hazardous and Solid Waste Amendments of 1984), major disposal practices have included use of landfills, surface impoundments, and deep-well injection. Storage of noncontainerized, bulk liquid, regulated hazardous wastes in landfills and disposal on land are prohibited. However, researchers have suggested efficient means of simultaneously treating and disposing of some types of hazardous wastes on land[38], and innovative treatment technologies are being researched and developed as alternatives to landfills.[43]

Adverse Human Health Impact Due to Hazardous Waste Exposure

Contributing Factors

Hazardous wastes, in most cases, exhibit a degree of heterogeneity relative to their constituents. The variations in composition and hazardous properties differ from one operation to another, and to a greater extent, from one generator to another. The waste materials may be in the form of a solid, liquid, gas, or combination. The associated hazards may be radiological, chemical, biological, or a mixture. In addition, exposure to the associated hazards may be via direct or indirect pathways and result in adverse human health impact.

The risks associated with hazardous waste exposure may be related to 1) whether

Table 48.9 — Major Methods for Long-Term Storage and Disposal of Hazardous Wastes

Media Classification	*Long-Term Storage and Disposal Method and Summary of Concept*
Air	**Combustion:** Thermal processes (e.g., incineration and pyrolysis, combustion engines, boilers and furnaces, manufacturing processes) that vent airborne emissions into the atmosphere for dispersal and disposal. Waste streams may be altered by natural physical and chemical processes.
	Evaporation: Intentinal or unintentional volatilization of hazardous liquids and sublimation of hazardous solids into the atmosphere.
Water	**Ocean dumping:** Transportation of wastes for dispersal and disposal on the ocean floor.
	Surface water discharge: Waste streams are discharged directly into surface waters or indirectly via sewer systems for dilution and disposal; original waste stream may be altered by natural biological, physical, and chemical treatment.
Soil	**Landfilling:** The placement of wastes, exclusive of liquid wastes, into an engineered land burial site. Landfills consist of impervious sides and bottoms to minimize horizontal and vertical leaching into the substrata. Leachate collection and monitoring wells are installed as an extra precaution. Wastes are buried and periodically covered to form discrete compartments or cells. The sites are eventually capped with a final impervious layer on closure. In many respects, landfilling is simply another form of long-term storage.
	Deep-well injection: Liquid wastes are pumped into underground geologic cavities (i.e., vacant aquifers) within the earth for long-term storage.
	Repository storage: Applies predominantly to high-level radioactive wastes. The wastes are placed in engineered steel-lined concrete tanks designed to shield emanating ionizing radiation. An alternative is storage in natural geologic formations within the earth's surface and subsurface.
	Surface impoundment: Discharge and discarding of wastes into anthropogenic reservoirs for storage.
	Land application: Liquid and semiliquid wastes are applied via spraying on or injecting into the soil surface in anticipation of degradation and immobilization due to combined biological and physicochemical interaction. The process could be viewed as a combined treatment and disposal process.

the wastes contain pure substances or compounds, which may be present in high concentrations; 2) whether they contain mixtures of substances that individually might not be as hazardous, but when combined present an increased risk; 3) whether they have properties that in small volumes and masses are innocuous, but are hazardous in larger volumes and masses; 4) whether they are in solid, semisolid, liquid, or gaseous form; and 5) the manner in which the wastes are generated, treated, and disposed.

The hazards encountered may be due to direct exposure to a given waste stream or indirect exposure via contact with by-products or residuals. Indirect exposures also include contact with contaminated food, air, or water along with impact associated with fires and explosions. In addition, the risk of toxicity depends on the mode of exposure and may be exacerbated by simultaneous exposures to multiple contaminants. Thus, to categorize, a waste 1) may be hazardous as generated; 2) may subsequently combine with other contaminants and react to produce magnified and secondary hazards; 3) may pose a greater hazard depending on mode of exposure and subsequent synergistic, potentiation, and additive effects; and 4) may pose a greater hazard by reason of location or method of handling or processing. As a result, stringent precautionary measures and controls should be implemented and maintained during all phases of hazardous waste management. This involves control of waste streams from the source of generation to the point of ultimate treatment, long-term storage, or disposal.

Impact on Human Health

Given an understanding of the generic classes of hazardous wastes, it is apparent that flammable, corrosive, and reactive waste materials may cause obvious, immediate effects (e.g., burns and explosions) due to acute or short-term exposures. Toxic wastes, however, may cause both immediate effects (e.g., asphyxiation and irritation) due to acute exposure and insidious, delayed effects (e.g., physiological dysfunction, mutagenesis, and carcinogenesis) due to chronic or long-term exposures.

There is public concern over both kinds of effects. It appears, however, that the public is more intimidated by the threat of delayed adverse effects resulting from exposure to toxic, radiological, and biologic wastes. This is apparently due to the mystery surrounding the potential for delayed effects, as opposed to the more obvious threat of immediate adverse effects one might associate with flammables and reactives. Because of this perception, wastes that should be classified generically as hazardous are often incorrectly qualified from a public perspective as being only toxic. Therefore, part of hazardous waste management is to develop a risk communication plan to deal with community-perceived risks. This plan includes determining who your target audience is, deciding which topics are most important to your audience, and developing messages that will adequately explain all perceived and real risks.(44)

However, the risk of injury and illness from flammable and reactive waste materials is very real. For example, there have been reported fires and explosions at hazardous waste sites due to flammables and reactives.

Studies also have investigated increased cancer mortality near hazardous waste sites(45) and the effects of hazardous waste on reproductive health.(46) Other studies report that exposure to low-level concentrations of airborne contaminants generated from hazardous waste sites may increase the prevalence of illness complaints from the surrounding neighborhood.(47) Another study suggested that residents exposed to higher levels of waste-site chemicals exhibited more adverse neurologic effects than residents with lower exposure.(48) The illnesses experienced also include psychological effects, as shown by demonstration of mental distress related to concern over perceived exposure to hazardous waste sites.(49) Equally important for consideration are studies suggesting an influence of reporting biases and possible hypochondriasis among individuals located in the vicinity of hazardous waste sites.(50) Unfortunately, epidemiologic studies suggest that there is no model to establish simple cause-and-effect relationships for these psychosocial issues.(51) Regardless, the threat of exposure has resulted in voluntary and involuntary emigration of residents from their neighborhoods.(52)

Risk Factors

The risk associated with hazardous wastes focuses on four major factors: 1) the hazards inherent to the wastes; 2) the release of wastes from facilities, sites, and vehicles; 3) direct and indirect exposure of humans; and 4) the variability of response and susceptibility to illness, if any, among those humans exposed. The first three factors apply to hazardous wastes in general, regardless of classification. The fourth factor, however, applies only to hazardous wastes subclassified as radioactive, toxic, or infectious. There is minimal or no variation in human susceptibility and vulnerability to the primary injuries from events involving flammable, corrosive, or reactive wastes.

Studies conducted on human volunteers continue to demonstrate variation among human responses and susceptibility to toxic, radioactive, and infectious waste exposures.(53) Basic toxicological and pathological concepts recognize several contributing factors, including age, weight, gender, health, mode of exposure, and entry path of toxicants. In addition, the problem is complicated by the potential presence of mixtures of components at a given waste site.(54)

Despite the perceived and real risks of occurrence, the number of published health effects related to exposures to hazardous wastes are low.(55) This may be attributable to inaccurate and incomplete assessment.(56) Although some studies concede that there is no demonstration of serious health effects, these studies are influenced by two major factors: 1) Many were based on a low number of studies at actual sites; and 2) most focus only on cancer, birth defects, and other clinically defined illness, so subtle health effects may go undetected. Improved mechanisms such as biomarkers to identify changes associated with toxic exposures may allow for earlier and more accurate assessment.(57)

Thus, qualitatively, there are inherent risks to health in relation to hazardous wastes. Quantitatively, however, it is often difficult to assess these risks, especially with regard to toxic, radioactive, and infectious exposures and impact. Risk assessment for these types of substances involves several factors: 1) estimating dosage and exposure; 2) considering each entry route to the body to obtain total dose; and 3) accounting for variations of concentrations generated at facilities and sites.[58] In addition, risk assessment must consider variables related to the collective contribution to exposure from multiple sources, including contaminated soil, water, and air. This task, however, is often based on estimation and speculation.

The Role of Occupational Hygiene in Hazardous Waste Management

Overview

Federal regulations such as RCRA influenced the evolution of new industries in the form of controlled hazardous waste treatment, storage, and disposal (TSD) facilities. The enactment of CERCLA, as amended by SARA, influenced the expansion of other related phases of hazardous waste management, such as emergency response to environmental releases and the investigation, characterization, remediation, and restoration of abandoned and mismanaged hazardous waste sites. This increase in hazardous waste facilities and mitigation activities resulted in greater risk of exposure due to the concomitant increased need for human interaction with the facilities and sites.

Environmentally sound operations and accurate assessment at hazardous waste facilities and sites involve a coordinated effort by several disciplines, including environmental scientists, occupational hygienists, toxicologists, health physicists, hydrogeologists, engineers, and safety specialists. Each of these disciplines involves some component of recognition, evaluation, and control of hazards to the environment, human health, or human safety.

The scope of occupational hygiene includes recognition, evaluation, and control of all stressors arising from the workplace that may have an effect on workers or members of the community. The role occupational hygiene plays in the area of hazardous waste management has been clearly defined.[59,60] The occupational hygienist becomes involved in hazardous waste management primarily through the existence of: 1) RCRA hazardous waste generator programs; 2) RCRA/OSHA TSD facility programs; 3) OSHA HAZWOPER remedial investigation/feasibility study/risk assessment (RI/FS/RA) activities; and 4) emergency response activities. When occupational hygiene is applied to hazardous waste management activities, the workplace includes hazardous waste TSD facilities; spill sites; and abandoned or indiscriminately managed disposal sites. Workers include any personnel, including investigators, involved at the facilities or sites. Members of the community include any people in the area that may be impacted by the hazardous waste site.

Recognition

The recognition phase includes anticipation and identification of potential and actual hazards. This phase commences prior to entering a facility or site and continues throughout investigations, evaluations, and general operations as additional data are compiled. Investigation and characterization involve gathering qualitative and quantitative data regarding a given TSD facility or abandoned site. These data include combinations of information, such as 1) the identification, hazardous characteristics, and quantity of wastes spilled, contained, stored, treated, and disposed; 2) the types of unit processes and standard operating procedures; 3) the number of operating personnel actually and potentially exposed; 4) topographic, geologic, and hydrologic features; 5) distance relative to off-site waterways (surface and ground), neighborhoods, or residences; and 6) any historical records.

Knowledge of several waste-handling processes can provide insight into potential exposures. Hazardous waste operations present an environment that is more diversified than a traditional industrial setting, mainly due to the uncertainty and heterogeneity of the wastes and secondary by-products. At abandoned sites, it is sometimes a challenge even to locate the wastes since they may have been disposed in bulk quantities onto the soil or disposed of in containers distributed above ground, underground, in surface water, and in structures. Wastes also may have dispersed via evaporation, run-off, and leaching. Accordingly, exposures in the hazardous waste industry are often more difficult to recognize, and, in turn, to evaluate and control.

Assessment of waste facilities and sites can be relatively complex.[61] As much information as feasible is gathered during the recognition phase and is reviewed and evaluated to design the strategy necessary for preliminary on-premise survey and evaluation. In addition, the information is useful in developing preliminary health and safety plans.

Evaluation

Initially, a preliminary survey that includes visual and instrumental monitoring of a facility or site is conducted. Visual monitoring refers to the observation of processes and/or conditions and subjectively and objectively identifying potential and actual hazards related to the completion of any possible exposure pathways between the hazardous waste and people. Instrumental monitoring involves the use of monitoring equipment to record qualitative and quantitative environmental surveillance data.

The evaluation of active TSD facilities essentially follows standard occupational hygiene protocol. Preliminary screening is necessary at some spill and abandoned disposal sites because of the increased uncertainty regarding the wastes and conditions present. Nonetheless, the instruments used to evaluate exposures at hazardous waste facilities and sites are the same as those used for general occupational hygiene and ambient environmental surveillance.[62–67]

Preliminary instrumental monitoring focuses on atmospheric screening for combustible gases and vapors, organic and inorganic gases and vapors, ionizing radiation, and oxygen.[68] Due to the uncertainty of the hazards that may be encountered by personnel during initial entry to a site, automated robotic assessment has been suggested[69] and continues to be studied.[70] Indeed, perhaps the safest way to evaluate contaminated hazardous waste sites is via remote sensing technologies that permit evaluation from off-site perimeter locations.[71]

The results of the preliminary screening data, in combination with other information, are used to 1) modify health and safety plans; 2) determine appropriate types and levels of controls; 3) designate support, decontamination, and exclusion zones; and 4) plan subsequent monitoring strategy for comprehensive environmental surveillance. Comprehensive environmental surveillance involves monitoring for air-, water-, and soil-borne contaminants, plus characterization of waste streams present. In addition, meteorological data such as temperature, relative humidity, barometric pressure, and wind speed and direction are collected. A summary of common monitoring instrumentation is presented in Tables 48.10 and 48.11.[72]

Characterization of a site can be influenced by randomness of distribution of wastes in the area and how the wastes will be handled by workers.[73] Sampling objectives must be clearly established to collect representative and interpretable samples.[74] Indeed, established protocols, advanced instrumentation, data processing, and quality assurance are essential for compilation of accurate monitoring data.[75]

Inhalation is considered the major mode of entry for contaminants at hazardous waste sites and facilities. As a result, personal external exposures to airborne contaminants are determined by using instantaneous or real-time plus integrated monitoring instruments and methods. Dermal absorption is a secondary mode of exposure and is difficult to evaluate accurately. A method for estimating dermal absorption via dermal patches impregnated with activated carbon, however, has been suggested.[76] Thermal stress is another major factor that should be evaluated during hazardous waste activities to determine the impact of temperature extremes on workers.[77]

Inhalation exposures due to airborne contaminants should be measured inside and outside of the source of generation within the site. There is a potential for contaminants to migrate off site due to volatilization and disturbance of soil. As a result, monitoring is also conducted at and outside of the site perimeter to determine migratory patterns. The concentrations measured, however, may vary depending on the nature of the operations.

Environmental surveillance, which can provide some data regarding external exposures, is augmented by medical surveillance.[78] Medical surveillance can provide data regarding the impact of external

Table 48.10 — Major Instrumentation for Evaluation of Atmospheric and Meteorologic Parameters at Hazardous Waste Facilities and Sites

Monitored Parameter	*Monitoring Instrument*	*Collection Medium*	*Type of Monitoring*	*Analytical Instrument*
Combustible Gases/Vapors	Combustible Gas Meter		Instantaneous/Area	Direct-reading
Oxygen	Oxygen Meter		Instantaneous/Area	Direct-reading
Organic Gases/Vapors	Analyzer w/ Flame Ionization Detector (FID)		Instantaneous/Area	Direct-reading
	Analyzer w/ Photoionization Detector (PID)		Instantaneous/Area	Direct-reading
	Analyzer w/ Infrared Radiation Detector (IR)		Instantaneous/Area	Direct-reading
	Manual Piston/ Bellows Pump	Detector Tubes	Instantaneous/Area	Direct-reading
	Low-/High-Flow Pump	Charcoal/ Silica Gel Adsorbent Tubes Tenax/ChroMosorb Solid Adsorbents	Integrated Personal/Area	Gas Chromatograph/ GC Mass Spectrometer/ High-Pressure Liquid Chromatograph
	High-Flow Pump	Impinger/ Bubbler w/ Liquid Absorbents	Integrated Personal/Area	UV/Vis Spectrophotometer
Organic Aerosols	High-Flow Pump	Fiberglass/ Teflon Filters	Integrated Personal/Area	Gas Chromatograph/ High-Pressure Liquid Chromatograph
Inorganic Gases/Vapors (e.g., Acids)	Manual Piston/ Bellows Pump	Detector Tubes	Instantaneous/Area	Direct-reading
	Low-/High-Flow Pump	Silica Gel Adsorbent Tubes	Integrated Personal/Area	Ion Chromatograph
	High-Flow Pump	Impinger/ Bubbler w/ Liquid Absorbent	Integrated Personal/Area	UV/Vis Spectrophotometer
Inorganic Aerosols (e.g., Metals; Asbestos)	Fibrous Aerosol Monitor (Asbestos/Total Fibers)		Instantaneous/Area	Direct-reading
	X-ray Fluorescence Monitor (Metals)		Instantaneous/Area	Direct-reading
	High-Flow Pump	Cellulose Ester Fiber Filter	Integrated Personal/Area	Atomic Absorption Spectrometer/Inductively Coupled Plasma

(continued on the next page.)

Table 48.10 — Major Instrumentation for Evaluation of Atmospheric and Meteorologic Parameters at Hazardous Waste Facilities and Sites (cont.)

Monitored Parameter	*Monitoring Instrument*	*Collection Medium*	*Type of Monitoring*	*Analytical Instrument*
Emission Light				(Metals); Electron (TEM) or (PLM/PCM) Microscope (Asbestos)
Biological Aerosols	High-Flow Pump	Cellulose Ester Fiber Filter/Impinger w/ Water/Cascade Impactor	Integrated Personal/Area	Incubator/ Light Microscope

(continued on next page.)

Monitored Parameter	*Monitoring Instrument*	*Collection Medium*	*Type of Monitoring*	*Analytical Instrument*
Total/ Respirable Aerosols	Suspended Particle Analyzer		Instantaneous/Area	Direct-reading
	High-Flow Pump	Polyvinyl Chloride Filter	Integrated Personal/Area	Gravimetric Electrobalance
Ionizing Radiation	Geiger-Mueller Counter		Instantaneous/Area	Direct-reading
	Integrated Personal Dosimeter		Integrated	Direct-reading
	Film Badges	Film + Filters	Integrated Personal	Densitometer
Noise	Sound Level Meter		Instantaneous/Area	Direct-reading
	Noise Dosimeter		Integrated/Personal	Direct-reading
Thermal Stress	WBGT Index Meter		Instantaneous/Area	Direct-reading
	Physiological Index Dosimeters		Instantaneous/Area	Direct-reading
Temperature	Thermometer		Instantaneous	Direct-reading
Atmospheric Pressure	Barometer		Instantaneous	Direct-reading
Wind Speed and Direction	Anemometer		Instantaneous	Direct-reading
Relative Humidity	Psychrometer		Instantaneous	Direct-reading

exposures on the contribution to absorbed doses. As suggested previously, hazardous waste operations and activities present a relatively unique occupational setting and source of potential adverse impact to the public, and a medical surveillance program must be designed accordingly.[79] The combination of environmental and medical surveillance data increases the probability of minimizing exposures and establishing a correlation between cause and effect.

The comprehensive set of data is used for several purposes: 1) to determine the extent of contamination and peripheral (horizontal and vertical) migration into the environment; 2) to determine potential and actual exposures to workers engaged in hazardous waste operations; 3) to determine potential and actual exposures to the public; and 4) to design strategy for control and remediation.

Table 48.11 — Major Instrumentation for Evaluation of Water, Soil, and Waste Parameters at Hazardous Waste Facilities and Sites

Monitored Parameter	*Type of Sample*	*Analytical Instrument(s)*
Organic chemical compounds	Grab/composite	GC/GC mass spectrometer/high-pressure liquid chromatograph/Fourier transform infrared (FTIR) spectrometer
Total organic halide	Grab/composite	Microcoulometric titrator/neutron bombardment gamma-ray detector
Total organic carbon	Grab/composite	Carbonaceous analyzer
Total and amenable cyanide	Grab/composite	UV spectrophotometer
Sulfide	Grab/composite	Titration apparatus
Total oil and grease	Grab/composite	Gravimetric electrobalance
Inorganic chemical compounds (e.g., metals)	Grab/composite	Atomic absorption spectrometer/Inductively coupled plasma atomic emission spectrometer
Biological agents (e.g., total coliform)	Grab/composite	Membrane filter apparatus + incubator + microscope
Solubility (hexane: water partition)	Grab/composite	Separatory funnel
pH	Grab/composite	pH meter
Specific conductance	Grab/composite	Conductivity meter
Flammability (i.e., ignitability)	Grab/composite	Pensky-Martens closed-cup tester/Setaflash closed-cup tester/Bureau of Explosives closed-drum tester
Corrosivity	Grab/composite	Resin-flask apparatus + SAE 1020 steel
Reactivity	Grab/composite	Cyanide release apparatus + UV spectrophotometer
Radioactivity (i.e., gross alpha and beta)	Grab/composite	Gas-flow proportional counter/scintillation counter

Control

Measures for controlling exposures to personnel involve implementation of administrative and engineering controls as well as the use of personal protective equipment (PPE). The implementation of administrative controls, such as development of a health and safety plan and standard operating procedures, including medical surveillance, should be a primary focus. Even if engineering and personal protective equipment controls are used, their full protective benefit is often compromised by poor work practices.

Engineering controls are most applicable to active TSD facilities and have been shown to reduce airborne levels of air contaminants at waste facilities.[80] They can include controlled process design, automation, and ventilation. Engineering controls are not always feasible, especially at uncontrolled spill or disposal sites. As a result, personal protective equipment must be used in conjunction with or as an alternative to engineering controls.

Personal protective equipment provides a relatively impermeable, but less than 100% efficient, barrier between an individual and the contaminated surroundings. A variety of equipment is available to protect the respiratory, dermal, and ocular systems. Procedures have been established[65,73] that recommend four levels of personal protection depending on specific environmental surveillance data or perceived conditions (Table 48.12). In the absence of certainty, full-body encapsulation is sometimes warranted. This practice sometimes creates a secondary health hazard, due to the increased potential for heat stress.[81]

Measures for Controlling Exposures of Workers on Hazardous Waste Sites

Prevention of Heat Stress

Often workers on a hazardous waste site are exposed to heat stress due to full-body encapsulation. Proper training and preventive measures can help prevent serious illness and loss of worker productivity. To avoid heat stress, management can take the following administrative steps: adjust work schedules to allow for modifying work/rest schedules according to monitoring requirements; allow work slowdowns as needed; rotate personnel and alternate job functions to minimize overstress or overexertion; add additional personnel to work teams; and perform work during cooler hours of the day. Also, management can provide air-conditioned shelter or shaded areas to protect personnel during rest periods; provide water to maintain workers' body fluids at normal levels; encourage workers to maintain good physical fitness; and train workers to recognize and treat heat stress. Management can provide cooling devices to help natural body heat exchange during work or severe heat exposure. Cooling devices can include field showers or hose-down areas (to reduce body temperature and/or to cool off protective clothing) and cooling jackets, vests, or suits.[82]

Administrative Controls

Site control includes compiling an accurate site map; preparing the site for work activities; establishing work zones; using the buddy system; establishing and enforcing decontamination procedures for personnel and equipment; establishing site security measures; setting up communication networks; enforcing safe work practices (standard operating procedures); and planning for emergencies. A site map shows prevailing wind direction, drainage, location of buildings, and all containers of hazardous materials. This will allow for the identification of areas requiring the use of PPE, access and evacuation routes, and problems areas. Preparing a site for remediation can be as hazardous as site cleanup, since it may include the movement of equipment and people. To help implement good work

Table 48.12 — Levels of Personal Protective Equipment for Hazardous Waste Operations and Activities

Level of Protection	*General Criteria for Use*	*Major Personal Protective Equipment*
A	Highest level of respiratory, dermal, and ocular protection is warranted.	• Supplied-air respirator • Fully encapsulating chemical-resistant suit + boots + gloves
B	Highest level of respiratory protection is warranted, but a lower level of dermal protection is needed.	• Supplied-air respirator • One- or two-piece chemical-resistant suit + boots + gloves
C	Criteria for wearing air-purifying respirators are met; non-immediately dangerous to life or health (IDLH) atmospheres; concentration of oxygen >19.5%	• Full or half-facepiece respirator (note: ocular protection is required if half-facepiece is worn) • One- or two-piece chemical-resistant suit + boots + gloves
D	No risk of respiratory or dermal exposure; non-IDLH atmospheres; concentration of oxygen >19.5%	• Ocular protection • Coveralls + boots

practices, such as the use of the proper level of PPE, site work zones should be established. Three frequently used zones are the Exclusion Zone, the area where contamination is suspected or known to be present; the Contamination Reduction Zone, the area where decontamination takes place; and the Support Zone, the uncontaminated area where workers should not be exposed to hazardous substances. The buddy system should be used during most activities in contaminated or hazardous areas. A buddy is able to provide his or her partner with assistance, observe his or her partner for signs of chemical exposure or heat stress, check the integrity of PPE; and notify the supervisor or others if emergency help is needed. To prevent exposure of unauthorized, unprotected people to site hazards, site security should be provided during working hours and during off-duty hours. To maintain good site control and pass along safety information and changes in tasks or work methods, internal communication must be established among personnel on-site and external communication between on-site and off-site personnel. To maintain strong safety awareness, standard operating procedures and hazardous substance information from material safety data sheets (MSDSs) should be developed and consistently provided employees through training and safety meetings.[82]

A Site Health and Safety Plan (HASP) establishes policies and procedures to protect workers and the public from potential hazards that may exist at the site. It should be developed before site activities begin. The HASP anticipates potential accident scenarios and provides measures to minimize accidents or injuries that might occur. It should address every work task to be performed at the hazardous waste site. The HASP includes a description of the risks associated with each operation; training required for personnel to handle specific hazardous situations; PPE and equipment necessary for various operations; site-specific medical surveillance and services necessary, including the location of the nearest medical treatment facility; air monitoring, personal monitoring, and environmental sampling; site control measures; decontamination procedures; a contingency plan for safe and effective response to emergencies; and a list of all standard operating procedures for activities that can be standardized, such as decontamination and respirator fit testing.[82] Table 48.13 is provided as a HASP checklist.[83] It represents the minimum regulatory requirements for a site-specific health and safety plan primarily according to the OSHA HAZWOPER standard. It cannot take the place of knowledgeable and experienced professional safety specialists and occupational hygienists.

Decontamination is the process of removing or neutralizing contaminants that have accumulated on personnel and equipment. Decontamination protocols have been developed to protect workers from hazardous substances that may contaminate protective clothing, respiratory equipment, tools, vehicles, and other equipment used on the site. They minimize the transfer of harmful materials into clean areas and help prevent the mixing of incompatible chemicals. They protect the community by preventing the uncontrolled transportation of contaminants from the site. It is necessary to decontaminate before personnel move from "dirty" to "clean" work areas; prior to eating, drinking, smoking, or using restroom facilities; and before transport trucks or equipment leave the site. Decontamination methods include physical removal of contaminants or by deactivation by chemical detoxification, disinfection or sterilization, or a combination of both physical and chemical means.[82]

Medical monitoring is used in addition to other administrative and engineering controls as well as appropriate PPE and decontamination procedures to provide adequate protection to workers. A program is needed to assess and monitor worker health and fitness prior to, during, and at the end of employment.[84] Employees may be monitored and/or placed under surveillance for having contact with hazardous substances. This may occur during clean-up operations or any processes that are conducted at TSD facilities; and during emergency response to hazardous substances releases. Also, workers who are or who may be exposed to hazardous substances above the established permissible exposure limit for 30 days or more a year; workers who wear a respirator for 30 days or more a year; and workers who are injured, become ill, or develop signs or symptoms due to possible overexposure should be covered by a medical surveillance program. It involves preplacement screening, periodic medical examinations, exposure-specific examinations, and termination

Table 48.13 — Site Health and Safety Plan (HASP) Checklist

1. Names of key personnel and health and safety personnel. Regulatory Reference: 1910.120(b)(2) and 1926.65(b)(2)

a. Are key personnel identified in the HASP? Comment:

b. Are health and safety personnel, including alternates, identified in the HASP? Comment:

2. Has a site-specific safety & health risk analysis been accomplished for each site task and operation found in the work plan? Regulatory Reference: 1910.120(b)(4)(ii)(A) and 1926.65(b)(4)(ii)(A)

a. Does the HASP address methods to deal with potential safety problems on the site? Comment:

b. Has an adequate risk analysis for each site task and operation been provided? Comment:

c. Does the risk analysis include as a minimum?
   Chemical contaminants
   Affected media
   Concentrations
   Potential routes of exposure
   Associated health effects
   Comment:

d. Are appropriate levels of PPE identified for each site task and operation? Comment:

3. Employee Training Regulatory Reference: 1910.120(b)(4)(ii)(B) and 1926.65(b)(4)(ii)(B) — refers to specific requirements found in 1910.120(e), 1926.65(e)

a. Does the HASP indicate that all on-site employees meet appropriate training requirements? Regulatory Reference: Certificates are to be provided per 1910.120(e)(6) and 1910.65(e)(6) Comment:

b. Have all on-site employees received initial 40-hour training? Are certificates either provided or available upon request? Regulatory Reference: 1910.120(e)(3) and 1926.6 Comment:

c. Do all supervisory personnel have 8-hour supervisory training? Are certificates provided or provisions for the certificates being provided on-site? Regulatory Reference: 1910.120(e)(4) and 1926.65(e)(4) Comment:

d. Do all employees working on-site have a minimum of three days of actual field experience under the direction of a skilled supervisor? Regulatory Reference: 1910.120(e)(3)(i) and 1926.65(e)(3)(i) Comment:

e. Is refresher training current? Are certificates provided or provisions made for the certificates to be provided on-site? Regulatory Reference: 1910.120(c)(8) and 1926.65(e)(8) Comment:

f. Have employees been trained to recognize the symptoms and signs of over exposure to chemical hazards? Regulatory Reference: 1910.120(c)(8) and 1926.65(c)(8) Comment:

g. Have employees been trained in first aid/CPR as necessary? Regulatory Reference: 1926.50(c) Comment:

Table 48.13 — Site Health and Safety Plan (HASP) Checklist (cont.)

h. Have the chemical/physical/toxicological properties of each substance been identified and communicated to the employee? Regulatory Reference: 1910.120(c)(8) and 1926.65(c)(8) Comment:

4. Personnel Protective Equipment Regulatory Reference: 1910.120(b)(4)(ii)(C), 1926.65(b)(4)(ii)(C) — refers to more specific requirements found in .120(g)(5), 65(g)(5). A written program must address the following:

a. Has the PPE been selected based upon the site hazards? Regulatory Reference: 1910.120(g)(5)(i) and 1926.65(g)(5)(i) Comment:

b. Have the use and limitations of the PPE been described? Regulatory Reference: 1910.120(g)(5)(ii) and 1926.65(g)(5)(ii) Comment:

c. Has the work mission duration been described? Regulatory Reference: 1910.120(g)(5)(iii) and 1926.65(g)(5)(iii) Comment:

d. Have decontamination and disposal procedures been established? Regulatory Reference: 1910.120(g)(5)(iv) and 1926.65(g)(5)(v) Comment:

e. Have employees been properly fitted with the PPE and trained in its use? Regulatory Reference: 1910.120(g)(5)(vi) and 1926.65(g)(5)(vi) Comment:

f. Have employees been trained in proper donning and doffing procedures? Regulatory Reference: 1910.120(g)(5)(vii) and 1926.65(g)(5)(vii) Comment:

g. Have inspection procedures been established? Regulatory Reference: 1910.120(g)(5)(viii) and 1926.65(g)(5)(viii)Comment:

h. Are procedures established to monitor the effectiveness of the PPE program? Regulatory Reference: 1910.120(g)(5)(ix) and 1926.65(g)(5)(ix) Comment:

i. Are provisions for limitations of use of the PPE in temperature extremes and for heat stress described? Are other appropriate medical considerations included, such as heart disease or claustrophobia? Regulatory Reference: 1910.120(g)(5)(x) and 1926.65(g)(5)(x) Comment:

5. Medical Surveillance Regulatory Reference: 1910.120(b)(4)(ii)(D) and 1926.65(b)(4)(ii)(D) — refers to specificrequirements found in .120(f) and .65(f). The HASP must include site-specific medical monitoring provisions. This should include respirator clearance exams as well as other specific tests specified by the examining physician after he/she reviews the site-specific information.

a. Have site-specific medical surveillance requirements been included in the HASP? Has all necessary information been provided to the physician? Regulatory Reference: 1910.120(f)(6) and 1926.65(f)(6) Comment:

b. Was the examination performed by or under the supervision of a board-certified occupational medicine physician? Comment:

6. Air Monitoring Regulatory Reference: 1910.120(b)(4)(ii)(E) and 1926.65(b)(4)(ii)(E) — refers to more specific comments found in 1910.120(h) and 1926.65(h)

a. Does the HASP include the frequency and types of air monitoring? Regulatory Reference: 1910.120(b)(4)(ii)(E), (h)(3) and 1926.65(b)(4)(ii)(E) and (h)(3) Comment:

Table 48.13 — Site Health and Safety Plan (HASP) Checklist (cont.)

b. Does the HASP describe methods for personal monitoring? Regulatory Reference: 1910.120(b)(4)(ii)(E) and 1926.65(b)(4)(ii)(E) Comment:

c. Does the HASP describe environmental monitoring? Regulatory Reference: 1910.120(b)(4)(ii)(E) and 1926.65(b)(4)(ii)(E) Comment:

d. Are the various types of instrumentation for site sampling described as well as methods for maintenance and calibration? Regulatory Reference: 1910.120(b)(4)(ii)(E) and 1926.65(b)(4)(ii)(E) Comment:

7. Site Control Regulatory Reference: 1910.120 (b)(4)(ii)(F) and 1926.65(b)(4)(ii)(F) — refers to specific requirements found in 1910.120(d) and 1926.65(d). The following items must be contained in the site control section of the HASP:

a. Is a site description and map provided to include size, location, etc.? Regulatory Reference: 1910.120(d)(3) and 1926.65(d)(3) Comment:

b. Have site work zones been established? Regulatory Reference: 1910.120(d)(3) and 1926.65(d)(3)Comment:

c. Is a "buddy system" established? Regulatory Reference: 1910.120(d)(3) and 1926.65(d)(3)Comment:

d. Have type(s) of site communications, including alerting means for emergencies, been described? Regulatory Reference: 1910.120(d)(3) and 1926.65(d)(3)Comment:

e. Are safe operating procedures or safe work practices described? Regulatory Reference: 1910.120(d)(3) and 1926.65(d)(3) Comment:

f. Has the nearest medical assistance source been described (as appropriate)? Regulatory Reference: 1910.120(d)(3) and 1926.65(d)(3) Comment:

8. Emergency Response Plan Regulatory Reference: 1910.120(b)(4)(ii)(H) and 1926.65(b)(4)(ii)(H) — refers to specific requirements found in .120(l), and .65(1). The plan should provide sufficient detail to ensure prompt, safe mitigation of potential site emergencies. The plan should indicate how emergencies would be handled at the site and how the risks associated with a response would be minimized.

a. Has pre-emergency planning been completed?
State/Local Emergency Planning Committee
On-Scene Coordinator
Hazardous Materials Team
Medical Treatment Facility
Ambulance
Medical Department
Regional Poison Control Center
Agency for Toxic Substances & Disease Registry
Other
Regulatory Reference: 1910.120(l)(2)(i) and 1926.65(1)(2)(i) Comment:

b. Have personnel roles, lines of authority, and communications been established? Regulatory Reference: 1910.120(l)(2)(ii) and 1926.65(1)(2)(ii) Comment:

Table 48.13 — Site Health and Safety Plan (HASP) Checklist (cont.)

c. Is emergency recognition and prevention discussed? Regulatory Reference: 1910.120(l)(2)(iii) and 1926.65(1)(2)(iii) Comment:

d. Have safe distances and places of refuge been described by specific maps and written descriptions provided for each site? Regulatory Reference: 1910.120(l)(2)(iv) and 1926.65(1)(2)(iv) Comment:

e. Have site security and control measures been described? Regulatory Reference: 1910.120(l)(2)(v) and 1926.65(1)(2)(v) Comment:

f. Have evacuation routes and procedures been described by specific maps and written descriptions provided for each site? Does this include the route to the Medical Treatment Facility? Regulatory Reference: 1910.120(l)(2)(vi) and 1926.65(l)(2)(vi) Comment:

g. Are decontamination measures, not discussed elsewhere in the HASP, described? Is the priority for field decontamination vice emergent medical assistance discussed? Regulatory Reference: 1910.120(l)(2)(vii)and 1926.65(1)(2)(vii) Comment:

h. Have provisions for emergency medical treatment and first aid been established?Who is providing the assistance? Medical treatment facility? Ambulance? Are these facilities equipped and personnel trained? Regulatory Reference: .120(l)(2)(viii) and 1926.65(1)(2)(viii) Comment:

i. Has information on the chemical hazard(s) been provided to the medical treatment facility/ ambulance personnel? Regulatory Reference: Comment:

j. Have emergency alerting and response procedures been established? Regulatory Reference: 1910.120(l)(2)(ix) and 1926.65(1)(2)(ix) Comment:

k. Are the telephone numbers listed for emergency response correct? Regulatory Reference: 1910.120(l)(2)(ix) and 1926.65(1)(2)(ix) Comment:

l. Are the site topography, layout, and prevailing weather conditions described? Regulatory Reference: 1910.120(l)(3)(i)(A) and 1926.65(1)(3)(i)(A) Comment:

m. Are PPE and emergency equipment provided and their location clearly indicated? Regulatory Reference: 1910.120(l)(2)(xi) and 1926.65(1)(2)(xi) Comment:

n. Are procedures to report incidents to local, state, and other authorities listed? Regulatory Reference: 1910.120(l)(3)(i)(B) and 1926.65(1)(3)(i)(B) Comment:

o. Are procedures to rehearse the plan included? Regulatory Reference: 1910.120(l)(3)(iv) and 1926.65(1)(3)(iv) Comment:

p. Are procedures to review and update the plan included? Regulatory Reference: 1910.120(l)(3)(v) and 1926.65(1)(3)(v) Comment:

q. Are procedures to evaluate and critique emergency response and follow-up included? Regulatory Reference: 1910.120(l)(2)(x) and 1926.65(1)(2)(x) Comment:

Table 48.13 — Site Health and Safety Plan (HASP) Checklist (cont.)

r. Are procedures for employers and employees to take to ensure employee safety from fire and other emergencies included? Regulatory Reference: 1910.38(a)(1) Comment:

9. Confined Space Entry Procedures Regulatory Reference: 1910.120(b)(4)(ii)(I) and 1926.65(b)(4)(ii)(I). If these are required, they must be in accordance with 1910.120(j)(9), 1910.146 and 1926.65(j)(9) Comment:

10. Spill Containment Program Regulatory Reference: 1910.120(b)(4)(ii)(J), 1926.65(b)(4)(ii)(J) — refers to specific requirements in 1910.120(j), 1926.65(j), IR 12.1, and EM-385-1-1, Sect 28.G & 28.H Elements to be potentially addressed include:

Drum and container handling
Opening of drums
Material handling equipment
Radioactive wastes, shock-sensitive wastes
Laboratory waste packs
Sampling drum and container contents
Shipping and transport of drums and containers
Appropriate procedures for tank and vault entry

a. Does the HASP contain a section discussing site-specific spill containment procedures? Comment:

11. Decontamination Procedures Regulatory Reference: 1910.120(k) and 1926.65(k)Decontamination procedures should be chosen based on site-specific contaminants.

a. Does the HASP contain site-specific decontamination methods for personnel and for equipment? Regulatory Reference: 1910.120(k)(2)(i), .120(k)(2)(ii), 1926.65(k)(2)(i) and .65(k)(2)(ii) Comment:

b. Are the decontamination methods appropriate for the site conditions and contaminants? Regulatory Reference: 1910.120(k)(i) and 1926.65(k)(i) Comment:

c. Are decontamination methods monitored by the site safety and health supervisor to determine their effectiveness? Regulatory Reference: 1910.120(k)(iv) and 1926.65(k)(iv) Comment:

12. Bloodborne Pathogens

a. Is there a Bloodborne Pathogens Program? Regulatory Reference: 1910.1030(e) Comment:

---

examinations. Blood tests, urine tests, and pulmonary function testing are often performed, and detailed written records are maintained.[82]

Personal Protective Equipment

After identifying contaminants of concern from all possible sources (e.g., soil, groundwater) and estimating possible exposure concentrations, determine the initial level of PPE based on the work to be conducted and your professional judgment.[85] PPE is always essential at uncontrolled spill or disposal sites. It must not only protect the respiratory, dermal, and ocular systems, but the entire body. Most situations at hazardous waste sites require skin protection for chemical or physical hazards. Hard hats, safety shoes, and eye protection are other forms of common protective equipment. Respiratory protection is required in IDLH or oxygen deficient atmospheres, in concentrations of specific chemicals at or above the action limits, in confined space entry with unknown atmospheres, and in the presence of skin or eye absorption of irritation hazards. No single combination of PPE is capable of protecting against all hazards. Therefore, PPE should be used with other protective methods. The use of PPE can create worker hazards such as heat stress, physical and psychological stress, impaired vision, impaired mobility, and impaired communication. For any given situation, equipment and clothing should be selected that provides an appropriate level of protection. As listed in Table 48.12, there are four levels of personal protection depending on specific data or perceived conditions. Level A is for the highest level of respiratory, dermal, and ocular protection; level D is essentially a work uniform and is used on any site where potential respiratory or skin hazards do not exist. Levels A through D ensembles can be used as a starting point for worker protective equipment. Each ensemble must be tailored to the specific situation to provide the most appropriate level of protection. The type of equipment used and the overall level of protection should be re-evaluated periodically as information about the site increases and as workers are required to perform different tasks.[82,86]

Engineering Controls

In the hierarchy of ways in which health hazards could be corrected, engineering controls have been designated first, with administrative controls second and personal protective equipment third. Engineering controls are to be implemented first unless they are not feasible for technical and/or economic reasons. Engineering controls are applied primarily at active TSD facilities, including process design, automation, and ventilation. Since working conditions at hazardous waste sites can vary greatly, the scope of engineering controls that might be found will be broad. Each separate job situation may benefit from engineering controls that have been developed specifically for them. The following is a list of possible engineering controls: machine guards, dust collection systems, local exhaust ventilation systems, scaffolding designs, hoist designs, stairway designs, automatic sprinkler systems, fall protection, trench shoring, two hand controls for presses and cutters, using non-metallic safety devices to prevent sparking, rollover protection for vehicles, sound-deadening designs, and proper wiring/grounding receptacles for electrical equipment. Engineering controls will only be effective if allowed to perform their designated tasks and are not defeated by individuals.[82]

References

1. **Wilson, D.G.:** *Handbook of Solid Waste Management.* New York: Van Nostrand Reinhold, 1977.
2. **U.S. Environmental Protection Agency (EPA):** *A History of Land Application as a Treatment Alternative,* by W.J. Jewell and B.L. Seabrook (EPA/430/9-79-012). Cincinnati, Ohio: U.S. EPA Document Distribution Center, 1979.
3. **Harris, C., W.L. Want, and M.A. Ward:** *Hazardous Waste: Confronting the Challenge.* New York: Quorum Books, 1987.
4. "General Index." *United States Code Annotated (USCA).* St. Paul, Minn.: West Publishing Co., 2001.
5. **Moore, E.B.:** *An Introduction to the Management and Regulation of Hazardous Waste.* Columbus, Ohio: Battelle Press, 2000.
6. **Wagner, T.P.:** *The Complete Guide to the Hazardous Waste Regulations—RCRA, TSCA, HMTA, OSHA, and Superfund.* New York: John Wiley & Sons, 1999.
7. **Ember, L.:** Pollution prevention: study says chemical industry lags. *Chem. Engin. News 73*:6–7 (1995).
8. **Johnson, J.:** New Jersey pilot program eases permit path for companies that cut toxics. *Environ. Sci. Technol. 30*:72A–73A (1996).
9. **Staines, J.:** Tips for managing and reducing waste. Adhesives Age 38:44–46 (1995).
10. **U.S. Environmental Protection Agency (EPA):** *RCRA Orientation Manual.* Washington, D.C.: EPA Office of Solid Waste/Communications, Information, and Resources Management Division, 2002.
11. "Resource Conservation and Recovery Act." *U.S. Code Annotated* Title 42, Part 6901 et seq. (1995).
12. "Hazardous Waste Management System." *Code of Federal Regulations* Title 40, Part 260 (1995).
13. **Dutkkiewicz, J., L. Jablonski, and S.A. Olenchock:** Occupational biohazards: a review. *Am. J. Ind. Med.14*:605–623 (1988).
14. **U.S. House of Representatives:** "The condition of information on hazardous waste," by E. Chelimsky. 2nd session, Sept. 24, 1986. Washington, D.C.: U.S. Government Printing Office, 1987. [Congressional subcommittee testimony]
15. **The Conservation Foundation:** *America's Waste: Managing for Risk Reduction.* Washington, D.C.: The Conservation Foundation, 1987.
16. **Lindgren, G.F.:** *Managing Industrial Hazardous Waste: A Practical Handbook.* Chelsea, Mich.: Lewis Publishers, 1989.
17. **Royston, M.G.:** Pollution Prevention Pays. New York: Pergamon Press, 1979.

18. **Burch, W.M.:** Process modifications and new chemicals. *Chem. Engin. Prog. 82*:5–8 (1986).
19. **Gibbs, W.W.:** Ounce of prevention: cleaner chemicals pay, but industry is slow to invest. *Sci. Am. 271*:103–105 (1994).
20. **Freeman, H.M.:** Industrial pollution prevention: a critical review. *J. Air Waste Mgmt. Assoc. 42*:618–656 (1992).
21. **Van Valkenburgh, G.:** Storing hazardous wastes safely. *Chem. Engin. 98*:203–204 (1991).
22. **Chemical Manufacturers Association (CMA):** *Guidance for Containers.* Arlington, Va.: CMA, 1995.
23. **Bouley, J.:** Drums & containers. *Poll. Engin. 25*:37 (1993).
24. **Muschett, F.D., and M.E. Enowitz:** The changing pollution control industry. *Poll. Engin. 18*:44–47 (1986).
25. **Wiedemann, P.M., and S. Femers:** Public participation in waste management decision making: analysis and management of conflicts. *J. Haz. Mat. 33*:355–368 (1993).
26. **Belhateche, D.H.:** Choose appropriate wastewater treatment technologies. *Chem. Eng. Progress 91*:32–51(1995).
27. **Kilduff, J., S. Komisar, and M. Nyman:** *Hazardous and Industrial Wastes—Proceedings of the Thirty-Second Mid-Atlantic Industrial and Hazardous Waste Conference.* Lancaster, Pa.: Technomic Publishing Co., 2000.
28. **LaGrega, M.D., P.L. Buckingham, and J.D. Evans:** *Hazardous Waste Management.* Boston: McGraw Hill, 2001.
29. **Congress of the United States, Office of Technology Assessment:** *Superfund Strategies* (OTA-ITE-252). Washington, D.C.: U.S. Government Printing Office, 1985.
30. **Hartenstein, R.:** Buffering acid precipitation, reducing soil erosion, and reclaiming toxic soil in the advent of global human carrying capacity. *Int. J. Environ. Studies 30*:287–300 (1986).
31. **Dempsy, C.R., and E.T. Oppelt:** Incineration of hazardous waste: a critical review. *J. Air Waste Mgmt Assoc. 43*:25–73 (1993).
32. **Manji, J.F.:** Pressure cooking could solve some hazardous waste problems in industry. *Automation 38*:26 (1991).
33. **Atlas, R.M.:** Bioremediation. *Chem. Engin. News 73*:32–42 (1995).
34. **Garg, S., and D.P. Garg:** Genetic engineering and pollution control. *Chem. Eng. Progress 86*:46–51 (1990).
35. **Stroo, H.F.:** Biotechnology and hazardous waste treatment. *J. Environ. Qual. 21*:167–175 (1992).
36. **Brubaker, G.R.:** In situ bioremediation. *Civil Engin. 65*:38–41 (1995).
37. **Bisesi, M.S.:** Vermial and microbial management of biological sludges under conditions of dynamic temperature and seasonal changes. *Bio. Wastes 32*:99–109 (1990).
38. **Collett, T.L.:** Enhance hazardous waste treatment using specialty chemicals. *Chem. Engin. Progress 87*:70–74 (1991).
39. **Trowbridge, T.D., and T.C. Holcombe:** Refinery sludge treatment/hazardous waste minimization via dehydration and solvent extraction. *J. Air & Waste Mgmt. Assoc. 45*:782–788 (1995).
40. **Stinson, S.C.:** Waste recycling plant uses molton metal baths. *Chem. Engin. News 71*:9 (1993).
41. **Gioia, F.:** Detoxification of organic waste liquids by catalytic hydrogenation. *J. Haz. Mat. 26*:243–260 (1991).
42. **Kittel, J.:** Nuclear waste management: issues and progress. *J. Environ. Sci. 27*:34–41 (1984).
43. **Krukowski, J.:** Alternatives to landfilling hazardous waste. *Poll. Engin. 26*:54–56 (1994).
44. **Johnson, B.L.:** *Impact of Hazardous Waste on Human Health—Hazard, Health Effects, Equity, and Communications Issues.* Boca Raton, Fla.: Lewis Publishers, 1999.
45. **Griffith, J., R.C. Duncan, W.B. Riggan, and A.C. Pellom:** Cancer mortality in U.S counties with hazardous waste sites and ground water pollution. *Arch. Environ. Health 44*:69–74 (1989).
46. **Johnson, B.L.:** A review of the effects of hazardous waste on reproductive health. *Am. J. Obstet. Gynecol. 181(1S)*:12S–16S (1999).
47. **Ozonoff, D., M.E. Colten, A. Cupples, T. Heeren, et al.:** Health problems reported by residents of a neighborhood contaminated by a hazardous waste facility. *Am. J. Ind. Med. 11*:581–597 (1987).
48. **Dayal, H., S. Gupta, N. Trieff, D. Maierson, et al.:** Symptom clusters in a community with chronic exposure to chemicals in two Superfund sites. *Arch. Environ. Health 50*:108–111 (1995).
49. **Edwards, F.L., and A.H. Ringleb:** Exposure to hazardous substances and the mental distress tort: trends, applications, and a proposed reform. *Columbia J. Environ. Law 11*:119–139 (1986).
50. **Kaye, W.E., H.I. Hall, and J.A. Lybarger:** Recall bias in disease status associated with perceived exposure to hazardous substances. *Ann. Epidemiol 4*:393–397 (1994).
51. **Elliot, S.J., S.H. Taylor, S. Walter, D. Steib, et al.:** Modeling pschosocial effects of exposure to solid waste facilities. *Soc. Sci. Med. 37*:791–804 (1993).
52. **Jacobson, J.L.:** *Abandoning Homelands, Worldwatch Institute Report: State of the World 1989.* New York: W.W. Norton, 1989.

53. **Hattis, D., L. Erdreich, and M. Ballew:** Human variability in susceptibility to toxic chemicals-a preliminary analysis of pharmacokinetic data from normal volunteers. *Risk Anal. 7*:415–426 (1987).
54. **Johnson, B.L., and C.T. DeRosa:** Chemical mixtures released from hazardous waste sites: implications for health risk assessment. *Toxicology 105(2–3)*:145–156 (1995).
55. **Betsinger, G., L. M. Brosseau, J. Golden:** Occupational health and safety in household hazardous waste management facilities. *AIHAJ 61*:575–583 (2000).
56. **Smith, M.T., C.S. Lea, and P.A. Buffler:** Human populations changes caused by hazardous waste. *Central Euro. J. Pub. Health 3*:77–79 (1995).
57. **Indulski, J.A., and W. Lutz:** Biomarkers used for the assessment of health hazards in populations living in the vicinity of communal and industrial waste dump sites. *Int. J. Occ. Med. Environ. Health 8*:11–16 (1995).
58. **Corn, M., and P.N. Breysse:** Human exposure estimates for hazardous waste site risk assessment. In *Risk Quantitation and Regulatory Policy* (19 Banbury Report), D.G. Hoel, R.A. Merrill, and F.P. Perea, eds. New York: Cold Spring Harbor Laboratory, 1985.
59. **Martin, W.F., and M. Gochfeld:** *Protecting Personnel at Hazardous Waste Sites.* Boston: Butterworth-Heinemann, 2000.
60. **National Institute for Occupational Safety and Health (NIOSH), Occupational Safety and Health Administration, United States Coast Guard, and United States Environmental Protection Agency:** *Occupational Safety and Health Guidance Manual for Hazardous Waste Site Activities* (NIOSH 85-115). Washington, D.C.: U.S. Government Printing Office, 1985.
61. **Sara, M.N.:** *Standard Handbook for Solid and Hazardous Waste Facility Assessments.* Boca Raton, Fla.: Lewis Publishers, 1994.
62. **U.S. Environmental Protection Agency (EPA):** *Test Methods for Evaluating Solid Waste* (EPA/SW-846). Washington, D.C.: U.S. Government Printing Office, 1995.
63. **Bisesi, M.S., and J.P. Kohn:** *Industrial Hygiene Evaluation Methods.* Boca Raton, Fla.: Lewis Publishers/CRC Press, 1995.
64. **Bishop, E.:** Air monitoring at hazardous waste sites. In *Protecting Personnel at Hazardous Waste Sites,* W.F. Martin and M. Gochfeld, eds. Boston: Butterworth-Heinemann, 2000.
65. **Koren, H., and M.S. Bisesi:** *Handbook of Environmental Health and Safety, Principles, and Practices.* Vols. I and II. Boca Raton, Fla.: Lewis Publishers/CRC Press, 1996.
66. **Simmons, M.S. (ed.):** *Hazardous Waste Measurements.* Chelsea, Mich.: Lewis Publishers, 1991.
67. **Pedersen, B.A., and G. M. Higgins:** Evaluation of chemical exposures in the hazardous waste industry. *J. Air Waste Mgmt. Assoc. 45*:89–94 (1995).
68. **U.S. Environmental Protection Agency (EPA):** *Standard Operating Safety Guides* (9284.01C). Cincinnati, Ohio: EPA Document Distribution Center, 1992.
69. **Bisesi, M.S.:** "Remote Control Robotic Assessment (RCRA) of Hazardous Waste Sites." Paper presented at the American Industrial Hygiene Conference, Detroit, Mich., May 1983.
70. **U.S. Environmental Protection Agency (EPA):** *Demonstration of Autonomous Air Monitoring Through Robotics,* by R.J. Rancatore and M.L. Philips (EPA/600-S2-89-055). Cincinnati, Ohio: Risk Reduction Laboratory, 1990.
71. **Leis, W.M., and F. Bopp III:** Hazardous waste dumps: dangerous as battlefields. *I & CS 66*:43–46 (1993).
72. **Hee, S.S.H.:** *Hazardous Waste Analysis.* Rockville, Md.: ABS Group Inc., Government Institutes Division, 1999.
73. **Parkhurst, D.F.:** Optimal sampling geometry for hazardous waste sites. *Environ. Sci. Tech. 18*:521–523 (1984).
74. **Sedman, R.M., S.D. Reynolds, and P.W. Hadley:** Why did you take that sample? *J. Air Waste Mgmt. Assoc. 42*:1420–1423 (1992).
75. **Almich, B.P., W.L. Budde, and R.W. Shobe:** Waste monitoring. *Environ. Sci. Tech. 20*:16–21 (1986).
76. **Cohen, B.M., and W. Popendorf:** A method for monitoring dermal exposure to volatile chemicals. *Am. Ind. Hyg. Assoc. J. 50*:216–223 (1989).
77. **Goldman, R.F.:** Heat stress in industrial protective encapsulating garments. In *Protecting Personnel at Hazardous Waste Sites,* W.F. Martin and M. Gochfeld, eds. Boston: Butterworth-Heinemann, 2000. pp. 295–355.
78. **Schaub, E.A., and M.S. Bisesi:** Medical and environmental surveillance. *N.J. Med. 91(10)*:715–718 (1994).
79. **American Industrial Hygiene Association/American Conference of Governmental Industrial Hygienists Joint Hazardous Waste Committee:** Proposed criteria for the selection of appropriate medical resources to perform medical surveillance for employees engaged in hazardous waste operations. *Am. Ind. Hyg. Assoc. J. 50*:A870–A872 (1989).
80. **Pederson, B.A.:** Evaluation of chemical exposures in the hazardous waste industry. *J. Air Waste Mgmt. Assoc.45*:89–94 (1995).
81. **Paull, J.M., and F.S. Rosenthal:** Heat strain and heat stress for workers wearing protective suits at a hazardous waste site. *Am. Ind. Hyg. Assoc. J. 48*:458–463 (1987).

82. **Barth, R.C., P.D. George, and R. H. Hill:** *Environmental Health and Safety for Hazardous Waste Sites.* Fairfax, Va.: American Industrial Hygiene Association, 2002.
83. **Simmons, M.A., and D. Coons:** *Health and Safety Plan Checklist.* Portsmouth, Va.: Navy Environmental Health Center, 2002.
84. **Andrews, L.P. (ed.):** *Worker Protection During Hazardous Waste Remediation.* New York: Van Nostrand Reinhold, 1990.
85. **Marlowe, C.S.E.:** *Safety Now! Controlling Chemical Exposures at Hazardous Waste Sites With Real-Time Measurements.* Fairfax, Va.: American Industrial Hygiene Association, 1999.
86. **Woodside, G.:** *Hazardous Materials and Hazardous Waste Management.* New York: John Wiley & Sons, 1999.

Outcome Competencies

After completing this chapter, the reader should be able to:

1. Define underlined terms used in this chapter.
2. Describe important differences that distinguish laboratories from other workplaces that use hazardous materials.
3. Describe the process used to design and implement a laboratory health and safety program.
4. Explain established risk assessment methods to plan experiments.
5. Assess the hazards associated with various classes of laboratory chemicals and various laboratory techniques.
6. Recognize unsafe acts and situations in laboratories.
7. Use established risk assessment methods to plan experiments, including selection of appropriate controls.
8. Describe training objectives that comply with regulations.
9. Implement the cradle-to-grave concept to purchase, store, and dispose of chemicals.
10. Describe key elements of OSHA's laboratory standard.

Key Topics

- I. Hazardous Materials
  - A. Flammable Chemicals
  - B. Corrosive Chemicals
  - C. Oxidizing Chemicals
  - D. Reactive Chemicals
  - E. Toxic Chemicals
  - F. Hazardous Waste
  - G. Radioactive Materials
- II. Physical Hazards
  - A. Hazardous Processes and Equipment
  - B. Modified Pressure Techniques
  - C. Modified Temperature Techniques
  - D. Energy Hazards
  - E. Separation Techniques
  - F. Anticipation/Recognition
  - G. Evaluation/Assessment
- III. Survey/Sampling Strategies
- IV. Controls
  - A. Engineering Controls
  - B. Chemical Storage Areas
  - C. Facility Design
  - D. PPE
  - E. Administrative Controls
- VI. Training
- VII. Regulations and Guidelines
  - A. OSHA Regulations
  - B. Related Regulations

Key Terms

chemical hygiene officer • chemical hygiene plan • Material Safety Data Sheets (MSDSs) • National Fire Protection Association • performance-oriented standard

Prerequisite Knowledge

College chemistry, any textbook.

Prior to beginning this chapter, the user should review the following chapters:

Chapter Number	Chapter Topic
3	Legal Aspects of Industrial Hygiene
4	Occupational Exposure Limits
5	Occupational Toxicology
7	Principles of Evaluating Worker Exposure
8	Occupational and Environmental Health Risk Assessment/Risk Management
9	Comprehensive Exposure Assessment
34	Prevention and Mitigation of Accidental Chemical Releases
35	General Methods for the Control of Airborne Hazards
37	Local Exhaust Ventilation
39	Personal Protective Clothing
43	Hazard Communication
48	Hazardous Waste Management
52	Occupational Safety

Laboratory Health and Safety

49

By Stefan Wawzynieci, Jr., CIH, NRCC-CHO, CHMM

Introduction

The chemical laboratory differs in significant ways from many other work sites. It is important to recognize these differences when evaluating health and safety conditions in the laboratory.

- Laboratories are likely to contain a very large variety but very small quantities of chemicals. Hundreds of chemical compounds, representing many different hazard classes, may be present in a laboratory; however, typical quantities of individual chemicals range from a few milligrams to a kilogram, or perhaps up to 5 kg of organic solvents. Laboratory equipment is small, in keeping with the quantity of chemicals being used.
- The processes carried out in laboratories change frequently, perhaps several times a day. Particularly in research laboratories, processes change rapidly as experimental results lead to decisions to try different materials or techniques. For example, a researcher in a synthetic organic chemistry laboratory may, in a single day, use distillation, crystallization, and several separation techniques, either concurrently or sequentially.
- The physical hazards associated with chemical laboratory work vary from insignificant to highly hazardous, including high-pressure and high-vacuum techniques, very high and very low temperatures, and highly reactive or explosive compounds.
- Individual laboratory workers are often intimately involved in designing the processes they carry out, giving them an unusual level of control over the safety practices associated with their work. Laboratory workers routinely make their own decisions about personal protective equipment (PPE) and engineering control needs associated with individual processes.
- Many standard hazard information sources—in particular, material safety data sheets (MSDSs)—report hazards and recommend controls based on operations with quantities of material that are orders of magnitude larger than quantities used in the laboratory, making direct application of the information to the laboratory difficult.

Occupational hygienists responsible for laboratory safety programs have several unusual challenges as a result of these unique laboratory workplace characteristics. The foremost challenge is determining what activities are actually being carried out at various times in a particular laboratory. Direct contact with laboratory workers is essential to this information collection process.

Additionally, evaluating the overall risk associated with highly variable use of chemicals and chemical byproducts is extremely problematic, especially if the hazards are unknown or ill defined. Actual exposures are difficult to measure because of limited periods and quantities of use. Another complicating factor is that hazard and toxicity information is not always available for the chemicals used in laboratories. Many specialty chemicals used in laboratories do not have established safe exposure levels. Other parameters for evaluation need to be found.

The following sections of this chapter describe the types of chemicals, processes, and controls that are most likely to be found in chemical laboratories. An understanding of this background information will assist the occupational hygienist in recognizing and evaluating the safety of a laboratory workplace. Appropriate controls can then be specified and implemented.

Hazardous Materials

The chemicals commonly found in laboratories exhibit a number of hazardous characteristics that need to be understood by the occupational hygienist; these include flammability, corrosivity, oxidizing power, reactivity, and toxicity.

Flammable Chemicals

Flammable chemicals occur in both liquid and gaseous states. Flammable liquids are typically present in a laboratory to be used as solvents for chemical reactions or as cleaning agents; therefore, the quantity of flammable liquid may be in the 1-quart to 5-gallon range, enough to present a significant fire hazard. (See section on Controls for recommended storage limits.) The most common solvents are listed in Table 49.1.

Both the flash point and boiling point of a flammable liquid should be reviewed in determining the hazard. This information should be available on the MSDS. The National Fire Protection Association (NFPA) has established a useful classification system for flammable liquids. A Class I flammable liquid is defined as having a flash point below 100°F (37.8°C) and having a vapor pressure not exceeding 40 psi. Subcategories include Class IA, those liquids having flash points below 73°F (22.8°C) and boiling points below 100°F; Class IB, those having flash points below 73°F and boiling points at or above 100°F; and Class IC, those having flash points at or above 73°F and below 100°F. Class II includes those combustible liquids having flash points at or above 100°F and below 140°F. Class IIIA includes those having flash points at or above 140°F and below 200°F, and Class IIIB includes those having flash points at or above 200°F. Because fire hazard decreases with increasing flash point and boiling point, Class IA contain most of chemicals of concern.

Flammable gases are typically present in a laboratory for use as fuels or possibly as reactants. Hydrogen, propane, natural gas, and acetylene are the most common fuel gases. Be aware that the flammability characteristic of some gases (hydrogen sulfide, ammonia, arsine) may be overlooked because of the emphasis on their toxicity.

Table 49.1 — Flammable Liquid Solvents

Solvent Class	*Examples*
Aliphatic hydrocarbons	hexane, cyclohexane, pentane, petroleum ether (an alkane, not an ether)
Aromatic hydrocarbons	toluene, xylenes (benzene, once very common, is rarely used as a solvent)
Alcohols	ethanol, methanol, isopropyl alcohol, ethylene glycol
Ethers	diethyl ether, diisopropyl ether, tetrahydrofuran
Ketones	acetone, methylisobutyl ketone, methyl-n-butyl ketone
Esters	ethyl acetate, butyl acetate

Corrosive Chemicals

Corrosive chemicals include a variety of acids and bases and are used in laboratories as reactants, titrants, and occasionally as cleaning chemicals. Highly concentrated acids and bases can readily cause serious damage to skin and eyes, whereas dilute solutions of the same materials may be quite innocuous. Hydrochloric, sulfuric, nitric, and acetic acids are commonly found in laboratories, as are sodium and potassium hydroxide. In concentrated form both acids and bases have significant potential for generating large amounts of heat when mixed with water or other reagents. Caution must be exercised to avoid splashing or spraying of corrosive materials.

It is important to note that some acids and bases, such as nitric acid and sodium oxide, are also strong oxidizers. Also, acetic acid, which is a weak organic acid, is actually a flammable liquid and should be stored as such.

Oxidizing Chemicals

Oxidizing chemicals are capable of providing oxygen (or chlorine or fluorine) in a reaction. Oxidizers must be used under carefully controlled conditions to avoid a fire or other extreme reaction. A solution of potassium dichromate in sulfuric acid has been used as a very strong cleaning solution for glassware; difficulty in disposing of chromium waste has reduced this practice, but old solutions can still be found in some laboratories. Perchloric acid is a strong oxidizer used to digest organic material prior to metals analysis. Peroxides, permanganates, periodates, and perborates also are used as oxidizers in laboratory work, providing a wide range of oxidizing power.

Reactive Chemicals

Reactive chemicals are those materials that are inherently unstable (e.g., explosives) or that react with air or moisture to produce toxic or unstable products, heat, or rapidly expanding gases. These materials need to be handled very carefully, with full cognizance of the conditions that must be avoided. The reader is encouraged to review Bretherick's *Handbook of Reactive Chemical Hazards*(1) for additional information on this subject. The following chemicals are some of the many reactive materials that may be used in the laboratory.

Concentrated (>10%) Solutions of Azides. These can be dangerously explosive; initiation of the explosion can be from heat, friction, or impact. Examples are acetyl azide, benzoyl azide, and benzenesulfonyl azide.

Acyl Halides. As a group, acyl halides tend to react violently with proton-donating solvents such as water, as well as aprotic solvents (dimethylformamide, dimethyl sulfoxide). The group includes acetyl chloride, benzoyl chloride, and methylchloroformate.

Alkali Metals. This group includes lithium, sodium, and potassium, their alloys, oxides, and hydrides; their reactivity with water has entertained many a high school chemistry class, yet the inherent danger must be recognized. This group is also incompatible with many other chemicals. Reference to the MSDSs is strongly recommended.

Alkyl Metals. Members of this group such as butyl lithium are highly exothermically reactive to atmospheric oxygen at ambient temperatures, water vapor (even 70% relative humidity conditions in air will cause ignition), and carbon dioxide.

Aqua Regia. A 1:4 or 1:3 mixture by volume of nitric and hydrochloric acids, aqua regia is a powerful oxidant, used for cleaning glassware. It decomposes with evolution of gases, and, if stored in tightly capped bottles, will explode.

Peroxidizable Compounds. These include diisopropyl ether (the most notorious) and diethyl ether, but also include less recognizable solvents such as 1,3-dioxane and tetrahydrofuran. Ethers by nature are not particularly reactive, but they react with air to form peroxides that are sensitive to shock and heat. Convenient test strips are available for periodic checking.

Metal Fulminates. This group is explosive, with fulminating silver being the most violent member. It is primarily silver nitride; it will explode in solution if stirred.

Metal Azides. These are sensitive explosives on their own, yet, in contact with acids, produce hydrogen azide, a highly toxic and explosive low-boiling liquid.

Perchlorates. In their heavy metal form as well as the organic salts, perchlorates are extremely sensitive explosives. Perchloric acid digestions should never be permitted in conventional chemical fume hoods, where the formation of perchlorates could occur. Hoods designed with a wash-down option are required.

Nitric Acid. This chemical deserves special mention, as it is both a corrosive and an oxidizer and reacts explosively with certain aromatic hydrocarbons, acetone, dimethylsulfoxide, and thiols.

Phosphorous (White). This chemical autoignites at ambient temperatures in air, with resulting irritating vapors to the eyes and respiratory tract.

Picric Acid. Also known as 2,4,6,-trinitrophenol, picric acid is a close relative of TNT (trinitrotoluene). It must be stored wet, as it is explosive when dry. The metal picrates (lead, mercury, copper, and zinc) are sensitive to heat, friction, and impact.

Toxic Chemicals

To quote from the Occupational Safety and Health Administration (OSHA) laboratory standard(2) section (3)(ii)(B)(b) definitions, "Hazardous Chemical":

> The term "health hazard" includes chemicals that are carcinogens; toxic or highly toxic agents; reproductive toxins; irritants; corrosives; sensitizers; hepatotoxins; nephrotoxins; neurotoxins; agents that act on the hematopoietic systems; and agents

that damage the lungs, skin, eye, or mucous membranes. In the case of formaldehyde, lab employees should be made aware of its use, even in neighboring labs. Sensitization to latex may be an issue for workers who are in the presence of latex gloves.

All of these toxic characteristics can be found in chemicals used in the laboratory. MSDSs are of some benefit in evaluating the toxicity of particular chemicals, but many of the chemicals used in laboratories have not been even minimally studied. Even when the toxicity of a particular chemical is well understood, the potential exposure to that chemical must be reviewed to make an estimate of the hazard associated with its use. This is also a major challenge, because exposures are highly dependent on how and where the chemical is used and how long the procedure takes. It is often very difficult to sample for airborne chemicals because of the very short period of use.

The National Academy of Sciences/National Research Council addressed this issue in detail in its 1995 report, *Prudent Practices in the Laboratory: Handling and Disposal of Chemicals*.[3] Chapter 3 of this publication describes a risk assessment process for laboratory chemical use. Briefly, the process includes the following steps.

(1) Identify chemicals to be used and how they will be used.
(2) Consult sources of information.
(3) Evaluate type of toxicity. If no information is available for a compound, it may be necessary to look for chemical similarities with other compounds of known toxicity.
(4) Consider possible routes of exposure.
(5) Evaluate quantitative information on toxicity. Classify as highly toxic, moderately toxic, slightly toxic, etc.
(6) Select appropriate procedures to minimize exposure.
(7) Prepare for contingencies.

Because potential exposure to chemicals in the laboratory is so variable, Point 6 above becomes the critical safety factor; chemical procedures should always be designed to keep exposure as low as reasonably possible.

Chapter 3 of *Prudent Practices* is also useful for evaluating laboratory chemicals for many other potential hazards.

Laboratory employees should be made aware of exposure from routes other than inhalation, such as from contaminated surfaces and equipment, and should receive training in decontamination procedures.

Hazardous Waste

Chemical laboratories produce hazardous waste. In general, the hazards associated with this waste are similar to the hazards of the chemicals that make up the waste, with a few notable exceptions. Chemical reactions produce intended products, plus a variety of byproducts. The products are likely to be anticipated and reasonably well understood, whereas there may be very little characterization of the byproducts. Whether product or byproduct, the new materials may be either more or less toxic or hazardous than the original starting materials. Procedures for handling hazardous waste should accommodate the fact that toxicity and hazard may be more significant than anticipated from knowledge of the original chemical components.

Mixing waste from different sources in the same container may also yield unexpected results. Caution is necessary to ensure that incompatible chemicals are not mixed inadvertently.

A third problem to be aware of, both for waste and reagent chemicals, is unlabeled containers. A reasonably common cause of laboratory accidents is opening and emptying an old, unlabeled bottle of waste or unstable chemical. Unlabeled containers should always be handled with extreme caution. Every effort should be made to avoid having unlabeled containers at all. (See Chapter 48, Hazardous Waste Management.)

Radioactive Materials

Radioactive materials used in laboratories, in most cases, fall under the purview of U.S. Nuclear Regulatory Commission (NRC) rules, or their counterparts in "agreement states," which serve to control the radiation hazard through detailed regulatory requirements. NRC has established guidelines or dose limits for exposure to radiation, and laboratories handling licensed materials must be posted as having radioactive materials within. One should realize, however, that laboratory workers who concentrate on controlling radiation hazards sometimes tend to forget that their radioactive isotopes are also chemicals that may also have associated chemical hazards. For example, radiolabeled PCBs (polychlorinated biphenyls) or dioxin may require more control for their chemical toxicity than for their radioactivity. Mixed wastes present another problem when the time comes for disposal. Waiting for a number of half-lives to pass may remove the radioactive characteristic, but not the hazard characteristic.

Physical Hazards

In some instances a laboratory worker may be subject to noise, via the following examples. Certain preparation techniques (grinding, blending, sonicating) may emit annoying frequencies. An instrumentation room may have a constant hum or pitch that may be irritating to a worker. Ventilation systems, especially older fume hoods, may be the source of a constant noise. An assessment should be made of the source, and/or monitoring of the employee using a noise dosimeter may be appropriate (see Chapter 24).

Physical constraints on the lab worker include such activity as lifting and repetitive motion. Many solvents are purchased in 5-gallon containers, and dispensing from a full drum, with back bent and knees locked, can lead to injury. Twisting motions with heavy containers can lead to back strain. Many analytical labs with high throughput of samples may require analysts to inject samples constantly, or pipette, requiring repetitive hand motion.

Cuts become a special concern if chemicals are involved, due to the direct contact with the bloodstream. Typical is the example of a mercury thermometer breaking while being handled. Forcing glassware assemblies is another source of cuts and punctures.

Slips and falls due to spills are a physical hazard, yet can be compounded if a chemical is either the spilled entity, or if the worker is carrying an open container of a chemical solvent or solution. The reflex to reach out and grab something may result in laboratory equipment or chemicals being knocked from benches.

Eye strain, leading to fatigue, may occur through constant monitoring of instruments, extensive microscope use, or through the repeated action of taking readings from a burette. Poor or harsh lighting impacts these activities further.

Hazardous Processes and Equipment

Accidents in laboratories involving equipment may be a result of misuse or may occur even with proper use, if the equipment has not been well-maintained. As part of a laboratory's internal inspection checklist, one should review the schedule of maintenance procedures required for pieces of equipment. This could be as simple as checking the oil level in a pump or inspecting electrical cords for fraying. After electrical hazards, probably the next most common hazards are those involving working with high pressure (compressed gases), vacuum systems, and extreme temperatures. Ionizing and nonionizing radiation hazards also exist in laboratories, potentially associated with X-ray equipment, lasers, nuclear magnetic resonance instruments, electron microscopes, and so forth. These hazards are covered in Chapters 25 and 26. Other physical hazards may be from the use of tools (cutting, drilling, mixing), and preventive measures would be similar to those in industry. The reader is encouraged to refer to those chapters addressing such hazards within this text. Instances of long hair being caught in rotating paddle mixers have been documented, and any laboratory using water-cooled equipment always faces the potential of a flood, with the resultant slippery conditions. The remainder of this section focuses on modified pressure techniques, modified temperature techniques, energy hazards, and potential problems associated with separation techniques.

Modified Pressure Techniques

Some processes, such as distillation of a high-boiling liquid, are more effective when carried out at reduced pressure, because the reduced pressure also decreases the boiling point. Greatly reduced pressure (high-vacuum) systems are also necessary for processes requiring very low concentrations of chemicals (such as vapor deposition). Reduced pressure equipment must be constructed to withstand a large pressure differential between the inside and outside of the system and must be shielded to avoid injury if implosion should occur.

High pressure reaction systems (e.g., hydrogenation cylinders) must also be constructed to hold the pressure that will be developed. In this case barriers against an explosion should be in place.

Modified Temperature Techniques

It is frequently important to control temperature when working with chemicals. Heat may be added to initiate a reaction or increase a reaction rate. Cooling may be used to condense a reaction product so that it can be collected or to keep the reaction from getting out of hand. Heating devices include electric heating mantles, infrared lamps, oil and sand baths, hot air guns, and even warm water. Cooling systems include cold water, ice baths, dry ice-solvent traps, cryogenic liquids, and mechanical refrigeration systems. In the case of a walk-in cold room, if dry ice is used as supplemental cooling inside the enclosure, there is the added hazard of potential asphyxiation due to the buildup of carbon dioxide, coupled with the lack of or limited fresh air supplied to the room. The bigger the deviation from ambient temperature, the more potential there is for an extreme reaction to occur; therefore, close monitoring of such processes is important. Very rapid temperature changes are also more likely to cause problems than will slow warming or cooling processes. Of special note with cryogenic liquids (e.g., liquid nitrogen) is the fact that they may condense oxygen from the air and cause an explosion if they contact combustible materials.

Energy Hazards

This section does not attempt to detail specific hazards of each powered piece of equipment used in the laboratory. The main thing to recognize is that electric shock can be a major hazard. As little as 10 mA can result in personal damage, and a current of 80 mA can be fatal. High-voltage lines may also be encountered, especially with instruments such as atomic absorption spectrophotometers and inductively coupled plasma units.

Electrical safety is governed by the National Electrical Code, sections of which OSHA has adopted in Code of Federal Regulations (CFR) Title 29, Part 1910, Subpart S. Although this code is geared to industrial applications, OSHA recognized that any piece of equipment that, through malfunction, disrepair, or poor maintenance, may present a shock hazard or initiate a fire, should be guarded through prudent measures. These measures may include signs, lockout/tagout procedures, and special enclosures.

Basic electrical safety begins with proper insulation, wiring to code by a licensed electrician, grounding, and adequate mechanical devices such as panels and breakers. Extension cords do not meet these requirements and should not be used in laboratories. A particularly important device for laboratory settings is the ground fault interrupter (GFI). A GFI protects an individual by means of creating an imbalance in the circuit if an individual's body and the live wires make contact. This imbalance is detected by the GFI and causes it to break the circuit. Response time by a GFI is measured in milliseconds, which limits the duration of the flow of current. One of the factors for the potential of electrical shock is the duration of the flow of current, and therefore, by minimizing this factor, the hazard is minimized. Other factors include the voltage, the actual current, and the amount of resistivity encountered. Any moisture, including perspiring hands, in contact with live wires decreases resistivity, thereby increasing the likelihood of shock.

OSHA's lockout/tagout standard(4) is based on common sense—do not work on electrical systems unless they are shut off and de-energized. Many laboratory instruments warn users of the presence of high voltage beneath the instrument's covers. Only trained or qualified staff should attempt repairs. If maintenance requires that the power remain on, the prudent thing to do is ensure that no circuit can be completed through an individual's body. Appropriate tools should be used, but the mere presence of tools for electrical repair does not give anyone the go-ahead to attempt the work.

Instruments that use or generate various types of hazardous radiation include lamps and lasers, X-ray generators, and microwave ovens and furnaces. Along with specific hazards associated with the type of radiation involved (e.g., eye injury from lasers), electrical hazards are always a possibility. Nuclear magnetic resonance instruments, which generate large static magnetic fields, have also become common analytical and research tools.

Separation Techniques

Distillation, extraction, and chromatography techniques are all employed to purify a reaction product or to increase the purity of a solvent. Traditionally, these techniques have involved large quantities of solvents, which are often flammable. Although many refinements have taken place in the past 25 years, greatly reducing the scale on which these techniques are carried out, they still account for a large portion of flammable chemical use in the laboratory.

Anticipation/Recognition

The ability to anticipate or recognize hazard potential can be learned, gained through experience, or may be innate in the health and safety officer as well as a worker. Just as a construction worker might anticipate slippery conditions along a muddy path at an outdoor site, he or she might also recognize the potentially hazardous condition of setting up a scaffold in mud. A laboratory worker must also be able to anticipate and recognize dangers in the work setting.

A formal hazard recognition program would incorporate the elements shown in flowchart format in Figure 49.1. The preliminary survey would reveal the obvious hazards. The next two steps on the figure are interconnected-a collection of MSDSs does not necessarily list which chemicals are being stored, nor does an inventory necessarily reveal what MSDSs are on hand. It is important to note that, as part of a laboratory's chemical hygiene plan, a collection of MSDSs could make up one appendix (taking into account space limitations), and a second appendix could be the inventory list. Developing a health and safety plan basically means setting up standard operating procedures (SOPs)—in what manner are the chemicals going to be used, and in what form or concentration? Next, a sampling strategy must be formed, based on number of laboratory workers using the chemicals, their work locations, and whether other factors have an effect on the possible route of exposure. Finally, a baseline survey can be performed, and based on the outcome, controls incorporated as necessary. For related material, see Chapter 7, Principles of Evaluating Worker Exposure, and Chapter 42, Surveys and Audits.

Evaluation/Assessment

In laboratory operations evaluation of hazards can be defined as the decision-making procedure that results in an opinion of the degree of hazard found in the laboratory after the recognition process has been completed. On occasion this assessment becomes a judgment call. For instance, if a laboratory's inventory shows only one severe health hazard (poison, or highly toxic by definition), in a single container, is it necessary to provide the "secure" storage area recommended? Or, knowing the premium placed on shelf storage space in labs, would it be allowable to simply provide secondary containment for the one bottle and store it with other chemicals that are known not to be incompatible with the poison? Factors such as laboratory accessibility, number or workers, and variables such as personalities that cannot be measured become factors in the evaluation equation. Determining the existence of a hazard is based on observation and measurement of contaminants arising from the laboratory procedures, in addition to assessment of how well any controls are working. Basic occupational hygiene practice teaches one to compare the results of monitoring with the established guidelines published.

A structured approach to evaluating laboratory hazards follows:

- What are the end-products of any experiments or analyses?
- Where are the exits?
- What are the starting materials?
- What chemicals or external variables (heat, light, irradiation) may be added?
- What is the duration of the procedure?
- Are written experimental procedures in place?
- Are written spill procedures or general cleanup procedures in place?

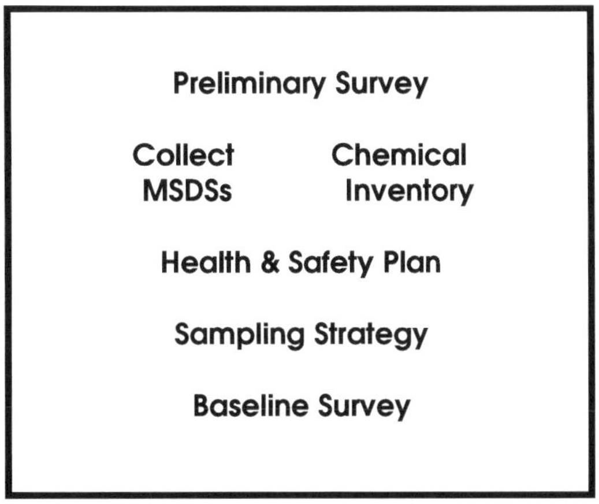

Figure 49.1 — Elements of a formal hazard recognition program.

- Are engineering controls adequate?
- Are safety appliances (showers, eyewash stations) available?
- How are chemicals stored?
- What are the potential routes of exposure? (splash, inhalation)
- How is the laboratory laid out (aisle space)?
- Do chemicals need to be transported outside of the laboratory?

These questions could be incorporated as part of an internal audit overseen by the laboratory supervisor. Laboratory employees, by knowing the audit parameters, can play an active role by requesting that assessment results be addressed.

Survey/Sampling Strategies

Ideally, the occupational hygienist or health and safety officer would attempt to work with the laboratory workers to identify which procedure or experiment causes discomfort or releases contaminants. The difficulty lies in the fact that single room laboratories may be large enough to house many simultaneous experiments, each with its own unique hazard. Alternatively, there may be an exposure that cannot be easily addressed by typical engineering controls, which for laboratories usually is a fume hood. For example, viewing slides under a microscope, which may also require addition of minute volumes of a volatile solvent, may not be possible under a fume hood because of the vibration of the blower. The exposure may not be extreme, it may not be for a duration approaching 8 hours or even the short-term exposure limit, but it may affect the worker. The strategy may be to try to sample the worst case and recommend numerous breaks if the results warrant such action. Another example involves weighing out toxic chemicals that, either because of their potential to become airborne as dust particles or because of their volatility, may pose an inhalation hazard. Again, a fume hood may not solve the problem because of the mechanical vibration, interfering with the sensitive balance. The weighing procedure may occur only once a day; it may last only 5 minutes. The strategy may be not to sample at all, but to relocate the weighing operation to a dedicated room, under negative pressure, with the room exhaust located such that the worker is not subject to turbulence that could direct the contaminants toward him or her.

Surveys should take into account peak exposures. In an environmental or analytical laboratory, sample throughput may be maximized in late morning or early afternoon. Sampling should reflect these peaks as well as the daily averages. Note whether there are multiple shifts. The reader is encouraged to review Chapter 8 for a more detailed discussion of exposure assessment strategies.

Controls

The primary control for limiting exposure to chemicals in laboratories is the fume hood. This is but one of the methods under the category of engineering controls. Typically these are mechanical devices that reduce or eliminate the hazards by isolation, ventilation, or enclosure, or substitution of a material, piece of equipment, or process. Engineering controls, including adequate provision for chemical storage and basic facility design, are the first line of defense for managing exposures. A second important control parameter is PPE. Certain basic PPE should be used by all laboratory workers; however, the need for more extensive equipment, such as respirators, should be avoided through use of engineering controls whenever possible. A third control mechanism, administrative control, also plays an important role in laboratory safety.

Engineering Controls

Fume Hoods/Laboratory Ventilation

The laboratory fume hood is the critical control technology for laboratories. When properly designed and used, it will control exposure to toxic, flammable, or odorous chemicals. It should be noted that many substance-specific regulations from OSHA require engineering controls to reduce and maintain employee exposures below the time-weighted average. The position of the sash on the hood is critical to provide optimal containment. Note that many new installations are fitted with alarms and continuous flow monitors.

Chemical fume hoods are of four basic types. Each meets the purpose of a hood, namely, (1) to provide a ventilated enclosure, containing, capturing, and exhausting hazardous chemicals; and (2) to provide a ventilated workplace to protect personnel from overexposure to those chemicals. (See chapter 37 for an expanded discussion of local exhaust systems; see also the American Conference of Governmental Industrial Hygienists' *Industrial Ventilation: A Manual of Recommended Practice*.[5])

The four types of hoods and their brief descriptions follow.

(1) Conventional fume hood—the simplest in design and, therefore, the least expensive to purchase. This fume hood moves a constant high volume of air. Operating costs are high, and the face velocities are non-uniform and often excessive. The principal mechanism is that, with the sash fully open, there is a minimum face velocity and, as the sash is lowered, the face velocity increases. The increased velocity can create turbulence inside the hood.

(2) Bypass fume hood—also simple in operating principle, with face velocities more maintainable, yet still variable across the hood. Above the sash is the bypass area, which allows air into the hood as the sash is lowered. There is still appreciable wasted energy, because of the relatively large volume of air being exhausted at all times.

(3) Auxiliary/make-up air fume hood—having an auxiliary air supply duct positioned above the working area in front of this hood reduces the amount of conditioned room air that is exhausted, resulting in lower operating costs. A disadvantage occurs in regions of temperature extremes if the make-up air is unconditioned, creating worker discomfort, and possible unacceptable conditions inside the hood.

(4) Variable air volume hood—controls drive up the initial costs of these hoods, yet the operating costs may be significantly lowered. These hoods are designed to maintain a constant average face velocity as the sash open area changes. The hood only exhausts enough air to meet actual needs.

Fume hood performance can be affected adversely by factors that cause air to be drawn out of the hood into the laboratory or that create turbulence within the hood. Thus, improperly located air diffusers, doors, windows, and traffic patterns reduce hood effectiveness, as does storage of chemicals and equipment within the hood that block the direction of airflow.

The basic ventilation design premise for the laboratory itself is that the room must be negatively pressurized with respect to the adjacent corridors. This minimizes the potential for contaminants generated within the laboratory space to affect neighboring spaces. Balancing such a ventilation system requires gathering data from all the fume hoods in the building, the room exhausts, windows that may be operable, and make-up (supply) air. The air required for negative room pressurization is the difference between the higher total exhausted air quantity and the lower supply air quantity. In general, laboratory air should never be recirculated. Newer laboratories being built now can continuously track the total exhaust and the total supply and make adjustments, with the result that more air leaves the lab than enters the lab.

Some general recommendations that involve laboratory ventilation include:

- Comfort ventilation, 20 ft^3/min per person in offices (American Society of Heating, Refrigerating and Air-Conditioning Engineers [ASHRAE]);[6]
- Laboratory ventilation, 6 air changes per hour (ac/hour) (ASHRAE),[6] 4–12 ac/hour (OSHA);[2]
- Chemical storage rooms, 6 ac/hour (OSHA);[7]
- Fume hood face velocity, 60–100 linear feet per minute (OSHA)[2]

Chemical Storage Areas

Because of the large number of individual chemicals typically found in a laboratory, it is tempting to arrange the containers alphabetically on shelves. This inevitably brings incompatible chemicals into close proximity to each other, which must not be allowed. A primary consideration for chemical storage is providing for segregation of chemicals by hazard class. NFPA defines segregation to mean storage within the same room, but physically separated by space. Spacing includes secondary containment (e.g., trays), sills on shelves, or curbs (berms) on floor storage.

In addition to providing for segregation, many other factors must be taken into consideration when designing or evaluating storage space. The construction of the room itself (i.e., its fire rating), existence of a fire suppression system, activities in nonlaboratory spaces (hospital, school, etc.), the type and severity of hazards associated with the chemicals to be stored, the size and number of containers to be stored, provision for secondary containment, and availability of specialized storage cabinets all play roles in determining what constitutes safe storage (see Tables 49.2 and 49.3).

A number of schemes exist for storing chemicals within a laboratory. For example, the National Institute for Occupational Safety and Health (NIOSH) *Manual of Safety and Health Hazards in the School Science Laboratory* includes a "Suggested Shelf Storage Pattern" (see Figure 49.2). Chemical distributors also have devised color-coding schemes for their labels, in which the color code corresponds to a particular hazard class (see Figure 49.3). The NFPA 704 fire diamond[8] is used by some laboratories as an additional labeling method, both for individual bottles and for posting at the entrances to laboratories, indicating the hazard potential to be found within. Fire department personnel and emergency responders may find this useful; however, they are more likely to assume the worst in the event of an emergency.

Local building and fire codes determine limitations for various types of chemical storage; laboratory managers and designers must remain in close contact with their local authorities to assure that laboratory facilities meet the applicable regulations. Local codes are generally based on one of three existing regional code publications. Also, NFPA offers guidance on laboratory design

Table 49.2 — Maximum Quantities of Flammable and Combustible Liquids in Sprinklered Laboratory Units Excluding Flammable Liquid Inside Liquid Storage Areas

		Excluding Quantities in Storage Cabinets or Safety Cans		*Including Quantities in Storage Cabinets or Safety Cans*	
Laboratory Unit Fire Hazard Class	*Flammable Combustible Liquid Class*[A]	*Maximum Quantity per 9.3 m² (100 ft²) of Laboratory Unit*	*Maximum Quantity per Laboratory Unit*	*Maximum Quantity per 9.3 m² (100 ft²) of Laboratory Unit*	*Maximum Quantity per Laboratory Unit*
A	I	38 L (10 gal)	2270 L (600 gal)	76 L (20 gal)	4540 L (1200 gal)
	I, II, and IIIA	76 L (20 gal)	3028 L (800 gal)	150 L (40 gal)	6060 L (1600 gal)
B	I	20 L (5 gal)	1136 L (300 gal)	38L (10 gal)	2270 L (600 gal)
	I, II, and IIIA	38 L (10 gal)	1515 L (400 gal)	76 L (20 gal)	3028 L (800 gal)
C	I	7.5 L (2 gal)	570 L (150 gal)	15 L (4 gal)	1136L (300 gal)
	I, II, and IIIA	15 L (4 gal)	757 L (200 gal)	30 L (8 gal)	1515 L (400 gal)
D	I	4 L (1.1 gal)	284 L (75 gal)	7.5 L (2 gal)	570 L (150 gal)
	I, II, and IIIA	4 L (1.1 gal)	284 L (75 gal)	7.5 L (2 gal)	570 L (150 gal)

[A]Includes Class I flammable liquids and liquified flammable gases.

Table 49.3 — Maximum Quantities of Flammable and Combustible Liquids in Nonsprinklered Laboratory Units Excluding Flammable Liquid Inside Liquid Storage Areas

		Excluding Quantities in Storage Cabinets or Safety Cans		*Including Quantities in Storage Cabinets or Safety Cans*	
Laboratory Unit Fire Hazard Class	*Flammable Combustible Liquid Class*[A]	*Maximum Quantity per 9.3 m² (100 ft²) of Laboratory Unit*	*Maximum Quantity per Laboratory Unit*	*Maximum Quantity per 9.3 m² (100 ft²) of Laboratory Unit*	*Maximum Quantity per Laboratory Unit*
A	I	38 L (10 gal)	1136 L (300 gal)	76 L (20 gal)	2270 L (600 gal)
	I, II, and IIIA	76 L (20 gal)	1515 L (400 gal)	150 L (40 gal)	3028 L (800 gal)
B	I	20 L (5 gal)	570 L (150 gal)	38L (10 gal)	1136 L (300 gal)
	I, II, and IIIA	38 L (10 gal)	757 L (200 gal)	76 L (20 gal)	1515 L (400 gal)
C	I	7.5 L (2 gal)	284 L (75 gal)	15 L (4 gal)	570 L (150 gal)
	I, II, and IIIA	15 L (4 gal)	380 L (100 gal)	30 L (8 gal)	760 L (200 gal)
D	I	4 L (1.1 gal)	140 L (37 gal)	7.5 L (2 gal)	284 L (75 gal)
	I, II, and IIIA	4 L (1.1 gal)	140 L (37 gal)	7.5 L (2 gal)	284 L (75 gal)

[A]Includes Class I flammable liquids and liquified flammable gases.

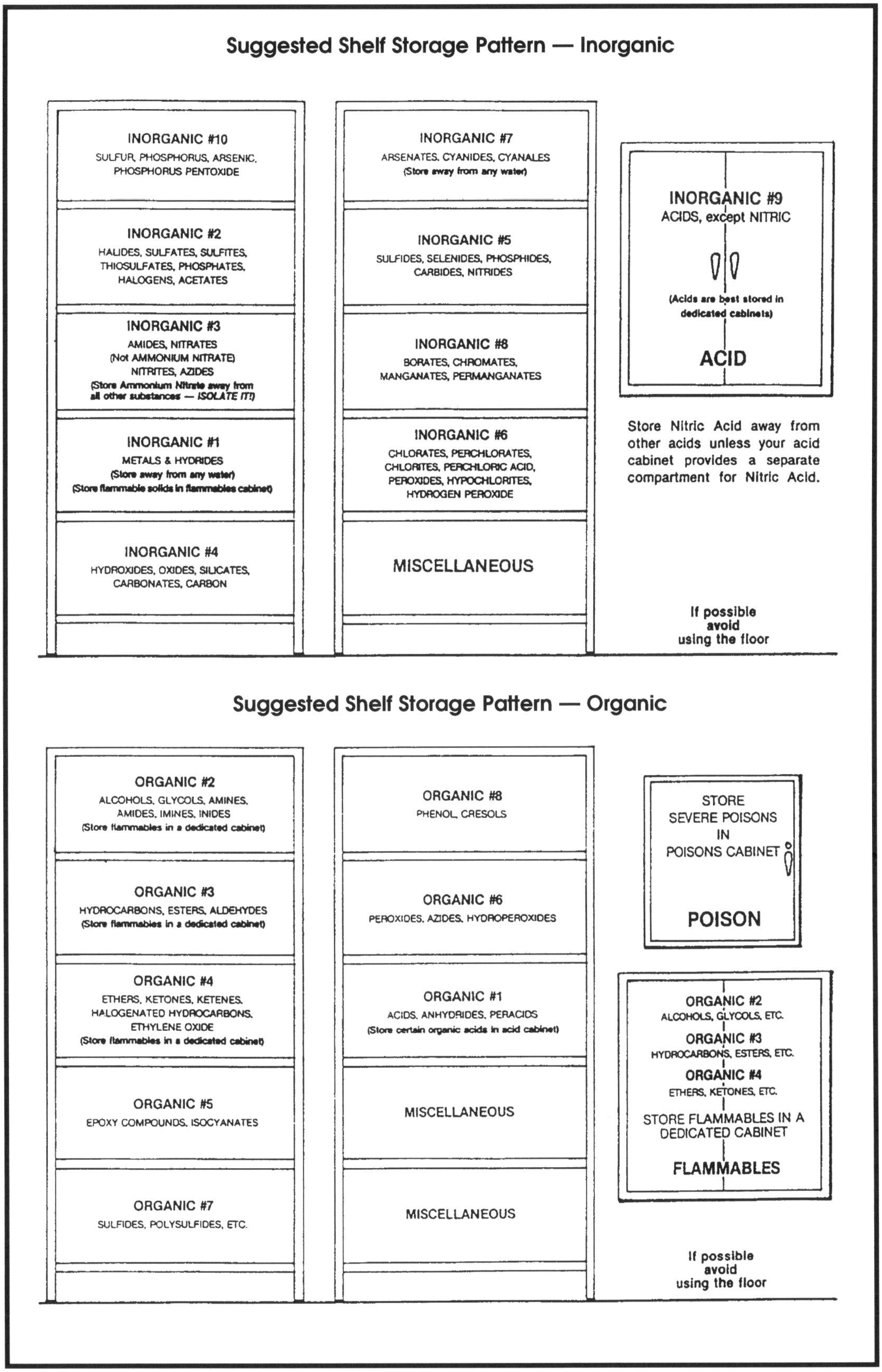

Suggested Shelf Storage Pattern — Inorganic
INORGANIC #10
SULFUR, PHOSPHORUS, ARSENIC, PHOSPHORUS PENTOXIDE
INORGANIC #2
HALIDES, SULFATES, SULFITES, THIOSULFATES, PHOSPHATES, HALOGENS, ACETATES
INORGANIC #3
AMIDES, NITRATES (Not AMMONIUM NITRATE) NITRITES, AZIDES
(Store Ammonium Nitrate away from all other substances — ISOLATE IT!)
INORGANIC #1
METALS & HYDRIDES
(Store away from any water)
(Store flammable solids in flammables cabinet)
INORGANIC #4
HYDROXIDES, OXIDES, SILICATES, CARBONATES, CARBON
INORGANIC #7
ARSENATES, CYANIDES, CYANALES
(Store away from any water)
INORGANIC #5
SULFIDES, SELENIDES, PHOSPHIDES, CARBIDES, NITRIDES
INORGANIC #8
BORATES, CHROMATES, MANGANATES, PERMANGANATES
INORGANIC #6
CHLORATES, PERCHLORATES, CHLORITES, PERCHLORIC ACID, PEROXIDES, HYPOCHLORITES, HYDROGEN PEROXIDE
MISCELLANEOUS
INORGANIC #9
ACIDS, except NITRIC
(Acids are best stored in dedicated cabinets)
ACID
Store Nitric Acid away from other acids unless your acid cabinet provides a separate compartment for Nitric Acid.
If possible avoid using the floor
Suggested Shelf Storage Pattern — Organic
ORGANIC #2
ALCOHOLS, GLYCOLS, AMINES, AMIDES, IMINES, INIDES
(Store flammables in a dedicated cabinet)
ORGANIC #3
HYDROCARBONS, ESTERS, ALDEHYDES
(Store flammables in a dedicated cabinet)
ORGANIC #4
ETHERS, KETONES, KETENES, HALOGENATED HYDROCARBONS, ETHYLENE OXIDE
(Store flammables in a dedicated cabinet)
ORGANIC #5
EPOXY COMPOUNDS, ISOCYANATES
ORGANIC #7
SULFIDES, POLYSULFIDES, ETC.
ORGANIC #8
PHENOL, CRESOLS
ORGANIC #6
PEROXIDES, AZIDES, HYDROPEROXIDES
ORGANIC #1
ACIDS, ANHYDRIDES, PERACIDS
(Store certain organic acids in acid cabinet)
MISCELLANEOUS
MISCELLANEOUS
STORE SEVERE POISONS IN POISONS CABINET
POISON
ORGANIC #2
ALCOHOLS, GLYCOLS, ETC.
ORGANIC #3
HYDROCARBONS, ESTERS, ETC.
ORGANIC #4
ETHERS, KETONES, ETC.
STORE FLAMMABLES IN A DEDICATED CABINET
FLAMMABLES
If possible avoid using the floor

Figure 49.2 — Suggested shelf storage patterns for inorganic and organic chemicals.

ChemAlert* storage codes

A color-coded bar on the label of every Fisher chemical provides an instant guide to storage. The storage code color is also denoted by its initial, and spelled out for additional clarification. The five storage colors and their descriptions are as follows:

RED (R): Flammable. Store in area segregated for flammable reagents.

BLUE (B): Health hazard. Toxic if inhaled, ingested or absorbed through skin. Store in secure area.

YELLOW (Y): Reactive and oxidzing reagents. May react violently with air, water or other substances. Store away from flammable and combustible materials.

WHITE (W): Corrosive. May harm skin, eyes, mucous membranes. Store away from red-, yellow-, and blue-coded reagents above.

GRAY (G): Presents no more than moderate hazard in any of categories above. For general chemical storage.

STORAGE CODE STOP **EXCEPTION**: Denoted by the word "STOP." Reagent incompatible with other reagents of the same color bar. Store separately.

Figure 49.3 — Color-code storage system.

and construction through a wide variety of laboratory-related standards, including NFPA 30, Flammable and Combustible Liquids Code; NFPA 45, Fire Protection Standard for Laboratories Using Chemicals (including reference to more than 20 other standards); NFPA 49, Hazardous Chemicals Data; NFPA 43A, Code for Storage of Liquid and Solid Oxidizing Materials; NFPA 43C, Code for Storage of Gaseous Oxidizing Materials; and NFPA 56C, Safety Standard for Laboratories in Hospitals.

Facility Design

Safety features should be designed into the laboratory. Safety showers, eyewashes, fire extinguishers or extinguishing systems, general and fume hood ventilation, sinks and ample space for chemical storage, and waste handling are all part of a safe laboratory. Evacuation routes from the laboratory are also important. Laboratories should have two exits that are easily accessed through uncluttered aisles. OSHA, the American National Standards Institute, NIOSH, NFPA, and building/fire codes all have specifications for location and construction of these various safety features. Figure 49.4 demonstrates several basic laboratory designs.

Some laboratories require additional safety features based on the operations intended to be carried out in the space. Local exhaust for certain instruments (e.g., gas chromatographs or atomic absorption units), wash-down hoods for perchloric acid digestions, explosion-proof refrigerators or freezers, walk-in fume hoods, glove boxes, and constant-temperature rooms all may be required at various times. In rare instances even a blow-out, pressure-relief panel may be a necessary feature of an isolated laboratory facility.

PPE

Because some hazards cannot be completely avoided through engineering, a minimum level of PPE is essential for all work with chemicals. Eye protection is the most important piece of safety equipment and should not be limited to goggles, but can include face shields for splash protection. Basic protective clothing includes lab coats or aprons, gloves and closed-toe shoes (no bare feet or open-toed sandals). Although canvas or nylon footwear may be popular, impermeable (e.g., leather) materials are preferred. Because of the variety of chemicals used in the laboratory setting, several types of gloves with different permeation characteristics need to be available.

Face shields and heavy leather coats and gloves may be appropriate for work where high-energy chemicals or processes increase the potential for serious injury. In some cases respiratory protection may be appropriate, such as during change-out of toxic gas cylinders in a central storage vault, but in general it should be possible to use engineering controls to avoid the need for a respirator. One exception may be in laboratories where research animals are held. There, respiratory protection may be necessary for those researchers who have allergies.

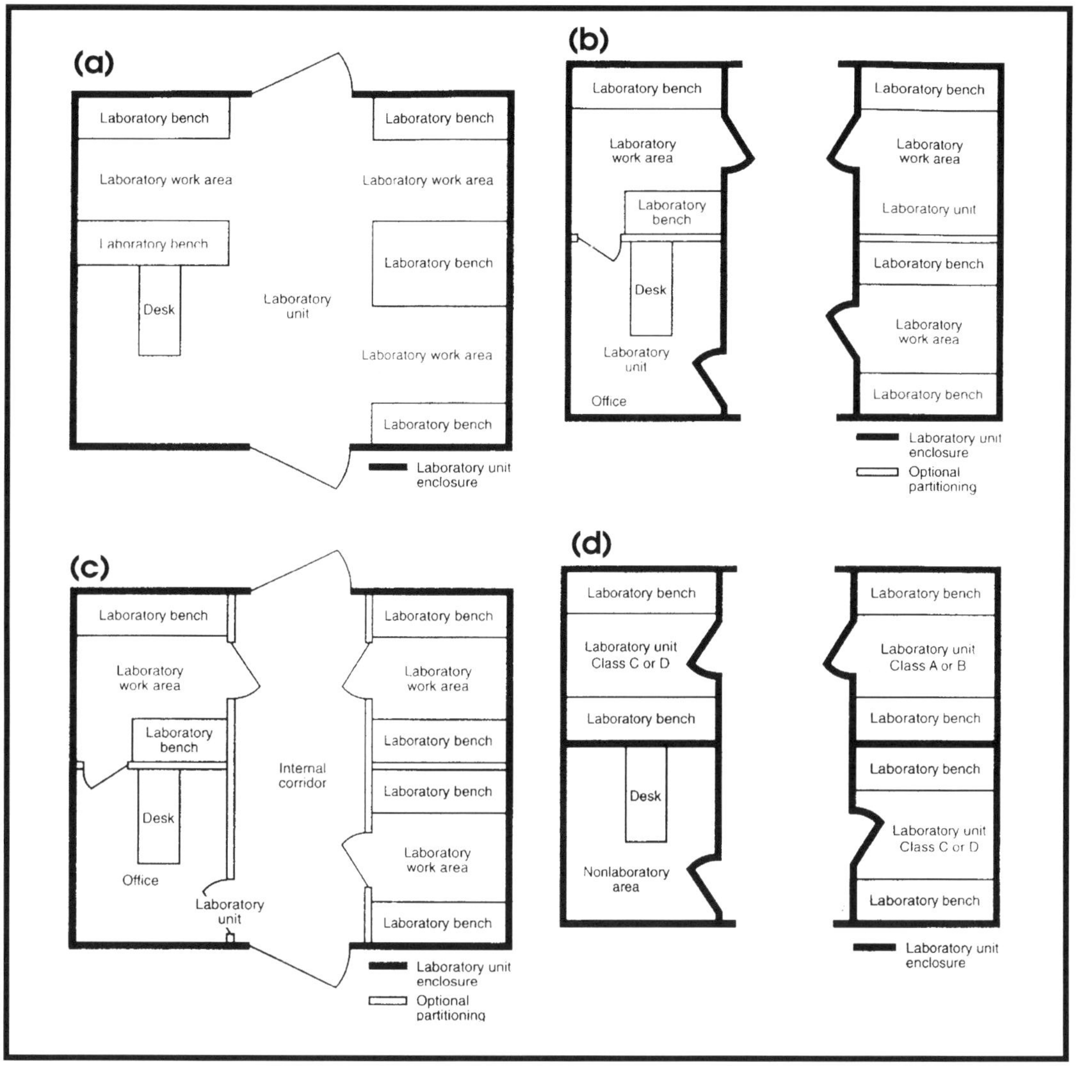

Figure 49.4 — Separation of laboratory areas: (a) laboratory unit without partitioning; (b) laboratory units separated by a required exit corridor; (c) laboratory unit with partitioning; (d) separation of laboratory units and nonlaboratory areas (plans not to scale).

Administrative Controls

Certain types of administrative controls can add considerable assurance that the laboratory provides a safe working environment. These include establishing basic safety rules, instituting an experiment planning process, establishing restricted areas for certain higher hazard activities, and maintaining an inventory of laboratory chemicals (in some jurisdictions, chemical inventories are required). These administrative controls should be a priority, as they set the ground rules for working in a lab. Posting specific hazards associated with certain laboratories is not only prudent, it also is required in some cases (biohazards, radioactive substances). These controls may all be considered SOP.

Safety Rules

Basic safety rules are useful for all laboratories. These include good housekeeping practices; routine safety inspections; special arrangements for working alone; no practical jokes or horseplay; no unaccompanied visitors; and no eating, drinking, or smoking in the laboratory.

Planning Laboratory Experiments

Experiment planning includes establishing goals for the experiment, evaluating hazards and assessing risks, and determining safe working procedures for the chemicals and equipment involved. Provision for acquisition and storage of chemicals and final disposal of waste should be included in the review. For high hazard work the institution may choose to require specific approval before work can begin. More advanced programs have developed an experimental process review procedure, especially for work with particularly hazardous substances.

Establishing Restricted Areas

Restricted areas may be useful or required for work with select carcinogens (defined in the OSHA laboratory standard) or with chemicals exhibiting a high degree of acute toxicity. The restricted area may be an entire laboratory, a portion of a lab, a fume hood, or a glove box. Special signs should be used to notify laboratory occupants of the hazards involved.

Chemical Inventories and Inspections

An inventory of laboratory chemicals has several advantages and is required in some states and jurisdictions. In general, an up-to-date inventory allows the chemist or analyst to determine quickly what is on hand. Sharing of resources is another reason for maintaining an inventory, as many chemicals remain on shelves unused, yet may be needed in a neighboring laboratory. A recurring inventory also shows which chemicals are not being used and can facilitate decisions to recycle or dispose of unnecessary material, in some cases significantly reducing potential hazard. With bar coding, computerization, and networking all readily available, keeping an inventory up-to-date is no longer the onerous task it once was.

The inventory process, if performed regularly, works hand in hand with safe storage procedures. By checking dates of receipt, dates of opening, together with condition of container and legibility of labels, one can demonstrate control over the chemicals. Short shelf-life chemicals can be identified before they deteriorate or become hazardous. The amount of dust on a container brings up the question of usefulness of the chemical and whether it should be stored in active or archival storage. The latter must also be inventoried regularly, as chemicals should not be stored indefinitely. Deterioration of specific compounds cannot always be predicted; however, the characteristics of possible degradation reactions of groups of compounds can be recognized. For example, chemicals that are packed under nitrogen for shipment are susceptible to oxidation when opened, and dehydration affects those compounds with bonded water molecules. Polymerization may occur over time, as in the case of styrene, and it is only through periodic checks that the determination of the viability of a compound can be made. Visual inspection of stored chemicals should be based on the following criteria.

- Change in color/opaqueness of contents
- Caking of anhydrous materials
- Solid residue in a liquid or liquid in a solid
- Bulging containers (over pressurization)
- Questionable container integrity (rusting, corrosion, etc.)
- Obvious error in labeling
- Layering in liquids

Reporting requirements under the Community Right-To-Know Act(9) are a driving force for inventorying chemicals and hazardous materials, because some of the reportable quantities and threshold planning quantities are for chemicals and amounts that can be found in some laboratories. Local authorities, such as fire departments, working through their local emergency planning committees, may require inventories for their files in the event of a chemical release or other accident involving the laboratory.

Training

One of the most important preventive measures that can be taken to ensure safety in the laboratory is a formal training and information program. Just as laboratory employees need to be trained properly on how to operate an instrument, they must also be familiar with the proper means of handling hazardous materials. No one would feel comfortable running an instrument without first becoming familiar with how to optimize its parameters, yet many laboratory workers approach chemicals without first looking at the MSDS or reviewing the safety information for the material. Ultimate responsibility for offering and implementing training programs lies with the management of the laboratory, but ultimate responsibility for ensuring a safe laboratory environment on a daily basis rests with the laboratory supervisor and worker. These individuals must put laboratory safety into practice.

A comprehensive training program begins with orientation. In some states, supervisors are responsible under law for ensuring the safety of their employees. High throughput laboratories emphasizing the number of analyses produced daily are courting danger if their orientation focuses primarily on analytical techniques and not on safe operating procedures. A new employee's observation that safety is secondary in a laboratory establishes the wrong mindset at the very beginning.

The initial training should cover these basics:

- The organization's safety policies and procedures
- Emergency procedures, first aid, and accident reporting
- Location of the MSDSs
- Identity of the chemical hygiene officer and how to contact him or her
- Location of the chemical hygiene plan

After the orientation, the employee's responsibilities are outlined, and specific training can be given pertaining to the hazards inherent in the instrumental techniques used and the chemical reactions that may be faced. An ongoing safety training program can be incorporated into part of routine weekly staff meetings, or monthly/quarterly corporate-level meetings. In a university setting small research groups usually hold seminars highlighting research progress, and safety should become a part of these talks. Departmental safety meetings should be called by the health and safety officer. In either case topics that should be addressed include what new experiments may be started and what new chemicals may be ordered, followed by distribution and discussion of corresponding MSDSs.

These are ideal opportunities for the laboratory workers to provide input, ask questions, and resolve concerns regarding hazards in the laboratory. If accidents have occurred, answers should be found to the inevitable inquiries about what happened, and how it happened, and most important, how it can be prevented from ever happening again. Training should occur every time a new procedure is introduced. Training on the proper use of safety showers and eyewashes can be combined with discussion of routine maintenance procedures (e.g., flushing the lines).

Training is required under OSHA's hazard communication standard, the laboratory standard, and hazardous waste operations and emergency response regulations. Commercially available programs can be purchased to address the requirement, videos can supplement (but not replace) in-house training, or professionals can be brought in to train large groups. Whatever combination of training techniques is used, some method of evaluation should be part of the program. Safety quizzes may not be popular, but they have the benefit of providing documentation, as do sign-in sheets at safety seminars. A measure of the level of comprehension is especially necessary due to the multicultural, multitalented work force of today.

Regulations and Guidelines

OSHA Regulations

As is the case in many occupations, one of the driving forces that brings attention to health and safety in a laboratory is the regulations. In 1986 OSHA suggested that when chemists work with established health and safety programs, they do not experience any additional occupational risks when compared with the general public; but when working without such a program, they are subject to a higher incidence of occupational diseases, such as cancer. Soon after, OSHA promulgated the laboratory standard, officially known as "Occupational Exposure to Hazardous Chemicals in Laboratories."[2] Unlike many other OSHA regulations, this is a performance-oriented standard and is predicated on the expectation that laboratory workers, through education and experience, have at least some level of knowledge about the hazards of chemicals. Laboratory work is also recognized as a very individual activity, affording each worker a greater level of control over safety than is likely to be found in the industrial setting.

OSHA recognizes the unique nature of laboratory work in its definition of "laboratory use of hazardous chemicals" as an occupation in which

(1) containers used for reactions, transfers, and other handling of substances are designed to be easily and safely manipulated by one person;

(2) multiple chemical procedures or chemicals are used;
(3) the procedures involved are not part of a production process; and
(4) protective laboratory practices and equipment are available and in common use to minimize the potential for employee exposure to hazardous chemicals.

With the exception of the permissible exposure limits (PELs), the laboratory standard supersedes most of the other standards in Subpart Z of 29 CFR 1910. Thus, the list of substance-specific standards (1910.1001-1048) is applicable to laboratories only for the associated PELs and action levels. The provisions on monitoring and medical surveillance for those specific substances do not apply. The laboratory standard covers monitoring and medical surveillance in general terms for all hazardous chemicals, when the PEL or action level is routinely exceeded. The exception would be a laboratory specializing in anatomy, for example, where substantial amounts of formaldehyde may lead to potential exposure. In this case the formaldehyde standard (29 CFR 1910.1048) would be applied. Laboratories with only incidental use of formaldehyde would abide by the lab standard. There may be instances in which there is no PEL or when the MSDS may cite only the threshold limit value. Lab employees should be trained to recognize both types of occupational exposure limits and the differences between them.

A chemical hygiene plan (CHP) must be developed to guide laboratory work. It must be a written document that sets forth procedures, equipment, PPE, and work practices that assure a safe work environment. The CHP must be accessible to all laboratory employees and must be implemented by the employer.

Following are the key elements required in the CHP and further discussion from a practitioner's approach.

SOPs. These are mandatory for all laboratory activities involving hazardous chemicals. In practice, such procedures can be generalized (e.g., safety glasses must be worn in the lab) and should state the obvious. If safety goggles are not specified for wear when acid is being used, and an accidental splatter injures a laboratory worker, the lack of an SOP is evidence of noncompliance with a performance-based standard.

Designation of a Chemical Hygiene Officer (CHO). This individual is charged with implementing the CHP. The practitioner's approach is to assign names to various responsibilities, including ultimate responsibility being given to upper management, thereby keeping CEOs and presidents involved and committed to a health and safety program. One CHO may suffice for an organization, or many can be named for individual laboratories of diverse research. In addition, a chemical hygiene committee may be formed, which may be already in place as a safety committee.

Employee Training and Provisions for Accessing Safety Information. In practice, a health and safety office is the key for implementation of this element. A well-established health and safety office can be staffed by experts to train laboratory workers in all aspects of the CHP. These professionals can be the consultants on staff who can answer inquiries, evaluate exposures, stay abreast of regulations, interact with regulators, conduct laboratory inspections, and act as intermediaries between laboratories and management.

Provisions for Medical Attention and Consultation for Laboratory Employees. In real life it is imperative that health care providers, whether they are on-site doctors or nurses or outside medical facilities, be made aware of laboratory hazards, and to provide them with MSDSs as necessary. Special care is sometimes required, as in the case of hydrofluoric acid burns. Interaction between the health care providers, the health and safety office, the CHO, and laboratory supervisors can be helpful in diagnosing and treating occupational diseases.

Methods of Fume Hood Operation Evaluation and Measures to Ensure the Presence of Safety Equipment. The health and safety office (or officer) is instrumental in this element as well. Monitoring fume hood performance can be part of a comprehensive laboratory inspection program. Such a program can be placed into a database and can be used for compliance purposes. Internal inspections (within each laboratory) are encouraged and should be on-going. The responsibility can be shared among laboratory workers.

Control Measure Criteria to Minimize/ Eliminate Hazardous Chemical Exposure. In practice, this requires cooperation among the workers, the supervisors, and the CHO. Training plays a big part here, because to set criteria, knowledge of PELs must be considered when evaluating experimental procedures, and thus addressing whether the potential for exposure exists and whether controls are warranted.

Provisions for Prior Approval Before Attempting Unfamiliar Laboratory Operations, or Other Circumstances Requiring a Supervisor's Approval. The approach best suited to address this element is for the laboratory supervisor or CHO to know the limits of each laboratory worker's expertise in laboratory operations and to oversee those operations, which, because of inherent hazards, require prior notification or approval. Employees must realize that such approval is necessary, and that they are subject to reprimands if it is not acquired.

Provisions for Extra Protective Measures for Employees Working with Particularly Hazardous Chemicals, or "Select Carcinogens." Application of this element to an active laboratory requires everyone in the lab to identify and recognize those reproductive toxins, substances of acute toxicity, and cancer-causing chemicals that are being considered for purchase or are already in the laboratory stockroom.

Because laboratories that use chemicals are likely to generate chemical waste (hazardous waste), it is possible that OSHA's Hazardous Waste Operations and Emergency Response (HAZWOPER) regulation is applicable to some employees, especially if an emergency response team has been designated for the facility.

Related Regulations

There are many other regulations covering laboratory operations; they are not discussed in this chapter, but any student or practicing occupational hygienist should become at least somewhat familiar with them. It is frequently the occupational hygienist who is given responsibility for these regulations. These include the Clean Air Act; the Clean Water Act; the Toxic Substances Control Act; the Emergency Planning and Community Right-To-Know Act; radioactive material use regulations (Nuclear Regulatory Commission Title 10); and transportation regulations (Department of Transportation Title 49). Also, the occupational hygienist should be familiar with additional OSHA regulations such as 1910.20, Access to Employee Exposure and Medical Records; 1910.133, Eye and Face Protection; and 1910.134, Respiratory Protection.

Summary

The chemical laboratory work environment differs significantly from other work sites. Laboratories are likely to contain a very large variety but very small quantities of chemicals; laboratory equipment is small in scale, in keeping with the quantity of chemicals being used; processes carried out in laboratories change frequently, perhaps several times a day; physical hazards associated with chemical laboratory work vary from insignificant to highly hazardous; and laboratory workers routinely make their own decisions about PPE and engineering control needs. All of these differences are important in evaluating health and safety conditions in the laboratory.

Chemicals routinely found in laboratories exhibit a number of hazardous characteristics that need to be understood by the occupational hygienist; the most common of these characteristics are flammability, corrosiveness, oxidizing power, reactivity, and toxicity. Also of concern are the unique hazards associated with the chemical waste produced in every laboratory, as well as radioactive materials, which may be present in some locations.

Notice should also be taken of physical hazards, such as heavy lifting, sharp or protruding objects, slips and falls, eye strain, and noise when evaluating the laboratory workplace.

Hazardous processes and equipment may also be a significant source of injury in a laboratory. Processes may involve unusually high or low temperatures and pressures, deviating significantly from ambient conditions. Electrical hazards may also be associated with equipment, and many devices have moving parts that need to be guarded for safe use.

The primary control for limiting exposure to chemicals in laboratories is the fume hood. Other appropriate engineering controls include adequate provision for chemical storage and basic facility design. A second important control parameter is PPE.

Certain basic PPE should be used by all laboratory workers; however, the need for more extensive equipment, such as respirators, should be avoided through use of engineering controls whenever possible. Administrative controls also help ensure the safety of the laboratory workplace; these include basic safety rules, an experiment planning process, restricted areas for certain higher hazard activities, inventories of laboratory chemicals, and routine inspections.

One of the most important preventive measures that can be taken to ensure safety in the laboratory is a formal training and information program. At a minimum, training should include the organization's safety policies and procedures, location of hazard information, identification of the organization's CHO, and information about the CHP.

The most relevant OSHA regulation is the laboratory standard, officially known as "Occupational Exposure to Hazardous Chemicals in Laboratories." Unlike many other OSHA regulations, the lab standard is performance-oriented and is predicated on the expectation that laboratory workers, through education and experience, have at least some level of knowledge about the hazards of chemicals. Under the standard a CHP must be developed to guide laboratory work.

Key elements of the CHP include standard operating procedures for all laboratory activities involving hazardous chemicals; designation of a CHO; employee training and provisions for accessing safety information; provisions for medical attention and consultation for laboratory employees; methods to be used to evaluate fume hood operation and measures to ensure that other equipment designed for safety are in place; criteria for the use of control measures to minimize or eliminate exposure to hazardous chemicals; provisions for prior approval before attempting unfamiliar laboratory operations or other circumstances requiring a supervisor's approval; and provisions for extra protective measures for employees working with particularly hazardous chemicals or select carcinogens.

References

1. **Bretherick, L.:** *Handbook of Reactive Chemical Hazards*, 4th ed. London: Butterworth, 1990.
2. "Occupational Exposure to Hazardous Chemicals in Laboratories," *Code of Federal Regulations* Title 29, Part 1910.1450. 1990.
3. **National Research Council: Prudent Practices in the Laboratory:** *Handling and Disposal of Chemicals.* Washington, D.C.: National Academy Press, 1995.
4. "The Control of Hazardous Energy (Lockout/Tagout)," *Code of Federal Regulations* Title 29, Part 1910.147. 1989.
5. **American Conference of Governmental Industrial Hygienists (ACGIH):** Laboratory ventilation. In *Industrial Ventilation: A Manual of Practice*, 22nd ed. Cincinnati, Ohio: ACGIH, 1995.
6. **American Society of Heating, Refrigeration and Air Conditioning Engineers (ASHRAE):** Laboratories. In *Applications Handbook.* Atlanta: ASHRAE, 1978.
7. "Flammable and Combustible Liquids," *Code of Federal Regulations* Title 29, Part 1910.106(d).
8. **National Fire Protection Association (NFPA):** Fire Protection Guide to Hazardous Materials. Quincy, Mass.: NFPA, 1991.
9. "Hazardous Chemical Reporting: Community Right-to-Know," *Code of Federal Regulations* Title 40, Part 370. 1987.

Outcome Competencies

After completing this chapter, the reader should be able to:

1. Define underlined terms used in this chapter.
2. Understand the key objectives of an occupational health program.
3. Describe the elements of medical surveillance programs.
4. Explain the role of the occupational hygienist in a medical surveillance program.
5. List criteria for selecting health care providers and the core competencies.

Key Topics

- I. Objectives of an Occupational Health Program
- II. Selecting Health Care Professionals
- III. Preventive Care—Medical Surveillance
- IV. Integrating the Occupational Hygienist Into the Medical Surveillance Program
  - A. Evaluate Workplace Exposures
  - B. Identify Individuals at Risk
  - C. Conduct Medical Examinations for Early Health Effects
- V. Report Medical Findings to Employees
- VI. Determine Employee Medical Restrictions
  - A. Accommodate Medical Restrictions
  - B. Analyze Potential Relationships Between Medical Results and Occupational Exposure
  - C. Implement and Maintain Effective Workplace Controls
- VII. Acute Medical Care — Medical Treatment
  - A. Preparing for Emergency Treatment
  - B. Disability Management — Managing Medical Cases
- VIII. Implementing Management Systems to Sustain the Occupational Health Program

Key Terms

Americans with Disabilities Act (ADA) • detectable preclinical phase • health history • management system • medical treatment • medical surveillance • occupational history • periodic medical examination • preplacement examination • primary prevention • pulmonary function tests • recommended accommodations • secondary prevention measures • sentinel health event • symptom questionnaires • tertiary prevention measures • work restrictions

Prerequisite Knowledge

Prior to beginning this chapter, the user should review the following chapters:

Chapter Number	Chapter Topic
1	History and Philosophy of Industrial Hygiene
3	Legal Aspects of the Occupational Environment
4	Occupational Exposure Limits
5	Environmental and Occupational Toxicology
6	Occupational Epidemiology
7	Principles of Evaluating Worker Exposure
8	Occupational and Environmental Health Risk Assessment/Risk Management
9	Comprehensive Exposure Assessment
10	Modeling Inhalation Exposure
19	Biological Monitoring
35	General Methods for the Control of Airborne Hazards
37	Local Exhaust Ventilation
41	Program Management
42	Surveys and Audits
43	Hazard Communication
44	Emergency Planning and Crisis Management in the Workplace

Developing An Occupational Health Program

50

By Thomas D. Polton and George Mellendick, MD, MPH

Introduction

Industrial hygiene is most commonly associated with efforts to control exposures to the chemical, physical, and biological causes of occupational disease. Indeed, these so-called primary prevention programs employ the control methods discussed throughout this book to eliminate or reduce employee exposures (i.e., substitution, engineering, administrative, and personal protective equipment). These approaches, which include substituting water-based materials for more toxic chemicals, constructing sound-attenuating barriers around noisy equipment, and establishing administrative controls for handling infectious agents, form the cornerstones of any occupational health program.

Primary prevention alone is often not sufficient to eliminate workplace illnesses. Instead, a comprehensive occupational health program must also include secondary and tertiary prevention measures. These are programs designed to identify individuals who are affected by exposures in the workplace, to prevent further exposure, and to provide medical treatment, if necessary. The medical department may bring to light health concerns among the work force that were not recognized or not adequately controlled.

A classic case in occupational medicine was the work performed by the medical team at the BF Goodrich plant near Louisville, Kentucky. Between September 1967 and December 1973, four cases of angiosarcoma of the liver, an exceedingly rare tumor, were diagnosed among men in the polyvinyl chloride polymerization section.[1] The recognition that vinyl chloride monomer exposure was the cause of this sentinel health event led to more restrictive regulations. In many cases, responsibility for secondary and tertiary prevention is put solely in the hands of occupational physicians and other health care professionals. But the occupational hygienist needs to be involved to make certain that the examinations performed by the health care professional are focused on the relevant workplace risks and to ensure that the appropriate controls are implemented to address work-related illnesses.

A comprehensive occupational health program consists of three efforts:

- Medical surveillance — to identify employees exhibiting signs or symptoms of the early stages of an illness (medical surveillance involves questionnaires, physical examinations, and testing that directly relates to the hazards of the workplace and associated risks);
- Medical treatment — to provide prompt medical care for all work-related injuries and illnesses and manage the medical care to expedite the employee's return to work; and
- Management systems — to ensure the necessary documentation is available and accessible, to periodically assess the program's effectiveness, and to implement improvements.

The remainder of this chapter will provide a more detailed explanation of these key elements of an occupational health program, provide guidance on selecting a qualified occupational health professional, and discuss the complementary roles of the medical staff and the occupational hygienist.

Objectives of an Occupational Health Program

The first step in establishing an occupational health program is to define the program's objectives. The scope of the program can range from the bare bones minimum of caring for injured employees to promoting improved health with elaborate wellness programs. The objectives vary depending upon the type of industry, its potential hazards, the work force, the resources within the community, and the level of support from the employer. A comprehensive medical program will often consist of three levels of medical services: acute medical care, disability management, and preventive care (see Table 50.1).

Acute medical care, the treatment of workplace injuries and illnesses that occur as a result of emergencies and non-emergencies, is the most fundamental level of medical service. At a minimum, the employer provides first aid services, but often the level of service extends to include treating many other medical conditions that are reported by employees. The medical department manages the treatment and care of employees to ensure they receive effective medical care. In some instances this involves referring employees to a medical professional to confirm a diagnosis or to treat the individual.

The next level of service is disability management. Prolonged absence from one's normal routine can have a devastating impact to one's recovery, affecting one physically and psychologically. The workplace's disability management program needs to be structured to encourage a patient's return to function and work as soon as possible after an illness or injury, yet without endangering the individual. The occupational health care professional must ensure that patients receive prompt diagnoses and proper treatment to aid their recovery and return to work. Offering employees flexible work assignments or restricting them from performing specific activities that are part of their normal responsibilities can lead to quicker recoveries. The medical department can assist in the early return to work regardless of whether the original injury or illness was work-related or non-work-related.

Preventive care is the third level of service and involves screening for the early signs and symptoms of disease. The preventive medical programs instituted by employers need not be limited to preserving the health of workers, but may also focus on promoting proper health practices. Many employers offer health promotion and wellness programs that feature nutritional counseling, exercise programs, and screening efforts for nonoccupational risk factors, such as high cholesterol and diabetes.

At a minimum, the occupational health program must address all relevant regulatory requirements imposed by federal, state, and local authorities. The occupational hygienist or safety professional needs to keep abreast of local, state, and national regulations as well as professional standards and practices. For example, governmental standards require medical surveillance and medical services when employees are exposed to particular hazards[2], use certain types of protective equipment[3], or perform specific tasks.[4] The specific requirements of these standards must be incorporated into the occupational health program; see Table 50.2 for OSHA regulated medical surveillance requirements.[5]

Table 50.1 — Elements of an Occupational Health Program—Possible Levels of Service

Medical Treatment

Acute Medical Care: Treating workplace injuries and illnesses that occur as a result of emergencies and nonemergencies.

Disability Management: Providing timely treatment and encouraging the prompt return to work.

Medical Surveillance

Preventive Care: Screening for the early signs and symptoms of disease.

Health Promotion: Worksite programs extending beyond preserving health to include promoting proper health (e.g., nutritional counseling, smoking cessation, and wellness program).

At a minimum, the occupational medical program must address all regulatory requirements. See Attachment A for guidance.

Table 50.2 — OSHA Regulated Medical Surveillance Requirements

	OSHA Regulated Toxic and Hazardous Substances	
Chemical	*Regulatory Reference*	*Medical Surveillance Criteria*
2-Acetylaminofluorene CAS #53-96-3	Title 29.CFR.1910.1014	Prior to assignment to enter a regulated area.
Acrylonitrile CAS #107-13-1	Title 29.CFR.1910.1045	Exposure at or above the Action Level without regard to respirator use.
4-Aminodiphenyl CAS #92-67-1	Title 29.CFR.1910.1011	Prior to assignment to a regulated area.
Arsenic - inorganic CAS #7440-38-2	Title 29.CFR.1910.1018	Exposure at or above the Action Level without regard to respirator use.
Asbestos CAS #1332-21-4	Title 29.CFR.1910.1001 Title 29.CFR.1915.1001 Title 29.CFR.1926.1101	Exposures at or above the Time Weighted Average and/or excursion limit.
Benzene CAS #71-43-2	Title 29.CFR.1910.1028	Employees exposed at or above the Action Level 30 days/year; at or above the Permissible Exposure Limit 10 days/year; at or above 10 ppm 30 days/year prior to 1987; to >0.1% benzene solvent as tire building machine operators.
Benzidine CAS #92-87-5	Title 29.CFR.1910.1010	Prior to assignment to enter a regulated area.
1,3 Butadiene CAS #106-99-0	Title 29.CFR.1910.1051	Before the time of initial assignment.
Cadmium CAS #7440-43-9	Title 29.CFR.1910.1027	Employees who are or may be exposed at or above the Action Level 30 days/year or previous exposure above Action Level total of 60 months.
Bis-Chloro-Methylether CAS #542-88-1	Title 29.CFR.1910.1008	Prior to assignment to enter a regulated area.
Coke Oven Emissions	Title 29.CFR.1910.1029	Employed in a regulated area 30 or more days/year.
1,2-Dibromo-3-Chloropropane CAS #107-13-1	Title 29.CFR.1910.1044	Employed in a regulated area and emergency exposures.
3,3'-Dichloro-Benzidine CAS #91-94-1	Title 29.CFR.1910.1007	Prior to assignment to enter a regulated area.
4-Dimethylaminoazobenzene CAS #60-11-7	Title 29.CFR.1910.1015	Prior to assignment to enter a regulated area.
Ethyleneimine CAS #151-56-4	Title 29.CFR.1910.1012	Prior to assignment to enter a regulated area.
Ethylene Oxide CAS #75-21-8	Title 29.CFR.1910.1047	For all employees who or may be exposed at or above the Action Level > 30 days/year
Formaldehyde CAS #50-00-0	Title 29.CFR.1910.1048	All employees exposed at or above the Action Level or exceeding the STEL
Lead CAS #74-39-1	Title 29.CFR.1910.1025 Title 29.1926.62	Employees who are or may be exposed above the Action Level for 30 days/year
Methylenedianiline CAS #101-77-9	Title 29.CFR.1910.1050	Before the time of initial assignment
Methyl Chloro Ether CAS #107-30-2	Title 29.CFR.1910.1006	Prior to assignment to a regulated area.
Methylene Chloride CAS #75-09-2	Title 29.CFR.1910.1052	Initially prior to initial assignment.
Alpha-Naphthylamine CAS #134-32-7	Title 29.CFR.1910.1004	Prior to assignment to a regulated area.
Beta-Naphthylamine CAS #91-59-8	Title 29.CFR.1910.1009	Prior to assignment to a regulated area.
4-Nitrobiphenyl CAS #92-93-3	Title 29.CFR.1910.1003	Prior to assignment to a regulated area.
N-Nitrosodimethylamine CAS #62-75-9	Title 29.CFR.1910.1016	Prior to assignment to a regulated area.
Beta-Propiolactone CAS #57-57-8	Title 29.CFR.1910.1013	Prior to assignment to a regulated area.
Vinyl Chloride CAS #75-01-4	Title 29.CFR.1910.1017	Exposure at or above the Action Level without regard to respirator use.

(continued on next page.)

Table 50.2 — OSHA Regulated Medical Surveillance Requirements (continued)

OSHA Regulated Physical and Biological Substances		
Agent	*Regulatory Reference*	*Medical Surveillance Criteria*
Bloodborne Pathogens	Title 29.CFR.1910.1030	All employees "reasonably anticipated" to be at risk for exposure.
Noise	Title 29.CFR.1910.95	When noise exposure is 85 dBA 8-hour Time Weighted Average or greater.
OSHA Regulated Occupational Groups		
Task	*Regulatory Reference*	*Medical Surveillance Criteria*
Hazardous Waste / Emergency Response	Title 29.CFR.1910.120	All employees at risk for exposure above PEL for 30 days or more a year without regard to the use of respirators. All employees who wear a respirator for 30 days or more a year. All employees who are injured, become ill or develop signs or symptoms due to possible overexposure or from an emergency response or hazardous waste operation.
Respiratory Protection	Title 29.CFR.1910.134	All workers wearing respirators.

There are many situations for which employers may decide to provide medical surveillance or establish medical treatment protocols, even though there are not any governmental requirements. For instance, workers may experience heat stress from performing physically demanding work while wearing protective equipment, face the potential for life-threatening emergencies because of accidental chemical releases, or endure continual shoulder pain caused by repetitive tasks. In each of these situations, the governmental standards do not contain specific provisions to address these risks to employee health, yet medical surveillance and, on occasion, medical treatment are indicated. For this reason, the occupational physician and the occupational hygienist are likely to include provisions in the employer's occupational health program to address these situations as well.

After determining the details of the medical surveillance and medical treatment programs, the occupational hygienist and health care provider should develop a written program defining the responsibilities of all of the participants and the procedures for maintaining important medical records (see Table 50.3). The program should be periodically reassessed, and improvements should be made to address deficiencies. The participants may identify the need for new work site programs or decide to discontinue programs that are no longer effective.

Selecting Health Care Professionals

A variety of health care professionals may implement the specific objectives of the medical program. For instance, occupational health care nurses assess and manage illnesses and injuries. Their primary role in surveillance activities is to assist the occupational physician. Nurse practitioners may perform examinations. Other health care professionals (including physician assistants, licensed practical nurses, and emergency medical technicians/paramedics) can be used to augment occupational health programs. When they identify health problems, they may provide first aid or emergency care under the direction or supervision of a physician or an occupational health nurse. It is imperative that the roles and responsibilities assigned to the health care professionals comply with the specific state's legal scope of practice[6] The individual state's licensing or certification board should be contacted with any concerns.

Before hiring a health care staff, the employer or the consultant designing the program should assess the availability and quality of the emergency medical care services and medical specialists within the community. For hazards requiring immediate attention, the company medical plan may specify having a physician or nurse on site or provide trained first-responder teams (also

Table 50.3 — Responsibilities of Health Care Professional and Occupational Hygienist in a Comprehensive Occupational Health Program

Program Element	*Health Care Professional*	*Occupational Hygienist*
Medical surveillance	• Perform medical screening to identify early symptoms of occupational disease at a reversible or treatable phase. • Analyze the medical data to identify and communicate medical trends for individuals and groups of workers. • Determine medical restrictions. • Advise on appropriate accommodations for workers to aid their prompt return to work. • Develop and implement wellness and health promotion activities for nonoccupational disorders.	• Characterize employee exposures to hazardous agents. • Identify employees to be offered medical evaluations because exposures exceed designated trigger levels. • Develop and implement appropriate accommodations for workers to aid their prompt return to work.
Medical treatment	• Treat work-related illnesses and injuries. • Coordinate emergency and nonemergency treatment with physicians and hospitals in the community. • Direct the recovery and rehabilitation of employees who have prolonged or complex illnesses or injuries.	• Integrate medical preparedness into emergency response plan. • Develop and implement appropriate accommodations for workers to aid their prompt return to work.
Program Management	• Maintain accessible and confidential individual employee medical and exposure records. • Periodically reassess the medical program and modify it according to revised needs.	

known as medical emergency response teams). This option might not be necessary if medical care is located nearby.

It is often advantageous to provide occupational health services on site, either full-time or on a part-time basis. In so doing the occupational health professional — nurse and/or physician — tends to develop a much better understanding of the occupational setting, the employees, and their work; thus, the professional inherently becomes more involved in the day-to-day operation of the medical program. On-site service providers tend to be more accessible to management for rendering medical opinions on many health matters-even some that are not strictly occupational. Regardless of whether the medical staff is situated on or off site, it is important that the medical professional become familiar with the workplace, the job requirements, and the occupational hazards. It may be beneficial for the occupational hygiene staff to organize periodic walk-throughs for medical professionals to tour the workplace.

Even more important than where the staff is located is the quality of the staff involved in the program. The competence of the occupational health nurse or physician is the most critical determinant of the value provided. The American College of Occupational and Environmental Medicine (ACOEM) has established core competencies for occupational physicians. These competencies define specific areas for judging knowledge and competence of candidates. Physicians who are trained in the field of occupational medicine must successfully pass a written examination to become board-certified in occupational medicine by the American Board of Preventive Medicine. However, physicians who are not board-certified in occupational medicine can develop competencies and proficiencies in those areas that are required for good practice through independent study and course work. Appendix A contains an abridged list of core competencies for occupational and environmental medicine developed by ACOEM.

For those in the nursing profession, the American Board for Occupational Health Nurses Inc. (ABOHN) sets the criteria for certification and administers the certification examinations. Occupational and environmental health nursing is the specialty practice for delivering cost-effective health and safety services to employees. Although voluntary, certification indicates that a nurse has met certain eligibility requirements and demonstrates knowledge of the specialty. Even in the absence of certification in occupational medicine and occupational health nursing, competency should be expected in core areas such as health promotion, medical case management, injury and illness prevention, and familiarity with occupational health hazards.

In hiring the appropriate health care professionals, the occupational hygiene professional should review the education and training of each candidate to make sure his or her credentials match the requirements of the position. It is also helpful to evaluate the experiences of the candidate to ensure he or she is familiar with the types of hazards encountered in the workplace and that he or she is knowledgeable in the relevant regulatory issues. Knowledge of workers' compensation laws, relevant regulatory issues, and the American with Disabilities Act may be important for those professionals involved in managing rehabilitative cases.

Preventive Care — Medical Surveillance

Medical surveillance is designed to detect illness or organ dysfunction at an early phase[7], during which intervention in the form of removal from the exposure and/or treatment would be effective. Medical examinations are typically offered before employees begin an assignment (preplacement), at a predetermined frequency during that assignment (periodic), and at the conclusion of employment or the end of the expected latency period of the materials to which workers have been exposed (termination).

The primary goal of the preplacement physical examination is to reveal any medical condition that might put the worker at an increased risk to himself or to others because of work exposures or activities.[8] It should not be used to exclude "unsuitable workers" from work opportunities. Instead, the employer is responsible for providing suitable workplace accommodations whenever feasible. The results of the preplacement examination also provide a baseline for comparing future examinations in order to assess the impact of subsequent exposures on the development of illnesses. Some employers also include screening for nonoccupational diseases such as hypertension or breast cancer. Others use the preplacement exam to direct workers to health promotion activities, such as smoking cessation programs.

The preplacement examination also offers an opportunity to educate workers about the potential hazards of the new job and about the health and safety measures being used to avoid illnesses and injuries. Another goal of the exam is to establish a rapport between the worker and the health care professional so that if a work-related problem does arise, the employee will feel comfortable discussing it with the health professional.

The periodic medical examination begins with questions concerning any changes in the job, work processes, or exposures that might increase the risk of occupational illness. Medical examinations and testing procedures are designed to detect changes in the health of the employee since the last examination that might indicate a need for a change in the work process or in job placement.[9] The examination may include biological monitoring and a variety of other surveillance techniques.

Employees should have an updated medical examination at the end of their employment or at the end of the disease latency period associated with past exposures. This is a decision that must come from both the occupational physician and the occupational hygienist. Employees may require an exit medical examination or an examination at the end of the disease latency period.

Medical surveillance includes a second important element. This is the analysis of medical data to identify changes in the health status of individual workers, as well as to identify any patterns or trends among groups of workers.[10] When performed properly, this analysis benefits both the individual worker and groups of workers who share common exposures and risks.

Individuals benefit when early detection is followed by appropriate intervention (e.g., reducing workplace exposures or providing medical treatment to the employee). Groups of workers benefit when analyses of their aggregate data uncover a link between exposures and illnesses and provide insight into how this link might be broken.

In many cases, analyzing the medical surveillance data may uncover the need for improved primary prevention controls. For example, the employer may re-evaluate the effectiveness of workplace controls or replace hazardous materials with less toxic substances, thereby preventing occupational illness. Medical surveillance, when designed as being part of an occupational health program, should be directly related to the hazards of the workplace and based on a careful risk assessment. The general screening programs that take place in the majority of occupational settings are most appropriately considered preventive medicine or wellness initiatives — not strictly medical surveillance. The basis for health surveillance based on exposure is appropriately defined in the United Kingdom regulation known as COSHH, the Control of Substances Hazardous to Health.[11] This regulation states that health surveillance is appropriate only when:

- An identifiable disease or adverse health effect may be related to the exposure;
- There is a reasonable likelihood that the disease or effect may occur under the particular conditions of work; and
- There are valid techniques for detecting indications of the disease or the effect.

Integrating the Occupational Hygienist Into the Medical Surveillance Program

An effective medical surveillance program requires cooperation between the occupational hygienist and the occupational physician. All too often the occupational hygiene and medical programs operate independently, such that the two entities fail to coordinate their efforts. A common experience is for the medical and occupational hygiene departments to communicate with each other, but not to have a true dialogue. The two groups talk to each other, but do not exchange the relevant information that each other needs to perform their jobs better.

After all, the occupational hygienist performs exposure assessments characterizing the workplace hazards encountered by employees. This information is needed by the occupational physician so that he or she may perform a medical evaluation targeted to the health risks of the employee, but all too often it is not available. Following the medical evaluation, the occupational hygienist should be notified if any medical findings may be the result of workplace exposure. The occupational physician should work with the occupational hygienist and the safety professional to accommodate any new work restrictions. The occupational hygienist plays a key role in altering the job to accommodate the workers' restrictions.

Inserting two additional steps in the tasks performed by these professionals can break the barriers between the two independently operating programs. It is incumbent upon the occupational hygienist to identify individuals at risk based upon their workplace exposures. These individuals may require specialized medical examinations because of the exposures they have (use of specific chemicals or elevated noise levels) or because of the tasks they perform (respirator use or confined space entry). The second important step to integrating these two programs is to have the occupational hygienist and the occupational physician, with the possible assistance of an epidemiologist, review the medical data for potential trends or patterns of disease. The relationship between the occupational hygienist and occupational physician is composed of eight steps described in the following sections (see Figure 50.1).

Evaluate Workplace Exposures

A well-designed medical surveillance program begins with a thorough characterization of the hazards encountered by workers. For each work area, process, or occupation, the occupational hygienist completes a workplace exposure assessment. This assessment identifies potential chemical, physical, and biological hazards in the workplace. Each of these types of stressors may impact the health of the employee, so it is important that the information is reported to the examining physician. For instance, when the workplace exposure assessment indicates that an employee's job involves

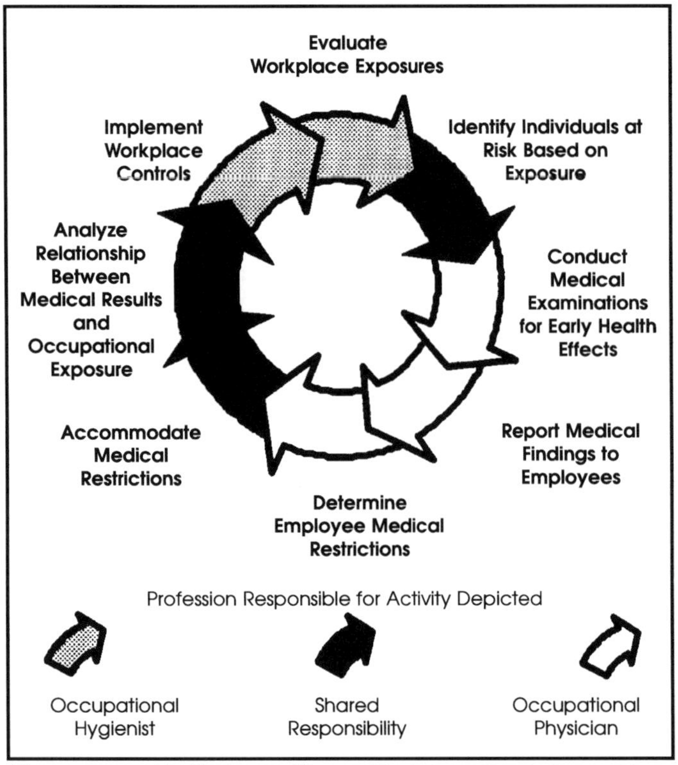

Figure 50.1 — Medical surveillance: The interaction between the occupational hygienist and the occupational physician.

highly repetitive tasks, it alerts the physician that the employee encounters ergonomic risks. The workplace exposure assessment should contain information describing the conditions in the workplace that relate to the intensity and duration of these exposures, with specific details on:

- Likely routes of exposure (inhalation, ingestion, and skin absorption or contact);
- Duration (length of the exposure during a typical work shift);
- Frequency (approximate number of times per day, month, or year this exposure occurs); and
- Intensity (average and peak concentrations of contaminant to which the worker is exposed).

The occupational hygienist and the occupational physician review the anticipated health effects, the likely target organs, and the expected disease latency periods associated with these exposures. The occupational physician then uses the information to develop a physical examination program containing all relevant questions that can be added to the basic occupational and health history. The surveillance examination will include appropriate diagnostic studies including biological monitoring or biomonitoring tests in a program of biological monitoring. The designated latency period influences the schedule for further medical evaluations.

The workplace exposure assessment should also contain information on government requirements for medical surveillance. Occupational physicians should be familiar with these regulatory requirements.

It is also important to report information about the workplace controls (engineering, administrative, or personal protective equipment) used to limit worker exposures. This information is not only critical in analyzing any group trends; as is the case with respirators, it also initiates required examinations.[3]

Identify Individuals at Risk

The occupational hygienist and the occupational physician use the findings of the workplace exposure assessments to decide which employees require medical surveillance. Often, the action level or trigger level for initiating an employee medical surveillance program is based on the airborne concentration of contaminants measured in the work areas. The most common trigger levels are as follows:

- *For acutely toxic materials:* a single episode exceeding the ceiling or the 15-minute short-term exposure limit (STEL); and
- *For chronic hazards:* employee exposure to one-half the full shift exposure limit (permissible exposure limit [PEL] or ACGIH threshold limit value [TLV®]) for the contaminant for 30 days or more. (Note that some specific regulations may differ from these general guidelines.)

Excessive exposure through routes other than inhalation may also jeopardize the employee's health. Workers may ingest toxic materials on their hands while eating or smoking in the workplace; they may also absorb solvents directly through the skin. For these situations, the occupational physician may use the results of biological monitoring (analysis of blood, urine, or expired air samples for elevated concentrations of workplace contaminants or their metabolites) as a trigger level for initiating more frequent medical examinations and for the occupational hygienist to intercede with primary prevention measures (see Chapter 19, Biological Monitoring).

Reports of health complaints or employee symptoms consistent with workplace exposures may be another reason for initiating a medical surveillance program.[12] For instance, employees working with coatings or adhesives containing diisocyanates may suddenly complain about wheezing or dry cough. The medical surveillance program also should include workers exposed to hazardous materials from accidental process releases, chemical spills, or other workplace incidents.

Conduct Medical Examinations for Early Health Effects

The cornerstone of the medical examination is the occupational health history. The initial occupational history for a new employee should consist of the following: risk assessment and/or job description; review of symptoms, any illnesses, or injuries related to past jobs; questions relevant to the requirements or potential hazards of the new job; and a listing of significant community and home exposures.[13] The medical history during the periodic examination focuses on changes in health status, illnesses, and possible work-related symptoms. Once the history is completed, it is followed by the medical examination and by appropriate medical and laboratory tests.

The selection of medical tests should also take into account both the occupational hygienist's workplace exposure assessments and the availability of reliable measures. Despite the fact the worker's occupational history indicates that he or she has had significant exposure to workplace contaminants, reliable medical tests are not always available. Biological monitoring is advancing rapidly, but it is still able to monitor only a limited number of occupational exposures.

Laboratory analysis of blood or urine, clinical procedures (audiometry, chest X-rays, or pulmonary function tests), symptom questionnaires, and the physical examination are not always definitive. They do, however, represent the best available technology for exercising secondary preventive measures.

The time it takes for symptoms to emerge is crucial in determining whether surveillance tests are feasible. For instance, surveillance testing is inappropriate for acute toxic effects like cyanide poisoning since the onset of symptoms is so rapid. However, conditions involving a longer onset period may be well-suited to a surveillance program that periodically evaluates a worker's health. The schedule (periodicity) of medical examinations should be based on the expected timing of health effects in relation to exposure. In this regard, both the induction period (the period between first exposure and first manifestation) and the duration of the "detectable preclinical phase" of a health effect are important considerations. Conditions with long induction periods often have long detectable preclinical phases during which testing will be beneficial. Testing, however, is inappropriate before sufficient time has lapsed for the health effect to be detected by the test being used.

The health professional designing the medical surveillance program should develop a plan for how medical data will be interpreted and acted on. Again, the occupational physician and the occupational hygienist should work together. This plan should include criteria used to determine when action will be taken in response to medical test results and what that action will be. Workers should be given a written summary of the action plan, in easily understandable terms, before they are asked to provide informed consent for participation in medical surveillance. It is important to remember that for medical surveillance covered by OSHA regulations, the medical surveillance is mandatory. All other medical surveillance, however, is essentially voluntary and generally benefits the individual worker and ultimately the workplace itself.

The following steps are highly recommended or required when the action threshold for a medical test is exceeded: employee notification; test confirmation either through retesting with the same method or using a more accurate method; medical evaluation and treatment if indicated; and evaluation and control of the occupational exposure. No plan can anticipate every situation that will arise during a surveillance program, and interpretation of individual test results often requires the judgment of the occupational physician.

Report Medical Findings to Employees

Notifying workers is considered mandatory by case law and in writing is considered current standard of care. It is critical that notification to workers regarding the findings of medical surveillance in the workplace be qualified to assure that the employee understands that these examinations in almost all cases are not comprehensive and provide no guarantee of current or future health. Most important of all, such occupational examinations do not replace ongoing care by a primary care physician. The worker should be told the potential significance of the test result; the risk, if any, from continued exposure to the work environment; the recommended changes in work practices or personal habits; and the necessary medical treatment. Nonoccupational medical findings (such as elevated blood pressure) should be referred to the employee's personal physician for treatment.

Determine Employee Medical Restrictions

The occupational physician should inform the employer of an employee's work restrictions and any recommended accommodations. It is important that the medical findings include a specific description of the employee's functional capabilities so that the individual does not perform tasks that jeopardize his or her health. Imprecise recommendations may lead an employer to reassign a worker, taking him or her off a job he is fully capable of performing. For instance, when a physician broadly declares that an employee is "unfit to wear a respirator," the worker will most often be reassigned from any job involving the use of a respirator. Yet, the medical examination may actually have indicated that the employee can work at a job requiring a respirator, provided it is worn occasionally for short periods or only for an emergency escape. This is another example of the necessity for the occupational physician and the occupational hygienist to work together.

The employee must be confident that the medical information will be kept strictly confidential, will be used only for the stated purposes, and will not adversely affect salary or other benefits. Employers may require access to personal information when considering requests for job accommodation or reviewing claims for workers' compensation benefits. The physician should avoid providing the employer with specific details or diagnoses without the worker's permission. The worker's health information also may have to be disclosed to other employees in certain situations.[14] Supervisors and managers may be informed of any necessary work restrictions, and, when appropriate, first aid and safety personnel may be notified if the worker's medical condition might require emergency treatment.

Personnel involved in the occupational health program need to recognize the special confidential status of HIV positivity and drug and alcohol treatment information.[14] They should be aware that a general consent for disclosure of medical records will often be insufficient in these situations and that specific written consent for release of this information must be obtained. This information should only be disclosed in compliance with federal and state law. It is important for workers to feel that their disclosures will be treated in a dignified and confidential manner to assure their agreement with this disclosure of sensitive information.

Accommodate Medical Restrictions

On returning certain employees to work it is sometimes necessary for the occupational hygienist to design reasonable accommodations to compensate for the worker's medical restrictions. This may mean implementing workplace controls; developing administrative recommendations to limit the duration, frequency, or intensity of workplace exposures; or providing personal protective equipment to eliminate contact with or exposure to a hazardous agent. If an employer rejects a disabled worker's request to return to work, the burden of proof is on the employer to mount a well-documented defense that proves at least one of the following:[15]

- The worker cannot perform the essential functions of the job, even with reasonable accommodation;
- The employer cannot accommodate the worker by redistributing the work among other employees or by restructuring the job;

- The employer cannot afford the cost of reasonable accommodation;
- Accommodation would substantially change the nature of the business; and/or
- The worker would be a "direct threat" to his or her health and safety or to other workers.

Throughout this process, the employer must verify compliance with the Americans with Disabilities Act (ADA) and state laws. Medical removal from a specific job should be considered as an interim measure when all other feasible actions are considered inadequate to protect the affected worker. In most instances, a physician will be required to determine whether an individual should be removed from the job while workplace evaluation and modification are being undertaken. In some circumstances, with frequent clinical monitoring, the individual may safely remain at his or her job during this process. Whenever the occupational physician recommends that a worker should be removed from a specific job, the worker should be informed of the basis for such a recommendation (e.g., the risk and severity of an adverse outcome if the worker remains in the job in question). Wages and benefits should be protected when individuals are removed from a job because of a medical determination.

Analyze Potential Relationships Between Medical Results and Occupational Exposure

The physician and the occupational hygienist should work together, sometimes with the aid of an epidemiologist, to examine patterns or trends from the occupational hygiene and the medical evaluation data. To gain the most insight, both individual and group trends should be examined.

Examining groups often uncovers links between illness and workplace exposures. The occupational hygienist's workplace exposure assessments are the starting point for this process. By categorizing workers according to their exposures, it may be possible to uncover a relationship between low-level exposures and early health effects.

Such analyses cannot be based on a small number of workers. The statistical power of larger groups makes it possible to uncover the impact of exposure to toxic agents at an early stage, where findings may be subtle, but intervention can have its greatest impact.

The medical surveillance program may also reveal that workers within a small group of employees have similar complaints about their health or that they have been diagnosed with similar illnesses. This is known as a disease cluster.[16] It is often the case that these workers also shared something else in common (such as the same occupational or nonoccupational exposure) or that they shared the same work area. Examples of clusters include a group of individuals with cancer, all of whom work in the same location.

The number of cases might be too small to be statistically significant, but the situations require a detailed investigation to determine potential causes. The occupational hygienist may be called on to work with the occupational physician to investigate these situations. Accurate information surrounding the onset of symptoms, the frequency and range of symptoms, symptom intensity and consistency, and pre-existing conditions may help in identifying the source of noncancer clusters. For cancer clusters it is important to gather information on commonality of the organ and cell type and to identify the latency periods.

Implement and Maintain Effective Workplace Controls

All these efforts to identify trends will be meaningless, unless the occupational hygienist acts on his or her findings. To prevent occupational disease, the occupational hygienist must implement workplace controls that will prevent similar problems from occurring in the future. In some cases, workplace evaluation may verify the effectiveness of some controls while discovering deficiencies in others. For instance, the medical surveillance program may confirm that inhalation exposures are adequately controlled for solvents. Reports of reddening of the skin, however, may indicate that a different type of glove is needed to better protect workers' hands and to prevent skin absorption.

To ensure that any improvements are sustained, the occupational hygienist should periodically verify the effectiveness of the workplace controls. Exhaust ventilation systems and other engineering controls must be inspected to measure the adequacy of the face velocities or to maintain the exhaust fans. For administrative controls to work, workers must be supervised to ensure that they follow recommended work practices or adhere to limitations on the maximum duration of an exposure. The occupational hygienist should also test the reliability of any personal protective equipment. This may mean establishing respirator cleaning procedures and schedules for replacing respirator cartridges at the end of their service life or performing fit-testing studies for respirator users. It is important to document the maintenance practices performed to demonstrate that the controls are properly serviced.

Occupational illnesses are prevented by controlling exposures. As a corollary to this maxim, we can only be assured that exposures are being controlled when controls are verified.

Acute Medical Care — Medical Treatment

Even with the best prevention programs, occupational injuries and illnesses will occur. To minimize the consequences and disruption associated with these events, it is important to establish protocols for handling emergencies and for providing nonemergency medical care to employees. These plans often involve the use of community medical services (hospitals and physicians) to supplement the employer's own resources. Off-site health care professionals should be taken on plant tours to make them familiar with the employer's operations. The management system includes the necessary preparation for both emergency and nonemergency situations.

Preparing for Emergency Treatment

Timely medical treatment is crucial in emergency situations, such as an accidental chemical release involving toxic chemicals, an employee overcome by heat stress, or an explosion with burn injuries. An emergency treatment plan must address situations that involve not only employees but also contractors, visitors, and community residents who may be affected by an untoward event.[17] The plan should be integrated with the overall site emergency response program designating the roles and responsibilities for both onsite and off-site personnel. Also, it should contain procedures, equipment lists, emergency contacts, and signs and symptoms of exposures. A designated emergency/first aid station should be selected and equipped with supplies that can be used to stabilize patients and treat injuries that require only first aid. Site personnel assisting emergencies should be trained to handle these situations.

The occupational hygienist may be assigned responsibility for briefing off-site medical personnel on the hazardous chemicals used at the operation and for keeping the chemical emergency information files up-to-date. Regulatory authorities in many jurisdictions require employers to provide material safety data sheets (MSDSs) to local emergency planning authorities or emergency personnel (e.g., U.S. EPA Emergency Planning and Community Right-To-Know Act of 1986 (EPCRA).[18] Advanced planning is required for emergency transportation to nearby medical facilities and for having health care professionals available around the clock.

Disability Management — Managing Medical Cases

Medical management programs are important for chronic conditions, especially cumulative trauma disorders and other work disorders due to ergonomic hazards. Like the medical surveillance program, the medical management program is not meant to replace the hazard prevention and control programs, but is a necessary complement to them. An occupational physician or occupational health nurse with training in the prevention and treatment of occupational disorders should supervise the program. The medical management program should address the following issues: early recognition and reporting of injuries and illnesses; careful maintenance and interpretation of medical records to identify trends; medical referral to specialists to ensure that workers receive appropriate treatment; and return-to-work and restricted-duty policies to aid the rehabilitation of employees.[19]

Implementing Management Systems To Sustain the Occupational Health Program

Maintenance of complete medical records is essential to comprehensive medical care, and occupational health programs are no exception. Medical records must be maintained individually, confidentially, and completely apart from personnel records. Medical records should include not only the results of medical examinations but also personal exposure and biological monitoring results provided to the physician, the purpose of the medical tests given, the interpretation of test results, and the plan for responding to the results. Notifications provided to employers of examination results indicating a need to evaluate the work environment should be maintained in the medical record, as should copies of any notification to the employee, either as an individual, or as a member of a group. If the employer retains off-site occupational health services, then the employer should also make certain that the results of medical surveillance examination can be retrieved and made available for independent review. This is also important because the employer may opt to change occupational health providers, or the provider himself or herself may change locations. It is critical that the information be retrievable and transferable to another independent medical examiner.

Records containing the results of the medical examinations must be maintained according to law. These records might be needed to compare with future test results for an individual or to further evaluate a suspected toxic effect using aggregate data. According to OSHA, employers must preserve worker medical records for the duration of employment plus 30 years.[20] The records must be made available, on request, to workers, their representatives, and authorized regulatory officials.

Under the OSHA recordkeeping standards, employers must record all work-related injuries that meet the severity criteria by the agency. The criteria include deaths, cases involving days away form work or restricted work activity, transfer to another job, medical treatment (beyond first aid), loss of consciousness, and significant injury or illness diagnosed by a licensed health care professional, as well as specific conditions. The specific conditions highlighted by OSHA are bloodborne pathogen cases, needlesticks and cuts from sharp objects, if contaminated with another person's blood or other potentially infectious material, splashes, or other exposures (if exposure results in a diagnosis of a bloodborne illness). OSHA requires the recording of medical removal cases performed to meet the requirements of an OSHA standard and occupational hearing loss.[21] In these cases, the company must file an Injury and Illness Report, OSHA 301, identifying the details of the incident. The employer must also maintain and post in the workplace an OSHA 300 log of work-related injuries and illnesses.

The records of health and safety incidents form the core information that should be reviewed to assess the effectiveness of the occupational health program. To promote continuous program improvement, the occupational hygienist and health care professional should, at least annually:[22]

- Ascertain that each injury or illness was promptly investigated to determine the cause and make necessary changes in health and safety conditions or procedures;
- Evaluate the efficacy of specific medical testing in the context of potential employee exposures;
- Add or delete medical tests as suggested by current occupational hygiene workplace exposure assessments;
- Review emergency treatment procedures and update lists of emergency contacts and hazardous chemical information files (MSDSs); and
- Evaluate the effectiveness of the medical case management programs and performance of referral physicians.

Summary

The primary objective of the occupational health program is to integrate occupational hygiene and occupational health, thus leading to the important union of primary and secondary preventive measures. The specific contents of the program vary depending on regulatory requirements, hazards of the workplace and its operations, the resources within the community, and the support of the employer. The level of medical care to be considered for a comprehensive occupational medicine program are acute, rehabilitative, and preventive services.

To maximize the effectiveness of the occupational health program, the occupational hygienist and the health care professional should work as a team. In a well-organized medical surveillance program, the occupational hygienist characterizes the hazardous exposures. The physician then uses this information to design effective medical evaluations for individuals with significant exposure to chemical, physical, or biological agents. Through preplacement, periodic, and termination examinations, the health care professional uncovers deficient workplace controls and employees with medical restrictions requiring accommodation. Together, the occupational hygienist and occupational physician develop medical treatment programs to minimize the consequences of emergency and nonemergency situations and to ensure that employees receive proper medical care so they can return to work as quickly as possible.

The occupational hygienist and health care professional should periodically review the medical and incident records to identify opportunities to improve the occupational health program. Hazard surveillance is the preferred prevention method over medical surveillance. Eliminating occupational illness relies on effective occupational hygiene programs to recognize, evaluate, and control occupational hazards.

Additional Sources

"The Americans with Disabilities Act of 1990," 42 USC 12113.

Conway, H., J. Simmons, and T. Talbert: The purposes of occupational medical surveillance in U.S. industry and related health findings. *J. Occup. Med. 35(7)*:670–686 (1993).

Harris, J.S. (ed.): *Occupational Medicine Practice Guidelines: Evaluation and Management of Common Health Problems and Functional Recovery in Workers.* Beverly Farms, Mass.: OEM Press, 1997.

Ellis, J.: Medical monitoring: can we do better? *Occup. Health, Safety 65(5)*:19–25 (1996).

LaDou, J. (ed.): *Occupational and Environmental Medicine*, 2nd ed. Stamford, Conn.: Appleton & Lange, 1997.

McCunney, R., P.P. Rountree, and J.L. Levin: *A Practical Approach to Occupational and Environmental Medicine*, 2nd ed., Phila-delphia: Lippincott Williams & Wilkins, 1994.

Murphy, L., and W.E. Halperin: Medical screening and biological monitoring: a guide to the literature for physicians. *J. Occup. Environ. Med. 37(2)*:170–184 (1995).

Newman, L.S.: Occupational illness: essential elements of the occupational history. *N. Eng. J. Med. 333(17)*:1128–1132 (1995).

Polton, T.: Critical roles for industrial hygienists in medical surveillance and the prevention of occupational disease. *The Synergist 6(1)*:24–25 (1995).

Silverstein, M.: Analysis of medical screening and surveillance in 21 Occupational Safety and Health Administration: support for a generic medical surveillance standard. *Am. J. Ind. Med. 26*:283–295 (1994).

Stave, G.M.: Recommended library and electronic resources for occupational and environmental physicians. *JOEM 39(5)*:469–472 (1997).

U.S. Department of Defense (DOD): *Occupational Medical Surveillance Manual* (Instruction 6055-M). Washington, D.C.: DOD. May 1998.

U.S. Department of Labor, Occupational Safety and Health Administration (OSHA): *Guidelines for First Aid Programs* (CPL 2-2.53). Washington, D.C.: OSHA. Jan. 7, 1991.

References

1. Epidemiologic notes and report : angiosarcoma of the liver among polyvinyl chloride workers-Kentucky. *Morbidity and Mortality Weekly Report*, Feb. 9, 1974; reprinted in *MMWR, 46(5)*:97–101.
2. *Code of Federal Regulations* Title 29, Parts 1910.1001, 1003, 1017, 1018, 1025, 1027, 1028, 1029, 1043, 1044, 1045, 1047, 1048, 1050, 1051, 1052.
3. "Respiratory Protection." *Code of Federal Regulations* Title 29, Part 1910.134.
4. "Hazardous Waste Operations and Emergency Response." *Code of Federal Regulations* Title 29, Part 1910.120.
5. **Occupational Safety and Health Administration (OSHA):** *Screening and Surveillance: A Guide to OSHA Standards* (OSHA 29CFR1910 and 29CFR1926). Washington, D.C.: OSHA, 2000 (reprinted).
6. **Occupational Safety and Health Administration:** *The Occupational Health Professional's Services and Qualifications: Questions and Answers.* Washington, D.C.: U.S. Government Printing Office, 1999 revised. p. 3.
7. **Baker, E.L.:** Role of medical screening in the prevention of occupational disease. *J. Occup. Med. 32(9)*:788 (1990).
8. **Goldman, R.H.:** General occupational health history and examination. *J. Occup. Environ. Med. 28(10)*:967 (1986).
9. **Goldman, R.H.:** General occupational health history and examination. *J. Occup. Environ. Med. 28(10)*:971 (1986).
10. **Baker, E.L.:** Role of medical screening in the prevention of occupational disease. *J. Occup. Med. 32(9)*:787 (1990).
11. **United Kingdom Health and Safety Commission (UKHSC):** Control of substances hazardous to health. In *General COSHH Approved Codes of Practice* (Regulation 11, Health surveillance (2)(b)). UKHSC, 2002.

12. **Silverstein, M.:** Medical screening, surveillance, and the prevention of occupational disease. *J. Occup. Med 32*:1035 (1990).
13. **National Institute for Occupational Safety Health (NIOSH):** *Occupational Safety and Health Guidance Manual for Hazardous Waste Site Activities* (DHHS/NIOSH Pub. No. 85-115). Washington, D.C.: U.S. Government Printing Office, 1985. pp. 5–7.
14. **American College of Occupational and Environmental Medicine (ACOEM), Committee on Ethical Practice in Occupational Medicine:** ACOEM position on the confidentiality of medical information in the workplace. *J. Occup. Environ. Med. 37(5)*:595 (1995).
15. **Equal Employment Opportunity Commission (EEOC):** *A Technical Assistance Manual on the Employment Provisions (Title I) of the ADA* [EEOC-M-1A]. EEOC, 1992.
16. **Sandler, H.M.:** Do you have a cluster? *Occup. Hazards 58(7)*:49–50 (1996).
17. **National Institute for Occupational Safety Health (NIOSH):** *Occupational Safety and Health Guidance Manual for Hazardous Waste Site Activities* (DHHS/NIOSH Pub. No. 85-115). Washington, D.C.: U.S. Government Printing Office, 1985. pp. 5-8.
18. **U.S. Environmental Protection Agency:** Emergency Planning and Community Right to Know Act (40CFR part 370). U.S. EPA, 1986.
19. **Occupational Safety and Health Administration (OSHA):** *Ergonomics Program Management Guidelines for Meatpacking Plants.* 1993 reprint. p. 6.
20. "Access to Employee Exposure and Medical Records Standard." *Code of Federal Regulations* Title 29, Part 1910.1020.
21. "Annual Summary." *Code of Federal Regulations* Title 29, Part 1904.5.
22. **National Institute for Occupational Safety Health (NIOSH):** *Occupational Safety and Health Guidance Manual for Hazardous Waste Site Activities* (DHHS/NIOSH Pub. No. 85-115). Washington, D.C.: U.S. Government Printing Office, 1985. pp. 5–10.

Appendix A — Core Competencies for Occupational Physicians

The American College of Occupational and Environmental Medicine (ACOEM) published core competencies of occupational physicians. The following is an abbreviated list of the 2008 version of the 10 core competencies and skills. Additional descriptions and definitions can be obtained through the ACOEM website.

Clinical Occupational and Environmental Medicine

The physician has the knowledge and skills to provide evidence based clinical evaluation and treatment for injuries and illnesses that are occupationally or environmentally related. The physician provides clinical care with an understanding of the workplace, work exposures, and relevant statutes, such as workers' compensation. Throughout the course of care, the physician seeks to maximize the patient's functional recovery.

(Note: Separate competencies have been developed for all of the following clinical subareas: general, cardiology, dermatology, emergency medicine and surgery, hematology/oncology, infectious disease, musculioskeletal, neurology, ophthalmology, otolaryngology, psychiatry, pulmonary, and reproductive medicine.)

OEM Related Law and Regulations

The OEM physician complies with and has the knowledge and skills to help bring organizations into compliance with state and federal regulations relating to OEM, as well as general public health laws. The physician is further able to effectively utilize the services of government agencies to facilitate the protection of worker and public health. The OEM physician is a recognized expert on issues relating to the causation of occupational and environmental injuries and illnesses, as well as the ability to perform work with or without reasonable accommodations. As a result, the physician is frequently called upon to provide expert testimony, to draft reports that render an unbiased expert opinion on contested cases, and to provide peer review.

Environmental Health

The physician has the knowledge and skills necessary to recognize potential chemical, physical, and biological environmental causes of health concern to the individual as well as to community health. Environmental issues most often include air, water, or ground contamination by natural or artificial pollutants. The physician has knowledge of the health effects of the broad physical and social environment, which includes housing, urban development, land-use and transportation, industry, and agriculture.

Work Fitness and Disability Integration

The physician has the knowledge and skills to determine if a worker can safely be at work and complete required job tasks. The physician has the knowledge and skills necessary to provide guidance to the employee and employer when there is a need for integration of an employee with a disability into the workplace. The OEM physician has the expertise to determine work fitness based upon the work capacity of the worker and the functional requirements of the job.

Toxicology

The physician has the knowledge and skills to recognize, evaluate, and treat exposures to toxins at work or in the general environment. This most often includes interpretation of laboratory or environmental monitoring test results as well as applying toxicokinetic data. Hazardous material exposures occur at work, at home, and in the general environment. Clinical acumen as well as knowledge of hazardous material databases equip the OEM physician to identify, manage, and prevent occupational and environmental toxicity. General principles of clinical toxicology underlie emergency, nonurgent, and target organ-specific medical management.

Hazard Recognition, Evaluation, and Control

The physician has the knowledge and skills necessary to assess if there is risk of an adverse event from exposure to physical, chemical, or biological hazards in the workplace or environment. If there is a risk with exposure, then that risk can be characterized with recommendations for control measures. The OEM physician has the knowledge and skills to evaluate the impact of such exposures on the health of individual workers, patients, and the public. The physician may collaborate with other professionals, such as industrial hygienists, safety engineers, ergonomists, and occupational health nurses, on such efforts.

Disaster Preparedness and Emergency Management

The physician has the knowledge and skills to plan for mitigation of, response to, and recovery from disasters at specific worksite as well as for the community at large. Emergency management most often includes resource mobilization, risk communication, and collaboration with local, state, or federal agencies.

Health and Productivity

A physician will be able to identify and address individual and organizational factors in the workplace in order to optimize the health of the worker and enhance productivity. These issues most often include absenteeism, presenteeism, health enhancement, and population health management.

Public Health, Surveillance, and Disease Prevention

The physician has the knowledge and skill to develop, evaluate, and manage medical surveillance programs for the work place as well as the general public. The physician has the knowledge and skills to apply primary, secondary, and tertiary preventive methods.

OEM Related Management and Administration

The OEM physician has the administrative and management knowledge and skills to plan, design, implement, manage, and evaluate comprehensive occupational/environmental health programs, projects, and protocols that enhance the health, safety, and productivity of workers, their families, and members of the community. The spectrum of activities may vary substantially depending upon the physician's practice setting and the characteristics of the organization(s) served.

chapter 51

Outcome Competencies

After completing this chapter, the reader should be able to:

1. Define underlines terms used in this chapter.
2. Apply the basic elements of effective report writing.
3. Apply the basic elements of effective graphic presentation
4. Develop strategies for presenting technical information to divergent audiences and levels of expertise.
5. Implement accepted standards of usage and style to achieve clarity and consistency in all written documents.

Prerequisite Knowledge

None

Key Terms

primary reader • informational report • interpretive report • rewriting • stand-alone graphics

Key Topics

I. Introduction
II. Advance Preparation
III. Defining the Purpose
IV. Defining the Primary Reader
V. Developing an Outline
VI. Writing Techniques
VII. Presenting Graphs, Tables, and Diagrams
VIII. Summary
IX. References

Report Writing

51

By Susan M. McDonald, CIH

Introduction

The ability to write effective reports helps occupational hygienists achieve their goals of preventing and controlling workplace hazards. Conversely, the occupational hygienist's failure to communicate accurately and completely may have severe consequences: a worker's health or a company's livelihood could be at risk. This chapter describes a report writing process that will assist occupational hygienists in communicating their knowledge and expertise effectively.

Occupational hygiene reports serve a variety of purposes and readers. They may be used to document worker exposures to hazardous materials, to justify capital expenditures for protective measures such as ventilation systems, to support litigation, or to provide a record for regulatory compliance. Further, reports may contain findings applicable elsewhere, such as risk assessment, epidemiology, or health surveillance. Readers come from divergent backgrounds, including workers, supervisors, union representatives, other occupational hygienists, nurses, physicians, engineers, government officials, lawyers, business executives, and the general public. In the age of e-mail and the Internet, it is important to keep in mind that any report may be circulated well beyond the audience for whom it was originally intended. Given this wide range of audiences and purposes, it is critical that occupational hygiene reports convey pertinent information clearly and accurately and at the same time strike a balance between brevity and detail. Today's professionals are inundated with information, and reports that are overly technical or take too long to get to the point will not be read. This chapter emphasizes presenting the most important information at the beginning of the report, providing supporting details in a logical, organized manner, and writing in a clear, direct style.

Occupational hygiene field work frequently involves gathering large amounts of information and numerical data. Preparing a well-organized, readable report from such research may seem daunting. Overcoming obstacles to effective communication may be accomplished by approaching writing as a series of steps. To produce effective reports, the writer should 1) prepare in advance; 2) define the purpose; 3) define the primary reader; 4) follow an outline; 5) draft the report; and 6) revise the draft.

Advance Preparation

Much of the work involved in report writing usually takes place well before the actual writing begins. Advance preparation can save time by eliminating the need for laborious revisions or additional field work. The occupational hygienist should have the final report in mind even while developing the data collection strategy. Further, scrupulous note taking in the field will serve the occupational hygienist well when writing the report. Nothing should be left to memory. All potentially important observations should be recorded at the time they are originally noted.

Defining the Purpose

In preparation for writing, the occupational hygienist should consider the purpose of the report. Is the report simply an update of an ongoing project? Will it include an interpretation of the findings? Will the report be used to provide justification for changing a practice or policy? Defining the report's purpose assists the writer in determining the scope and format of the report.

Reports usually are intended either to inform or to persuade through interpretation. The informational report simply presents the facts and generally requires less time and effort than an interpretive report. Examples of informational reports include status reports on a continuing project and survey reports that list findings without developing conclusions or recommendations.

In the interpretive report, the writer not only presents findings but also critically evaluates the results, draws conclusions, and offers recommendations. The purpose of such reports is not merely to inform but also to persuade the reader to accept the writer's viewpoint, to take action, or to make a change in policy or practice. Examples of interpretive reports include feasibility studies and comprehensive work site evaluations. The interpretive report is distinguished by its inclusion of expert opinion to guide the reader in making decisions.

The writer must understand at the outset what type of report is expected. If the primary audience does not expect a detailed analysis, the writer should simply present the facts rather than interpret them. For instance, a physician may seek information on an employee's potential workplace exposures to determine the need for medical surveillance. In this case the occupational hygienist should simply provide a brief report listing the potential exposure hazards, perhaps attaching relevant exposure monitoring data. If, on the other hand, the physician seeks the occupational hygienist's expertise in interpreting the findings of an exposure assessment, the report should include a detailed evaluation, including an informed analysis correlating the worker's exposures with potential or known health effects. In this case the occupational hygienist applies experience and knowledge to guide the physician.

In addition to considering the primary purpose of the report, the writer should consider the report's possible other uses or ultimate fate, such as an exhibit in a lawsuit or a public media outlet. Given the widespread use of e-mail, the Internet, and electronic distribution systems, it is prudent to keep in mind that a report may end up far from its original recipient. Ensuring the technical validity of the data, documenting all findings, and making clear distinctions between facts and professional opinions are the best methods for developing a report that will withstand legal or public scrutiny. For guidance on preparing reports as legal documents, the occupational hygienist should consult an attorney.

Defining the Primary Reader

The primary reader is the person empowered to take action based on the report. Identifying the report's purpose and determining the primary reader usually go hand in hand, since it is the primary reader who explicitly or implicitly establishes the purpose of the report. Knowing the expectations and background of the primary reader is essential to effective report writing. Trying to write for a generalized or nonspecific audience is likely to be a futile endeavor. Without a specific audience in mind, the occupational hygienist will not know how to present technical information, what terminology to use, or what level of detail to provide.

Identifying the audience assists the writer in determining the report's tone and language. For example, if the primary reader is another occupational hygienist, the writer may freely use occupational hygiene terms and notations. However, if the primary reader does not have an occupational hygiene background, the writer should use non-technical terms and provide explanations of concepts that are integral to occupational hygiene work. For instance, a reader unfamiliar with the concept of time-weighted average exposures may benefit from an explanation of the calculations involved in determining these results. Instead of simply presenting exposure results, the writer should also assist the reader's understanding by including a glossary or other method of explaining the occupational hygiene concepts used in the report. The challenge is to provide sufficient technical detail without confusing or losing the reader.

The writer needs to be alert to the expectations and background of the reader, to consider what the reader already knows and needs to know. Is the reader knowledgeable about the report's subject? Does the reader expect a detailed analysis or a one-page summary? What action is the reader likely to take as a result of the report?

Consider the case of the occupational hygienist who must convince an upper-level manager to spend thousands of dollars to install a local exhaust ventilation system to reduce workers' exposures to an airborne hazardous substance. The occupational hygienist must select the most pertinent information and write a report that is brief, convincing, and to the point, perhaps highlighting the hidden costs of not installing the system. Detailed technical analysis may be included as background, but the first page should summarize the occupational hygienist's position. The writer should proceed under the assumption that the primary reader, in this case a business executive seeking the bottom line only, may not read past the first page of the report. However, a report on the same topic written for another occupational hygienist or a ventilation engineer would likely include much more technical detail.

Developing an Outline

Identifying the purpose and primary reader assists the writer in determining the scope, format, and language of the report. The next step in the report-writing process is developing an outline, which provides an organization for presenting information in a logical manner. A well-organized report guides the reader effortlessly through even the most complex information. A poorly organized report may never be read before it is filed away indefinitely.

The occupational hygienist who has collected a large amount of data may feel overwhelmed by the prospect of presenting such information in a logical and readable manner. Using an outline allows the writer to approach the report one section at a time, thus helping the writer get started.

Depending on the purpose of the report, the level of detail in the outline may be minimal or extensive. The occupational hygienist may wish to develop a series of outlines or formats to be used for different types of reports that are required on a regular basis. However, in all cases, the basic approach to organization is the same: put the most important information first and provide supporting details in a logical manner.

A standard outline that may be applied to all types of reports has the following sections:

- Summary — Provides a synopsis of the most important information about the current project. It tells the primary reader what was done and why, provides a synopsis of the results, and conveys what comes, or should come next.
- Background —Brings the reader up to date, explaining what led to the current project. Depending on the type of report, this section may be subdivided to include an introduction, a further description of the project's purpose, a description of the research methodology, and other information not directly related to the findings or conclusions.
- Findings — This section summarizes the results of the current project. Depending on the report's scope and purpose, this section may contain a detailed description of findings or may simply list the results. This section is distinguished by the factual nature of the information presented, as opposed to the interpretation of findings in the Conclusions section.
- Conclusions — This section correlates the findings presented in the previous section with proposed actions. Depending on the report's purpose, this section may be brief or extensive. For example, a brief informational report may not include detailed interpretations but may propose follow-up work. An interpretive report draws conclusions from the findings and makes recommendations. The amount of detail and degree of analysis in this section depends on the report's scope and the primary reader's expectations. This section presents the occupational hygienist's conclusions and recommendations, which are opinions and should be presented in a way that distinguishes them from facts.

A suggested outline is shown in Figure 51.1 for a generic occupational hygiene survey report, intended as an interpretive report and written for another occupational hygienist. The purpose of the report is to summarize the occupational hygienist's comprehensive work site evaluation, presenting the exposure assessment findings and developing recommendations to improve health and safety conditions at the site. This outline should be seen not as a rigid structure but as an approach to organizing information. Each report, as each occupational hygiene project, is unique, and the report outline should allow for flexibility. The goal is to present the most important information in a way that achieves the desired results. An example of an executive summary is shown in Figure 51.2.

Writing Techniques

Once the report's purpose, audience, and outline have been established, the writer is

Executive Summary

This section is a one-page summary of the purpose, main activities, findings (e.g., exposure monitoring results), and conclusions. It summarizes critical information for the primary reader, such as conclusions correlating workers' health symptoms to exposures and recommended actions for exposure control. The executive summary is written after the rest of the report has been prepared.

Background

Introduction. This section includes a more detailed description of the purpose of the survey, a description of the work site and workers, and a summary of previous surveys and findings at the site. It may include subsections covering such information as the health effects associated with identified exposures. It may also be useful to include figures such as process flow diagrams or illustrations depicting the location of workers and engineering controls.

Survey Methods. This section summarizes the industrial hygienist's sampling strategy (e.g., number and types of workers monitored) as well as sampling and calibration methods. It may need to be subdivided depending on the extent of the monitoring or other survey methods. Methods for other exposure assessment (such as sound level measurements) as well as methods for control measure assessment are included here.

Analytical Methods. Methods for laboratory analysis of collected samples are described here (including information on limits of detection), as well as any other pertinent analytical methods.

Findings

Exposure Monitoring Results. Such results may be presented in both text and tabular formats. Information such as analytical limits of detection should be repeated here if necessary to assist the reader in understanding the data presented.

Control Measure Assessments. Results of engineering control measurements, such as local exhaust ventilation airflow measurements, are included here. Tables and diagrams may be useful in illustrating the location of ventilation systems and processes with respect to airflow measurements.

Results of Statistical Analysis. Statistical analyses of the sampling results and other findings are presented in this section, along with any associated graphs or tables.

Conclusions

Discussion of Findings. This section contains the occupational hygienist's interpretation of the findings. For instance, this section may present a discussion of the identified correlations between exposures and controls, or between exposures and potential health effects. This section may compare the findings with applicable regulations and professional consensus standards.

Recommendations. This section proposes actions based on the interpretation of the findings. For example, recommendations for additional control measures, medical evaluation of workers, and further exposure monitoring are included here.

Figure 51.1 — Report Outline for an Occupational Hygiene Survey.

ready to prepare a first draft. In this draft the writer should not be overly concerned about exact wording or organization. The point of the first draft is to get down all the pertinent information, and then reorganize as necessary to create a logical flow of ideas. (The outline should assist in this regard.)

It is good practice to take a break between writing the draft and completing the final report. Leaving the draft alone for a day or two allows the writer to bring a fresh perspective to the project. Many writers also find it helpful to have colleagues review their reports before preparing the final versions. Such peer readers provide an objective view of the material and may have suggestions for making the report clearer or better organized.

Every good writer knows that the secret to good writing is rewriting. One of the paradoxes of writing is that it takes longer to write a succinct report than it does to write a wordy one. Revising helps to ensure that the final report is free of awkward language or unnecessary words that distract from the content. In addition, thorough proofreading helps to eliminate technical and typographical errors.

This section presents some advice on writing techniques but is not intended as a complete guide to grammar or usage. Every occupational hygienist's library should contain reference manuals on grammar and usage as well as scientific communication methods (see the bibliography following this chapter). In addition, the Internet is an invaluable resource that provides ready online access to guidance on grammar, usage, and the entire range of writing techniques.

The principles of effective communication outlined below apply to all kinds of writing, whether a brief memo or a large technical document:

- Use plain English. Resist the urge to use flowery language or technical jargon. One of the most common writing pitfalls is to use overly technical language in an effort to impress the reader. Rather than impress, the writer may confuse or lose the reader altogether.
- Never use a long word when a short one will do. However, in some cases a long word expresses an entity much more eloquently and precisely than a series of short words. Eloquence should prevail. This advice comes from *The Elements of Style*, by William Strunk, Jr. and E.B. White, a brief publication with indispensable advice about writing.
- Use the active voice whenever possible. For example, rather than write, "It was stated by the safety officer," write, "The safety officer said."
- Eliminate unnecessary words. For example, instead of "call your attention to the fact that," say "remind you"; instead of "emergency situation," say "emergency"; instead of "to provide protection," say "to protect."
- Vary sentence structure and length to avoid sounding choppy or monotonous.
- Be alert to the appearance of the printed page. Reading long stretches of text without paragraph breaks is tedious. Short paragraphs help to make even a complex technical report easier to read.
- Be consistent in the use of abbreviations and notations standard to the occupational hygiene profession. The first use of a term should always be written out, followed by the appropriate abbreviation in parentheses, for example, "0.1 part per million (ppm)."

> A preliminary occupational hygiene evaluation of the XYZ Microscopy Unit has determined that the laboratory hood is not working properly and the technicians have been advised to stop all work with glutaraldehyde until the hood is repaired. The Unit supervisor asked the Division of Environmental Health and Safety (EH&S) to conduct an assessment of the lab after a microscopy technician reported experiencing skin rashes and respiratory problems, effects that may be associated with glutaraldehyde exposure. The occupational hygienist observed the technician's work practices and obtained hood face velocity measurements. The results indicated that airflow across the hood's opening was extremely erratic and in the very low range (less than 25 feet per minute) at some points. In addition to the hood repair, EH&S recommends that all microscopy technicians working in the area receive refresher training in the safe handling of glutaraldehyde. The affected employee should be referred to the on-site occupational health unit for follow-up medical evaluation. After the hood is repaired, EH&S will conduct monitoring to assess the technicians' exposure to glutaraldehyde.

Figure 51.2 — Sample of an Executive Summary for a Brief Report.

- Use gender-neutral language. For instance, instead of "man," use "people" or "humans." Instead of "man-made," use "synthetic" or "constructed," depending on your meaning. Instead of "he/his," use the plural, "they/theirs."
- All statements of opinion or fact not directly attributable to the author should be appropriately referenced. Opinions should be presented as such, distinct from facts. In general, conclusions and recommendations are opinions and not facts.
- Avoid generalizations or vague statements. Be as specific as possible and use examples when necessary to illustrate an idea or principle.
- All information not directly attributable to the author must be properly cited. Follow the citation style that is standard for your organization. Currently there is no universal standard for citing electronic sources, which tend be less reliably available than hard-copy references such as journals and books. When citing the electronic source, provide as much information as possible to direct the reader to the original source, and be sure to include the date that the site was accessed.
- Make the report perfect. There should be no misspellings, no typographical errors, and no errors in calculations. The occupational hygiene report in particular must be technically accurate to be accepted as a legal or historical record.

The widespread use of the personal computer, e-mail, and the Internet has wrought major changes in how professionals, including occupational hygienists, communicate. This technology has made it easier to generate and transmit copious amounts of information via electronic networks. The word processor in particular has accelerated the editing process by allowing a writer to quickly insert, delete, and move text. Yet, effective communication still takes time and effort, and writing improvement comes only with practice. The challenge is using technology to communicate essential information rather than to generate information simply because it is easy to do so.

Presenting Graphs, Tables, and Diagrams

Occupational hygiene information is often presented most clearly in a table, graph, or diagram. A well-chosen illustration can greatly enhance the effectiveness of a report. For instance, tables provide a summary of complex data in a form that is more succinct and illustrative than text. Graphs can illustrate relationships between variables much more efficiently than text. Schematic diagrams can provide a visual guide to process flow or other procedures. However, as with the written portion of the report, the writer must be alert to the expectations and needs of the primary reader when selecting illustrations.

For example, the reader should not have to flip back and forth through the report's pages to view the referenced table or graph. In general, figures should be numbered sequentially and should follow immediately the text in which they are first referenced, rather than being placed in an appendix at the back of the report. The exception is an unusually large table that is not mentioned frequently or only supports the text indirectly. In such a case the information should be placed in an appendix or made available to the reader on request.

All visual displays should be self-explanatory. A good rule of thumb is to consider whether the graph or table would be understandable if it were to become separated from the rest of the report. This practice is particularly important for reports that may ultimately serve as historical or legal documents. Tables and graphs may be copied and circulated separately, another reason to ensure that the figure is self-explanatory. The following guidelines are presented to assist the report writer in preparing stand-alone graphics:

- A complete title must be included on every graph, table, or diagram.
- Each axis on a graph must be labeled clearly and completely.
- A legend containing information pertinent to understanding the data should be provided on the same page as the graph. For example, laboratory conditions such as temperature, pressure, and relative humidity should be included in a legend accompanying a calibration curve.

- Data presented in a table should be appropriately labeled, including units with standard abbreviations.
- Tables that summarize air sampling results should list the analytical method employed and the method's limit of detection. Other information, such as air volume sampled as well as each sample location, should be included wherever necessary to allow the reader to interpret the data presented.

In addition to writing reports, occupational hygienists frequently are expected to make oral presentations of their work. Some guidelines for oral presentations are given in Figure 51.3.

Summary

The method for preparing occupational hygiene reports presented in this chapter may be summarized as follows:

- The occupational hygienist should begin to prepare for the final report at the beginning of the project.
- The writer should identify the report's purpose and primary reader and should work from an outline.
- The writer should begin with a draft and revise it to produce the final report.
- The report should present the most important information first.
- The report should be neat, succinct, readable, and error-free.
- The occupational hygienist should be ever alert to the possibility that any written report may become a legal or historical record.

References

1. **Blicq, R.S.:** *Guidelines for Report Writers.* Englewood Cliffs, NJ: Prentice-Hall, Inc., 1982.
2. **Dodd, J.S. (ed.):** *The ACS Style Guide.* Washington, DC: American Chemical Society, 1997.
3. **Perelman, L.C., J. Paradis, and E. Barrett:** *The Mayfield Handbook of Scientific and Technical Writing.* Mountain View, California: Mayfield Publishing Company, 1998.
4. **Roman, K. and J. Raphaelson:** *Writing that Works.* New York: HarperPerennial, 1992.
5. **Rubens, P. (ed.):** *Science and Technical Writing*, 2nd edition. New York: Henry Holt, 2001.

Guidelines for Preparing Oral Presentations

General Tips

- Do not use slides that require an apology for their quality.
- Do not use slides that require you to say, "You probably can't read this from where you're sitting, so I'll read it to you."
- Do not use slides that require you to say, "Ignore the other five columns on this slide and only look at Column C." If the five columns are not necessary to the presentation, do not include them on the slide.

Your presentation should:

- Present data that is readily understandable.
- Use information that is current, accurate, and objective.
- Adequately convey ideas.
- Keep the message on target.
- Coordinate commentary with audiovisuals.
- Be CLEAR and SIMPLE!

Developing the presentation

- Begin with a title slide containing the name of the presenter, company, telephone and e-mail.
- Create "word slides" in a precise outline; the audience has about 20 seconds to absorb the message.
- Use a maximum of six text lines and no more than 30 characters per line on a single slide.
- Maintain consistent graphic elements including color, font, and text size.
- Use a dark background (blue, black) and light colors (white, light blue) for text and graphics.
- Avoid intensely bright or saturated colors such as red and yellow for text; use only as main headings.
- Text size should be at least 24 points; headings should be no less than 36 points. Use no more than two fonts per slide. Avoid using all capital letters or underlining. **Bold** and *italic* should be used sparingly.
- When possible, use horizontal slides, which fill the screen better than vertical slides.
- Clearly label charts and graphs and include legends; proofread, spell check, and correct errors.
- **Inserting Images** — Use images and graphics from digital cameras, scanners, and the Internet. In general, images that project well on a 17-inch monitor will project well in electronic presentations.
- Mix images and text on a single frame or alternate frames; import the images as background.

From AIHCE Speaker's Handbook, American Industrial Hygiene Association, Fairfax, VA, 1996; AIHCE 09 Speakers' Corner, accessed June 2009 at www.aiha.org.

Figure 51.3 — Guidelines for slide presentations.

6. **Sabin, W.A.:** *The Gregg Reference Manual*, 5th edition. New York: Gregg Division/McGraw Hill, 1977.

7. **Strunk, W., Jr., and E.B. White:** *The Elements of Style*. New York: Macmillan, 1959.

Outcome Competencies

After completing this chapter, the reader should be able to:

1. Define underlined terms used in this chapter.
2. Distinguish "occupational safety" from "occupational health."
3. Identify important historical events in the evolution of occupational safety.
4. Review common methods for measuring safety performance.
5. Review safety program elements.
6. Identify main OSHA standards that overlap safety and health.
7. Review qualifications for safety professionals.

Prerequisite Knowledge

The user is also referred to the following chapters:

Chapter Number	Chapter Topic
1	History of IndustrialHygiene
3	Legal Aspects of Industrial Hygiene
30	Ergonomics
32	Upper Extremities
38	Testing, Monitoring, and Troubleshooting of Existing Ventilation Systems
46	Confined Spaces
49	Laboratory Health and Safety

Key Terms

common exposure base • continuous improvement • employee involvement • hazard prevention and control • incident rate • instantaneous • management commitment • recordable injury • safety and health training • Standard Industrial Classification (SIC) • Voluntary Protection Program (VPP) • work site analysis

Key Topics

I. Key Historical Events

II. Measuring Safety Performance
   A. Business Measurements for Safety

III. Safety Management Systems
   A. Management Commitment and Employee Involvement
   B. Work Site Analysis
   C. Hazard Prevention and Control
   D. Safety and Health Training

IV. OSHA Standards that Overlap Safety and Health

V. Qualifications for Becoming a Safety Professional

Occupational Safety

52

By Daniel S. Markiewicz, CIH, CSP, CHMM

Introduction

This chapter provides an overview of occupational safety. To better understand *occupational safety,* we must first distinguish that term from occupational health. The distinction between occupational safety and occupational health is linked to the definition of occupational injury and occupational illness. The terms *safety* and *injury* have been used primarily the work domain of safety professionals, whereas the terms health and illness have been used primarily the work domain of occupational hygienists.

In 1986 the Bureau of Labor Statistics (BLS) published *Recordkeeping Guidelines for Occupational Injuries and Illnesses,* which distinguishes an injury from an illness by one word: instantaneous.[1] Instantaneous may be defined as the point in time it takes to snap one's fingers and refers to a single event. Occupational safety, therefore, is focused primarily on preventing unwanted and unplanned events (i.e., incidents that are instantaneous in nature and that might lead to an employee suffering an injury).

Although on the surface this distinction is clear, there still may be confusion. An example would be a nurse who contracts hepatitis—a classical "illness"—from a needle stick. Because the hepatitis developed from a single instantaneous event, by BLS definition it is an injury. Following this concept, a back problem caused by a single lift would be an injury. Carpal tunnel syndrome caused by the repetitive use of a poorly designed tool would be an illness. Chemical exposures, depending on circumstances, may result in either an injury or illness. These examples help illustrate why there is a blurring of the distinction between a safety professional and an occupational hygienist. There are many areas where the professions meet and overlap; as such, for both professions to be successful they must be complementary.

Occupational safety is a broad topic that encompasses both conditions and acts (e.g., behavior that might lead to injuries). "Conditions" may be viewed as everything except acts. Major categories for safety conditions include mechanical, thermal, electrical, and chemical energies. In 1931 Heinrich found that 88% of occupational injuries were caused by acts and 10% of occupational injuries were caused by conditions.[2] DeReamer, with a more current view, showed that conditions and acts are equally responsible for causing occupational injuries.[3] Whether conditions or acts cause more injuries will continue to be debated, and both areas will need to be addressed fully for injury prevention efforts to be effective. This overview of occupational safety is not intended to make the reader proficient at preventing or reducing occupational injuries. This chapter's main focus is to highlight key safety concepts and identify areas in which safety professionals and occupational hygienists must work together to help eliminate and minimize worker injury and illness.

Key Historical Events

There are many milestones in safety's long history. This chapter can briefly cover only a few of the many important historical events that have created and developed the field of occupational safety. Chapter 1 in this book discusses the history of occupational hygiene and to a limited extent occupational safety.

Because injury and death have occurred since the beginning of mankind, it is interesting to consider when safety regulations first became a part of society. Grimaldi and Simonds describe the Code of Hammurabi (circa 2100 B.C.) as one of the earliest known of the bodies of law that addressed the injured or killed worker.[4] The Code of Hammurabi contained specifications only for indemnification and punishment for causing injury or death to a worker. The code did not address prevention, but because it was based on the principle of an "eye for an eye" the code likely acted as a strong motivator for those who controlled workers to engage in injury prevention efforts (i.e., safety activities).

Specific legislation aimed at preventing injury to workers—primarily children—is believed to have arisen in England in the late 18th century. Children who worked were made part of an apprentice system that provided instruction on how to do their jobs, including how to avoid injuries while they worked. In 1784 an outbreak of fever in the cotton mills in the Manchester area of England drew special attention to the hazards and long hours being worked by children. Following this event a number of laws were passed to further protect children at work. The most notable act that followed was the Health and Morals Act of 1802, which provided regulations governing sanitary and safety conditions and hours worked by children. Taking a lead from English law, the state of Massachusetts in 1877 developed laws concerning employment and safety of children in factories.

Ferguson provides a good review of safety's history in the United States, beginning with the first two decades of the 20th century.[5] In Ferguson's opinion there is always a desire for people to expect a new century to surpass the last. This is why the early period of the 20th century is labeled the "Progressive Era"; it is a period in which the "Safety First" movement was allowed to grow, according to Ferguson. The Safety First movement recognized the waste created by injuries to employees and sought means to eliminate these injuries.

Events that capture the public's attention, such as the outbreak of fever in the English cotton mills, are precursors for better controls for a problem. The major event that prompted a cry for better worker safety early in the 20th century was the Triangle Shirtwaist Factory fire in 1911. The fire resulted in the death of 146 workers who could not escape the fire because management at the factory had blocked or locked exits. This event influenced the creation and improvement of many codes, standards, and regulations to prevent a similar occurrence. Still, in 1991 a fire at a chicken processing plant in Hamlet, N.C., resulted in 25 employee deaths because management had also blocked or locked exits. These events separated by time serve to demonstrate that attention to safety, even for obvious and well-known hazards, must be a continuous process.

Since the creation of the Code of Hammurabi, many employers have been required to indemnify injured workers. Early in the 20th century, however, a very restrictive indemnification process covered workers in the United States. This process would not allow an injured worker to prevail against his or her employer if (1) the employee "contributed" to his or her injury; (2) the employee "assumed" the risk associated with the work; or (3) the injury was caused through the "negligence" of a fellow employee. These restrictions prevented most injured workers from obtaining compensation from their employers.

Following the Triangle Shirtwaist Factory fire there were changes in laws that made it easier for injured employees to obtain compensation from their employers. In 1911, New Jersey, Wisconsin, and the state of Washington passed the first workers' compensation laws in the United States. Today, every state has a workers' compensation law. Although the application varies from state to state, these laws generally are in the form of an insurance policy in which the employer pays a premium for coverage. Because it is financially beneficial for both the company that issues the policy and the company that purchases the policy to have few or preferably no compensable injuries, workers' compensation laws have done much to foster and encourage the implementation of injury prevention activities. Smitha et al. illustrates how the reform of many state workers' compensation laws in the 1980s and 1990s resulted in the adoption of workplace safety and health regulations at the state level.[6] These regulations include the requirement for safety committees, safety and health programs, insurance carrier loss control services, and targeting initiatives for extra hazardous employer programs.

Arguably the greatest event to shape the field and profession of occupational safety has been the implementation of the Occupational Safety and Health (OSH) Act of 1970. Before the Occupational Safety and Health Administration (OSHA) was created as part of the OSH Act, laws protecting workers were only found on a state-by-state basis or were limited to narrow populations of workers. The OSH Act provided a federal mandate, backed by substantial investigative powers and penalty incentives, for employers to provide and maintain a safe and healthy working environment for nearly every working man and woman in the nation. The act codified national consensus standards for worker safety and health that were in effect prior to 1973. These voluntary standards were developed by organizations such as the American Conference of Governmental Industrial Hygienists (ACGIH), American National Standards Institute (ANSI), and American Petroleum Institute. The OSH Act also created the National Institute for Occupational Safety and Health (NIOSH). NIOSH provided for the first time a concerted effort on a national scale to study and find solutions to hazards that might cause injuries to employees.

Few would argue that OSHA has not made substantial progress toward making employers more attentive to safety. Some people nevertheless have questioned whether OSHA has had a significant impact in reducing employee injury and illness. Peterson, after evaluating national occupational injury and illness statistics and subjecting the data to statistical control tests, found there was (1) no significant change from 1981 to 1991 in total (injury and illness) cases; (2) no significant change from 1981 to 1991 in lost-time cases; and (3) a significant deterioration in lost workday statistics from 1983 through 1992.[7] Peterson argues that regulatory compliance and preventing occupational injuries have little to do with each other. Roughton and Grabiak agree that OSHA has weaknesses, but indicate that beginning with changes implemented in 1995 it can build itself into an organization that will place the highest premium on real results rather than reactive activities and processes.[8] Blair and Geller offer recommendations to improve OSHA's framework and strategy to optimally improve safety performance.[9] These recommendations include the vision that OSHA should (1) benchmark innovative practices established by other countries, (2) continue the trend toward performance-based standards, (3) emphasize the development and appropriate use of simple procedures such as job safety analysis to identify and control risks, and (4) attain more expertise in the person-based and behavior-based aspects of safety.

Measuring Safety Performance

Safety performance can be measured in many ways. The most basic safety performance measures used by employers are those that were mandated by OSHA shortly after promulgation of the OSH Act. These performance measures are explained and demonstrated in the BLS *Recordkeeping Guidelines for Occupational Injuries and Illnesses*.[1] These guidelines are subject to change, and the latest record-keeping requirements by OSHA should always be referenced.

The heart of the record-keeping guidelines is a strict adherence to definitions as to what is a recordable injury and what is not. It has already been pointed out in this chapter how the guidelines distinguish between an injury and an illness. Determining whether an injury is work related and whether it is recordable have been points of considerable confusion among employers who are required to keep injury and illness records.

The "incident rate" is the numerical performance measure required by OSHA. The incident rate is the number of injuries and illnesses or lost workdays related to a common exposure base of 100 full-time workers. The common exposure base provides for accurate industry comparisons, trend analysis over time, or comparisons among firms regardless of size. The incident rate is calculated as follows:

$$N / EH \times 200{,}000 \qquad (1)$$

where

N = number of injuries and illnesses or lost workdays

EH = total hours worked by all employees during a calendar year

200,000 = the base for 100 full-time equivalent workers (working 40 hours/week, 50 weeks/year)

In addition to OSHA requirements for employers to record occupational injuries and illnesses, employers also are required to make periodic reports of deaths, injuries, and illnesses. This periodic reporting becomes part of the Annual Survey of Occupational Injuries and Illnesses.

Occupational injury statistics can be found at the OSHA and BLS homepages on the Internet (see Appendix A at the end of this chapter). In 2000 the total cases for nonfatal occupational injury incident rates per 100 full-time workers in all establishments was 5.8. This number is an average, so some employers have a lower rate and some have a higher rate. The incident rate may also be viewed as a percentage of employees who suffer the degree of injury for which the rate was calculated. As an example, an incidence rate of 5.8 means that nearly 6% of all employees experienced a recordable injury in 2000.

OSHA recordable injury rates for all establishments reached an all-time low in 2000. The total lost workday cases (that involve days away from work, or days of restricted activity, or both) for all establishments in 2000 was 2.8. This measure for the severity of injuries was also an all-time low. For comparison, the total recordable injury cases and lost workday cases for all establishments in 1973 were, respectively, 10.6 and 3.3. Although record low injury rates are a proud accomplishment, we must not lose sight of the actual number of nonfatal cases of injuries occurring to workers in private industry. More than 5 million workers suffered an OSHA recordable injury in 2000.

Business Measurements for Safety

Drivers to prevent injuries to employees include cost savings and cost avoidance, compliance with regulations, meeting laudable goals, and as the president of Jones and Laughlin Steel said in 1948 when asked to justify safe working conditions, "it is the right thing to do."(10)

Although safety may be the right thing to do, it also must compete against other business priorities for management's time, attention, and its fair share of limited resources (e.g., time and money). The basic safety measure of recordable cases and lost workdays is insufficient to demonstrate the value of safety to an organization. This is especially so when injury rates are at record low levels. A variety of safety metrics have been developed that are more familiar to management. O'Brien devised business metrics for safety that include leading indicators (measurements for prevention of injuries) and trailing indicators (measurements of injuries, e.g., number of injuries, lost workday case rate).(11) Jervis and Collins developed a decision tool to help determine which safety program elements offer the best return on investment.(12) And Esposito described how to sell safety to business managers using metrics.(13)

OSHA also addressed the business cost and savings from safety. In 1996 the assistant secretary of labor for OSHA claimed that occupational injuries and illnesses cost American business $100 billion a year. In August 1998 OSHA developed a free software program, "$AFETY PAYS," to assist employers in assessing the impact of occupational injuries and illness (with lost workdays) on their profitability. The software uses a company's profit margin, the average cost of an injury or illness, and an indirect cost multiplier to project the amount of sales a company would need to generate to cover those costs. In early 2002, OSHA stated that each avoided occupational fatality saved $910,000; each prevented injury or illness resulting in time away from work saved $28,000; and, each serious injury or illness avoided saved $7000.

Johnson called the year 2002 "The Year of Business of Safety."(14) Johnson points to numerous examples showing why safety is more about business than regulatory compliance. His examples include the 2002 American Industrial Hygiene Conference holding 18 professional development courses relating to management and only 5 for regulatory issues. Johnson reports that the modern drivers for safety investments include organizational values and liabilities, global management systems, new performance metrics, and competitive contributions from safety.

Safety Management Systems

Simple activity-based safety, such as just complying with regulations, may not be effective in preventing and substantially reducing worker injuries. To accomplish this a process, system, or program approach must be taken. These approaches to safety stress the comprehensive nature of the challenge, often setting forth a step-by-step pathway, to prevent and reduce injuries to workers. Brown, in describing a systems approach to safety, acknowledges "more than a knowledge of the principles is necessary to bring about a safe environment. A 'procedure' must be followed whereby principles on paper become a reality."[15, pp. 3,4]

Figure 52.1 provides an example of a system approach to safety. In this example a potentially catastrophic safety hazard exists. The hazard, if left unabated, may result in a fire or explosion. The hazard has a seemingly simple fix—ensure that the bonding strap is always properly affixed and in good repair. But to assure that the fix is promptly and consistently made other conditions and actions must be part of the system.

Although there have been many recommendations for ways to prevent and reduce injuries to employees, there is no one best solution.

OSHA, through its enforcement and other activities, has the most experience in seeing which workplace safety programs have been the most effective in achieving low injury incident rates. In 1982, OSHA developed its Voluntary Protection Programs (VPP) to recognize and promote outstanding safety programs. One of the initial reasons for developing VPP included helping OSHA conserve resources by exempting outstanding safety programs from routine inspections. OSHA could then target its limited resources and attention to work sites with poor safety performances. The early VPP participants were showing lost workday case rates that ranged from one-fifth to one-third the rates experienced by average work sites.

Using knowledge gained from VPP participants and other experiences, OSHA in 1989 issued its voluntary Safety and Health Program Management Guidelines.[16] These guidelines represent a distillation of OSHA's view of the most effective practices to protect employees from injuries. These guidelines cover four main elements: (1) management commitment and employee involvement; (2) work site analysis; (3) hazard prevention and control; and (4) safety and health training. Each of these elements is briefly described in the following paragraphs.

Management Commitment and Employee Involvement

This element recognizes that management commitment provides the motivating force and resources for organizing and controlling activities within an organization. In effective safety programs, management regards worker safety as a fundamental value no less important than any other organizational value. Management commitment can be demonstrated by the following activities:

- Clearly state a work site policy on safety and health so that all personnel understand the priority of safety and health protection in relation to other organizational values.
- Establish and communicate a clear goal for the safety program and objectives for meeting that goal.
- Provide for and encourage employee involvement in the structure and operation of the safety program.
- Assign and communicate responsibility for all aspects of the safety program.
- Provide adequate authority and resources to responsible parties so that assigned responsibilities can be met.

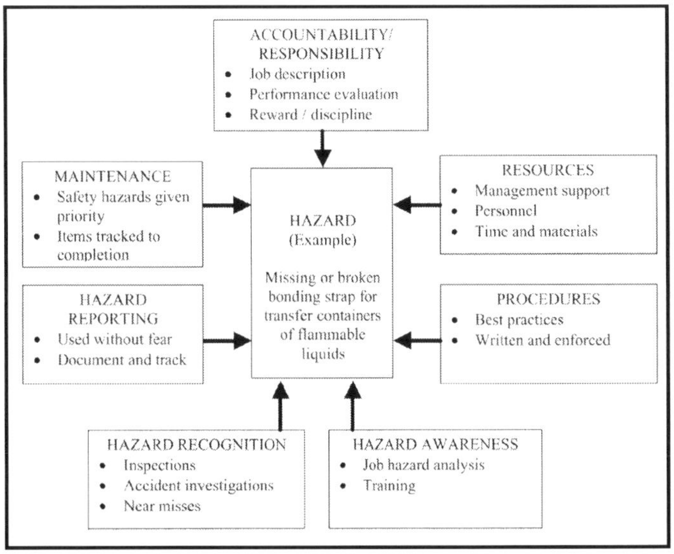

Figure 52.1 — Example: System approach to safety.

- Hold people accountable for meeting responsibilities.
- Review program operations at least annually to evaluate successes and identify deficiencies that should be corrected.

Work Site Analysis

This element involves a variety of work site evaluations to identify not only existing hazards but also conditions, operations, and changes that might create future hazards. Effective management actively analyzes the work and the work site to anticipate and prevent dangerous situations.

To ensure that all hazards are identified, management and employees must:

- Conduct comprehensive baseline work site safety surveys with periodic updates;.
- Analyze planned and new facilities, processes, and equipment for safety hazards.
- Perform routine job hazard analyses, including investigation of accidents.
- Provide a reliable system for employees to notify management about conditions that seem hazardous without fear of reprisal.
- Analyze injury and illness trends over time so that accidents and incidents with common causes can be identified and prevented.

Hazard Prevention and Control

Where feasible, hazards are eliminated by effective design of the job site or job. When it is not feasible to eliminate hazards, they are controlled to prevent unsafe exposure. Elimination or control is accomplished in a timely manner once a hazard or potential hazard is recognized. Hazard prevention and control utilizes the following techniques:

- Engineering controls, when feasible and appropriate, are used to eliminate or control the hazard.
- Procedures for safe work are established, understood, and followed by all affected parties.
- Provisions are made for personal protective equipment and administrative controls.

Safety and Health Training

Training must address the safety and health responsibilities of all personnel concerned with the work site. Safety training is most often effective when incorporated into other training about performance requirements and job practices. Training is conducted to:

- Ensure that all employees understand the hazards to which they might be exposed and how to prevent harm to themselves and others from exposure to these hazards.
- Assist supervisors in carrying out their jobs effectively.
- Ensure that managers understand their safety and health responsibilities.

From a regulatory viewpoint OSHA does not require these safety program elements as of 2002. However, OSHA is considering rulemaking that would, at the least, encourage employers to develop and follow basic safety program elements.

Other organizations have developed or are developing safety and health management systems that may be applied internationally. The British BS 8800:1996 *Guide to Occupational Health and Safety Management Systems* was one of the first systems considered for global use. BS 8800 and several other systems were combined in 1999 to create the Occupational Health and Safety Assessment Series (OHSAS) specification, OHSAS 18001. OHSAS 18001 was developed to be compatible with the systems approach to management by the International Organization for Standardization (ISO) through its series ISO 9001:1994 (Quality) and ISO 14001:1996 (Environmental). The International Labour Organization (ILO) developed guidelines on occupational safety and health management systems: ILO-OSH 2001. The safety program elements in the ILO standard include:

- Policy
- Worker participation
- Responsibility and accountability
- Competence and training
- Management system documentation
- Communication
- Initial review
- System planning, development, implementation
- Objectives
- Hazard prevention and control measures such as management of change,

emergency prevention, preparedness and response, procurement, and contracting
- Performance monitoring and measurement
- Investigation of worker-related injuries, illness, disease, and incidents and their impact on safety and health performance
- Audit
- Management review
- Prevention and corrective action
- Continual improvement

OSHA Standards that Overlap Safety and Health

Some OSHA standards clearly fall into the safety domain (e.g., machine guarding and lockout and tagout requirements). Others, such as chemical-specific standards (asbestos, benzene, cadmium), more clearly align with occupational health and occupational hygiene concerns. Several standards, however, overlap safety and health concerns in more or less equal proportions. These standards more than any others should be understood and appreciated by safety professionals and occupational hygienists alike. These standards bring the two professions close together and help demonstrate why both professions must work together if each is to be successful. For purposes of simplicity the standards, with just a few exceptions, are cited here by their general industry (29 CFR 1910) notations. The brief explanation for each standard that follows emphasizes the safety and health connections within that standard. This is not an inclusive list; only the most important and significant standards are covered.

Employee Emergency Plans and Fire Prevention Plans (1910.38). Emergency action plans are required to ensure employee safety in the event of a fire or other emergency. The plan must be prepared in writing and reviewed with affected employees. Employers must apprise employees of the fire hazards of the materials and processes to which they are exposed. Fire is predominately a safety issue because burns are, with few exceptions, readily viewed as injuries. Fire also creates noxious and poisonous decomposition products that cross over into health concerns. Therefore, the properties of flammable and combustible materials, how they burn, how they are extinguished, and what byproducts burning material may create are key overlapping safety and health concerns. Other emergencies may include spills of materials that may be explosive and/or corrosive, indicating safety concerns and also health concerns due to toxicity. Safety professionals and occupational hygienists must work together to create effective emergency action plans.

Ventilation (1910.94). Ventilation is used to keep particulates, gases, vapors, and other forms of hazardous materials at safe levels. "Safe" includes the concept of not allowing the concentration of materials to reach flammable or combustible levels (safety issue) as well as keeping exposures below toxic levels (health issue). Ventilation also improves housekeeping because it can keep dust or other potentially hazardous debris off the floor.

Occupational Noise Exposure (1910.95). Although most hearing loss is the result of long-term exposure to excessive noise, and thus is a health concern, loud noise also should be controlled for safety reasons. Loud or distracting sounds may hinder an employee's ability to hear warning signals or to clearly understand and communicate with fellow workers.

Subpart H - Hazardous Materials (1910.101-1910.120). For reasons identified previously—the fire, corrosive and toxic nature of hazardous materials—this whole category is a strong cross-over for safety and health concerns. Two standards are particularly important, however: process safety management of highly hazardous chemicals (1910.119) and hazardous waste operations and emergency response (1910.120). The standard on process safety management of highly hazardous chemicals incorporates all of the safety program elements previously discussed. Although the standard addresses only employers with more than a "threshold quantity" of the most hazardous chemicals, this standard sets the tone for proper management regardless of the amount of the chemical or the significance of its hazardous properties. The standard on hazardous waste operations and emergency response clearly is a joint safety and health effort. Safety and health concerns are stressed as being equally important.

Permit-Required Confined Spaces (1910.146). This is another example of needing to be aware of atmospheric conditions that might be combustible or toxic. Additional safety concerns include lighting, lockout/tagout, and communications.

Subpart L - Fire Protection (1910.155-1910.165). The safety and health connection associated with fire has already been explained. In the standard on portable fire extinguishers (1910.157) safety professionals must define when fighting a fire has gone beyond the "incipient" stage. In other words, when does the smoke from a fire become toxic? Beyond the incipient stage of a fire, employees need to be better trained and know when and how to wear personal protective equipment. This may then require the creation of fire brigades (1910.156) with appropriate training. Also, because extinguishing materials such as water may be used to put out a fire, basic electrical safety hazards and precautions must be considered.

Subpart Z - Toxic and Hazardous Substances (1910.1000-1910.1500). Although most of the standards in this category fall more toward occupational hygiene, there are some notable areas in which safety plays a key role. The introduction to this chapter provided the example that hepatitis contracted from a needle stick would be viewed as an injury. Given this example, the entire bloodborne pathogens (1910.1030) standard should be treated as mostly a safety issue. The far-reaching standard on hazard communication (1910.1200) fits both a safety and health pattern. It is fitting that the main vehicle to communicate hazards is identified as a "material safety data sheet." Last, the occupational exposure to hazardous chemicals in laboratories (1910.1450) standard also incorporates many safety functions (e.g., injury prevention principles).

Many other hazards within workplaces are hard to define as being either a safety or health hazard. Is an ill-fitting glove worn by an employee mostly a safety hazard or a health hazard? From a safety point of view the ill-fitting glove may prevent a proper grip and result in an employee dropping a heavy weight onto his or her foot, causing an injury. The ill-fitting glove may also require an employee to squeeze harder to hold parts. Over time carpal tunnel syndrome, an illness, might result.

OSHA's standard on lockout and tagout, which addresses prevention of unexpected start-up or operation of equipment, may seem to be entirely a safety issue. But the standard actually is about controlling energy, including energy in the form of stored fluids, pressurized gases; and unstable or reactive materials.

The inadvertent release of these energies also could cause health consequences. Thus, there is another overlap. If all that separates an injury from an illness-and thus safety and health—is the point in time needed for a short snap of one's fingers, then safety professionals and occupational hygienists have much in common.

Qualifications for Becoming a Safety Professional

According to McLean, because safety is a multidisciplinary profession it draws its workers from many different areas, including education, engineering, psychology, medicine, and biophysics.[17] In many facilities safety activities are managed and performed by the human resource manager, maintenance engineer, or security guard. It is still not uncommon today to find an injured employee who, unable to return to his or her normal job, has taken on safety responsibilities and has become the workplace "safety professional." The term *safety professional*, then, is a generic term for other titles such as safety engineer, safety manager, safety representative, safety contact, or some other semidescriptive term that addresses the performance of safety activities. The American Society of Safety Engineers defines *safety professional* as "an individual who, by virtue of his specialized knowledge, skill and educational accomplishments, has achieved professional status in the safety field."[18]

Which backgrounds are best suited to safety will be open to debate for a long time. An engineering background may be best suited if prevention and control of physical hazards (i.e., conditions) is a primary objective. If it were true that 80% or more of injuries are the result of unsafe acts, perhaps a person with primarily an education or psychology background would be better suited for the job. Manuele[19] believes that before the practice of safety can be considered a profession, it must have a sound theoretical and practical base for the practice, but safety professionals have not yet agreed on these fundamentals. Because safety professionals are not all cut from the same cloth, qualifications for who is a safety professional and who can practice and manage safety activities are situation-by-situation decisions made by employers.

Employers looking to hire someone with demonstrated competence in the field of occupational safety can check to see whether the safety professional is certified. The most demanding of the certifications is the Certified Safety Professional® designation (CSP®) issued by the Board of Certified Safety Professionals (BCSP). BCSP was organized in 1969 to evaluate the academic and professional experienced qualifications of safety professionals, administer examinations, and issue certificates of qualification to those professionals who meet BCSP's criteria and successfully pass its examination.

As of 2002 about 10,000 people hold the CSP. About 95% of current CSPs have a bachelor's degree or higher, and more than 44% have advanced degrees.

To become a CSP, a candidate must complete the following steps.[20]

- Complete and submit application material.
- Register for and take the examination(s) leading to the CSP.
- Make an appointment to take the examination at a testing center and sit for the examination at the scheduled time.
- Complete all requirements for the CSP.
- Pay an annual renewal fee.
- Meet continuance of certification requirements.

DeClue described a number of changes made by BCSP to upgrade the quality of the certification.(21) The first change, in mid-1996, was for BCSP to become accredited by the National Commission for Certifying Agencies. Beginning in January 1997 applicants for the CSP were required to have an associate degree in safety and health, or a bachelor's degree in any field that has minimum qualification for the academic requirement. The degrees must be from U.S. academic institutions accredited by a regional accrediting body recognized by the Commission on Recognition of Post-Secondary Accreditation. BCSP periodically evaluates the relevance of questions on the CSP examination, and questions are improved as appropriate. Quality improvements by BCSP distinguish the CSP as the premier credential among the many credential designations (legitimate, bogus, or "in between") that are available to people working in the safety field.

Conclusion

Occupational safety defies a simple description. Its main focus is on prevention of worker injuries. Overlap with occupational hygiene is clearly evident. BCSP interprets safety practice in broad terms, and CSP examination questions now cover safety, health, fire protection, ergonomics, environmental, and related topics. BCSP indicates that:[20]

- Only 13% of CSPs deal solely with safety as a job function.
- Eighty-seven percent deal with some of the other topics.
- Forty percent have responsibility for safety, health, and environmental matters.

What occupational safety is or may become is not so much a matter of definition or functions but of performance in preventing or limiting harm to people from workplace hazards.

References

1. **Bureau of Labor Statistics:** *Recordkeeping Guidelines for Occupational Injuries and Illnesses.* Washington, D.C.: U.S. Department of Labor, 1986.
2. **Heinrich, W.W.:** *Industrial Accident Prevention.* New York: McGraw-Hill, 1931.
3. **DeReamer, R.:** *Modern Health and Safety Technology.* New York: John Wiley & Sons, 1980.
4. **Grimaldi, J.V., and R.H. Simonds:** *Safety Management.* Homewood, Ill.: Irwin, 1989.
5. **Ferguson, D.S.:** Snapshots of safety's history: What will they think of next? *Prof. Safety 41(12)*:22–26 (1996).
6. **Smitha, M.W., K.R. Oestenstad, and K.C. Brown:** State workers' compensation reform & workplace safety regulations. *Prof. Safety 46(12)*:45–50 (2001).

7. **Petersen, D.:** The Occupational Safety and Health Act of 1970: 25 years later. *Prof. Safety 41(12)*:27–28 (1996).
8. **Roughton, J.E., and L.J. Grabiak:** Reinventing OSHA: Is it possible? *Prof. Safety 41(12)*: 29–33 (1996).
9. **Blair, E.H., and Geller, E.S.:** Does OSHA need a new paradigm? *Prof. Safety 45(9)*:27–32 (2000).
10. **Andrews, E.W.:** Basics of safety. In *Accident Prevention Manual for Industrial Operations*, 4th ed., pp. 6–7. Chicago: National Safety Council. 1959.
11. **O'Brien, D.P.:** Business metrics for safety: A quantitative measurement approach to safety performance. *Prof. Safety 43(8)*:41–44 (1998).
12. **Jervis, S., and T.R. Collins:** Measuring safety's return on investment. *Prof. Safety 46(9)*:18–23 (2001).
13. **Esposito, P.A.:** "Selling Safety to Management Using Metrics." Paper presented at ASSE Seminar, Dallas, Tex., March 7-8, 2001.
14. **Johnson, D.:** Can you prove safety & health's bottom line? Is it necessary? *Ind. Safety Hyg. News 36(5)*:26–29 (2002).
15. **Brown, D.B.:** *Systems Analysis & Design for Safety*. Englewood Cliffs, N.J.: Prentice-Hall, 1976.
16. "Safety and Health Program Management Guidelines; Issuance of Voluntary Guidelines." *Federal Register 54*:3904 (26 January 1989).
17. **McLean, W.T.:** The safety professional. In B.A. Plog, editor, *Fundamentals of Industrial Hygiene*, 3rd ed., pp. 585–589. Chicago: National Safety Council, 1988.
18. **American Society of Safety Engineers:** About ASSE. [Online] Available at www.asse.org (Accessed May 2002).
19. **Manuele, F.A.:** Principles for the practice of safety. *Prof. Safety 42(7)*:27–31 (1997).
20. **Board of Certified Safety Professionals:** *CSP Application Guide*. [Online] Available at www.bcsp.com/exam_guide/exam_guide1.html (Accessed 2002).
21. **DeClue, M.C.:** "The future is now," BCSP declares. *Prof. Safety 41(12)*:21 (1996).

Appendix A

The occupational safety professional should have access to a basic library of safety textbooks. The following books are recommended.

Ashfal, C.R.: *Industrial Safety and Health Management*. Englewood Cliffs, N.J.: Prentice-Hall, 1990.

Brauer, R.: *Safety and Health for Engineers*. New York: Van Nostrand Reinhold, 1994.

Brown, D.B.: *Systems Analysis & Design for Safety*. Englewood Cliffs, N.J.: Prentice-Hall, 1976.

Chemical Manufacturers Association: *Resource Guide for Employee Health and Safety Code: Program Performances Measures*. Washington, D.C.: Chemical Manufacturers Association, 1995.

DeReamer, R.: *Modern Safety and Health Technology*. New York: John Wiley & Sons, 1980.

Geller, S.: *Psychology of Safety: How to Improve Behaviors and Attitudes in the Job.* Boca Raton, Fla.: CRC Lewis, 1996.

Goetsch, D.: *Occupational Safety and Health*. Englewood Cliffs, N.J.: Prentice-Hall, 1996.

Grimaldi, J.V., and R.H. Simonds: *Safety Management*. Homewood, Ill.: Irwin, 1989.

Hammer, W.: *Occupational Safety Management and Engineering*. Englewood Cliffs, N.J.: Prentice-Hall, 1989.

Krause, T.: *Employee-Driven Systems for Safe Behavior*. New York: Van Nostrand Reinhold, 1995.

Manuele, F.: *On the Practice of Safety*, 2nd ed. New York: Van Nostrand Reinhold, 1997.

Marshall, G.: *Safety Engineering*. Monterey, Calif.: Brooks/Cole Engineering Division, 1982.

National Safety Council: *Accident Prevention Manual for Industrial Operations*, 11th ed. Itasca, Ill.: National Safety Council.

Slote, L.: *Handbook of Occupational Safety and Health*. New York: John Wiley & Sons, 1987. [2-volume set].

Outcome Competencies

After completing this chapter, the reader should be able to:

1. Understand the rationale for Industrial Hygienists and other Health Safety and Environmental (HSE) professionals to develop a business case for implementing occupational illness and injury preventions.
2. Explain the financial and non-financial value and benefits that HSE interventions can bring to a business or organization.
3. Describe and apply the steps needed to develop a value proposition for an HSE intervention.
4. Develop and present a basic business case for the implementation of HSE interventions within a business or organization.

Prerequisite Knowledge

Prior to beginning this chapter, the reader should review the following chapters:

Chapter Number	Chapter Topic
8	Occupational and Environmental Health Risk Assessment/Risk Management

Key Terms

The Value Strategy • Value proposition • financial analysis • non-financial analysis • forced pairs comparison • SIPOC

Key Topics

I. Introduction
   A. The Approach
   B. The Value of Health, Safety, and Environmental Interventions
   C. Fundamental Concepts Incorporated into the Value Strategy
   D. The Value Strategy Process

II The Steps of the Value Strategy Process
   A. Step 1: Identify Key Business Objectives and Hazards
   B. Step 2: Conduct Risk Assessment
   C. Step 3: Align Value Opportunities
   D. Step 4: Identify Impacts
   E. Step 5: Measure Impact
   F. Step 6: Determine Value
   G. Step 7: Value Presentation

III. Summary

IV. References

The AIHA® Value Strategy

53

By Michael T. Brandt, DrPH, CIH, PMP and Bernard D. Silverstein, CIH

Introduction

Each year millions of American workers suffer injuries and illnesses. The economic and financial impact of occupational illnesses and injuries is significant to employers because the annual total direct and indirect costs have been reported to be as high as $171 billion dollars in the U.S.[1–3] These costs positively and negatively affect the bottom line of both for-profit and non-profit organizations. In order to cover the increased of illnesses and injuries resulting from worker exposure to health hazards, companies will need to produce and sell more products and services, and non-profit organizations will need to reallocate funding from one cost account to another. In either case, injured and ill workers cost organizations large sums of money. The basic economics of labor management will drive organizations to assure that the supply of labor is well managed in terms of performance and productivity, which affects the quality of the work performed, and in terms of operational excellence, which affects the worker attendance and the ultimate cost of labor.

Health and safety hazard control measures are taken to protect employees from illness and injury, reduce health care costs, improve productivity, and contribute to organizational success. The extent to which any organization allocates staff and financial resources to industrial hygiene programs and health hazard control measures is often driven by a combination of social, ethical, technical, compliance, and economic arguments.[4] In many organizations, particularly in for-profit enterprises, loss control and cost management are fundamental drivers for investing in industrial hygiene beyond the prevailing cultural norm of HSE professionals that protecting worker health is "the right thing to do."

The Approach

The Value Strategy[5] is a process for Industrial Hygienists and other health, safety and environmental (HSE) professionals to use to develop a business case for companies or other organizations to invest in preventing occupational or environmental injury or illness. It provides an approach for determining and illustrating the business value of health, safety and environmental projects, programs and activities (interventions). Many times the industrial hygiene, safety or environmental (HSE) professional is faced with designing and implementing programs or activities to mitigate a specific risk, exposure, or compliance issue and may not entirely appreciate other values that the intervention brings to the business. The Value Strategy is a comprehensive, multi phase approach developed to assist HSE professionals in identifying, assessing, and presenting a complete business value proposition to support HSE programs and projects.

The Value Strategy has three phases:

I. Preliminary Investigation and Study Prioritization;
II. Value Assessment; and
III. Value Presentation.

Within these phases are seven model components; each component includes the specific steps and approaches in a sequential construct. The Value Strategy represents a flexible approach that allows users multiple entry points and allows them to substitute their own existing information and methods of analysis whenever possible. The Value Strategy is easily modified to meet the specific or unique requirements for demonstrating value to corporations, government and non-profit organizations.

The Value of Health, Safety and Environmental Interventions

Phil Crosby, a well-respected thought leader in the quality movement, defined the cost of quality as the "cost of conformance", that is, the cost of a company's quality assurance program plus the "cost of nonconformance", the cost of quality defects.[6] The Value Strategy corollary is the cost of HSE-related losses plus the cost of HSE projects, programs and activities. Therefore, gross cost savings from HSE interventions would be the cost of HSE-related losses before the intervention minus the cost of HSE-related losses after the intervention, as depicted in Figure 53.1.

The HSE value framework, in addition to tracking cost savings and cost avoidance, captures the total value added to a business or organization, including non-financial value. Since there are many situations where HSE interventions may result in new revenue for the business, there must be a mechanism to capture revenue generation. There should also be a means for capturing key impacts on the business process.

Fundamental Concepts Incorporated into the Value Strategy

Existing concepts and models form the basis for The Value Strategy. In general, a model is an abstraction of a real-life system with the purpose of increasing understanding of that system. It is also a representation of a system, which provides a means for investigating the components of the system. Of particular importance to this endeavor is a specific type of model — the business model — which has been described in varied ways.

Peter Drucker, the father of modern management,[7] suggests that the business model must identify who the customer is, what the customer values, and how a company makes money in the business. In other words, what is the underlying logic that explains how value can be delivered to the customer? Business models have been promoted as a way to explain how a firm or enterprise works — i.e., how the individual pieces of the business fit together. Business modeling has also been characterized as the managerial equivalent of the scientific method; it starts with a hypothesis, tests that hypothesis, and revises actions as needed.[8]

Models can be presented in physical, graphical, or mathematical terms. Graphical models consist of lines, symbols, shapes, or charts and include Pareto Diagrams, Ishikawa Diagrams, and break-even charts. Formulas and equations are the mainstay of mathematical models and are frequently used in business to aid in decision making or planning activities. Examples include linear programming, cost benefit analysis, and return on investment calculations.

A strategy is a method or plan that combines a set or series of activities to accomplish a specific predetermined goal or result. Using a business model that accurately describes the operation of the business process and how various components of the business interact (including HSE interventions), a strategy can be developed that enables HSE professionals to identify and present the value of HSE within the context of that business operation.

A successful business strategy must create a common sense reason that connects technical potential with the attainment of value. To accommodate this need, The Value Strategy provides both mathematical and graphical models that define the principal customer as the business enterprise, government or other non-profit organization and examines the relationship between the technical role of the HSE professional and the financial and non-financial economic value of their contributions.

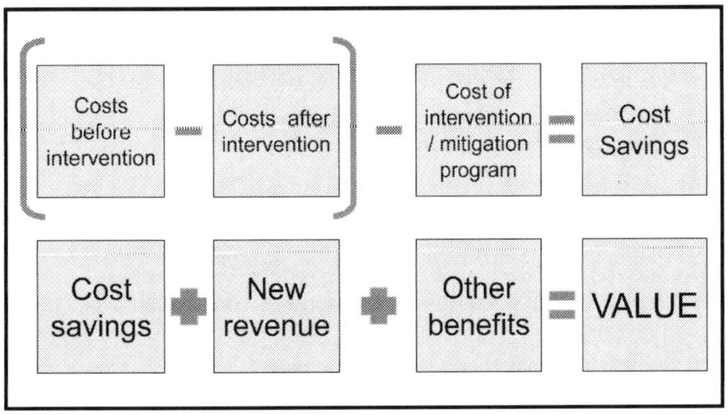

Figure 53.1 — The HSE Value Framework.

The Value Strategy Process

The Value Strategy enables managers and HSE professionals to develop a business case for the purposes of determining and illustrating the business value of HSE interventions.

Funding of projects for worker health and safety projects, new products, increasing productivity, or any other business activity, is a competitive activity. Business decisions may be made for a variety of reasons, such as regulatory requirements or corporate policy; however, the main driver is often the value a project brings to the company. How much money will a given project return on the investment? The Value Strategy uses generally accepted business economics to create the business case that investing in occupational health, safety or environmental protection makes sound business sense and will provide a sound return on that investment.

The Value Strategy allows the user to demonstrate value using both financial and non-financial analysis, as appropriate to meet the needs of the organization and key decision makers. The *financial analysis* allows the user to calculate generally-accepted financial business metrics by capturing detailed business data that demonstrate the impact of cost avoidance, cost savings, revenue generation, and other financial aspects of a business or organization. The *non-financial analysis* allows the user to demonstrate the value of the HSE contribution by evaluating the impact of interventions on non-financial business goals and objectives.

The Steps of The Value Strategy Process

The Value Strategy consists of seven sequential model components (steps). An overview of the model is shown in Figure 53.2.

1. Identify Key Business Objectives and Hazards
2. Conduct Risk Assessment
3. Align Value Opportunities
4. Identify Impacts
5. Measure Impact
6. Determine Value
7. Value Presentation

Step 1: Identify Key Business Objectives and Hazards

Completing an assessment of business goals and objectives is important in order to have a broad perspective of how HSE projects, programs and activities may support the overall business goals. The business objectives to assess depend entirely on what the organization has developed. The HSE professional needs to consider corporate and local goals and objectives, depending on what level of management will be making the business decision. In addition, mission statements, strategic plans, and annual operating plans should be evaluated. Key performance indicators, shown in Figure 53.3, associated with each objective should be captured in this inventory.

The Value Strategy recognizes that all business values are not created "equal."[9] That is, all business managers routinely make decisions based on a "Value Priority", where some business objectives have more weight or importance than others.

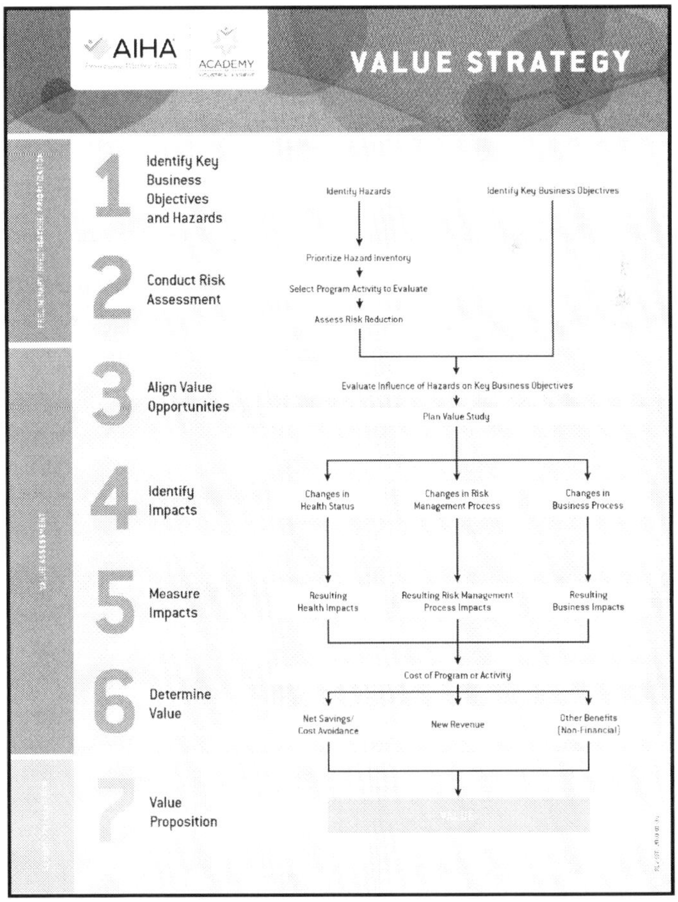

Figure 53.2 — The Value Strategy.

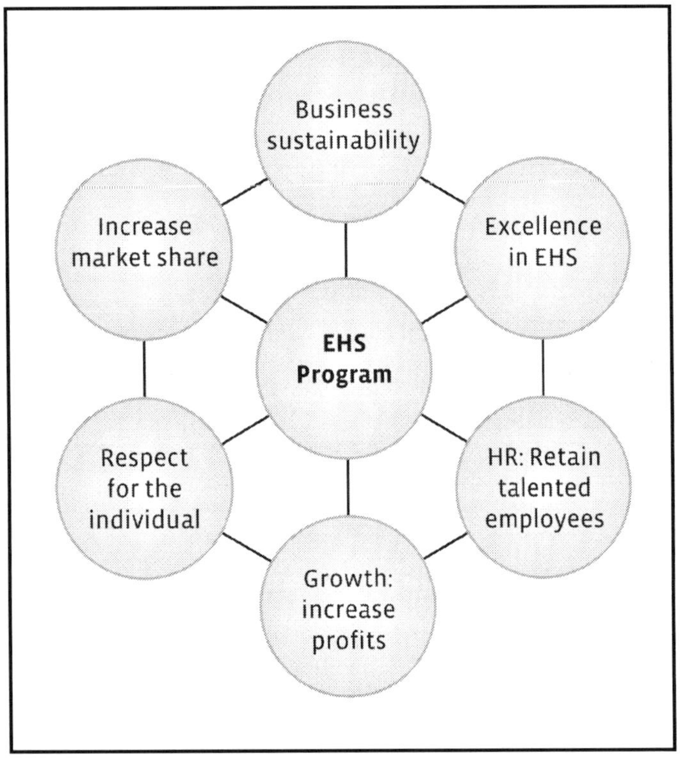

Figure 53.3 — Key Performance Indicators.

This chapter presents a tool, "Forced Pairs Comparison"[10] (see figure 53.4) that can be used to quantify this priority based on input from the business management or leadership team. In Forced Pairs Comparison, a representative group of managers will compare pairs of key performance indicators. The indicator that is more important will get ranked a five, the less important indicator will receive a one. The results of this assessment will be used later in the process to help prioritize potential risk and align interventions with business objectives.

As part of the first step of The Value Strategy, the HSE professional identifies occupational and environmental health and safety hazards. The Value Strategy allows for a flexible approach for hazards identification. Several classical approaches are can be employed such as the American Industrial Hygiene Association (AIHA®) publication, *A Strategy for Assessing and Managing Occupational Exposures, Third Edition*[11] and the American National Standard Institute (ANSI)/AIHA® Standard Z10–2005 *Occupational Health and Safety Management Systems.*[12] Other criteria for hazard identification may include actual illnesses, claims or allegations, known or

Business Value Prioritization (Forced-pairs comparison method)	Business sustainability	Excellence in HSE	Retain talented employees	Increase profits	Respect for the individual	Increase market share	TOTAL
Business sustainability		3	3	5	5	5	21
Excellence in HSE	3		5	5	1	1	15
Retain talented employees	3	1		3	1	5	13
Increase profits	1	1	3		1	1	7
Respect for the individual	1	5	5	5		1	17
Increase market share	1	5	1	1	5		13

Figure 53.4 — Forced Pairs Comparison.

suspected employee overexposures, known or suspected compliance issues, emerging regulatory issues, new or uncertain health impacts and special interests by the public, non-government organizations (NGOs), and other stakeholders. This approach of screening hazards by specific criteria helps the HSE professional narrow down which interventions are likely candidates to contribute value to the overall business.

Step 2: Conduct Risk Assessment

The hazard inventory developed in Step 1 can be a long list of potential hazards to address. The next step in The Value Strategy is to conduct risk prioritization to reduce this list to a manageable short list of workplace hazards that may require intervention. This can be conducted using one of several existing methods[4,5] or an internal method adopted for this use. The desired result is a relative risk ranking that allows the HSE professional to concentrate on the most significant risks to the business.

The HSE professional conducts a pre-intervention (see Figure 53.5) or baseline risk assessment and follows it up with a post-intervention risk assessment (see Figure 53.6) later in the process. The health, safety or environmental risk reduction that results from this intervention becomes part of the overall value proposition. The risk assessment process may be visited many times in *The Value Strategy*, to identify key projects, the best solutions for employee protection.

Step 3: Align Value Opportunities

In this step, the HSE professional identifies and prioritizes value opportunities that can be further evaluated. Once the company-specific business objectives inventory is built in Step 1, The Value Strategy directs the user to evaluate how the HSE project, program or activity under consideration influences those identified business objectives — either favorably or unfavorably. For example, an Industrial Hygiene program of periodic monitoring employee exposures strongly supports and aligns with an overall Human Resource business objective of "creating a great place to work." By thoughtfully considering how a program or activity influences each business objective, the industrial hygienist begins to identify potential value streams to the overall enterprise. While this analysis can be completed by the individual HSE professional, it is recommended that a small cross-functional team of internal stakeholders work together to complete the influence ratings. A team approach can help to ensure full identification of value opportunities and a balanced evaluation. Then the HSE Professional can plan a more thorough study of the selected HSE project, programs and activities with the strongest favorable influence on business objectives.

Once the value opportunities are assessed, the selection of the project work area can be made and the HSE professional can plan The Value Strategy. While there will have been interactions with business

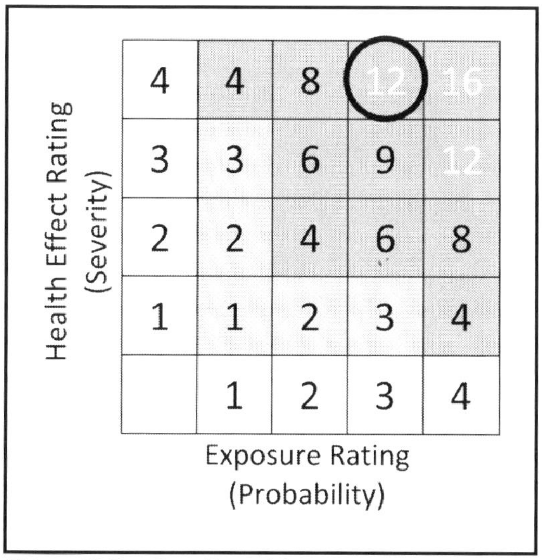

Figure 53.5 — Baseline Risk Assessment.

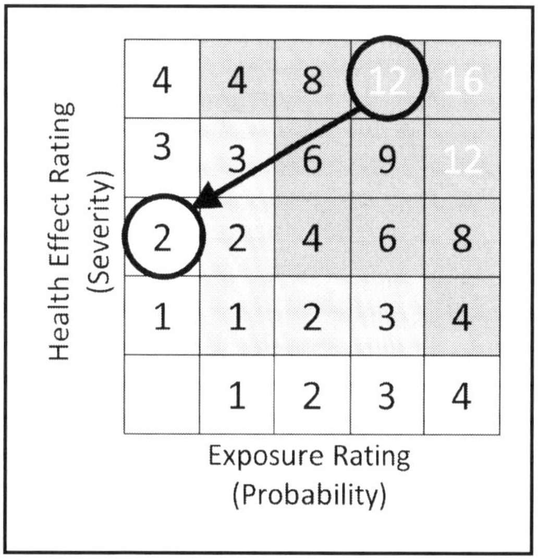

Figure 53.6 — Post-intervention Risk Assessment.

managers and other stakeholders previously, at this point it is imperative to engage and involve all the key stakeholders. To achieve the objective of worker protection, the project team will analyze the advantages of various process interventions. This will include the different options, normally based on using different levels in the "Hierarchy of Controls"(13) (see Figure 53.7). When using alternatives such as material substitution and process enclosure, emphasis is placed on working closely with engineering and process development personnel.

Finally, the plan is developed using a project tool such as the Strategy Map process, MS Project, Visio, Mind Manager, etc. These tools are useful in developing the required project steps, responsibilities and time frames for completion of the steps.

Step 4: Identify Impacts

Based on the Value Strategy plan, the next step for the HSE professional is to identify the impacts or anticipated changes resulting from the HSE intervention. The intent of this step is to simply identify or "flag" impacts; the magnitude of each change is measured in the next step. Impacts are categorized into three areas:

- Health status
- Risk management
- Business process

Identification of impacts in these three areas helps to understand and build the value proposition for the HSE intervention. One process widely used for the identification of impacts is the Six Sigma method called SIPOC(14) (see Figure 53.9) where **S**upport **I**nputs for a **P**rocess are used to identify **O**utputs or impacts to the **C**ustomer. Using process mapping as a guide, the project team can systematically identify project related health, risk management and business process impacts.

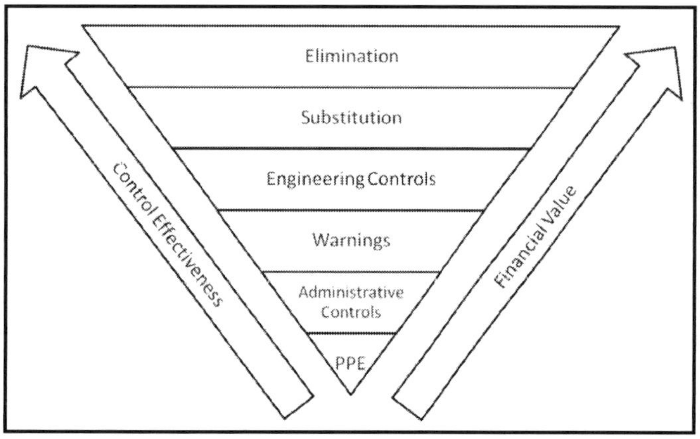

Figure 53.7 — Hierarchy of Controls.

The value of the HSE profession is determined by what the organization gets from their work; it is this impact or the effect they have on the organization. By reducing risk, the principle function of the HSE profession, three changes will occur: (1) the health of the employees will change; (2) the business process will change; and (3) the work of the HSE professional will change and constitute the intermediate outcomes of intervention.

These three categories of change are incorporated into the financial and non-financial analysis. In the analysis they were used to identify steps in the thinking process that translated operational changes and risk reduction that impact business value. That effort is done by using a sequential cause and effect analysis to translate reductions in risk to changes in health, the risk reduction process, or the business process. The business impacts resulting from those changes are then isolated and a value case is then made for those impacts.

Step 5: Measure Impact

In this step of The Value Strategy, the HSE professional measures the impacts associated with identified changes in health status, risk management, and business processes. In the *financial approach*, impacts are entered into The Value Strategy as costs in dollars (or other denomination). It is important in this step to capture as many impacts as possible associated with the changes from HSE projects, programs, and activities. Impacts may be positive or negative.

Resulting Health Impacts. From a health status viewpoint, impacts may include workers' compensation and other illness related costs, as well as other impacts such as changes in absenteeism, presenteeism, insurance premiums, labor turnover, medical removal, job transfer, training/re-training, worker productivity and other factors. Where exact costs are not available, defensible estimates or the non-financial approach can be used.

Resulting Risk Management Impacts. From risk management viewpoint, costs are captured in the categories of HSE duties and

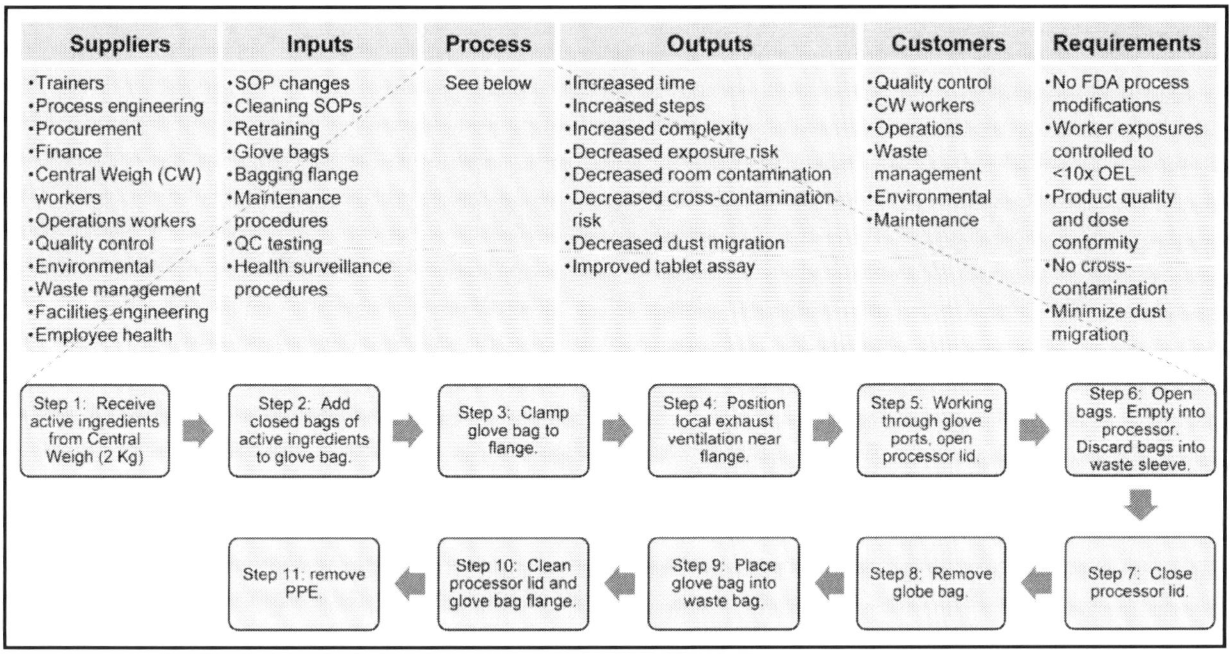

Figure 53.9 — SIPOC.

responsibilities, administrative load/recordkeeping, hierarchy of controls, monitoring/medical surveillance, and other HSE risk management processes. For example, an intervention may reduce the need for personal protective equipment (PPE) and reduce downtime associated with donning and doffing PPE, employee training, and medical approvals. These cost impacts can often be directly measured or estimated.

Resulting Business Impacts. From a business process point of view, impacts are measured across the previously identified change categories such as process design, inputs, equipment, materials, management, flow, pace, and other process changes. For example, if an HSE intervention reduces or eliminates process steps, the costs savings in terms of improved cycle time can be measured or estimated.

At this point in the process, individual cost impacts have been collected and assessed by the project team for consideration.

Step 6: Determine Value

The HSE professional must determine the overall value of their intervention. Considerations include the cost of the intervention (investment cost) and cost savings/avoidances, new revenue generation, and any other benefits resulting from the intervention. Results are used to prepare a value presentation in the final step of The Value Strategy.

The financial analysis of The Value Strategy focuses on guiding the user through a series of calculations to define intervention costs and to capture the costs before and after a particular HSE intervention. These before and after costs should be determined across the categories of health status, risk management process, and business process. In addition, the financial analysis (see Figure 53.10) may capture, as required, a number of parameters and business assumptions, such as depreciation, corporate tax rate, inflation rate, discount rate, loaded wages, and others. These data are used to calculate financial metrics such as Return on Investment, Payback Period, Internal Rate of Return, and Net Present Value in the financial analysis.

The Financial analysis can also capture other benefits such as improvements in product ordering, time to market, protection of revenue/market share, utilization of people, employee morale, product and service reliability, and company reputation. While many of these parameters are difficult to quantify exactly, the project team may be asked to make credible estimates where possible.

Non-financial benefits play an important role in “selling” a HSE business case. Non-financial benefits are “soft” or “intangible”

Net Cash Flow	Year 0	Year 1	Year 2	Year 3	Year 4	Year 5
Net cash flow	($1,000)	$350	$350	$350	$350	$350
Present values	($1,000)	$318	$289	$263	$239	$217
NPV = $326			Simple payback = 1.33 years			
IRR = 11%			Discounted payback = 3.06 years			
Simple ROI = 75%			Simple unit cost impact = ($0.15)			
Discounted ROI = 32.7%			Discounted unit cost impact = ($0.065)			

Figure 53.10 — Financial Analysis.

business impacts that cannot be directly quantified. Even though these benefits are difficult to quantify and explain, they remain very important to HSE professionals. Increasingly managers are beginning to feel traditional financially oriented benefits are no longer the only deciding factor. Successful managers emphasize not only financial benefits such as cash flows and returns, but also, include value drivers such as customer and employee satisfaction, innovation, sustainability, reputation, and lower attrition rates to mention a few. In the non-financial assessment, the value of the actual or proposed HSE interventions is tied to business goals and objectives (see Figure 53.11). These are often the key to success of projects where direct costs are outweighed by the intangible benefits to the organization.

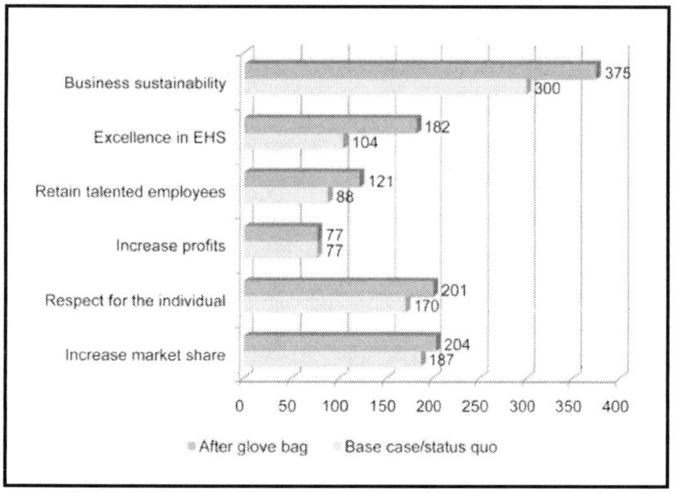

Figure 53.11 — Impact of non-financial benefits before and after project intervention.

Step 7: Value Presentation

In the final step of The Value Strategy, the HSE professional assembles the Business Case Study, to document all methods and assumptions, inputs and outcomes. An executive summary presentation that describes the value of the HSE project, program or activity can be prepared and used to promote the intervention. Areas of focus include financial and non-financial analyses that address cost savings/avoidance, new business revenue, business goals and objectives and other benefits.

The value presentation is a critical termination of both the underlying financial and non-financial approaches within *The Value Strategy*. Key components of the presentation are:

- Executive summary
- Hazard Identification
- Methods and assumptions
- HSE intervention description
- Hazard and risk reduction
- Business opportunities
- Changes and impacts
- Costs of HSE intervention
- Value determination
  - financial metrics
  - non-financial metrics
- Summary statement and recommendations.

Summary

The Value Strategy was developed to assist users in understanding, measuring, demonstrating, and communicating how health, safety and environmental investments improve employee protection and business performance by answering the following questions:

- Which HSE hazard has the greatest impact on employee health and safety and business goals and objectives?
- How do health, safety and environmental investments compare to operational and other business investments?
- To which projects should we allocate financial and human resources?
- Which HSE investment creates the greatest value for the organization?

Health, Safety and Environmental related process improvements that are designed to reduce or eliminate employee and environmental exposures often result in significant business improvements and savings. Health, Safety and Environmental professionals can be the catalysts to drive management actions, and to enable organizations to make process or business changes that not only protect employees but also result in significant business improvements that can save money and enhance an organization's competitive advantage.

References

1. **Leigh, J.P., S. Markowitz, M. Fahs, and P. Landrigan:** *Cost of Occupational Injuries and Illnesses.* Ann Arbor, MI: The University of Michigan Press, 2003.
2. **Leigh, J.P., S. Markowitz, M. Fahs, C. Shin, and P. Landrigan:** Occupational Injury and Illness in the United States: Estimates of Costs, Morbidity, and Mortality. *Arch. Intern. Med. 157(14)*:1557–1568 (1997).
3. **Leigh, J.P., J.E. Cone, and R. Harrison:** Costs of Occupational Injuries and Illnesses in California. *Prev. Med. 32*:393–406 (2001).
4. **Miller, P. and C. Haslam:** Why Employers Spend Money on Employee Health: Interviews with Occupational Health and Safety Professionals from British Industry. *Safety Sci. 47*:163–169 (2009).
5. **American Industrial Hygiene Association (AIHA®):** *The AIHA® Value Strategy Manual.* Fairfax, VA: AIHA®, 2010.
6. **Crosby, P.B.:** *Quality is Free.* New York: Mentor, 1980.
7. **Drucker, P.:** *The Practice of Management.* New York: Harper Collins, 1993.
8. **Magretta, J.:** *Why Business Models Matter.* Boston, MA: Harvard Business Review, May 2002; Reprint R0205F; Pages 3–8.
9. **Downs, D.E.:** "All Values Are Not Created Equal." *The Synergist.* Fairfax, VA: AIHA®, October 2, 2006.
10. **Thurstone, L.L.:** A Law of Comparative Judgment. *Psych. Rev. 34*:273–286 (1927).
11. **American Industrial Hygiene Association (AIHA®):** *A Strategy for Assessing and Managing Occupational Exposures,* 3rd edition. Ignacio, J.L. and W.H. Bullock (eds.). Fairfax, VA: AIHA®, 2006.
12. **American Industrial Hygiene Association (AIHA®):** *ANSI/AIHA Z10-2005 Occupational Health and Safety Management Systems.* Fairfax, VA: AIHA®, 2005.
13. **National Institute for Occupational Safety and Health (NIOSH):** *Prevention through Design — Plan for the National Initiative. Department of Health and Human Services.* Cincinnati, OH: NIOSH, March 2009.
14. **Pande, P.S., R.P. Neuman, and RR. Cavanaugh:** *The Six Sigma Way.* New York: McGraw-Hill, 2002.

Glossary

Terms included in this glossary are taken principally from the text in this book, and from the following AIHA publications: *Direct-Reading Colorimetric Indicator Tubes Manual*, 2nd Edition (edited by Janet B. Perper and Barbara J. Dawson; published 1993); the *Emergency Response Planning Guidelines and Workplace Environmental Exposure Level Guides Handbook* (updated and published annually); *Extremely Low Frequency (ELF) Electric and Magnetic Fields* (by R. Timothy Hitchcock, Sheri McMahan, and Gordon C. Miller; published 1995); and *Particle Sampling Using Cascade Impactors* (AIHA Aerosol Technology Committee; edited by John Y. Young; published 1995).

The following books were also used in compiling this glossary: *Calculation Methods for Industrial Hygiene* (by Salvatore R. DiNardi; published 1995 by Van Nostrand Reinhold); *Illustrated Dictionary of Environmental Health and Occupational Safety* (by Herman Koren; published 1996 by CRC Press-Lewis Publishers); *McGraw-Hill Dictionary of Scientific and Technical Terms*, 4th Edition (Sybil P. Parker, editor in chief; published 1989 by McGraw-Hill, Inc.); *Terminology of Heating, Ventilation, Air Conditioning, and Refrigeration* (published 1986 by ASHRAE); *Webster's Medical Desk Dictionary* (published 1986 by Merriam-Webster Inc.); *Webster's New World College Dictionary*, 4th Edition (published 2001 by IDG Books Worldwide, Inc.); and *The Work Environment, Volume Three — Indoor Health Hazards* (edited by Doan J. Hansen; published 1994 by CRC Press-Lewis Publishers).

A

A/V: Standard abbreviation for antivibration.

AAIH: See *American Academy of Industrial Hygiene, Academy of Industrial Hygiene.*

AAOM: See *American Academy of Occupational Medicine.*

ABC: See *activity-based costing.*

abduction: Movement of an extremity or other body part away from the axis of the body.

ABIH: See *American Board of Industrial Hygiene.*

absolute gain: A ratio of the actual transmitted power density in the main beam to the power density transmitted from an isotropic radiator.

absolute pressure: It is never less than zero. The absolute pressure in a system can approach zero, but for the pressure to be negative it would first have to pass through zero which is like absolute temperature on a thermodynamic scale. It is possible to approach but not reach absolute zero pressure.

absolute temperature: Temperature as measured above absolute zero. (Also known as "thermodynamic temperature.")

absolute zero: The temperature at which all molecular motion stops. Either -273.15°C (0 K) in the SI system of units, or -459.67°F (0°R) in the English system. (See also *Kelvin temperature, Rankine temperature.*)

absorbed dose: 1. The mass or moles of exposing compound that actually enters the bloodstream through any external routes of exposure; the absolute bioavailability. 2. Amount of a substance penetrating the exchange boundaries of an organism after contact. Calculated from intake and absorption efficiency and expressed as mg/kg/day.

absorbing medium: A collection medium that allows for the penetration of airborne chemicals into the material where the chemicals will either physically dissolve or chemically react with the collection medium.

absorption: To take in a substance across the exchange boundaries of an organism (skin, lungs, or gastrointestinal tract) and ultimately into body fluids and tissues. (See also *uptake*.)

Academy of Industrial Hygiene (AIH): A professional association of certified industrial hygienists, formerly known as the American Academy of Industrial Hygiene, but was dissolved in 1999 and since reformed as the AIH with AIHA®. AIH requires maintenance of certification and active practice of the profession.

acceleration: Any gradual speeding up of a process. The time rate of change of velocity.

acceleration due to gravity: The rate of increase in velocity of a body falling freely in a vacuum; value varies with latitude and elevation. The International Standard at sea level and 45 latitude is 9.80665 meters per second squared (m/sec^2) or 31.174 feet per second squared (ft/sec^2).

accelerometer: An instrument that measures acceleration or gravitational force capable of imparting acceleration.

acceptable air quality: Air in which there are no known contaminants at harmful levels as determined by occupational hygienists, and air with which 80%–90% of the people do not express dissatisfaction based on comfort criteria: temperature, relative humidity, nonhazardous odors, and air movement (draftiness/stuffiness).

acceptable risk: Risk level deemed acceptable by an individual, organization, or society as a whole.

acceptance sampling: The procedures by which decisions to accept or reject a sampled lot or population are made based on the results of a sample inspection. In air pollution work, acceptance sampling could be used when checking a sample of filters for certain measurable characteristics such as pH, tensile strength, or collection efficiency to determine acceptance or rejection of a shipment of filters, or when checking the chemical content of a sample of vials of standard solutions from a lot of vials to be used in an interlaboratory test.

acceptance testing: A systematic procedure to test as-received materials before use to determine whether they are contaminated.

acclimatization: Adaptation of a species or population to a changed environment over several generations. (Also known as "acclimation.")

accuracy: 1. The degree of agreement of a measurement, X, with an accepted reference or true value, T, usually expressed as the difference between the two values, X – T, or the difference as a percentage of the reference or true value, 100(X – T)/T, and sometimes expressed as a ratio, X/T. 2. Measure of the correctness of data, as given by differences between the measured value and the true or specified value. Ideal accuracy is zero difference between measured and true value. 3. Conformity of an indicated value to an accepted standard value, or true value. Quantitatively, expressed as an error or an uncertainty. The property is the joint effect of method, observation, apparatus, and environment. Accuracy is impaired by mistakes, by systematic bias (e.g., abnormal ambient temperature), or by random errors (imprecision). 4. The degree of freedom from error (i.e., the degree of conformity to truth or to a rule). Accuracy is contrasted with precision (e.g., four-place numbers are less precise than six-place numbers; nevertheless, a properly computed four-place number might be more accurate than an improperly computed six-place number). (See also *precision, repeatability*.)

acfm: See *actual cubic feet per minute.*

ACGIH®: See *American Conference of Governmental Industrial Hygienists.*

acid: A compound that reacts with an alkali to form a salt and water. It turns litmus paper red and has pH values of 0 to 6.

ACIL: See *American Council of Independent Laboratories.*

acne: A pleomorphic, inflammatory skin disease involving sebaceous follicles of the face, back, and chest and characterized by blackheads, whiteheads, papules, pustules, and nodules.

acoustic trauma: The temporary or permanent hearing loss due to a sudden intense acoustic event such as an explosion.

acoustical absorption: Material added to a workspace environment to reduce noise above 300 Hz.

acrid: Sharp, bitter, stinging, or irritating to the taste or smell.

ACS: See *American Chemical Society*.

action level: 1. In general, the level of a pollutant at which specified actions or counter measures are to be taken. 2. A term used by OSHA in several chemical standards. A level of exposure at which the employer must initiate some actions such as medical monitoring and training. The action level is generally set at 50% of the PEL. 3. This is the concentration or level of an agent at which it is deemed that some specific action should be taken. The action can range from more closely monitoring the exposure atmosphere to making engineering adjustments. In general practice the action level is usually set at one-half of the ACGIH® TLV®.

action potential (AP): A transient change in electric potential at the surface of a nerve or muscle cell occurring at the moment of excitation.

activated carbon: Activated carbon is commonly used in gas adsorption. (Also known as "activated charcoal.")

active sampling: The collection of airborne contaminants by means of a forced movement of air by a sampling pump through an appropriate collection device.

activity-based costing: A method of identifying and allocating costs based on measurable activities. There are two elements of ABC: activity analysis and cost object analysis.

actual cubic feet per minute (acfm): Actual cubic feet per minute of gas flowing at existing temperatures and pressure. (See also *scfm*.)

acuity: Pertains to the sensitivity of a bodily organ to perform its function.

acute: Severe, often dangerous effect used to denote an exposure to high concentrations of a contaminant for short duration.

acute effect: An adverse effect (usually) arising from a short exposure (minutes to hours) to a chemical.

acute exposure: Large dose/short time.

Acute Exposure Guideline Levels (AEGLs): Developed by the EPA, these guidelines are developed based on an assessment of the health risks in extensive peer-review processes and are published regularly in the United States *Federal Register*.

acute intake: Intake averaged over a period of less than two weeks.

acute mountain sickness (AMS): Refers to high altitude pulmonary edema and/or high altitude cerebral edema. Symptoms (severe breathlessness and/or chest pain) can rapidly become life-threatening if not treated by an immediate descent to a lower altitude. AMS is subdivided into benign and malignant. (See also *high altitude pulmonary edema, high altitude cerebral edema*.)

acute toxicity: The adverse effects resulting from a single dose or single exposure to a substance. Ordinarily refers to effects occurring within a short time following administration. Terminology and units used for different descriptive categories of toxicity vary. Examples of toxicity classifications as defined by different organizations are:

- LC50 inhalation (ppm): extremely toxic = <10; highly toxic = 10–100; moderately toxic = 100–1000; slightly toxic = 1000–10,000; practically nontoxic = 10,000–100,000; relatively harmless = >100,000. [**Hodge, H.C., and J.H. Sterner:** Tabulation of Toxicity Classes. *Am. Ind. Hyg. Quarterly 10*:93 (1949).]
- LC50 inhalation (ppm): highly toxic = <200; toxic = 200–2000. [29 CFR 1910.1200, Appendix A — Health Hazard Definitions.]
- LC50 inhalation (ppm): extremely toxic = <10; highly toxic = 10–100; moderately toxic = 100–1000; slightly toxic = 1000–5000; practically nontoxic = >5000. [Adapted from E.I. du Pont de Nemours & Co., Haskell Laboratory.]

acute toxicity study: Toxicity study durations of less than five days exposure.

adduct: The product of a reaction between an endogenous macromolecule and an exposing chemical or its metabolite.
adenoma: A benign tumor with glandular structure or of a glandular organ.
administered dose: Mass of a substance given to an organism and in contact with an exchange boundary, expressed as mg/kg/day.
administrative controls: The use of management involvement, training of employees, rotation of employees, air sampling, biological sampling, and medical surveillance to protect individuals.
administrative solution: A managerial rather than an engineering solution to reduce work-related stress.
adsorbent: A material that causes molecules of gases, liquids, or solids to adhere to its internal surfaces without physical or chemical changes to the adsorbent material. Solid materials, such as silica gel and activated alumina, have this property.
adsorbing medium: A collection medium that traps airborne chemicals onto the surface of the material.
adsorption: 1. Surface adherence of a material, which extracts one or more substances present in an atmosphere or mixture of gases and liquids, unaccompanied by physical or chemical change. Condensation of gases, liquids, or dissolved substances on the surfaces of solids. 2. The attachment of molecules or atoms to the surface of another substance; a process whereby one or more components of an interfacial layer between two bulk phases are either enriched or depleted.
aerobic: In presence of air.
aerodynamic diameter: Diameter of a unit-density sphere having the same gravitational settling velocity (terminal velocity) as the particle in question. (See also *cutoff particle diameter, mass median aerodynamic diameter.*)
aerodynamic equivalent diameter: The diameter of a unit density sphere that would exhibit the same settling velocity as the particle in question.
aerosol: Solid or liquid particles of microscopic size dispersed in a gaseous medium, solid or liquid, suspended in air (e.g., dust, fumes, fog, and smoke). The diameter of the particles may vary from micrometers (µm) down to less than 0.01 micrometers, and are fine enough to remain so dispersed for a period of time. (See also *fume.*)
aerosol photometer: The most popular of direct-reading aerosol monitors. They operate by illuminating an aerosol as it passes through a chamber (sensing volume) and by measuring the light scattered by all the particles at a given scattering angle relative to the incident beam. As the number of particles increases, the light reaching the detector increases. The detector can be a solid-state photodiode or a photomultiplier tube.
agent: A chemical, radiological, mineralogical, or biological entity that may cause deleterious effects in an organism after the organism is exposed to it.
agglomerate: a group of nanoparticles held together by relatively weak forces, including van der Waals forces, electrostatic forces, and surface tension.
agreement states: Regulates reactor-produced radionuclides within their borders and must provide at least as much health and safety protection as under Nuclear Regulatory Commission.
Agricola: In De Re Metallica (1556), this German scholar described every facet of mining, smelting, and refining, noting prevalent diseases and accidents. He suggested means of prevention including mine ventilation and protective masks. In 1912 his work was translated into English by Herbert Clark Hoover and Lou Henry Hoover.
AHU: See *air-handling unit.*
AIChE: See *American Institute of Chemical Engineers.*
AIHA®: See *American Industrial Hygiene Association.*
AIHA® Value Strategy: a process for Industrial Hygienists and other health, safety and environmental (HSE) professionals to use to develop a business case for companies or other organizations to invest in preventing occupational or environmental injury or illness.
AIME: See *American Institute of Mining, Metallurgical, and Petroleum Engineers.*
air: The atmosphere: the mixture of invisible, odorless, tasteless gases, such as nitrogen and oxygen, that surrounds the earth.

air change: 1. New, cleansed, or recirculated air introduced to a space. 2. A method of expressing the amount of air movement into or out of a building or room, in terms of the number of building volumes, or room volumes, exchanged in unit time.

air cleaner: 1. A device used to remove airborne impurities from air. (See also *air filter.*) 2. A device for removing a chemical hazard from an airstream before discharge to the ambient air. 3. A device to separate contaminants from an airstream. Examples include filters, scrubbers, electrostatic precipitators, cyclones, and afterburners.

air conduction: The process by which sound is transmitted through air from one point to another.

air contaminant: A substance (solid, liquid, or gaseous) not found in the normal composition of the atmosphere.

air ducts: A system of ducts to carry conditioned air to and from rooms.

air exfiltration: Air leaking outward. (See also *air infiltration.*)

air filter: A mechanical device that removes contaminants from an airstream.

air-handling unit (AHU): A device to move and condition (heat, cool, filter, and humidify) air in a central location.

air infiltration: Uncontrolled inward air leakage through cracks and interstices in any building element, and around windows and doors of a building, caused by the pressure effects of wind or the effect of differences in the indoor and outdoor air density.

air monitoring: The sampling for and measuring of contaminants in the air.

air quality: ASHRAE defines acceptable indoor air quality as "air in which there are no known contaminants at harmful concentrations and with which a substantial majority (usually 80%) of the people exposed do not express dissatisfaction." The problem with this definition is that in nonindustrial environments measurable contaminants are rarely present in levels known to be harmful, even when complaints of discomfort and adverse health effects are considerably in excess of the "acceptable" 20%. Until health risks have been established for chronic low-level exposures to both known and currently unrecognized pollutants, one must rely on the second part of this definition for guidance. Indoor air must meet standards that provide for the health and comfort of the majority of occupants.

air sampling: The collection and analysis of samples of air to measure the amounts of various pollutants or other substances in the air or the air's radioactivity.

air temperature: See *dry bulb temperature.*

air velocity: 1. The rate of motion of air in a given direction, measured as distance per unit time. 2. The axial velocity of the air entering or leaving a given effective face area. 3. Units for air velocity are meters per second (m/sec), feet per min (ft/min), or miles per hour (mph).

airborne particles: Impurities as solid or liquid particulate matter from natural or manmade sources. (Also known as "airborne particulates.")

airborne particulate matter: The ACGIH® TLV® committees have divided this general category into three classes based on the likely deposition within the respiratory tract. Although past practice was to provide TLVs® in terms of total particulate mass, the recent approach is to take into account the aerodynamic diameter of the particle and its site of action. Inhalable particulate mass (IPM) TLV®s are designated for compounds that are toxic if deposited at any site within the respiratory tract. The typical size for these particles can range from sub-micrometer size to approximately 100 micrometers (μm). Thoracic particulate mass (TPM) TLV®s are designated for compounds that are toxic if deposited either within the airways of the lung or the gas-exchange region. The typical size for these particles can range from approximately 5–15 μm. Respirable particulate mass (RPM) TLV®s are designated for those compounds that are toxic if deposited within the gas-exchange region of the lung. The typical size for these particles is approximately 5 μm or less. It should also be noted that the term "nuisance dust" is no longer used since all dusts have biological effects at some dose. The term "particulates," not otherwise classified, is now being used in place of nuisance dusts; however, the time-weighted average (TWA) of 10 mg/m^3 for IPM is still used, while a value of 3 mg/m^3 for RPM is now recommended.

air-line respirator: An atmosphere-supplying respirator in which the respirable gas is not designed to be carried by the wearer (listed by NIOSH as Type C and CE supplied air respirators).

air-purifying respirator: A respirator in which ambient air is passed through an air- purifying element that removes the contaminant(s). Air is passed through the air-purifying element by means of the breathing action of the respirator wearer or by a blower.

aliphatic: Usually applied to petroleum products derived from a paraffin base and having a straight or branched chain, or saturated or unsaturated molecular structure.

aliquot: Of, pertaining to, or designating an exact divisor or factor of a quantity, especially of an integer; contained exactly or an exact number of times.

alkali: A compound that has the ability to neutralize an acid and form a salt. Turns litmus paper blue and has pH values of 8 to 14. (Also known as "base, caustic.")

allergen: Any antigen (such as pollen, a drug, or food) that induces an allergic state in humans or animals.

allergic reaction: 1. Reaction of the body to chemical and/or biological agents, characterized by bronchoconstriction, nasal congestion, tearing, sneezing, wheezing, coughing, itching rash, and eruptions. 2. Immune response following exposure to a foreign agent or substance in an individual who is hypersensitive to that substance as a result of prior exposures. Examples are some types of skin rashes and asthma.

allergy: A response of a hypersensitive person to chemical and physical stimuli.

alpha particle: A nucleus consisting of two protons and two neutrons at nuclear distances. (Also known as "doubly charged helium ion.")

alveoli: Tiny air sacs of the lungs at the end of a bronchiole, through which gas exchange takes place by which the blood takes in oxygen and gives up its carbon dioxide in the process of respiration.

ambient: Surrounding, encircling, or pertaining to the environment.

ambient air: The air outdoors.

ambient air conditions: Characteristics of the environment (for example, temperature, relative humidity, pressure motion).

ambient noise: Ambient noise is the total noise within a given environment, being usually a composite of sounds from many sources near and far.

ambient temperature: 1. The temperature of the medium surrounding an object. In a domestic or commercial system having an air-cooled condenser, it is the temperature of the air entering this condenser. 2. The temperature of the medium such as air, water, or earth, into which the heat of equipment is dissipated: (a) For self-ventilated equipment, the ambient temperature is the average temperature of the air in the immediate neighborhood of the equipment; (b) For air or gas-cooled equipment with forced ventilation or secondary water-cooling, the ambient temperature is taken as that of the ingoing air or cooling gas; (c) For self-ventilated enclosed (including oil-immersed) equipment considered as a complete unit, the ambient temperature is the average temperature of the air outside the enclosure in the immediate neighborhood of the equipment.

ambient total pressure: The atmospheric pressure at a given location that varies with local weather conditions and altitude; the pressure that would be read by a barometer at that location.

American Academy of Industrial Hygiene (AAIH): See *Academy of Industrial Hygiene.*

American Academy of Occupational Medicine (AAOM): A professional association of physicians working in occupational medicine full time to promote maintenance and improvement of health in the workplace.

American Board of Industrial Hygiene (ABIH): Founded in 1960 by AIHA® and ACGIH®, ABIH offers a voluntary certification program for industrial hygienists. ABIH considers education, experience, and performance on a two-part examination in granting the titles Industrial Hygienist in Training (IHIT) and Certified Industrial Hygienist (CIH).

American Chemical Society (ACS): A scientific, educational, and professional society of chemists and chemical engineers. Headquarters are in Washington, D.C.

American Conference of Governmental Industrial Hygienists (ACGIH®): An organization founded in 1938, whose members typically are industrial hygienists working in government or at universities. Many of the ACGIH technical committee publications (threshold limit values [TLVs®] and *Industrial Ventilation: A Manual of Recommended Practice*) are recognized worldwide as authoritative sources.

American Council of Independent Laboratories (ACIL): Headquarters are in Washington, D.C.

American Industrial Hygiene Association (AIHA®): An organization founded in 1939, whose membership includes industrial hygienists and other OEHs professionals from the private and public sectors. AIHA is recognized for its technical committee publications, its proactive role in governmental affairs, and for promoting the profession of industrial hygiene.

American Institute of Chemical Engineers (AIChE): A member of the Accreditation Board for Engineering and Technology, the American National Standards Institute (ANSI), and related organizations. Headquarters are in New York, N.Y.

American Institute of Mining, Metallurgical, and Petroleum Engineers (AIME): This professional organization, founded in 1871 as the American Institute of Mining Engineers, is dedicated to the exploration, extraction, and production of the Earth's minerals, materials, and energy resources. AIME comprises five separately incorporated units with a combined membership of more than 90,000. Headquarters are in New York, N.Y.

American National Standards Institute (ANSI): A voluntary membership organization that develops consensus standards. Headquarters are in New York, N.Y.

American Public Health Association (APHA): Represents health professionals in more than 40 disciplines in the development of health standards and policies. Headquarters are in Washington, D.C.

American Society for Testing and Materials (ASTM): A nonprofit organization that develops standard testing methods through consensus of volunteers (manufacturers, users, etc.) Headquarters are in West Conshohocken, Pa.

American Society of Heating, Refrigerating and Air-Conditioning Engineers (ASHRAE): A professional society committed to the establishment of standards in heating, refrigeration, and air-conditioning. Headquarters are in Atlanta, Ga.

American Society of Mechanical Engineers (ASME): A technical society of approximately 123,000 members committed to developing safety codes, equipment standards, and educational guidance. Headquarters are in New York, N.Y.

American Society of Safety Engineers (ASSE): A society of safety professionals of approximately 31,000 members committed to improving the workplace through promotion of standards and education. Headquarters are in Des Plaines, Ill.

Ames Test: A test for mutagenicity conducted in the bacterium *Salmonella typhimurium*. (Also known as the "Ames assay.")

amplitude: 1. Angular distance north or south of the prime vertical; the arc of the horizon, or the angle at the zenith between the prime vertical and a vertical circle, measured north or south from the prime vertical to the vertical circle. 2. The maximum absolute value attained by the disturbance of a wave or by any quantity that varies periodically.

ampoule: A small sealed glass vial filled with liquid.

ampoule detector tube: A detector tube consisting of one or more filling layers and a reagent ampoule. The ampoule contains part of the reagent system, which for reasons of stability cannot be placed in a single tube. During use, the ampoule is broken and the contents liberated.

AMS: Acute mountain sickness. See *high altitude pulmonary edema, high altitude cerebral edema.*

AMU: See *atomic mass unit.*

anaerobic: In absence of air.

analogue: Compound of the same structural type.

analytical blank: A blank used as a baseline for the analytical portion of a method. For example, a blank consisting of a sample from a batch of absorbing solution used for normal samples but processed through the analytical system only, and used to adjust or correct routine analytical results. (Also known as "reagent blank.")

analytical limit of discrimination: A concentration above which one can, with relative certainty, ascribe the net result from any analysis to the atmospheric particulate and below which there is uncertainty in the result. One approach to determining a statistical limit is to use a one-sided tolerance limit for the analytical discrimination limit (that is, a level [limit] below which a specified percentage [e.g., 99%] of blank filters analyses fall with a prescribed confidence [e.g., 95%]). [**Note:** "Limits for Qualitative Selection and Quantitative Determination," by L.A. Currie, *Analytical Chemistry 40(3)*:586-593, 1968, contains a detailed discussion of limits of detection.]

analytical methods: Detailed laboratory procedures that specify how to measure the amount of chemicals collected on the sampling media.

anemia: A condition in which the blood is deficient in red blood cells, hemoglobin, or total volume.

anesthetic effect: The loss of the ability to perceive pain and other sensory stimulation.

angstrom (Å): A unit of length equal to 10-10 meters or 0.1 nanometers used primarily to express wavelengths of optical spectra. (See also *nanometer.*)

annoyance: A sound level of an intermittent broad-band noise is about 10 dBA above the background sound levels. Tonal sounds and other "attention-getting" sounds might cause annoyance at lower levels.

anoxia: The lack of oxygen (or a significant reduction in oxygen).

ANSI: See *American National Standards Institute* (formerly titled USA Standards Institute; American Standards Association).

antagonists: Skeletal muscles that act to brake or decelerate a limb.

anthropometry: The science of measurement of the body's mass, size, shape, and inertial properties.

anthropometry: The science of measurement of the body's mass, size, shape, and inertial properties.

antibody: The protein that a living organism is stimulated to make from its B lymphocytes when a foreign antigen is present.

anticipation: One of four primary responsibilities of the industrial hygienist. The anticipation of what health hazard problems may occur before a plant, process, or product is introduced. Anticipation depends on and extends the ability to recognize, coupled with a broad and current awareness of developments in the organization and its business, in scientific developments and new technologies, in regulatory areas bearing on the organization's activities, and in other activities that have an impact on the health of workers. (See also *recognition, evaluation, and control.*)

antigen: A large macromolecule that triggers an immune response.

antiparticle: A particle with the same mass and spin as the particle itself but an opposite charge and mag-netic field.

AP: See *action potential.*

APF: See *assigned protection factor.*

APHA: See *American Public Health Association.*

aphake: Absence of the ocular lens.

apnea: The temporary cessation of breathing.

apparent temperature: An index of heat discomfort during the summer months. It includes the amplifying effect of increasing humidity on the discomfort level. (Also known as "heat index.")

appearance: A description of a substance at room temperature and normal atmospheric conditions.

appendage: Any subordinate or external organ or part of a plant or animal as a branch, tail, or limb.

applied dose: Amount of a substance given to an organism, especially through dermal contact.

aquatic toxicity: The adverse effects to marine life that result from being exposed to a toxic substance.

aqueous: Relating to or resembling water.

area: The cross-sectional area (e.g., duct, window, door, or any space) through which air moves. Units used are square feet (ft^2) or square meters (m^2).

area free: The total minimum opening area in an air inlet or outlet through which air can pass.

area sampling: The collection of airborne chemicals at a fixed position in the work area.

arithmetic mean: The most commonly used measure of central tendency, commonly called the "average." Mathematically, it is the sum of all the values of a set divided by the number of values in the set. (Also known as "average.")

aromatic: Applied to a group of hydrocarbons and their derivatives characterized by a molecular ring structure.

artery-vein differential: The difference in the oxygen content of the artery and the vein. For example, the artery may have 19 mL of oxygen/100 mL of blood and the vein may have 15, giving a differential of 4.

arthrogram: X-ray image of a joint after the injection of a dye or contrast medium.

arthroscope: Lighted surgical tube used to examine the interior of a joint.

ASA: Acoustical Society of America

asbestosis: Pneumoconiosis caused by breathing asbestos dust.

ASHRAE: See *American Society of Heating, Refrigerating and Air-Conditioning Engineers.*

ASME: See *American Society of Mechanical Engineers.*

aspect ratio: A ratio of length to width, greater than 3:1.

asphyxia: Suffocation from lack of oxygen. Chemical asphyxia is produced by a substance, such as carbon monoxide, that combines with hemoglobin to reduce the blood's capacity to transport oxygen. Simple asphyxia is the result of exposure to a substance, such as carbon dioxide, that displaces oxygen.

asphyxiant: 1. A vapor or gas that can cause unconsciousness or death by suffocation (lack of oxygen). Most simple asphyxiants are harmful to the body only when they become so concentrated that they reduce oxygen in the air (normally about 21%) to dangerous levels (18% or lower). Asphyxiation is one of the principal potential hazards of working in confined and enclosed spaces. 2. A chemical that displaces oxygen in the air, potentially resulting in insufficient oxygen to sustain life, especially in poorly ventilated areas. A chemical asphyxiant chemically interferes with the body's ability to take up and transport oxygen; a physical asphyxiant displaces oxygen in the environment.

assay: The quantitative or qualitative evaluation of a hazardous substance; the results of such an evaluation.

ASSE: See *American Society of Safety Engineers.*

assigned protection factor (APF): The expected workplace level of respiratory protection that would be provided by a properly functioning respirator or a class of respirators to properly fitted and trained users.

asthma: A condition marked by recurrent attacks of labored breathing and wheezing resulting from spasms of the upper airways of the lung.

ASTM: See *American Society for Testing and Materials.*

asymptomatic: The lack of identifiable signs or symptoms.

ataxia: A loss of balance with an unsteady gait; a failure of muscular coordination, total or partial.

atm: See *atmosphere.*

atmosphere (atm): A unit of pressure equal to 760 mmHg (mercury) at sea level.

atmosphere-supplying respirator: A class of respirators that supply a respirable atmosphere, independent of the workplace atmosphere.

atmospheric pressure: The pressure exerted in all directions by the atmosphere. At sea level, mean atmospheric pressure is 29.92 inches Hg, 14.7 psi, 407 inches wg, or 760 mmHg.

atom: The smallest unit of an element that still maintains the physical and chemical properties of the element.

atomic mass: The number of protons plus the number of neutrons in the nucleus (the sum of the nucleons).

atomic mass unit (AMU): One-twelfth the mass of the 12-carbon nucleus.

atomic number: The number of protons in the nucleus of a nuclide. (Also known as the "Z number.")

atomic weight: 1. The (weighted) average mass of naturally occurring isotopes of an element. 2. The relative mass of the atom on the basis of ^{12}C 12.

atrophy: Wasting of muscles or other tissues in the body caused by a decrease in the number of cells or shrinkage of the cells. Some cases of carpal tunnel syndrome can lead to muscle atrophy.

attendant: An individual stationed outside one or more permit spaces who monitors the authorized entrants and performs all attendant's duties assigned in the employer's permit space program. (See *OSHA 1910.146.*)

attenuation (sound): The reduction, expressed in decibels, of the sound intensity at a designated first location as compared with sound intensity at a second location, which is acoustically farther from the source.

attitude: Manner, disposition, feeling, or position toward a person or thing.

audible range: The frequency range over which normal ears hear — approximately 20 Hz through 20,000 Hz. Above the range of 20,000 Hz, the term "ultrasonic" is used. Below 20 Hz, the term "subsonic" is used.

audiogram: A record of hearing loss or hearing level measured at several different frequencies — usually 500–6000 Hz. The audiogram may be presented graphically or numerically.

audiologist: A person trained in the specialized problems of hearing and deafness.

audiometer: A signal generator or instrument that can be operated manually or automatically for measuring objectively the sensitivity of hearing in decibels referred to audiometric zero. Pure tone audiometers are standard instruments for occupational use.

audiometric testing program: Test records that provide the only data that can be used to determine whether the program is preventing noise-induced permanent threshold shifts (NIPTS). It is an integral part of the hearing conservation program. (See also *noise-induced permanent threshold shift.*)

audit: A systematic check to determine the quality of operation of some function or activity. Audits may be of two basic types: 1) performance audits in which quantitative data are independently obtained for comparison with routinely obtained data in an air pollution measurement system; or 2) system audits are of a qualitative nature and consist of an on-site review of a laboratory's quality assurance (QA) system and physical facilities for air pollution sampling, calibration, and measurement.

auditory: Pertaining to, or involving, the organs of hearing or the sense of hearing.

authoritative occupational exposure limit: An occupational exposure limit set and recommended by credible organizations, such as ACGIH® or AIHA®. (See also *occupational exposure limit.*)

authority: The power to judge, act, or command.

authorized entrant: An employee who is authorized by the employer to enter a permit space. (See *OSHA 1910.146.*)

autoignition temperature: The lowest temperature at which a flammable gas- or vapor-air mixture will ignite from its own heat source or a contacted heated surface without necessity of spark or flame. Vapors and gases will spontaneously ignite at a lower temperature in oxygen than in air, and their autoignition temperature may be influenced by the presence of catalytic substances.

autoimmunity: An immune state in which antibodies are formed against the person's own body tissues.

automation: See *mechanization.*

autonomic nervous system: A subdivision of the central nervous system (CNS) that transmits signals to the smooth and cardiac muscles associated with the viscera or organ systems.

autoxidation: Slow reaction with air.

availability: The fraction or percentage of time that an item performs satisfactorily (in the reliability sense) relative to the total time the item is required to perform, taking into account its reliability and its maintainability, or the percentage of "up time" of an item or piece of equipment, as contrasted with its percentage of inoperative or "down time."

averaging time: The period over which a function is measured, yielding a time-weighted average (e.g., average concentration of an air pollutant).

aversion response: Blink reflex of the eye.

Avogadro's number: The number of molecules (6.02 × 1023 molecules/mole) contained in one gram molecular weight or one gram molecular volume. (e.g., 28.001 grams of CO = 6.02 × 1023 molecules of CO).

A-weighted response: The simulation of the sensitivity of the human ear at moderate sound levels.

B

backpressure: See *pressure drop.*

backup layer: The secondary layer of sorbent material in a sorbent tube that adsorbs chemicals that are not effectively trapped onto the primary collection layer.

bacteria: Small, relatively simple organisms found in soil, water, and the alimentary tract of animals and man. Some cause diseases in man.

baffle: A surface, usually in the form of a plate or wall, used to deflect fluids.

balanced system: A system in which the static pressure of each branch entering a junction is equal or balanced at the junction.

band pressure level: The sound pressure level for the sound contained within a specified frequency band. The reference pressure must be specified.

bandwidths (BW): 1. The difference between the frequency limits of a band containing the useful frequency components of a signal. 2. The range between the low and high cutoff frequencies of an acoustic filter. For measurement of sound the bandwidths generally used are octaves, 1/3 and 1/10 octaves.

bar: 1. A unit of pressure equal to 10^5 pascals or 10^5 newtons per square meter or 10^6 dynes per square centimeter (cm^2). 2. A unit of pressure equal to 10^6 dynes/cm^2 (part of the SI system of units).

barometer: A device for measuring atmospheric pressure using a working fluid, usually mercury. Fabricated from a long glass tube, closed at one end, evacuated, filled with mercury and inverted in a cistern of mercury. The height of the column of mercury is a measure of atmospheric pressure.

barometric effect: Variations in barometric pressure caused by altitude or weather changes.

barometric hazard: From an occupational hygiene perspective, barometric hazards can be categorized as: 1) hypobaric (low pressure) hazards; 2) hyperbaric (high pressure) hazards; and 3) hazards from changes in pressure, predominantly — but not exclusively — decreases in pressure.

barometric pressure: See *atmospheric pressure.*

barotrauma: Injury to air-containing structures (such as the middle ears, sinuses, lungs, and the gastrointestinal tract) due to unequal pressure differences across their walls.

basal cell carcinoma: A locally invasive, rarely metastatic nevoid tumor of the epidermis.

base: A substance that 1) liberates hydroxide (OH) ions when dissolved in water; 2) receives hydrogen ions from a strong acid to form a weaker acid; and 3) neutralizes an acid. Bases react with acids to form salts and water. Bases have a pH greater than 7 and turn litmus paper blue.

baseline survey: The initial evaluation of a health and safety parameter that will be used as the basis for all future comparisons.

basic characterization: The first step of the exposure assessment process. The basic information needed to characterize the workplace, work force, and environmental agents is collected and organized. Information is gathered that will be used to understand the tasks that are being performed, the materials being used, the processes being run, and the controls in place so that a picture of exposure conditions can be made.

batch method: A static generation method for preparing a known mixture of gas or vapor for verification testing of detector tubes. The method uses a volatile liquid to produce a known concentration in a container of known volume. A pure gas, or vapor of known volume and concentration, could be used also.

batch mixture: A fixed quantity of mixture prepared in an appropriate container.

BCSP: See *Board of Certified Safety Professionals.*

Beer-Lambert law: See *Bouguer-Lambert-Beer law.*

behavior: The aggregate of observable responses of an organism to internal or external stimuli.

behavior based observation and feedback: See person-based.

BEI®: See *biological exposure index.*

bellows pump: A sampling pump that draws a fixed volume of air using an air chamber with flexible sides (i.e., a bellows).

belonging: Someone or something that belongs.

benchmark (BM): A relatively permanent natural or artificial object bearing a marked point with an elevation above or below an adopted datum (e.g., "sea level" is known).

benign: Not malignant or recurrent; often used to describe tumors that might grow in size but do not spread throughout the body.

benign acute mountain sickness (benign AMS): A constellation of symptoms (highlighted by frontal headaches) that can range from discomforting to incapacitating and is precipitated by a rapid ascent but will generally resolve spontaneously within 3 to 5 days.

beta: High speed particle with characteristics of an electron emitted from a nucleus in beta decay.

beta-glucan: Beta-glucans (or β-glucans) form the major portion of most fungal cell walls and may be chemically bound to chitin (and hence insoluble) or may form a soluble matrix in which the chitin fibrils are embedded. Most fungi that are common in indoor environments contain beta-glucans.

bias: A systematic (consistent) error in test results. Bias can exist between test results and the true value (absolute bias or lack of accuracy), or between results from different sources (relative bias). For example, if different laboratories analyze a homogeneous and stable blind sample, the relative biases among the laboratories would be measured by the differences among the results from the different laboratories. If the true value of the blind sample were known, however, the absolute bias or lack of accuracy from the true value would be known for each laboratory. (See also *systematic error.*)

bilateral: Condition that affects both sides of the body. Bilateral carpal tunnel syndrome occurs in both hands.

billion: In the United States, 10^9. In the United Kingdom and Germany, 10^{12}.

bioaccumulation: The accumulation or concentration of material in the body over a period of time.

bioassay: A test to determine the potency of a substance at producing some adverse health effect on a biological system.

biochemical epidemiology: The correlation of chemical markers measured in bodily media with epidemiological variates.

biohazardous waste: Byproducts containing blood, body fluids, or recognizable body parts that present a substantial or potential hazard to human health or the environment when managed improperly.

biological agents: Any of the viruses, microorganisms, and toxic substances derived from living organisms and used as offensive weapons to produce death or disease in humans, animals, and growing plants.

biological exposure index (BEI®): ACGIH's procedures for estimating the amount of a material contained in the human body by measuring it (or its metabolic products) in tissue, body fluids, or exhaled air.

biological extrapolation: Assumption that results of toxicological studies on animals are applicable to humans.

biological half-life: The time required for a living tissue, organ, or organism to eliminate one-half of a substance that has been introduced into it.

biological monitoring: 1. The measurement of chemical markers in body media that are indicative of external exposure to chemical and physical agents. 2. An assessment of overall exposure to chemicals and other materials that are present in the workplace through measurement of the appropriate determinant(s) in biological specimens collected from the worker at a specified time. The determinant can be the chemical itself or its metabolite(s) or a characteristic reversible biochemical change induced by the chemical.

biological safety cabinet: Containment equipment that prevents the release and transmission of biological agents.

biological time constant: The time required for a portion of an absorbed chemical to undergo metabolic changes in the body.

biological wastes: Pathogenic or infective wastes that, if introduced into the human body, might disrupt biochemical and physiological function through infectivity or toxicity.

biologically effective dose: The absolute mass or moles of exposing compound that actually exposes a target organ internally after absorption.

biomarker: The determinant to be measured in a biological system.

biomechanics: A discipline that deals with the mechanical aspects of body motion. This term has been defined by the American Society of Biomechanics as "the application of the principles of mechanics to the study of biological systems." Biomechanics thus uses the knowledge base of anatomy, physiology, and mechanical engineering. The studies of muscle activity and the forces on and within the body are points of interest to the biomechanist.

biopsy: The removal and examination of tissue, cells, or fluids from a living body for examination.

biosafety: The art and science of maintaining a broken chain of infection.

biosafety level (BSL): The rating of biohazard potential described in four degrees of severity: 1) BSL1 agents are low risk and not known to cause disease in healthy adult humans; 2) BSL2 agents are associated with agents known to cause human disease that can be moderately serious, and for which preventive or therapeutic interventions are often available; 3) BSL3 agents are indigenous or exotic with potential for infection following aerosol transmission. Agents are associated with serious or lethal human disease for which preventive or therapeutic interventions may be available; 4) BSL4 organisms are dangerous/exotic agents that pose a high risk of life-threatening disease, and for which preventive or therapeutic interventions are not usually available.

biotechnology: Techniques that use living organisms or parts of organisms to produce a variety of products (from medicines to industrial enzymes) to improve plants or animals or to develop microorganisms to remove toxics from bodies of water, or act as pesticides.

bioterrorism: The use of biological agents, such as pathogenic organisms or agricultural pests, for terrorist purposes.

biotransformation: Biotransformation is the process through which toxicants are chemically converted, generally reducing their lipophilicity and increasing their hydrophilicity. (See also *metabolism.*)

blank sample: A sample of a carrying agent (gas, liquid, or solid) that is normally used to selectively capture a material of interest, and that is subjected to the usual analytical or measurement process to establish a zero baseline or background value, which is used to adjust or correct routine analytical results. (Also known as "blank.")

bitter aerosol fit-test: A respirator fit test using a bitter compound (such as solution of sodium chloride, water and denatonium benzoate) instead of saccharine (sweet) or irritant smoke (stannous oxychloride).

blast gate damper: See *damper, blast gate.*

blood: The red fluid contained in arteries and veins.

blood-brain barrier: A barrier postulated to exist between brain capillaries and brain tissue to explain the relative inability of many substances to leave the blood and cross the capillary walls into the brain tissues.

bloodborne pathogen(s): Pathogenic organism(s) present in human blood, or other potentially infectious body fluids, that can cause disease in humans. These pathogens include, but are not limited to, the hepatitis B virus (HBV) and the human immunodeficiency virus (HIV).

Board of Certified Safety Professionals (BCSP): A professional board establishing minimum academic and experience attainments needed to qualify as a safety professional. The BCSP issues certificates to qualified individuals.

blood distribution: The distribution of blood to different parts of the body. For example, during exercise more blood is distributed to the muscles.

body burden: The total amount of a chemical retained in the body.

boiling point (BP): 1. The temperature at which a liquid changes to a vapor. 2. The temperature at which the vapor pressure of a liquid equals the atmospheric pressure. The temperature at which the vapor pressure of a liquid equals the absolute external pressure at the liquid-vapor interface.

bone conduction: Transmission of sound vibrations to the internal ear via the bones of the skull.

boredom: In the workplace, too little information, which might lead to fatigue.

Bouguer-Lambert-Beer law: The intensity of a beam of monochromatic radiation in an absorbing medium decreases exponentially with penetration distance.

Boyle's law: At a constant temperature the volume of a given quantity of any gas varies inversely as the pressure to which the gas is subjected.

BP: See *boiling point.*

Bragg-Gray principle: The amount of ionization produced in a small gas-filled cavity surrounded by a solid absorbing material that is proportional to the energy absorbed by the solid.

brainstorming: A procedure used to find a solution for a problem by collecting all ideas, without regard for feasibility that occurs from a group of people meeting together.

brake horsepower: Brake power expressed in horsepower.

brake power: The actual power delivered by or to a shaft (from the use of a brake to measure power).

branch: 1. In ducts, piping, or conduit another section of the same size or smaller at an angle with the main. Also, the section of pipe from a main to a register or radiator. 2. (computer) A set of instructions that are executed between two successive decision instructions.

branch line: An air supply line connecting the controller and controlled device.

breakthrough: Significant sample loss that occurs when chemicals are not effectively trapped by the collection media.

breakthrough time: The time elapsed from the initial contact of the chemical on the outside surface until detection on the inside surface.

breakthrough volume: That volume of an atmosphere containing two times the permissible exposure limit (PEL) for a specific contaminant that can be sampled at the recommended flow rate before the efficiency of the sampler degrades to 95%.

breathing zone (BZ): The volume surrounding a worker's nose and mouth from which he or she draws breathing air over the course of a work period. This zone can be pictured by inscribing a sphere with a radius of about 10 inches centered at the worker's nose.

breathing zone sampling: Air samples that are collected in the breathing zone. NIOSH sometimes uses this term to describe the sample collection technique in which a second individual collects a sample in an employee's breathing zone.

BRI: See *building-related illness.*

British thermal unit (Btu): The amount of heat energy needed to raise the temperature of 1 pound of water 1°F from 59°F to 60°F. It is defined by the British Standards Institution as 1055.06 joules.

brick and mortar structure: A major barrier to dermal penetration consisting of densely packed dead cells, called corneocytes.

broad-band: A band with a wide range of frequencies.

bronchial tubes: Branches or subdivisions of the trachea (windpipe) that carry air into and out of the lungs. (Also known as "bronchioles.")

bronchoconstriction: Constriction of the bronchial air passages.

browser: A software application used to locate and display Web pages. Three of the most popular browsers are Netscape Navigator®, Microsoft Internet Explorer®, and Spyglass Mosaic®. All of these are graphical browsers, which means that they can display graphics as well as text. Also, most modern browsers can present multimedia information, including sound and video.

BSL: See *biosafety level.*

Btu: See *British thermal unit.*

bubble flowmeter: A device used to calibrate pumps for airflow rate. Air sampled by the pump is measured by the displacement of a soap bubble in a burette. The volume displacement per unit time (i.e., flow rate) can be determined by measuring the time required for the soap bubble to pass between two scale markings that enclose a known volume.

buffer: Any substance in a liquid that tends to resist the change in pH when acid or alkali is added.

building envelope: The outer shell, or the elements of a building, that encloses conditioned spaces, through which thermal energy may be transferred to, or from, outdoors.

building-related illness (BRI): Infectious, allergic, or toxin-induced disease with objective clinical findings related to building occupancy. (Also known as "building-related disease.")

building wake: The zone around a building's envelope.

burn: The visible destruction (or permanent change) in skin, eyes, tissue, etc., at the site of contact.

BW: See *bandwidths.*

BZ: See *breathing zone.*

C

c: See *ceiling.*

CA: See *corrective action.*

calibrate: To check, adjust, or systematically standardize the graduations of a quantitative measuring instrument.

calibration: Establishment of a relationship between various calibration standards and the measurements of them obtained by a measurement system, or portions thereof. The levels of the calibration standards should bracket the range of levels for which actual measurements are to be made.

calibration standard: A standard used to quantitate the relationship between the output of a sensor and a property to be measured. Calibration standards should be traceable to a standard reference material (SRM), certified reference material (CRM), or a primary standard.

calorie: Heat required to raise the temperature of 1 gram of water 1°C, specifically from 4°C to 5°C. Mean calorie = 1/100 part of the heat required to raise 1 gram of water from 0°C to 100°C. Great calorie or kilocalorie = 1000 calories.

calorimeter: 1. A device for measuring heat quantities, such as machine capacity, combustion heat, specific heat, vital heat, heat leakage, etc. 2. A device for measuring quality (or moisture content) of steam or other vapor. 3. Equipment for measuring emitted or absorbed heat quantities.

cancellation: A method for reducing radiation exposure levels. The general principle involves having wires in proximity carry current, and produce fields, that are opposite in phase. The field from one wire then effectively cancels the field from the other at locations removed from the two.

cancer: A cellular tumor that is usually associated with spread throughout the body and can be fatal.

cancer slope factor: See *slope factor.*

canister/cartridge: A container with a filter, sorbent, or catalyst — or combination of these items — which removes specific contaminants from the air passed through the container.

canopy hood: A one- or two-sided overhead hood that receives rising hot air or gas. (See also *receiving hood.*)

capitalism: An economic system in which all or most of the means of production and distribution, as land, factories, communications, and transportation systems, are privately owned and operated in a relatively competitive environment through the investment of capital to produces profits.

capture hood: A ventilation system hood that captures contaminants that are released from a process. A slot-plenum hood is an example of a capture hood.

capture velocity (V_c): 1. Air velocity at any point in front of a capture hood opening necessary to overcome opposing air currents and to capture contaminated air at that point and cause it to flow into the hood and prevent the contamination from reaching the workers' breathing zone. 2. The velocity of air flowing past a contaminant source that is necessary to overcome the opposing air currents and capture or entrain the contaminant at that point and move it into the hood. (Also known as "control velocity.")

carbon dioxide toxicity: Carbon dioxide becomes toxic when it suppresses respiration. The combination of the accumulation of exhaled carbon dioxide at increased pressure (either in the breathing system's dead space or due to a malfunction) can rapidly cause toxic effects.

carcinogen: A substance or agent capable of causing or producing cancer in mammals, including humans. A chemical is considered to be a carcinogen if: a) it has been evaluated by IARC and found to be a carcinogen or potential carcinogen; b) it is listed as a carcinogen or potential carcinogen in the Annual Report on Carcinogens published by the National Toxicology Program (NTP); or c) it is regulated by OSHA as a carcinogen.

carcinogen classification systems: Several different carcinogen classifications have been developed by organizations such as EPA, IARC, and ACGIH®. The system used by ACGIH® can be summarized as follows: (A1) Confirmed Human Carcinogen — To have this designation a chemical must have human data to support its classification. Examples are nickel subsulfide, bis(chloromethyl) ether, and chromium VI compounds; (A2) Suspected Human Carcinogen — This designation requires relevant animal data in the face of conflicting or insufficient human data. Examples are diazomethane, chloromethyl methyl ether, and carbon tetrachloride; (A3) Animal Carcinogen — To have this designation a chemical must have caused cancer in animal studies by nonrelevant routes of exposure or mechanisms (e.g., kidney tumors produced in male rats from many hydrocarbons, paradichlorobenzene, d-limonene, etc.; hormone-mediated thyroid tumors from compounds such as the ethylene bisdithiocarbamates) or at excessive doses, etc. Furthermore, there are human data available that are in contradiction to the results in animals. Examples are nitrobenzene, crotonaldehyde, and gasoline; (A4) Not Classifiable as a Human Carcinogen — This classification is given to chemicals for which there is inadequate data to say whether it is a potential human carcinogen. It is typically applied to chemicals for which an issue of carcinogenicity has been raised but for which there are insufficient data to answer the question. Examples are pentachloronitrobenzene, phthalic anhydride, and acetone; (A5) Not Suspected as a Human Carcinogen — This classification is given to chemicals that have strong supporting data in humans to show that they are not carcinogens. Data from animals can also be used to support this classification. To date, the only example of a chemical receiving this designation is trichloroethylene.

carcinogenesis: The development of malignant tumors or neoplasms composed of abnormal cells exhibiting uncontrolled growth, invasiveness, and metastasis.

carcinogenic: A substance or material capable of producing cancer.

carcinoma: A malignant tumor of epithelial cell origin (e.g., skin, lung, breast), tending to infiltrate the surrounding tissue and give rise to metastases (tumors at distant sites).

cardiovascular system: See *CVS.*

carpal tunnel: Bony, narrow passage at the intersection of the hand and wrist through which the median nerve and many tendons pass.

carpal tunnel syndrome (CTS): Compression of the median nerve caused by the swelling of tendons in the carpal tunnel. CTS is characterized by numbness, pain, and tingling in the fingers; and clumsiness and loss of grip strength in the hand.

CAS: See *Chemical Abstracts Service.*

cascade impactor: A sampling device that uses a series of impaction stages with decreasing particle cut size so that particles can be separated into relatively narrow intervals of aerodynamic diameter. It is used for measuring aerodynamic size distribution of an aerosol sample.

case control study: A study that evaluates groups that are divided by their disease status to compare the level(s) of exposure between the groups.

catalyst: A substance that changes the speed of a chemical reaction but undergoes no permanent change itself.

catchball: The continuing two-way communication at all levels of the policy deployment process, to evaluate lower-level plans and the continuing utility of the original policies.

cavitation: The formation of cavities on a surface of a solid by liquid moving over it with velocity high enough to induce erosion of the surface when the cavity collapses.

cc: Cubic centimeter, a volume of measurement in the metric system that is equal in capacity to one milliliter (mL). One quart is about 946 cc.

CEGL: See *continuous exposure guidance level.*

ceiling (c): 1. The maximum allowable human exposure limit for an airborne substance, not to be exceeded even momentarily. Used in OSHA PELs, ACGIH® TLVs®, and NIOSH RELs. 2. The concentration that should not be exceeded during any part of the working exposure. In conventional occupational hygiene practice, if instantaneous monitoring is not feasible, then the ceiling can be assessed by sampling over a 15-minute period, except for chemicals that may cause immediate irritation, even with exposures of extremely short duration.

ceiling limit: Control of exposure to fast-acting substances by value placing a limit on their concentration. Such substances are marked with a "C" in the ACGIH threshold limit value (TLV®) table. The concentration of these substances cannot at any time in the work cycle (except for a 15-minute period) exceed the TLV®. Also known as "ceiling value." (See also *threshold limit value.*)

ceiling value: See *ceiling limit.*

Celsius temperature: Temperature scale used with the SI system of units in which the freezing point of water is 0°C, the triple point is 0.01°C, and the boiling point is approximately 100°C. (Formerly referred to as the "centigrade scale.")

center of gravity: A fixed point in a material body through which the resultant force of gravitational attraction acts.

centigrade temperature: See *Celsius temperature.*

central nervous system (CNS): The brain and spinal cord.

central-fan system: A mechanical indirect system of heating, ventilating, or air conditioning in which the air is treated or handled by equipment located outside the rooms served, usually at a control location, and is conveyed to and from the rooms by a fan and distributing ducts.

Certified Industrial Hygienist (CIH): A professional industrial hygienists who by education, experience, and demonstration of knowledge has satisfied the requirements of ABIH and has been designated as a CIH in either the comprehensive practice or chemical aspects of the profession. The CIH designation builds on the IHIT requirements in recognizing long experience and proven professional ability.

certified reference material (CRM): Standards prepared by gas vendors in quantities of at least 10 cylinders for which 1) the average concentration is within 1% of an available standard reference material (SRM); and 2) 2 cylinders are selected at random and audited by the U.S. EPA.

CET: See *corrected effective temperature.*

CFR: See *Code of Federal Regulations.*

chain of custody: A procedure for preserving the integrity of a sample or of data (e.g., a written record listing the location of the sample/data at all times).

channeling: Uneven flow of sampled air through a detector tube because of improper packing.

Charles-Gay-Lussac law: Gases increase in volume for each 1°C rise in temperature. This increase is equal to approximately 1/273.15 of the volume of the gas at 0°C.

chemical: A single molecule or a mixture of molecules.

Chemical Abstracts Service (CAS): An organization under the American Chemical Society. CAS abstracts and indexes chemical literature from throughout the world in "Chemical Abstracts." "CAS Numbers" are used to identify specific chemicals or mixtures.

Chemical Abstracts Service (CAS) number: A concise, unique means of material identification. Each chemical may have more than one synonym but only one CAS number.

chemical agent: Dust, gas vapor, or fume that acts on or reacts with the human physiologic system.

chemical asphyxiant: See *asphyxiant.*

chemical asphyxiation: Toxic reaction wherein chemicals reaching the bloodstream react in such a way as to deprive the body of oxygen.

chemical family: A group of single elements or compounds with a common general name. Example: acetone, methyl ethyl ketone (MEK), and methyl isobutyl ketone (MIBK) are of the "ketone" family; acrolein, furfural, and acetaldehyde are of the "aldehyde" family.

chemical hazard: Exposure to any chemical which, in acute concentrations, has a toxic effect.

chemical name: The name given to a chemical in the nomenclature system developed by the International Union of Pure and Applied Chemistry (IUPAC) or the CAS. The scientific designation of a chemical or a name that will clearly identify the chemical for hazard evaluation process.

chemical pneumonitis: Inflammation of the lungs resulting from inhalation of chemical vapors and characterized by an outpouring of fluid in the lungs.

chemical waste: Chemical waste is either organic (hydrocarbons or substituted hydrocarbons) or inorganic (metallic or nonmetallic elements). The hydrocarbons are composed solely of carbon and hydrogen; substituted hydrocarbons also include functional groups composed of elements such as chlorine, nitrogen, phosphorous, sulfur, or oxygen. Inorganic waste materials are typically in the form of salts, hydrides, and oxides. The hazards associated with organic compounds and the fate of the compounds in the environment depend mainly on their chemical compositions and associated physical properties.

chemicals of potential concern (CoPC): Chemicals that are potentially site-related and whose data are of sufficient quality for use in the quantitative risk assessment.

cholestasis: An acute reaction within the liver where the production and/or secretion of bile is impaired. It is caused by exposure to environmental and occupational agents.

chromatograph: An instrument that can separate and analyze mixtures of chemical substances.

chromosomal aberrations: A change in the normal number, size, or shape of chromosomes.

chromosomes: One of several structures in the nucleus of eukaryotic cells. They contain the genes (or hereditary material) in the form of threads of DNA.

chronic: Applies to persistent, prolonged, repeated exposures and their effects.

chronic daily intake: Intake averaged over a long period of time (seven years to lifetime).

chronic effect: Disease symptom or process of long duration, usually frequent in occurrence, and almost always debilitating.

chronic exposure: Small dose/long time.

chronic mountain sickness: A rare response to prolonged stays at elevation. Its symptoms include those of benign AMS (perhaps also of HACE but not HAPE), but occur only after several years of exposure. This condition is hypothesized to be the cascading result of very high increases in hematocrit. Because the time of response of chronic mountain sickness is so delayed relative to industrial personnel transfers, it is considered herein to be outside the occupational hygienist's realm. (Also known as "Monge's disease.")

chronic reference dose: Applicable for periods of seven years to lifetime.

chronic symptom: Symptom that persists for a long period.

chronic toxicity: Adverse health effects that can occur from prolonged, repeated exposure to relatively low levels of a substance; might have a chronic effect from an acute exposure.

chronic toxicity study: Refers to toxicity study durations of greater than 6 months.

CIH: See *Certified Industrial Hygienist.*

cilia: Tiny hair-like "whips" in the bronchi and other respiratory passages that normally aid in the removal of dust trapped on these moist surfaces.

circadian effects: The routine alterations in physiology related to time of day.

cirrhosis: A condition in which the liver has become hardened and its physiological functions are highly impaired.

class: Collection of related chemical groups or topics.

Class 1: Classification of a laser product's output power and potential hazard during normal use under the Federal Laser Product Performance Standard (See 21 CFR Subchapter J, Part 1040.10). Class 1 lasers cannot emit laser radiation at known hazard levels.

Class 2: Classification of a laser product's output power and potential hazard during normal use under the Federal Laser Product Performance Standard (See *21 CFR Subchapter J, Part 1040.10*). Class 2 lasers are low-powered devices that emit visible radiation above Class 1 levels but do not exceed 1 mW.

Class 2a: Classification of a laser product's output power and potential hazard during normal use under the Federal Laser Product Performance Standard (See *21 CFR Subchapter J, Part 1040.10*). Class 2a is a special designation based on a 1000-second (16.7- minute) exposure and applies only to lasers that are not intended for viewing such as supermarket laser scanners. The emission from a Class 2a laser is defined such that the emission does not exceed the Class 1 limit for an emission duration of 1000 seconds.

Class 3a: Classification of a laser product's output power and potential hazard during normal use under the Federal Laser Product Performance Standard (See *21 CFR Subchapter J, Part 1040.10*). Class 3a lasers have intermediate power levels (CW = 1 to 5 mW). Class 3a emissions may be "low" or "high" irradiance.

Class 3b: Classification of a laser product's output power and potential hazard during normal use under the Federal Laser Product Performance Standard (See *21 CFR Subchapter J, Part 1040.10*). Class 3b includes moderately powerful lasers (e.g., CW = 5 to 500 mW). In general, Class 3b lasers are not a fire hazard, nor are they generally capable of producing a hazardous diffuse reflection except for conditions of staring at distances close to the diffuser.

Class 4: Classification of a laser product's output power and potential hazard during normal use under the Federal Laser Product Performance Standard (See *21 CFR Subchapter J, Part 1040.10*). Class 4 lasers are high-powered devices (e.g., CW >500 mW). These are hazardous to view under any condition (direct or scattered radiation) and are potential fire and skin hazards.

Clean Air Act: The original Clean Air Act was passed in 1963, but the U.S. national air pollution control program is actually based on the 1970 version of the law. The 1990 Clean Air Act Amendments are the most far-reaching revisions of the 1970 law. In this text, the 1990 amendments are referred to as the 1990 Clean Air Act.

clean room: An enclosed space environmentally controlled, within specified limits, of airborne particles, temperature, relative humidity, air pressure, and air motion. (Also known as "white room.")

clean space: An open area environmentally controlled as in a clean room.

clean workstation: An open or enclosed work area environmentally controlled as a clean room.

cleanup level: Remedial target for concentration of contaminant in air, water, or soil.

clinical chemistry: Analytical testing of the blood and other body fluids to determine the functioning of various organs and systems.

cluster: A small group of employees have similar complaints about their health or they may have been diagnosed with similar illnesses, generally sharing something in common (such as the same job, exposure, or area of employment).

CMM: Cutaneous malignant melanoma. See *nonmelanoma skin cancer.*

CNS: See *central nervous system.*

CNS depression: A reversible state of stupor or unconsciousness.

CNS effects: Signs and symptoms include drowsiness, dizziness, loss of coherence, and other signs or symptoms of toxic effects on the central nervous system (CNS).

cochlea: The auditory part of the inner ear that contains the nerve cells that when damaged results in hearing impairment.

cocoon: Remaining in a facility during a hazardous situation with air intake equipment to the building turned off.

Code of Federal Regulations (CFR): A collection of the regulations that have been promulgated under U.S. Law.

Code of Professional Ethics for the Practice of Industrial Hygiene: This code provides standards of ethical conduct to be followed by industrial hygienists as they strive toward the goals of protecting employees' health, improving the work environment, and advancing the quality of the profession.

coefficient of entry: A dimensionless factor that describes how efficient a given hood is at converting static pressure (SP) into velocity pressure (VP).

coefficient of variation (CV): A measure of precision calculated as the standard deviation of a set of values divided by the average. It is usually multiplied by 100 to be expressed as a percentage.

cognition: The conscious faculty or process of knowing, of becoming, or of being aware of thoughts or perceptions, including understanding and reasoning.

cohort study: A longitudinal study that follows groups that are divided by their exposure status to compares the risk for an outcome between the groups.

cold trap: A sampling vessel that has been immersed in a cooling system, such as dry ice or liquid nitrogen, to extract the contaminants from the airstream for subsequent analysis.

collaborative tests: The evaluation of a new analytical method under actual working conditions through the participation of a number of typical or representative laboratories in analyzing portions of carefully prepared homogeneous samples. (Also known as "collaborative studies.")

colonization: The state in which infection and establishment of an organism within a host has occurred without resulting in subclinical or clinical disease.

color density tube: A detector tube that uses color intensity (or density) to determine the amount of compound present.

colorimetric (colorimetry): A measuring method that uses a change in color as an indication of the concentration of a compound.

colorimetric detector tube: See *detector tube.*

colorimetric indicator tube: See *detector tube.*

coma: A state of unconsciousness from which the person cannot be aroused by physical stimulation.

combustible: Capable of catching fire or burning; usually a liquid with a flash point at or above 37.8°C (100°F) but below 93.3°C (200°F).

combustible gas indicator: A general survey instrument capable of measuring a wide range of air contaminants but cannot distinguish among them. They are usually used as area samplers to measure concentrations that are immediately dangerous to life and health, and concentrations that are within occupational exposure limits, in the ppm range. (See also *flame ionization detector, photoionization detector [PID].*)

commissioning: The acceptance process in which an HVAC system's performance is determined, identified, verified, and documented to assure proper operation in accordance with codes, standards, and design intentions.

common exposure base: The unit of 100 full-time workers used to calculate the incident rate. (See also *incident rate.*)

communications plan: The communications plan defines the individuals who must be informed during the evaluation. It is intended to comply with all of the facility security and notification procedures. It includes the team roster that identifies the team members by name and the tasks each is to perform.

comparability: A measure of the confidence with which one data set can be compared to another.

completeness: The amount of valid data obtained from a measurement system compared with the amount that was expected to be obtained under correct normal operations, usually expressed as a percentage.

compliance: Compliance with health and safety regulations.

compliance strategy: One of two general exposure assessment strategies. It usually uses worst-case monitoring with a focus on exposures during the time of the survey. An attempt is made to identify the maximum-exposed worker(s) in a group. One or a few measurements are then taken and simply compared with the occupational exposure limit (OEL). If the exposures of the maximum-exposed workers are sufficiently below the OEL, then the situation is acceptable. This strategy provides little insight into the day-to-day variation in exposures levels and is not amenable to the development of exposure histories that accurately reflect exposures and health risk. (See also *comprehensive strategy.*)

compound: A substance composed of two or more elements joined according to the laws of chemical combination. Each compound has its own characteristic properties different from those of its constituent elements.

compound hood: A hood that has two or more points of significant energy (i.e., static pressure) loss. Examples include slot hoods and multiple opening, lateral draft hoods.

comprehensive exposure assessment: The systematic review of the processes, practices, materials, and division of labor present in a workplace that is used to define and judge all exposures for all workers on all days.

comprehensive strategy: One of two general exposure assessment strategies. It is directed at characterizing and assessing exposure profiles that cover all workers, workdays, and environmental agents. These exposure profiles are used to picture exposures on unmeasured days and for unmeasured workers in the similarly exposed group. In addition to ensuring compliance with OELs, this strategy provides an understanding of the day-to-day distribution of exposures. (See also *compliance strategy.*)

comprehensive survey: A multifaceted examination of all recognized health and safety hazards in a defined work environment. It encompasses a wall-to-wall evaluation of the health and safety factors that may place an employee at increased risk of developing an adverse effect from working in a specific setting.

compressibility: The relative variation of volume with pressure; depends on the process to which a gas is subjected.

computed tomography: A technique in which measurements to create both spatially and temporally resolved concentration distribution maps are generated when a network of intersecting open-path FTIR spectrometers are used in a room.

concentration: 1. The amount of a given substance in a stated unit of measure. Common methods of stating concentration are percent by weight or by volume; weight per unit volume; normality; etc. 2. The quantity of a chemical per unit volume (see ppm, mg/m^3); 10,000 ppm = 1%. In air, the relationship between ppm and mg/m^3 is as follows: ppm × MW = 24.45 × mg/m^3 where ppm = the volume ratio of a chemical in air expressed in parts per million; MW = the chemical's molecular weight; 24.45 = the number of liters occupied by 1 mole of any gas at STP (i.e., 298 K or 25°C [77°F]) and 760 mmHg or 1 atm; mg/m^3 = the chemical's concentration in air expressed in milligrams of chemical per cubic meter of air.

concentration–time (C–T): Two factors on which dosage is based. (See also *dose.*)

concentric: A muscle contraction where the muscle shortens while developing tension.

conceptus: The whole product of conception at any stage of development, from fertilization of the ovum to birth.

condensation: Act or process of reducing from one form to another denser form such as steam to water.

conduction: 1. Transmission of energy by a medium that does not involve movement of the medium itself.
2. Conductive heat transfer when there is direct contact between a hotter and a colder substance.

conductive hearing loss: Any condition that interferes with the transmission of sound to the cochlea.

confidence coefficient: The chance or probability, usually expressed as a percentage, that a confidence interval has of including the population value. The confidence coefficients usually associated with confidence intervals are 90%, 95%, and 99%. For a given sample size, the width of the confidence interval increases as the confidence coefficient increases.

confidence interval: A value interval that has a designated probability (the confidence coefficient) of including some defined parameter of the population.

confidence level: The probability that a stated confidence interval will include a population parameter.

confidence limits: The upper and lower boundaries of a confidence interval.

configuration control: A system for recording the original equipment configuration, physical arrangement, and subsequent changes thereto.

confined space: 1. A space that 1) is large enough and so configured that an employee can bodily enter and perform assigned work; 2) has limited or restricted means for entry or exit (for example, tanks, vessels, silos, storage bins, hoppers, vaults, and pits are spaces that may have limited means of entry); and 3) is not designed for continuous employee occupancy. (See *OSHA 1910.146.*) 2. An enclosure that contains an oxygen deficiency, where the oxygen concentration is less than 19.5%. Examples are underground utility vaults, storage tanks, and large diameter pipes.

congener: Compound with related but not identical structure.

conjugate: The product of reaction of an exposing single chemical or a single metabolite with the endogenous biochemical pathways of the body.

conjunctiva: The delicate membrane that lines the eyelids and covers the exposed surface of the eyeballs.

conjunctivitis: Inflammation of the membrane (conjunctiva) that lines the eyelids and covers the front of the eyeball.

consensus standard: Any generally accepted standard of environmental quality established through input from a number of experts and professional groups knowledgeable about matters pertaining to the subject of the standard.

Conservation of Energy law: Energy can neither be created nor destroyed, and therefore the total amount of energy in the universe is constant.

conservation of mass: In all ordinary chemical changes, the total mass of the reactants is always equal to the total mass of the products.

constant flow: A feature available on air sampling pumps whereby the flow rate will automatically compensate for flow restrictions, thereby ensuring that the flow rate is held constant throughout the sampling period.

constant volume pump: A sampling pump designed to draw a fixed volume of air with each full pump stroke. Examples are the simple squeeze bulb, the bellows pump, and the piston pump.

constrained-layer damping: The use of a laminated construction consisting of one or more sheet metal layers, each separated by and bonded to a viscoelastic layer.

contact dermatitis: An acute or chronic inflammation of the skin resulting from irritation by or sensitizing to some substance coming in contact with the skin.

contact rate: Amount of medium (e.g., water, soil) contacted per unit of time or event.

continuity equation: An equation obeyed by any conserved, indestructible quantity such as mass, electric charge, thermal energy, electrical energy, or quantum-mechanical probability, which is essentially a statement that the rate of increase of the quantity in any region equals the total current flowing into the region.

continuous exposure guidance level (CEGL): Established by the Committee on Toxicology of the National Research Council (NRC) for the U.S. Department of Defense. CEGLs are intended for normal, long-lasting military operations. CEGLs are ceiling concentrations designed to avoid adverse health effects, either immediate or delayed, for exposure periods up to 90 days. (See also *EEGL, SPEGL.*)

continuous flow respirator: An atmosphere-supplying respirator that provides a continuous flow of respirable gas to the respiratory inlet covering.

continuous improvement: See *kaizen.*

continuous operation: Industrial operation in which the final product is produced at or near a continuous rate.

continuous wave (CW): A laser that operates continuously.

control: One of four primary responsibilities of the occupational hygienist. It is the culmination of the effort in addressing the primary objective of the occupational hygienist: providing a healthful work environment. Current occupational hygiene practice recognizes a hierarchy of controls; in priority order, these are engineering controls, work practices, administrative controls, and as a last resort use of personal protective equipment. (See also *anticipation, recognition, and evaluation.*)

control chart: A graphical chart with statistical control limits and plotted values (usually in chronological order) of some measured parameter for a series of samples. Use of the charts provide a visual display of the pattern of the data, enabling the early detection of time trends and shifts in level. For maximum usefulness in control, such charts should be plotted in a timely manner (that is, as soon as the data are available). (Also known as "Shewhart control chart," "statistical control chart.")

control measures: The overall strategy for controlling the environment as well as the specific components that make up that strategy. These include local exhaust and general ventilation, process isolation or enclosure, shielding from heat, ionizing radiation, ultraviolet light, or any other forms of radiant energy, protective clothing, and respiratory protective devices, and other controls.

control velocity: See *capture velocity.*

convection: 1. The transfer of heat by the flow of some liquid or gas. 2. Motion resulting in a fluid from the difference in density and the action of gravity; heat loss or gain by the body to the surrounding atmosphere.

conversion: 1. The process of changing information from one form of representation to another, such as from the language of one type of machine to that of another, or from magnetic tape to the printed page. 2. The process of changing from one data processing method to another, or from one type of equipment to another. 3. To change from use of one fuel to another.

convulsions: An abnormal, and often violent, involuntary contraction or series of contractions of the muscles.

cooling probe: A probe used in high temperature applications to cool the sample before entry into the detector tube. It sometimes is called a "hot air probe."

CoPC: See chemicals of potential concern.

cornea: The transparent structure that forms the exposed surface of the eyeball and allows light to enter the eye.

corneal opacity: A density, spot, or opaque shadow in the cornea.

corrected effective temperature (CET): Amendment to the ET scale that includes allowances for radiation. This scale uses the globe temperature instead of the dry bulb temperature.

corrective action (CA): 1. The act of varying the manipulated process variable by the controlling means in order to modify overall process operating conditions. 2. CA should consist of identifying the problem; designation of a person or persons to correct the problem; identifying appropriate corrective actions; instituting the corrective action; evaluating the correction to determine if the CA did, in fact, correct the problem; and, finally, placing the previously nonconforming system back on-line.

corrosive: 1. A chemical that causes visible destruction of, or irreversible alterations in, living tissue by chemical action at the site of contact. 2. A chemical that causes necrosis of biological tissues.

corrosive waste: Materials that can induce severe irritation and destruction of human tissue on contact due to accelerated dehydration reactions.

cosine law: The law that the energy emitted by a radiating surface in any direction is proportional to the cosine of the angle which that direction makes with the normal.

coughing: To expel air from the lungs suddenly with a harsh noise, often involuntarily.

counter-control: When individuality or perceived personal control is made scarce with top-down control, some people will exert contrary behavior in an attempt to assert their freedom. (Also known as "psychological reactance.")

CPS: cycles per second. See *hertz.*

crepitus: Crackling or grating noise or sensation sometimes made by a joint.

criteria: Standard on which a judgment or decision may be based.

criteria document: Publication of NIOSH-related research on which standards can be based. Documents contain essential parts of a standard, including environmental limits, sampling requirements, labeling, monitoring requirements, medical examinations, compliance methods, protective equipment, record keeping requirements, and other recommendations to OSHA for establishment of a standard.

Criteria for Fatigue Decreased Proficiency (FDP): Boundaries that represent the ability of a person to work at tasks under vibration exposure without the vibration interfering with the worker's ability to perform.

critical temperature: Saturation temperature corresponding to the critical state of the substance at which the properties of the liquid and vapor are identical; the temperature above which a gas cannot be liquefied by pressure alone.

CRM: See *Certified Reference Material.*

cross-sectional study: A study that examines the relationship between diseases (or other health-related characteristics) and other variables of interest as they exist in a defined population at one particular time.

cross-sensitivity: The tendency of detector tubes to respond to more than one compound.

C–T: See *concentration–time.*

CTD: Cumulative trauma disorder. See *repetitive strain injury.*

CTS: See *carpal tunnel syndrome.*

cubic meter: See *m^3.*

cumulative dose: Total dose resulting from repeated exposures.

cumulative trauma disorder (CTD): See *repetitive strain injury.*

current density: The basic exposure limit at the lowest radio frequencies (less than 100 kHz).

customer: Anyone who may be affected by the information developed though sampling or other analysis of the work environment. Customers may be internal or external (e.g., regulatory agencies, employees, purchasers of services/products, and company management).

cutaneous: Pertaining to the skin.

cutaneous malignant melanoma (CMM): See *nonmelanoma skin cancer.*

cutoff particle diameter: Diameter of a particle that has 50% probability of being removed by the device or stage and 50% probability of being passed through. Also known as "50% cutpoint," "d_{50}," or the "effective cutoff diameter." (See also *aerodynamic diameter, mass median aerodynamic diameter.*)

50% cutpoint size (d_{50}): The parameter used to characterize impactor performance. It is the particle size captured by the impactor with 50% efficiency.

CV: See *coefficient of variation.*

CVS: Cardiovascular system; the heart and blood vessels.

CW: See *continuous wave.*

C-weighted response: The simulation of the sensitivity of the human ear at high sound levels.

cyanosis: Blue appearance of the skin, especially on the face and extremities, indicating a lack of sufficient oxygen in the arterial blood.

cycle time: The time required to carry out a cycle; used principally for time and motion studies.

cycles per second (CPS): See *hertz.*

D

d: See *density correction factor.*

d50: See *50% cutpoint size.*

Dalton's law: Also known as Dalton's Law of Partial Pressure. According to this law, at constant temperature the total pressure exerted by a mixture of gases in a definite volume is equal to the sum of the individual pressures that each gas would exert if occupying the same total volume above. Each constituent of a mixture of gases behaves thermodynamically as if it alone occupied the space. The sum of the individual pressures of the constituents equals the total pressure of the mixture.

damage risk criterion: The suggested baseline of noise tolerance. A damage risk criterion may include in its statement a specification of such factors as time of exposure; noise level and frequency; amount of hearing loss that is considered significant; percentage of the population to be protected; and method of measuring the noise.

damaging wrist motion: 1. A bent wrist involving a force. 2. 1000 damaging wrist motions per hour is an upper ergonomic limit. Also, all pinch grips requiring more than eight pounds of pressure are considered dangerous.

damper, blast gate: A sliding damper used in an air-handling system.

data validation: A systematic effort to review data to identify any outliers or errors and thereby cause deletion or flagging of suspect values to ensure the validity of the data for the user. This "screening" process may be done by manual and/or computer methods, and may use any consistent technique such as pollutant concentration limits or parameter relationships to screen out impossible or unlikely values.

dB: See *decibel.*

DC: See *duty cycle.*

de minimis risk: A risk that is so low as to be negligible (i.e., one case of disease per million persons exposed).

deQuervain's disease: A repetitive strain injury (RSI) characterized by inflammation of the tendons and their sheaths that often causes pain at the base of the thumb and the inside of the wrist. (Also known as "deQuervain's syndrome.")

decibel (dB): A dimensionless unit used to express a logarithmic ratio between a measured quantity and a preference quantity. It is commonly used to describe the levels of acoustic intensity, acoustic power sound pressure levels, and hearing threshold when a reference quantity is specified.

decision tree: A flow chart designed to assist detector tube users in determining sampling strategies and interpreting results.

decomposition: Breakdown of a material or substance (by heat, chemical reaction, electrolysis, decay, or other process) into parts, elements, or simpler compounds.

decompression sickness: A condition marked by the presence of nitrogen bubbles in the blood and other body tissues resulting from a sudden fall in atmospheric pressure. (Also known as "decompression illness," "evolved gas dysbarism," "compressed air sickness," "caisson worker's syndrome," "aeroembolism," and "air embolism.")

decontamination: Removal of harmful substances such as noxious chemicals, harmful bacteria or other organisms, or radioactive material from exposed individuals, rooms, and furnishings in buildings, or the exterior environment.

defatting: The removal of fat or oils; defatting the skin results in dryness, flakiness, and a whitish appearance.

default value: Standard numbers used in exposure assessment when more specific data is not available (e.g., body weight, media intake).

degradation: A deleterious change in one or more physical properties of a protective material caused by contact with a chemical.

delayed hypersensitivity: Occurs as a result of an allergy to one or more specific substances (antigens) through type IV cell-mediated immunity. (Also known as "allergic contact dermatitis.")

***Delphi Technique:** The Delphi Technique was developed by the RAND Corporation in the late 1960s as a forecasting methodology. Later, the U.S. government enhanced it as a group decision-making tool with the results of Project HINDSIGHT, which established a factual basis for the workability of Delphi. That project produced a tool in which a group of experts could come to some consensus of opinion when the decisive factors were subjective, and not knowledge-based.

demand respirator: An atmosphere-supplying respirator that admits respirable gas to the facepiece only when a negative pressure is created inside the facepiece by inhalation.

demyelination: Destruction of myelin; loss of myelin from nerve sheaths or nerve tracts.

density: 1. The mass (weight) per unit volume of a substance. For example, lead is much more dense than aluminum. The density of a material (solid, liquid, gas, or vapor) is given by the relationship between the mass of the material and the volume the mass occupies. 2. The ratio of mass to volume of a material, usually expressed in grams (g) per cubic centimeter (cc). At 4°C (39.2°F), 1 cc of water weighs 1 g.

density correction factor (d): A factor to correct or convert air density at any temperature and pressure to equivalent conditions at ACGIH ventilation-defined standard conditions (STP) and vice versa. For example: Actual air density = (0.075 lb/ft^3) × d, where d = 530/460 + T * BP/29.92 in.-Hg. [Note: T = degrees Fahrenheit; BP = pressure in in.-Hg.]

deoxyribonucleic acid (DNA): The molecules in chromosomes that contain genetic information in most organisms.

depressant: A substance that diminishes bodily functions, activity, or instinctive desire.

derivitization: The process of trapping an airborne chemical onto a sorbent material or filter that has been pretreated with a chemical reagent, thereby causing a chemical reaction that produces a stable compound for analysis.

dermal: Pertaining to the skin.

dermal absorption: The transfer of contaminant across the skin and subsequent incorporation into the body.

dermal exposure: Contact between a chemical and the skin.

dermatitis: Inflammation of the skin from any cause. There are two general types of skin reaction: primary irritation dermatitis and sensitization dermatitis.

desiccant: Material that absorbs moisture.

desiccate: Dry intensively.

desorption: Removal of a substance from the surface at which it is absorbed.

desorption efficiency: A measure of how much of a specific analyte can be recovered from a sorbent; typically expressed as a percent of analyte spiked onto the sorbent.

detector tube: A hermetically sealed glass tube containing an inert solid or granular material such as silica gel, alumina, pumice, or ground glass. The most widely used direct-reading devices. (Also known as "colorimetric detector tube," "colorimetric indicator tube," or "length-of-stain tube.")

detector tube system: A measuring device that consists of a pump and a detector tube. Accessories such as stroke counters, hoses, and probes also might be included. The exception to this is a passive dosimeter, which does not use a pump.

determinant: The substrate or indicator to be measured in a biological system.

detonable: Capable of detonation.

developmental reference dose: Likely to be without appreciable risk of developmental effects, applicable to a single exposure event.

developmental toxicity: A harmful effect on the embryo or fetus; embryotoxicity, fetotoxicity, or teratogenicity.

dew point temperature (T_{dp}): 1. The temperature and pressure at which a gas begins to condense to a liquid. 2. The temperature at which air becomes saturated when cooled without addition of moisture or change of pressure; any further cooling causes condensation.

differential diagnosis: The assessment of a patient, including the skin condition as it first appears, what it looks like and what symptoms were initially associated with it, how the skin disease may have changed, and what is being done to treat the condition.

diffuse reflection: A reflection of light, sound, or radio waves from a surface in all directions according to the cosine law.

diffusion: Aerosol particles in a gaseous medium are bombarded by collisions with individual gas molecules that are in Brownian motion. This causes the particles to undergo random displacements known as diffusion. The particle parameter that describes this process is the particle diffusivity (or diffusion coefficient), D_B.

diffusion system: A flow-metering system based on diffusion through a defined space.

diffusive sampling: Passive samplers that rely on the movement of contaminant molecules across a concentration gradient that for steady-state conditions can be defined by Fick's first law of diffusion.

dilution ventilation: A form of exposure control that relies on the dilution of airborne contaminants into workplace air.

dimensional analysis: Dimensional analysis is a technique to manipulate units as numbers.

dimensions of risk: Attributes of risk that affect perception of that risk (e.g., familiarity or voluntariness of exposure).

direct-reading instruments: A tool available to occupational hygienists for detecting and quantifying gases, vapors, and aerosols. (Also known as "real-time monitors.")

disaster: A calamitous event, especially one occurring suddenly and causing great damage or hardship.

disease cluster: An apparent increase in specific outcomes (disease) among individuals linked in time or space (cluster) or by exposure characteristics.

disinfection: The killing of infectious agents (except bacterial spores) below the level necessary to cause infection.

Sanitizers are used on inanimate surfaces; antiseptics are used on skin.

dispersion model: A mathematical model to calculate the dispersion or spread of a pollutant from a source.

displacement: 1. The linear distance from the initial to the final position of an object moved from one place to another, regardless of length of path followed. 2. The distance of an oscillating particle from its equilibrium position.

disposal: Final placement or destruction of toxic, radioactive, or other wastes; surplus or banned pesticides or other chemicals; polluted soils; and drums containing hazardous materials from removal actions or accidental releases. Disposal may be accomplished through use of approved secure landfills, surface impoundments, land farming, deep-well injection, ocean dumping, or incineration.

dissipative muffler: A device that absorbs sound energy as the gas passes through it; a duct lined with sound-absorbing material is the most common type.

distress: Acute physical or mental suffering.

distribution: Once a chemical has entered the body, it might need to be transported to other sites to induce toxic effects.

divergence: Laser beam spread.

DMF: Abbreviation of dimethylformamide.

DMSO: Abbreviation of dimethylsulfoxide.

DNA: See *deoxyribonucleic acid*.

document control: A systematic procedure for indexing the original document (i.e., Revision No. 0) and subsequent revisions (i.e., Revision No. 1, 2, 3...) by number and date of revision.

dominant-lethal study: A mutagenicity study designed to detect an increase in the incidence of embryo lethality related to exposure of a parent to a test agent.

dosage: Mass of substance per mass of body weight (e.g., mg/kg, where mg represents the amount of substance administered and kg is the body weight of the test animal).

dose: A term used interchangeably with dosage to express the amount of energy or substance absorbed in a unit volume of an organ or individual. dose adjustment: Modification of doses used in animal experimentation to equivalent levels for human beings. The usual method is to calculate the ratio of body weights raised to some power, which is roughly equivalent to the ratio of surface areas; a simple ratio of body weights has also been used.

dose rate: The dose delivered per unit of time. Concentration of a contaminant multiplied by the duration of human exposure ($D = C \times T$).dose response: In general, the relationship between dose and biological change in organisms; the relationship between administered dose or exposure and the biological change in organisms.

dose-effect study: Laboratory experiment in which animals are given varying doses of known or potentially harmful substances over varying periods of time, and the physical effects are measured in order to set exposure limits for these substances in the occupational environment.

dose-response assessment: See *toxicity assessment*.

dose-response curve: 1. Graphic representation relating biologic response to concentration of contaminant and time of exposure. By multiplying these factors, dose is determined. 2. A mathematical relationship between the dose administered or received and the incidence of adverse health effects in the exposed population; toxicity values are derived from this relationship.

dose-response relationship: With increasing dose, greater biological effects (i.e., responses) will be elicited; that is to say a dose-response relationship can be demonstrated.

dosimeter: 1. Instrument used to detect and measure an accumulated dose of radiation. It is usually a pencil-sized chamber with a built-in self-reading meter, used for personnel monitoring. 2. An instrument that measures the accumulated energy to which one might be exposed (i.e., noise, radiation, etc.). (Also known as "dose meter.")

dosimetry: Accurate measurement of doses.

draft: A current of air, when referring to: 1. The pressure difference that causes a current of air or gases to flow through a flue, chimney, heater, or space. 2. A localized effect caused by one or more factors of high air velocity, low ambient temperature, or direction of airflow, whereby more heat is withdrawn from a person's skin than is normally dissipated.

draft coefficient: A coefficient expressing the resistance encountered by a body when moving in a fluid.

Draize Test: Animal testing to assess the potential irritation or corrosion of a material to skin or eyes.

drug: 1. Any substance used internally or externally as a medicine for the treatment, cure, or prevention of disease. 2. A narcotic preparation.

dry bulb temperature (T_{db}): Temperature of air as determined by a standard thermometer. Temperature units are expressed in degrees Celsius (°C), Kelvin (K) (K = Celsius + 273), or degrees Fahrenheit (°F) (F = 9/5 Celsius + 32).

duct: 1. A passageway for conveying gases. 2. A passageway made of sheet metal or other suitable material, not necessarily leak-tight, used for conveying air or other gas at low pressures. 3. The component of the local exhaust ventilation system that carries contaminants from the hood, through the ventilation system, out of the workroom, through an air-cleaning device, and into the ambient environment.

duct distribution: Distribution of air into a room or a building by ductwork.

duct sizing, equal-friction method: A method of calculating duct size so that frictional resistance per unit length is constant.

duct sizing, static-regain method: A method of calculating duct size so that the regain in static pressure between two draw-off points equals the frictional resistance between the points.

duct sizing, velocity-reduction method: A method of calculating duct size so that selected velocities occur in specific duct lengths.

duct system: A series of ducts, elbows, and connectors to convey air or other gases from one location to another.

duct transition section: A section of duct, breeching, or stack used to connect these elements with structures of different cross-sectional dimensions.

duct velocity: Air velocity through the duct cross section. When solid material is present in the airstream, the duct velocity must be equal to the minimum design duct velocity or transport velocity.

duplicate sample: A sample collected in the same location and manner as an actual sample and used to evaluate the entire sampling/analysis method.

dust: 1. Solid particles that are capable of temporary suspension in air or other gases. Usually produced from larger masses through the application of physical forces (for example, handling, crushing, grinding, rapid impact). Typical dusts are rock, ore, metal, coal, wood, and grain. Size ranges are usually between 0.1 µm and 30.0 µm. Particles may be up to 300–400 µm, but those above 20–30 µm usually do not remain airborne. 2. Air suspension (aerosol) of solid particles, usually particle size less than 100 µm. 3. Fine, solid particles; small dust particles may be respirable (less than 10 µm).

duty cycle (DC): The ratio of on-time RF emissions to the total time of operation (on-time plus off-time).

duty cycling (electric): The process of turning off electrical equipment for predetermined periods during operating hours to reduce consumption and demand.

duty factor: See *duty cycle*.

dying back: The condition in which prolonged or repeated exposure to toxics can cause the neural axon to continue to degenerate from the distal to the proximal end.

dynamic blank: A blank that is prepared, handled, and analyzed in the same manner as normal carrying agents except that it is not exposed to the material to be selectively captured. For example, an absorbing solution that would be placed in bubbler tube, stoppered, transported to a monitoring site, left at the site for the normal period of sampling, returned to the laboratory, and analyzed. (Also known as "field blank.")

dynamic calibration: Calibration of a measurement system by use of calibration material having characteristics similar to the unknown material to be measured. For example, the use of a gas containing carbon dioxide of known concentrations in an air mixture could be used to calibrate a carbon dioxide sensor system.

dynamic load: Muscle (local) fatigue is divided into static and dynamic. When muscles are loaded but do not move, it is a static load; when loaded muscles move, it is dynamic.

Dynamic System: A calibration system in which the standard gas solution is generated continually and is flowing.

dyne: The centimeter-gram-second unit of force, equal to the force required to impart an acceleration of 1 centimeter per second (cm/sec) to a mass of 1 gram. An arcane term.

dysbaric osteonecrosis: Causes detectable lesions most commonly on the body's long bones. Although its etiology is unknown, this chronic disease might be related to the evolution of gas bubbles that may or may not be diagnosed as decompression sickness.

dysbarism: A condition of the body resulting from the existence of a pressure differential between the total ambient pressure and the total pressure of dissolved and free gases within the body tissues, fluids, and cavities.

dyspnea: Labored or difficult breathing; a symptom.

E

E: See *electric-field strength.*

EAP: See *emergency action plan.*

ear: The entire hearing apparatus, consisting of three parts: the external ear, the middle ear, and the inner ear.

ear protectors: Plugs or muffs designed to keep noise from the ear to preserve hearing acuity.

ear wax: The waxy discharge in the outer ear canal.

earmuff: A type of hearing protector worn outside the ear.

eaters: Organic compounds that may be made by interaction between an alcohol and an acid, and by other means, and includes solvents and natural fats.

eccentric: A muscle contraction where the muscle lengthens while developing tension.

ECD: See *electron capture detector.*

EC_X: See *effective concentration "X."*

eczema: A disease of the skin characterized by inflammation, itching, and the formation of scales.

edema: An excessive accumulation of fluid in the cells, tissue spaces, or body cavities due to a disturbance in the fluid exchange mechanism.

E_{eff}: See *effective irradiance.*

EEGL: See *emergency exposure guidance level.*

effective concentration "X" (EC_X): The concentration of a material that has caused a biological effect to X percent of the test animals.

effective irradiance: 1. Measured values of irradiance weighted by a response (action) spectrum, in this case the relative spectral effectiveness normalized to the most biologically effective wavelength (for eye effects), 270 nm. 2. Ultraviolet irradiance weighted (adjusted) for biological efficacy (relative spectral effectiveness).

effective temperature (ET): The sensation of warmth or cold felt by the human body.

EHS: See *extremely hazardous substance.*

EL: See *explosive limits.*

electric field: 1. One of the fundamental fields in nature, causing a charged body to be attracted to or repelled by other charged bodies. Associated with an electromagnetic wave or a changing magnetic field. 2. Specifically, the electric force per unit test charge.

electric-field strength (E): The force on a stationary positive charge per unit charge at a point in an electric field. (Also known as "electric vector," "electric field intensity.")

electrochemical detector: Responds to compounds (such as phenols, aromatic amines, ketones, aldehydes, and mercaptans) that can be readily oxidized or reduced. Electrode systems use working and reference electrodes to quantify analytes over a range of six orders of magnitude.

electrochemical sensors: Sensors used by a variety of instruments dedicated to monitoring specific single gas and vapor contaminants. Electrochemical sensors are available for up to 50 different individual gases, including oxygen, carbon monoxide, nitric oxide, nitrogen dioxide, hydrogen sulfide, hydrogen cyanide, and sulfur dioxide.

electrogoniometer: A device that measures joint angles. An electrogoniometer is a potentiometer that is placed at the joint center and two extensions that are attached to the limbs that intersect at the joint. The electrogoniometer is generally interfaced to a computer via an analog-to-digital converter and may be sampled at a very high rate. These devices can be designed to measure rotations about one, two, or three axes at a joint.

electrolyte: A chemical compound that when molten or dissolved in certain solvents, usually water, will conduct an electric current.

electromagnetic radiation: The propagation, or transfer, of energy through space and matter by time-varying electric and magnetic fields.

electromagnetic spectrum: The total range of wavelengths or frequencies of electromagnetic radiation, extending from the longest radio waves to the shortest known cosmic rays. Any location on the spectrum may be characterized by wavelength, frequency, and photon energy.

electromagnetic susceptibility: A problem experienced with sampling equipment due to electromagnetic fields in the environment that might result in errors or malfunctions in operation.

electromyogram (EMG): The detected electrical signal of a muscle contraction.

electromyograph: An instrument that converts the electrical activity of muscles into visual records or sound. electromyography: The study of the electrical signal associated with a muscle contraction. Electromyography is used to diagnose carpal tunnel syndrome and other repetitive strain injuries.

electron: A subatomic particle that carries a negative charge.

electron capture detector (ECD): Extremely sensitive gas chromatography detector that is a modification of the argon ionization detector, with conditions adjusted to favor the formation of negative ions.

electron equilibrium: A point or area in a radiation detector in which the number of electrons entering equals the number of electrons leaving the local point volume.

electronic mail (e-mail): The transmission of messages over communications networks. The messages can be notes entered from the keyboard or electronic files stored on disk. Most mainframes, minicomputers, and computer networks have an e-mail system. Some electronic-mail systems are confined to a single computer system or network, but others have gateways to other computer systems, enabling users to send electronic mail anywhere in the world.

element: Solid, liquid, or gaseous matter that cannot be further decomposed into simpler substances by chemical means.

ELF: See *extremely low frequency*.

elimination: Internal clearance of a marker from an internal organ.

Ellenbog, Ulrich: An Austrian physician who in 1473 described the symptoms of poisoning from lead and mercury and suggested preventive measures.

elutriator: A device used to separate respirable and nonrespirable particulates such as the cyclone or horizontal types.

e-mail: See *electronic mail*.

embryo: The early or developing stage of any organism. In animals, the period of development beginning when the long axis is established and continuing until all major structures are represented.

embryogenesis: During early human development, several cellular phases occur during a process known as embryogenesis. The phases include cell proliferation, cell differentiation, cell migration, and organogenesis.

embryotoxin: A material harmful to the developing embryo.

emergency: 1. A sudden, urgent, usually unforeseen occurrence or occasion requiring immediate action. 2. Any occurrence (including any failure of hazard control or monitoring equipment) or event internal or external to the permit space that could endanger entrants. (See *OSHA 1910.146*.)

emergency action plan (EAP): The basis for identifying and assessing the risks associated with potential emergencies, planning for appropriate response and recovery, and training those who would be involved or affected should the emergency occur. Facilities that depend solely on the local community fire, police, and emergency medical services to handle an emergency without including them in emergency response planning might later find an increase in injuries, deaths, and economic losses while time is lost struggling to determine the proper course of action. An EAP provides knowledge to everyone affected so that they may react and respond quickly and safely.

emergency exposure guidance level (EEGL): Established by the Committee on Toxicology of the National Research Council (NRC) for the U.S. Department of Defense. EEGLs provide guidelines for military personnel operating under emergency conditions in which circumstances are peculiar to military operations. The EEGL is a ceiling guidance level for single emergency exposures usually lasting 1 hour to 24 hours — an occurrence expected to be infrequent in the lifetime of an individual. (See also *CEGL, SPEGL.*)

emergency planning: Planning for an unintended event.

emergency response: Responding to an unintended event.

Emergency Response Planning Guideline 1 (ERPG–1): The maximum airborne concentration below which nearly all individuals could be exposed for up to 1 hour without experiencing more than mild, transient adverse health effects or without perceiving a clearly defined objectionable odor.

Emergency Response Planning Guideline 2 (ERPG–2): The maximum airborne concentration below which nearly all individuals could be exposed for up to 1 hour without experiencing or developing irreversible or other serious health effects or symptoms that could impair an individual's ability to take protective action.

Emergency Response Planning Guideline 3 (ERPG–3): The maximum airborne concentration below which nearly all individuals could be exposed for up to 1 hour without experiencing or developing life-threatening health effects.

Emergency Response Planning Guidelines (ERPGs): Values intended to provide estimates of concentration ranges above which one could reasonably anticipate observing adverse health effects (see *ERPG–1; ERPG–2; ERPG–3*). The term also refers to the documentation that summarizes the basis for those values. The documentation is contained in a series of guides produced by the Emergency Response Planning Committee of AIHA.

EMF: Acronym for "electric magnetic fields" or "electromagnetic fields."

EMG: See *electromyogram.*

emission: 1. Material released into the air either by a primary source or a secondary source, as a result of a photochemical reaction or chain of reactions. 2. Any radiation of energy by means of electromagnetic waves, as from a radio transmitter. 3. A discharge of fluid from a living body.

emphysema: A lung disease resulting from the enlargements of the alveoli accompanied by destruction of normal tissue.

employee: A worker who might be exposed to hazardous chemicals under normal operating conditions or in foreseeable emergencies. Workers such as office workers or bank tellers who encounter hazardous chemicals only in unusual isolated instances are not covered.

encephalopathy: 1. Any disease of the brain. 2. Acute toxic encephalopathy is characterized by headaches, irritability, poor coordination, seizures, coma, and death. Causative agents include carbon monoxide, organic solvents such as carbon disulfide, and metals (including lead and manganese). 3. Chronic toxic encephalopathy is characterized by a gradual loss of memory and psychomotor control, dementia, and motor disorder. Associated toxicants include arsenic, lead, manganese, and mercury.

enclosing hood: A hood that either completely or partially encloses the contaminant emission source.

end-exhaled breath: The exhaled breath forced from the lungs after natural exhalation. (Also known as "alveolar exhaled breath.")

endogenous: Intrinsic; found naturally in the living system under study.

endotherm: Absorption of heat.

endotoxin: 1. A toxin that is produced within a microorganism and can be isolated only after the cell is disintegrated. 2. A lipopolysaccharide that forms the outer cell wall of gram-negative bacteria.

energy: 1. The capacity to do work. 2. Having several forms that may be transformed from one to another, such as thermal (heat), mechanical (work), electrical, and chemical.

engineered nanoparticle: intentionally produced; designed with very specific properties or compositions (e.g., shape, size, surface properties, and chemistry).

engineering controls: Process change, substitution, isolation, ventilation, source modification.

engineering solution: The use of machines to reduce work-related stress.

entry: The action by which a person passes through an opening into a permit-required confined space. Entry includes ensuing work activities in that space and is considered to have occurred as soon as any part of the entrant's body breaks the plane of an opening into the space. (See *OSHA 1910.146.*)

entry loss: Loss in pressure caused by a fluid stream flowing into a pipe, duct hood, or vessel.

entry personnel: Any individuals directly involved in a confined space entry. This may include the entrant, attendant, and entry supervisor. The designated attendant does not actually enter the space. (Also known as "entry crew.")

entry supervisor: The person (such as the employer, foreman, or crew chief) responsible for determining whether acceptable entry conditions are present at a permit space where entry is planned, for authorizing entry and overseeing entry operations, and for terminating entry as required by this section. (See *OSHA 1910.146.*)

environmental conditions: Natural or controlled conditions of air and radiation prevailing around a person, an object, a substance, etc.

environmental monitoring: Program in which samples of air contaminants or energy measurements are taken and which establishes the level of worker exposure to such agents.

environmental quality: Any standard specifying lower limits for contaminants, chemical or physical agents, and/or resulting stresses to the human body in order to maintain a particular, healthful, and safe environment in which to work.

enzyme: An agent that catalyzes a biological reaction that is not itself consumed in the reaction.

EPA's Risk Management Program: Requires community exposure risk assessments and hazard communication, specifying the process and required outcomes.

epicondylitis: A repetitive strain injury (RSI) characterized by swelling and pain in the tendons and muscles around the elbow joint. (Also known as "tennis elbow.")

epidemiological surveillance: An ongoing systematic analysis and interpretation of the distribution and trends of illness, injury, and/or mortality in a defined population, relative to one or more indicators of workplace hazards or risks. (Also known as "rate-based surveillance.")

epidemiology: The science that deals with the incidence distribution and control of disease in a population.

equation of state: An equation that relates pressure (P), volume (V), and thermodynamic temperature (T), with an amount of a substance (n). The simplest form is the Ideal Gas law: $PV = nRT$.

equilibrium: Condition in which a particle or all the constituent particles of a body are at rest or in unaccelerated motion in an inertial reference frame. (Also known as "static equilibrium.")

equivalent chill temperature: The expression of wind-chill reflecting the cooling power of wind on exposed flesh.

equivalent length: The resistance of an appurtenance in a conduit through which the fluid flows; expressed as the number of feet of straight conduit of the same diameter that would have the same resistance.

ergonomics: The application of human biological sciences with engineering sciences to achieve optimum mutual adjustment of people and their work, the benefits measured in terms of human efficiency and well-being. (Also known as "human factors engineering.")

ERPGs: See *Emergency Response Planning Guidelines.*

error: The difference between an observed or measured value and the best obtainable estimate of its true value.

erythema: Redness of the skin.

escape: The act of entrants exiting the space by their movement during an emergency condition.

eschar: A dry scab that forms as a result of a burn or other corrosive action.

estimated risk: Prediction of risk level.

ET: See *effective temperature.*

etiology: The study or knowledge of the causes of disease.

evaluation: One of four primary responsibilities of the occupational hygienist. The examination and judgment of the amount, degree, significance, worth, or condition of something. Evaluation perhaps uses more "art" in its implementation and than any of the other occupational hygiene responsibilities. (See also *anticipation, recognition, and control.*)

evaporation rate: 1. The ratio of the time required to evaporate a measured volume of a liquid to the time required to evaporate the same volume of a reference liquid under ideal test conditions. The higher the ratio, the slower the evaporation rate. 2. The rate at which a material is converted from the liquid or solid state to the vapor state; may be expressed relative to the evaporation rate of a known material, usually n-Butyl acetate (with an evaporation rate of 1.0 by definition). Faster evaporation rates are >1, and slower evaporation rates are <1.

excretion: Appearance of a marker outside the body.

excursion: Deviation from a definite path. A movement above or below a norm.

excursion factor: Maximum extent to which an ACGIH threshold limit value (TLV®) can be exceeded.

exfoliation: Peeling or flaking of skin.

exhaust air: Air discharged from any conditioned space.

exotherm: Liberation of (reaction) heat.

expiration date: The date beyond which the manufacturer will no longer assure the stability and reliability of the tube.

explosive: A chemical that causes a sudden, almost instantaneous release of pressure, gas, and heat when subjected to sudden shock, pressure, or high temperature.

explosive limits: See *flammable limits.*

exposure: 1. As it pertains to air contaminants, it is the state of being exposed to a concentration of a contaminant. 2. Subjection of an employee in the course of employment to a chemical that is a physical or health hazard, and includes potential (e.g., accidental or possible) exposure. "Subjected" in terms of health hazards includes any route of entry (e.g., inhalation, ingestion, skin contact, or absorption). 3. Contact of an organism with a chemical or physical agent, quantified as the amount of chemical available at the exchange boundaries of the organism and available for absorption. Usually calculated as the mean exposure and some measure of maximum exposure. 4. The amount of an environmental agent that has reached the individual (external dose) or has been absorbed into the individual (internal dose or absorbed dose).

exposure assessment: Determination or estimation (qualitative or quantitative) of the magnitude, frequency, duration, and route of exposure.

exposure event: An incident of contact with a chemical or physical agent. It can be defined by time or incident.

exposure limit: A limit established to prevent an adverse health effect.

exposure limit value: General term designating any standard or measurement restricting human exposure to harmful or toxic agents.

exposure modeling: A mathematical model used to compute a worker's exposure.

exposure pathway: Path a chemical or physical agent takes from source to exposed organism. Consists of 1) source or release; 2) transport medium (possible); 3) exposure point; and 4) exposure route.

exposure point: Location of potential contact between an organism and a chemical or physical agent.

exposure profile: Graphic presentation of data on exposure of workers to contaminants in industry.

exposure rating: An estimate of exposure level relative to the occupational exposure limit (OEL).

exposure route: The way an organism comes into contact with a chemical or physical agent (e.g., ingestion, inhalation, dermal contact, etc.).

exposure surveillance: The systematic and ongoing characterization of chemical or physical agents in the occupational setting, often to determine how many employees have been exposed and to what extent over time. This approach may be especially useful in those instances where there is an absence of health outcomes known to be associated with potential hazardous exposures in the workplace. (Also known as "hazard surveillance.")

extensor: Muscle that straightens (extends) a limb.

exterior hood: A hood that is located adjacent to a contaminant source but does not enclose it.

external quality control: The activities that are performed occasionally, usually initiated and performed by persons outside of normal routine operations (such as on-site system surveys, independent performance audits, interlaboratory comparisons) to assess the capability and performance of a measurement process.

extrapolation: The process of estimating unknown values from known values.

extremely hazardous substance (EHS): As defined by the U.S. Environmental Protection Agency in the Superfund Amendment and Reauthorization Act (SARA) Title III.

extremely low frequency (ELF): An order of magnitude band designation usually applied to the part of the electromagnetic spectrum between 30 Hz and 300 Hz.

extrinsic safety: Plants that require external features to control hazards. The features should be arranged to minimize the undesirable consequences of a release.

F

F: See *frequency.*

face velocity: See *hood face velocity.*

factor of safety: Ratio of a normal working condition to the ultimate conditions, such as, in strength of materials, ratio of working stress to ultimate strength.

Fahrenheit temperature: The temperature scale in which, at standard atmospheric pressure, the boiling point of water is 212°F and the freezing point is 32°F. (See also *Rankine temperature.*)

fail-safe: Redundant engineering designed to prevent loss in case of a disaster.

FAM: See *fibrous aerosol monitor.*

fan: 1. A device for moving air by two or more blades or vanes attached to a rotating shaft. Provides the energy to move air through the system. 2. The local exhaust ventilation system component that provides the energy required by a specific design to move air through the system.

far field: In noise measurement, this refers to the distance from the noise source where the sound pressure level decreases 6 dB for each doubling of distance. (Also known as "free field," "Inverse Square law.")

fate: Destiny of a chemical or biological pollutant after release into the environment. It involves temporal and spatial considerations of transport, transfer, storage, and transformation. (Also known as "environmental fate.")

Fatigue Decreased Proficiency (FDP): See *Criteria for Fatigue Decreased Proficiency.*

fault tree analysis: A graphical method of performing a failure modes and effects analysis.

FDP: See *Criteria for Fatigue Decreased Proficiency.*

feces: Solid/liquid waste excreted from the anus.

feedback: The reaction of some results of a process serving to alter or reinforce the character of that process.

fempto: A prefix meaning 10^{-15}.

fetotoxin: A material harmful to the fetus.

fetus: The unborn offspring of an animal in the postembryonic period, after all major structures are represented.

FFT spectrum analyzer: Divides the audible frequency spectrum into even smaller bands. This type of analysis can be used to identify tones that can be traced to specific pieces of equipment.

fiber: An elongated particle having an aspect ratio (i.e., a ratio of length to width of greater than 3:1). A fiber may be naturally occurring (such as plant fibers and asbestiform silicate minerals) or synthetic (such as vitreous or graphite fibers).

fibrillation: Rapid, uncoordinated contractions of the heart that are ineffective in pumping blood.

fibrosis: The development in an organ of excess fibrous connective tissue usually as a reparative or reactive process.

fibrous: Made up of fibers or fiber-like tissue.

fibrous aerosol monitor (FAM): Modified light-scattering monitor that is a direct-reading device designed to measure airborne concentrations of fibrous materials (such as asbestos and fiber glass) with a length-to-diameter aspect ration greater than three. Results are reported as a fiber count rather than mass concentration.

FID: See *flame ionization detector.*

field data sheets: A marked-up floor plan or system schematic to show where the field data is to be collected, the methodology for collecting the data, and the individual responsible for collecting the data. The use of field data sheets ensures that the field data is collected in a concise manner, that all of the data required to meet the project objectives are recorded, and that future data are collected in a similar manner for trend analysis and correlation purposes.

filter: 1. A device to remove solid material from a fluid.
2. A capacitor and/or inductor placed in a series/parallel combination across a DC line to remove the effects of the AC signal or to decrease the ripple voltage in a DC power supply. 3. A component used in respirators to remove solid or liquid aerosols from the inspired air.

filter bank: Interchangeable frame or cylinder containing a filtering material. Most HVAC system filters remove solid material (particles) from the air stream. (Also known as "filter cell," "filter cartridge," "filter unit," "filter element.")

fire point: The lowest temperature at which a volatile, combustible material can evolve enough vapors to support combustion.

first-pass metabolism: The ability of tissues, in particular liver, skin, and lung, to render chemicals foreign to the organism less or more toxic, or to transform them into a more water-soluble state, with the help of specific enzymes (Phase I and Phase II enzymes).

fit factor: A quantitative measure of the fit of a particular respirator to a particular individual.

fit-test: The use of a challenge agent to evaluate the fit of a respirator on an individual.

fixators: Skeletal muscles that generally stabilize and control the bony structures that constitute the joint.

flame ionization detector (FID): A device in which the measured change in conductivity of a standard flame (usually hydrogen) due to the insertion of another gas or vapor is used to detect the gas or vapor.

flame photometric detector (FPD): The flame photometric detector is used to measure phosphorus- and sulfur-containing compounds such as organophosphate pesticides and mercaptans. The FPD measures these compounds by burning the column effluent in a hydrogen-air flame with an excess of hydrogen. The compounds emit light above the flame. A filter optimized to pass light at 393 nm is used to detect sulfur compounds; a filter optimized to pass light at 535 nm is used to detect phosphorus compounds. A photomultiplier tube is then used to quantify the amount of light passing through the selective filter.

flammable: The capability of a substance to be set on fire or support combustion easily. Flammable is not synonymous with "inflammable."

flammable limits: 1. The range of flammable vapor or gas-air mixture between the upper and lower flammable limits. 2. The minimum and maximum concentrations in air of a flammable gas or vapor at which ignition can occur. Concentrations below the lower flammable limit (LFL), also referred to as the lower explosive limit (LEL), are too lean to burn; concentrations above the upper flammable limit (UFL), also referred to as the upper explosive limit (UEL), are too rich to burn.

flammable liquid: Any liquid having a flash point below 37.8°C (100°F).

flammable waste: Materials that serve as fuels that can ignite and sustain a chain reaction when combined in a suitable ratio with oxygen in the presence of an ignition source.

flange: A surface at and parallel to the hood face that provides a barrier to unwanted airflow from behind the hood.

flash blindness: A temporary effect in which visual sensitivity and function is decreased severely in a very short period. (Also known as "blinding glare.")

flash point: 1. Minimum temperature to which a product must be heated for its vapors to ignite momentarily in a flame when operating under standardized conditions. (See also *fire point*). 2. In a vacuum cooling chamber, the pressure corresponding to the vapor pressure at the product temperature and below which water vaporizing commences. 3. The temperature at which the vapor above a volatile liquid forms a combustible mixture with air.

flat response: A response that looks at the entire audible frequency spectrum without applying any weighting.

flat-file database: A relatively simple database system in which each database is contained in a single table. In contrast, relational database systems can use multiple tables to store information, and each table can have a different record format. Relational systems are more suitable for large applications, but flat databases are adequate for many small applications.

flatus: Sudden excretion of internal gas/vapor from the mouth or the anus.

flexion: Act of bending, especially of a joint.

flexor: Muscle that bends (flexes) a limb.

flow chart: A graphical representation of the progress of a system for the definition, analysis, or solution of a data-processing or manufacturing problem in which the symbols are used to represent operations, data or material flow, and equipment, and lines and arrows represent interrelationships among the components. (Also known as a "control diagram," "flow diagram," "flow sheet.")

flow rate standards: Measurements based on discrete standards, such as the platinum kilogram (known as "K-20") for mass and the platinum meter bar for length. For flow rate measurements there is no off-the-shelf identity standard such as gallons per minute or liters per second. To supply a fundamental basis for any flow rate measurement, the identity standard must be one that is derived.

flow-dilution system: A system that continuously mixes accurately metered flows of a test component with a diluent (e.g., clean air).

fluids: A state of matter that flows under pressure (i.e., gas and liquid states).

fluorescence detector: Measures the emission of light produced by fluorescing eluents and is extremely sensitive to highly conjugated aromatic compounds such as PAHs. Some analytical methods use derivitization reagents to fluoresce the analyte. In these methods a light source raises the fluorescent analyte to an unstable higher energy level, which quickly decays in two or more steps, emitting light at longer wavelengths. The basic detector components are a lamp; a flow cell with windows at a 90° angle for the column effluent; filters or diffraction gratings to select the excitation and emission wavelengths; and a photomultiplier tube or other light-measuring device.

flux: The absorption rate per unit area.

fog: General term applied to visible aerosols in which the dispersed phase is liquid; formation by condensation is implied.

foot candle: A unit of illumination. The illumination at a point on a surface that is one foot from, and perpendicular to, a uniform point source of one candle.

force: An interaction of two objects that produces a change in the state of motion of an object. A force may cause an object to move, accelerate or decelerate, change direction, or stop from moving.

force couple: The pair of forces arranged to produce pure rotation (angular motion).

force platform: A force platform measures the ground reaction force (GRF) applied to the body by the surface of the platform.

force ratio: See *mechanical advantage*.

formable earplug: A type of hearing protector that is formed by the user prior to being inserted in the ear canals.

formative evaluation: Gathering information on adequacy and using this information as a basis for further development. (Also known as "process evaluation.")

formula: The scientific expression of the chemical composition of a material.

Fourier transform infrared spectrometry: A spectroscopic technique in which all pertinent wavelengths simultaneously irridate the sample for a short period and the absorption spectrum is found by mathematical manipulation of the Fourier transform so obtained.

FPD: See *flame photometric detector*.

free-body diagram: A conceptual drawing of the forces and moments acting on the system.

free-layer damping: A layer of nonhardening viscoelastic material (usually in the form of tapes, sheets, mastics, or sprays) is adhered to the surface. (Also known as "extensional damping.")

freezing point: For a particular pressure, the temperature at which a given substance will solidify or freeze upon removal of heat. The freezing point of water is 32°F (0°C).

frequency (F): The time rate of repetition of a periodic phenomena. The frequency is the reciprocal of the period and is sometimes called pitch.

frequency of sound: Rate of oscillation or vibration; units are 1 cycle per second or 1 hertz.

fresh air: Air taken from the outside ambient environment. The fresh air must satisfy the EPA Ambient Air Quality Standards. (Also known as "outdoor air," "outside air.")

fresh-air make up: The volume of outside air introduced into an occupied space to replace the air removed from a space. (Also known as "replacement air.")

friction factor: 1. A coefficient used to calculate friction forces due to fluid flow. 2. Quotient of the tangential force exerted by a fluid on a surface (per unit area) by half the product of the density and the square of the velocity.

friction loss: Pressure loss due to friction between a flowing fluid and its contact surface.

frictional resistance: The resistance of fluid flow due to friction between the fluid and the contact surface it flows past.

fritted glass bubblers: In fritted glass bubblers, air passes through formed porous glass plates and enters the liquid in the form of small bubbles.

frostbite: Injury to skin and subcutaneous tissues, and in severe cases also to deeper tissues, from exposure to extreme cold.

full work cycle: Amount of time required to complete a task or process; may be less or more than an 8-hour shift.

full-shift sampling: The collection of survey information over the course of an 8-hour day to determine the actual 8-hour time-weighted average (TWA) exposure concentration. It is the preferred method to use to accurately characterize an operation for the gathering of baseline and routine monitoring data and to document regulatory compliance.

fume: 1. Minute solid particles generated by condensation from the gaseous state, generally after volatilization (evaporation) from melted substances, such as welding, and often accompanied by a chemical reaction, such as oxidation. Examples are iron oxide from welding; lead oxide from soldering; and copper oxide from smelting. Size ranges are usually between 0.001 μm and 1.0 μm. 2. Very small, airborne particles commonly formed by condensing vapors from burning or melting materials. (See also *aerosol, dust.*)

functional analysis: A mathematical analysis that examines each aspect of the measurement system (sampling and analysis) in order to quantitate the effect of sources of error. A functional analysis is usually performed prior to a ruggedness test to determine those variables that should be studied experimentally.

fundamental unit: Mass, length, and time.

G

g: See *gram.*

g/kg: Grams per kilogram body weight; an expression of dosage.

gage: 1. An instrument for measuring pressure, flow, or level. 2. A scale of measurement for sheet metal thickness, wire and drill diameters, etc. (Also known as "gauge.")

gamma ray: A photon emitted from a nucleus.

gas: Any material in the gaseous state at 25°C and 760 mmHg. Normally, a formless fluid, it expands to fill the space or enclosure. Gases can be changed to the liquid or solid state only by the combined effect of increased pressure and decreased temperature. Examples are welding gases, internal combustion engines exhaust gases, and waste gases from refining or sewage (such as hydrogen sulfide, waste anesthesia gases, hydrogen, and ammonia). Size ranges are usually less than 0.0005 μm. Within acceptable limits of accuracy, satisfies the perfect gas law.

gas chromatograph (GC): Highly sophisticated instrument that identifies the molecular composition and concentrations of various chemicals in water and soil samples. (Also known as "mass spectrometer.")

gas chromatography: A separation technique involving passage of a gaseous moving phase through a column containing a fixed adsorbent phase; it is used principally as a quantitative analytical technique for volatile compounds.

gas constant (R): The coefficient (R) in the Ideal Gas law equation given by PV = nRT; the constant factor in the equation of state for ideal gases. In the SI system of units, R = 0.08205 liters * atmosphere/mole (K); in the I-P system, 21.85 cubic feet * inches mercury/pounds mole (°R).

gas narcosis: Gas narcosis is caused by nitrogen in normal air during dives of more than 120 feet (35 meters). Helium, substituted for nitrogen in "mixed gas diving," can cause an effect called "high pressure nervous syndrome" beyond 500 fsw.

gas solubility: The extent that a gas dissolves in a liquid to produce a homogenous system.

gas toxicities: Gas toxicities caused by oxygen and carbon dioxide. The damage of lack of oxygen to the lung and brain (central nervous system [CNS]) will vary with time of exposure and depth. While a carbon dioxide partial pressure of 15–40 mmHg will stimulate the central respiratory sensor, concentrations >80 mmHg suppress respiration.

gaseous exchange: In the alveoli, the absorption of oxygen and concomitant removal of waste gases.

gastrointestinal tract: The mouth, esophagus, stomach, intestines, and related organs.

gauge pressure: The difference between two absolute pressures, one of which is usually atmospheric pressure.

gauss: The cgs (centimeter-gram-second) unit of magnetic flux density.

gavage: Introduction of a test agent through a tube passed into the stomach.

GC: See gas chromatograph.

general duty clause: Section 5(a)(1) of the Administrative Procedures Act (see *29 CFR 1905*) imposes the following general duty: "Each employer—(1) shall furnish to each of his employees employment and a place of employment which are free from recognized hazards that are causing or are likely to cause death or serious physical harm to his employees."

general motion: A combination of both translation and rotation. (See also *rotation, translation.*)

general reliability: The capability of an item or system to perform a required function under stated conditions for a stated period of time.

general ventilation: Ventilation systems designed primarily for temperature, humidity, and odor control; health hazard protection is secondary. (Also known as "comfort ventilation.")

generation: A group of organisms having a common parent or parents and comprising a single level in line of descent.

genetic engineering: A process of inserting new genetic information into existing cells in order to modify any organism for the purpose of changing one of its characteristics.

genetic mutation: A mutation that involves expression of the aberration in the offspring of the exposed individual due to alteration of germ or sex cells (male spermatozoa and/or female ova).

genotoxic chemical: An electrophilic (i.e., electron-deficient) compound that has an affinity for genetic information, specifically the electron-dense (i.e., nucleophilic) DNA.

genotoxin: A material harmful to the genetic material.

geometric mean (σ_g): Mathematically, the geometric mean (σ_g) can be expressed in two equivalent ways or in words, the nth root of the product of all values in a set of n values, or the antilogarithm of the arithmetic mean of the logarithms of all the values of a set of n values.

geometric standard deviation (GSD): A measure of dispersion in a lognormal distribution. The value will always be greater than or equal to one. Typically, lognormal distribution is used to describe particle size distribution of an aerosol sample. (See also *lognormal distribution.*)

geometry: The physical orientation of a detector to the radiation source.

globe temperature (T_g): The measure of radiant heat.

GLR: See *graphic level recorder.*

going into debt: In normal exercise, enough oxygen is supplied to the blood from the lungs. But in maximal exercise or underwater, the lungs cannot furnish enough oxygen and the "emergency" supply of anaerobic oxygen is used — that is, there is an oxygen debt.

good samaritan doctrine: A legal theory in which persons who bring a personal injury action against a defendant, who normally does not owe a duty of care to the plaintiff, show that the defendant owed a duty to the plaintiff, that they negligently failed to discharge that duty, and that the plaintiff's injury was caused by such negligence.

grab sample: A sample taken within a short time period, generally to determine the contaminants at a specific time or during a specific event.

grab sampling: The direct collection of an air-contaminant mixture into a device such as a sampling bag, syringe, or evacuated flask over a few seconds or minutes.

gram (g): A unit of mass; defined as the mass of 1 cc of water at 4°C (39.2°F).

gram mole: The amount of substance represented by one gram molecular weight or one gram molecular volume (mole).

gram molecular weight: The sum of the individual atomic weights of all the atoms in a molecule (express mass in units of grams, g).

graphic level recorder (GLR): An instrument for providing a written record of the sound levels of particular events as a function of time.

gravimetric: Of or pertaining to measurement by weight.

gravimetric analysis: A process in which a known volume of aerosol-laden air is drawn through a filter of known initial weight, then reweighing the filter to determine the mass captured.

GSD: See *geometric standard deviation.*

H

H: See *magnetic-field strength.*

HSI: See *heat stress index.*

Haber's law: The Haber relationship expresses the constancy of the product of exposure concentration and exposure duration (Ct = K, where C represents exposure concentration, t is time, and K is constant). The Haber relationship does not hold over more than small differences in exposure time.

HACE: See *high altitude cerebral edema.*

hair: The flexible shaft of distinct coloring that protrudes from the skin surface.

half-time (pseudo first order): $t_{0.5} = 0.693/k$ where k is the pseudo first-order process rate constant in units of time.

halo formation: A visible ring or line of excess particles that are deposited on the substrate or around the nozzle. The presence of the halo formation indicates incorrect sample flow through the nozzle and is very undesirable.

halocarbon: Partially or fully halogenated hydrocarbon.

Hamilton, Dr. Alice: An American physician and social reformer. She entered the field of industrial medicine in 1910 and not only presented substantial evidence of the relationship between toxins and ill health, but also provided solutions to the problems she encountered. In 1919 she became the first woman faculty member at Harvard University and in 1943 wrote her autobiography "Exploring the Dangerous Trades." She has been called the "Mother of American occupational medicine."

hand-arm vibration syndrome (HAVS): A condition contracted after prolonged exposure to hand-arm vibration with symptoms that include intermittent tingling and/or numbness of the fingers and finger blanching (turning white). With additional vibration exposure, the symptoms of HAVS become more severe and include increasing stiffness of the finger joints, loss of manipulative skills, and loss of blood circulation, which can lead to gangrene and tissue necrosis.

HAPE: See *high altitude pulmonary edema.*

hapten: A simple substance that reacts like an antigen *in vitro* by combining with antibody; may function as an allergen when linked to proteinaceous substances of the tissue.

hardware: Hardware is the electronic and physical apparatus necessary to run computer programs (i.e., software).

HAVS: See *hand-arm vibration syndrome.*

Hawthorne Effect: A tendency for employees to do the job in a nonroutine manner while being observed.

HAZAN: See *hazard analysis.*

hazard: Source of risk.

hazard analysis (HAZAN): A generic term for a variety of quantitative hazard and risk analysis methods. A logical sequence for the systematic examination of a facility is to use hazard identification and ranking techniques first. If there are possible scenarios that could lead to unacceptable consequences, then qualitative techniques (HAZOP) can be applied next. When there is a qualitative hazard, HAZAN methods can be used to estimate the quantitative probability of adverse events. How much analysis is worthwhile is a function of the consequence of the adverse event and the difficulty in preventing it.

hazard and operability (HAZOP) survey: One of the most common and widely accepted methods of systematic qualitative hazard analysis. It is used for both new and existing facilities and can be applied to a whole plant, a production unit, or a piece of equipment. It uses as its database the usual sort of plant and process information and relies on the judgment of engineering and safety experts in the areas with which they are most familiar. The end result, therefore, is reliable in terms of engineering and operational expectations, but it is not quantitative and might not consider the consequences of complex sequences of human errors.

hazard distance: The linear distance from the antenna at which the field intensity is reduced to the exposure limit.

hazard evaluation: Evaluation based on data concerning concentration of a contaminant and duration of exposure.

hazard identification: Determining whether a chemical can cause adverse health effects in humans and what those effects might be.

hazard index: Sum of more than one hazard quotient for multiple substances and/or multiple exposure pathways. Calculated separately for chronic, subchronic, and shorter-duration exposures.

hazard prevention and control: Applies the following measures: 1) engineering techniques are used when feasible and appropriate; 2) procedures for safe work are established, understood, and followed by all affected parties; and 3) provisions are made for personal protective equipment and administrative controls.

hazard quotient: Ratio of a single substance exposure level over a specified period to a reference dose (RfD) for that substance derived from a similar exposure period.

hazard ratio: A number obtained by dividing the airborne concentration of a contaminant by its exposure limit.

hazard warning: Any words, pictures, symbols, or combinations thereof appearing on a label or other appropriate form of warning that convey the specific physical or health hazard(s) — including target organ effects — of the chemical(s) in the container(s). (See the definitions for *physical hazard* and *health hazard* to determine the hazards that must be covered.)

hazardous waste: Bi-products of society that can pose a substantial or potential hazard to human health or the environment when improperly managed. Possesses at least one of four characteristics (ignitability, corrosivity, reactivity, or toxicity), or appears on special EPA lists.

HazMat: Universally recognized abbreviation for hazardous materials. HAZMAT is also used.

HAZOP: See *hazard and operability survey.*

HAZWOPER: Acronym for hazardous waste operations and emergency response.

head: 1. Historically, a unit of pressure. 2. In fluid statics and dynamics, a vertical linear measure.

Health Advisories (1-day or 10-day): Concentrations of contaminants in drinking water at which adverse, noncarcinogenic health effects would not be expected to occur to a child exposed for one or 10 days. [**Note:** Issued by the U.S. EPA Office of Drinking Water.]

health care professional: Occupational physicians are qualified to design, manage, supervise, and deliver health care in occupational settings. Some services may be provided by other practitioners such as occupational health nurses, physician assistants, licensed practical nurses, or emergency medical technicians.

Health Effects Assessment Summary Table (HEAST): Tabular presentation of toxicity information and values for certain chemicals that have been evaluated by different U.S. EPA programs. As data in HEAST might not have received the level of validation required by IRIS, some chemicals not listed in IRIS may appear in HEAST.

health hazard: A chemical for which there is statistically significant evidence, based on at least one study conducted in accordance with established scientific principles, that acute or chronic health effects might occur in exposed employees. The term "health hazard" includes chemicals that are carcinogens, toxic or highly toxic agents, reproductive toxins, irritants, corrosives, sensitizers, hepatotoxins, nephrotoxins, neurotoxins, agents that act on the hematopoietic system, and agents that damage the lungs, skin, eyes, or mucous membranes. Appendix A of the OSHA hazard communication standard provides further definitions and explanations of the scope of health hazards covered by this section, and Appendix B describes the criteria to be used to determine whether a chemical is to be considered hazardous for purposes of this standard.

health inspections: An inspection conducted by those who are classified as occupational hygienists.

health surveillance: The measurement of chemical markers in body media that are indicative of adverse and nonadverse health effects.

healthy worker effect: A phenomenon observed initially in studies of occupational diseases; workers usually exhibit lower overall death rates than the general population because severely ill and disabled are ordinarily excluded from employment.

hearing conservation: The program for preventing or minimizing noise-induced deafness through audiometric testing, measurement of noise, engineering control, and ear protection.

hearing level: A measurement of hearing acuity. The deviation in decibels of an individual's threshold from the zero reference of the audiometer.

hearing loss: The deviation of hearing acuity from normal.

hearing protection device (HPD): Equipment worn to reduce the sound exposure of persons either before engineering or administrative noise controls can be administered or when these controls are not yet feasible. (See also *earmuff, formable earplug, preformable earplug, semi-insert.*)

HEAST: See *Health Effects Assessment Summary Table.*

heat: Energy transferred by a thermal process.

heat balance: A statement that shows the changes in a system from heat and work input to output losses.

heat capacity: The amount of heat necessary to raise the temperature of a given mass 1 degree; numerically, the mass multiplied by the specific heat.

heat strain: The body's response to heat stress.

heat stress: 1. The external heat load placed on the body due to the characteristics of the environment. 2. The burden, or load of heat, that must be dissipated if the body is to remain in thermal equilibrium.

heat stress index (HSI): A composite measure used for the quantitative assessment of heat stress.

hedonic tone: A category judgment of the relative pleasantness or unpleasantness of an odor. Perception of hedonic tone is influenced by subjective experience, frequency of occurrence, odor character, odor intensity, and duration. (See also *odor threshold.*)

helium oxygen saturation diving: A decompression schedule specifying a set rate of feet per hour. For example, an ascent from saturation diving at 340 ft would require 120 hours (or five days). On the other hand, saturation diving allows more working time per day, greatly reducing the total time for long jobs in addition to avoiding the hazards of multiple compressions and decompressions.

helmet: A hood that offers head protection against impact and penetration.

hematopoietic: Pertaining to or affecting the formation of blood cells.
hematuria: The presence of blood or blood cells in the urine.
hemoglobin: The red coloring matter of the blood which carries the oxygen.
Henry's law: The equilibrium concentration of a gas dissolved into a liquid will equal the product of the partial pressure of the gas times its solubility in the liquid.
HEPA filter: High efficiency particulate air filter; a filter capable of removing very small particles from the airstream. A HEPA filter is capable of trapping particulate material in the size of 0.3 microns (or greater) from the air with a minimum efficiency of 99.97%.
hepatic: Pertaining to the liver.
hepatitis: The inflammation of the liver; commonly of viral origin but also occurring in association with syphilis, typhoid fever, malaria, toxemias, and parasitic infestations.
hepatotoxicant: A material harmful to the liver.
hertz (Hz): Unit of frequency equal to one cycle per second. (See also *frequency of sound*.)
high altitude cerebral edema (HACE): A sickness with symptoms that include many benign AMS symptoms but are differentiated by disturbed consciousness (irrationality, disorientation, and even hallucinations), abnormal reflex and muscle control (ataxia, bladder dysfunction, and even convulsions), and/or perhaps most characteristically papilloedema (swelling of the optic disc). (See also *acute mountain sickness*.)
high altitude pulmonary edema (HAPE): The edema in HAPE is characterized by the release of large quantities of a high protein fluid into the lung. Differential symptoms, which are often denied by the patient, include severe breathlessness and chest pain, with or without the above symptoms of benign AMS. Symptoms of patients with HAPE will rapidly progress to a dry cough, production of a foamy pink sputum, audible bubbling and gurgling sounds while breathing, and cyanosis of the lips and extremities. (See also *acute mountain sickness*.)
high performance liquid chromatography (HPLC): Laboratory method used to separate organic molecules using a liquid phase.
homeotherm: An endotherm that maintains a constant body temperature as do most mammals and birds.
homolog: 1. One of a series of compounds, each of which is formed from the one before it by the addition of a constant element; any chemical structurally similar to another chemical. 2. Compound of the same (organic) series. (Also known as "homologue.")
hood: 1. A device that encloses, captures, or receives emitted contaminants. 2. A respiratory inlet covering that completely covers the head and neck and may cover portions of the shoulders.
hood centerline: A line from the center or the hood face extending perpendicularly outward.
hood face velocity (V_f): Air velocity at the hood face opening of an enclosing hood (e.g., a laboratory hood).
horizontal entry: A confined space entry that requires the entrant to enter through an opening in the side of the confined space.
horsepower: The unit of power in the I-P system indicating work done at the rate of 550 foot-pounds per second, or 745.7 watts. (See also *brake horsepower*.)
House of Quality: A tool that correlates customer needs with process design requirements.
HPD: See *hearing protection device*.
HPLC: See *high performance liquid chromatography*.
human factors: Plants that are designed so that human operators can affect or control hazards.
human health risk assessment: The evaluation by occupational hygienists of the potential risk of exposure to the health of workers.
humidity: Water vapor within a given space.
HVAC system: HVAC (heating, ventilation, and air-conditioning) is the distribution system that heats, ventilates, cools, humidifies, dehumidifies, and cleanses air in a building or building zone, principally for the comfort, health, and safety of the occupants.
hydration: To combine with water.

hydrocarbons: The basic building blocks of all organic chemicals which are composed solely of carbon and hydrogen.

hygrometer: An instrument to measure humidity in the atmosphere.

hygroscopic: Readily absorbing or retaining moisture.

hygroscopicity: The tendency to absorb water vapor.

hyperbaric: Pertaining to an anesthetic solution with a specific gravity greater than that of the cerebrospinal fluid.

hyperemia: An increased blood flow or congestion of blood anywhere in the body.

hypergolic: Ignites on contact.

hyperplasia: An abnormal increase in the number of normal cells composing a tissue or organ.

hypersensitivity: A state of heightened responsiveness in which the body reacts to a foreign agent or substance more strongly than normal; generally results from prior exposures to the agent or substance.

hypersensitivity diseases: Diseases that result from specific immune system responses to environmental challenges. There are two general categories: 1) the IgE-mediated diseases (asthma, allergic rhinitis, or hayfever); 2) hypersensitivity pneumonitis, which is mediated by IgG and the cellular immune system. All hypersensitivity diseases require an initial series of sensitizing exposures during which the immune system becomes activated. Symptoms occur on subsequent exposures in response to stimulation of the previously activated immune response. Most cases of hypersensitivity disease are caused by proteins or glycoproteins, although some highly reactive chemicals can bind to larger molecules to cause hypersensitivity pneumonitis.

hypersusceptibility: Greater than normal sensitivity to certain substances.

hypobaric: Pertaining to an anesthetic solution with a specific gravity lower than that of the cerebrospinal fluid.

hyponatremia: Subnormal or reduced blood sodium levels.

hypothermia: Condition of reduced body temperature in homeotherms.

hypotonic: 1. Pertaining to subnormal muscle strength or tension. 2. Referring to a solution with a lower osmotic pressure than physiological saline.

hypoxia: Occurs when there is an insufficient amount of oxygen delivered to the tissues.

Hz: See *hertz.*

I

IARC: See *International Agency for Research on Cancer.*

I_c: See *contact current.*

IC: See *ion chromatography.*

ice point: 1. Equilibrium temperature of ice and water (usually at standard atmospheric pressure). 2. Temperature at which water freezes under normal atmospheric pressure, 14.696 psig, 32°F (101.325 kPA, 0°C).

ideal gas: A gas with internal energy and enthalpy that depends solely on temperature and that is defined by the perfect gas equation, Pv = nRT. (Also known as "perfect gas.")

Ideal Gas law: An equation of state, a relationship between the pressure, volume, and thermodynamic temperature of a gas (PV = nRT). (Also known as the "Perfect Gas law.")

identity: Any chemical or common name indicated on the material safety data sheet (MSDS) for a chemical. The identity used permits cross-references to be made among the required list of hazardous chemicals, the label, and the MSDS.

IDLH: See *immediately dangerous to life and health.*

IDP: See *integrated product development.*

IHIT: See *Industrial Hygienist in Training.*

I_I: See *induced current.*

illuminance: The luminous flux crossing a surface of a given area.

immediately dangerous to life and health (IDLH): Any atmosphere that poses an immediate hazard to life or poses immediate irreversible debilitating effects on health.

immune response: Chemical/cellular response of the body to an antigen.

immunosuppression: Suppression of an immune response by the use of drugs or radiation. Toxic interactions also can cause suppression of the immune response. Immunosuppression decreases an individual's resistance and increases vulnerability to infection and proliferation of neoplastic or other mutated cells.

impact: A forceful collision between two bodies that is sufficient to cause an appreciable change in the momentum of the system on which it acts. (Also known as "impulsive force.")

impaction: The state of impacting.

impaction plate: A supporting surface on which a substrate is placed for collection of certain cutoff size particles. (See also *impactor stage, substrate, substrate coating*.)

impactor stage: One in a series of intercepting devices in the cascade impactor to collect certain cutoff size particulates. The stage includes the impaction plate, a support surface where a substrate can be placed, the nozzle for the subsequent stage, and an O-ring for sealing gaps around the edge of the stage. (See also *impaction plate, substrate, substrate coating*.)

impeller: The rotating part of a device (fan, blower, compressor, or pump).

impervious: Incapable of being passed through or penetrated.

impinge: To impact, hit, strike, collide, or push against.

impingement: Method of measuring air contaminants in which particulates are collected by their collision against some other material; also refers to the way in which particulate matter collects inside the respiratory tract.

impingers: Small glass bottles normally filled with a specific liquid that will absorb airborne chemicals when air containing the contaminant is bubbled through it.

incentive/reward programs: A program designed to achieve a desired outcome in worker behavior by rewarding an individual or group.

incidental ultrafine particle: used in the context of nanometer-diameter particles that have not been intentionally produced but are the incidental products of processes involving combustion, welding, or diesel engines.

Inch-Pound System of Units: The I-P system is the de facto engineering standard set of units used in the United States.

inch-pound units: See *Inch-Pound System of Units*.

incident rate: The numerical performance measure required by OSHA. It is the number of injuries, illnesses, or lost workdays related to a common exposure base of 100 full-time workers. It is calculated as N/EH × 200,000 where N = number of injuries and/or illnesses or lost workdays; EH = total hours worked by all employees during a calendar year; and 200,000 = the base for 100 full-time equivalent workers (working 40 hours/week, 50 weeks/year).

index of suspicion: Knowledge of the signs and symptoms of the agents of a covert act.

indicating layer: The colorimetric reactive portion of the detector tube.

induced current (Ii): A current produced in a conductor by a time-varying magnetic field.

industrial hygiene survey: Systematic analysis of a workplace to detect and evaluate health hazards and recommend methods for their control.

industrial hygienist: Professional hygienist primarily concerned with the control of environmental health hazards that arise out of or during the course of employment. (See also *Certified Industrial Hygienist, Qualified Industrial Hygienist*.)

Industrial Hygienist in Training (IHIT): A degree indicating partial fulfillment of CIH certification. The IHIT designation recognizes special education in and knowledge of the basic principles of industrial hygiene.

industrial ventilation (IV): The equipment or operation associated with the supply or exhaust of air, by natural or mechanical means, to control occupational hazards in the industrial setting.

inert chemical: Not having active properties.

inert dust: Dust that does not chemically react with other substances.

inert gas: A gas that neither experiences nor causes chemical reaction, nor undergoes a change of state in a system or process (e.g., nitrogen or helium mixed with a volatile refrigerant).

infection: 1. Invasion of the body by a pathogenic organism with or without disease manifestation. 2. Pathological condition resulting from invasion of a pathogen.

inflammation: A form of tissue reaction to injury that is often marked by pain, heat, redness, and swelling.

informational report: A simple presentation of the facts that generally requires less time and effort than an interpretive report. Examples of informational reports include status reports on a continuing project and survey reports that list findings without developing conclusions or recommendations.

infrared: The region of the electromagnetic spectrum including wavelengths from 0.78 microns to about 300 microns.

infrared gas analyzer: A direct-reading instrument that is versatile, can quantify hundreds of chemicals, and is capable of being used for continuous monitoring, short-term sampling, and bag sampling. It is often used in indoor air investigations to measure the buildup of carbon dioxide. (Also known as "infrared gas monitor.")

infrared radiation (IR): Wavelengths of the electromagnetic spectrum that are longer than those of visible light and shorter than radio waves; infrared wavelengths measure 10^{-4} cm to 10^{-1} cm.

ingestion: Introduction of substances into the digestive system.

inhalable fraction: The fraction of total workplace aerosol actually entering the respiratory tract.

inhalation: The breathing in of a substance in the air (e.g., gas, vapor, particulate, dust, fume, mist).

inhibitor: A chemical added to another substance to prevent an unwanted chemical change.

initiation: 1. Triggering off explosion or decomposition. 2. The formation of the DNA-carcinogen adduct is the first step of carcinogenesis.

innervation ratio: The number of muscle fibers innervated by a single motor neuron, which varies from 1:1900 (1 neuron per 1900 muscle fibers) as in the gastrocnemius to 1:15 (1 neuron per 15 muscle fibers) as in the extraocular muscles. The lower the innervation ratio, the finer the control of the muscle force.

inorganic: Term used to designate compounds that generally do not contain carbon.

inspired air: Air drawn in during the breathing process.

inspiring: A management method in which leaders share authority and acknowledge contributions of others, enabling others to feel and act like leaders. This facilitates as sense of ownership for the team members and helps the group achieve peak performance.

instantaneous: Instantaneous may be defined as equivalent to the time it takes to snap one's fingers and refers to a single event. Occupational safety, therefore, is focused primarily on preventing unwanted and unplanned events (i.e., accidents that are instantaneous in nature that might lead to an employee suffering an injury).

instantaneous sampling: Sampling done at one particular time either by a direct-reading instrument or by trapping a definite volume of air for analysis.

instructional objectives: A road map for the development of training content and what training format should be used. They are also a means of measurement that allows for the evaluation of whether performance does, or does not, reach the desired goal.

instructional systems design: The systematic approach to instructional technology that emphasizes the importance of a training needs assessment, the specification of instructional objectives, precisely controlled learning experiences to achieve these objectives, and criteria for performance; and evaluative information based on performance measures.

instructional technology: The theory and practice of design, development, utilization, management, and evaluation of processes and resources for learning.

intake: Measure of exposure expressed as mass of substance in contact with the exchange boundary per unit body weight per unit time (i.e., mg/kg/day).

integrated product development (IPD): A systematic approach to the multifunctional, concurrent design of products and their related processes. It includes manufacturing and support of the products through their life cycle.

Integrated Risk Information System (IRIS): U.S. EPA database containing verified reference doses (RfDs), slope factors, and current health and regulatory information. It is the EPA's preferred source of toxicity information for Superfund.

integrated sampling: The passage of a known volume of air through an absorbing or adsorbing medium to remove the desired contaminants from the air during a specified period.

interactive multimedia: Software that allows or requires the user to press keys or "click" the mouse to control the actions of the software. (See also *multimedia.*)

interception: The state of intercepting.

interference: The term applied when a contaminant, other than the target gas or vapor, reacts with a reagent in the detector tube to produce erroneous results.

interlaboratory quality control (QC): A systematic procedure for selecting interlaboratory participants, analyte, duration, and frequency of interlaboratory testing, and evaluating statistics and reporting of test data to ensure the quality of test results.

internal occupational exposure limit: An occupational exposure limit (OEL) formally set by an organization for its private use. (See also *occupational exposure limit.*)

internal quality control: The routine activities and checks (such as periodic calibrations, duplicate analyses, and use of spiked samples) included in normal internal procedures to control the accuracy and precision of a measurement process. (See also *quality control.*)

International Agency for Research on Cancer (IARC): Headquarters are in Geneva, Switzerland.

International System of Units: Le Systeme International d'Unites (the SI system) divides units into three categories: base units, supplementary units, and derived units. The base units consist of seven well-defined and dimensionally independent quantities. These include length, mass, time, thermodynamic temperature, electric current, amount of a substance, and luminous intensity.

Internet: The Internet is a series of interconnected networks of computers. Unlike online services, which are centrally controlled, the Internet is decentralized by design. Each Internet computer, called a host, is independent. Its operators can choose which Internet services to provide to its local users and which local services to make available to the global Internet community.

Internet service provider (ISP): A company that provides and manages connections from users to the Internet.

interpreting: A management skill in which a leader sifts through all available data to choose that which is most important to the organization's future.

interpretive report: A report that presents findings and also critically evaluates the results, draws conclusions, and offers recommendations. The purpose of such a report is not merely to inform but also to persuade the reader to accept the writer's viewpoint, to take action, or to make a change in policy or practice. Examples of interpretive reports include technological feasibility studies and comprehensive work site evaluations. The interpretive report is distinguished by its inclusion of expert opinion to guide the reader in making decisions.

interstitial: Situated between the cellular components of an organ or structure.

intrabeam viewing: The viewing condition in which the eye is exposed to all or part of a laser beam.

intralaboratory quality control (QC): A systematic procedure for evaluating the precision and accuracy for within analyst and between analyst data, constructing and using control charts, and using duplicate, replicate, and/or spiked samples to ensure the quality of test results.

intrinsic safety: Plants that are designed so that departures from the norm tend to be self-correcting or at most lead to minor events rather than major disasters. Plants designed to be forgiving and self-correcting are inherently safer than plants where equipment has been added to control hazards or where operators are expected to control them.

intrinsically safe: A feature available on air sampling equipment that ensures that pumps are not an explosive hazard in specific environments.

inverse dynamics: Since all of the forces and moments that cause the moment are calculated by evaluating the resulting motion itself, the technique generally used for this calculation is known as an inverse dynamics approach.

Inverse Square law: The propagation of energy through space is inversely proportional to the square of the distance it must travel. An object 3 feet away from an energy source receives 1/9 the energy as an object 1 foot away.

***in vitro*:** Literally means "in glass;" experimental work done on cell cultures.

***in vivo*:** Literally means "in life;" an experiment that was conducted in the living organism.

ion chromatography (IC): A chromatographic technique that separates mixtures of ions.

ionization potential: The energy per unit charge needed to remove an electron from a given kind of atom or molecule to an infinite distance; usually expressed in volts. (Also know as "ion potential.")

I-P units (inch-pound units): Units using inches, pounds, and other designations; as opposed to SI units in the metric system. Examples are foot, Btu, horsepower, and gallon.

IR: See *infrared radiation.*

IREQ: See *required clothing insulation.*

IRIS: See *Integrated Risk Information System.*

irradiance: The amount of radiant power per unit area that flows across or on to a surface. (Also known as "radiant flux density.")

irreversible injury: An injury or effect that is not reversible once the exposure has been terminated.

irritant: A chemical, which is not corrosive, that causes a reversible inflammatory effect on living tissue by chemical action at the site of contact.

irritation: An inflammatory response or reaction of tissues resulting from contact with a material.

isobar: Two or more nuclides with the same atomic mass but different atomic numbers.

isokinetic sampling: A sampling condition in which air flowing into an inlet has the same velocity and direction as ambient airflow. (See also *subisokinetic sampling, superisokinetic sampling, stack sampling.*)

isolation: Separating employees from hazardous operations, processes, equipment, or environments (e.g., use of control rooms, physically separating employees and equipment, and barriers placed between employees and hazardous operations.)

isomer: 1. A metastable state of a nucleus that exists longer than 10^6 sec and decays by gamma emission to a nuclide with the same atomic number and same atomic mass. 2. A molecule that has the same number and kind of atoms as another molecule, but has a different arrangement of the atoms.

isometric: A muscle contraction in which the muscle remains at the same length while developing tension.

isothermal: A process at constant temperature.

isotope: 1. Two or more nuclides with the same atomic number but different atomic mass. 2. Atoms of the same element that differ in atomic weight.

ISP: See *Internet service provider.*

iterative risk assessment: A process in which increasingly complex and data-rich risk assessments are conducted.

IV: See *industrial ventilation.*

J

J: See *joule.*

jaundice: A yellow discoloration of the skin, mucous membranes, and eyes most often due to abnormalities of the liver or rapid destruction of blood cells.

jet: See *nozzle, jet.*

job rotation: In job-rotation, people shift jobs periodically during the day.

joule (J): In the SI system of units, the unit of energy equal to the work done when a current of 1 ampere is passed through a resistance of 1 ohm for 1 second; a unit of energy equal to the work done when the point of application of a force of 1 newton is displaced 1 meter in the direction of the force. (See also *newton.*)

K

kaizen: The philosophy of total quality requires a paradigm shift, away from a reluctance to tamper with processes that appear to be working to one stating that all processes are imperfect and an organization must strive for continuous improvement. This philosophy ensures that the organization will never be satisfied with less than optimal performance in any of its processes. Kaizen indicates that every process can and should be continually evaluated and improved, in terms of time required, resources used, resultant quality, and other aspects relevant to the process.

kcal: See *kilocalorie.*

Kelvin scale (absolute): The fundamental temperature scale, also called the absolute or thermodynamic scale, in which the temperature measure is based on the average kinetic energy per molecule of a perfect gas. The zero of the Kelvin scale is -273°C.

Kelvin temperature: The SI system of units absolute temperature scale (K), on which the triple point of water is 273.16 K and the boiling point is approximately 373.15 K (1 K = 1°C). The Kelvin is the fraction 1/273.16 of the temperature of the thermodynamic triple point of water.

kg: Kilogram, or 1000 grams.

kilocalorie (kcal): Amount of heat required to raise the temperature of 1000 grams 1°C.

kilogram: See *kg.*

kilogram mole: The amount of substance represented by 1 kilogram molecular weight or 1 kilogram molecular volume (mol).

kilogram molecular weight: The sum of the individual atomic weights of all the atoms in a molecule (express mass in units of kilograms [kg]).

kinematics: A branch of mechanics that concerns the description of a body's motion in space without an explanation of the cause of the observed motion.

kinesiology: The study of movement.

kinetic energy: Energy due to motion.

kinetics: A branch of mechanics that concerns the underlying causes of movement rather than the result of the movement.

K_m: See *partition coefficient.*

L

L: See *liter.*

laboratory quality control (QC) plan: A written plan that details the processes by which data generated by the laboratory will be evaluated, corrected (if necessary), and reported to the customer.

lacrimation: The excessive secretion and discharge of tears.

lagging: Asbestos and magnesia plaster that is used as a thermal insulation on process equipment and piping.

Lambertian surface: An ideal, perfectly diffusing surface for which the intensity of reflected radiation is independent of direction.

laminar flow: Gas flow with a smooth non-turbulent pattern of streamlines, with no streamline looping back on itself; usually occurs at very low Reynolds numbers. (See also *turbulent flow.*)

laminar flow biological safety cabinet: Containment equipment used to prevent the release and transmission of biological hazards via the airborne route.

LAN: See *local area network.*

laser: Light amplification through stimulated emission of radiation resulting when the rate at which energy is added to a monochromatic beam is greater than that at which it is extracted and light amplification results.

laser radiation: Optical radiation that propagates in the form of a beam and has various special properties, including low divergence, monochromaticity, and coherence.

Laser Safety Officer (LSO): The LSO, as described in *American National Standard for the Safe Use of Lasers* (ANSI Z136.1–1993), is one who administers the overall laser safety program. ANSI Z136.1 defines the LSO as one with "the authority to monitor and enforce the control of laser hazards and effect the knowledgeable evaluation and control of laser hazards."

latency: A delay between the onset of exposure to a hazardous agent and the onset of illness attributable to that agent.

latency period: The time that elapses between exposure and the first manifestation of damage. (Also known as the "latent period.")

LC: See *lethal concentration*.

LC_{50}: The airborne concentration of a given substance that when inhaled over a period of time will kill 50% of the animals under test.

LC_{Lo}: See *lowest lethal concentration*.

LC_X: See *lethal concentration "X."*

LD: See *lethal dose*.

LD_{50}: The oral dose required to produce death in 50% of the exposed species, usually within the first 30 days.

LD_{Lo}: See *lowest lethal dose*.

LD_X: See *lethal dose "X."*

leak test: A procedure to determine whether the pump or the detector tube is leaking.

***Legionella*:** A genus of bacteria, some species of which have caused a type of pneumonia called "Legionnaires' Disease."

LEL: Lower explosive limit. See *lower flammable limit*.

length of stain: The length of color change in a detector tube. The length of stain is proportional to the concentration of the contaminant in the sampled atmosphere.

length-tension relationship: This relationship describes the maximal force that a muscle, muscle fiber, or sarcomere can exert and its length.

lesion: A structural or functional alteration due to injury or disease.

lethal concentration "X" (LC_X): The concentration that was lethal to X percent of test animals. It may be expressed, for example, as LC_{50}, LC_{10}, etc.; these would represent the concentrations producing deaths in 50%, 10%, etc., of the exposed animals, respectively.

lethal concentration (LC): LC_{50} indicates atmospheric concentration of a substance at which half of a group of test animals die after a specified exposure time. LC0 indicates atmospheric concentration at which no deaths occur.

lethal dose "X" (LD_X): The dose that was lethal to X percent of test animals. The amount of a chemical, per unit of body weight, that will cause death in X percent of test animals. Most commonly used as LD_{50}, the dose producing deaths in 50% of the dosed animals.

lethal dose (LD): LD_{50} indicates a dose that kills half of a group of test animals. LD_0 indicates a dose at which no deaths occur.

leukopenia: A decrease below normal in the amount of leukocytes in the blood.

LEV: See *local exhaust ventilation*.

level: Logarithm of the ratio of one quantity to a reference quantity of the same kind. The base of the logarithm, the reference quantity, and the kind of level must be specified.

levers: Levers consist of a resisting load, a fulcrum (axis of rotation), and a motive force. The musculoskeletal system is a system of levers in which the bones are rigid bodies and the muscles are the force actuators.

LFL: See *lower flammable limit*.

L_I: See *sound intensity level*.

lifetime cancer risk estimate: The result of the exposure and toxicity assessments of a carcinogen. Represents the upper bound of the probability of an individual developing cancer as a result of lifetime exposure to the chemical.

ligament: 1. Cord-like tissue that connects bone to bone. 2. A flexible, dense, white fibrous connective tissue joining, and sometimes encapsulating, the articular surfaces of bones.

limit of detection (LOD): A stated limiting value designating the lowest concentration that can be detected and that is specific to the analytical procedure used. (See also *minimum detectable level*.)

limit of quantification (LOQ): A stated limiting value designating the lowest concentration that can be quantified with confidence and that is specific to the analytical procedure used.

liquid: A state of matter in which the substance is a formless fluid that flows in accord with the law of gravity.

liter (L): An SI unit of volume limited to capacity in dry measure and fluid measure (both liquids and gases). No prefixes except milli- (mL) or micro- (μL) should be used. (Also known as "litre," "cubic decimeter.")

LOAEL: See *lowest observable adverse effect level*.

local area network: A local area network (LAN) usually serves a limited area such as a building, department, or office. The LAN has a central computer called a server that runs the network software and controls access to the files and peripherals, such as printers.

local effects: Actions of chemicals that occur in a tissue only at the site of exposure, without being distributed into the organism. The opposite are systemic effects, actions of chemicals that occur in tissues other than the site of exposure, and require that the chemical be absorbed (via ingestion, inhalation, or dermal penetration) and transported to its target(s) via the blood stream.

local exhaust ventilation (LEV): An industrial ventilation system that captures and removes emitted contaminants before dilution into the workplace ambient air can occur.

LOD: See *limit of detection.*

logic chart: A flow chart designed to assist detector tube users in interpreting the results of a series of measurements.

lognormal distribution: 1. Particle size distribution characterized by a bell-shaped or Gaussian distribution shape when plotted on a logarithmic size scale. (See also *geometric standard deviation.*) 2. The distribution of a random variable that has the property that the logarithms of its values are normally distributed.

loose-fitting facepiece: A respiratory inlet covering that is designed to form a partial seal with the face, does not cover the neck and shoulders, and may or may not offer head protection against impact and penetration.

LOQ: See *limit of quantification.*

loss: Usually refers to the conversion of static pressure to heat in components of the ventilation system (i.e., "the hood entry loss").

low-dose extrapolation models: Mathematical models used to extend a dose-response curve beyond known data points representing higher dose levels. A number of models, including the single-hit, multihit, multistage, and linearized multistaged models, seem to fit the known data points equally well but result in widely varying estimates of response at lower dose levels.

lower boundary of working range: Refers to the contaminant concentration that may be quantitated at a specific air volume when the mass of contaminant is equal to the LOQ.

lower explosive limit (LEL): See *flammable limits, lower flammable limit.*

lower flammable limit (LFL): The minimum concentration, as a percentage, of flammable gas or vapor mixed with air that can be ignited. Also referred to as the lower explosive limit (LEL). See *flammable limits, upper flammable limit.*

lowest lethal concentration (LC_{Lo}): The lowest concentration of a substance in air that has been reported to have caused death in test animals.

lowest lethal dose (LD_{Lo}): The lowest dose of a substance reported to have caused death in test animals.

lowest toxic concentration (TC_{Lo}): The lowest concentration of a substance shown to have produced an adverse health effect in humans or test animals.

lowest toxic dose (TD_{Lo}): The lowest dose reported to cause toxic effects in humans or test animals.

lowest observable adverse effect level (LOAEL): Lowest exposure level at which there are statistically or biologically significant increases in frequency or severity of adverse effects between the exposed population and its appropriate control group.

L_p: See *sound pressure level.*

LSO: See *Laser Safety Officer.*

lumen: The light flux on 1 square foot (ft^2) of an area, every part of which is 1 foot from a point source having a luminous intensity of one candle.

luminance: 1. Brightness as perceived by the eye (just visible wavelengths). 2. The ratio of the luminous intensity in a given direction of an infinitesimal element of a surface containing the point under consideration, to the orthogonally projected area of the element on a plane perpendicular to the given direction.

M

m^3: Cubic meter; 1 cubic meter of air is equal to 1,000 liters of air.

MA: See *mechanical advantage*.

macromolecules: High molecular weight biochemicals such as proteins, phospholipids, glycosides, nucleic acids, and their mixed analogs like glycolipids, lipoproteins, and chromatin (nuclear protein/DNA complex).

magnetic field: One of the elementary fields in nature; it is found in the vicinity of a magnetic body or current-carrying medium and, along with electric field, in a light wave.

magnetic flux density: A vector quantity that is used as a quantitative measure of magnetic field. The force on a charged particle moving in the field is equal to the particle's charge times the cross product of the particle's velocity with the magnetic induction. (Also known as "magnetic displacement," "magnetic induction," "magnetic vector.")

magnetic-field strength (H): An auxiliary vector field, used in describing magnetic phenomena, whose curl, in the case of static charges and currents, equals the free current density vector, independent of the magnetic permeability of the material. (Also known as "magnetic field intensity," "magnetic force.")

main: 1. Pipe or duct for distributing or collecting flowing fluid from various branches. 2. The regulated compressed air piped to pneumatic controls.

mainframe computer: A mainframe computer is a very large, powerful computer with extensive data storage and processing capabilities that can support many simultaneous users. They are the largest computers made today, followed by minicomputers, and then by personal computers.

maintainability: The probability that an item that has failed (in the reliability sense) can be restored (i.e., repaired or replaced) within a stated period of time.

MAK: Maximum allowable concentration.

malformation: Defective or abnormal formation.

malignant: Tending to become progressively worse and to lead to death; often used to describe tumors that grow in size and also spread throughout the body.

management commitment: Management commitment can be demonstrated by the following activities: 1) clearly state a work site policy on safety and health so that all personnel will understand the priority of safety and health protection in relation to other organizational values; 2) establish and communicate a clear goal for the safety program and objectives for meeting that goal; 3) provide for and encourage employee involvement in the structure and operation of the safety program; 4) assign and communicate responsibility for all aspects of the safety program; 5) provide adequate authority and resources to responsible parties so that assigned responsibilities can be met; 6) hold people accountable for meeting responsibilities; and 7) review program operations at least annually to evaluate successes and identify deficiencies that should be corrected.

management of hazardous waste: The implied control and environmentally sound handling of hazardous waste during the phases of generation, storage, processing for recovery or reuse, transporting, treating, and discharging into the air and water or discarding onto the soil.

manifold: A holder for more than one detector tube. When attached to the sampling pump, it permits simultaneous sampling.

man-made mineral fibers (MMMF): amorphous fibers made from rock, ceramic, slag, or glass. Short term exposure effects of these agents are mostly skin related and involve itching, rashes, or burning. MMMFs may also irritate the upper respiratory system (nose and throat) and may result in bronchitis. Long term effects involve scarring of the lung.

manometer: An instrument for measuring pressure; essentially a U-tube partially filled with a liquid (usually water, mercury, or a light oil), so constructed that the amount of displacement of the liquid indicates the pressure being exerted on the instrument.

marker: The determinant to be measured in human body media.

maser: Microwave amplification by stimulated emission of radiation. When used in the term "optical maser," it is often interpreted as molecular amplification by stimulated emission of radiation.

mass: A quantitative measure of a body's resistance to being accelerated. Equal to the inverse of the ratio of the body's acceleration to the acceleration of a standard mass under otherwise identical conditions.

mass loading: The situation in which an accelerometer that is too heavy will weigh down the surface and give inaccurate results. To avoid mass loading, the general rule is that the accelerometer's mass should be no more than one-tenth (1/10) of the effective mass of the surface to which it is mounted. (See also *accelerometer.*)

mass median aerodynamic diameter (MMAD): Aerodynamic diameter of the particles that falls in the middle of the distribution of mass, the size of the particles for which half of the total mass is contributed by smaller particles and half by larger particles. (See also *aerodynamic diameter, cutoff particle diameter.*)

mass spectrometer: See *gas chromatograph.*

material safety data sheet (MSDS): A document containing information on a specific chemical substance's hazardous ingredients, their properties, and precautions for use.

maximally exposed individual (MEI): The single individual with the highest exposure in a given population.

McCready, Benjamin W.: American physician who wrote *On the Influence of Trades, Professions, and Occupations in the United States in the Production of Disease* (1837). His monograph is generally recognized as the first work on occupational medicine in the United States

MCS: See *multiple chemical sensitivity.*

mean: A statistical description of the "average." Mathematically, it is the sum of the results divided by the number of results. (See also *arithmetic mean, geometric mean.*)

mean free path: The average distance traveled between collisions by the molecules in a gas or vapor.

mean radiant temperature: The mean radiant temperature is the temperature of an imaginary black enclosure, of uniform wall temperature, that provides the same radiant heat loss or gain as the environment measured. It can be approximated from readings of globe temperature, dry bulb temperature, and air velocity.

measures of central tendency: Measures of the tendency of values in a set of data to be centered at some location. Measures of central tendency are, for example, the median, the mode, the arithmetic mean, and the geometric mean.

measures of dispersion or variability: Measures of the differences, scatter, or variability of values of a set of numbers. Commonly used measures of the dispersion or variability are the range, the standard deviation, the variance, and the coefficient of variation (or relative standard deviation).

mechanical advantage: The ratio of the force produced by a machine such as a lever or pulley to the force applied to it. (Also known as "force ratio.")

mechanization: 1. The replacement of human or animal labor by machines. 2. To produce or reproduce by machine.

MED: See *minimum erythemal dose.*

median: The middle value of a set of data when the data are ranked in increasing or decreasing order. If there are an even number of values in the set, the median is the arithmetic average of the two middle values.

median nerve: The nerve that runs down the center of the front of the arm and through the carpal tunnel. Swollen tendons pressing on the median nerve cause the symptoms of carpal tunnel syndrome.

Medical Literature Analysis and Retrieval System (Medlars®): The computerized system of databases and data banks offered by the National Library of Medicine. It is comprised of two computer subsystems: ELHILL® and TOXNET®.

medical monitoring: The measurement of chemical markers in body media known to be indicative of adverse health effects.

medical removal: Transfer of employees from jobs entailing exposures until they are sufficiently recovered to return to the work area without risk of impairment to health. Medical removal should never be used to avoid correction of excessive exposures.

medical screening: The performance of tests or procedures aimed at the early identification of subclinical or clinical disease. Usually, medical screening consists of the application of tests or procedures that provide an indication of the presence or absence of disease but are not as sensitive or specific as diagnostic tests.

medical surveillance: 1. A system for the identification and management of individual cases of illness, as well as for the early recognition of latent disease (screening) and for the provision of health promotion activities. 2. The measurement of chemical markers in body media that may be indicative of external exposure to chemical and physical agents and/or of potentially adverse effects. 3. The systematic collection, analysis, and evaluation of health data in the workplace to identify cases, patterns, or trends suggesting an adverse effect on workers' health. Medical surveillance can be used to evaluate the effectiveness of control activities.

medical testing: The medical testing of workers to detect organ dysfunction or disease before an individual would normally seek medical care and while intervention is still beneficial. Tests may indicate the presence of a disease, or an early sign of illness, and the need for additional testing.

medical treatment: The medical care given to work-related injuries or illnesses.

MEI: See *maximally exposed individual.*

melting point (MP): For a given pressure, the temperature at which the solid and liquid phases of the substance are in equilibrium.

menses: The discharge from the vagina during menstruation.

metabolic heat: Heat generated by the body's physical and chemical processes.

metabolism: Energy resulting from physical and chemical changes that are constantly occurring in the body. Term used for heat stress evaluation. (See also *heat stress.*)

metabolite: The stable reduction/oxidation (redox) product of catabolism of an exposing chemical.

metallic oxide semiconductor (MOS) sensor: A solid-state sensor used to detect ppm and combustible concentrations of gases. It can be used to detect a variety of compounds including nitro, amine, alcohol, and halogenated hydrocarbons, as well as a limited number of inorganic gases.

metastable: An excited state of a nucleus, indicated with a letter "m" in the mass number, which will decay by an isomeric transition with the emission of a gamma.

meter: A basic unit of length or distance in the SI system of units. (Also known as "metre.")

methemoglobinemia: The presence of hemoglobin in the oxidized state in the blood.

methods study: An analysis of the methods in use, of the means and potentials for their improvement, and of reducing costs.

mg: See *milligram.*

mg/kg: Milligrams per kilogram body weight; an expression of dosage.

mg/m^3: Air sampling measurement in milligrams (of contaminant) per cubic meter (of air).

microbar: A unit of pressure, commonly used in acoustics, which equals 1 micropascal (μPa). A reference point for the decibel is 20 micronewtons per meters squared (mN/m^2).

microbe: A microorganism, especially a bacterium of a pathogenic nature.

microbiology: The study of microorganisms, including algae, bacteria, fungi, viruses, and protozoa.

microclimate: The conditions such as temperature, humidity, and motion of air within an enclosure or outdoor limited area.

microenvironment: A well-defined place (such as a home, office, or car) in which a chemical or biological agent is present in a uniform manner.

micrometer: A unit of length, one millionth of a meter (one thousandth of a millimeter). (Also known as "micrometre.")

micron: 1. Greek mu (μ); often used interchangeably for micrometer, but micrometer is the preferred usage. 2. A unit of length equal to 10-4 centimeters, approximately 1/26,000 of an inch.

micronucleus: A small nucleus; in eukaryotic organisms, micronuclei are produced when chromosomes are broken and the fragments are left in the cytoplasm following cell division.

microsecond: One-millionth of a second.

microwave: Any electromagnetic radiation having a wavelength in the approximate range of from 1 millimeter to 1 meter; the region of the electromagnetic spectrum between infrared and short wave-radio lengths.

microwave radiation: A subset of RF radiation that occupies the spectral region between 300 GHz and 300 MHz.

midstream urine: A urine sample taken with the first couple of mL discarded to eliminate potential microorganisms or semen.

MIG: Metal inert gas; a type of welding.

milestones: Interim goals in the process of eliminating a problem that help evaluate the success of the solution.

milliamp: One-thousandth of an amp.

milligram (mg): One-thousandth of a gram.

milliliter (mL): One-thousandth of a liter.

millimeter (mm): One-thousandth of a meter, or one-tenth of a centimeter.

Mine Safety and Health Administration (MSHA): Established by the Mine Safety and Health Act of 1977, this agency is part of the U.S. Department of Labor. MSHA has the responsibility to set standards for and conduct inspections of working conditions in mines and mining-related industries.

minimum detectable level: The limit of detection for an analytical method is the minimum concentration of the constituent or species of interest that can be observed by the instrument and distinguished from instrument noise with a specified degree of probability. For example, one approach used is to make repeated measurements of the extractant liquid (trace metal analyses) and calculate the standard deviation of the results and hence the desired statistical tolerance limit for instrumental noise (e.g., an upper 99% limit at 95% confidence). (See also *limit of detection.*)

minimum duct transport velocity: According to the ACGIH *Industrial Ventilation Manual*, "When solid material is present in the airstream, the duct velocity must be equal to or greater than the minimum air velocity required to move the particles in the air stream."

minimum erythemal dose (MED): The lowest dose of ultraviolet (UV) light to cause an erythemal response (skin reddening). From 250–304 nanometers (nm) ranged from 14–47 millijoules per cubic centimeters (mJ/cm^2) and increased dramatically above 313 nm.

miscible: Susceptible to being mixed; soluble in all proportions.

mismanagement of hazardous waste: The uncontrolled and environmentally unsound or indiscriminate handling of hazardous wastes, whether intentionally or unintentionally.

mist: A dispersion of suspended liquid particles, many large enough to be individually visible to the unaided eye. Generated by condensation from the gaseous to the liquid state or by breaking up a liquid into a dispersed state, such as splashing, foaming, or atomization. Mist forms when a finely divided liquid is suspended in the atmosphere. Examples are the oil mist produced during cutting and grinding operations, acid mists from electroplating, acid or alkali mist from picking operations, and paint spray mist from spraying operations. Particle size ranges are between 0.01 µm and 10.0 µm.

mixed exhaled breath: The breath that is naturally exhaled without forcing.

mixing box: A compartment in which two air supplies mix before being discharged. (Also known as "blending box" or "mixing unit.")

mixing factor: A dimensionless quantity used to adjust the volume of air moving in a space for poor air distribution.

mixture: Any combination of two or more chemicals if the combination is not, in whole or part, the result of a chemical reaction.

mL: See *milliliter.*

mm: See *millimeter.*

MMAD: See *mass median aerodynamic diameter.*

mmHg: Abbreviation for millimeter(s) of mercury.

mobilizing: Enlisting available resources to reach an identified goal and ultimately achieve the organization's vision.

mode: The value or values occurring most frequently in a sample of data.

modifying factor: Used in converting NOAELs/LOAELs to reference doses

(RfDs). Range from >0 to 10, reflects professional judgment of uncertainties not addressed by uncertainty factors.

moist air: ASHRAE defines moist air as "a binary (or two component) mixture of dry air and water vapor. The amount of water vapor varies from zero (dry air) to a maximum that depends on temperature and pressure."

molar gas volume: The volume (usually liters) occupied by 1 mole (usually gram mole) of gas.

mold: A downy or furry growth on the surface of organic matter, caused by fungi, especially in the presence of dampness or decay.

mole: Mass of a substance represented by 1 molecular weight or 1 molecular volume. If the mass is in pounds, the unit is a pound mole; in grams, the unit is a gram mole, in kilograms the unit is a kg mole or mol.

molecular volume: The volume occupied by 1 molecular weight of a gas (either kilogram molecular weight or gram molecular weight).

molecular weight: Weight (mass) of a molecule based on the sum of the atomic weights of the atoms that make up the molecule.

molecule: Generally the smallest particle of an element or a compound capable of retaining the physical properties and chemical identity of the substance in mass.

moment arm: The distance from the fulcrum to each force. (See also *levers*.)

moment of force: See *torque*.

moment of inertia: The measure of resistance to rotational change.

monitor: Periodic or continuous determination of the amount of contamination present in an occupied region; used as a safety measure for purposes of health protection.

monitoring instruments: A broad range of scientific equipment used for the purposes of collecting and/or measuring chemical levels.

monodisperse: Composed of particles with a single size or a small range of sizes. (See also *polydisperse*.)

monodisperse aerosol: An aerosol with a uniform size distribution having a geometric standard deviation of less than 1.1.

Monte Carlo: A repeated random sampling from the distribution of values for each of the parameters in a generic exposure or dose equation to derive an estimate of the distribution of exposures or doses in the population.

Monte Carlo analysis: A method that obtains a probabilistic approximation to the solution of a problem by using statistical sampling techniques.

MOS: See *metallic oxide semiconductor.*

motor neuron: An efferent nerve cell. For a muscle to reach its active state it must receive a signal from the nervous system via a nerve referred to as a motor neuron, at which time the muscle exerts tension on its skeletal attachments.

motor unit: A single motor neuron and the muscle fibers that it innervates. A muscle may have many motor units, ranging from a few hundred to up to a thousand per muscle.

mottling: Colored spots or blotches.

MP: See *melting point.*

mppcf: Million particles per cubic foot (of air).

MS: Mass spectrometer. See *gas chromatograph.*

MSDS: See *material safety data sheet.*

MSHA: See *Mine Safety and Health Administration.*

mucous membrane: The mucous-secreting membranes lining the hollow organs of the body (i.e., eyes, nose, mouth, etc.).

multilayer detector tube: A detector tube construction containing several filling layers. In addition to the indicating layer, the tube contains one or more prelayers, which act as a filter to remove interfering substances or for chemical conversion of the gas or vapor being measured. Such tubes may be used to determine qualitatively the classes of compounds present in the atmosphere sampled.

multimedia: Software that incorporates sound, video, text, and sometimes animation.

multiple chemical sensitivity (MCS): A condition resulting from exposure to toxic chemicals that affect the immune system, leading to multiple sensitivities to other chemicals and/or foods. Symptoms of MCS, which may be similar to those of sick building syndrome

(SBS), are often attributed to exposure to trace amounts of chemicals (especially those with perceptible odor) in indoor air.

multiple particle optical monitor: A real-time dust monitor used to measure aerosol concentrations.

mutagen: A substance or agent capable of altering the genetic material in a living cell.

mycotoxins: Secondary products of fungal metabolism. The chemical structures of mycotoxins are quite diverse, ranging from that of moniliformin ($C_4H_2O_3$) to complex polypeptides with molecular weights higher than 2,000.

N

N: See *newton.*

nail: The horny covering at the upper tip of fingers and toes.

nanofiber: a nano-object with two external dimensions at the nanoscale with a nanotube defined as a hollow nanofiber and a nanorod as a solid nanofiber.

nanometer: Unit of measurement for radiation wavelengths. One nanometer (nm) equals 10-6 millimeters or 10 angstrom units. (See also *angstrom.*)

nano-object: material with one, two, or three external dimensions in the size range from approximately 1–100 nm.

nanoparticle: a nano-object with all three external dimensions at the nanoscale.

nanoplate: a nano-object with one external dimension at the nanoscale.

nanotechnology: the manipulation of matter on a near-atomic scale to produce new structures, materials, and devices.

narcosis: Stupor or unconsciousness produced by chemical substances.

NAS: See *National Academy of Sciences.*

nasopharyngeal region: The space behind the posterior nasal orifices, above a horizontal plane through the lower margin of the palate.

National Academy of Sciences (NAS): A private, honorary organization of scholars in scientific and engineering research serving as advisory agency to the federal government.

National Cancer Institute (NCI): One of the National Institutes of Health, designed to expand existing scientific knowledge on cancer causes and prevention as well as on the diagnosis, treatment, and rehabilitation of cancer patients.

National Fire Protection Association (NFPA): An international organization that promotes fire protection and prevention. NFPA establishes safeguards (standards, etc.) against loss of life and property by fire. Headquarters are in Quincy, Mass.

National Institute for Occupational Safety and Health (NIOSH): Established by the Occupational Safety and Health Act of 1970, NIOSH is part of the Centers for Disease Control and Prevention within the U.S. Department of Health and Human Services. NIOSH, based in Cincinnati, Ohio, traces its origins to 1914 when the U.S. Public Health Service organized a division of Industrial Hygiene and Sanitation. NIOSH's responsibilities include research and recommending occupational health and safety standards.

National Institute of Standards and Technology (NIST): An agency of the U.S. Department of Commerce's Technology Administration. Originally established by Congress in 1901 as the National Bureau of Standards; its name was changed in 1988. NIST's primary mission is to promote U.S. economic growth by working with industry to develop and apply technology, measurement, and standards. Headquarters are in Gaithersburg, Md.

National Research Council (NRC): Develops and publishes emergency exposure limits such as CEGLs, EEGLs, and SPEGLs. Headquarters are in Washington, D.C.

National Safety Council (NSC): A nonprofit, international public service organization dedicated to improving the safety, health, and well-being of populations throughout the world. Total membership exceeds 18,500. Headquarters are in Itasca, Ill.

National Toxicology Program (NTP): Overseen by the U.S. Department of Health and Human Services.

natural wet bulb temperature (T_{nwb}): The temperature measured when the wetted wick covering the sensor is exposed only to naturally occurring air movements.

NCEL: New chemical exposure limit.

NCI: See *National Cancer Institute.*

near field: In noise measurement, this refers to a field in the immediate vicinity of the noise source where the sound pressure level does not follow the Inverse Square law.

necrosis: 1. Death of a cell or group of cells as a result of injury, disease, or other pathological state. 2. Tissue death.

negative-pressure device: See *negative-pressure respirator.*

negative-pressure respirator: A respirator in which the air pressure inside the respiratory inlet covering is negative during inhalation with respect to the ambient air pressure.

neoplasm: See *tumor.*

nephrotoxicant: A substance harmful to the kidney.

net force: The sum of all concurrent forces.

neural: Relating to the nervous system.

neuropathy: Functional disturbance or pathology of the nervous system; may be central (affecting the brain or spinal cord) or peripheral (affecting nerves outside the brain and spinal cord).

neurotoxicant: A substance harmful to nerves or the brain.

neurotransmitter: A substance (such as norepinephrine or acetylcholine) that transmits nerve impulses across a synapse.

neutral (handshake) position: Keeping the wrist straight to avoid joint deviation.

neutrino: Massless particle traveling at the speed of light; created in isobaric decay.

newton (N): In the meter-kilogram-second system, the unit of force required to accelerate a mass of 1 kilogram 1 meter per second; equal to 100,000 dynes. (See also *dyne.*)

NFPA: See *National Fire Protection Association.*

NHZ: See *nominal hazard zone.*

NIC: See *notice of intended change.*

NIOSH: See *National Institute for Occupational Safety and Health.*

NIPTS: See *noise-induced permanent threshold shift.*

NIR: See *nonionizing radiation.*

NIST: See *National Institute of Standards and Technology.*

nitrogen narcosis: Narcosis caused by gaseous nitrogen at high pressure in the blood. Produced in divers breathing air at depths of 100 ft (30 m) or more.

nitrogen-phosphorus detector: Highly sensitive and selective for nitrogen and phosphorous compounds, including amines and organophosphates. The detector is similar in principle to the flame ionization detector (FID), except that ionization occurs on the surface of an alkali metal salt, such as cesium bromide, rhobidium silicate, or potassium chloride. (Also known as a "thermionic" or "alkali flame detector.")

NITROX: Enriched oxygen mixtures used to increase total dive time.

NITTS: See *noise-induced temporary threshold shift.*

nm: See *nanometer.*

NMSC: See *nonmelanoma skin cancer.*

no observable adverse effect level (NOAEL): Exposure level at which there are no statistically or biologically significant increases in frequency or severity, or any adverse effects between the exposed population and its appropriate control group.

no observable effect level (NOEL): That quantity of a chemical to which laboratory animals are chronically exposed (expressed in parts per million [ppm] in their diets or mg/kg of body weight) that produces no effect when compared with control animals.

NOAEL: See *no observable adverse effect level.*

NOEL: See *no observable effect level.*

noise: Unwanted sound; unwanted because it can cause annoyance, interfere with speech or communication, and/or cause hearing impairment.

noise enclosure: Equipment that reduces the noise of a sound source by completely surrounding the source with a barrier material.

noise level: For airborne sound, unless specified to the contrary, noise level is the weighted sound pressure level called sound level; the weighting must be indicated.

noise reduction: See *attenuation.*

Noise Reduction Rating (NRR): A single-number rating of hearing protection. The higher the NRR, the higher the attenuation for a specific ideal situation (laboratory-fit of HPD).

noise-induced hearing loss: Hearing loss due to excessive exposure to noise.

noise-induced permanent threshold shift (NIPTS): A permanent loss in hearing sensitivity due to the destruction of sensory cells in the inner ear. This damage can be caused by long-term exposure to noise or by acoustic trauma.

noise-induced temporary threshold shift (NITTS): A temporary loss in hearing sensitivity. This loss can be a result of the acoustic reflex, short-term exposure to noise, or simply neural fatigue in the inner ear. With NITTS, hearing sensitivity will return to the pre-exposed level in a matter of hours or days (without continued excessive exposure).

nominal hazard zone (NHZ): Zone around the laser where the beam intensity exceeds the exposure limit.

nonbeam hazard: A hazardous agent, other than the beam, generated by the use of lasers (e.g., electricity, airborne contaminants, plasma radiation, fires, and explosions).

noncarcinogen: A chemical that exerts adverse health effects other than cancer.

noncompliance: Noncompliance with health and safety regulations.

nonflammable: Not easily ignited, or if ignited, not burning rapidly.

nongenotoxic chemicals: Toxic substances that do not interact directly with DNA.

nonionizing radiation (NIR): Photons with energies less than 12.4 eV are considered to have insufficient energy to ionize matter, and are nonionizing in nature. The nonionizing spectral region includes the ultraviolet (UV), visible, infrared (IR), radio-frequency (RF), and extremely low frequency (ELF) spectral regions.

nonmandatory guidelines: OSHA standards for fire protection (29 CFR 1910.156 through .165) reference many of the NFPA's national consensus standards as nonmandatory guidelines that would be considered acceptable in complying with requirements of Title 29, Part 1910, Subpart L.

nonmelanoma skin cancer (NMSC): A type of skin cancer and basal cell carcinoma. Four variables have been implicated in NMSC: 1) lifetime sun exposure; 2) the intensity and duration of the UV-B component in sunlight; 3) genetic predisposition; and 4) other factors unrelated to sunlight, such as exposure to ionizing radiation and polycyclic aromatic hydrocarbons. (Also known as "cutaneous malignant melanoma.")

nonstochastic effect: The effect of radiation exposure on a population in which there is an assumed threshold dose that increases in effect with an increase in severity with an increase in dose. (See also *stochastic effect*).

nonthreshold: Characterizes a dose-response curve that passes through the origin of the graph indicating that any exposure will increase the probability of cancer occurrence. Used by the U.S. EPA for carcinogens. (See also *threshold*.)

nontraditional workplace: Usually typical offices, schools, shopping malls, and other public places. They are not normally considered workplaces where exposure occurs. These are locations that often suffer poor indoor air quality. Domestic residential environments may also be considered a nontraditional workplace.

normal distribution: An important symmetric continuous probability distribution characterized completely by two parameters: the mean and the standard deviation.

normal temperature and pressure (NTP): 298.15 K and 1 atmosphere, 760 mmHg.

notice of intended change (NIC): This term is unique to ACGIH. Chemicals appearing on the NIC list for at least one year serve as notice that a chemical has a TLV® proposed for the first time or that a current TLV is being changed. This procedure allows ample time for those with data or comments to come forth.

noxious: Harmful to health.

nozzle, jet: The opening through which aerosol particles travel during sampling. Nozzles or jets restrict or confine the flow of air carrying the aerosol; nozzle sizes affect the airstream velocities (and the collection efficiency of the cascade impactor).

NRC: See *National Research Council.*

NRR: See *Noise Reduction Rating.*

NSC: See *National Safety Council.*

NTP: See *National Toxicology Program.*

NTP: See *normal temperature and pressure.*

nuclear binding force: That amount of energy required to separate the nucleus into its individual nucleons beyond the nuclear distance.

nuclear force: Short-range fundamental force in nature that is attractive and holds nucleons together at nuclear range.

Nuclear Regulatory Commission: An independent agency established by the Energy Reorganization Act of 1974 to regulate civilian use of nuclear materials. NRC is headed by a five-member Commission.

nucleon: Particle found in the nucleus; either a proton or a neutron.

nuclide: General term referring to any nucleus plus the orbital electrons (number of protons plus number of neutrons) in each energy state.

nuisance dust: Generally innocuous dust, not recognized as the direct cause of a serious pathological condition.

numerical extrapolation: Extension of dose-response relationship to dose levels below those observed in toxicological or epidemiological studies.

O

o.d.: Outside diameter.

occluded: Closed, shut, or blocked.

occupational cancer: Cancer caused by exposure to chemical or physical agents in the work environment.

occupational disease: Disease associated with a work environment, usually caused by a specific agent.

occupational exposure limit (OEL): A health-based workplace standard to protect workers from adverse exposure (e.g., PELs, TLVs®, RELs, WEELs, etc.).

occupational health: A discipline of environmental health. The profession specializes in the art and science of recognition, evaluation, and control of chemical, physical, and biological stressors or factors arising in or from the workplace that may cause discomfort or adverse health effects to workers or members of the community.

Occupational Health Psychology (OHP): the application of psychological principles to improving the quality of work-life and promoting the safety, health, and well being of people at work. OHP is multidisciplinary and draws upon public health, preventive medicine, nursing, industrial engineering, law, epidemiology, sociology, gerontology, and psychology to promote worker safety, health, and well being.

occupational health and safety (OHS) plan: A plan that at minimum should include specific instructions on personal protective equipment (PPE); lockout/tagout (LO/TO); confined space entry (CSE); security; spills and contingency plans; emergency procedures; phone numbers of the facility emergency coordinator, police, fire, ambulance and nearest hospital; locations of first aid kits; eye washes and showers; and the facility contractor OHS policy.

occupational hygiene audit: A process used to evaluate periodically the existence and the effectiveness of biological, chemical, ergonomic, and physical health and safety program elements present in a workplace.

occupational hygiene survey: An activity carried out by a qualified individual to measure and evaluate various biological, chemical, ergonomic, and physical parameters in the workplace or environment to determine their standings in relation to established health and safety standards.

Occupational Safety and Health Act (OSH Act) of 1970: In 1970, the U.S. Congress passed the OSH Act "to assure safe and healthful working conditions for working men and women by authorizing enforcement of the standards developed under the Act; by assisting and encouraging the states in their efforts to assure safe and healthful working conditions; by providing for research, information, education, and training in the field of occupational safety and health; and for other purposes" (Public Law 91–596).

Occupational Safety and Health Administration (OSHA): Established by the OSH Act of 1970, OSHA is located within the U.S. Department of Labor. The agency's responsibilities include promulgating occupational safety and health standards and inspecting workplaces to ensure compliance with these standards.

Occupational safety and health standards: Defined in §3(8) of the OSH Act to mean standards that require the adoption of "practices, means, methods, operations, or processes, reasonably necessary or appropriate to provide safe or healthful employment and places of employment."

occupied space: Any space inside a building occupied at various times.

octave bands: 1. A frequency range in which the ratio of upper to lower frequency is 2:1. 2. A measurement of the broad range of frequencies humans can hear. Frequencies are normally divided into nine octave bands. An octave is defined as a range of frequencies extending from one frequency to exactly double that frequency. Each octave band is named for the center frequency (geometric mean) of the band.

OD: See *optical density.*

odor character: Used to describe a substance's odor (e.g., "fishy," "rancid," "bananas").

odor threshold: In general, the lowest concentration of gas or a material's vapor that can be detected by odor. The detection threshold is the lowest concentration of odorant that will elicit a sensory response in the olfactory receptors of a specified percentage of a given population. The recognition threshold is the minimum concentration that is recognized as having a characteristic odor quality by a specified percentage of a given population. (See also odor character, hedonic tone.)

OEL: See *occupational exposure limit.*

off-specification: Low quality. (Also known as "off-spec.")

ohm (W): The unit of electrical resistance in the rationalized meter-kilogram-second system of units, equal to the resistance through which a current of 1 amphere will flow when there is a potential difference of 1 volt across it.

Ohm's law: The current, I, through an electrical circuit is related directly to the difference in potential, V, and inversely related to the resistance, R, or I (amperes) = V/R (volts/ohms).

OHS: Occupational health and safety. See *occupational health and safety plan.*

olfactory: Relating to the sense of smell.

OPC: See *optical particle counter.*

operating plan: A plan that generally describes where the organization would like to be in one to two years.

operating system: The operating system is a piece of software that forms the interface between the user's program and the computer hardware.

optical density (OD): The quantity used to specify the ability of protective eyewear to attenuate optical radiation, where OD = $\log_{10}$ (ML/EL).

optical particle counter (OPC): A single-particle, direct-reading instrument that uses monochromatic light such as a laser or light-emitting diode or a broad band light source such as a tungsten filament lamp to illuminate aerosols.

optical radiation: A broad category of radiation that includes ultraviolet (UV), visible, and infrared (IR).

optimism: A disposition or tendency to look on the more favorable side of happenings or possibilities.

optimum risk: A risk level that balances the cost of the risk with the cost of risk mitigation.

organic: Term used to designate chemicals that contain carbon. To date nearly 1 million organic compounds have been synthesized or isolated. Many occur in nature; others are produced by chemical synthesis.

organic peroxide: An organic compound that contains the bivalent -O-O structure and may be considered a structural derivative of hydrogen peroxide where one or both of the hydrogen atoms has been replaced by an organic radical.

orifice: A small opening that controls flow rate of gases or liquids. Orifices are used in some hand-held detector tube pumps.

orifice plate: A plate with a relatively sharp-edged opening or orifice used to measure fluid flow rates based on pressure difference between the two sides of the plate.

origin: The point on a graph that represents zero on both the vertical and horizontal axes or lines.

O-ring: A ring made of rubber or latex to seal gaps around the impaction stages and to facilitate proper seating of the stage in the cascade impactor.

oscillate: To move back and forth in a steady uninterrupted rhythm; to vary between alternate extremes, usually within a definable period.

OSH Act (of 1970): See *Occupational Safety and Health Act of 1970.*

OSHA: See *Occupational Safety and Health Administration.*

OSHA compliance: Sampling being done for the purpose of ensuring that airborne chemical levels in the workplace are within allowable limits specified by the Occupational Safety and Health Administration.

OSHRC: Occupational Safety and Health Review Commission.

otologist: A physician who specializes in diseases of the ear.

outlier: An extreme value that questionably belongs to the group of values with which it is associated. If the chance probability of its being a valid member of the group is very small, the questionable value is thereby "detected" and may be eliminated from the group based on further investigation of the data.

overload: In the workplace, too much information, which might lead to fatigue.

oxidant: Oxidizing agent (Also known as "electron sink").

oxidation: In a literal sense, a reaction in which a substance combines with oxygen provided by an oxidizer or oxidizing agent.

oxidizer: A chemical other than a blasting agent or explosive that initiates or promotes combustion in other materials, causing fire either by itself or through the release of oxygen or other gases.

oxidizing agent: A chemical that produces oxygen readily and gains electrons during the reaction; may start or assist the combustion of other materials.

oxygen deficiency: An atmosphere having less than the percentage of oxygen found in normal air. Normally, air contains about 21% oxygen at sea level. When the oxygen concentration in air is reduced to approximately 16%, many individuals become dizzy, experience a buzzing in the ears, and have a rapid heartbeat. OSHA indicates 19.5% as the lower limit of oxygen acceptable in industry.

oxygen toxicity: Harmful effects of breathing oxygen at pressures greater than atmospheric.

oxygen-deficient atmosphere: An atmosphere containing less than 19.5% oxygen by volume. (See *OSHA 1910.146.*)

oxygen-enriched atmosphere: An atmosphere containing more than 23.5% oxygen by volume. (See *OSHA 1910.146*)

ozone: A colorless gas with a characteristic odor that is produced in ambient air during the photochemical oxidation of combustion products such as nitrogen oxides and hydrocarbons. It can also result from the operation of electrical motors, photocopy machines, and electrostatic air cleaners in occupational environments.

P

Pa: See *pascal.*

PAH(s): See *polycyclic aromatic hydrocarbons.*

parameter: Limit of consideration in a study or investigation.

pareto analysis: An analysis tool based on the ratio that often 80% of the problems in a process are the result of only 20% of the potential causes. Pareto analysis is used to isolate and identify areas of significant concern from a group of many potential concerns.

partial pressure: Pressure of a gas in a mixture equal to the pressure that it would exert if it occupied the same volume alone at the same temperature. (See also *Dalton's law.*)

particle: A small discrete object, often having a density approaching the intrinsic density of the bulk material. It may be chemically homogenous or contain a variety of chemical species. It may consist of solid or liquid material or both. (See also *aerosol.*)

particle bounce: Rebound of particles that fail to adhere after impacting on a collecting surface.

particle diffusivity (D_B): Aerosol particles in a gaseous medium are bombarded by collisions with individual gas molecules that are in Brownian motion. This causes the particles to undergo random displacements known as diffusion. The particle parameter that describes this process is the particle diffusivity, DB. (Also known as "diffusion coefficient.")

particle size distribution: A relationship expressing the quantity of a particle property associated with particles in a given size range.

particulate: Particle of solid or liquid matter.

partition coefficient (K_m): 1. In the equilibrium distribution of a solute between two liquid phases, the constant ratio of the solute's concentration in the upper phase to its concentration in the lower phase. 2. The ratio at equilibrium of penetrant concentration in the SC to that in the vehicle.

parts per billion by volume (ppb): Sometimes written as ppbv or ppb v/v; an expression of concentration as a volume ratio, usually parts of contaminant per billion parts of air. It may also be used to express dietary exposure concentration as a weight ratio.

parts per million by volume (ppm): Sometimes written as ppmv or ppm v/v; an expression of concentration as a volume ratio, usually parts of contaminant per million parts of air. It may also be used to express dietary exposure concentration as a weight ratio.

part-time work: Where a job is split among several people, each of whom works part of the shift.

PAS: See *photoacoustic spectroscopy.*

pascal (pa): 1. A unit of pressure equal to the pressure resulting from a force of 1 newton acting uniformly over an area of 1 square meter (m^2). 2. A unit of pressure equal to kg/m sec^2 (part of the internationally adopted SI system of units).

passive dosimeter: A sample collection device based on the mass transport of the air contaminant to the sorbent by gaseous diffusion. It can incorporate direct-reading colorimetry to determine the concentration of a chemical in the air.

passive sampling: The collection of airborne gases and vapors at a rate controlled by a physical process such as diffusion through a static air layer or permeation through a membrane without the active movement of air through an air sampler.

pathogenicity: The act of producing disease.

pathway: The course a chemical or pollutant takes from the source to the organism exposed.

PCB: Polychlorinated biphenyl.

PEL: See *permissible exposure limit.*

PEL–C: See *permissible exposure limit–concentration.*

PEL–STEL: See *permissible exposure limit–short-term exposure limit.*

PEL–TWA: See *permissible exposure limit–time-weighted average.*

penetration: The flow of a chemical through zippers, weak seams, pinholes, cuts, or imperfections in the protective clothing on a nonmolecular level.

perceived risk: The risk that the individual believes exists.

percent volatile: Percent volatile by volume is the percentage of a liquid or solid (by volume) that will evaporate at an ambient temperature of 70°F (unless some other temperature is specified). Examples such as butane, gasoline, and paint thinner (mineral spirits) are 100% volatile; their individual evaporation rates vary, but in time each will evaporate completely.

performance audit: A quantitative analysis or check with a material or device with known properties or characteristics. The audit is performed by a person different from the routine operator/analyst using audit standards and audit equipment different from the calibration equipment. Such audits are conducted periodically to check the accuracy of a project measurement system. Some performance audits might require the identification of specific elements or compounds, in lieu of, or in addition to, a quantitative analysis. For some performance audits it may be impractical or unnecessary to have a person different than the routine operator/analyst; in these cases the routine operator/analyst must not know the concentration or value of the audit standards until the audit is completed. The other conditions of the audit must still be met (that is, the audit standards must be different from the calibration standards, and the audit device must be different from the calibration device).

performance measures: The observable demonstration that the individual has learned a desired instructional objective.

performance standards: 1. Regulatory requirements limiting the concentrations of designated organic compounds, particulate matter, and hydrogen chloride in emissions from incinerators. 2. Operating standards established by the U.S. EPA for various permitted pollution control systems, asbestos inspections, and various program operations and maintenance requirements. 3. Performance standards state the object to be obtained or the hazard to be abated.

perfusion: The pumping of a fluid through a tissue or organ by way of an artery.

periodic motion: Any motion that is repeated at regular intervals. (See also *oscillate*.)

periodic vibration: Vibration is considered periodic if the motion of a particle repeats itself considerably over time.

periodicity: The frequency at which tests are given.

peripheral nervous system (PNS): The autonomic nervous system, the cranial nerves, and the spinal nerves including their associated sensory receptors.

peripheral neuropathy: Any disease affecting the peripheral nervous system.

permeability: A factor, characteristic of a material, that is proportional to the magnetic induction produced in a material divided by the magnetic-field strength; it is a tensor when these quantities are not parallel.

permeation: The movement of a chemical through a protective clothing barrier that has no visible holes.

permeation method: A method for preparing a known mixture of a low concentration gas for verification testing of detector tubes. Gas permeates the walls of a gas permeable vessel (permeation tube) into a mixing solution, where it is combined with the diluent gas (usually purified air). The test gas concentration is calculated from the permeation rate, the flow rate of the diluent gas, and the thickness of the walls of the permeation tube.

permeation rate: The rate of movement (mass flux) of the chemical through the barrier. The permeation rate is normally reported in mass per unit area per unit time (e.g., µg/cm/min) after equilibrium is reached and may be normalized for thickness.

permeation tube: A plastic tube in which is sealed a liquefied gas or volatile liquid that slowly permeates through the walls at a constant rate.

permissible concentration: Official term that replaces "threshold limit value." (See also *threshold limit value*.)

permissible dose: Amount of radiation that may be received by an individual within a specified period with expectation of no significantly harmful result.

permissible exposure limit (PEL): Established by OSHA (see *29 CFR 1910.1000, Subpart Z*). The permissible concentration in air of a substance to which nearly all workers may be repeatedly exposed 8 hours a day, 40 hours a week, for 30 years without adverse effects. (See also *PEL–C, PEL–STEL, PEL–TWA*.)

permissible exposure limit–concentration (PEL–C): An acceptable ceiling concentration. An employee's exposure to any material in 29 CFR 1910.1000, Table Z1 — the name of which is preceded by a C — shall at no time exceed the ceiling value given for that material in the table.

permissible exposure limit–short-term exposure limit (PEL–STEL): The employee's 15-min time-weighted average (TWA) exposure that shall not be exceeded at any time during a workday unless another time limit is specified in a parenthetical notation below the limit.

permissible exposure limit–time-weighted average (PEL–TWA): An 8-hour time-weighted average. An employee's exposure to any material listed in 29 CFR 1910.1000, Table Z2, in any 8-hour work shift of a 40-hour workweek shall not exceed the 8-hour time-weighted average limit given for that material in the table.

permissible heat exposure threshold limit values: A limit designed to provide a work temperature and wet bulb globe temperature (WBGT) combination so that 95% of the workers would not have a deep body temperature exceeding 38°C. Work load categories are light work, <200 kcal/hour (233 watts); moderate work, 200–350 kcal/hour (233–407 watts); and heavy work, 350–500 kcal/hour (407–581 watts).

permit-required confined space: A confined space that has one or more of the following characteristics: 1) contains or has the potential to contain a hazardous atmosphere; 2) contains a material that has the potential for engulfing an entrant; 3) has an internal configuration such that an entrant could be trapped or asphyxiated by inwardly converging walls or by a floor that slopes downward and tapers to a smaller cross section; or 4) contains any other recognized serious safety or health hazard. Also known as a "permit space." (See *OSHA 1910.146.*)

permittivity: A fundamental quantity that describes the interaction of matter with the electric field. Permittivity of tissue depends on the water content of the tissue and the frequency of the electric field.

person-based: One of two basic approaches used to produce beneficial change in people, the other being behavior-based.

personal computer: The basic personal computer consists of a central processing unit (CPU), random access memory (RAM), a hard disk drive, a floppy disk drive, CD-ROM (computer disk, read-only memory), a video card, and a monitor (often called a VDT [video display terminal] or VDU [video display unit]).

personal mastery: An employee's commitment to one's own learning, as demonstrated by a desire to focus one's energies by continually aligning one's personal growth activities with the needs of the organization.

personal protective equipment (PPE): Equipment (e.g., gloves, eye protection, respirators) designed to protect individuals from biohazards.

personal sampler: Air-sampling instrument developed in the United States for estimating exposure of individual workers to air contaminants.

personal sampling: The collection of airborne chemicals in the worker's breathing zone by having the worker wear sampling equipment throughout the workday.

personnel enclosure: When there are multiple noisy sound sources in a room and a low number of operators, it is sometimes useful to enclose the employees instead of the equipment.

perturbation: Any effect that makes a small modification in a physical system.

PF&ID: See *process flow and instrumentation diagram.*

pH: 1. The symbol relating the hydrogen ion (H+) concentration to that of a given standard solution. A pH of 7 is neutral. Numbers increasing from 7 to 14 indicate greater alkalinity. Numbers decreasing from 7 to 0 indicate greater acidity. 2. Means used to express the degree of acidity or alkalinity of a solution with neutrality indicated as 7.

phosphenes: The sensation of flashes of light within the eye caused by EMF.

photoacoustic spectroscopy (PAS): A spectroscopic technique for investigating solid and semisolid materials, in which the sample is placed in a closed chamber filled with a gas such as air and illuminated with a monochromatic of any desired wavelength, with intensity modulated at some suitable acoustic frequency; absorption of radiation results in a periodic heat flow from the sample, which generates sound that is detected by a sensitive microphone attached to the chamber.

photoconjunctivitis: See *photokeratitis.*

photoionization detector (PID): A portable, general survey instrument used for detecting leaks, surveying plants to identify problem areas, evaluating source emissions, monitoring ventilation efficiency, evaluating work practices, and determining the need for personal protective equipment for hazardous waste site workers.

photokeratitis: An injury to the eye that results from acute, high-intensity exposure to UV-B and UV-C. Commonly referred to as "arc eye" or "welder's flash" by workers, this injury results from exposure of the unprotected eye to a welding arc or other artificial sources rich in UV-B and UV-C. Sunlight exposure produces these sequelae only in environments where highly reflective materials are present, such as snow ("snow blindness") or sand. (Also known as "photoconjunctivitis.")

photometer: An instrument used in measuring the intensity of light, especially in determining its relative intensity from different sources.

photon energy: Photon energy describes the energy possessed by electromagnetic energy when characterized as discrete bundles, as described by quantum theory.

The unit of photon energy is the Joule (J) or the electron volt (eV).

photosensitivity: Reaction to light that causes the skin to become sensitive. Photosensitivity includes two types of reactions: phototoxicity and photoallergy. Phototoxicity is more common and affects all individuals if the UV dose or the dose of the photosensitizer is high enough. Photoallergy is an acquired altered reactivity in the exposed skin resulting from an immunologic response. An agent, such as many medications, some sunscreen agents, plants (e.g., figs, parsley, limes, parsnips, and pinkrot celery), and industrial photosensitizers (including coal tar, pitch, anthracene, naphthalene, phenanthrene, thiophene, and many phenolic agents) can instigate photosensitivity.

physical asphyxiant: See *asphyxiant.*

physical hazard: A chemical for which there is scientifically valid evidence that it is a combustible liquid, a compressed gas, explosive, flammable, an organic peroxide, an oxidizer, pyrophoric, unstable (reactive), or water-reactive.

physical work capacity (PWC): The maximum amount of oxygen that an individual can consume per minute.

physiological heat exposure limit: An exposure limit based on a physiological response.

physiology: The science and study of the functions or actions of living organisms.

PID: See *photoionization detector.*

piezoelectric mass sensor: A sensor based on the principle that when crystalline materials are mechanically stressed by compression or tension they produce a voltage proportional to the stress. When these crystals are subjected to an electric current, they oscillate, and the natural vibrational frequency depends on the thickness and density of the crystal.

pion: The exchange particle in a nucleus.

piston pump: A hand-held sampling pump that draws a fixed volume of air. It operates by pulling and locking a piston into position while the sample is drawn into the detector tube. The piston is released after the sampling time has elapsed.

pitch: See *frequency.*

pitot tube: A small bore tube inserted into a flowing stream with its orifice facing the stream to measure total pressure. The term is often used for a double tube instrument from which the flow velocity can be calculated with one orifice facing the flowing stream to register total pressure and the other perpendicular to the stream to register static pressure.

Planck's constant: Constant of proportionality relating the quantum of energy that can be possessed by radiation to the frequency of that radiation; value is approximately 6.625×10^{-27} erg/sec. (See also *quantum.*)

plane wave: 1. Wave in which the wavefront is a plane surface; a wave whose equiphase surfaces form a family of parallel planes. 2. To understand a plane wave, consider an ideal point-source antenna that emits radiation in an isotropic pattern. The radiation pattern would be spherical (uniform in all directions), so near this antenna a receiver detects curvature in the approaching field. However, if removed sufficiently far from the source, some distance into the far field, a receiver would sample only a very small area of an immense curved wavefront. In the local region of space occupied by the receiver, it would detect a flat, or planar front; hence, the name, plane wave.

plasma: The liquid that does not contain the cellular components of blood on sitting or mild centrifugation of a blood sample.

plenum: A large air compartment or chamber connected to the slot that functions to distribute the static pressure (i.e., suction) evenly across the slot area.

plenum chamber: 1. An air compartment at a pressure slightly above atmospheric. 2. In an air distribution system, that part of the casing, or an air chamber attached to the furnace, from which the air duct system or direct discharge heat outlet delivers heated or cooled air.

plenum velocity: Air velocity in the plenum. If you provide a uniform air distribution with slot-type hoods, the maximum plenum velocity should be one-half the slot velocity or less.

Pliny the Elder: A Roman scholar who in 50 A.D. identified the use of animal bladders to prevent the inhalation of lead dust and fume.

pneumoconiosis: A chronic disease of the lungs resulting from the inhalation of various kinds of dusts. The pneumoconioses that include siderosis (iron oxide), silicosis (free silica), asbestosis (asbestos), etc., generally require a period of years for development.

PNS: See *peripheral nervous system.*

policy deployment: The process by which a company develops policies, including improvement targets, and deploys them throughout the organization. This deployment is performed in a manner that permits the operating organizations to establish supporting goals and targets, along with a method to measure performance.

pollutants (air): 1. Generally, any substance introduced into the environment that adversely affects the usefulness of a resource. 2. Any substance in air that could, in high enough concentration, harm man, other animals, vegetation, or material. Pollutants may include almost any natural or artificial composition of airborne matter capable of being airborne. They may be in the form of solid particles, liquid droplets, gases, or in combination thereof. Generally, they fall into two main groups: 1) those emitted directly from identifiable sources; and 2) those produced in the air by interaction between two or more primary pollutants, or by reaction with normal atmospheric constituents, with or without photoactivation. Exclusive of pollen, fog, and dust, which are of natural origin, about 100 contaminants have been identified and fall into the following categories: solids, sulfur compounds, volatile organic chemicals, nitrogen compounds, oxygen compounds, halogen compounds, radioactive compounds, and odors.

polycyclic aromatic hydrocarbons (PAHs): Organic compounds, usually formed from incomplete combustion, that might pose a risk of cancer.

polydisperse: Composed of particles with a range of sizes.

polymerization: A chemical reaction in which one or more small molecules combine to form larger molecules. A hazardous polymerization is a reaction that takes place at a rate that releases large amounts of energy. If hazardous polymerization can occur with a given material, it will be cited in the material safety data sheet (MSDS).

poor warning properties: A substance with odor, taste, or irritation effects that are not detectable or not persistent at concentrations at or below the exposure limit.

popliteal height: The distance from the floor to the joint in back of the knee.

portal of entry: See *route of entry.*

positive beta ray: The high-speed particle with characteristics of a positron emitted from a nucleus in positive beta decay.

positive-pressure device: See positive-pressure respirator.

positive-pressure respirator: A respirator in which the pressure inside the respiratory inlet covering is normally positive with respect to ambient air pressure.

positron: The positive electron.

Pott, Sir Percival: English physician who in 1775 described the relationship between scrotal cancer and work as a chimney sweep as related to the lack of hygiene measures.

power density: The amount of power per unit area in a radiated microwave or other electromagnetic field, usually expressed in units of watts per square centimeter.

powered air-purifying respirator (PAPR): An air-purifying respirator that uses a blower to force the ambient atmosphere through air-purifying elements to the inlet covering.

ppb: See *parts per billion by volume.*

PPE: See *personal protective equipment.*

PPE controls: The use of PPE to protect individuals.

ppm: See *parts per million by volume.*

precautionary principle: See prudent avoidance.

precision: The degree of agreement of repeated measurements of the same type using a specified sampling device; usually expressed as the coefficient of variation or relative standard deviation of replicate measurements.

pre-classifier: A device that removes particles ahead of a particle sensor or sampler, often similar to the particle removal occurring ahead of the respiratory region of interest. (Also known as "pre-collector," "pre-cutter," or "pre-separator.")

pre-collector: See *pre-classifier*.

pre-cutter: See *pre-classifier*.

prelayer: A layer in a detector tube preceding the indicating layer. Prelayers usually are nonindicating and are used to remove humidity, control interferences, or provide actual reaction components.

premolded earplug: A type of hearing protector that is preformed and simply inserted in the ear.

presbycusis: The hearing loss normally occurring due to age because of the degeneration of the nerve cells due to the ordinary wear and tear of the aging process.

pre-separator: See *pre-classifier*.

pressure: 1. Thermodynamically, the normal force exerted by a homogeneous liquid or gas, per unit of area, on the wall of the container. 2. Force exerted per unit area.

pressure drop: 1. Loss in pressure (as from one end of a refrigerant line to the other) from friction, static, heat, etc. 2. The differential pressure across some element of a system, such as a valve or orifice. (Also known as "backpressure.")

pressure-demand respirator: A positive-pressure atmosphere-supplying respirator that admits respirable gas to the facepiece when the positive pressure is reduced inside the facepiece by inhalation.

preventive maintenance: A systematic procedure by which laboratory components that are most likely to fail are replaced and instruments recalibrated to ensure that the laboratory operates at maximum efficiency.

primary barriers: Protection of the worker and environment in the immediate area of potential exposure. Biosafety cabinets, sealed centrifuge rotors, glove boxes, high efficiency particulate aerosol (HEPA)-filtered animal enclosures, and PPE (especially gloves, eye protection, and sometimes respirators) are important primary barriers.

primary prevention: Actions taken to prevent initiation of the disease process by removing or reducing risk factors.

primary reader: The person empowered to take action based on the report.

primary standard: 1. A measurement device that is directly traceable to the National Institute of Standards and Technology (NIST). Examples of traceable primary standards for volume are soap bubble flow meters and spirometers. 2. A material having a known property that is stable, that can be accurately measured or derived from established physical or chemical constants, and that is readily reproducible. 3. Devices such as flowmeters that base their calibration on direct and measurable linear dimensions such as the length and diameter of a cylinder.

primary prevention: preventing disease before it develops, for example, through changing stressful job characteristics, organizational changes, or changes in the economic or political context in which people work.

prime movers: Skeletal muscles that are responsible for the primary action at the joint.

prion: Any of a group of tiny infectious agents composed mainly or entirely of protein: though lacking in demonstrable nucleic acid, prions are capable of self-replication and are thought to be the cause of various degenerative diseases of the nervous systems of vertebrates.

process: All activities that produce an output for a customer.

process change: Changing a process to make it less hazardous (e.g., paint dipping in place of paint spraying).

process controls: Emission control devices installed as a part of a process or on a piece of equipment.

process hood: A device to capture, enclose, or receive hazards from a process. Hoods enclose a process and capture or receive contaminants.

procurement quality control (QC): A systematic procedure by which supplies, materials, and capital equipment are procured and tested to certify the specified quality of those materials.

proficiency testing: Special series of planned tests to determine the ability of field technicians or laboratory analysts who normally perform routine analyses. The results may be used for comparison against established criteria or for relative comparisons among the data from a group of technicians or analysts.

progeny of 222-radon: The first four decay products — ^{218}Po, ^{214}Pb, ^{214}Bi, and ^{210}Po.

program management: The keeping of records and program assessment efforts to evaluate the effectiveness of the comprehensive occupational health program.

promotion: The mutated precancerous cell divides and proliferates in the second step of carcinogenesis.

promulgated standard: Standard that has been enacted or otherwise made into law or regulation by authority.

pronation: 1. Turning the palm downward or toward the back. 2. Eversion of the foot.

propagation: Spread or transmission of decomposition, flame, or explosion.

protocol: In science, the rules and outline of an experiment.

prudent avoidance: An approach in which one chooses a low-cost, easily accomplished method to reduce exposure but makes no concerted effort in this regard. An example is the choice between walking in the vicinity of a high-strength field source or taking an equally effective, alternative route farther away from the source.

psi: Pounds per square inch.

psychology: The science that deals with the functions of the mind and the behavior of an organism in relation to its environment.

psychosocial stressors: Threats to working people that influence health through psychological pathways, such as uncertainty, anxiety, and loss of control or physiological pathways, such as sympathetic nervous system arousal or immune system responses, or influence safety through fatigue and production pressure.

psychosomatic: A physical disorder that is caused by or notably influenced by the emotional state of the patient.

psychrometer: An instrument consisting of wet and dry bulb thermometers for measuring relative humidity.

psychrometric: One of two types of wet bulb measurement that relies on artificial ventilation. (See also *natural wet bulb, wet-bulb globe temperature.*)

psychrometric chart: A graphical representation of the properties of moist air, usually including wet and dry bulb temperatures, specific and relative humidities, enthalpy, and density.

psychrometric wet bulb temperature (Twb): Temperature measured by a thermometer on which the sensor is covered by a wetted cotton wick that is exposed to forced movement of the air. Accuracy of wet bulb temperature measurements requires using a clean wick, distilled water, and proper shielding to prevent radiant heat gain. (Also known as “wet bulb temperature.”)

PTS: Permanent threshold shift. (See also *temporary threshold shift.*)

pulmonary: Relating to or associated with the lungs.

pulmonary irritation: Irritation of the lungs.

pulmonary region: The region containing the respiratory bronchioles, alveolar ducts, and alveolar sacs across which gas exchange occurs.

pulmonary system: A subsystem of the cardiovascular system (CVS) in which blood from the right ventricle is pumped to the lungs, where carbon dioxide is removed and oxygen is added before the blood is returned to the left side of the heart.

pulvation: The act of particles being emitted or induced to become airborne. (**Note:** This term was coined by Hemeon.)

pump: A mechanical device used in air monitoring to draw the sample gas through a collection device.

pure tone: Sound energy characterized by its singleness of frequency.

PWC: See *physical work capacity.*

pyrolyzer: A device that thermally decomposes certain gases and vapors, releasing constituents that then can react with the indicating layer in the detector tube.

pyrophoric: A chemical that will ignite spontaneously in air (and occasionally friction) at a temperature of 13°F or below.

Q

Q: See *volume flow rate.*

QA: See *quality assurance.*

QC: See *quality control.*
QCM: See *quartz crystal microbalance.*
QFD: See *quality function deployment.*
Qualified Industrial Hygienist: A person qualified to practice industrial hygiene by virtue of educational qualifications and examination by the American Board of Industrial Hygiene (ABIH).
qualitative: Pertaining to kind or type (name).
qualitative fit-test: A pass/fail fit-test that relies on the subject's sensory response to detect the challenge agent.
quality: The totality of features and characteristics of a product or service that bear on its capability to satisfy a given purpose. For air pollution measurement systems, the product is air pollution measurement data, and the characteristics of major importance are accuracy, precision, completeness, and representativeness. For air monitoring systems, "completeness," or the amount of valid measurements obtained relative to the amount expected to have been obtained, is a very important measure of quality. The relative importance of accuracy, precision, and completeness depends on the particular purpose of the user.
quality assurance: A system for integrating the quality planning, quality assessment, and quality improvement efforts of various groups in an organization to enable operations to meet user requirements at an economical level. In air pollution measurement systems, quality assurance (QA) is concerned with all of the activities that have an important effect on the quality of the air pollution measurements, as well as the establishment of methods and techniques to measure the quality of the air pollution measurements. The more authoritative usage differentiates between "quality assurance" and "quality control" — quality control being "the system of activities to provide a quality product" and quality assurance being "the system of activities to provide assurance that the quality control system is performing adequately."
quality assurance program plan: An orderly assembly of management policies, objectives, principles, and general procedures by which an agency or laboratory outlines how it intends to produce data of acceptable quality.
quality assurance project plan: An orderly assembly of detailed and specific procedures by which an agency or laboratory delineates how it produces quality data for a specific project or measurement method. A given agency or laboratory would have only one quality assurance program plan, but would have a quality assurance project plan for each of its projects (group of projects using the same measurement methods; for example, a laboratory service group might develop a plan by analytical instrument since the service is provided to a number of projects).
quality audit: A systematic examination of the acts and decisions with respect to quality in order to independently verify or evaluate compliance to the operational requirements of the quality program or the specification or contract requirements of the product or service, or to evaluate the adequacy of a quality program.
quality control (QC): The system of activities designed and implemented to provide a quality product.
quality control reference sample: A material used to assess the performance of a measurement or portions thereof. It is intended primarily for routine intralaboratory use in maintaining control of accuracy and would be prepared from or traceable to a calibration standard. (Also known as "working standard.")
quality function deployment (QFD): A systematic means of ensuring that the demands of the customer are accurately translated into action within the supplier organization.
quantitative: Pertaining to the amount (mass).
quantitative analysis: The branch of chemistry dealing with the accurate measurement of the amounts or percentages of the various components of a compound or mixture.
quantitative fit-test: A fit-test that uses an instrument to measure the challenge agent inside and outside the respirator.
quantum: Invisible unit of energy equal for radiation of frequency to the product h, where h is Planck's constant. (See also *Planck's constant.*)
quartz: Crystalline silicone dioxide. The main constituent in sandstone and

some igneous rocks. (Also known as "free silica.")

quenching: The repressing of optical radiation in a detector caused by heat or ultraviolet and not by radiation.

queue time: On a flowchart, the amount of time for each step and time between steps.

R

R: See *gas constant.*

radiance: Radiometric brightness (all optical wavelengths).

radiant exposure: The photobiological dose of radiant energy.

radiant temperature: The temperature resulting from the body-absorbing radiant energy.

radiation: The transmission of energy in the form of electric and magnetic fields (i.e., electromagnetic waves). Also known as "radiant energy."

radio frequency (RF): A frequency at which coherent electromagnetic radiation of energy is useful for communication purposes. Roughly the range from 10 kilohertz (kHz) to 100 gigahertz (gHz).

radioactivity: The spontaneous change in nucleonic configuration and/or energy content of a nucleus.

radiological wastes: Wastes that consist of radioactive components that emit ionizing radiation.

radionuclide: An unstable nucleus.

radiowave: An electromagnetic wave produced by reversal of current in a conductor at a frequency in the range from about 10 kilohertz (kHz) to about 300,000 megahertz (mHz).

radius of gyration: The square root of the ratio of the moment of inertia of a body about a given axis to its mass.

radon: A noble gas that emits alpha particles with a half-life of 3.8 days. It is a decay product of radium 226, which is a decay product of the uranium 238 series. Radon equilibrates rapidly with its decay products so that without a replenishing source, significant concentrations cannot be maintained.

radon daughters: Radon daughters, two of which emit alpha particles, have half-lives of less than 30 min.

Ramazzini, Bernardino: Italian physician and educator and author of *De Mobis Artificum Diatriba (Disease of Workers)* visited shops and workplaces to study the working conditions and health problems of various trades. He suggested that physicians ask their patients, "Of what trade are you?" He is recognized as the "father of occupational medicine."

random error: Variations of repeated measurements that are random in nature and individually not predictable. The causes of random error are presumed to be indeterminate or nonassignable. The distribution of random errors is generally presumed to be normal (Gaussian).

random noise: Random noise is an oscillation in which instantaneous magnitude is not specified for any given instant of time.

random sample: A sample obtained in such a manner that all items or members of the lot, or population, have an equal chance of being selected in the sample. In air pollution monitoring the population is usually defined in terms of a group of time periods for which measurements are desired. For 24-hour samplers, the population is usually considered as all of the 365 (or 366) 24-hour calendar day periods in a year. For continuous monitors, the population is often considered as all of the hourly average values obtained (or that could have been obtained) during a particular period, usually a calendar year. For either 24-hour or continuous monitors, a single air pollution result from a site could be a sample of the conceptually infinite population of values that might have been obtained at the given site for all possible combinations of equipment, materials, personnel, and conditions that could have existed at that site and time.

random vibration: A varying force acting on a mechanical system, which may be considered to be the sum of a large number of irregularly timed small shocks, induced typically by aerodynamic turbulence, airborne noise from rocket jets, and transportation over road surfaces.

range: The difference between the maximum and minimum values of a set of values. When the number of values is small (i.e., 8 or less), the range is a relatively sensitive (efficient) measure of variability. As the number of values increases above 8, the efficiency of the range (as an estimator of the variability) decreases rapidly. The range or difference between two paired values is of particular importance in air pollution measurements, since in many situations duplicate analyses or measurements are performed as a part of the quality assurance program.

Rankine temperature: An absolute temperature scale conventionally defined by the temperature of the triple point of water equal to 491.68°R, with 180 divisions between the melting point of ice and the boiling point of water under standard atmospheric pressure (1°R = 1°F).

Raynaud's Phenomenon of Occupational Origin: See hand-arm vibration syndrome.

Raynaud's syndrome: A type of repetitive strain injury (RSI) considered to be caused by persistent heavy vibration (for example, from a jackhammer or bicycle handlebars) or exposure to extreme cold, characterized by pain, tingling, numbness, and pale skin on the fingers or toes. (Also known as "constitutional cold fingers," "dead finger.")

RC: Reduced comfort. See *reduced comfort (RC) resonance.*

reaction: A chemical transformation or change. The interaction of two or more substances to form new substances.

reactive waste: Waste consisting of chemically unstable materials typically characterized as either strong oxidizing or reducing agents.

reactivity: Chemical reaction with the release of energy. Undesirable effects (such as pressure buildup, temperature increase, formation of noxious, toxic, or corrosive byproducts) may occur because of the reactivity of a substance to heating, burning, direct contact with other materials, or other conditions in use of in storage.

reagent grade: A chemical reagent that meets standards for purity set by the American Chemical Society. These reagents are produced for laboratory use.

real-time monitors: See *direct-reading instruments.*

reasonable maximum exposure (RME): Used in conservative exposure assessment calculations. Based not on worst-case scenario, but on 90% or 95% upper confidence limits on input parameters.

receiving hood: 1. A ventilation system hood that receives contaminants that are thrown or directed into the hood. A canopy hood is an example of a receiving hood. 2. A hood designed and positioned to take advantage of any initial velocity or motion imparted to the contaminant by the generating process.

reciprocity: Mutual exchange.

recognition: One of four primary responsibilities of the industrial hygienist. The line separating "anticipation" and "recognition" is not always a clear one. Some have distinguished them on the basis of whether the situation being examined actually exists. If it is still in a conceptual phase, the process being applied is considered to be "anticipation." Then it is assumed that, in the recognition phase, the facility exists. This is a somewhat arbitrary distinction; anticipation of hazards can and does occur with existing facilities, and recognition of hazards can take place when the facility is in a planning stage. (See also *anticipation, evaluation, and control.*)

recognition process: A process used to recognize workplace hazards.

recombinant DNA: The new DNA that is formed by combining pieces of DNA from different organisms or cells.

recommended alert limits: Heat exposure limits for unacclimatized workers.

recommended exposure limit (REL): An occupational exposure limit recommended by NIOSH as being protective of worker health and safety over a working lifetime. The REL is used in combination with engineering and work practice controls, exposure and medical monitoring, labeling, posting, worker training, and personal protective equipment. It is frequently expressed as a TWA exposure for up to 10 hours/day during a 40-hour work week; may also be expressed as 1) a short-term exposure limit (STEL) that should never be exceeded and is to be determined in a specified sampling time (usually 15 minutes); or 2) a ceiling (C) limit that should never be exceeded even instantaneously unless specified over a given time period.

recommended standard: A standard that has been recommended to authority for promulgation or enactment into law.

recordable injury: A work-related injury reported by an employer under the OSH Act of 1970.

redox compound: Compound with reducing and oxidizing features.

reduced comfort (RC) resonance: The boundaries concerned with preservation of comfort during vibration exposure.

reducing agent: In a reduction reaction (which always occurs simultaneously with an oxidation reaction) the reducing agent is the chemical or substance that 1) combines with oxygen; or 2) loses electrons to the reaction. (See also *oxidation.*)

reductant: Reducing agent (electron source).

re-entrainment: Resuspension of particles after they have been settled onto a collecting surface.

reference dose (RfD): U.S. EPA toxicity value for evaluating noncarcinogenic effects resulting from exposures at Superfund sites. An estimate (with uncertainty spanning an order of magnitude or greater) of daily exposure level for humans, including sensitive subpopulations, that is likely to be without an appreciable risk or deleterious effects during a lifetime.

reflective listening: A management tool by which one summarizes and repeats the position of the other party.

regulatory occupational exposure limit: An occupational exposure limit set and recommended by government agencies. (See also *occupational exposure limit.*)

regulatory standards: Regulatory standards are issued by a governmental body that is authorized by law to issue, and usually enforce compliance with, such standards; there is no voluntary or discretionary option for the user to determine whether or not to comply.

REL: See *recommended exposure limit.*

relational database: A type of database that stores data in the form of a table. Relational databases are powerful because they require few assumptions about how data is related or how it will be extracted from the database. As a result, the same database can be viewed in many different ways. Another feature of relational systems is that a single database can be spread across several tables. This differs from flat-file databases, in which each database is self-contained in a single table. Nearly all full-scale database systems for personal computers use a relational database. Small database systems, however, use other designs that provide less flexibility in posing queries.

relative error: An error expressed as a percentage of the true value or accepted reference value. All statements of precision or accuracy should indicate clearly whether they are expressed in absolute or relative sense. (This gets complicated when the absolute value is itself a percentage as is the case for many chemical analyses.)

relative humidity (RH): The ratio of the quantity of water vapor present in the air to the quantity that would saturate it at any specific temperature.

relative permittivity: Permittivity values that have been normalized to a fundamental constant, the permittivity of space, 8.85 × 10-12 farads/meter. Sometimes called the "dielectric constant." (See also *permittivity.*)

relative standard deviation (RSD): See *coefficient of variation.*

renal: Relating to or associated with the kidney.

repeatability: The precision, usually expressed as a standard deviation, measuring the variability among results of measurements at different times of the same sample at the same laboratory. The unit of time should be specified, since within a day repeatability would be expected to be smaller than between day repeatability.

repetitive strain injury (RSI): A general term for a group of soft-tissue injuries caused by overuse of the hand, wrist, and arm experienced by people who regularly work on computers, play certain musical instruments, or work in construction, mining, clerical, and food preparation jobs. RSIs result when repetitive motions damage the nerves of the hands, arms, shoulders, or neck, or affect the joints, muscles, ligaments, tendons, or tendon sheaths of these areas. Some common types of RSI are carpal tunnel syndrome, thoracic outlet syndrome, tendinitis, tenosynovitis, and deQuervain's disease. Symptoms range from tingling, numbness, and pain in the neck, shoulders, arms, or hands to reduced grip strength and clumsiness. (Also known as "repetitive motion injury," "cumulative trauma disorder," or "overuse injury.")

replacement air: Air supplied to a space to replace exhausted air. (Also known as "compensating air" or "make-up air.")

replicability: The precision, usually expressed as a standard deviation, measuring the variability among replicates.

replicates: Repeated but independent determinations of the same sample, by the same analyst, at essentially the same time and same conditions. Care should be exercised in considering replicates of a portion of an analysis and replicates of a complete analysis. For example, duplicate titrations of the same digestion are not valid replicate analyses, although they may be valid replicate titrations. Replicates may be performed to any degree (e.g., duplicates, triplicates).

representative sample: A sample taken to represent a lot or population as accurately and precisely as possible. A representative sample may be either a completely random sample or a stratified sample depending on the objective of the sampling and the conceptual population for a given situation.

reproducibility: The precision, usually expressed as a standard deviation, measuring the variability among results of measurements of the same sample at different laboratories.

reproductive toxicity: A harmful effect on the adult reproductive system.

required clothing insulation (IREQ): An index that assumes a minimal cold tolerance level for skin temperature of 30°C and skin wetness of 0.06 in a stationary standing man. With these assumptions the amount of insulation required to obtain thermal balance can be calculated.

required sweat rate: The international standard (ISO 7933) for the amount of sweat required to maintain thermal balance.

rescue: The activities associated with a trained rescue crew entering a confined space to retrieve an injured or incapacitated entrant.

resorption: In mammalian species that give birth to litters, the intrauterine tissue remaining at the site of death of an embryo or fetus.

respirable dust: Term used to indicate particulate matter that can be inhaled. Generally considered to be 5 μm or less in aerodynamic diameter.

respirable fraction: Particles that penetrate the pulmonary region.

respiratory inlet covering: That portion of a respirator that connects the wearer's respiratory tract to an air-purifying device or respirable gas source, or both. It may be a facepiece, helmet, hood, suit, or mouthpiece/nose clamp.

respiratory system: The breathing system (including mouth, nose, larynx, trachea, lungs, etc.) and associated nerves and blood supply.

responsible party: Someone who can provide additional information on the hazardous chemical and appropriate emergency procedures, if necessary.

retention time: In gas chromatography, the time at which the center, or maximum, of a symmetrical peak occurs on a gas chromatogram.

retinal hazard region: The spectral region where the retina is at greatest risk.

return air: Air extracted from a space and returned to that space, usually after passing through filters and the air-handling unit.

reverberant field: An area where sound levels will remain constant regardless of additional distance from the source. The sound level in the reverberant field depends on the sound power level of the sound source and the amount of sound absorption in the room.

reversible behavior disruption: A sensitive measure of RF exposure. In general, behavioral changes are thermal effects attributed to significant increases in body temperature due to absorbed RF energy.

rework: The portion of the output that must undergo additional processes to correct any unacceptable characteristics introduced during initial production.

rewriting: The process of revising a report to ensure that the final version is free of awkward language or unnecessary words that distract from the content.

Reynolds number: A dimensionless number proportional to pipe or duct diameter, velocity, and density of fluid, and inversely proportional to the viscosity of the fluid. A Reynolds number greater than 2500 indicates turbulent flow; less than 2500, it indicates streamlined flow.

RfD: See *reference dose.*

RH: See *relative humidity.*

risk: Probability and magnitude of harm. For exposures to chemicals, risk is a function of both exposure and toxicity.

risk agent: The chemical or physical agent that is the source of the risk.

risk analysis: A quantitative analysis used to determine risk.

risk assessment: The process of determining, either quantitatively or qualitatively, the probability and magnitude of an undesired event and estimating the cost to human society or the environment in terms of morbidity, mortality, or economic impact.

risk characterization: The last step in the risk assessment process characterizes the potential for adverse health effects and evaluates the uncertainty involved.

risk communication: The exchange of information about health or environmental risks among risk assessors and managers, the general public, news media, interest groups, etc.

risk estimate: Different expressions of risk may have different implications: 1) individual lifetime risk — the risk of an individual developing the adverse health effect sometime during the remaining lifespan; 2) population or societal risk – the integration of the individual lifetime risk over the exposed population; 3) relative risk – the probability of developing a specific adverse health effect given exposure to a risk agent compared with the same probability given no exposure to the agent; 4) standardized mortality ratio (SMR) – death rate due to a specific cause in an exposed population compared with the death rate in the general population; used often in occupational epidemiology studies; 5) loss of life expectancy — individual lifetime risk multiplied by 36 years equals the average remaining lifetime.

risk factor: Characteristic (e.g., race, sex, age, obesity) or variable (e.g., smoking, occupational exposure level) associated with increased probability of a toxic effect.

risk management: Control of risks to acceptable levels through the application of various remediation techniques.

risk perception: The level of risk an individual, organization, or society associates with a risk agent.

RME: See *reasonable maximum exposure.*

rms: See *root-mean-square.*

robust design: A technique for making the utility of the final product insensitive to variations in the manufacturing process. In EHS terms this might mean that no matter how different the input chemicals are the final product will have no increased exposure potential from one batch to the next.

root cause: The activity that, if corrected or eliminated, will solve the identified problem.

root-mean-square (rms): The square root of the arithmetic mean of the squares of a set of values.

rotameter: A flowmeter, consisting of a precision-bored, tapered, transparent tube with a solid float inside.

rotation: Angular motion.

roughness factor: The ratio of size of projections from the surface of a pipe or duct, to the diameter of the pipe or duct.

route of entry: Means by which a chemical enters the body (e.g., ingestion, inhalation, dermal absorption, or injection).

routinely collected data: Various types of exposure and health data that are collected routinely in the occupational setting for use in surveillance programs.

RPE: Rating of Perceived Exertion.

RSD: Relative standard deviation. See *coefficient of variation.*

RSI: See *repetitive strain injury.*

ruggedness testing: A special series of tests performed to determine the sensitivity (the desired result is to confirm the insensitivity) of a measurement system to variations of certain factors suspected of affecting the measurement system.

S

SA: See *specific absorption.*

safe: In occupational health, when a situation is safe it is meant that it is free from an unacceptable amount of risk rather than free from all risk. Something is safe if its actual risk is judged to be acceptable.

Safety Equipment Institute (SEI): An organization that conducts a voluntary third-party certification program of safety equipment, including detector tubes and pumps.

safety and health training: Addresses the safety and health responsibilities of all personnel concerned with the work site. Training is often most effective when incorporated into other training about performance requirements and job practices. Training is conducted to 1) ensure that all employees understand the hazards to which they might be exposed and how to prevent harm to themselves and others from exposure to these hazards; 2) permit supervisors to carry out their jobs effectively; and 3) ensure that managers understand their safety and health responsibilities.

safety inspections: An inspection conducted by those who are classified as safety specialists.

Safety Triad: Triangle of safety-related factors encompassing (1) environment factors (including equipment, tools, physical layout, procedures, standards, management systems, and temperature); (2) person factors (including people's attitudes, beliefs, and personalities); and (3) behavior factors (including safe and at-risk work practices and going beyond the call of duty to intervene on behalf of another person's safety).

saliva: Watery fluid secreted into the the mouth from the salivary glands.

sample: A subset or group of objects or things selected from a larger set, called the "lot" or "population." The objects or things may be physical such as specimens for testing or they may be data values representing physical samples. Unless otherwise specified, all samples are assumed to be randomly selected. Usually, information obtained from the samples is used to provide some indication or inference about the larger set. Samples, rather than the population, are usually examined for reasons of economy — the entire population under consideration is usually too large or too inaccessible to evaluate. In cases in which destructive testing is performed, sampling is a must — otherwise the entire population would be consumed. In many situations, the population is conceptually infinite and therefore impossible to check or measure.

sample breakthrough: Most commercially available sampling tubes consist of two sections of sorbent separated by glass wool or polyurethane. In charcoal tubes the second or backup section is usually one-third of the total weight of the charcoal. These two sections are desorbed and analyzed separately in the laboratory. As a guideline, if 25% or less of the amount of contaminant collected on the front section is found on the backup section, significant loss of the compound (breakthrough) has probably not occurred. If greater than 25% is detected, breakthrough is evident and results should be reported as "breakthrough, possible sample loss."

sampler capacity: A predetermined conservative estimate of the total mass of contaminant that can be collected on the sampling medium without loss or overloading; typically two-thirds of the mass of contaminant on the sorbent at the breakthrough volume.

sample volume: The amount of air pulled through the collection device by a pump during sampling.

sampling media: Devices used to collect airborne chemicals for subsequent analysis, such as sorbent tubes, bags, and filters.

sampling strategy: A sampling plan that includes, but is not limited to, an assessment of the type and number of samples to be collected, the methods to be used, the accuracy of the methods, and the overall objectives for sampling.

SAR: See *specific absorption rate.*

sarcoma: A malignant tumor that develops from connective tissue cells.

SC: See *stratum corneum.*

SCBA: See *self-contained breathing apparatus.*

SCE(s): See *sister-chromatid exchange(s).*

scenario building: A method that forces both planners and managers to think outside the traditional comfort zone. It is a group process involving many organizational levels.

scfm: Air volume flow rate at standard conditions.

scope of practice: The legal specifications for credentials, responsibilities, and limitations of health care practitioners generally developed by state authorities.

SE: See *shielding effectiveness.*

search engine: A program that searches documents for specified keywords and returns a list of the documents where the keywords were found. Although search engine is really a general class of programs, the term is often used to specifically describe systems that enable users to search for documents on the World Wide Web. Typically, a search engine works by sending out a spider to fetch as many documents as possible. Another program, called an indexer, then reads these documents and creates an index based on the words contained in each document. Each search engine uses a proprietary algorithm to create its indices such that, ideally, only meaningful results are returned for each query.

sebum: The waxy excretion on the skin surface.

secondary barriers: Protection of the external environment, including nonlaboratory work areas and the outside community. Secondary containment is achieved by a combination of facility design (differential pressurization of work areas, HEPA-filtered exhaust ventilation, sterilization of effluent liquids, etc.) and work practices and procedures.

secondary prevention: involves early detection and prompt efforts to correct the beginning stages of illness, for example, reversing high blood pressure, buildup of plaque in the arteries, or chronic insomnia, before a heart attack occurs through health promotion, stress management or Employee Assistance Programs.

secondary standard: Devices such as flowmeters that trace their calibration to primary standards and maintain their accuracy with reasonable care and handling in operation.

sedimentation: The movement of an aerosol particle through a gaseous medium under the influence of gravity.

SEG: See *similar exposure group.*

self-contained breathing apparatus (SCBA): An atmosphere-supplying respirator in which the respirable gas source is designed to be carried by the wearer.

self-efficacy: The self-confidence that a person can successfully accomplish what he or she sets out to do. (Also known as "self-effectiveness.")

semi-insert: A type of hearing protector that is a cross between earplugs and earmuffs; earplug-like devices attached to the ends of a headband that are pressed into the ear canal.

sensation: A mental condition or physical feeling resulting from stimulation of a sense organ or internal bodily changes.

sensitive volume: The part of a radiation detector that actually detects radiation.

sensitivity: The proportion of individuals with the disease that a test measure identifies correctly.

sensitivity analysis: In uncertainty analysis, comparison of risk estimates based on the means and upper bounds of the probability distributions of the input variables.

sensitization: The phase (usually 10 days) in which a person becomes allergic to an antigen.

sensitizer: A foreign agent or substance that is capable of causing an immune response in an individual. In most cases, initial exposure results in a normal response, but repeated exposures lead to progressively strong and abnormal responses.

sensorineural hearing loss: The type of hearing loss that affects the inner ear.

Sentinel Health Event: A Sentinel Health Event (SHE) is a preventable disease, disability, or untimely death whose occurrence serves as a warning signal that the quality of preventive and/or therapeutic medical care may need to be improved. A SHE (Occupational) is a disease, disability, or untimely death which is occupationally related and whose occurrence may: 1) provide the impetus for epidemiologic or industrial hygiene studies; or 2) serve as a warning signal that materials substitution, engineering control, personal protection, or medical care may be required. The present SHE (O) list encompasses 50 disease conditions that are linked to the workplace. Included are only those conditions for which objective documentation of an associated agent, industry, and occupation exists in the scientific literature. (Source: http://www.cdc.gov/NIOSH/sheoabs.html.)

serum: The liquid that does not contain the cellular components of blood on coagulation.

server: A computer or device on a network that manages network resources. For example, a file server is a computer and storage device dedicated to storing files. Any user on the network can store files on the server. A print server is a computer that manages one or more printers, and a network server is a computer that manages network traffic. A database server is a computer system that processes database queries.

shaping: Using the interpreted data, leaders shape a vision for the future that reflects the organization's values and goals. (See also *interpreting*.)

shared vision: A level beyond simply signing onto the personal vision of a charismatic leader. It is the ability to translate such a vision throughout the organization in a manner that fosters a genuine commitment.

shelf life: The period in which detector tubes remain stable when stored in accordance with a manufacturer's specifications.

shelter in place: An action plan where a facility determines the appropriate action would be to remain in the building with air intake equipment turned off, rather than evacuating.

shielding effectiveness (SE): Shielding effectiveness is used to describe the capability of a material as a shield. SE is a function of losses resulting from absorption, reflection, and internal reflection.

shock: 1. Clinical manifestations of circulatory insufficiency, including hypertension, weak pulse, tachycardia, pallor, and diminished urinary output. 2. A pulse or transient motion or force lasting thousandths to tenths of a second that is capable of exciting mechanical resonances.

short-term exposure limit (STEL): 1. Maximum concentration for continuous 15-minute period. Allowed four times a day, with at least 60 minutes between exposures. 2. Used in reference to the OSHA PEL–STEL and ACGIH's TLV–STEL. The STEL represents a time-weighted average (TWA) exposure that should not be exceeded for any 15-minute period. 3. STELs are recommended when exposures of even short duration to high concentrations of a chemical are known to produce acute toxicity. It is the concentration to which workers can be exposed continuously for a short period of time without suffering from 1) irritation; 2) chronic or irreversible tissue damage; or 3) narcosis of sufficient degree to increase the likelihood of accidental injury, impaired self-rescue, or reduced work efficiency. A STEL is defined as a 15-minute TWA exposure that should not be exceeded at any time during a workday, even if the overall 8-hour TWA is within limits, and it should not occur more than four times per day. There should be at least 60 minutes between successive exposures in this range. If warranted, an averaging period other than 15 minutes can also be used.

short-term public emergency guidance level (SPEGL): Established by the Committee on Toxicology of the National Research Council (NRC) for the U.S. Department of Defense. The SPEGL is a suitable concentration for unpredicted, single, short-term, emergency exposure of the general public. In contrast to the EEGL, the SPEGL takes into account the wide range of susceptibility of the general public. (See also *EEGL, CEGL*.)

SI metric units: 1. Le Systeme International d'Unites; the international metric system. 2. An internationally accepted system of metric units based on mass in kilograms, length in meters, and time in seconds.

SIC: See *Standard Industrial Classification Code.*

sick building syndrome: The term "sick building syndrome" has come into common use for those problems where excessive comfort and health-related symptoms are present that are clearly related to building occupancy, but that are not associated with objective clinical signs.

significance: Importance; consequence. Part of the evaluation process. (See also *evaluation.*)

significant figures: Numerical figures containing as many digits (other than location zeroes) as are contained in the least exact factor used in their determination. [**Note:** Do not confuse significant figures with the 10 to 16 decimal places that appear on the display of scientific and engineering calculators.]

SIL: See *speed interference level.*

silica gel: A regenerative absorbent consisting of the amorphous silica. Used in dehydrating and in drying and as a catalyst carrier.

similar exposure group (SEG): A group of workers having the same general exposure profile for the agent(s) being studied because of the similarity and frequency of the tasks they perform, the materials and processes with which they work, and the similarity of the way they perform the tasks.

simple asphyxiation: Coating or blockage of passageways in the lungs so that oxygen cannot reach the alveoli or be absorbed into the bloodstream.

SIPOC: a Six Sigma method where Support Inputs for a Process are used to identify Outputs or impacts to the Customer.

sister-chromatid exchange(s) SCE(s): An exchange of genetic material between the chromatid pairs of a chromosome during cell division.

site control: Consists of compiling an accurate site map; preparing the site for work activities; establishing work zones; using the buddy system; establishing and enforcing decontamination procedures for personnel and equipment; establishing site security measures; setting up communication networks; enforcing safe work practices (standard operating procedures); and, planning for emergencies.

Site Health and Safety Plan: Establishes policies and procedures to protect workers and the public from potential hazards that may exist at the site.

skeletal variant: A minor alteration of the skeletal structure that will not adversely affect function or length of life of the organism and that occurs normally in a small proportion of animals.

skin: When used with an exposure guideline such as an OSHA PEL or ACGIH® TLV®, it indicates that the substance may be absorbed in toxic amounts through the skin or mucous membranes.

SKIN designation: A designation that emphasizes the role of the skin in contributing to overall exposures to chemicals and does not denote toxic effects on the skin.

skin notation: Denotes the possibility that dermal absorption may be a significant contribution to the overall body burden of the chemical (that is, the airborne OEL might not be adequate to protect the worker because the compound also readily penetrates the skin. Other toxicity endpoints on skin such as irritation, dermatitis, and sensitization are not sufficient to warrant the skin notation. In practice, the skin notation is given to compounds with a dermal LD_{50} less than 1000 mg/kg, or if there are other data indicating that repeated dermal exposure results in systemic toxicity.

SLM: See *sound level meter.*

slope factor: Plausible upper-bound estimate of the probability of a response per unit intake of a chemical over a lifetime. Used to estimate an upper-bound probability of an individual developing cancer as a result of a lifetime of exposure to a particular level of a potential carcinogen.

slot: See *slot hood.*

slot hood: A hood that has an opening (i.e., a slot) that has a width to length ratio of 0.2 or less; used to provide uniform air distribution and adequate capture velocity over a finite length of contaminant generation.

slot velocity: Air velocity through the openings into a slot-plenum hood. Primarily used to obtain a uniform air velocity across the edge of a tank. The correct selection of the slot velocity will produce a uniform capture velocity.

slurry: Pourable mixture of solid and liquid.

smog: Smoke and fog: extensive atmospheric contamination by aerosols arising from a combination of natural and anthropogenic sources.

smoke: 1. Carbon or soot particles less than 1.0 µm in size. These small, gas-phase particles created by incomplete combustion, consist predominantly of carbon and other combustible materials. Smoke generally contains droplets and dry particles. Size ranges are usually between 0.01 µm and 1.0 µm. 2. A mixture of dry and liquid particles generated by incomplete combustion of an organic material, combined with and suspended in the gases from combustion.

soap bubble burette: A tube with a defined volume in which a soap film (bubbles) are injected to measure flow rate. It is a flow calibration device for sampling pumps. Modern technology has computerized the measurement of a flow rate with electronic timing sensors in the bubble burette/meter. (Also called a "bubble meter.")

social psychology: The study of the manner in which the attitudes, personality, and motivations of the individual influence, and are influenced by, the structure, dynamics, and behavior of the social group with which the individual interacts.

software: Computer instructions or data. Anything that can be stored electronically is software. The storage devices and display devices are hardware. Software is often divided into two categories: 1) systems software — includes the operating system and all the utilities that enable the computer to function; 2) applications software — includes programs that do real work for users. For example, word processors, spreadsheets, and database management systems fall under the category of applications software.

solubility in water: Susceptible of being dissolved; may be expressed as the percentage of a material (by weight) that will dissolve in a solvent. The following terms are used to express solubility: negligible = <0.1%; slight = 0.1%–1.0%; moderate = 1.0%–10.0%; appreciable = 10.0%–99.0%; complete = soluble in all proportions.

solution: Mixture in which the components lose their identities and are uniformly dispersed. All solutions are composed of a solvent (water or other fluid) and the substance dissolved called the "solute." Air is a solution of oxygen and nitrogen. A true solution is homogeneous as salt in water.

solvent: A substance that dissolves other substances, most commonly water but often an organic compound.

solvent extraction: The process of extracting adsorbed chemicals from sorbent material through the use of solvents.

somatic mutation: A mutation that is characterized by manifestation of the damage in the exposed individual due to alteration of somatic or body cells.

somatic nervous system: A subdivision of the central nervous system (CNS) that transmits signals to the skeletal muscles for movement.

SOP: See *standard operating procedure.*

sorbent tube: A small glass tube normally filled with two layers of a solid sorbent material that will adsorb specific chemicals for subsequent elution and laboratory analysis.

sound absorption coefficient: The ratio of sound energy absorbed to that arriving at a surface or medium. (Also known as "acoustic absorption coefficient" or "acoustic absorptivity.")

sound analyzer: A device for measuring the band pressure or pressure-spectrum level of a sound as a function of frequency.

sound intensity analyzer: Analyzers used to identify specific noise sources and to determine compliance with purchase specifications limiting the sound power level.

sound intensity level (Li): A vector quantity having both magnitude and direction. Although the Li does not correspond to the loudness of a sound, it is useful as an analytical measurement and is necessary to determine accurately the sound power level.

sound level meter (SLM): An instrument used to measure noise and sound levels in a specified manner; the meter may be calibrated in decibels or volume units and includes a microphone, an amplifier, an output meter, and frequency-weighting networks.

sound power level: The sound pressure level or sound intensity level data can be used to calculate the sound power level of a sound source. Sound power is analogous to the electrical power rating of a light bulb and is measured in watts.

sound pressure level (L_p): The level, in decibels, of a sound that is 20 times the logarithm to the base 10 of the ratio of the measured pressure of this sound to the reference pressure. The reference pressure is 0.0002 dynes/cm^2.

sound shadow: Noise that slips through sound-blocking barriers.

source modification: Changing a hazard source to make it less hazardous (e.g., wetting dust particles or lowering the temperature of liquids to reduce off-gassing and vaporization).

SP: See *static pressure*.

span gas: The concentration of a calibration gas mixture needed to span a desired concentration range of a chemical specific detector.

span vapor: The concentration of a calibration vapor mixture needed to span a desired concentration range of a chemical specific detector.

spatial averaging: A method of estimating average exposure of the whole body by collecting densitometric data across the vertical dimension of a simple linear model of the body.

specific absorption (SA): A quantity that represents RF exposure within tissues. The SA is the time integral of the sound absorption rate (SAR) and, is the RF dose. It is the energy absorbed per unit mass of tissue, with units of joules per kilogram (J/kg). (See also *specific absorption rate.*)

specific absorption rate (SAR): A quantity that represents RF exposure within tissues. The SAR is the rate at which energy is absorbed per unit mass, or dose rate. It is the fundamental quantity of the exposure criteria, and the dosimetric quantity of choice in studies of biological effects. It is generally expressed in units of watts per kilogram (W/kg), representing the power deposited in a unit mass. The unit, W/kg, is also used for metabolic rate, where the resting metabolic rate of an adult human being is about 1 W/kg. The SAR depends on the electric-field strength in tissues (Ei), the electrical conductivity of tissues, and the density of tissues.

specific activity: The activity per unit mass of a radio-nuclide.

specific gravity: 1. The ratio of the mass of a unit volume of a substance to the mass of the same volume of a standard substance at a standard temperature. Water at 39.2°F (4°C) is the standard usually referred to for liquids; for gases, dry air (at the same temperature and pressure as the gas) is often taken as the standard substance. 2. The weight of a material compared with the weight of an equal volume of water is an expression of the density (or heaviness) of a material. Insoluble materials with specific gravity of less than 1.0 will float in (or on) water. In soluble materials with a specific gravity greater than 1.0 will sink in water. Most, but not all, flammable liquids have specific gravity less than 1.0 and, if not soluble, will float on water — an important consideration for fire suppression.

specific reliability: The probability that an item will perform a required function under stated conditions for a stated period of time.

specification standards: Description of the specific means of hazard abatement. (See also *performance standards.*)

specificity: The proportion of people without the disease that a test measure identifies correctly.

spectrophotometer: An instrument used for comparing the relative intensities of the corresponding colors produced by chemical reactions.

spectrophotometry: A procedure to photometrically measure the wavelength range of radiant energy absorbed by a sample under analysis; can be visible light, ultraviolet light, or X-rays.

spectrum (noise): The distribution in frequency of the magnitudes (and sometimes phases) of the components of the wave. Spectrum also is used to signify a continuous range of frequencies, usually wide in extent, within which waves have some specified common characteristics.

specular reflection: Reflections may be specular or diffuse, or a combination of the two. Specular reflection, which may be regarded as a type of direct viewing, occurs when the beam is incident on a mirror-like surface. This depends on the wavelength and the dimension of the surface irregularities of the reflector (i.e., it is a wavelength-dependent phenomenon). Specular reflections occur when the size of the surface irregularities of the reflecting surface are smaller than the incident wavelength.

speed interference level (SIL or PSIL): The speech interference level of a noise is the arithmetic average, in decibels, of the sound pressure levels of the noise in the three octave bands of frequency 600–1200, 1200–2400, 2400–4800 Hz for SIL and the preferred center frequencies of 500, 1000, and 2000 Hz for PSIL.

SPEGL: See *short-term public emergency guidance level.*

spiked sample: A normal sample of material (gas, solid, or liquid) to which is added a known amount of some substance of interest. The extent of the spiking is unknown to those analyzing the sample. Spiked samples are used to check on the performance of a routine analysis or the recovery efficiency of a method.

spontaneously combustible: A material that ignites as a result of retained heat from processing, or that will oxidize to generate heat and ignite, or that absorbs moisture to generate heat and ignite.

spot cooling: Cooling the air of a limited portion of an enclosed space.

sprain: Injury in which some fibers of a ligament are overstretched or torn but not completely severed. When the ligament is torn in two, the injury is called a severe sprain.

sputum: Watery fluid with solids excreted from the throat and upper lungs on expectoration.

squamous: Scaly or plate-like.

squamous cell carcinoma: A carcinoma of epithelial origin.

squeeze bulb pump: A sampling pump that draws a fixed volume of air using a squeeze bulb.

SRM: See *standard reference material.*

SRS: See *standard reference sample.*

stack: 1. A structure that contains a flue, or flues, for the discharge of gases. 2. The vertical train of a system of soil, waste, or vent piping extending through one or more stories. 3. A device used to discharge air into the ambient environment and away from the building wake.

stack sampling: A collection of aerosol samples in exhaust air ducts such as stacks or chimneys. (See also *isokinetic sampling, subisokinetic sampling, superisokinetic sampling.*)

stand-alone graphics: Visual displays in a report that are self-explanatory.

standard: Any rule, principle, or measure established by authority.

standard air: In ventilation, dry air at 70°F, 29.92 in. Hg (21°C, 760 mmHg) [ACGIH]; air at 68°F, 29.92 in. Hg, 50% relative humidity (20°C, 760 mmHg) [ASHRAE]. [**Note:** Chapter 33 in this book uses the ACGIH STP in all calculations.]

standard air decompression: A schedule applicable to either scuba or surface air-supplied divers who completely decompress in the water, in a diving bell, or chamber before reaching surface pressures. The maximum recommended air dive is 190 ft for 40 minutes with emergency dives to 300 ft for 180 minutes.

standard ambient temperature: Datum condition for the rating of equipment (usually 20°C).

standard atmosphere: Standard atmospheric pressure is the barometric pressure at standard conditions, 25°C and sea level.

standard conditions: 1. A set of physical, chemical, or other variables of a substance or system that defines an accepted reference state or forms a basis for comparison. 2. Operating conditions of a refrigeration system corresponding to some standard (e.g., evaporating temperature, condensing temperature, subcooling temperature, superheat).

standard deviation: 1. The positive square root of the variance of a distribution; the parameter measuring the spread of values about the mean. 2. The positive square root of the expected value of the square of the difference between a random variable and its mean.

standard error: The standard deviation of the distribution of a sample statistic.

Standard Industrial Classification (SIC) Code: A classification system used to identify places of employment by major types of activity.

standard operating procedure (SOP): A written document that details an operation, analysis, or action in which mechanisms are thoroughly prescribed and that is commonly accepted as the method for performing certain routine or repetitive tasks.

standard reference material (SRM): A material produced in quantity, of which certain properties have been certified by the National Institute of Standards and Technology (NIST) or other agencies to the extent possible to satisfy its intended use. The material should be in a matrix similar to actual samples to be measured by a measurement system or be used directly in preparing such a matrix. Intended uses include 1) standardization of solutions; 2) calibration of equipment; and 3) auditing the accuracy and precision of measurement systems.

standard reference sample (SRS): A carefully prepared material produced from or compared against an SRM (or other equally well-characterized material) such that there is little loss of accuracy. The sample should have a matrix similar to actual samples used in the measurement system. These samples are intended for use primarily as reference standards 1) to determine the precision and accuracy of measurement systems; 2) to evaluate calibration standards; and 3) to evaluate quality control reference samples. They may be used "as-is" or as a component of a calibration or quality control measurement system. Examples: An NIST-certified sulfur dioxide permeation device is an SRM. When used in conjunction with an air dilution device, the resulting gas becomes an SRS. An NIST-certified nitric oxide gas is an SRM. When diluted with air, the resulting gas is an SRS.

standard temperature and pressure (STP): 1. Measured volumes of gases are generally recalculated to 0°C and 760 mm pressure. 2. Standard temperature and pressure; 298 K (25°C) and 760 mmHg (1 atm).

standardization: A physical or mathematical adjustment or correction of a measurement system to make the measurements conform to predetermined values. The adjustments or corrections are usually based on a single-point calibration level.

standards in naturally occurring matrix: Standards relating to the pollutant measurement portions of air pollution measurement systems may be categorized according to matrix, purity, or use. Standards in a naturally occurring matrix include Standard Reference Materials and Standard Reference Samples.

standing wave: A wave in which the ratio of an instantaneous value at one point to that at any other point does not vary with time. (Also known as "stationary wave.")

static: Without motion or change.

static calibration: The artificial generation of the response curve of an instrument or method by use of appropriate mechanical, optical, electrical, or chemical means. Often a static calibration checks only a portion of a measurement system. For example, a solution containing a known amount of sulfite compound would simulate an absorbing solution through which has been bubbled a gas containing a known amount of sulfur dioxide. Use of the solution would check out the analytical portion of the pararosaniline method but would not check out the sampling and flow control parts of the bubbler system.

static load: Muscle (local) fatigue is divided into static and dynamic. When muscles are loaded but do not move, it is a static load; when loaded muscles move, it is dynamic.

static pressure (SP): 1. The potential pressure exerted in all directions by a fluid at rest. For a fluid in motion, it is measured in a direction normal (at right angles) to the direction of flow; thus, it shows the tendency to burst or collapse the pipe. When added to velocity pressure, it gives total pressure. 2. The pressure developed in a duct by a fan; SP exerts influence in all directions; the force in inches of water measured perpendicular to flow at the wall of the duct; the difference in pressure between atmospheric pressure and the absolute pressure inside a duct, cleaner, or other equipment. 3. The fan-generated differential pressure between the inside of the local exhaust ventilation (LEV) system and the outside ambient pressure; represents the energy that is continually delivered to the system by the fan.

static pressure (SP) loss: The amount of kinetic energy to overcome an obstruction or fitting in a ventilation system.

statistical control chart: See *control chart.*

statistical control chart limits: The limits on control charts that have been derived by statistical analysis and are used as criteria for action or for judging whether a set of data does or does not indicate lack of control.

steatosis: An acute reaction within the liver where lipid droplets may accumulate and produce what is known as fatty liver.

STEL: See *short-term exposure limit.*

sterilization: The removal or destruction of all microorganisms, including pathogenic and other bacteria, vegetative forms, and spores.

stochastic effect: 1. Biological effect from radiation exposure on a population based on random statistics in which there is assumed no threshold with an increase in the probability of occurrence with an increase in dose. 2. Effect for which the probability of occurrence depends on the absorbed dose. Heredity effects and cancer induced by radiation are considered to be stochastic effects. This means that, even for an individual, there is no threshold of dose below which the effect will not appear, but the chance of experiencing the effect increases with increasing dose. (See also *nonstochastic effect.*)

Stokes diameter: In measuring aerosol sedimentation behavior, the shape, size, and density of particles is often unknown. It is convenient to discuss particle size in terms of the diameter of a spherical particle of the same density that would exhibit the same behavior as the particle in question, or the Stokes diameter (d_{Stk}).

storage: Temporary holding of waste pending treatment or disposal, as in containers, tanks, waste piles, and surface impoundments.

STP: See *standard temperature and pressure.*

strain: 1. Change in length of an object in some direction per unit undistorted length in some direction, not necessarily the same; the nine possible strains from a second-rank tensor. 2. Injury in which some of the fibers of a muscle are overstretched or torn but not completely severed. When the muscle is torn in two, the injury is called a severe strain. Also, a general term used to describe a minor tear in a ligament or tendon.

strategic plan: A plan that generally describes where an organization would like to be in three to five years.

stratified sample: A sample consisting of various portions that have been obtained from identified subparts or subcategories (strata) of the total lot, or population. Within each category or strata, the samples are taken randomly. The objective of taking stratified samples is to obtain a more representative sample than that which might otherwise be obtained by a completely random sampling. The idea of identifying the subcategories or strata is based on knowledge or suspicion of (or protection against) differences existing among the strata for the characteristics of concern. The identification of the strata is based on knowledge of the structure of the population, which is known or suspected to have different relationships with the characteristic of the population under study. Opinion polls or surveys use stratified sampling to ensure proportional representation of the various strata (e.g., geographic location, age group sex, etc.). Stratified sampling is used in air monitoring to ensure representation of different geographical areas, different days of the week, and so forth. (Also known as "stratified random sample.")

stratum corneum (SC): The outer layer of flattened keratinized cells of the epidermis.

strength-of-evidence: A method of evaluating the evidence of carcinogenicity of a chemical in which both positive and negative evidence are considered. (See also *weight-of-evidence*.)

stresses: Environmental stimuli that represent potential adverse impacts on the health of workers. Stresses may include chemical and physical agents as well as ergonomic and psychological stress.

stressors: Stimuli that disrupts the homeostasis of an organism.

stroke volume: The amount of blood pumped by the left ventricle of the heart for each heartbeat. It is given in mL of blood per beat or L/beat.

subacute toxicity study: Toxicity study durations of five days to 14 days.

subchronic intake: Intake averaged over a period of two weeks to seven years.

subchronic reference dose: Applicable for time periods of two weeks to seven years.

subchronic toxicity study: Toxicity study durations of 15 days to six months.

Subcommittee on Consequence Assessment on Protective Actions (SCAPA): A Subcommittee of the Department of Energy (DOE) that developed Temporary Emergency Exposure Limits (TEELs) to fill the gaps where there are no ERPGs or AEGLs.

subcutaneous: Beneath the skin.

subharmonics: A sinusoidal quantity having a frequency that is an integral submultiple of the frequency of some other sinusoidal quantity to which it is referred; a third subharmonic would be one-third the fundamental or reference frequency.

subisokinetic sampling: A sampling condition in which the air flowing into an inlet has a lower velocity than the ambient airflow. Subsequently, the sample collected tends to be biased with larger particles. (See also *isokinetic sampling, stack sampling, superisokinetic sampling*.)

substitution: Substituting a less hazardous material, equipment, or process for a more hazardous one (e.g., use of soap and water in place of solvents, use of automated equipment in place of manually operated equipment).

substrate: A collection element that is placed onto the impaction stage for collection of aerosol samples. It can be glass plate, aluminum foil, plastic film, or membrane filter. (See also *impaction plate, impactor stage, substrate coating*.)

substrate coating: Materials that are applied onto certain substrates to capture or stabilize particles that are impacted during sampling. (See also *isokinetic sampling, stack sampling, superisokinetic sampling*.)

SUMMA® canister: A pre-evacuated stainless steel canister that acts as an air collection vessel; the interior surface is electrochemically passivated using the SUMMA process to prevent reaction of the sample with the canister.

summative (product) evaluation: Gathering information on adequacy and using this information to make decisions about utilization.

superisokinetic sampling: A sampling condition in which the air flowing into an inlet has a higher velocity than the ambient airflow. Subsequently, the sample collected tends to be biased with smaller particles. (See also *isokinetic sampling, stack sampling, subisokinetic sampling*.)

supination: 1. Turning the palm upward. 2. Inversion of the foot.

supplier: The provider of that output for a customer.

supply air: Air supplied through ducts to an occupied space.

surface supplied helium-oxygen decompression: A schedule that can involve stops breathing either the bottom supplied mixture, a 40% oxygen mixture, or pure oxygen. The maximum dive on this schedule is 380 ft for 120 minutes.

survey: An episodic investigation of a particular situation and, usually, for a specific purpose.

Sustainability Group Index: Indicates that companies generate added value by integrating economic, environmental, and social growth potentials into their business strategies.

sweat: The watery fluid excreted on the skin surface during high physical activity or in hot, humid environments.

symptom: Any condition accompanying or resulting from an exposure, a disease, or a disorder.

synergism: Cooperative action of substances whose total effects is greater than the sum of their separate effects.

synergists: Skeletal muscles that generally stabilize and control the bony structures that constitute the joint.

system: 1. An organized collection of parts united by regular interaction. 2. A heating or refrigerating scheme or machine, usually confined to those parts in contact with a heating or refrigerating medium. 3. An arbitrarily chosen group of materials and devices set apart for analytical study.

system audit: A systematic on-site qualitative review of facilities, equipment, training, procedures, record keeping, data validation, data management, and reporting aspects of a total (QA) system 1) to arrive at a measure of capability of the measurement system to generate data of the required quality; and/or 2) to determine the extent of compliance of an operational QA system to the approved QA Project Plan.

systematic error: The condition of a consistent deviation of the results of a measurement process from the reference or known level. The cause for the deviation, or bias, may be known or unknown, but is considered "assignable." By assignable it is meant that if the cause is unknown, it should be possible to determine the cause. (See also *bias.*)

systemic: Spread throughout the body, affecting all body systems and organs, not localized in one spot or area.

systemic effects: Adverse effects other than at the site of contact.

systemic system: A subsystem of the cardiovascular system (CVS) in which blood from the left ventricle is pumped to the body arteries. Oxygen and nutrients are removed and carbon dioxide and metabolic waste products are added before the blood is returned in the veins to the right side of the heart. Nutrients are added from the intestines. Fat-soluble wastes are biotransformed in the liver into water-soluble wastes and put back into the blood. The kidney then eliminates water-soluble wastes through urine. Some wastes are eliminated in the intestines (feces).

systems thinking: The ability to see all processes as a system of interrelated events. It allows for the identification and correction of unacceptable patterns.

T

Taguchi experiments: A method for evaluating several different elements of a process at the same time, as opposed to classic experimental design, which focuses on time- and resource-consuming technical analysis of one factor at a time.

tapered-element oscillating microbalance (TEOM): An instrument that determines aerosol mass using resonance oscillation.

tare: A deduction of weight, made in allowance for the weight of a container or medium; for example, the initial weight of a filter.

target: Either the nucleus of the nuclide to be bombarded by a subatomic particle or photon or an anode of an X-ray producing machine.

target concentration: A preliminary estimate of the airborne concentration of the contaminant of interest relative to the purpose of testing.

target organs: 1. The organ of the body most affected by exposure to a particular substance. 2. The body organs that are affected by exposure to a hazardous chemical, physical, or biological agent.

target velocity: The target velocity is the average of the range of transport velocity and is used at the beginning of a transport design problem. Once a duct diameter is selected, the precise actual velocity is then calculated.

TC_{Lo}: See *lowest toxic concentration.*

T_{db}: See *dry bulb temperature.*

TD_{Lo}: See *lowest toxic dose.*

T_{dp}: See *dew point temperature.*

team learning: The situation in which a team develops the ability to think as a group.

teams: Groups associated in a joint action.

temperature: That property of a body that determines the flow of heat. Heat will flow from a warm body to a cold body.

temporal effect: An effect over time.

Temporary Emergency Exposure Limits (TEELs): Values intended to provide estimates of concentration ranges above which one could reasonably anticipate observing adverse health effects. The term also refers to the documentation that summarizes the basis for those values. The four levels of TEEL values are based on a 15-minute time-weighted average (similar to a short-term exposure limit) for a total of four values.

temporary threshold shift (TTS): The hearing loss suffered as the result of noise exposure, all of which is recovered during an arbitrary period of time. (The loss that is not recovered is called permanent threshold shift [PTS].)

tendinitis: Inflammation of a tendon and some of the adjacent muscle tissue.

tendon: Fibrous tissue, similar to a ligament, that attaches muscle to bone.

tenosynovitis: A type of repetitive strain injury (RSI) characterized by swelling of the outside sheath of a tendon. (Also known as "synovitis.")

TEOM: See *tapered-element oscillating microbalance.*

teratogen: A substance that causes birth defects in the offspring.

teratogenesis: The process by which toxic compounds called teratogens can induce perinatal aberrations in an exposed embryo or fetus, yet because of relatively low concentrations may pose no significant hazard of toxicity to the mother.

tertiary prevention measures: consists of measures to reduce or eliminate long-term impairments and disabilities and minimize suffering after illness has occurred, for example, rehabilitation and return-to-work after a heart attack.

T_g: See *globe temperature.*

Thackrah, Charles T.: English physician who published *The Effects of the Principal Arts, Trades, and Professions and of Civic States and Habits of Living on Health and Longevity* in 1831. His views on disease and prevention helped stimulate factory and health legislation in England. The British Factories Acts of 1864, 1878, and 1901 were the forerunners of modern occupational safety and health legislation.

thenar eminence: The ball of flesh at the base of the thumb.

thermal balance: The heat exchange between the human body and the environment.

thermal conductivity: The heat flow across a surface per unit area per unit time, divided by the negative of the rate of change of temperature with distance in a direction perpendicular to the surface.

thermal conductivity detector: The thermal conductivity detector is the most universal gas chromatographic detector because it can measure most gases and vapors. It has low sensitivity compared with the other detectors and is used primarily for analysis of low molecular weight gases such as carbon monoxide, carbon dioxide, nitrogen, and oxygen. This detector measures the differences in thermal conductivity between the column effluent and a reference gas, made of uncontaminated carrier gas. The most common carrier gas for this detector is helium because it is inert and has a very low molecular weight. The column effluent and the reference gas pass through separate detector chambers that contain identical electrically heated filaments. Energy is transferred from the filament when analyte molecules strike the heated filament and rebound with increased energy. Heat loss will therefore be directly proportional to the number of collisions per unit time. Differences in thermal conductivity between gases is proportional to the rate of diffusion to and from the filament. Since diffusion is inversely proportional to molecular weight, lighter molecules will have higher thermal conductivities. Compounds with molecular weights greater than the reference gas will conduct more heat away from the filament than the pure, low molecular weight reference gas, thereby reducing the electrical resistance to the filament. The difference in resistance between the two filaments is amplified and recorded.

thermal desorption: The process of extracting adsorbed chemicals from sorbent material through the use of heat.

thermal drift: Drift caused by an internal heating of equipment during normal operation or by changes in external ambient temperature.

thermal effects on safety behavior: The relationship between unsafe work behavior and ambient temperatures, described as a U-shaped curve, with the minimum unsafe behavior rate occurring in the preferred temperature zone of 17°C (63°F) to 23°C (73°F) wet bulb globe temperature (WBGT), and with the unsafe behavior rate increasing when ambient temperatures increase or decrease from this range.

thermal stress: A combination of air temperature, radiant heat exchange, air movement, and the partial pressure of water vapor that makes the environment stressful.

thermodynamic properties: Basic qualities used to define the condition of a substance (e.g., temperature, pressure, volume, enthalpy, entropy).

thermodynamics: The science of the relation of heat to other forms of energy.

thermoluminescent dosimetry (TLD): The method of quantifying radiation dose by use of material that stores the radiation energy in electron traps. The material is later subjected to heat that releases the energy in the form of optical photons.

thermometer: An instrument that measures temperature.

THF: Abbreviation for Tetrahydrofuran.

thoracic fraction: Particles that enter the tracheobronchial region generally smaller than 10 μm.

thoracic outlet syndrome: A type of repetitive strain injury (RSI) that occurs when both the arteries and nerves going from the neck to the arms are compressed. Signs include coldness and weakness in the forearm, hand, and fingers, and numbness and pain in the entire arm.

threshold: Characterizes a dose-response curve that does not pass through the origin of the graph, indicating there is an exposure level that will not result in an increase in the probability of occurrence of an adverse health effect. Used by the U.S. EPA for noncarcinogens and developmental toxins. (See also *non-threshold*.)

threshold concentration: The minimum concentration of a given substance that is sufficient to just initiate an observable effect.

threshold limit value (TLV®): Used by the American Conference of Governmental Industrial Hygienists (ACGIH®) to designate degree of exposure to contaminants and expressed as parts of vapor or gas per million parts of air by volume at 25°C and 760 mmHg pressure, or as approximate milligrams of particulate per cubic meter of air (mg/m^3). (See also *permissible concentration*.) An exposure level under which most people can work consistently for 8 hours a day, daily, with no harmful effects. TLVs® are listed as either an 8-hour TWA or a 15-minute STEL.

threshold limit value–time-weighted average (TLV®–TWA): The time-weighted average concentration for a normal 8-hour workday and a 40-hour workweek to which nearly all workers may be exposed repeatedly, day after day, without adverse effects.

tidal movement: Volume of air inspired of expired during each respiratory cycle.

tiered risk assessment: See *iterative risk assessment*.

tight-fitting facepiece: A respiratory inlet covering that is designed to form a complete seal with the face. A half facepiece (includes quarter-masks, disposable masks, and masks with elastomeric facepieces) covers the nose and mouth; a full facepiece covers the nose, mouth, and eyes.

time-response relationship: When a particular toxic effect is closely monitored as a function of time, it is possible to develop a time-response relationship. This curve, like the dose-response curve, contains valuable information that can reveal the onset of response, the time of maximum response, the duration of the response (i.e., sustained or transient), and possible recovery from the exposure.

time-weighted average (TWA): 1. Average exposure for an individual over a given working period, as determined by sampling at given times during the period. 2. The most frequently used exposure guideline term; the average concentration over a workday (8 hours for OSHA PELs and ACGIH® TLVs®, up to 10 hours in a 40-hour workweek for NIOSH RELs). 3. This is the fundamental concept of most occupational exposure limits (OELs). It is usually presented as the average concentration over an 8-hour workday for a 40-hour workweek; however, this implies that concentrations will be both above and below the average value. The ACGIH® TLV® committee has recommended excursion limits to prevent concentrations from severely exceeding the average value. The proposed excursion limits are that exposures should typically not exceed the TWA by more than threefold and for a period not exceeding 30 minutes during the workday. Even if the TWA is not exceeded for the work shift, in no case should the excursion be more than fivefold the TWA value.

time-weighted average (TWA) concentration: Refers to concentrations of contaminants that have been weighted for the time duration of sample. A sufficient number of samples are needed to permit a time-weighted average concentration throughout a complete cycle of operations or throughout the work shift.

time-weighted exposure: Average over a given working period of a person's exposure, as determined by sampling at given times during the period.

tinnitus: A ringing, roaring, or hissing sound in one or both ears.

tissue equivalent: A material with an effective Z equal to that of tissue.

TLD: See *thermoluminescent dosimetry.*

TLD chip: The dosimeter made from thermoluminescent material, either CaF^2 or LiF.

TLV®: See *threshold limit value.*

TLV–C: A ceiling exposure limit that should not be exceeded for even an instant.

TLV–STEL: A short-term exposure limit; a 15-minute time-weighted average exposure that should not be exceeded.

TLV–TWA: An 8-hour time-weighted average (TWA) exposure limit.

TNT: Abbreviation for Trinitrotoluene.

T_{nwb}: See *natural wet bulb temperature.*

tolerance: An adaptive state characterized by diminished responses to the same dose of a chemical.

tolerance limits: A particular type of confidence limit used frequently in quality control work in which the limits apply to a percentage of the individual values of the population.

torque: The product of a force and the perpendicular distance from the line of action of the force to the axis of rotation. The unit of torque in the SI system is the newton-meter (Nm).

total absorption: The amount of sound absorption in an enclosure is quantified as its total absorption.

totally encapsulated chemical protective (TECP) suit: A full body garment that completely encloses the wearer by itself or in combination with a respirator, gloves, and boots. The suit is constructed of protective clothing material that isolates the body from direct contact with potentially hazardous chemicals.

total pressure (TP): The sum of the static pressure and the velocity pressure.

total quality: A management methodology that emphasizes the improvement of the processes by which businesses operate and products are produced.

Total Safety Culture: A critical mass of individuals who actively care for the safety and health of others cultivating constructive conformity and obedience.

toxic agent: Substance potentially or actually poisonous to the human body.

toxic reaction: Alteration of a biologic system or organ due to the action of toxic agents.

Toxic Substances List: Annual compilation of known toxic substances prepared by NIOSH and containing about 25,000 names representing some 11,000 different chemical substances.

toxic waste: Discarded or used materials that may induce biochemical and physiological changes in human systems following either systemic contact via absorption into blood and tissues, or local contact.

toxicity: A relative property of a chemical agent; refers to a harmful effect on some biologic mechanism and the condition under which this effect occurs.

toxicity assessment: Both qualitative and quantitative data are developed in a toxicity assessment: 1) a description of the types of health effects that might be expected to occur in humans; and 2) some estimate of toxicity, such as the dose required to cause these health effects. Conceptually, this estimate of toxicity is based on a dose-response curve. The outcome of the toxicity assessment may be a slope factor or an exposure limit. Slope factors are based on the slope of the dose-response curve and can be used to develop a probabilistic risk estimate.

toxicity value: Numerical expression of a substance's dose-response relationship.

The most common values used in Superfund risk assessments are reference doses (RfDs) for noncarcinogenic effects and slope factors for carcinogenic effects.

toxicologic effect: Harmful or poisonous effect of a chemical agent.

toxicologist: Specialist in the science that deals with poisons and their effects.

toxicology: Scientific study of poisons, their actions, their detection, and the treatment of conditions produced by them.

toxicoses: Toxicoses include cancer, asphyxiation, skin rash, and mucous membrane irritation. Most of the common pollutants are toxins that exert their effects in a dose-response way, for the most part without regard to host susceptibility. Many are inflammatory agents that act directly on the contacted cells. Some are absorbed and exert effects on organ systems distant from the site of exposure. Some cross the blood-brain barrier to cause central nervous system (CNS) effects.

TP: See *total pressure*.

traceability: A documented chain of comparisons connecting a working standard (in as few steps as practical) to a national (or international) standard such as a standard maintained by the National Institute of Standards and Technology (NIST).

tracheitis: Inflammation of the trachea.

tracheobronchial region: The region consisting of the trachea and conducting airways (bronchi and bronchioles).

traditional workplace: The traditional workplace as viewed from an occupational hygiene perspective, includes foundries, machine shops, chemical plants, manufacturing areas, assembly lines, and oil refineries.

training: The education or instruction of a person. Multimedia software is an effective training tool.

training needs assessment: The determination of an instructional need, triggered either by external or internal factors, leads to an analysis of the training task or training needs assessment. It includes identifying needs, determining to what extent the problem can be classified as instructional in nature, identifying constraints, resources and learner characteristics, and determining goals and priorities.

transducer: A device such as a microphone capable of being actuated by waves from one or more transmission system or media and of supplying related waves to one or more other transmission systems or media.

transient: Something lasting only a very short period of time.

translation: Straight line motion.

transmission loss: The ratio, expressed in decibels, of the sound energy incident on a structure to the sound energy that is transmitted. The term is applied both to building structures (walls, floors; etc.) and to air passages (muffler, ducts, etc.).

transport: The movement of chemicals within one environmental compartment or from one compartment to another.

transport velocity: The transport velocity or the minimum design transport velocity required to move particles in an air stream.

transportation: The removal of wastes from a plant to an off-site location.

treated filter: A filter that has been coated with a layer of chemical reagent to improve collection of specific chemicals for subsequent laboratory analysis.

treatment: 1. Any method, technique, or process designed to remove solids and/or pollutants from solid waste, wastestreams, effluents, and air emissions. 2. Methods used to change the biological character or composition of any regulated medical waste so as to substantially reduce or eliminate its potential for causing disease.

trigger-level: An exposure condition that, when exceeded, requires the affected employees to be offered medical surveillance.

Trilinear chart of the nuclides: The organization of nuclides by atomic number and number of neutrons to yield isotopes, isobars, and isotones.

triple bottom line: The systems-oriented judgment of companies assessing their financial, social, and environmental performance.

true risk: The actual value of the risk level.

TTS: See *temporary threshold shift*.

tumor: Abnormal mass of tissue that might be or might not be malignant.

turbulent flow: Chaotic flow with streamlines looping back on themselves; less "well-behaved" and predictable than laminar flow. (See also laminar flow.)

TWA: See *time-weighted average.*

8-hour TWA: Average concentration to which an employee is actually exposed over an 8-hour day. See *time-weighted average.*

T_{wb}: See *psychrometric wet bulb temperature.*

twin detector tube: A detector tube construction consisting of a combination of a pretube and an indicating tube, joined by an intermediate sleeve and a piece of shrunk-on tubing.

U

UEL: See *upper flammable limit.*

UFL: See *upper flammable limit.*

UL: Underwriters' Laboratories, Inc.

ultrafine particle: traditionally used by aerosol research and occupational and environmental health communities to describe airborne particles smaller than 100 nm in diameter.

ultrasonics: The technology of sound at frequencies above the audio range.

ultrasound: Sound with a frequency above about 20,000 Hz, the upper limit of human hearing.

ultraviolet (UV): Those wavelengths of the electromagnetic spectrum which are shorter than those of visible radiation and larger than X-rays, 10^{-5} cm to 10^{-6} cm wavelength. (Also known as "black light.")

ultraviolet (UV) absorbance detector: The ultraviolet (UV) absorbance detector measures the UV light absorbance of the column effluent. It is especially sensitive to aromatic hydrocarbons. The basic components of the UV detector are a UV lamp, a flow-cell with a UV-transparent window for the column effluent, and a photodiode or other light-measuring device. Some UV detectors can be operated at only one wavelength, typically 254 nm, while others can also operate at additional wavelengths using fluorescent waveplates. A variable UV detector can be tuned to any wavelength within its operating range.

ultraviolet radiation: Wavelengths of the electromagnetic spectrum that are shorter than those of visible light and longer than X-rays; wavelengths measure 10^{-5} cm to 10^{-6} cm.

uncertainty: Deviation in predicted values from the actual values. May result from lack of data or variability in the data.

unit: 1. A factory-made encased assembly of the functional elements indicated by its name, such as air-conditioning unit, room-cooling unit, humidifying unit, etc. 2. A portion or subassembly of a computer that accomplishes some operation or function.

Universal Precautions: Guidelines established by the Centers for Disease Control and Prevention (CDC) instructing health care professionals to take blood and body fluid precautions for all patients regardless of their bloodborne infection status. These guidelines, known officially as "Universal Blood and Body Fluid Precautions," are part of a 1987 CDC report titled "Recommendations for Prevention of HIV Transmission in Health-Care Settings."

unstable: Tending toward decomposition or other unwanted chemical change during normal handling or storage.

unstable reactive: A chemical that in the pure state, or as produced or transported, will vigorously polymerize, decompose, condense, or become self-reactive under conditions of shocks, pressure, or temperature.

upper explosive limit (UEL): See *upper flammable limit.*

upper flammable limit (UFL): The percentage by volume of a flammable gas or vapor that is the maximum level ignitable. Also referred to as "upper explosive limit."

upper measurement limit: The useful limit (mg of analyte per sample) of the analytical instrument.

upper respiratory tract: The mouth, nose, sinuses, and pharynx.

uptake: Mass potentially breathed in/out after a specific time period.

urine: The watery nonviscous excretion voided by the urethra.

urticarial reaction: 1. Hives or nettle rash. 2. A skin condition characterized by the appearance of intensely itching wheals or welts with elevated, usually white centers and a surrounding area of erythema.

user seal check: A test conducted by the wearer to determine whether the respirator is properly adjusted to the face.

UV: See *ultraviolet.*

UV-A: The UV divisions are named regions. UV-A is the blacklight region.

UV-B: The UV divisions are named regions. UV-B is the erythema region. UV-B and UV-C regions are often called actinic UV, because they are capable of causing chemical reactions.

UV-C: The UV divisions are named regions. UV-C is the germicidal region. UV-B and UV-C regions are often called actinic UV, because they are capable of causing chemical reactions.

V

vacuum: State in which the gas pressure is lower than atmospheric pressure.

vacuum UV: The 100–180 nm region is known as the vacuum UV region because these wavelengths are readily absorbed in air.

validated sampling and analysis method: A method that has met critical accuracy requirements when tested throughout the working range.

validity: See *accuracy.*

values: Ideals, customs, or institutions that arouse an emotional response in a given group or individual.

vapor: Gaseous phase of a substance ordinarily liquid or solid at 25°C and 760 mmHg. Evaporation is the process by which a liquid changes to a vapor state, and mixes with the surrounding atmosphere. Solvents with low boiling points volatilize readily. Examples of substances that emit vapors are trichloroethylene, methylene chloride, and mercury. Size ranges are usually less than 0.005 µm. It is near equilibrium with its liquid phase and for occupational hygiene calculations it follows the gas laws.

vapor density: 1. The ratio of the mass of a vapor or gas to the mass of an equal volume of air at the same temperature; an expression of the density of the vapor or gas. 2. The weight of a vapor or gas compared to the weight of an equal volume of air is an expression of the density of the vapor or gas. Materials lighter than air have vapor densities less than 1.0 (e.g., acetylene, methane, hydrogen). Materials heavier than air (e.g., propane, hydrogen sulfide ethane, butane, chlorine, sulfur dioxide) have vapor densities greater than 1.0. All vapors and gases will mix with air, but the lighter materials will tend to rise and dissipate (unless confined). Heavier vapors and gases are likely to concentrate in low places – along or under floors, in sumps, sewers, and manholes, in trenches and ditches – where they may create fire or health hazards.

vapor pressure (VP): 1. The pressure exerted by a vapor. If a vapor is confined and accumulates over its liquid or solid at a constant temperature, it reaches a maximum pressure called the saturated vapor pressure. [**Note:** For a specific liquid or solid with a constant volume of vapor above it, the vapor pressure depends only on the temperature.] 2. The pressure exerted by a saturated vapor above its own liquid in a closed container. When quality control tests are performed on products, the test temperature is usually 100°F, and the vapor pressure is expressed as pounds per square inch (psig or psia), but vapor pressures reported as MSDSs are in millimeters of mercury (mmHg) at 68°F, unless stated otherwise. Three facts are important to remember: a) vapor pressure of a substance at 100°F will always be higher than the vapor pressure of the substance at 68°F; b) vapor pressures reported as MSDSs in mmHg are usually very low pressures; 760 mmHg is equivalent to 14.7 pounds per square inch; c) the lower BP of a substance, the higher its vapor pressure. 3. A measure of the tendency of a liquid to form a gas (usually a function of temperature); the pressure exerted when a solid or liquid is at equilibrium with its own vapor; normally reported in mm of mercury (mmHg). The higher the vapor pressure, the more volatile the chemical.

variability: Source of uncertainty in risk assessment due to the fact that many parameters are best described not as point values but as probability distributions.

variance: 1. The square of the standard deviation. 2. Mathematically, the sample variance is the sum of squares of the differences between the individual values of a set and the arithmetic average of the set, divided by one less than the number of values.

V_c: See *capture velocity*.

velocity: 1. The time rate of distance moved. 2. A vector quantity that denotes the simultaneous time rate and direction of linear motion. The designer must fully understand the different velocities of importance in exhaust ventilation design. 3. The time rate of movement of air in meters per second (feet per minute).

velocity pressure (VP): The pressure created by moving air.

ventilation (control): The process of supplying or removing air by natural or mechanical means to or from any space. Such air may or may not have been conditioned.

verification: The establishment of the reliability of a measurement method by comparison with one or more reference methods.

vertical entry: A confined space entry that requires the entrant to descend into the confined space from above or below.

vertical standards: An industry-specific standard that regulates an industry in addition to OSHA general industry standards. For example the construction industry and the longshoring industry are subject to both general and vertical standards.

V_f: See *hood face velocity*.

vibration isolator: Decouples structures, such as a human hand from a pneumatic tool or a driver from a vehicle, by using "soft" connections. Vibration energy is absorbed by the isolator instead of being transmitted to the user.

vibration transmissibility ratio: The vibration transmissibility ratio is the ratio of the vibration output (vibration at the seat) to the vibration input (vibration at the floor of the vehicle). A transmissibility ratio of 1 means there is no change in the level of vibration between the input and output; a ratio >1 indicates an amplification of the original vibration; a ratio <1 indicates a reduction or attenuation of the original vibration.

vibration-induced damage: Bodily damage caused by excessive exposure to vibration.

vibration-induced white finger (VWF): See *hand-arm vibration syndrome*.

videography: A tool used to conduct a kinematic analysis that uses the digitization of key anatomical landmarks into Cartesian coordinates that are recorded on a storage device.

virulence: The quality of being virulent, or very poisonous, noxious, malignant; the relative infectiousness of a microorganism causing disease.

virus: A software program that attaches itself to another program in computer memory or on a disk, and spreads from one program to another. Viruses may damage data, cause the computer to crash, display messages, or lie dormant.

viscosity: The tendency of a fluid to resist internal flow without regard to its density.

visible radiation: Electromagnetic radiation with wavelengths capable of causing the sensation of vision, ranging approximately from 4000 angstroms (extreme violet) to 7700 angstroms (extreme red). (Also known as "light radiation.")

vision statement: A statement that identifies where an organization wants to be in the future. In broad terms it establishes the end point for an improvement process and allows the development of a plan to move from an unacceptable present to a beneficial future.

VOC: See *volatile organic compound*.

vol: See *volume*.

volatile organic compound (VOC): Any organic compound that participates in atmospheric photochemical reactions.

volatility: 1. The tendency or ability of a liquid to vaporize. Liquids such as alcohol and gasoline, because of their well-known tendency to evaporate rapidly, are called volatile liquids. 2. A measure of how quickly a substance forms a vapor at ordinary temperatures.

volatilize: Readily convertible to a vapor or gaseous state.

voltage: The electrical potential energy difference per unit charge between two points.

volume (vol): A measure of the size of a body or definite region in three-dimensional space. It is equal to the least upper bound of the sum of the volumes of nonoverlapping cubes that can be fitted inside the body or region, where the volume of a cube is the cube of the length of one of its sides.

volume flow rate (Q): The quantity of air flowing in cubic feet per minute (ft^3/min) or cubic meters per second (m^3/sec).

voluntary guidelines: Guidelines are published by consensus organizations and are published for general voluntary use; the decision to use the guidelines is totally a discretionary one considered by the user.

Voluntary Protection Program (VPP): Developed in 1982 by OSHA to recognize and promote outstanding safety programs.

VP: See *vapor pressure.*

VP: See *velocity pressure.*

VPP: See *Voluntary Protection Program.*

VWF: Vibration-induced white finger. See *hand-arm vibration syndrome.*

W

WAN: See *wide area network.*

waste: 1. Unwanted materials left over from a manufacturing process. 2. Refuse from places of human or animal habitation.

water vapor pressure: The pressure exerted by water vapor at a specific temperature.

water-reactive: A chemical that reacts with water to release a gas that is either flammable or presents a health hazard.

Watts per square meter (W/m²): A unit that expresses power density for nonionizing radiation.

wavelength (L): 1. The distance between the ends of one complete cycle of a wave. 2. Wavelength is the descriptor used for UV, visible, and IR radiation. 3. The distance in the line of advance of a wave from any point to a like point on the next wave. It is usually measured in angstroms, microns, or nanometers.

WBGT: See *wet bulb globe temperature.*

WEEL(s)™: See *workplace environmental exposure level(s).*

WEEL™ guides: See workplace environmental exposure level guides.

weighting network (sound): Electrical networks (A, B, C) that are associated with sound level meters. The C network provides a flat response over the frequency range 20–10,000 Hz of interest while the B and A networks selectively discriminate against low (below I KC) frequencies.

weight-of-evidence: U.S. EPA classification system for characterizing the evidence that an agent is a human carcinogen or developmental toxin. It relies mainly on positive evidence. (See also *strength-of-evidence*).

wet bulb globe temperature (WBGT): 1. The combination of the effect of the four main thermal components affecting heat stress: air temperature, humidity, air velocity, and radiation, as measured by the dry bulb (T_{db}), natural wet bulb (T_{nwb}), and globe (T_g) temperatures. 2. Temperature calculated as the sum of 0.7 natural wet bulb + 0.2 black globe + 0.1 dry bulb. (See also *natural wet bulb, psychrometric.*)

wet bulb temperature: See *psychrometric wet bulb temperature.*

wet globe temperature (WGT): A temperature reading that combines air temperature, humidity, air velocity, and radiation into a single reading.

WGT: See *wet globe temperature.*

Wheatstone bridge: A four-arm bridge circuit, all arms of which are predominantly resistive; used to measure the electrical resistance of an unknown resistor by comparing it with a known standard resistance.

white room: See *clean room.*

whole-body vibration: The exposure of the entire body to workplace vibrations. Whole-body vibration can cause both physiological and psychological effects ranging from fatigue and irritation to motion sickness (kinetosis) and to tissue damage.

wide area network (WAN): Two or more LANs linked together into a larger network form a wide area network (WAN). A WAN can be used to connect different divisions within a company, different plants in different cities, and so forth. The links between LANs to form a WAN can be made with modems, satellites, or telephone lines.

wind-chill index: The cooling effect of any combination of temperature and wind, expressed as the loss of body heat in kilogram calories per hour per square meter of skin surface; it is only an approximation because of individual body variations in shape, size, and metabolic rate.

window: The entry point on a radiation detector for radiation into sensitive volume.

WMSDs: See *Work-Related Musculoskeletal Disorders.*

work: Exertion or effort directed to produce or accomplish something.

work plan: A plan that ensures that all required data are efficiently collected and properly documented. It should include field data sheets and a communications plan.

work site analysis: Examination of the work site to identify not only existing hazards but also conditions and operations in which changes might occur to create hazards. Effective management actively analyzes the work and the work site to anticipate and prevent harmful occurrences. To ensure that all hazards are identified, management and employees must: 1) Conduct comprehensive baseline work site surveys for safety and periodic comprehensive update safety surveys; 2) Analyze planned and new facilities, processes, and equipment for safety hazards; 3) Perform routine job hazard analyses, including investigation of accidents; 4) Use a reliable system for employees, without fear of reprisal, to notify management about conditions that seem hazardous; and 5) Analyze injury and illness trends over time so that patterns with common causes can be identified and prevented.

working fluids: Pressure is indicated by the height of a working fluid in the barometer or manometer. The most commonly used working fluid for a barometer is mercury. Other fluids can be used but are not as convenient.

working occupational exposure limit: An informal occupational exposure limit set by a occupational hygienist based on whatever information may be available to differentiate acceptable from unacceptable exposures. Working OELs are sometimes stated in ranges (e.g., 0.1 to 1.0 mg/m^3) or incorporate large safety factors to account for uncertainty. (See also *occupational exposure limit.*)

working range: The range of contaminant concentration (mg/m^3) that may be accurately quantified at specified air volumes (liters) by a specific method.

workplace environmental exposure level (WEEL™) guides: Exposure guidelines developed by AIHA® intended to protect the health and safety of workers exposed to hazardous substances or conditions.

workplace exposure assessment: The exposure characterization of the worker's potential exposure to hazardous chemical, physical or biological agents. The information included should include the agents, their likely routes of exposure, and intensity, duration, and frequency of the exposure.

Work-Related Musculoskeletal Disorders (WMSDs): The specific term "work-related musculoskeletal disorders" refers to: 1) musculoskeletal disorders to which the work environment and the performance of work contribute significantly; or 2) musculoskeletal disorders that are made worse or longer lasting by work conditions. These workplace risk factors, along with personal characteristics (e.g., physical limitations or existing health problems) and societal factors, are thought to contribute to the development of WMSDs.

workstation: The computers linked to a server.

World Wide Web (WWW): A system of Internet servers that support specially formatted documents. The documents are formatted in a language called HTML (HyperText Markup Language) that supports links to other documents, as well as graphics, audio, and video files. This means you can jump from one document to another simply by clicking on hot spots. Not all Internet servers are part of the Web.

worst-case-scenario: A method of conducting an exposure assessment in which the most conservative value of each input parameter is selected. (See also *reasonable maximum exposure.*)

WWW: See *World Wide Web.*

XYZ

Youden plot: Large variations in results reported from different laboratories analyzing the same samples might be explained by random errors in the measurements or by systematic errors in the different laboratories. Practically speaking, it is highly probable that systematic errors made by the participating laboratories are the cause for these wide variations. This can be evaluated using another technique for analyzing interlaboratory variability — the "two-sample" or Youden plot. In this graphical technique each participating laboratory is sent two similar samples (A and B) and asked to perform one analysis on each sample. When the results are returned, the results obtained by a laboratory for Sample A are plotted with respect to the results obtained by the same laboratory for Sample B. Median lines are drawn, and outliers are identified and discarded from the data set. If there were no bias in the results, the plotted points should be randomly distributed around the intersection of the two median lines drawn. It is rare that this is observed. Generally what is observed is that the plotted points fall around a line drawn at 45° from the intersection of the two median lines, indicating that each participating laboratory has its own technique (an internal consistency) for analyzing the samples. (Laboratories who report one sample high are more likely to report the second sample high. The converse is true, also.) Through the use of two samples similar in concentration, an estimate of precision can be made. This is done by constructing a perpendicular line from the plotted point to the 45° line.

zero gas: A gas containing less than 1 ppm sulfur dioxide.

zoonoses: See *zoonotic infection.*

zoonotic infection: Disease transmissible from animals to man.

zygomycosis: Any infection caused by fungi of the class zygomycetes.

zygote: A cell produced by the joining of two gametes that are either sex or germ cells.

Index

A

B

D

E

F

G

H

I

M

N

O

P

Q

R

S

T

U

W

X

Y

Z